T0181217

REHABILITATION
A Post-critical Approach

Rehabilitation Science in Practice Series

Series Editors

Published Titles

Ambient Assisted Living, *Nuno M. Garcia and Joel J.P.C. Rodrigues*

Assistive Technology Assessment Handbook, *edited by Stefano Federici and Marcia J. Scherer*

Assistive Technology for Blindness and Low Vision, *Roberto Manduchi and Sri Kurniawan*

Computer Access for People with Disabilities: A Human Factors Approach, *Richard C. Simpson*

Computer Systems Experiences of Users with and Without Disabilities: An Evaluation Guide for Professionals, *Simone Borsci, Maria Laura Mele, Masaaki Kurosu, and Stefano Federici*

Devices for Mobility and Manipulation for People with Reduced Abilities, *Teodiano Bastos-Filho, Dinesh Kumar, and Sridhar Poosapadi Arjunan*

Human–Computer Interface Technologies for the Motor Impaired, *edited by Dinesh K. Kumar and Sridhar Poosapadi Arjunan*

Multiple Sclerosis Rehabilitation: From Impairment to Participation, *edited by Marcia Finlayson*

Neuroprosthetics: Principles and Applications, *edited by Justin Sanchez*

Paediatric Rehabilitation Engineering: From Disability to Possibility, *edited by Tom Chau and Jillian Fairley*

Quality of Life Technology Handbook, *Richard Schultz*

Rehabilitation: A Post-critical Approach, *Barbara E. Gibson*

Rehabilitation Goal Setting: Theory, Practice and Evidence, *edited by Richard J. Siegert and William M. M. Levack*

Rethinking Rehabilitation: Theory and Practice, *edited by Kathryn McPherson, Barbara E. Gibson, and Alain Leplège*

REHABILITATION
A Post-critical Approach

Barbara E. Gibson
University of Toronto
Ontario, Canada

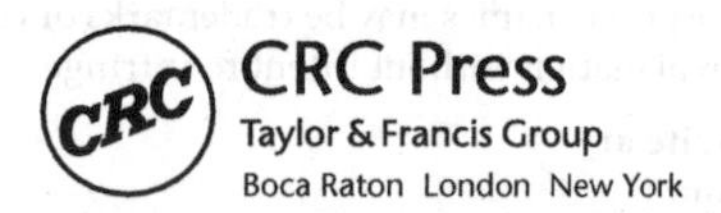

CRC Press is an imprint of the
Taylor & Francis Group, an **informa** business

CRC Press
Taylor & Francis Group
6000 Broken Sound Parkway NW, Suite 300
Boca Raton, FL 33487-2742

Printed on acid-free paper
Version Date: 20151130

International Standard Book Number-13: 978-1-4822-3723-8 (Paperback)

Visit the Taylor & Francis Web site at
http://www.taylorandfrancis.com

and the CRC Press Web site at
http://www.crcpress.com

Contents

Foreword

Doing Disability Studies of Rehabilitation

Disability studies, as I will define it, aims to uncover the cultural emergence of human ability and difference, with the overall aim of democratic social change. This definition is extremely broad and, accordingly, has numerous advantages. I will outline two of them (and gloss over the deficits). First, it means that we can expand the scope of inquiry from those classified as different, medically or otherwise, to any cultural location where personhood is distributed. The object of inquiry, then, is not *deviance from* but *ability*.* The basic question: how is the *ability-to* culturally allocated? A second, and closely related, advantage of this definition is that we can do disability studies of, well, almost anything—capitalism, medicine, bureaucracy—so long as these or other institutions shape agency, capacity, or ability, then we can do disability studies of them. The book before you is more than simply a case for reflexivity in, and theoretical reflections on, rehabilitation: it is an important contribution to a burgeoning space of inquiry, to disability studies of rehabilitation.

"Disability studies of rehabilitation" is an intentionally ugly name for an extremely important project.† The point is not only to analyze business-as-usual rehabilitation through a predefined theoretical lens, as in "the application of theory to practice," but to transform the practice of rehabilitation itself. This book makes clear that rehabilitation does more than simply making people's lives better. Gibson demonstrates that clinical practices and practicing clinicians outline, in whole or in part, what a better life is. It is the responsibility of those who are defining life to admit

* Here I have Becker's classic definition of deviance in mind, from his *Outsiders* (1963), particularly the movement from deviant *actors* to the reception of deviant *acts*. For a comparison of the classic deviance scholarship on disability and the (newer) field of disability studies, see Titchkosky (2000).

† Following Peirce's "pragmaticism" (1972), the term is ugly enough that nobody will want to steal it.

as much. "Mobility," "independence," or "quality-of-life" (Chapters 6, 5, and 3, respectively): these professional concepts do not simply measure patients; they chart the horizons of patient*hood*. Admitting the world-making potential of rehabilitation practice, the unending goal of Gibson's "post-critical" approach is to think of ways in which patients, practitioners, and their allies can define The Good—and achieve it together.

This book is littered with insights drawn from works of philosophy and social theory, together used to excavate the tacit underpinnings of rehabilitation science. One is left asking: do we *need* to do theory to do post-critical rehabilitation in the first place? While the sociological theorist in me wants to exclaim "of course!" the disabled person cannot. To require that anyone participating in a life-affirming rehabilitation practice have a firm grounding in abstract theory is to replace one professional prerequisite with another. We are trying to eliminate needless barriers, not create new ones. Theoretical exploration is one kind of language in which this inquiry can take place. It is not the only one; we can do it theoretically, or we can do it in plain English. The important point, once again, is that we do it together.

To admit that "theory" is one of the motley ways of expressing ourselves is not to argue that it is useless. This would be plain hypocrisy on my part: I have used theoretical and philosophical concepts to make sense of what disability might be, how it is made up, and what shape it might take in the future. I found Heidegger's *Being and Time* to be an excellent tool for coming to terms with my own experiences of disability and rehabilitation, and, reciprocally, I used those same experiences to make sense of that difficult book. Reading *Being and Time* through my experience of disability—perhaps more aptly, "doing disability studies of Heidegger"—gave me a way of coping with my own experience of rehabilitation.* In that book, Heidegger pursues a fundamental ontology of *Dasein* (German for "existence," literally "there-being"), outlining how the structures that make human experience possible are fundamentally different than the presence of objects. Heidegger (1982, 1996) calls the distinction between these forms of being the "ontological difference." By examining our practical engagement with the world in daily tasks, we can illuminate what is unique to our own mode of existence, being-in-the-world. "Disability" and "ability" are simply descriptions of this more basic kind of Being, the being of Dasein.

Heidegger's ontological difference came to life during my personal experience of rehabilitation. Throughout my career as a rehabilitation

* I document the experience in far more detail in Abrams (2014b).

patient, I quickly learned that there is a stark difference between life as a disabled person and being the object of clinical intervention. In my case, this stems from my diagnosis of Becker muscular dystrophy. In my daily life, falls are an expected problem, say, once or twice a week. To explain the post hoc mechanics of a fall and to direct one's life around the possibility of falling—this demonstrates Heidegger's ontological difference. Nonreflexive rehabilitation thinks only in terms of present entities, falling bodies, and atrophied muscles, and not of disability as a way of life. By developing a common theoretical tongue, we are able to think about these experiences in new ways, to stand outside the routine, to retreat, and then to address the mundane anew.

Disability studies of rehabilitation do not draw their strength from the ability to crunch numbers. If this is the rubric against which research is judged, then regression analysis has us beat. We are not, however, only seeking horsepower. The true strength of theoretical exploration is to provide a new conceptual currency to those who would care to listen. Barbara Gibson's book is a primer in an emerging patois, where we, bound by common goals and not professional designation, can make sense of rehabilitation as a communal effort. Admitting the dangers of needless jargon, this communal effort is based not in terminological adequacy, but a shared politics of experience. A goal of Gibson's book reflects that of critical health research more generally: to hear the voices of those who have not yet been heard. It was this same language that brought me into contact with Dr. Gibson in the first place, and her book will be successful if it brings any more experiences in collaborative dialogue. While statistically insignificant, this task is both noble and necessary.

There is, of course, more than one method of thinking theoretically. I am a monist—not because I believe in the unity of The One Being: I lack the attention span to entertain too much at once. Gibson's book does not suffer from this monism. As in Wittgenstein's (1958, p. 87) metaphor of an old nautical rope, Gibson's exploration gains its strength from the assemblage of various threads of theoretical inquiry rather than extending a singular system of thought throughout. Thus, she asks us not to subscribe to any *one* individual account of existence, but to explore rehabilitation's formation of "the real" instrumentally. Many (and I count myself among this many) will find themselves caught between the various strands at one time or another. But this is the very point of the book—to unsettle the everyday, to make strange what is before us, to experiment with the real. It is discomforting—and intentionally so. The benefits of the journey are worth the occasional headache for the systematic thinker, to be sure.

For me, to cast Gibson's book on rehabilitation as a contribution to the disability studies canon will surely ruffle some feathers. The conventional approach is as follows. Disability studies and medicine don't mix.* Medicine does the medical model, focusing on broken bodies; we disabled persons are to emancipate ourselves from oppressive social order through activist research. When medicine does address disability, it does so through the "individual tragedy model" (Oliver, 1986), failing to address the social and material conditions that reproduce the real tragedy: a culture that does not accommodate human difference. The medical model cannot see social exclusion. In fact, it perpetuates it.

This book does nothing of the sort. On the contrary, Gibson does a great service to disability studies by directing an abstract critique of medicine to the particular practices that actively constitute the body as an objective *thing*. She isolates the very measures, practices, and discourses that give rehabilitation the *ability to* judge the body biomechanically possible in the first place. The focus shifts from deviance to capacity. This is where we must combat business-as-usual medicine's aesthetic invalidation of disabled people (Hughes, 2000). A dedicated empirical focus on medical *practices* is a marked improvement over the tired critique of medicine in the abstract—what I have elsewhere called the "biomedical boogeyman" (Abrams, 2014a, p. 754), a lazy sociological fabrication, at once everywhere and yet nowhere. By moving from sociological abstraction to concrete practices, from medi*calization* to medi*cine*, we can do disability politics more effectively.

Thomas Abrams

References

Abrams, T. 2014a. Boon or bust? Heidegger, disability aesthetics and the thalidomide memorial. *Disability & Society* 29(5): 751–762.

Abrams, T. 2014b. Flawed by Dasein? Phenomenology, ethnomethodology, and the personal experience of physiotherapy. *Human Studies* 37(3): 431–446.

Barnes, C. 2000. A working social model? Disability, work, and disability politics in the 21st century. *Critical Social Policy* 65: 441–457.

Becker, H.S. 1963. *Outsiders: Studies in the Sociology of Deviance.* New York: The Free Press.

Heidegger, M. 1982. *The Basic Problems of Phenomenology* (A. Hofstader, trans. revised ed.). Bloomington, IN: Indiana University Press.

* Here I am thinking of the social model of disability: see Oliver (1992) and Barnes (2000).

Heidegger, M. 1996. *Being and Time* (J. Stambaugh, trans.). New York: State University of New York Press.

Hughes, B. 2000. Medicine and the aesthetic invalidation of disabled people. *Disability & Society* 15(4): 555–568.

Nicholls, D.A. and Gibson, B.E. 2010. The body and physiotherapy. *Physiotherapy Theory and Practice* 26(8): 497–509.

Oliver, M. 1986. Social policy and disability: Some theoretical issues. *Disability, Handicap & Society* 1(1): 5–17.

Oliver, M. 1992. Changing the social relations of research production? *Disability, Handicap & Society* 7(2): 101–114.

Peirce, C.S. 1972. *Charles S. Peirce: The Essential Writings*. New York: Harper & Row.

Titchkosky, T. 2000. Disability studies: The old and the new. *Canadian Journal of Sociology* 25(2): 197–224.

Wittgenstein, L. (1958). *Preliminary Studies for the "Philosophical Investigations", Generally Known as the Blue and Brown Books*. Oxford, U.K.: Oxford Blackwell.

Acknowledgments

This book would not have been possible without the assistance and support of many people. I owe a world of gratitude to David Nicholls, whose insights can be found on every page of the book. Thank you for your generosity, wisdom, and support. My heartfelt thanks to Thomas Abrams for the inspired foreword and to my indefatigable collaborators on Chapter 4, Gail Teachman and Yani Hamdani. To Patrick Jachyra, Bhavnita Mistry (Queen Bee), and Kelly O'Brien, thank you for lending a hand when it was most needed. Finally, to Richard Smith, who makes everything possible, thank you for keeping things sweet, light, and crude.

Author

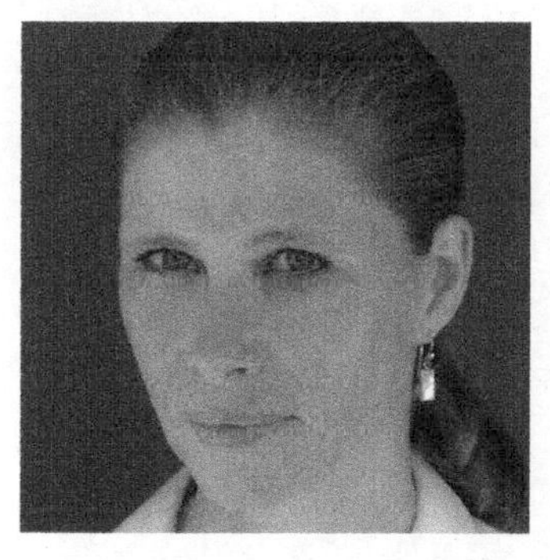

Barbara E. Gibson is an associate professor in the Department of Physical Therapy, University of Toronto, Ontario, Canada, and a senior scientist at the Bloorview Research Institute at the Holland Bloorview Kids Rehabilitation Hospital in Toronto, Ontario, Canada. She holds the Bloorview Children's Hospital Foundation chair in childhood disability studies. She is a physical therapist and bioethicist, whose research examines the sociopolitical dimensions of childhood disability and rehabilitation. She holds cross appointments at the Person Centred Research Centre, AUT University, Auckland, New Zealand, and the CanChild Centre for Childhood Disability Research, McMaster University, Hamilton, Ontario, Canada. She is an academic fellow at the Centre for Critical Qualitative Health Research and a member of the Joint Centre for Bioethics at the University of Toronto.

Contributors

Thomas Abrams
Department of Social Justice Education
Ontario Institute for Studies in Education
University of Toronto
Toronto, Ontario, Canada

Barbara E. Gibson
Department of Physical Therapy
University of Toronto
and
Bloorview Research Institute
Holland Bloorview Kids Rehabilitation Hospital
Toronto, Ontario, Canada

Yani Hamdani
Dalla Lana School of Public Health
University of Toronto
Toronto, Ontario, Canada

Gail Teachman
Graduate Department of Rehabilitation Sciences
University of Toronto
and
Bloorview Research Institute
Holland Bloorview Kids Rehabilitation Hospital
Toronto, Ontario, Canada

1

Moving Rehabilitation

The meaning of movement is the very movement of meaning

José Gil (2005, p. 125)

The task of this book is to foment revolution by inciting a "movement movement:" to perturbate, instigate, agitate, disorder, and disturb. I use movement as a point of departure to re-examine the core concepts and philosophical foundations of rehabilitation. Throughout I discuss the possibilities of engaging in multiple ideas of movements, not only physical, but also social, emotional, and political movements to suggest new approaches to care and practice. Engaging with questions common to critical and postmodern approaches to research, I explore the limitations of biomedicine as the organizing framework in rehabilitation and explore new directions to diversify and re-imagine practice. In so doing, this book outlines a reconfigured ethics of rehabilitation.

Rehabilitation is its own movement that has a history, a logic, a rhythm, and an arc. My goal is to unearth this movement with a series of post-critical displacements, not to destroy rehabilitation but to paradoxically (re)build it through a dismantling. Movement is a metaphor for change that I employ to examine ways to re-*form* rehabilitation.* Doing so requires a kind of dislodging of some of the core tenets of rehabilitation and a broader examination of its philosophical and political moorings. I approach this task by drawing on postmodern and critical ideas to deconstruct and reconstruct some root(ed) concepts. Think of it as a kind of re-action, doing and then doing again, but differently and in multiple directions. Such a move requires different modes of talking about what rehabilitation is and does. Etymologically speaking, when we develop we

* In this effort, I owe a tremendous debt to David Nicholls who, in 2009, first proposed to me the idea of applying a postmodern reading of movement to rehabilitation. Our initial explorations of this idea have been published elsewhere (Nicholls and Gibson 2010; Nicholls et al. 2015), and its antecedents can be found in Nicholls' other works (2006, 2012).

undo what has previously been wrapped up. We re-move, that is, we move again and again in order to rethink, re-imagine, and re-open worlds of possibility for rehabilitation recipients.

Movement is central to rehabilitation; it is an outcome, a practice, and an ideology. It can also be mobilized to foster connectivities, to re-form, re-consider, re-fuse, re-figure, re-collect, and re-assemble care, research, and education practices. Rehabilitation clinicians, researchers, and educators mostly discuss movement in terms of the physical movements of joints and limbs, and in relation to the anatomy, physiology, and biomechanics of the biological body. Collectively, we may speak of gross and fine motor function, or more recently in our history, how movement facilitates participation in activities and social roles. Despite this growing interest in the social and human aspects of persons' lives, movement remains primarily focused on the mechanical: on mobilizing material bodies. This reduces rehabilitation to kinematics and pathologies, a "biomechanical discourse" (Nicholls and Gibson 2010). But movement as metaphor serves a broader function in rehabilitation. As Nicholls et al. (2015, p. 106) note, "(w)hen we speak of momentum, goals or progress, or growth and development, we are often speaking of the material objective reality of a person's physical aptitude or performance, but we are also keeping one eye on the more ethereal aspects of these phenomena, and thus drawing on the power of metaphor to give the particular notion additional weight of meaning." Movement thus has multiple meanings and a discursive power that can be mobilized to re-form rehabilitation.

Movements are everywhere and take multiple forms in the world. There are kinematic movements—displacements with speed and direction, but other forms of movement also abound in talk and action. They can be seen in a visual artist's use of line and positioning to suggest flows and kinetics. Art engages the eye to produce an emotional change in the perceiver who is transformed. Musical movements do the same. A movement in music is both a part of a symphony and a change in tempo; the music moves through movements and, together with the listener, creates new experiences. *Emotions* in everyday life tether experience and motivate action, with emotional adjustments involving the transformation of perceptions into actions and actions into perceptions (Winance 2006a, p. 60). There are also social movements (reforms, revolutions), economic change, fashion trends, and military deployments. People are spiritually moved (transcendence) and participate in movements—marches, demonstrations, transitions, displacements, maneuvers, campaigns, crusades, and drives. Movement in its multiple expressions can be put to work in re-imagining and re-forming rehabilitation, to avoid stasis and inspire creative practices. As Nicholls et al. (2015, p. 105) note, movement can be deployed to stimulate creativity, which ultimately benefits care recipients:

> Somehow we seem to have lost the ability to see the metaphorical significance of notions like detachment and dislocation in physical rehabilitation, preferring instead to reduce these ideas down to the level of bones and joints, muscles and tendons. And while we would argue these are entirely valid ways of thinking about structural integrity, we might also gain something from thinking about how these words carry cultural, existential, philosophical, political, social, and spiritual significance for individuals and communities that, if acknowledged, could open up entirely new dimensions to our rehabilitation practices.

In this book, I draw from postmodern and post-critical theories to stimulate movement. In doing so, the book contributes to addressing a sustained call from leading rehabilitation scholars for a greater focus on theory development in the field (e.g., Gibson et al. 2010; McPherson et al. 2015; Siegert et al. 2005; Whyte 2008; Whyte and Hart 2003). There is a significant gap in the theoretical sophistication of rehabilitation literature, and much of the robust conceptual work that is available, with some notable exceptions, has been published in social science or methodology-focused journals. Despite an increasing focus on critical research in rehabilitation, to date there are no full texts that specifically develop and apply a critical reading of rehabilitation practices.

Rehabilitation as an enterprise dedicated to helping people to not only survive but thrive will always have to grapple with how to understand and support human flourishing. I argue throughout the book that this work cannot be achieved without surfacing some of the problems that arise within the limited biomedical framings of rehabilitation. I do so, however, not as a theoretical exercise, but to move toward better practices that help people to live well. In this regard, I am particularly focused on interrogating entrenched understandings of disability, the consequences for people labeled as disabled, and the possibilities for a reconfigured rehabilitation that draws on key strands of critical disability studies.

In this introductory chapter, I begin by delineating the "post-critical" approach that underpins the book and grounds the analysis in the subsequent chapters. I discuss the limits of positivist approaches to rehabilitation and unpack how they contribute to entrenching disciplinary divisions, including those between disability studies and rehabilitation sciences. In applying a post-critical lens to rehabilitation, I introduce the idea of re-forming rehabilitation via an "ethic of openness" that is further expanded on throughout the book. I then discuss some key terms that appear in the book and some of the controversies that surround them. I conclude with an overview of each of the chapters.

A Post-Critical Approach

Rehabilitation professionals are committed to helping to enhance people's lives, but may struggle with how to do so in light of some of the bigger questions regarding their roles in, for example, working to maintain hope for recovery, "normalize" impaired bodies, and/or promote greater acceptance of diverse abilities. A key problem is the lack of theoretical tools for working through the function of rehabilitation in the lives of disabled people. Rehabilitation has been critiqued for lacking theoretical grounding (McPherson et al. 2015; Siegert et al. 2005) and an under-appreciation of the social and political dimensions of disability (Hammell 2006; Magasi 2008b; Oliver 1996). Beyond the development and application of middle range theories and frameworks like the International Classification of Functioning, Disability, and Health (ICF) (World Health Organization 2001), or profession-specific concepts like occupation, there has been little scholarship that explores the philosophical moorings of rehabilitation as a sociopolitical enterprise. Unearthing the complexity of rehabilitation practices and the implications for care recipients cannot be accomplished without uniting empirical and theoretical investigations. Theories and methods from the social sciences and humanities are slowly making an entrée into rehabilitation studies, and many of these are reflective of the "relational turn" in theorizing across disciplinary fields of inquiry. The post-critical approach that I describe in the following is an extension of this work that consolidates key premises from critical and postmodern scholarship.

Divisions between "postmodern" and "critical" approaches are slippery and indeed each has a number of variants. For my purposes it is not necessary to draw neat borders around them, and doing so would actually be antithetical to a postmodern commitment to dynamism and openness. Moreover, this slippage or *bricolage* is consistent with the blurring of genres that is occurring across contemporary fields of inquiry (Kincheloe and McLaren 2011; Lincoln and Guba 2011, p. 97). Borrowing from Agger (1991), I use the term "post-critical" as shorthand to capture the commonalties among the traditions that inform my approach.

Post-critical approaches emerged historically to challenge prevailing notions about "the order of things" and the assumptions that underpin ingrained principles of Western science (Foucault 1970). This has been called the "relational" or "postmodern turn" in contemporary theorizing, and it can be traced across the history of thought and key philosophers such as Kant, Marx, Hegel, and Niestzche; the writings of social theorists such as Foucault, Habermas, Derrida, and Deleuze; and feminists such as Irigaray, Haraway, Butler, and Shildrick among others. These scholars question truth claims, and the apparently objective nature of science, emphasizing the mediating role of social contexts and structures. Post-critical approaches now cross every field of inquiry including art, architecture, literature, cultural studies, gender studies, anthropology, and sociology as well as those that have historically intersected with rehabilitation: health sciences, education, psychology, and disability studies. Rehabilitation as a cross-disciplinary field is surrounded by post-critical scholarship and yet to date has made few inroads in this direction.

The most central and enduring feature of both critical and postmodern approaches is a shared critique of the dominance of positivism (Agger 1991). The rational scientific project of positivism is deeply ingrained in Western society and fields such as the health sciences and has relegated other modes of understanding to the margins. Rationalist thought and the scientific method can be traced to the seventeenth-century Enlightenment and Descartes' separation of mind and body into two distinct substances, each with a different essential nature (Mehta 2011). The body was viewed as a physical material object, while the mind was positioned as the locus of knowledge. This mind–body separation laid the groundwork for a host of other dualisms (e.g., person/object, science/art, man/woman, gay/straight, disabled/able-bodied) and the positivist empirical science that continues its dominance in health care and other fields to the present day (Holmes et al. 2006).

Positivist bioscience assumes that there is a stable reality. It is assumed that phenomena such as, for example, health, depression, disability, or quality of life exist in exactly the same way whether we understand them "correctly" or not. The task of scientific research is to uncover this underlying reality and establish relationships of cause and effect. Positivism emphasizes that science is objective, rational, neutral, and value free and is separate from the particulars of time and place or emotional, subjective, or political viewpoints (Green and Thorogood 2009, p. 13; Mehta 2011). Most of the research in health care and rehabilitation draws on this framing through the use of the "scientific method" where phenomena, their properties, and mechanisms are objectively established and described in putatively neutral terms. In the health sciences and other areas of inquiry, these methods are promoted for keeping data free of values and biases. For example, questionnaires that purport to measure quality of life

(Chapter 3) assume a pre-existing entity with a stable set of properties that can be measured under discrete "domains" (physical, psychological, social). Quality of life however is a concept, not a material object. Like all concepts, it is a human construction and only one possible way of framing people's experiences of their worlds. The reification of quality of life that I further explore in Chapter 3 helps reveal how positivism and the scientific method are so dominant in health care that they are usually not recognized as a particular way of knowing, and other ways of knowing are seen as unthinkable (Holmes et al. 2006).

Post-critical work rejects the assumptions of an objective, neutral, and value-free science and posits that all knowledge is perspectival (i.e., we always observe something from a certain viewpoint). Knowledge and what counts as legitimate ways of knowing (epistemology) arise from the historical conditions that precede individuals, and there can be no neutral or objective epistemology—that is, there is never a view from nowhere (Danemark et al. 2002, pp. 8–9). Coming back to the example of quality of life with a post-critical approach, the concept of quality of life and its assigned properties are recognized as "constructions." While the concept may be useful for labeling outcomes that fall beyond the simple presence or absence of disease, cure versus quality of life could have been divided in a host of other ways, not divided at all, or conceived of in different ways entirely. Post-critical approaches thus are focused on uncovering what is taken for granted as true or given and, without necessarily rejecting these "truths," acknowledge that they are provisional and always open to revision.

Assumptions of a neutral science miss out on how knowledge has been produced, how it persists, and whose interests it serves. Instead, post-critical work traces the evolution of power and discourse (patterned ways of thinking in talk and text) to explain how knowledge emerges and changes over time, and how contingent explanations of phenomena are taken up as stable realities. Post-critical work uses the methods of "problematization" and "deconstruction" to reveal the foundations that underpin the apparent truth-value of dominant ideas. These methods challenge the ways that prevailing descriptions of the world appear as self-evident, natural, or "just the ways things are." For example, Holmes et al. (2006) illuminate how evidence-based practice and the knowledge hierarchy that it constructs rely on positivist "regimes of truth" that dictate what counts as evidence, while other forms of knowledge are denigrated or ignored. They note that the task of analysis is "to demonstrate how concepts or ideas are contingent upon historical, linguistic, social and political discourses… by attending to how they came to be constructed in the first place" (Holmes et al. 2006, p. 182).

Over the past five decades, there has been a sustained and growing critique that bioscience at a minimum runs the risk of incomplete understandings of the complexities of health and illness and their effects on persons (see Williams 2003 for a review). Mehta (2011) goes so far as to say that by adhering rigidly to scientific method, biomedicine "gave up its moral responsibility toward the real health concerns of human beings." The dominance of positivism reflects particular historical alignments of knowledge and power, and who has the power to speak and to silence. Foucault (1980), in particular, demonstrated how dominant ideas persist not because of any overt form of imposition of will, but because dominant forms become normalized, taken for granted, and understood as "the way things are," which re/produces actions that further sediment the ideas (Foucault 1980).

Power is a pivotal concept in post-critical work and particularly the relation between knowledge and power in producing truth claims. Following Foucault (1980, p. 52), "(i)t is not possible for power to be exercised without knowledge, it is impossible for knowledge not to engender power." Power for Foucault is not the overt power of one group over another but instead is hidden and unrecognized. He saw power as circulating among individuals who are "vehicles of power" rather than its "points of application" (Foucault 1980, p. 98). Instances of oppression are understood as effects of power that materialize on a grid of power relations (Powers 2007).

Foucault was interested in how dominant ideologies structure what is thinkable and doable and how discourses constitute objects of knowledge. Said differently, power is a relational process embedded in context-specific situations, and one that exerts particular effects (experienced as both/neither "positive" or "negative") in the lives of people. Discourses are ways of thinking, speaking about, or representing things that are specific to a given place and time. In the context of contemporary health care, the authority of the clinician can be understood as a discursive power that imbues the figure of the clinician with the moral and intellectual sanction to prescribe treatment. This authority "shapes the realm of the possible" (Holmes et al. 2006, p. 183) and concomitantly becomes the manner in which the recipients of care understand themselves (McLaughlin and Coleman-Fountain 2014).

As part of the critique of positivism and bioscience, post-critical approaches focus on unearthing and "making strange" the classifications and categories that we take for granted as "true" representations of an underlying reality. "Classificatory thinking" as Bauman (2007) explains assigns arbitrary labels that divide up the world in particular ways. These are sedimented over time and appear as real in their common usage. Language itself thus constitutes reality (Agger 1991). Classifications are world-making in that they impose the logic and order that orients human practice and thought:

> To classify means to set apart, to segregate. It means first to postulate that the world consists of discrete and distinctive entities; then to postulate that each entity has a group of similar or adjacent entities with which it belongs, and with which—together—it is opposed to some other entities; and then to make the postulated real by linking differential patterns of action to different classes of entities...To classify, in other words, is to give the world a structure: to manipulate its probabilities; to make some events more likely than some others; to behave as if events were not random, or to limit or eliminate randomness of events (Bauman 2007).

Post-critical analysis works to illuminate the historical antecedents of classifications, uncovering how categories and their contemporary meanings came into being and the consequences of dividing the world accordingly. The categories and classificatory schemes explored in this book include disability (Chapter 2), quality of life (Chapter 3), development and childhood (Chapter 4), and in/dependence (Chapter 5) among others.

Post-critical approaches reverse the positivist tendency to reduce and finalize categories and concepts by seeking a diversity of relational meanings. Static or closed definitions of concepts are eschewed and instead used as tools for analysis. As Bourdieu and Wacquant (1992, pp. 95–96) put it: "(C)oncepts have no definition other than systemic ones, and are designed to be put to work empirically in systemic fashion. (Concepts) can be defined but only within the theoretical system they constitute, not in isolation... And what is true of concepts is true of relations, which acquire their meaning only within a system of relations." Said differently, there is no absolute meaning of a concept but only how it is used within a particular context and what it comes to mean to the people who use it. Concepts like disability, science, health, research, and gender are used to understand and order the world but they also exert both expected and unanticipated effects. Critical and postmodern approaches use concepts reflexively, examining how key words came to be dominant, how they continue to shape how we think and what we do, and to discover opportunities for change.

The belief that the bioscientific method is the only legitimate path to knowledge is deeply ingrained in health and rehabilitation. Dominant views of rehabilitation and disability are taken up and reproduced over time. They underpin *the logics* of rehabilitation, that is, its processes, structures and policies, the kind of research that is considered valid, the objects of treatment, and the priorities of rehabilitation organizations. Rehabilitation largely reflects the key features of positivist biomedicine as outlined by Nicholls (2012a, p. 361):

> Biomedicine privileges certain ways of thinking (reason, objectivity, value neutrality) and certain ways of practicing (assessment, diagnosis, treatment), it defines what is normal and abnormal, who is sick and who is well, who is mad and who is sane. It is also largely responsible for the day-to-day working of the health system (the design of hospitals around medical sub-specialities), the language of health care, and the way that health care is taught.

Dominant ways of understanding disability and the goals of rehabilitation are produced and reproduced by professionals who have the power to define what constitutes good or poor outcomes for recipients of care. This produces a particular focus in rehabilitation that has been challenged by disability studies scholars (Finkelstein 1998; Oliver 1996; Rioux and Bach 1994; Wendell 1996) and increasingly from within rehabilitation (French and Swain 2001; Hammell 2006; Kielhofner 2005; Magasi 2008b; Papadimitriou 2008; Swain and French 2004; Yoshida 1993).

So far I have noted that post-critical approaches share a critique of positivism, an analytical focus on the relationship between power and knowledge and the effects of classificatory schemes, and a commitment to relational inquiry. These and other key features of a postmodern/post-critical scholarship that I have drawn from Shildrick (1997) and Kincheloe and Mclaren (2011) are listed in Box 1.1. These features and their implications will be further explored in each of the chapters. It is worth mentioning that while these ideas overlap, Shildrick positions herself as a postmodern (or "postconventional") scholar while Kincheloe and Mclaren identify as critical.

The common features of post-critical approaches sketch out a set of ready-to-hand ideas for rehabilitating rehabilitation. They highlight the importance of historical analyses in revealing how contemporary practices grew from assumptions that built upon other assumptions, and how "things could be otherwise." Power, politics, and ingrained discourses orient practices and, while we can never fully escape these contingencies, revealing their logic is a powerful tool for effecting meaningful change. A post-critical lens thus suggests alternative areas of inquiry, new ways of producing knowledge, and different ways of examining common issues in rehabilitation. Explicitly aimed at re-form, a post-critical lens can be mobilized to examine every day practices and ask why they persist, whose interests they serve, what power relations are at play, and what assumptions underpin their ongoing acceptance (Agger 1991; Eakin et al. 1996). Analysis is directed at uncovering the inherent instabilities in all assumptions and truth claims. Nothing is ever settled. The aim is not to falsify past claims so much as to disrupt them toward creating spaces for other possibilities (Shildrick 1997, p. 6). To move! Unsettle. Not to destroy but

BOX 1.1 COMMON FEATURES AND IMPLICATIONS OF POST-CRITICAL APPROACHES

Features:

- All thought is fundamentally mediated by power relations that are socially and historically constituted (K&M)
- Facts can never be isolated from the domain of values or removed from some form of ideological inscription (K&M)
- Certain groups in any society are privileged over others, and although the reasons for this privileging vary widely, the oppression that characterizes contemporary societies is most forcefully reproduced when subordinates accept their social status as natural, necessary, or inevitable (K&M)
- Language is central to the formation of subjectivity (K&M)

Implications:

- The human subject can no longer individually authorize knowledge claims, and the notion of subjectivity itself is deeply problematized (MS)
- The boundaries between discrete bodies of knowledge have blurred to challenge both the hierarchical organization of distinct disciplines and the division between theory and practice (MS)
- Rational/scientific notions of a coherent truth and knowledge give way to dispersed, competing, and conflicting discourses (MS)
- The appeal to unified rationality or morality is not plausible, nor are the teleological ideals of the "grand narratives" of liberal humanism and science (including medical discourse) (MS)

Note: K&M = Kincheloe and McLaren (2011, p. 164), MS = Margrit Shildrick (1997, p. 6)

to reconsider and reconfigure what has been sedimented as "just the way things are." In these efforts, critical disability studies have much to offer in informing and re-forming rehabilitation practices.

Critical Disability Studies

Critical disability studies align with other areas of post-critical inquiry aimed at illuminating concepts and issues such as autonomy, competence, wholeness, normalcy, independence/dependence, health, physical appearance, and notions of progress (Linton et al. 1995, p. 5). As an academic field closely aligned with political advocacy, critical disability studies examine cultural representations throughout history, and the policies and practices of all societies to understand the sociopolitical (rather than the physical or psychological) determinants of disability (Longmore 2003, p. 222). While there are many strands of disability studies, they hold in common a shared belief that biomedicine is overly concerned with biological, neurological, and physiological processes, to the exclusion of the moral, social, political, cultural, and discursive mediators of disablement. This philosophical shift does not entail a complete rejection of "impairment effects" (Thomas 1999, pp. 24–25) or the utility of intervention and treatment. Instead, it challenges the idea that the economic and social marginalization of people labeled as disabled are inevitably linked to their bodily impairments. Disablement is understood as a sociopolitical process that affects individuals, but not individualized within a solitary person (Goodley 2014, pp. 341–349).

Dis/ability like other categories of race, sexuality, and gender can be examined as a socially constructed and maintained division that labels individual and assigns them a particular identity that has consequences for their lives. Thus as Linton et al. (1995, p. 5) note, disability studies work to "analyze the construction of the category 'disability,' the impact of that construction on society, and on the content and structure of knowledge." The sociopolitical analysis of disability can thus serve as an exemplar that provides a broader understanding of society and the significance of human variation (see Chapter 2). Bringing critical disability studies into rehabilitation has the potential to not only raise awareness of the sociopolitical aspects of disability experience, but to radically transform the organizing principles of practice.

Critical disability studies have much to offer rehabilitation but maintain a rather marginal position in professional discourse and scholarship. Disability as "a problem to be fixed" remains a dominant idea in rehabilitation despite increased emphasis on "biopsychosocial" models of care (Chapter 2). Advocates working in disability studies have a long tradition of rejecting biomedical approaches to disability, and the field is replete with sophisticated research and scholarship debating the complex relations that intersect to produce disabled bodies. While it may be argued that rehabilitation has made great strides in moving away from the so-called medical model of practice through an increased interest in enabling activity and participation, it still largely constructs disability as an individual deficit that is addressed through individual interventions

(French and Swain 2001; Hammell 2006; Magasi 2008b). Helping persons is not in and of itself a problem, but the focus on individual bodies decontextualizes disability and off-loads responsibility for change onto disabled people. Magasi (2008a, p. 613) in her call for infusing disability studies into rehabilitation suggests:

> Even though client-centered practice is a laudable goal in service delivery, the emphasis on the individual can actually depoliticize the plight of people with disabilities and thereby obscure the role that larger social factors play in shaping the disability experience. Just as no man is an island, no person with a disability lives apart from the social context. Attitudes about disability frame how people see themselves and how others see them. Practitioners must be careful that, while they keep the person firmly in the center of their rehabilitation practice, they do not lose sight of the larger world in which that person lives.

In rehabilitation, a biomedical focus on individual deficits (whether at the level of body structures, activity, or participation) orients what counts as a "problem" to be fixed. The interdisciplinary lens of critical disability studies provides an avenue to integrate bioscientific and sociopolitical approaches to rehabilitation without privileging one over the other.

An Ethic of Openness

Throughout the book I sketch out a reconfigured ethics of rehabilitation that is congruent with a post-critical commitment to *openness*. Ethics in this sense is not focused on the mainstream bioethics of contemporary health care and its concerns with, for example, procedural research ethics, decision-making, or informed consent. Dominant forms of contemporary bioethics are grounded in analytical philosophy and a materialist ethic that reduces moral concepts to empirically (pre)determined outcomes arrived at through the rational application of principles. I problematize the assumption that only outcomes hold moral relevance for practice and question the normativities that govern rehabilitation and its constitution of "the good." Mainstream bioethics tends to universalize the subject as a bearer of rights devoid of history, particularity, relationships, or social location (Kelly 2003). Instead, my project builds from a relational ethics that particularizes experiences in the social and temporal contexts where they are constituted and reproduced. In so doing I examine ethical moments of radical openness, and how to disassemble habits of thought in rehabilitation. I explore ethical questions that are seldom asked about the object of rehabilitation rather than those concerned with the "proper conduct" of the ethical practitioner (Shildrick 1997, p. 7). They are ideas that appear and disappear in our peripheral vision: Why the focus on independence? Why privilege walking? How do we think about disability? What happens when we think differently?

This *ethic of openness* I describe draws from the work of Margrit Shildrick and her postmodern approach to disability and the body. An open approach is not an ethic of adherence to universal rules or principles, but rather one that seeks to challenge ingrained norms, avoiding stasis and opening up new possibilities for practice (Shildrick 1997, pp. 212–213). Shildrick's approach seeks to break down binary categories that form the basis of contemporary Western bioethics including normal/abnormal, health/illness, and self/other (Shildrick 2005, p. 4). Binaries are scrutinized to reveal their unreflective assumptions, not necessarily to discard them, but to accept that they are unstable and open to transformation. Shildrick insists that such an approach is necessary to deal with the full complexity of contemporary life (2005, p. 11):

> In light of the real confusions, complexities, and misunderstandings that characterize everyday experiences and decision making, subjecting the normative structures of modernity to a critique that exposes rather than covers over their shortcomings and inevitable aporias—in other words, places of paradox and impasse—seems well-conceived. But in postmodernist thinking, it is not only the evidently disordered contexts that clearly stretch our ability to impose predetermined rules, but the normative structure as a whole that is questioned. If nothing can be taken as given, then there is always an intrinsic undecidability at work.

An ethic of openness is thus the normative expression of a post-critical epistemology. While it is not intended to provide a prescriptive set of rules for determining action, it does provide a *method of analysis* that can be employed to understand the multiple effects of practices some of which are unintended, potentially harmful, and largely obscured from view. For example, practices focused on measuring and ameliorating impairments can contribute to social harms by marking the desirable or undesirable traits of individuals or populations (Chapter 2). As I explore throughout the book and summarize in Chapter 7, an ethic of openness is most clearly understood as an ethic of doubt. An open approach mobilizes and reforms existing conceptual orientations, not as some kind of finalized solution, but as an ongoing commitment to thinking against the grain.

Moving Bodies

Hand-in-hand with an ethic of openness is an examination of bodies, that is, how we think about bodies (or *the* body, but "the" assumes a universality which I want to avoid) and what we do in the name of rehabilitation *to* and *with* bodies and to what ends. My engagement with bodies extends beyond formulations of the "body as object" to consider how persons live through their bodies in an embodied relation with the world. This is the "lived body" described by phenomenologists who suggest that we perceive and act in the world through an integrated body with no distinction between the psychological and the material (Bullington 2013). Embodiment troubles the Cartesian split of mind/body, collapsing the distinction between subject and object (Merleau-Ponty 1962). Hughes and Patterson (1997, p. 335) suggest that: "To be a body (the body as subject) is a purely experiential ontological condition in which the body is as it is -in pain, pleasure, joy or tears. This is the body as sensibility, motility and kinesthetic…the realm of habitual, sensate being in which the body is the body-subject." Persons thus both *have* bodies and *are* bodies in the same moment—the social is embodied and the body is social (Crossley 1995). Bodies move in the world and "it is through the spatial and temporal extension of our bodies that we become our selves" (Shildrick 2002, p. 49). There is no subject without a body, or body without a subject.

In post-critical scholarship, bodies are understood as constructions or "effects of language." In other words, we do not have any direct knowledge of an essential or pre-existing body but rather we understand the body only through concepts and categories. As Donna Haraway states, "[B]odies are not born: they are made" (Haraway 1989, p. 10). Thus we can ask what kinds of bodies are produced and reproduced by rehabilitation. Bodies that deviate from pre-established norms are assessed as amenable to intervention, and these acts of assessment and intervention in turn reproduce "patient bodies," "fit bodies," "healthy bodies," "dysfunctional bodies," and/or "disabled bodies." Moreover, post-critical approaches trouble notions that inhere in contemporary health-care practices of the autonomous self contained within a material body. As I explore in Chapters 5 and 6, reconsidering bodies as connected, unbounded by the skin, and in a constant state of flux suggests other possibilities for new bodily forms and new ways of doing-in-the-world. Bodies extend into other bodies, machines, prosthetics, and animals that create functional assemblages. These configurations call into question where the body begins and ends, and expand the possibilities of what a body can do. Through these explorations, I suggest that the pervasive and reductive notions of "body as machine" in rehabilitation are limited and limiting.

So where does this talk of openness, ethics, and bodies lead? Not patient-centered or rehabilitation-centered but de-centered: moving together and apart. I consider that the task of rehabilitation is to foster connectivities, movement between bodies, and new dynamic technologies of body-worlds (re-form, re-consider, re-figure, re-collect, re-assemble). Movement for people ("clients") and movement as a basis for politico-ethical re-form. I ask how we think about disability: Is it a "problem" and of what or for whom? I explore movement as multiple tangled "lines of flight" rather than as a uniform, unidirectional trajectory. I identify constraints to movement (sociocultural and material, immediate and remote), and suggest both opportunities for ruptures in these constraints, and creative possibilities within relatively bounded systems.

Use of Terms

In this section, I provide preliminary explanations of key terms and concepts. This helps to ground the discussion and introduces some of the controversies and alternative epistemologies explored throughout the book.

Practice: My use of "practice" refers to the broad gamut of what rehabilitation professionals *do* in their day-to-day work. It is not limited to clinical practice (and certainly not to "best practices"), but rather includes all of the activities undertaken in research, scholarship, and education. Practice can refer to both a habitual way of doing something (an entrenched practice), as well as a process (to practice ethically). Practices are active in that they do things in the world; they are acts done *with* or *to* others and have consequences for recipients of care. In sociology, practices are conceived of as behaviors that are comprised of meanings, knowledge, materials, and competencies which interconnect elements of bodily and mental activities (Maller 2015, p. 57). Sociological examinations of practices look at the interplay between individual choices, actions, and their contextual mediators. Viewed this way, all of the doings of practice across research, education, and the clinic are organized according to particular "logics" and assumptions that are built into the social and institutional contexts of professional work. The mundane practices of individuals and groups can be said to exhibit a *practical logic* that integrates rational calculation and external structural mediators (Bourdieu 1980, p. 50). The origins of these local logics, how they shape practice, and their effects on individuals are explored in each of the chapters.

Biomedicine: The term biomedicine denotes the medical profession in Western nations and is meant to indicate its emphasis on biology, pathology, and the scientific method. Analogous terms are "Western medicine," "allopathic medicine," "bioscientific medicine," or simply "medicine" (Gaines and David-Floyd 2004). Biomedicine is grounded in objectivist scientific methods and particular understandings of the body and disease ("bioscience"). The underpinnings of biomedicine have been critiqued in favor of more holistic or humanistic approaches to care that treat the "whole person" rather than physical pathology. I expand on this discussion in greater depth in Chapter 3.

Neoliberalism: Neoliberalism refers to a political economic theory that emerged in the second half of the twentieth century and continues to dominate the contemporary landscape globally. Closely aligned with capitalism, neoliberalism proposes that human well-being can best be advanced through free market economies that are allowed to grow with minimal interference from governments. Neoliberal policies are responsible for pervasive changes in contemporary social life. These expand beyond the restructuring of public institutions, but as Harvey (2007, p. 3) notes, how people and societies understand "divisions of labour, social relations, welfare provisions, technological mixes, ways of life and thought, reproductive activities, attachments to the land and habits of the heart." Neoliberalism reflects and promotes particular values, which include rationality, self-sufficiency, autonomy, productivity, individualism, and self-interest. The emphasis on personal and economic freedom (which have been largely taken up as self-evident values) shifts the responsibility for prosperity onto individuals and away from the community or state (Harvey 2007). In health care and rehabilitation, these values are reproduced in notions of individual responsibility for health, and in the construction of outcomes oriented to independence, self-care, productivity, and economic self-sufficiency. I explore these ideas in more detail throughout the book.

Recipients of care: The usages of terms "patient," "client," or "consumer" are contentious in the health-care literature. Arguments in favor of the use of "client" or "consumer" (or other terms such as "service user") construct health care as form of service provision usually framed within a neoliberal discourse promoting individual rights and autonomy. The paternalism that has come to be associated with the use of "patient" is rejected in favor of terms that signal a leveling of power imbalances between the recipients of care and health professionals (Hammell 2006, p. 11). While there is much merit to these arguments, the assumption of the rational, autonomous, rights-bearing individual, and the reductionist views of power they rely on have also been the subject of much critique (McLaughlin 2009). Thus while I sometimes use the terms client or patient, I prefer to use "recipients of care," or simply "people" to avoid compounding some of the problems associated with classifying persons along these lines.

Disabled people/people with disabilities: Similar to the patient/client debate, disability terminology is also contested and at times divisive. Both of these terms are used widely but there are variations across disciplines, regions, and even age groups (Goodley 2011, p. 9). Each reflects a particular political stance that responds to the exclusion of people with physical, sensory, psychiatric, or cognitive impairments. The term "people with disabilities" uses what is called "people first" language that puts the person before the disability by describing "what a person has, not who a person is" (Snow 2008). "Disabled people," the terminology that I most often use, suggests that disability is not something a person has, but rather something experienced as a result of prejudice, discrimination, and social exclusion (Morris 2001; Titchkosky 2001). The function of locating disability *either* in the person *or* the environment, however, has also been challenged on a number of fronts that outline the co-constituting relationships between the two (Hughes and Paterson 1997). In Chapter 2, I problematize the category of "disability" and how it functions to separate one group of people (disabled) from another (so-called normal or non-disabled people). To underscore these acts of categorization, I frequently use the terminology "people labeled as disabled."

Mobilizing Post-Critical Methodologies: Book Outline

The project of the book is to draw on post-critical approaches to problematize taken-for-granted ideas that underpin practice, but also to suggest points of departure and "lines of flight" for a reconfigured rehabilitation. "Lines of flight," as described by Deleuze and Guattari (1987, p. 205), are creative thought-movements that produce cracks in the dominant reality and present new ways of thinking and doing. Such shifts are partly realized through language. Language is a way to get stuck in the taken for granted, but can also be a powerful tool to destabilize, move, and remake the world. Fraser and Gordon (1994, p. 310) remind us that "keywords typically carry unspoken assumptions and connotations that can powerfully influence the discourses they permeate in part by constituting a …taken-for-granted commonsense belief that escapes critical scrutiny."

The purpose is not to obfuscate by introducing sometimes challenging post-critical concepts (like "lines of flight"), but rather to capitalize on their explanatory power. As Bourdieu (1989, p. 24) said, "complexity lies within the social reality and not in a somewhat decadent desire to say complicated things." To help break what is taken for granted, in this book I engage with the complexity underlying key concepts and terms in rehabilitation through a number of entry points and overlaps.

This book builds on other nascent efforts in rehabilitation and its disciplines that draw on the relational turn in contemporary theorizing to invigorate health-care research, practice, and pedagogy. Karen Whalley Hammel's problematizations of the "sacred texts" and assumptions underpinning rehabilitation have been particularly groundbreaking and influential in this regard (2006, 2009a,b, 2015). Hammel, like other boundary crossers from within rehabilitation (e.g., French and Swain 2001; Kielhofner 2005; Magasi 2008b; Roush and Sharby 2011; Yoshida 1993), has drawn from disability studies to rethink the dominant constructions of normalcy that pervade rehabilitation practices. There is also a small but growing group of critical social scientists studying the social processes of rehabilitation and the implications for practice. I have been particularly influenced in this regard by the work of Christina Papadimitriou (2007, 2008), Brett Smith (2008, 2013; Smith and Sparkes 2005, 2008), and Myriam Winance (2006a,b, 2007, 2010, 2014). The work of these scholars and many others (e.g., Clark et al. 2007; Edwards et al. 2014; Fadyl et al. 2015; Kinsella and Whiteford 2009; Leplege et al. 2015; Manderson and Warren 2008, 2010; Nicholls and Cheek 2006; Parry 2004; Ravaud and Stiker 2001; Rudman 2014; Setchell et al. 2014; Shaw and DeForge 2012; Stiker 1999; Trede 2012; Wheatley 2005) signal that a post-critical rehabilitation movement is upon us. My hope in these pages is to build on the momentum of these individuals who, by resisting the status quo, propel rehabilitation into multiple lines of flight.

In my experience there is a clear need for post-critical scholarship to help guide trainees in critiquing rehabilitation practices and developing research ideas. To that end, the book is developed with graduate students in mind, but will be useful for anyone across disciplines who is new to post-critical thinking. As a transdisciplinary project, the book integrates research, scholarship, and theories from health sciences, social sciences, philosophy, and disability studies. In doing so, it will be of interest to readers looking to engage in boundary-crossing scholarship and has broader applications outside of rehabilitation to health, education, and social welfare.

Outline of Chapters

The book is designed to be read as an application of post-critical methodologies to the case of rehabilitation realized through the metaphor of movement. To that end, each of the chapters examines a core philosophical concept in rehabilitation, how it came to be dominant, its effects, and its consequences. In the final chapter, I explore the implications for reforming rehabilitation practices guided by a reflexive "ethic of openness" to promote new ways of thinking and doing rehabilitation.

Each of Chapters 2 through 6 works toward cultivating creative change by critically unpacking and destabilizing five of rehabilitation's most entrenched concepts: disability, quality of life, independence, development, and mobility. All follow a similar outline wherein I first work to unpack the concept by looking at some of its historical antecedents and tracing how current practices and understandings emerged over time. I then analyze how the concept is employed in health care and rehabilitation, the intended and unintended effects, and the possibilities for change. I chose to focus on disability, quality of life, independence, and mobility because they strike me as among the most deeply embedded, most used, and thus the most taken-for-granted concepts in the field. The choice of development is perhaps more personal as it stems from my experiences as a physiotherapist and childhood disability researcher exploring the linkages between developmental discourses and the therapeutic endpoints that are constructed for children labeled as disabled. Nevertheless, I argue that developmental discourses have effects that extend beyond children's rehabilitation.

While each chapter deals with a different rehabilitation concept, they are interconnected and overlapping in exploring the logics of rehabilitation practices and their effects. In Chapter 2, I examine the construction of disability in rehabilitation contexts. Because rehabilitation historically has been oriented to restoration and re/integration, I suggest that it inevitably relies on notions of normalization that efface differences and thus risks devaluing bodies labeled as disabled. I propose that practices oriented to helping people create new ways of doing and being in world do not have to be constructed in relation to preconceived bodily norms or modes of function. I extend this discussion in Chapter 3 through an exploration of the ordering of bodies through measures of quality of life. I examine the conceptual confusion that surrounds quality of life measurement, and how the measures themselves, in assessing functional abilities and symptoms outside of their social contexts, reproduce deeply held social biases about what constitutes a good life. Development (Chapter 4), because it is discussed as either "normal" or "delayed," provides another rich example for exploring the normative dimensions of rehabilitation. Developmental discourses, although most prominent in children's rehabilitation, have implications for all populations in terms of how categories of childhood, adulthood, and aging are conceived and reproduced.

Independence and quality of life are closely related in rehabilitation discourse with the former promoted as a key determinant of the latter, and both are intertwined with how disability is constructed and addressed. In Chapter 5, I problematize independence as a taken-for-granted goal of rehabilitation and explore the idea of movement in and out of various "dependencies" as being inherent to the human condition. Chapter 6 serves an integrative function with mobility practices used as exemplars to synthesize and apply the key ideas raised in the previous chapters. Mobility is a key intervention and outcome of rehabilitation both as an end in itself and for its therapeutic and preventative effects. The chapter surfaces the normative meanings of mobility and draws on the postmodern notion of "assemblages" to consider the examples of amputee mobilities, crawling mobilities, and wheelchair mobilities.

The concluding Chapter 7 reviews and consolidates the ideas presented in the book and draws on the movement metaphor to suggest new directions in practice, research, and scholarship. I suggest that the task of rehabilitation is to foster connectivities within a reconfigured ethics of rehabilitation that includes attention to political reform and breaking habits of thought. This includes a discussion of how rehabilitation could benefit from further immersion into the social and political determinants of disability, and the benefits of more cross-pollination between rehabilitation studies and critical disability studies.

The book should be read as an exposition of how to employ a theoretical methodology toward enacting practical change and not as a critique of particular areas of practice. Readers will note that the practice examples offered throughout are primarily oriented to physical rehabilitation, and that some patient groupings are represented more than others. Similarly, the concepts that are examined in each of the chapters provide points of departure for exploring how to do post-critical analyses, but there are numerous other concepts that also could be explored. To that end, the book provides an analytical methodology for reflexive scholarship that sees theory and practice as intimately intertwined and provides practical directions for change and re-forms toward a moving movement.

References

Agger, B. 1991. Critical theory, poststructuralism, postmodernism: Their sociological relevance. *Annual Review of Sociology* 17: 105–131.

Bauman, Z. 2007. *Modernity and Ambivalence.* Cambridge, U.K.: Polity Press.

Bourdieu, P. 1980. *The Logic of Practice.* Stanford, CA: Stanford University Press.

Bourdieu, P. 1989. Social space and symbolic power. *Sociological Theory* 7(1): 14–25.

Bourdieu, P. and Wacquant, L.J.D. 1992. *An Invitation to Reflexive Sociology.* London, U.K.: University of Chicago Press.

Bullington, J. 2013. *The Expression of the Psychosomatic Body from a Phenomenological Perspective* (*Springer Briefs in Philosophy*). New York: Springer.

Clark, A.M., MacIntyre, P.D., and Cruickshank, J. 2007. A critical realist approach to understanding and evaluating heart health programmes. *Health* 11(4): 513–539.

Crossley, N. 1995. Merleau-Ponty, the elusive body and carnal sociology. *Body and Society* 1(1): 43–63.

Danemark, B., Ekstrom, M., Jakobsen, L., and Karlsson, J.C. 2002. *Explaining Society.* London, U.K.: Routledge.

Deleuze, G. and Guattari, F. 1987. *A Thousand Plateaus: Capitalism and Schizophrenia.* Minneapolis, MN: University of Minnesota Press.

Eakin, J., Robertson, A., Poland, B., Coburn, D., and Edwards, R. 1996. Towards a critical social science perspective on health promotion research. *Health Promotion International* 11(2): 157–165.

Edwards, G., Noreau, L., Boucher, N. et al. 2014. Disability, rehabilitation research and post-Cartesian embodied ontologies—Has the research paradigm changed? In *Environmental Contexts and Disability,* eds. B. Altmana and S. Barnartt, 8th edn., pp. 73–102. Bingley, U.K.: Emerald Group Publishing Limited.

Fadyl, J., McPherson, K., and Nicholls, D. 2015. Re/creating entrepreneurs of the self: Discourses of worker and employee 'value' and current vocational rehabilitation practices. *Sociology of Health & Illness,* 37(4): 506–521.

Finkelstein, V. 1998. Disability: A social challenge or an administrative responsibility? In *Disabling Barriers—Enabling Environments,* eds. J. Swain, V. Finkelstein, S. French, and M. Oliver, pp. 34–43. London, U.K.: Sage.

Foucault, M. 1970. *The Order of Things: An Archaeology of Human Sciences,* 2nd edn. London, U.K.: Tavistock Publications.

Foucault, M. 1980. Power/knowledge: Selected interviews and other writings 1972–77. ed. C. Gordon. New York: Pantheon Books.

Fraser, N. and Gordon, L. 1994. A genealogy of dependency: Tracing a keyword of the U.S. welfare state. *Signs* 19(2): 309–336.

French, S. and Swain, J. 2001. The relationship between disabled people and health and welfare professionals. In *Handbook of Disability Studies,* eds. G.L. Albrecht, K.D. Seelman, and M. Bury, pp. 734–753. London, U.K.: Sage.

Gaines, A.D. and David-Floyd, R. 2004. Biomedicine. In *Encyclopedia of Medical Anthropology*, eds. M. Ember and C. Ember, pp. 95–109. Dordrecht, the Netherlands: Kluwer Academic Publishers.

Gibson, B.E., Nicholls, D.A., and Nixon, S. 2010. Critical reflections on the physiotherapy profession in Canada. *Physiotherapy Canada* 62(2): 98–103.

Gil, J. 2005. The dancer's body. In *A Shock to Thought: Expression after Deleuze and Guattari*, ed. B. Massumi, pp. 117–127. London, U.K.: Taylor & Francis (e-book).

Goodley, D. 2011. *Disability Studies: An Interdisciplinary Introduction*. London, U.K.: Sage.

Goodley, D. 2014. *Dis/ability Studies: Theorising Disablism and Ableism*. New York: Routledge.

Green, J. and Thorogood, N. 2009. *Qualitative Methods for Health Research*. London, U.K.: Sage.

Hammell, K.W. 2006. *Perspectives on Disability and Rehabilitation*. Edinburgh, U.K.: Elsevier.

Hammell, K.W. 2009a. Sacred tests: A sceptical exploration of the assumptions underpinning theories of occupation. *Canadian Journal of Occupational Therapy* 76(1): 6–13.

Hammel, K.W. 2009b. Self-care, productivity, and leisure, or dimensions of occupational experience? Rethinking occupational 'categories'. *Canadian Journal of Occupational Therapy* 76(2): 107–114.

Hammell, K.W. 2015. Client-centred occupational therapy: The importance of critical perspectives. *Scandinavian Journal of Occupational Therapy* 22(4): 237–243.

Haraway, D. 1989. The biopolitics of postmodern bodies: Determinations of self in immune system discourse. *Difference* 1: 3–43.

Harvey, D. 2007. *A Brief History of Neoliberalism*. Oxford, U.K.: Oxford University Press. ProQuest ebrary. http://site.ebrary.com/lib/alltitles/docDetail.action?docID=10180656&p00=brief%20history%20neoliberalism (accessed March 20, 2015).

Holmes, D., Murray, S.J., Perron, A., and Rail, G. 2006. Deconstructing the evidence-based discourse in health science: Truth, power, and fascism. *Integrated Journal Evidence Based Health* 4: 180–186.

Hughes, B. and Paterson, K. 1997. The social model of disability and the disappearing body: Towards a sociology of impairment. *Disability and Society* 12(3): 325–340.

Kelly, S.E. 2003. Bioethics and rural health: Theorizing place, space and subjects. *Social Science & Medicine* 56: 2277–2288.

Kielhofner, G. 2005. Rethinking disability and what to do about it: Disability studies and its implications for occupational therapy. *The American Journal of Occupational Therapy* 59(5): 487–496.

Kincheloe, J.L. and McLaren, P. 2011. Critical pedagogy and qualitative research: Moving to the bricolage. In *Handbook of Qualitative Research*, 3rd edn., eds. N.K. Denzin and Y.S. Lincoln, pp. 163–178. London, U.K.: Sage.

Kinsella, E.A. and Whiteford, G.E. 2009. Knowledge generation and utilisation in occupational therapy: Towards epistemic reflexivity. *Australian Occupational Therapy Journal* 56(4): 249–258.

Leplège, A., Barral, C., and McPherson, K.M. 2015. Conceptualizing disability to inform rehabilitation: Historical and epistemological perspectives. In *Rethinking Rehabilitation Theory and Practice*, eds. K.M. McPherson, B.E. Gibson, and A. Leplège. Boca Raton, FL: CRC Press.

Lincoln, Y.S. and Guba, E.G. 2011. Paradigmatic controversies, contradictions and emerging confluences. In *Handbook of Qualitative Research*, 2nd edn., eds. N.K. Denzin and Y.S. Lincoln, pp. 97–128. Thousand Oaks, CA: Sage.

Linton, S., Mello, S., and O'Neill, J. 1995. Disability studies: Expanding the parameters of diversity. *The Radical Teacher* 47(Fall): 4–10.

Longmore, P.K. 2003. *Why I Burned My Book and Other Essays on Disability*. Philadelphia, PA: Temple University Press.

Magasi, S. 2008a. Disability studies in practice: A work in progress. *Topics in Stroke Rehabilitation* 15(6): 611–617.

Magasi, S. 2008b. Infusing disability studies into the rehabilitation sciences. *Topics in Stroke Rehabilitation* 15(3): 283–287.

Maller, C.J. 2015. Understanding health through social practices: Performance and materiality in everyday life. *Sociology of Health and Illness* 37(1): 52–66.

Manderson, L. and Warren, N. 2008. Constructing hope dis/continuity and the narrative construction of recovery in the rehabilitation unit. *Journal of Contemporary Ethnography* 37(2): 180–201.

Manderson, L. and Warren, N. 2010. The art of (re)learning to walk: Trust on the rehabilitation ward. *Qualitative Health Research* 20(10): 1418–1432.

McLaughlin, H. 2009. What's in a name: 'client','patient','customer','consumer', 'expert by experience','service user'—What's next? *British Journal of Social Work* 39(6): 1101–1117.

McLaughlin, J. and Coleman-Fountain, E. 2014. The unfinished body: The medical and social reshaping of disabled young bodies. *Social Science and Medicine* 120: 76–84.

McPherson, K.M., Gibson, B.E., and Leplège, A. 2015. Rethinking rehabilitation: Theory, practice, history—And the future. In *Rethinking Rehabilitation Theory and Practice*, eds. K.M. McPherson, B.E. Gibson, and A. Leplege. Boca Raton, FL: CRC Press.

Mehta, N. 2011. Mind-body dualism: A critique from a health perspective. *Mens Sana Monographs* 9(1): 202–209.

Merleau-Ponty, M. 1962. *Phenomenology of Perception*. London, U.K.: Routledge.

Morris, J. 2001. Impairment and disability: Constructing an ethics of care that promotes human rights. *Hypatia* 16(4): 1–13.

Nicholls, D.A. 2012a. Postmodernism and physiotherapy research. *Physical Therapy Reviews* 17(6): 360–368.

Nicholls, D.A. 2012b. Foucault and physiotherapy. *Physiotherapy Theory Practice* 28(6): 447–453.

Nicholls, D.A. and Cheek, J. May 2006. Physiotherapy and the shadow of prostitution: The society of trained masseuses and the massage scandals of 1894. *Social Science & Medicine* 62(9): 2336–2348.

Nicholls, D.A. and Gibson, B.E. 2010. The body and physiotherapy. *Physiotherapy Theory Practice* 26(8): 497–509.

Nicholls, D.A., Gibson, B.E., and Fadyl, J. 2015. Rethinking movement: Postmodern reflections on a dominant rehabilitation discourse. In *Rethinking Rehabilitation: Theory and Practice*, eds. K.M. McPherson, B.E. Gibson, and A. Leplege, pp. 97–116. Boca Raton, FL: CRC Press.

Oliver, M. 1996. *Understanding Disability: From Theory to Practice*. New York: St. Martin's Press.

Papadimitriou, C. 2007. 'It was hard but you did it': The co-production of 'work' in a clinical setting among spinal cord injured adults and their physical therapists. *Disability & Rehabilitation* 30(5): 365–374.

Papadimitriou, C. 2008. Becoming en-wheeled: The situated accomplishment of re-embodiment as a wheelchair user after spinal cord injury. *Disability & Society* 23(7): 691–704.

Parry, R.R.H. 2004. The interactional management of patients' physical incompetence: A conversation analytic study of physiotherapy interactions. *Sociology of Health & Illness* 26(7): 976–1007.

Powers, P. 2007. The philosophical foundations of Foucaultian discourse analysis. *Critical Approaches to Discourse Analysis Across Disciplines* 1(2): 18–34.

Ravaud, J. and Stiker, H. 2001. Inclusion/exclusion: An analysis of historical and cultural meanings. In *Handbook of Disability Studies*, eds. G.L. Albrecht, K.D. Seelman, and M. Bury, pp. 490–514. Thousand Oaks, CA: Sage.

Rioux, M.H. and Bach, M. 1994. *Disability Is Not Measles: New Research Paradigms in Disability*. Toronto, Ontario, Canada: The Roeher Institute.

Roush, S.E. and Sharby, N. 2011. Disability reconsidered: The paradox of physical therapy. *Physical Therapy* 91(12): 1715–1727.

Rudman, D.L. 2014. Embracing and enacting an 'Occupational imagination': Occupational science as transformative. *Journal of Occupational Science* 21(4): 373–388.

Setchell, J., Watson, B., Jones, L., Gard, M., and Briffa, K. 2014. Physiotherapists demonstrate weight stigma: A cross-sectional survey of Australian physiotherapists. *Journal of Physiotherapy* 60(3): 157–162.

Shaw, J.A. and DeForge, R.T. 2012. Physiotherapy as bricolage: Theorizing expert practice. *Physiotherapy Theory Practice* 28(6): 420–427.

Shildrick, M. 1997. *Leaky Bodies and Boundaries: Feminism, Postmodernism and (Bio)ethics*. London, U.K.: Routledge.

Shildrick, M. 2002. *Embodying the Monster: Encounters with the Vulnerable Self*. London, U.K.: Sage Publications.

Shildrick, M. 2005. Beyond the body of bioethics: Challenging the conventions. In *Ethics of the Body: Postconventional Challenges*, eds. M. Shildrick and R. Mykitiuk, pp. 1–26. Cambridge, U.K.: MIT Press.

Siegert, R.J., McPherson, K.M., and Dean, S.G. 2005. Theory development and a science of rehabilitation. *Disability Rehabilitation* 27(24): 1493–1501.

Smith, B. 2008. Spinal cord injury, the body, and narratives of recovery in mental distress. *Spinal Cord Injury Psychosocial Process* 20(2): 18–30.

Smith, B. 2013. Sporting spinal cord injuries, social relations, and rehabilitation narratives: An ethnographic creative non-fiction of becoming disabled through sport. *Sociology of Sport Journal* 30(2): 132–152.

Smith, B. and Sparkes, A.C. 2005. Men, sport, spinal cord injury, and narratives of hope. *Social Science & Medicine* 61(5): 1095–1105.

Smith, B. and Sparkes, A.C. 2008. Changing bodies, changing narratives and the consequences of tellability: A case study of becoming disabled through sport. *Sociology of Health and Illness* 30(2): 217–236.

Snow, K. 2008. People first language. *Disability Is Natural*. Woodland Park, CO: BraveHeart Press. http://www.disabilityisnatural.com/images/PDF/pfl09.pdf (accessed March 2, 2015).

Stiker, H.J. 1999. The birth of rehabilitation. In *A History of Disability*, pp. 121–189. Ann Arbor, MI: University of Michigan Press.

Swain, J. and French, S. 2004. Physiotherapy: A psychosocial approach. In *Researching together: A participatory approach*, eds. S. French, J. Sim. 3rd ed., pp. 317–331. Oxford, U.K.: Butterworth-Heinemann.

Titchkosky, T. 2001. Disability: A rose by any other name? “People-First” Language in Canadian Society. *Canadian Review of Sociology and Anthropology* 38(2): 125.

Thomas, C. 1999. *Female Forms: Experiencing and Understanding Disability*. Buckingham, U.K.: Open University Press.

Trede, F. 2012. Emancipatory physiotherapy practice. *Physiotherapy Theory Practice* 28(6): 466–473.

Wendell, S. 1996. *The Rejected Body: Feminist Philosophical Reflections on Disability*. New York: Routledge.

Wheatley, E.E. 2005. Disciplining bodies at risk cardiac rehabilitation and the medicalization of fitness. *Journal of Sport & Social Issues* 29(2): 198–221.

Whyte, J. 2008. A grand unified theory of rehabilitation (we wish!). The 5th John Stanley Coulter Memorial Lecture. *Archives of Physical Medicine and Rehabilitation* 89(2): 203–209.

Whyte, J. and Hart, T. 2003. It’s more than a black box; it’s a Russian doll: Defining rehabilitation treatments. *American Journal of Physical Medicine and Rehabilitation* 82(8): 639–652.

Williams, S.J. 2003. Beyond meaning, discourse and the empirical world: Critical realist reflections on health. *Social Theory and Health* 1(1): 42–71.

Winance, M. 2006a. Trying out the wheelchair: The mutual shaping of people and devices through adjustment. *Science, Technology, & Human Values* 31(1): 52–72.

Winance, M. 2006b. Pain, disability and rehabilitation practices—A phenomenological perspective. *Disability and Rehabilitation* 28(18): 1109–1118.

Winance, M. 2007. Being normally different? Changes to normalization processes: From alignment to work on the norm. *Disability & Society* 22(6): 625–638.

Winance, M. 2010. Care and disability: Practices of experimenting, tinkering with, and arranging people and technical aids. In *Care in Practice: On Tinkering in Clinics, Homes and Farms*, eds. A. Mol, I. Moser, and J. Pols, pp. 93–117. Bielefeld, Germany: Transaction Publishers.

Winance, M. 2014. Universal design and the challenge of diversity: Reflections on the principles of UD, based on empirical research of people's mobility. *Disability & Rehabilitation* 36(16): 1334–1343.

World Health Organization. 2001. *International Classification of Functioning, Disability and Health.* Geneva, Switzerland: World Health Organization.

Yoshida, K. K. 1993. Reshaping of self: A pendular reconstruction of self and identity among adults with traumatic spinal cord injury. *Sociology of Health and Illness* 15(2): 217–45.

2
Disability/Normality

This chapter examines how rehabilitation risks reproducing the normative body and, in so doing, perpetuates the "othering" of people labeled as disabled. Rehabilitation focuses on assisting people to achieve or approximate normal: normal function, normal behaviors, normal movement patterns, normal activities, and normal roles. Normal in all of these instances focuses on techniques and technologies to encourage uniformity in body structures, how bodies move, and typical social roles. While these practices can have positive effects, the impulse toward normalization also contributes to sustaining negative attitudes toward disabled people and disavows the richness of human diversity. Rehabilitation recognizes the influences of "environmental factors" on individual abilities, but the larger sociopolitical themes that mediate disablement remain largely unacknowledged. In what follows I unpack the tension between disability and normality in contemporary social discourse and how it is reflected in rehabilitation practice and scholarship. I suggest that, through an "ethic of openness," rehabilitation can be mobilized to help people adjust to and create new ways of doing and being in the world that do not have to be constructed in relation to preconceived bodily norms or modes of function.

To begin, I consider the question of "What is disability?" and the meanings reflected in prominent models of disablement including the social model and the International Classification of Functioning, Disability, and Health (ICF). I then consider normality by tracing how the concept of "normal as ideal" evolved through nineteenth-and twentieth-century advancements in statistics and socio-medical applications of the bell curve that persist today. I conclude the chapter by drawing from post-critical scholarship to suggest a way forward that disturbs, perturbs, and moves the disability/normality divide toward acceptance of indeterminacy, which opens up new avenues for rehabilitation.

What Is Disability?

The lack of robust philosophical frameworks to work through the function of rehabilitation in the lives of disabled people can be problematic for rehabilitation practitioners. Researchers and clinicians are oriented to helping individuals but may hold conflicting visions of how to do so that reveal the crux of how disability is understood and addressed in the contemporary world. What differences count as needing of intervention and why? Are ameliorating impairments and/or pursuing participation in typical social roles the "right" paths? How can rehabilitation promote acceptance of diverse bodies and abilities?

Addressing questions like these reveals the philosophical commitments that pervade rehabilitation but are seldom discussed or critiqued. Rehabilitation is not oriented to cure but rather to reestablishing physical and social function, to reintegration and restoration. Following injury, this represents a return to previous function, or the closest possible approximation. For those with life-long impairments, it is also an approximation toward something. What? The answer can only be normal: normal bodies, normal activities, and/or normal social roles. It is not as simple as asking patients to state what they want in the narrowest sense of "client-centeredness" (Hammel 2007, 2013). "What are your goals?" the clinician asks. And s/he takes this seriously, explains how they may be achieved (or not) through a series of steps, broken down into long- and short-term goals aligned with the ICF framework, some oriented to the level of "body structures," others to enabling "activity and participation" (Holliday et al. 2005; Playford et al. 2009; Wade 2009). Techniques are applied, equipment ordered, home exercises assigned. But rehabilitation as part of a cultural and juridical set of norms is set up to accommodate some goals and not others. Some are declared unrealistic and unachievable. Others are required, deemed necessary: "You cannot go home unless/until you can get up those stairs." Sometimes patients do not have therapy goals. They are "not engaged" in their rehabilitation. Lack of engagement is also diagnosed, studied, and addressed in rehabilitation (Kortte et al. 2007; Lequerica and Kortte 2010). People are *sent* to rehabilitation, sometimes gladly, sometimes not. And rehabilitation has a program designed to address their problems *as defined by* rehabilitation: the amputee program, burns and plastics, stroke, traumatic brain injury, pediatric, geriatric, cognitive, physical, and vocational rehabilitation. Each program is part of a system and a society that understands disability a particular way, as a problem of one kind or another that can be labeled (diagnosed) and grouped according to set categories and admission criteria. Through these techniques of categorization, disability is made into an object of rehabilitation, something that can be addressed, helped, fixed, eased. Made normal. Normality as a goal is positioned in opposition to disability, which is constructed as the problem requiring intervention.

What is meant by disability? Disability is thought of in many different ways that are held in tension and form the basis of intense debates particularly in the interdisciplinary field of disability studies (Hughes and Paterson 1997; Oliver 1996; Shildrick 2009; Thomas 1999; Tremain 2001). Some questions from this field help to engage with these tensions: What does it mean to claim that all of us move in and out of disability? To be disabled and nondisabled at the same time? Can disability be desirable? The answers depend on how disability is defined, understood, and/or experienced. Function, one could say, occurs across a continuum without a bright line separating disability and ability. Desirable? Many in the deaf community would prefer not to hear, and claim deafness as a cultural identity not a deficit (Skelton and Valentine 2003). But then again deaf people would be unlikely to characterize the inability to hear as disability, so they are not claiming "disability" is desirable. A tension is thus revealed. What is disability? Is it the opposite of ability? Or something else? Disability is not equivalent to impairment (another slippery category) and not all impairments instigate interventions. Similarly, there are those who claim we are all "temporarily able-bodied" and becoming progressively more disabled with age (Zola 1991). True perhaps, but also incomplete, conceptually thin. "Temporary" suggests that some people are in one category and others are not, but this notion is contested (Shildrick 2002; Shildrick and Price 2002).

Another way to think about disability is to try to determine who "counts" as disabled. For example, is it Stephen Hawking, or the single mother living in a refugee camp, or perhaps both? There is no "right" answer to this question other than perhaps one, both, and neither. Dis/abled states are elusive, contingent, and never settled. Hawking can *do* (in multiple senses of the word: "make do," function) much because he has supports (physical, financial, social, etc.). Is he disabled without these supports? Yes. With them? Perhaps also yes. The woman can do little for herself and her children without supports but she (in my hypothetical case) has few. Ability/doing requires partnership, cooperation, money, food, and shelter. We all rely on these things. We have dependencies (see Chapter 5). The woman's children are not as disabled as they might be without their mother, and she without them.

But you might object: this is not disability but something else. The woman and her children do not have any impairments. If we accept that this is the case, then disability is related to bodies, to impairments. Bodies are marginalized because of their differences, but only people who have an impairment count as disabled. Disability advocates might bock at this suggestion, which seems to imply that disability is caused by impairments rather than exclusionary environments. Other problems arise because, as I discuss in the following, impairment is also not as stable as it seems, not a given biological reality, not natural but naturalized (Tremain 2001). This naturalization further complicates how disability is understood. Perhaps we can start with this: Those labeled as disabled have bodies that fall outside a presumed norm. They are prevented from "doing" because most places, spaces, and technologies are designed for bodies with typical morphologies and abilities, and because they are singled out for their differences and "othered."

Theorizing Disability

How disability is defined and understood has changed over time and varies across academic fields and disciplines. Biomedical views of disability, the so-called medical model, still hold tremendous sway in health care and rehabilitation (Hammell 2006; Kielhofner 2005). The medical model draws from disease theory to conceive of disability as an individual problem that arises because of a biologically dysfunctioning body part or system (Boorse 1975). This understanding underpins the study of how bodily functions affect a person's movement, mobility, activities, occupations, and social participation. Clinically, the focus is most often either on repairing/reshaping/restoring the biological body, and/or helping an individual to adapt through maximizing their existing abilities and modifying their immediate physical environments (French and Swain 2001; Magasi 2008a). While the role of the "environment" and "contextual factors" are acknowledged, biomedicine and rehabilitation remain largely silent on the politics of disablement.

Challenges to the causal linkages between impairment and disability are still rare and underdeveloped in rehabilitation. In other words, rehabilitation and health care more broadly reflect a dominant cultural belief that the social disadvantages that "disabled" individuals experience in daily life arise primarily from their impairments, even while acknowledging the influence of material and social "barriers" or "facilitators" that modify the degree of disability experienced by a given individual. Hammel (2006, p. 59) notes that the medical model of disability is so dominant in rehabilitation that the existence of competing ways of understanding disability is rarely acknowledged. I would modify this somewhat to suggest that the entrenchment of biomedical thinking over time makes other approaches not only unacknowledged but *unthinkable*, that is, biomedical views of disability are taken for granted as simply the "ways things are."

A couple of notes of caution should be raised here. Biomedical conceptions of disability have been the subject of much critique from several quarters including medical sociology, disability studies, and increasingly from within the health care and rehabilitation disciplines (e.g., Hammell 2006; Magasi 2008a; McRuer 2006; Oliver 1996; Phelan 2011; Skelton and Valentine 2003; Stiker 1999; Thomas 2007). Rehabilitation arguably preceded other health fields in recognizing disability in relation to a larger set of parameters than impairment alone. It has made substantial strides toward recognizing the social determinants of disability and in refocusing interventions away from "fixing" impairments toward enabling social participation, most notably through embracing the ICF as a guiding framework (Haglund and Henriksson 2003; Kjellberg et al. 2011; Steiner et al. 2002; Stucki et al. 2002, 2007). Nevertheless, along with others (Magasi 2008a; McRuer 2006; Oliver 1996; Stiker 1999), I would argue that the orientation toward differences (in body structures, activities, or participation) as problems to be fixed through intervention remain and are reflected in the very definitions ascribed to rehabilitation. For example, Miller-Keane and O'Toole's (2003) encyclopaedia defines rehabilitation as: *The process of restoring a person's ability to live and work as normally as possible after a disabling injury or illness.* The definition reflects a focus on social participation and normal life, and it also attributes disability to physical causalities. It is the *illness or injury* that is disabling, and the goal is to be as normal as possible. Statements like these are ubiquitous in rehabilitation and reveal how the socio-politics of disablement are still largely absent from the field.

A second caution is also needed. The so-called medical model has never been claimed as a guiding framework by medicine, rehabilitation, or any health discipline. Imrie (2004, p. 303), citing Kelly and Field, states that it is "actually very hard to find this medical model in practice. Few practitioners and no textbooks of any repute subscribe to uni-directional causal models and invariably interventions are seen in medical practice as contingent and multi-factorial." Disability may be largely conceived of as contiguous with impairments in health and rehabilitation fields, but there is also recognition of the larger contextual determinants of ability and disability. This recognition influences incremental changes in how rehabilitation is conceptualized, researched, and practiced. The adoption of the ICF is a case in point that I will return to in the following. Rehabilitation has moved away from a central focus on fixing the body as per a biomedical model and has steadily embraced more holistic health-care practices that focus on (re)integrating the person into society (Nordenfelt 2006).

The move toward holism, to seeing the patient in a context, however (still) relies on particular ideas of disability and normality. Rehabilitation seldom questions the notion of reintegration or reflects on its view that to live, be, and do "like everybody else" is the best possible outcome (Stiker 1999, pp. 178–179). Why is difference, by default, something to be avoided, repaired, or obliterated? To locate this discussion, I first consider the social model of disability, which is often considered the radical opposite to the biomedical model, and despite its influence, is still not well integrated into rehabilitation education, practice, or research.

The Social Model of Disability

In juxtaposition to biomedical perspectives, the social model squarely locates disability in the environment (Oliver 1983). The basic premise of the social model is that disability is the outcome of exclusionary social and material arrangements—including physical barriers, prejudice, discrimination, and segregation. Its proponents reject approaches that focus on individuals whether through adaptation or interventions, and instead draw attention to dominant "ableist" discourses, practices, and policies (Hahn 1988; Oliver 1983, 1996). Medicine and rehabilitation are critiqued for an "undersocialised" account of disability by failing to theorize the interrelationships between biology, personal biography, and the sociocultural order (Imrie 2004). Thus, disability is constructed entirely as an issue of social context, arising from ways in which particular human variations are dealt with in society (Amundson 2000).

The social model emerged in the 1970s as part of the disability movement, which paralleled the rise of other civil rights movements. Since then, it has been tremendously influential and remains the dominant framework in disability studies today (Goodley 2013). In focusing on the material and social production of disability, the model has contributed to shifting policy debates, public awareness, and legislative reform, including the landmark American with Disabilities Act (Hahn 1988; Silvers et al. 1999, pp. 74–76).

The social model has been criticized as inadequately accounting for multidimensional nature of disability (Corker 1999; Freund 2001; Imrie 2000; Kitchin 1998; Thomas 2007). In lifting the theoretical gaze away from the *individual* to locate the problem within the disabling *environment*, critics suggest that the body is rendered irrelevant. In his earlier work, Mike Oliver who spearheaded the model went so far as to say that the body and its impairments had *nothing* to do with disability (Oliver 1996, p. 35). A key critique suggests that the social model—or at least work advanced in its name—focuses too heavily on a materialist reading of disability and socio-material barriers, neglecting to theorize the body and bodily impairments and their relationships to disablement (Hughes and Paterson 1997; Thomas 1999, pp. 24–25). Imrie (2004, pp. 291–292) suggests that the exclusion of impairment from the social model mirrors the reductionism of medicine in treating the impaired body as an inert, physical object that is separate from the self and the disablement process. Despite efforts to the contrary, notions of the body-as-object persists in models of disablement like the ICF that have been widely embraced in rehabilitation practices.

International Classification of Functioning, Disability, and Health

These two ways of viewing disability, biomedical and sociopolitical, and the critiques of each helped pave the way for the development of disablement models that attempt to integrate the two (Nagi 1991; Verbrugge and Jette 1994; WHO 2001). The most widely adopted of these has been the World Health Organization (WHO)'s International Classification of Functioning, Disability and Health, or ICF (WHO 2001). The ICF attempts to integrate biomedical and social determinants of disability in a comprehensive classification scheme that recognizes the dialectical relationship between the two. Instead of reducing disability to either physiological or social causes, the model seeks to develop a relational understanding of the multiple mediators of disablement (Bickenbach et al. 1999; Imrie 2004).

The introduction of the International Classification of Impairment, Disability and Handicap (ICIDH) in 1980 (WHO 1980) followed by the ICF in 2001 helped accelerate changes to rehabilitation philosophy, practice, research, and education (Cerniauskaite et al. 2011; Darrah 2008; Peterson and Rosenthal 2005; Stucki et al. 2007). The ICF divides "functional performance" into three primary components of "body functions and structures," "activity limitations," and "participation" and asserts that function is the result of the dynamic interaction of myriad "personal" and "contextual" factors (WHO 2001). The multifactorial nature of the ICF addressed critiques that its precursor, the ICIDH, echoed the medical model in drawing a linear relationship between impairment and disability, and in locating the source of disability primarily within the malfunctioning of the biological body (Imrie 2004; Ravaud and Stiker 2001).

The ICIDH was critiqued for equating disability with abnormality by positioning disabled people as deviating from a preconceived norm (Bickenbach 2001; Imrie 2004; Ravaud and Stiker 2001). Arguably, these problems persist in the ICF, albeit in subtler forms. The developers of the ICF set out to remove the simplistic causal linkages made between impairment and disability through establishing a classification of "health and health-related states" that applied to all people not just those labeled as disabled (WHO 2001, p. 7). Thus, in the ICF, the presence of any impairment does not necessarily indicate that a person should be "regarded as sick" or disabled (WHO 2001, p. 13). Furthermore, the ICF acknowledges sociopolitical factors and removes the conflation of disability and impairment, for example, by suggesting that an individual with a condition such as HIV "may exhibit no impairments" but can still be disabled "because of the denial of access to services, discrimination or stigma" (WHO 2001, p. 16). Contra the ICIDH that under-theorized the relationship of disability to the environment, the ICF works to acknowledge this complexity and support the need for interventions aimed at sociopolitical change.

A persistent critique of the ICF, however, is the reliance on statistical norms to define human dysfunction and disability. This is seen across the three main classifications of function. Limitations or restrictions in *activities* and *participation* are "assessed against a generally accepted population standard...The expected performance is the population norm, which represents the experience of people without the specific health condition" (pp. 15–16). Similarly, *impairment* is described as "a deviation from certain generally accepted population standards in the biomedical status of the body and its functions...Abnormality here is used strictly to refer to a significant variation from established statistical norms...and should be used only in this sense (p. 213)." Presumably, the "only in this sense" qualification is meant to suggest that abnormality is value-neutral and should not be seen as a moral judgment of the individual. Rather "abnormality" is a statistical variation presented as an unassailable objective fact. In critiquing this assumption, Imrie (2004, p. 294) suggests:

> While the ICF notes that social and institutional relations (*i.e.* the interaction of body functions and structures with other domains) influence the meaning and consequences of impairment, the biological body, for the ICF, is "a fact," and impairment, at the level of body functions and structures, is seen as a "pre-social," biological, bodily difference.

Thus, while the ICF acknowledges a relationship between impairment and the sociomaterial environment, it retains certain problems. The first is a reproduction of discourses of normal versus abnormal with the latter as deviant and thus amenable to intervention. The ICF relies on statistical norms and "generally accepted" population standards to understand what constitutes a problem to be addressed. This is not inherently wrong but it exerts particular effects, not the least of which is the reproduction of a persistent view of disability as a (negative) form of deviance that gets acted upon and inscribed with social and cultural meanings.

A second problem with the ICF is an under-theorized notion of impairment that reduces it to a pre-given biological fact. Critics suggest that impairment is not a "natural" physical phenomenon but a contingent category that changes over time (Abberly 1996; Hughes and Paterson 1997; Shildrick 2009). Critical disability scholars note that the impaired body is a social construction that relies on particular classificatory schemes of intact/broken, healthy/unhealthy, and functional/dysfunctional that are not natural but constructed and change across time and place. Likening essentialist understandings of impairment to the naturalization of sexual characteristics, Tremain (2001, p. 632) states:

> Impairments are materialized as universal attributes (properties) of subjects through the iteration and reiteration of rather culturally specific regulatory norms and ideals about (for example) human function and structure, competency, intelligence and ability. As universalized attributes of subjects, furthermore, impairments are naturalized as an interior identity or essence *on which* culture acts in order to camouflage the historically contingent power relations that materialized them as natural.

Thus, far from constituting a biological given that is affected by context, Tremain suggests that the impaired body is materialized *through* social relations and powerful scientific discourses that are reproduced over time and place. Shildrick (2009, p. 7) similarly notes that the seemingly natural distinction made between diverse bodily forms is "at best convenient and at worst a violent imposition, both literally and metaphorically, of epistemic power."

These two critiques of the ICF, reliance on statistical norms to define dysfunction and a reductive understanding of impairment, are, of course, closely related issues—the recognition of deviance relies on a stable view of impairment as preexisting its measurement. These ideas pervade how disability is talked about and understood on a social scale that extends beyond rehabilitation and the ICF, but is reproduced in both. The normal/disabled division is a pervasive social "truth" with a far reach and a long history (Shildrick 2002; Stiker 1999). In what follows, I consider notions of normal and normality and how they mediate rehabilitation practices, and then discuss how post-critical approaches to the disability/normality divide can inform and move rehabilitation practices.

What Is Normal(ity)?

According to Lennard Davis (1997), the disabled body was invented in the nineteenth century alongside the development of the statistical norm. He notes that contemporary definitions of normal as "constituting or conforming to the standard," "regular," or "usual" (Davis 1997, p. 11) did not arise until the mid-nineteenth century. This conception of normal gave rise to a new constellation of terms including "normalcy," "average," and "abnormal." The idea of norms and averages grew directly from an increasing interest in statistically mapping the distribution of human characteristics. Davis attributes the invention of the "average man" to Adolphe Quetelet (1796–1847) who described *l'homme moyen* as representing the average of all human (presumably male) attributes in a given country. Notably, Quetelet's average man was a combination of both *physical* and *moral* attributes. Davis describes how, with the ability to map human characteristics in terms of averages and deviations from the norm, an insidious shift occurred whereby the average became the ideal, which was further transformed into a human imperative. Previously held notions of the ideal were associated with a mytho-poetic unattainable body that was not found in the human world but represented by mythological gods or through Christ (Davis 1997; Ravaud and Stiker 2001). The introduction of the concept of the norm, however, suggested that most of the population could and should be part of this norm, and that deviations could be addressed for the general betterment of a population. The statistical ideal thus contained an imperative toward attainment that was not present in the classical ideal. During this time the bell curve, which Francis Galton termed the "normal distribution" curve, was increasingly used to distinguish supposedly positive versus negative deviations in the population (e.g., higher versus lower intelligence) by dividing the curve into ranked quartiles. The quartiles established a *hierarchy* of traits whereby a new kind of ideal was created that could only be known in relation to a central norm. Human progress and the possibility of eliminating deviant morphologies and traits were driven by the possibilities written onto the normal curve.

The idea that the population could be "normalized" was expressed both in a mathematical and a social sense, and as such the early statisticians were also prominent eugenicists of their time. Eugenics, statistics, and evolutionary theories developed in parallel and together worked to define normal human development (see Chapter 4). Evolution suggested that the weakest "defectives" of a species would be weeded out by natural selection, and eugenicists looked for methods to identify and eliminate defective traits in other ways, for example, through the forced sterilization of "mentally defective" women. Conflations of physical and moral failings persisted as physical differences became synonymous with personal character and placement on the bell curve.

An example of how the ideal of normality was operationalized is provided by Amundson (2000) who describes how nineteenth-century educators relied on the concept of statistical normality to integrate deaf children into the population by forbidding them to sign. Instead, they were taught to lip-read and to speak aloud, skills that are extremely difficult for most profoundly deaf individuals. The goal was to "help" children to be like others, to achieve or approximate a "normal" way of communicating despite its limited utility. The educators of the time presumably had good intentions, but the point is how ideas regarding what was helpful versus harmful were driven by assumptions regarding the right and proper norm. Michalko (1998, pp. 90–91) provides a contemporary example in his description of how blind individuals are taught to make "eye contact" to mimic the gestures of sighted people and thus appear "normal." These examples suggest that without a space to allow for different ways of doing and being in the world, interventions designed to ameliorate disability can exacerbate it.

It is important to recall that eugenics was a common approach to social welfare that had more or less wide acceptance in Europe and North America and persisted well into the twentieth century. It was only through the horrors of Nazi Germany that eugenics fell out of favor. Nevertheless, remnants of these ideas persist today in different forms and inform how disability, impairment, and the need for interventions such as genetic counseling and rehabilitation are constructed. Ian Hacking has elegantly suggested that these processes use "a power as old as Aristotle to bridge the fact/value distinction, whispering in your ear that what is normal is also right" (Amundson 2000, p. 43).

This is the invention of the deviant body, the disabled body, the non-conforming body. Far from being conceived of in neutral terms as part of a spectrum of human variation, deviant bodies were and are constructed as problems to be fixed or eliminated. Ideas of normal versus deviant bodies are still deeply entrenched in the Western imaginary and are not easily dispelled with attempts at value-free language as per the ICF. Achieving or approximating normal drives much of what is done in the name of policies, services, and interventions designed to help disabled people. This includes rehabilitation interventions focused at helping individuals to reintegrate through normalization. Returning to the distinction between the ideal and the normal, Ravaud and Stiker (2001, p. 494) suggest that normalization "… is not a question of leading all members of a society to an ideal model of humanity… It is a question of defining the mean, comparing deviations from this mean, and trying to diminish such deviations to bring individuals closer to the mean."

The multiple meanings of normal used in medicine and rehabilitation tend to obscure how statistical statements and value judgments are conflated in practice. Normal is equated with good health, the responsibility of every citizen and the mandate of health-oriented enterprises. A return to or approximation of normal provides the underlying taken-for-granted rationale that reproduces itself in countless health interventions. As Leslie Butt (1999) suggests, numbers, and the positivist science that they are embedded within, create a veneer of value-free truths that constitute an unquestioned reality. Empirical measurement and classifications that appear as "objective" measures of difference construct the ideal outcomes that can be attained through intervention (see Chapter 3). Interestingly, Butt makes these points through a detailed examination of how pervasive views of normal development label indigenous infants as "small" and thus unhealthy. The supposedly value-free average body size becomes the standard, and deviations from this standard produce the "at-risk" infant requiring medico-social care. Her point, which can be equally applied to interventions against nonnormate morphologies, is that standards are created out of statistical norms that in turn sustain meanings. These meanings are not universal truths but historically, politically, and culturally contingent and open to revision. Deviations from the norm do not necessarily require intervention, and interventions do not necessarily have to be aimed at normalization. It is here that post-critical approaches can help to reconceptualize the normal/disabled binary.

Post-Critical Movements: Perturbing the Normal/Disabled Divide

The normal/disabled division is a constructed binary that mediates thought and practice, but it can also be deconstructed, dismantled, and re-formed. Post-critical perspectives suggest that so-called natural (biological) categories of human difference such as race, sex, and impairment cannot be understood except through discourse and are part of a set of contingent divisions and categories to which are assigned particular social judgments (Amundson 2000; Katz and Marshall 2004). Seen through a postmodern lens, the biological body can never be apprehended directly because understanding is always mediated by language and particular ways of knowing (Grosz 1994). Bodies are thus "materialized through discourse" (Shildrick and Price 1996, p. 176) and notions of natural, normal, or disabled bodies are revealed as highly problematic. To be clear, these approaches do not suggest that bodies "do not exist" in material form, but rather that we cannot understand bodies, or any phenomena, except through language—that is through talking, writing, and thinking with words and their meanings. Thus meanings, descriptions about what "the body" or a given body is or is not, are always imposed through discourse. What a body "is" is not self-evident or out there to be discovered, rather it is created and could be created differently (Nicholls and Gibson 2010).

The pervasive "classificatory style of reasoning," of dividing bodies under categories of gender, race, impairment, etc., both opens up and closes off ways of being and doing (Katz and Marshall 2004). Modes of classification not only provide a mooring that can lead to new insights and practices but, as Ian Hacking suggests, also provide their "own criteria of proof and demonstration" and are thus "self-authenticating" (Hacking 2002, p. 4). This closes down other ways of seeing the world and other forms of insight or practice. Far from neutral descriptors, the binaries of man/woman, white/of color, young/old, gay/straight, disabled/able-bodied each contain positions of relative privilege and power that are increasingly problematized in the postmodern era (Ravaud and Stiker 2001, p. 499). Even staying within the realm of positivist science, it has been demonstrated repeatedly that seemingly stable categories like race and sex do not fall into clear divisions and cannot be upheld (Amundson 2000). Nevertheless, disability studies scholars like Amundson (2000) note that although science has long ceased attributing the disadvantages experienced by certain races and genders to biological differences, the disadvantages experienced by those labeled as disabled are still primarily attributed to biology.

Emerging scholarship in critical disability studies has questioned the normal/disabled division that is reflected in both the medical and social models of disability (Goodley and Rapley 2001; Hughes and Paterson 1997; Paterson and Hughes 1999; Shildrick and Price 2002; Stiker 1999; Tremain 2001). While the social model emphasizes disabling environments and the biomedical model disabling impairments, both rely on the philosophical separation of impairment and disability, on bodies as natural pre-given biological entities onto which disability is written. Although the social model complicates and politicizes disability, it nevertheless leaves intact the notion of impairment as a biological given. Either through "adaptation" or "equal rights," the goal is for disabled persons to be as similar to nondisabled persons as possible, to be integrated into a dominant social order that valorizes social and biological norms (Gibson 2006). Such unreflective valorization of dominant modes of doing and being reproduces policies and practices of normalization that, instead of addressing disadvantage, threaten to preserve existing patterns of "functional dominance" and social privilege (Silvers et al. 1999, p. 108).

Disability and impairment are relational concepts in that each cannot be understood except in relation to some notion of normal. Their absence or presence assumes a point of deviation—to be categorized as disabled is to be marked out as an exception to an assumed norm (Shildrick 2009, p. 1). Deploying a post-critical approach, the impaired body is conceived of not as a biological entity but as a surface for the inscription of meanings. Thus, without denying that disability exerts very real effects on those labeled as disabled, or that pain and dysfunction can cause suffering, ideas of disability or impairment as stable and fixed categories are viewed as highly problematic. Any attempt to define disability is seen as closing down a shifting set of parameters that are historically contingent and resist closure (Shildrick 2009, p. 2).

Margrit Shildrick's "ethic of openness" that I introduced in Chapter 1 re-imagines the binary of disabled/nondisabled providing a point of departure for rethinking rehabilitation. Together with Janet Price, Shildrick has argued that the reliance on modernist notions of identity as difference does not allow for a recognition of irreducible multiple differences and connections among all persons (Price and Shildrick 1998; Shildrick 2000; Shildrick and Price 1996). I take up these ideas again in Chapter 5 in relation to in/dependence, but for my purposes here I note how an ethic of openness resists the binary structures of normal/disabled by placing "less emphasis on vulnerability as the dependency of others and more on the notion of vulnerability as the risk of ontological uncertainty for all of us" (Shildrick 2002, p. 78). An ethic of openness acknowledges the vulnerability of a person at the moment of engagement with an *uncategorized* other. It acknowledges a *multiplicity* of bodily differences without trying to contain differences within categories of disability/ability, normal/abnormal. As Shildrick notes (2002, p. 2):

> It is not that some bodies are reducible to the same while others figure as the absolute other, but rather that all resist full or final expression… The issue is not one of revaluing differently embodied others, but of rethinking the nature of embodiment itself.

In place of these binaries, Shildrick's ethic acknowledges both vulnerability to the other, and the vulnerability of the self, blurring the lines that separate and divide "us" and "them." This is a powerful idea that requires a philosophical shift, not to discard the norm but to deflect its power, to use it reflectively, and to see it as one way among others of thinking about differences. If normal/disabled is no longer taken as fact but only one way to characterize diverse bodies, then a world of possibilities, movements, and changes opens up for enhancing all our lives. It is no longer clear who is or is not disabled because the category itself is revealed as deeply problematic in the face of shared vulnerabilities. Disability is re-imagined as a fluid category that we all can/will/do move in and out of (Gibson 2006). Others' disabilities make each of us consider our own limitations and with that approach a liberation, an opening in the confines of the self (Kristeva 1998).

Rehabilitating Normal/Disabled

What does this troubling of the normal/disabled divide mean for rehabilitation? First of all there is a need to acknowledge that normal drives intervention; not to say it is "wrong" but rather to consider its effects, both positive and negative. As noted, ideas of statistical deviance from established norms are built into the ICF and other classificatory schemes used to determine what counts as a problem amenable to intervention. In rehabilitation, we can see examples from the level of body structures to participation in social roles. Rehabilitation professionals help people to achieve normal tone, normal range of motion, normal gait patterns, normal speech, normal occupations, to engage in typical activities of school or work, and to live normal lives. When normal is not possible or practical, then the goal is to approximate it, to get as close as possible. These ideas are reflected in common rehabilitation measures and how good and poor outcomes are defined (see Chapter 3).

Writing from a disability studies perspective, Colin Goble (2013, p. 33) makes the following observations regarding the rehabilitation process:

> Although there are variations, the general pattern of professional interventions is as follows. The functional capacity of the individual is assessed using scales and assessment tools that measure their performance against "normative" standards of functioning. Programmes or interventions are then designed which aim to reduce the gap between the performance of the impaired individual and the normative standard as far as possible. Success is achieved when the professional expert judges that the performance of the individual has moved as far as possible in the right direction… for a deaf child it might be to learn to lip read, for a child with cerebral palsy it might be to focus on walking or feeding themselves, or for an elderly person recovering from a stroke it might focus on reteaching them to wash themselves. The assumption usually remains, however, that the problem lies within the person, and the solution is a technical intervention from a professional expert who helps the person achieve a greater level of independence, and thus moves them closer to a more socially and culturally accepted level of normality.

Goble uses a rather accusatory tone in this quotation, so let me reiterate that I am not saying that rehabilitation efforts are necessarily misguided. Rehabilitation is oriented to helping people improve their health and well-being and does so in myriad ways, but that should not be the end of the conversation. Rehabilitation undoubtedly helps, but as part of a social system of normalizing practices, it may also harm in other ways. No person or group lives outside the dominant social order or is immune to its influence (Bourdieu and Wacquant 1992, pp. 120–121). Negative discourses of disability and the imperative to "overcome" differences are socially pervasive and internalized across individuals and fields of practice and are taken up by individuals as self-evident. Included are "patients" who often want to be normal or return to normal, as much as or more so than their clinicians (Amundson 2000; Gibson et al. 2014; Oliver 1996). These dominant practices are countered through points of resistance—alternative discourses, subversive practices, protests, displacements, and creative movements—that disrupt habits of thought and action. Nevertheless, the impetus toward normality is socially entrenched and continues to affect rehabilitation practice in ways that may be hidden and are seldom explored. This critique has been persistently leveled against rehabilitation by disability studies activists and scholars (French and Swain 2001; Goble 2013; McRuer 2006; Oliver 1996; Stiker 1999) and is gaining traction from within rehabilitation (Gibson 2014; Hammell 2006; Magasi 2008b; Phelan 2011; Roush and Sharby 2011).

IP Multicast Routing Protocols

This book discusses the fundamental concepts that are essential to understanding IP multicast communication. The material covers the well-known IP multicast routing protocols, along with the rationale behind each protocol. The book starts with the basic building blocks of multicast communications and networks, then progresses into the common multicast group management methods used, and finally into the various, well-known multicast routing protocols used in today's networks. IP multicast provides significant benefits to network operators by allowing the delivery of information to multiple receivers simultaneously with less network bandwidth consumption than using unicast transmission. Applications that can benefit greatly from multicast communications and multicast-enabled networks include audio and video conferencing, collaborative computing, online group learning and training, multimedia broadcasting, multi-participant online gaming, and stock market trading.

This book's goal is to present the main concepts and applications, allowing readers to develop a better understanding of IP multicast communication. *IP Multicast Routing Protocols: Concepts and Designs* presents material from a practicing engineer's perspective, linking theory and fundamental concepts to common industry practices and real-world examples.

The discussion is presented in a simple style to make it comprehensible and appealing to undergraduate- and graduate-level students, research and practicing engineers, scientists, IT personnel, and network engineers. It is geared toward readers who want to understand the concepts and theory of IP multicast routing protocols, yet want these to be tied to clearly illustrated and close-to-real-world example systems and networks.

IP Multicast Routing Protocols

Concepts and Designs

James Aweya

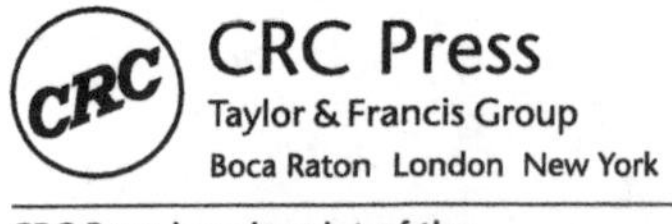

CRC Press is an imprint of the
Taylor & Francis Group, an **informa** business

Designed cover image: ©Shutterstock Images

First edition published 2024
by CRC Press
2385 NW Executive Center Drive, Suite 320, Boca Raton FL 33431

and by CRC Press
4 Park Square, Milton Park, Abingdon, Oxon, OX14 4RN

CRC Press is an imprint of Taylor & Francis Group, LLC

ISBN: 9781032701943 (hbk)
ISBN: 9781032701929 (pbk)
ISBN: 9781032701967 (ebk)

DOI: 10.1201/9781032701967

Typeset in Times
by codeMantra

Contents

Despite the move away from impairment-based to more participatory goals (e.g., Wiart and Darrah 2002), deeply ingrained assumptions about disability as a problem to be fixed still dominate every aspect of rehabilitation, including how programs are structured and funded, individual goal setting with patients, education of rehabilitation students, and which forms of research are funded. Stiker (1999), in his detailed exposition of the history and philosophical moorings of rehabilitation, discusses normalization in terms of an "integration of oblivion" (p. 133). He suggests that, in the name of equality, rehabilitation attempts a kind of erasure of disability that strives to *efface* differences. Promoting acceptance of diversity and difference are given short shrift when compared to the amount of time, energy, and money spent on achieving or approximating normal bodies, movement patterns, roles, and activities.

But things could be otherwise. Rehabilitation has the potential to provide a key sight for resistance to normalization. To counter the assumptions that disabled people want or should want to be "normal," Swain and French (2000) have proposed an "affirmation model of disability" wherein disabled individuals assert a positive identity of *impairment* (not, or not just, disability) and in so doing actively resist and repudiate discourses of normality and what disabled people should or should not want to be and do. These ideas, although theoretically divergent, echo the notions of respect for and celebration of diverse bodily forms suggested by Shildrick's ethic of openness. Ravaud and Stiker (2001) make a similar appeal. They suggest that the impulse toward normalization has multiple effects including sustaining negative attitudes toward disabled people and a rejection of the richness of human diversity.

Paradoxically, in working toward helping people live better lives, rehabilitation risks limiting possibilities and potentials when it adopts a too narrow notion of what constitutes a good life. As I discuss further in subsequent chapters, normalizing practices in rehabilitation and efforts to help people look and do like others can limit creative innovation in interventions and design. An example of an open approach to rehabilitation that does not rely on approximating the body normal comes from the work of Hugh Herr who designs cutting edge prosthetics and is himself a double amputee (see Gibson 2014). Herr has multiple sets of prosthetic legs that he uses for different purposes, for example, walking versus rock climbing, and as such each has different designs and functionalities. Some legs function and look more like biological legs while others deviate substantially from "normal legs" and are functionally superior in many respects. The design of these and similar innovative prostheses required a shift away from the notion of normal as ideal. Herr's collection of task-specific legs does not approximate a normal condition. The design imperative has moved away from how to make the amputee body look and function normally, to asking "What can this body do?" and "What technologies, interventions, and innovations can be mobilized to achieve these doings?" Such a move abandons the categories of disabled/nondisabled, normal/abnormal because they are no longer useful in determining practice.

Dominant ideas regarding disability are of course not limited to rehabilitation but are reflective of larger social discourses. These ideas are often reflected in the values and beliefs of people with newly acquired impairments as they struggle to make sense of their new bodily realities, or of new parents of children born with congenital conditions. Individuals come to rehabilitation with hopes that interventions like surgery, drugs, and intense therapies will cure or at least minimize their differences. Clinicians are placed in the position of managing high hopes with patients or family members willing to do "whatever it takes" and seeking as much intervention as they can get and/or afford (Gibson et al. 2012b). This raises tough questions about the role of rehabilitation and how best to help individuals seeking care. Practitioners struggle with these ideas on a daily basis—they want to support clients and families, do not want to destroy hope, and find ways of deflecting "unrealistic" goals (LeRoy et al. 2015). These struggles expose a tension. What to do when individuals want to pursue a kind of normal that they cannot attain? Does the "client-centred" practitioner respect these goals, or steer them toward other ways of being? How does this steering occur? How should it?

An unreflective pursuit of normal can paradoxically increase inclusion while amplify marginalization (Gibson 2014; Gibson et al. 2007). When persons with newly acquired bodily impairments only focus on returning to/approximating "normal life," other possibilities will be closed off. Instead of inclusion, persons can end up relegated to a netherworld of liminality, occupying the borders of social spaces without meaningful integration (Priestley 2000). A more open approach to rehabilitation partners with the recipients of care to reimagine what counts as a positive outcome. For example, in our research with young men with Duchenne muscular dystrophy, we have suggested that paid work may not always be possible or desirable, and other pursuits such as caring for others, sustaining relationships, or managing personal care needs may take on a greater significance (Aitchison 2003; Gibson et al. 2009). These kinds of considerations open up multiple additional pathways for rehabilitation that create spaces for different ways of living and contribute to the acceptance of differences.

Rehabilitation has an opportunity to illuminate and promote counter-narratives of disability, to assist individuals to pursue alternative life scripts, multiple ways of being and doing, that do not rely on an arbitrary construction of normality. Doing so requires deep reflection about the programs and services made available to clients, and what constitutes good or poor outcomes. It relies on providing space for reflective dialogue with clients and families whose values may shift in light of bodily changes and experiences. An important task is to recognize the many ways that people labeled as disabled are marginalized and to determine how best to assist individuals to attain or maintain a positive disability identity within the context of their therapeutic goals. To assist with these efforts, all rehabilitation professionals (clinicians, educators, researchers, administrators) need to develop a reflexive stance on their own assumptions and how these are reproduced in their practices.

Karen Whalley Hammel (2006, p. 50) has asserted that a core task for rehabilitation is to help people to live with pride and dignity—to resist rather than reproduce notions of disability as tragedy. She suggests rehabilitation focuses on helping people not to deny their difference but to see that difference "doesn't matter." I agree somewhat with the sentiment, but would approach it another way. Differences do matter but the meaning and significance attached to particular kinds of differences comes from discrete notions of "normal as good" that should be radically reformulated. Categories and concepts that carry the weight of tragedy—disability, dependency, and abnormality—need to be rehabilitated, rethought, and re-moved. Rehabilitation can be mobilized to help people adjust to and create new realities (Papadimitriou 2008), new ways of doing and being in world, that do not have to be constructed in relation to preconceived bodily norms or modes of function.

References

Abberly, P. 1996. Work, utopia and impairment. In *Disability and Society: Emerging Issues and Insights*, ed. L. Barton, pp. 61–82. New York: Longman Publishing.

Aitchison, C. 2003. From leisure and disability to disability leisure: Developing data, definitions and discourses. *Disability and Society* 18(7): 955–969.

Amundson, R. 2000. Against normal function. *Studies in History and Philosophy of Biology and Biomedical Sciences* 31(1): 33–53.

Bickenbach, J.E. 2001. Disability, human rights, law and policy. In *Handbook of Disability Studies*, eds. G.L. Albrecht, K.D. Seelman, and M. Bury, pp. 565–584. London, U.K.: Sage.

Bickenbach, J.E., Chatterji, S., Badley, E.M., and Ustun, T.B. 1999. Models of disablement, universalism and the international classification of impairments, disabilities and handicaps. *Social Science and Medicine* 48(9): 1173–1187.

Boorse, C. 1975. On the distinction between disease and illness. *Philosophy & Public Affairs* 49(1): 49–68.

Bourdieu, P. and Wacquant, L.J.D. 1992. *An Invitation to Reflexive Sociology.* London, U.K.: University of Chicago Press.

Butt, L. 1999. Measurements, morality, and the politics of "normal" infant growth. *Journal of Medical Humanities* 20(2): 81–100.

Cerniauskaite, M., Quintas, R.U.I., Boldt, C., Raggi, A., Cieza, A, Bickenbach, J.E., and Leonardi, M. 2011. Systematic literature review on ICF from 2001 to 2009: Its use, implementation and operationalisation. *Disability and Rehabilitation* 33(4): 281–309.

Corker, M. 1999. Differences, conflations and foundations: The limits to 'accurate' theoretical representation of disabled people's experience? *Disability & Society* 14(5): 627–642.

Darrah, J. 2008. Using the ICF as a framework for clinical decision making in pediatric physical therapy. *Advances in Physiotherapy* 10(3): 146–151.

Davis, L.J. 1997. Constructing normalcy. In *The Disability Studies Reader*, ed. L.J. Davis, pp. 9–28. New York: Routledge.

French, S. and Swain, J. 2001. The relationship between disabled people and health and welfare professionals. In *Handbook of Disability Studies*, eds. G.L. Albrecht, K.D. Seelman, and M. Bury, pp. 734–753. London, U.K.: Sage.

Freund, P. 2001. Bodies, disability, and spaces: The social model and disabling spatial organizations. *Disability and Society* 16(5): 689–706.

Gibson, B.E. 2006. Disability, connectivity and transgressing the autonomous body. *Journal of Medical Humanities* 27(3): 187–196.

Gibson, B.E. 2014. Parallels and problems of normalization in rehabilitation and universal design: Enabling connectivities. *Disability & Rehabilitation* 36(16): 1328–1333.

Gibson, B.E., Mistry, B., Smith, B. et al. 2014. Becoming men: Gender, disability, and transitioning to adulthood. *Health* 18(1): 93–112.

Gibson, B.E., Secker, B., Rolfe, D., Wagner, F., Parke, B., and Mistry, B. 2012a. Disability and dignity-enabling home environments. *Social Science & Medicine* 74(2): 211–219.

Gibson, B.E., Teachman, G., Wright, V., Fehlings, D., and McKeever, P. 2012b. Children's and parents' beliefs regarding the value of walking: Rehabilitation implications for children with cerebral palsy. *Child: Care, Health and Development* 38(1): 61–69.

Gibson, B.E., Young, N.L., Upsher, R.E.G., and McKeever, P. 2007. Men on the margin: A bourdieusian examination of living into adulthood with muscular dystrophy. *Social Science & Medicine* 65(3): 505–517.

Gibson, B.E., Zizelsoberger, H., and McKeever, P. 2009. 'Futureless persons': Shifting life expectancies and the vicissitudes of progressive illness. *Sociology of Health & Illness* 31(4): 554–568.

Goble, C. 2013. Independence, independence and normality. In *Disabling Barriers-Enabling Environments*, eds. J. Swain, S. French, C. Barnes, and C. Thomas. London, U.K.: Sage.
Goodley, D. 2013. Who is disabled? exploring the scope of the social model of disability. In *Disabling Barriers-Enabling Environments*, eds. J. Swain, S. French, C. Barnes, and C. Thomas, pp. 118–124, London, U.K.: Sage.
Goodley, D. and Rapley, M. 2001. How do you understand "learning difficulties"? Towards a social theory of impairment. *Journal Information* 39(3): 229–232.
Grosz, E.A. 1994. *Volatile Bodies: Toward a Corporeal Feminism. Bloomington and Indianapolis*. Bloomington, IN: Indiana University Press.
Hacking, I. 2002. Inaugural lecture: Chair of philosophy and history of scientific concepts at the collège de france. *Economy and Society* 31(1): 1–14.
Haglund, L. and Henriksson, C. 2003. Concepts in occupational therapy in relation to the ICF. *Occupational Therapy International* 10(4): 253–268.
Hahn, H. 1988. The politics of physical differences: Disability and discrimination. *Journal of Social Issues* 44(1): 39–47.
Hammell, K.W. 2006. *Perspectives on Disability and Rehabilitation*. Edinburgh, U.K.: Elsevier.
Hammell, K.W. 2007. Client-centred practice: Ethical obligation or professional obfuscation? *The British Journal of Occupational Therapy* 70(6): 264–266.
Hammel, K.W. 2013. Client-centred practice in occupational therapy: Critical reflections. *Scandinavian Journal of Occupational Therapy* 20(3): 174–181.
Holliday, R.C., Antoun, M., and Playford, E.D. 2005. A survey of goal-setting methods used in rehabilitation. *Neurorehabilitation and Neural Repair* 19(3): 227–231.
Hughes, B. and Paterson, K. 1997. The social model of disability and the disappearing body: Towards a sociology of impairment. *Disability and Society* 12(3): 325–340.
Imrie, R. 2000. Disabling environments and the geography of access policies and practices. *Disability and Society* 15(1): 5–24.
Imrie, R. 2004. Demystifying disability: A review of the international classification of functioning, disability and health. *Sociology of Health & Illness* 26(3): 287–305.
Katz, S. and Marshall, B.L. 2004. Is the functional 'normal'? Aging, sexuality and the bio-marking of successful living. *History of the Human Sciences* 17(1): 53–75.
Kielhofner, G. 2005. Rethinking disability and what to do about it: Disability studies and its implications for occupational therapy. *The American Journal of Occupational Therapy* 59(5): 487–496.
Kitchin, R. 1998. "Out of place", "knowing one's place": Space, power and the exclusion of disabled people. *Disability and Society* 13(3): 343–356.
Kjellberg, A, Bolic, V., and Haglund, L. 2011. Utilization of an ICF-based assessment from occupational therapists' perspectives. *Scandinavian Journal of Occupational Therapy* 19(3): 274–281.

Kortte, K.B., Falk, L.D., Castillo, R.C., Johnson-Greene, D., and Wegener, S.T. 2007. The Hopkins rehabilitation engagement rating scale: Development and psychometric properties. *Archives of Physical Medicine and Rehabilitation* 88(7): 877–884.

Kristeva, J. 1998. The limits of life. In *Taking action for human rights in the twenty-first century*, eds. F. Mayor and R. P. Droit, pp. 102–105. Paris, France: UNESCO.

Lequerica, A.H. and Kortte, K. 2010. Therapeutic engagement: A proposed model of engagement in medical rehabilitation. *American Journal of Physical Medicine & Rehabilitation/Association of Academic Physiatrists* 89(5): 415–422.

LeRoy, K., Boyd, K., De Asis, K. et al. 2015. Balancing hope and realism in family-centered care: Physical therapists' dilemmas in negotiating walking goals with parents of children with cerebral palsy. *Physical & Occupational Therapy in Pediatrics* 35(3): 253–264.

Magasi, S. 2008a. Disability studies in practice: A work in progress. *Topics in Stroke Rehabilitation* 15(6): 611–617.

Magasi, S. 2008b. Infusing disability studies into the rehabilitation sciences. *Topics in Stroke Rehabilitation* 15(3): 283–287.

McRuer, R. 2006. *Crip Theory: Cultural Signs of Queerness and Disability.* New York: New York University Press.

Michalko, R. 1998. The mystery of the eye and the shadow of blindness. Toronto: University of Toronto Press.

Miller-Keane, C. and O'Toole, M.T. 2003. *Miller-Keane Encyclopedia and Dictionary of Medicine, Nursing, and Allied Health*, 7th edn. Philadelphia, PA: Saunders.

Nagi, S.Z. 1991. Disability concepts revisited: Implications for prevention. In *Disability in America: Toward a National Agenda for Prevention*, eds. A. Pope and A. Tarlov, pp. 309–327. Washington, DC: National Academy Press.

Nicholls, D.A. and Gibson, B.E. 2010. The body and physiotherapy. *Physiotherapy Theory Practice* 26(8): 497–509.

Nordenfelt, L. 2006. On health, ability and activity: Comments on some basic notions in the ICF. *Disability & Rehabilitation* 28(23): 1461–1465.

Oliver, M. 1983. In *Social Work with Disabled People*, Basingstoke, U.K.: Palgrave Macmillan.

Oliver, M. 1996. A sociology of disability or a disablist sociology? In *Disability and Society: Emerging Issues and Insights*, ed. L. Barton, pp. 18–42. New York: Longman Publishing.

Papadimitriou, C. 2008. Becoming en-wheeled: The situated accomplishment of re-embodiment as a wheelchair user after spinal cord injury. *Disability & Society* 23(7): 691–704.

Paterson, K. and Hughes, B. 1999. Disability studies and phenomenology; the carnal politics of everyday life. *Disability and Society* 14(5): 597–610.

Peterson, D.B. and Rosenthal, D.A. 2005. The international classification of functioning, disability and health (ICF): A primer for rehabilitation educators. *Rehabilitation Education* 19: 81–94.

Phelan, S.K. 2011. Constructions of disability: A call for critical reflexivity in occupational therapy. *Canadian Journal of Occupational Therapy* 78(3): 164–172.

Playford, E.D, Siegert, R., Levack, W., and Freeman, J. 2009. Areas of consensus and controversy about goal setting in rehabilitation: A conference report. *Clinical Rehabilitation* 23(4): 334–344.

Price, J. and Shildrick, M. 1998. Uncertain thoughts on the dis/abled body. In *Vital Signs*, eds. M. Shildrick and J. Price. Edinburgh, U.K.: Edinburgh University Press.

Priestley, M. 2000. Adults only: Disability, social policy and the life course. *Journal of Social Policy* 29(3): 421–439.

Ravaud, J.F. and Stiker, H.J. 2001. Inclusion/exclusion. An analysis of historical and cultural meanings. In *Handbook of Disability Studies*, eds. G.L. Albrecht, K.D. Seelman, and M. Bury, pp. 490–514. London, U.K.: Sage.

Roush, S.E. and Sharby, N. 2011. Disability reconsidered: The paradox of physical therapy. *Physical Therapy* 91(12): 1715–1727.

Shildrick, M. 2000. Becoming vulnerable: Contagious encounters and the ethics of risk. *Journal of Medical Humanities* 21(4): 215–227.

Shildrick, M. 2002. *Embodying the Monster: Encounters with the Vulnerable Self.* London, U.K.: Sage.

Shildrick, M. 2009. *Dangerous Discourses of Disability, Subjectivity and Sexuality.* Basingstoke, U.K.: Palgrave Macmillan.

Shildrick, M. and Price, J. 1996. Breaking the boundaries of the broken body. *Body and Society* 2(4): 93–113.

Shildrick, M. and Price, J. 2002. Bodies together: Touch, ethics and disability. In *Disability/Postmodernity: Embodying Disability Theory*, eds. M. Corker and T. Shakespeare, pp. 63–75. London, U.K.: Continuum.

Silvers, A., Wasserman, D., and Mahowald, M.B. 1999. *Disability, Difference, Discrimination: Perspectives on Justice in Bioethics and Public Policy.* Lanham, MD: Roman and Littlefield.

Skelton, T. and Valentine, G. 2003. 'It feels like being deaf is normal': An exploration into the complexities of defining D/deafness and young D/deaf people's identities. *Canadian Geographer* 47(4): 451–466.

Steiner, W.A., Ryser, L., Huber, E., Uebelhart, D., Aeschlimann, A., and Stucki G. 2002. Use of the ICF model as a clinical problem-solving tool in physical therapy and rehabilitation medicine. *Physical Therapy* 82(11): 1098–1107.

Stiker, H.J. 1999. The birth of rehabilitation. In *A History of Disability*, pp. 121–189. Ann Arbor, MI: University of Michigan Press.

Stucki, G., Cieza, A., and Melvin, J. 2007. The international classification of functioning, disability and health: A unifying model for the conceptual description of the rehabilitation strategy. *Journal of Rehabilitation Medicine* 39(4): 279–285.

Stucki, G., Ewert, T., and Cieza, A. 2002. Value and application of the ICF in rehabilitation medicine. *Disability & Rehabilitation* 24(17): 932–938.

Swain, J. and French, S. 2000. Towards an affirmation model of disability. *Disability & Society* 15(4): 569–582.

Thomas, C. 1999. *Female Forms: Experiencing and Understanding Disability.* Buckingham, U.K.: Open University Press.

Thomas, C. 2007. *Sociologies of Disability and Illness: Contested Ideas in Disability Studies and Medical Sociology.* New York: Palgrave MacMillan.

Tremain, S. 2001. On the government of disability. *Social Theory and Practice* 27: 617–636.

Verbrugge, L.M. and Jette, A.M. 1994. The disablement process. *Social Science & Medicine* 38(1): 1–14.

Wade, D.T. 2009. Goal setting in rehabilitation: An overview of what, why and how. *Clinical Rehabilitation* 23(4): 291–295.

Wiart, L. and Darrah, J. 2002. Changing philosophical perspectives on the management of children with physical disabilities—Their effect on the use of powered mobility. *Disability and Rehabilitation* 24(9): 492–498.

World Health Organization (WHO). 1980. *International Classification of Impairments, Disabilities and Handicaps: A Manual of Classification Relating to the Consequences of Disease.* Geneva, Switzerland: World Health Organization.

World Health Organization (WHO). 2001. International classification of functioning, disability and health. Geneva, Switzerland: World Health Organization.

Zola, I.K. 1991. Bringing our bodies and ourselves back in: Reflections on a past, present, and future "medical sociology". *Journal of Health and Social Behavior* 32: 1–16.

3

Quality of Life

In Chapter 2, I argued that an unreflective pursuit of normal bodies, activities, and social roles organizes and sustains rehabilitation practices. In this chapter, I consider the ways in which the valorization of normality in rehabilitation is reflected in measures and judgments of quality of life. Intended to capture outcomes beyond the presence or absence of disease, quality of life terminology is now ubiquitous in contemporary health care, and improving quality of life is a pervasively stated goal of rehabilitation programs the world over. Myriad tools have been devised to measure the quality of life of populations, groups, and individuals, and quality of life arguments are advanced in momentous decisions such as withholding or withdrawing "futile" medical treatments. Quality of life research has emerged as a field of inquiry unto itself, with a 680% increase in the proportion of quality of life studies published from 1966 to 2005 (Moons et al. 2006).

As I explore further below, these developments have not only changed research and health-care practices, they have helped structure how we think about what it means to be "healthy" or "disabled" and ultimately what it means to be human (Rapley 2003). In so doing, I make a distinction between the lay concept of "quality of life" and its reductive manifestation as "QOL" in health measurement, because these terms have come to differ in their phenomenological reference and usage (Taylor 1994). Conceptual confusion abounds in QOL research and scholarship, not only in terms of the relevant "domains" of interest and how they interact, but also at a more fundamental philosophical level where there is very little agreement about "what it is" that is being measured or discussed. My approach in this chapter is to change the parameters of the discussion, not to ask what it is but what it *does*. Quality of life/QOL is a useful concept that has contributed to moving health care away from a disease model into a more expansive ways of understanding health and the experience of illness/impairment. However, as I discuss, quality of life judgments are always necessarily relational, reproducing social ideas of what constitutes a good or deficient life. These normative discourses coalesce with notions of disability/normality in shaping how impaired bodies are conceived and acted upon, not just by practitioners but also by the recipients of care. Shared notions of quality of life co-mingle with internalized presuppositions about the self that are embedded, as Rose (1992, p. 141) suggests, "in the very language that we use to make persons thinkable, and in our ideal conceptions of what people should be." In considering these effects, this chapter builds my argument for novel and creative ways of understanding difference as something other than a problem to be fixed. My goal is not to replace quality of life with something putatively "better," but to signal a need for ongoing scrutiny of the assumptions that underpin rehabilitation and their effects, opening up alternative possibilities.

Origins and Confusions

Quality of life terminology came into common usage after the end of World War II and initially referred to material wealth and the acquisition of goods, that is, care, housing, disposable income, etc. (Farquhar 1995). Over time, the term began to encompass other aspects of well-being. Farquhar (1995) traces this development in the United States where, in the 1960s, quality of life was increasingly associated with values of personal freedom, leisure, emotion, enjoyment, simplicity, and personal caring. At the same time, there was an increased interest in the measurement of these and other indicators of change in societal quality of life. Such developments were bound up in the emergence of the "interview society" and increasing interest in gathering people's opinions through public surveys, opinion polls, and focus groups (Gubrium and Holstein 2003). Capturing people's subjective judgments was increasingly viewed as valuable to social engineers, policy makers, marketers, and health practitioners since, it was argued, subjective judgments are "real and people act on them" (Farquhar 1995, p. 1439).

Measurement of quality of life in health-care research and practice paralleled these developments with the first patient-based questionnaires to assess symptoms emerging in the field of psychiatry during World War II and in the post-war years (Armstrong et al. 2007). These early measures lead to the development of other patient reporting tools in other fields that could be used for population screening and the monitoring of disease impact over time. Armstrong et al. (2007) trace the history of quality of life measurement in the health sciences and how it morphed from measurement of symptoms, to activities of daily living, and eventually to "health-related quality of life (HRQOL)" in the mid-1980s. They outline how measurement of quality of life functioned to detach "distal symptoms" (e.g., activities of daily living) from pathology and in so doing transformed the nature and meaning of symptoms in health care. No longer was it necessary to link, for example, physical functioning to a physiological process, rather the dysfunction itself became the problem to be treated. The amelioration of distal symptoms shifted the object of health care away from the biological body and effectively reoriented practices. These shifts are evident in the extensive work of the World Health Organization (WHO) and other bodies to develop holistic measures of quality of life (e.g., WHOQOL 1998) and sophisticated models of function (e.g., WHO 2001) that acknowledge that health and disability are not solely determined by pathology.

In contemporary usages, quality of life has been equated with life satisfaction, physical functioning, perceived health status, utility, health perceptions, symptoms, well-being, or different combinations of these dimensions (Hunt 1997). Moons et al. (2006) suggest there are at least eight different conceptual categories of QOL in the health literature: normal life, social utility, happiness/affect, satisfaction with life, achievement of personal goals, natural capacities, (economic) utility, and satisfaction with specific domains. The conceptual gaps between categories such as "natural capacity" and "happiness" are obviously so immense that it is difficult to imagine how they came to carry the same QOL label. Some measures derive from a single conceptual category, such as life satisfaction or function, while others from multiple categories that are organized into domains. Regardless of these distinctions, quality of life has become a kind of catch-all term with competing and conflicting meanings. As Dijkers (2007, p. 153) notes:

> (T)he term QOL is being used in a great number of ways, and… the differences between the various conceptualizations are far from superficial. They involve major discrepancies that tie in with epistemology, and other philosophical concerns. What is QOL in one conceptualization is at best a determinant of QOL in another. While the judgments of the persons whose life it is are core to some definitions of the concept, for others they are useless distractions.

These kinds of definitional problems are pervasive in the QOL literature and have persisted for decades with no sign of abating (for reviews, see Moons et al. 2006; Rapley 2003). Consensus on the definition of quality of life is perhaps not possible or even desirable. However, it is highly troubling that this single term refers to a bewildering range of concepts, and yet so much of rehabilitation research and practice claims to measure and/or improve it. Rapley (2003, p. 142) has gone so far as to state that "much HRQOL ... is based in dubious ethical practices and research design ... and/or is methodologically so flawed as to be worthless." These judgments nevertheless form the "evidence base" that drives interventions at individual, group, and population levels and have enormous impact on how health and social programs and services are funded.

QOL, Function, and Normalization

The conflation of QOL with function is a key source of conceptual confusion in the literature and has particular relevance for rehabilitation. Practitioners may disagree with my argument in Chapter 2 that rehabilitation is focused on normalization but are unlikely to dispute its goals of improving function. Rehabilitation is broadly concerned with optimizing "physical, sensory, intellectual, psychological and social" function (Barnes and Ward 2000; Tulsky and Rosenthal 2003; WHO 2014) and has been described as the "medicine of function" (Bethge et al. 2014). However, as I will argue, optimization of function (couched in the terminology of QOL) is a version of normalization dressed in different clothes.

The WHO (2011) defines rehabilitation as "a set of measures that assist individuals who experience, or are likely to experience, disability to achieve and maintain *optimal functioning* in interaction with their environments" (WHO 2011, p. 308, my italics). This definition of rehabilitation closely aligns with the WHO's broad definitions of quality of life and health, each of which includes physical, social, and psychological dimensions (WHO 1948; WHOQOL 1998). These expansive definitions are useful in assuring that the complexity of health and well-being is not reduced to questions of mortality and morbidity but also create challenges that translate into research and practice (Sullivan 2003). Some of these are around conceptual ordering. In other words, when considering health, function, and/or QOL, is any one a subset of another? Or are they equivalent? Separate? Overlapping? The notion of HRQOL now used extensively in health research suggests that health is only one aspect of QOL. HRQOL has been described as encompassing those aspects of overall QOL that can be clearly shown to affect health including "physical and mental health perceptions and their correlates, including health risks and conditions, *functional status*, social support, and socioeconomic status" (Centers for Disease Control and Prevention 2000). Nevertheless, no clear consensus has emerged regarding what is being measured with QOL or HRQOL instruments, or their relationship to functional abilities and/or health status (Sullivan 2003). Health, QOL, and HRQOL concepts and measures all refer to social, psychological and physical dimensions, capacities and functions, which get conflated in various ways to render them virtually indistinct.

A Case Example

The confusion surrounding health, function, and QOL are reflected in research employing standardized measures of these phenomena. Studies that purport to measure QOL commonly use "health status" and/or functional measures and vice versa and may or may not include research participants' subjective views (a point I return to later in this chapter). These diverse measures are often independently or collectively labeled as "QOL measures" and terms such as function, health status, and (HR) QOL may be used interchangeably. Moreover, despite calls to the contrary, quality of life is frequently not defined and/or gets reduced to particular functional abilities adding to rather than addressing conceptual confusion (Gill and Feinstein 1994; Tulsky and Rosenthal 2003).

To demonstrate this, it is useful to unpack published quality of life research, which I do here using the example of a study by Hetherington et al. (2006). My point is not to single out this paper or its authors, but to illustrate points of tension in quality of life research that are pervasive even within studies hailed as methodologically rigorous (Gill and Feinstein 1994). Two key issues are demonstrated in this paper, first quality of life is not defined, and second there is an assumed causal link between functional abilities and quality of life. The first few words of the title and abstract start to signal a conflation of concepts. The title of the paper refers to function: "*Functional* outcome in young adults with spina bifida and hydrocephalus," while the abstract refers to quality of life: "*Quality of life* was studied in 31 adult survivors of spina bifida (SBH)..." (p. 117). Already there is a disconnect, an assumption, the replacement of one concept with another. The authors go on to say that little is known about "adult function" with the population, and then link function to QOL by stating: "To the extent that physical and cognitive problems of SBH children (sic) persist into adulthood, the quality of life of adults with SBH would be compromised" (p. 118). A causal link is thus made between physical and cognitive dysfunction which *necessarily* diminishes QOL regardless of life stage (childhood vs adulthood) or other life circumstances. There is no evidence presented to establish this causal link, and no discussion of other potential influences on QOL. Nor is there any definition of quality of life offered. The authors acknowledge that conceptual clarity is "elusive," and suggest that quality of life is "commonly" focused on "four central domains" in the literature, three of which are categories of function: physical and occupational function, cognitive/psychological function, and social interaction (p. 118). The literature review is centered on reviewing impaired functions in this population. The study itself used a mixture of standardized physical and cognitive functional assessments and other instruments labeled as "QOL measures." The description of the analysis includes the following statement: "Under the assumption that overall independence and range of experiences contributes to QOL, a regression model was tested..." (p. 122). Two new causal links with QOL are thus made beyond the earlier links to function: range of experiences and independence.

I am not disputing the importance of researchers declaring the assumptions that underpinned their statistical analyses. The key point I want to make is the rather large conceptual leaps made between limitations in functional abilities/daily tasks and quantified judgments of QOL. The methods are sound, but the underlying premises in this paper do what much of QOL research does, assumes in some form or another that function is either equivalent to QOL or is one of its major determinants—not just any function, but *normal* function. So, for example, using a cane or wheelchair may reduce a quality of life domain score even though, depending on the circumstances, use of either may be more efficient and more enjoyable than independent walking (Amundson 2000; Metts 2001). Research in this vein perpetuates the view that life quality is directly determined by the degree of impairment and fails to acknowledge the interconnectedness of life quality with myriad other aspects of life such as personal relationships, security, expectations, spirituality, self-worth, emotional well-being, socioeconomic status, and/or civic and social inclusion (Amundson 2000; Koch 2000).

Links made between functional abilities and enjoyment, value, or quality of life are closely tied to notions of normalization. The ability to fulfill a "normal role" has been used extensively in conceptualizing QOL measures that compare the functioning of an individual with that of "healthy" persons. The closer an individual's life approximates the standard for normalcy, the better QOL is judged to be (Moons et al. 2006). The link to normality is further made in bioethicist Dan Brock's philosophical analysis where he states that "[Q]uality of life must always be measured against normal, primary functional capacities for humans..." (Brock 1993, p. 308 cited in Amundson 2000). This statement is consistent with Katz and Marshall's (2004) critical observation that function-oriented approaches in health care have replaced disease-oriented approaches. Function, they suggest, is the new normal in establishing what counts as "healthy," "successful," or "productive" (p. 63).

As I discussed in the previous chapter, we cannot sensibly talk about a loss or lack of function except in relation to some notion of normal function. Normal (or supra normal) outcomes do not drive intervention, but loss or lack of function does. So while it is not common to talk about "normal quality of life," all kinds of norms, standards, and thresholds are used to generate QOL scores on standardized measures. These effects are evident in other assessments and measures used in rehabilitation practice and multiply their effects. In cardiac rehabilitation, for example, Wheatley (2005) notes that commonly used tools assessing risks for a future cardiac event define bodies "as either *at-risk* (i.e., deviant) or *normal*" according to a boundary that dictates practice and interventions (p. 205, her italics).

Challenges from within the Health Sciences

There is a well-established body of empirical literature demonstrating that functional status is not correlated with individuals' ratings and perceptions of the quality of their lives. In my own field of childhood disability, research has demonstrated that subjective ratings of QOL do not correlate well with function (Livingston et al. 2007; Rosenbaum et al. 2007; Schneider et al. 2001; Young et al. 2007). Qualitative interviews with children with cerebral palsy revealed several elements important to the quality of their lives including social relationships with families and friends, the variety of opportunities provided by school and home environments, and the pursuit of recreational activities (Young et al. 2007). Children requiring moderate to maximum levels of assistance for self-care and mobility tasks were reported to be well satisfied with their school abilities and friendships. In a review, Livingston et al. (2007) reported that several studies have found similar discordance between function and life quality as defined by participants.

Research with adults has yielded similar findings. As examples, in qualitative interviews with over 150 disabled people, Albrecht and Devlieger (1999) found that 54.3% of the respondents with moderate to serious impairments reported having an excellent or good QOL. Robbins et al. (2001) found that HRQOL measured with patients with amyotrophic lateral sclerosis (ALS) did not correlate with physical function. They concluded that the ALS-specific HRQOL instrument used in their study was a measure of physical function only, and excluded important spiritual, religious, and psychological factors. Perhaps more striking, research findings have shown that some persons describe richer and more meaningful lives after disabling injuries or illnesses (Koch 2001; Parsons et al. 2008; Young and McNicoll 1998), and that loss of function had changed their lives for the better in a number of ways including stronger interpersonal ties, richer spirituality, or becoming a "better person" (Parsons et al. 2008).

Research studies like those discussed earlier support the arguments of disability scholars that the presumed link between function and life quality is dubious at best and reflects deeply held social biases regarding disability and disabled people (Amundson 2005; Metts 2001). The benefits of QOL measurement need to be considered alongside their potential harms in perpetuating notions that a life of reduced function is necessarily of lower quality. However, asking individuals to rate and/or describe their life quality still assumes that QOL is a stable pre-existing entity that can be accessed once the appropriate method of assessment is identified.

Directing asking people to assess their QOL may begin to deal with the presumed causal relationships between disability and life quality, but fails to address the more insidious effects of QOL discourses in re/producing shared social understandings of the good life. Attending to these effects requires more than refining operational definitions or domains of QOL research. Rather what is needed are efforts toward breaking of habits of thought, problematizing existing distinctions, and attending to how QOL discourses produce bodies for rehabilitation interventions. I begin to address these imperatives in the following sections, but first consider two additional areas of relevance to the discussion: the division of QOL measurement into subjective and objective domains or instruments, and the operation of quality of life judgments in clinical decision-making.

The Subjective/Objective Divide

In quality of life research, measures and subscales are categorized as either "subjective" or "objective." Subjective or "self-rated" measures are those where participants choose item responses from predetermined lists or scales. In most (but not all) cases, participants have no method of indicating whether particular items contribute to their quality of life and how, or to indicate what else might be of relevance that is not included in the measure. Objective scales on the other hand are those that are completed by an observer, usually a health professional, who assesses how well or poorly the individual performs on items such as activities of daily living (ADLs). Objective measures and scales are more likely to measure symptoms and functional abilities and are either not concerned with subjective correlates of quality of life, or presume these linkages. Some, however, would suggest that these scales are not "true" QOL measures, which further demonstrates the conceptual confusion in the field.

The subjective/objective division relies on particular formulations of subjectivity and objectivity, implying that subjective scales reflect individual perspectives and objective scales are value-neutral. Each, however, reduces quality of life to a set of predetermined parameters that trouble the subjective/objective distinction. Objective scales tend to measure functional abilities and inevitably reflect the subjective evaluations of clinical experts who bring their own values into their judgments of functional performance (Rapley 2003, p. 66). Far from being value-neutral, the development of the scales reflect *a priori* value judgments regarding what items and domains count as relevant in determining good or poor QOL outcomes. Subjective scales often reduce personal input to a set of forced responses that disregard the individual's perspective on the relevant significance of each of the items in relation to their lives. Furthermore, they assume that individuals have stable perspectives, judgments, and values about what constitutes a good life that remain constant across time, place, and cultural context (Amundson 2005; Gill and Feinstein 1994; Koch 2001; Sullivan 2003).

Changes to individual subjective ratings across time are termed "response shift" in measurement parlance and are considered a challenge to the validity of subjective scales (Sullivan 2003). But more is going on here than a shift in perspectives. Abrams (2014) has stated that "subjectivity is an artifice," noting that the act of transforming subjective experiences into ranked and ordered data for statistical analysis removes them from the phenomenological experience of the individual into a world of measurable, objective presence.

Apart from labels of objective or subjective, standardization unavoidably imposes particular normative ideas of what constitutes a good life for the person or group being measured. The reduction of a person's quality of life to a set of statistical correlates cannot help but lose any perspective on the ineffable nature of life quality. In the well-intentioned impetus to measure something other than presence or absence of disease, complex existential questions of whether life is of good or poor quality and why (which have been discussed and pursued across cultures since ancient times [Diener and Suh 1997]) get reduced to, for example, a "total QOL score" of −0.64 ± 1.2. QOL operates in the same way as other scientific terms to homogenize that which it purports to clarify (Rapley 2003, pp. 216–217). The goodness of life gets reduced to measurable variables and loses any sense of embodied interaction or context. Discrepancies between standardized tests of QOL and individuals' perceptions of the quality of their lives are dismissed, explained away (Brock 2005), or couched as paradox (Albrecht and Devlieger 1999).

To address the problems inherent in "objective" third-party assessments, some have suggested that subjective "satisfaction with life" is the only "correct" conceptualization of QOL (Dijkers 2007; Moons et al. 2006). Individual self-determinations however do not occur in a social vacuum and are shaped by prevailing normative discourses of disability, normality, and the good citizen in the same way that professionals' values are mediated. Personal judgments of the goodness of a life are formed within sociocultural environments across time and place, and—in the moment of contemplation—by immediate circumstances, emotions, and state of mind. Subjective judgments are furthermore shaped by the professional context at the time and place of assessment, that is, who is asking, for what purpose, and what do they expect to hear?

Research participants are likely to respond to the authority of experts by reinterpreting their functional abilities according to the standards of the research design (Katz and Marshall 2004; Jarvinen 2000). This may result in apparent inconsistencies in responses, but is part of a larger problem of asking people to know and describe themselves according to fixed measurable units. Rapley (2003, p. 215) notes:

> The provision by a research participant of an answer to a social scientist's question about their quality of life, under such an account, is not then the *act* of a *person* but the act of a being that may, more accurately, be likened to a gas meter. The "levels" of subjective well-being, satisfaction with relationships and the rest reported by persons are merely *readings* of objectified, "inner," psychical dials. This surely is a misunderstanding not only of what it means to be a *person*, but also of what it means to *act*.

Self-report measures inevitably look at what a person can do, not what they actually do, like to do, or avoid doing (Katz and Marshall 2004). Measures thus impose particular authoritative notions of ability, function, and quality of life that shape response. Perhaps more importantly, self-judgments are mediated by neoliberal ideologies of productivity, social contribution, and idealized notions of normal and good lives—a point I expand on in the following.

Quality of Life Judgments in Clinical Practices

I have focused primarily on problems with QOL measurement and research, but quality of life discourse also mediates rehabilitation practices and decision-making in a number of other ways with serious consequences. Unilateral quality of life judgments are on a daily basis used in, for example, life and death decision-making regarding life-sustaining interventions such as ventilation, and in the burgeoning field of genetic testing and counseling. In both of these fields, the clear messaging is that it is better not to exist than to live with disability (Gibson 2001; Scully 2005). Even though extensive research has shown that people labeled as disabled do not rate their lives any differently than other people (Albrecht and Devlieger 1999; Bach et al. 1991; Gerhart et al. 1994) quality of life judgments continue to be advanced in public arguments and the clinical reasoning of individual practitioners. For example, Ravenscroft and Bell (2000) in a survey examining decision-making in intensive care units found that professionals' judgments of "perceived quality of life" was one of the most common reasons for terminating individuals' life support. The presumption that a loss (or congenital lack) of physical or cognitive functioning necessarily equates with a life-not-worth-living is manifest in practices and policy debates regarding "futile" treatments, selective abortion, and euthanasia.

In the late 1990s when long-term ventilation had only recently become available as a life-extending option for people with chronic respiratory failure, I conducted a study of Canadian physicians working with youth with Duchenne muscular dystrophy (DMD) (Gibson 2001). This was before medical information was widely accessible on the Internet, and it meant that individuals and families primarily relied on their healthcare practitioners to share information about emerging treatment options. Few families were aware of the option of long-term ventilation as a lifesaving option for youth with DMD, and without it individuals would usually die of respiratory insufficiency by the time they were about 20 years old. In a national (Canadian) survey, I found that 25% of physicians were not discussing the option of long-term ventilation with families, and the most common reason for withholding information was perceived poor quality of life. In interviews with a subset of physicians, I discovered a range of practices from complete lack of disclosure to positive encouragement, including various ways of framing information in a positive or negative light creating a veneer of clinician "neutrality." This range of approaches, based almost exclusively on physicians' quality of life assumptions, meant that the geographical location of the young person with DMD (the region served by a physician) largely determined the possibility of living into adulthood. In the study, I argued that clinicians' judgments of quality of life should not be determining who lives or dies and at the very least physicians should be discussing their judgments with patients and families.

Practice has changed since the study was conducted and long-term ventilation is now routinely offered to individuals with DMD in North America and across the developed world (Finder et al. 2004). Nevertheless, the example serves to illustrate the potential dangers of rigid or unreflective quality of life judgments in clinical practice. In the study context, such judgments had life or death consequences, but quality of life beliefs are deeply embedded in how disability and disabled people are discussed and acted upon across everyday rehabilitation practices (education, research, and clinical). Seemingly mundane decisions may not have the same momentous consequences as life or death decisions but they can exert other, less obvious, harms. Clinicians are by and large motivated to do what is in the best interests of their patients and to provide support with difficult decisions. They may have legitimate concerns about interventions they feel may harm individuals, but also must remember that their quality of life judgments are always unavoidably value based. For example, individuals are not necessarily "in denial" when they choose to live with seemingly severe impairments, and attempting to convince them to comply with advice may be ill-advised. It is particularly telling that research demonstrates health professionals are likely to make treatment recommendations based on perceptions of quality of life that do not correlate with those of their patients (Bach et al. 1991; Gerhart et al. 1994; Schneiderman et al. 1993).

In writing about possible dangers of quality of life judgments, I am not suggesting we can or should try to eliminate them. For example, the clinician's perception of quality of life comes from the totality of their experience and can act as a resource in shared decision making with individuals. The dangers, rather, arise from unexamined assumptions about quality of life, mistaking contingent judgments for established facts, or becoming mired in particular ways of understanding. All health-care practitioners, whether in research, education, or clinical practice, share a responsibility to continually reflect on their own values and assumptions of what constitutes a good or poor life quality and how this is manifested in their practices.

The Object of Intervention

I have discussed problems with conceptualizing and measuring quality of life/QOL and how quality of life judgments can be problematic in the context of clinical practice. For the most part my discussion has focused on a critique of how quality of life is defined and understood, in other words, debates about what it *is*. I now turn to a post-critical reading of quality of life to consider what QOL discourses *do*, and particularly how the disabled body is *materialized* through practices. As noted, post-critical approaches can be used in to examine how the objects of health science are constructed and naturalized through associated practices and applications (Chapter 1). The dysfunctional body can be understood as an *effect* of cultural concepts, metaphors, and narratives, such that the various ways bodies are talked about brings them into being in particular ways that mediate actions. It follows from this reading that disability, impairment, and quality of life do not *precede* their measurement but rather are *constructed* in part by tools that reflect notions of "dysfunctional" lives and persons as necessarily flawed. The instruments and acts of assessment serve to bring into being and sustain a class of persons labeled as disabled.

The methods of measuring quality of life rely on a positivist epistemology to presuppose that quality of life is "real," that is a pre-existing stable object or "construct" that is discoverable and amenable to measurement. By assuming their object exists as a measurable entity, QOL instruments act to create the entity and sustain its existence. The acronym (QOL) takes on its own meaning with a stable set of measurable properties that de-coupled it from that which it purports to represent—the quality of a life or lives (quality of life). QOL is, however, but one way of describing a set of putatively related and contested phenomena, which could potentially comprise the totality of one's life. Moreover, QOL and HRQOL are part of broader, largely-negative social narratives of disability that not only guide professional practices but also mediate how individuals understand themselves, their lives, and their place in the world.

With the reductive shift from quality of life to QOL, scale scores become the object of care. Successes in treatment, programs, or policy are judged by improvements in scores, which no longer need to correlate with any subjective or objective state of the individual. In other words, the score itself becomes the object of care—the patient. Thus we can say that measurement constructs and sustains its object such that the patient is incidental to action. QOL scores mobilize actions in policy, programs, and treatment such that whatever the measure was trying to represent no longer *matters*, the measure is the matter. The measurable constructs the real. Whereas quality of life was meant to get at something beyond pathology, the measurement of "QOL" has changed that elusive something into another thing, one that can be measured, quantified, and statistically manipulated, which categorizes bodies according to which ones have good (normal) or poor (disabled) lives.

These acts of defining some lives as necessarily compromised, along with parsing and quantifying the amount and type of compromise, involve a mix of conceptual and material acts that actively shape and reshape disabled bodies. Rosengarten (2005) makes this argument in relation to viral load tests utilized in HIV health-care practices as a site of "material discursive activity" that presuppose particular bodily identities and acts to materialize them (p. 77). In the rehabilitation context, Abrams (2014) draws on Heidegger's concept of "ontological difference" and his personal experiences with physical therapy to demonstrate how the clinical encounter actively constitute the body as a therapeutic object:

> The most extreme example of the ontological difference emerged when I was asked to judge my "subjective" experience of muscle disease and its treatment according to the so-called "Patient-Specific Functional Scale" ... This and similar scales are the very stuff of objective presence: the individual subject is isolated from the times and spaces of care, and asked to rank their "functionality" qua daily comportment in a physically extended world. The scale deploys subjectivity as the baseline of healthy existence, to come up with a clear-cut trajectory for progress and further treatment, both in terms of clock-time. The difference between care and subjective measures is the ontological difference. Such scales are not, of course, the only measure employed in the therapeutic relationship, but their use supports my main argument well: both client and practitioner actively constitute the body as objectively present in the therapeutic relationship, as a living thing accountable to explicitly measurable criteria.

In Abrams account, measures as part of the repertoire of clinical tools convert the subjective and existential experience of living with muscular dystrophy into an ontologically different object available for rehabilitation. Similarly, QOL measures interact with the impaired body through acts of assessment, further materializing it in ways that seem to separate the measure and the lived body into distinct entities. The disabled body, pre-constructed through biomedical discourse, is made available to manipulations that can be further measured and modified if it fails to produce the desired scores. For example, a low score in a self-care domain such as dressing constructs the patient as disabled in a particular way that mobilizes a program of intervention. Dressing can then be re-measured to assess for change and to determine if further alterations to body practices are required. Independent dressing, that is, dressing without help from another person, receives the best possible score. In this way, the measurement tool constructs and controls the meanings of disability and life quality. The body that achieves action in particular ways, independent dressing, is functioning well and has better QOL. Moreover, individuals are obliged to turn a critical gaze on their own bodies, assess their limits according to these parameters, and work toward normal function. Reshaped by these interventions, the body becomes a personal and professional project, the site for improvement toward the normal, and available for new assessments, new interventions in a continual making of not only the material body, but a good life. This relational reading of the disabled body and the QOL measure emphasizes how the two are co-constituting rather than pre-given. There is no "disabled" body that exists prior to its evaluation by the measure, and the measure relies on the constructed disabled body for its legitimacy.

QOL assessment thus serves to produce bodies of a certain kind that are identified for rehabilitation. Measurement divides, ranks, and categorizes bodies into normative classes of good or poor quality of life, functioning, and health that determine a host of interventions. Measures, as Abrams (2014, p. 443) notes, "disclose 'the body for professional measurement' in orderable and categorizable form… that delivers clinical experience from the clinical encounter to the statistical table." Only through language and concepts are these divisions made, and they could have been made in myriad other ways or not at all. Labels and instruments that created functional versus dysfunctional bodies sustain the illusion of an objective, measurable, and valid reality through their pervasive use as outcome targets. The measure creates and affirms the phenomenon in a loop without the possibility of appeal. The body already constituted through medicine/rehabilitation is further materialized through interventions to reshape and correct the body, behaviors, and improve QOL. The goal is to get better, and better is a higher score, which is inevitably linked to more typical or normal function. QOL measurement is thus both normative and normalizing.

Armstrong et al.'s (2007) historical analysis discussed above demonstrates how the body is continually re-categorized, reshaped, and remade through health measurement, which is increasing understood in terms of QOL. By tracking how the Sickness Impact Profile (SIP) was discussed in published research between 1986 and 2004, they exemplify how quality of life emerged as the catch-all concept that pervades health care today. The SIP questionnaire includes items about symptoms, mental health states, physical function/activities, and social activities. Armstrong and colleagues track how earlier papers referred to the SIP as a measure of "symptoms" or "subjective health," but the frequency of referring to it as a "QOL measure" rose exponentially since 2000. This relatively recent development reflects how bodies are understood through health measures and also how measures themselves are shaped and materialized as of a certain type through how they are labeled and used. Thus far from being separate entities, bodies, tools, and language inevitably interact to produce and reproduce health-care objects and practices.

Through the materialization and measurement of the dysfunctional body, the possibility for closer-to-normal is constructed as a private responsibility both imposed on individuals and taken up by them. Nikolas Rose (1992) argues that particular presuppositions about the self and the purpose of life are embedded in language and have changed over time. He notes that the guidance of selves in contemporary society is

> ...no longer dependent upon the authority of religion or traditional morality; it has been allocated to "experts of subjectivity" who transfigure existential questions about the purpose of life and the meaning of suffering into technical questions about the most effective ways of managing malfunction and improving "quality of life" (Rose 1992, pp. 141–142).

QOL measurement exemplifies this transfiguration of existential questions about the meaning of life into discrete questions that incite the management of experts like rehabilitation professionals. But Rose's point is that these kinds of transformations pervasively change how *all* persons in contemporary societies view their bodies and their lives. The imperative for self-surveillance and personal improvement (reflected in notions such as "self-efficacy" and "self-management") is a dominant discourse that has become naturalized and in turn structures individual practices (Foucault 1991). Thus, the notion that typical bodies and functions are preferable is deeply ingrained in the social imaginary, and it pervasively structures individual practices and shared moral imperatives for self-improvement (see Chapter 2). The language of quality of life, and the disability/normality binary, act as powerful filters that structure the ways people understand, judge, and act upon themselves and their expectations of others. Practitioners, patients, family members, educators, researchers, and policy makers share these naturalized assumptions, which manifest in how they think and act toward themselves and others. Nevertheless, these understandings are not fixed; they have changed over time and could again be otherwise.

There is an extensive body of work on how commonly used classifications change the ways in which individuals experience themselves and affect their behaviors, goals, and values. Indeed, these explorations are a central theme in post-critical scholarship (Bourdieu 1991; Foucault 1980; Hacking 2002; Rose 1999). Hacking (2002) reminds us that classifications and people interact—persons become aware of being classified, if only because of being treated or institutionalized in a certain way, and so experiencing themselves in that way. These are aspects of the ways in which we "make up people." The newly impaired person is hyper-aware of joining a new classificatory group, "the disabled," and is likely to resist being so defined. But new or modified classifications also hold transformative possibilities. Witness the variations in terms used to refer to people with various impairments over time (e.g., handicapped, disabled, developmentally delayed, challenged, special) and how they are resisted through emerging terms such as crip-culture, d/Deaf culture, or neurodiversity. Hacking refers to this as "the looping effect" whereby classifications make people but are not static; they can be broken and reconstituted. New terms will make new groups and materialize bodies in new ways and close or open up different options.

In this discussion, I have highlighted how conceptual labels have multiple effects, to emphasize that my goal in examining quality of life/QOL and its measures is not to replace them with something supposedly "better," but to signal the need for caution and reflection as well as precision and specification where it is needed. QOL assessment in its goal of providing information beyond the absence or presence of disease has a number of uses including program evaluation, allocation of scarce resources and research funding, and monitoring clinical change (Rapley 2003, p. 76). In all of these endeavors, however, it is important to ask: What is being measured? What causal links are assumed and why? How does the measure operate to allow/promote certain identities and possibilities and close off others? Are there other ways of understanding the body, dis/abilities, and the patient that circumvent the negative effects of quality of life judgments?

Reforming Quality of Life

Early in this chapter, I stated that optimization of function is an extension of normalization dressed in different clothes. This chapter expands my argument against the theoretical inertia that keeps rehabilitation from *moving* to new ways of understanding difference as something other than a problem to be eradicated. Quality of life, like disability, is a relational term that contains within it a normative judgment. Quality of life can be good or poor, or described according to the myriad sliding scales, dimensions, and domains that constitute the weight of measures developed for its assessment. Normative judgments are always made in relation to something else, good relies on bad, abnormal relies on normal, and vice versa. We cannot think one without the other. All assessments of quality of life, whether they be formal measures or bedside clinical judgments, rely on preconceived notions of what constitutes a good life. And, as I have discussed here and in Chapter 2, these judgments have been shown repeatedly to be linked with notions of normal, whether they be statistical norms of functional ability, or common assumptions about the preferability of a narrowly conceived "normal" or "healthy" life.

Throughout this chapter, I have also suggested that the problems inherent in third-party judgments or the use of standardized measures to assess quality of life are not addressed solely by soliciting the "subjective" views of the individual being assessed. Subjective views are not stable truths that can be "accessed" at a single point in time but are rather formed and reformed in a continual process. Moreover, perceptions of life quality are not created in a vacuum but formed in relation to the geo-temporal social milieus in which people are immersed. Ideas of what constitutes a good or poor life are part of a larger repertoire of socially embedded ideas that mediate how persons come to understand themselves and others (Bourdieu 1977). Asking people about their quality of life is undoubtedly important in any situation where quality of life judgments dictate intervention, but it does not address some of the more insidious effects on thought and action.

Likely the greatest problems associated with the measurement of QOL are conceptual. No one can agree on what it is, but almost everyone agrees that we are not getting any closer to a consensus over time. Perhaps a first step is to uncouple the link between objective indicators of quality of life and any notion of life satisfaction. Doing so requires reigning in applications of QOL and HRQOL measurement and the relatively recent explosion in quality of life research—taking a turn, going backwards, re-moving the concepts. Rapley (2003, p. 222) has suggested that qualitative research approaches seem more amenable to exploring complex concepts like quality of life that have physical, social, and existential elements. I tend to agree, but my purpose is not to identify a "better" method for assessing QOL. The way out can only be to eliminate its catch-all, unreflective usage in health care; not to stop trying to improve people's lives in all the ways that matter but to stop trying to pin down, parse out, and measure something labeled QOL or HRQOL. We can continue to measure function, symptoms, activities of daily life, affective states, and all the other "domains" of interest. But we must cease to assume a direct relationship between these phenomena and the goodness of a life, to label diverse concepts as quality of life, or even assume that "together" they constitute quality of life. Because of its ineffable nature, we need to stop claiming we can measure life quality through a questionnaire. Ceasing to reify the score or assuming that "improving" (normalizing) function will necessarily affect quality of life opens up possibilities for different practices, movements, perturbations, and oscillations.

I am not suggesting the complete abandonment of quality of life but rather a return that paradoxically also provides a way forward, that is, retreating from the epidemiological notion of "QOL" and returning to a more open consideration of "quality of life." I agree with Rapley (2003) that quality of life could instead be used as a "sensitizing concept" to guide the design of programs or interventions, but one that would need to be unpacked, specified, debated, and researched in each application. Rapley (2003, p. 223) states that "there is no reason why we should not set about designing human services by asking ourselves about how this or that service process or this or that service structure might affect the quality of the lived experience of persons served in such a way or such a place." He notes that when we invoke quality of life we are unavoidably engaged in the weighing of normative moral questions of the goodness of a life and thus should avoid statistical abstractions. Rather, he suggests that quality of life can be conceptually useful to guide debate in the public forum and encourage transparency and engagement in decision-making. This seems to me to be a useful suggestion for opening up a concept that has become almost meaninglessness (yet incredibly powerful), but is still helpful in orienting practices to outcomes beyond the absence or presence of pathology.

The ideas of health, function, and quality of life are the bread and butter of rehabilitation. They are reflected in definitions and descriptions of rehabilitation, in foundational concepts and frameworks like occupation and the ICF, and in the measures used in rehabilitation research and clinical practices. It is therefore vital that we clarify how these concepts are understood, applied, and relate to one another in our practices and to critically assess how they construct and reproduce particular notions of bodies, patients, and preferred outcomes.

References

Abrams, T. 2014. Flawed by Dasein? Phenomenology, ethnomethodology, and the personal experience of physiotherapy. *Human Studies* 37: 431–446.

Albrecht, G.L. and Devlieger, P.J. 1999. The disability paradox: High quality of life against all odds. *Social Science & Medicine* 48(8): 977–988.

Amundson, R. 2000. Against normal function. *Studies in History and Philosophy of Science Part C: Studies in History and Philosophy of Biological and Biomedical Sciences* 31(1): 33–53.

Amundson, R. 2005. Disability, ideology, and quality of life: A bias in biomedical ethics. In *Quality of Life and Human Difference*, 1st edn., eds. D. Wasserman, J. Bickenbach, and R. Wachbroit, pp. 101–124. Cambridge, U.K.: Cambridge University Press.

Armstrong, D., Lilford, R., Ogden, J., and Wessely, S. 2007. Health-related quality of life and the transformation of symptoms. *Sociology of Health & Illness* 29(4): 570–583.

Bach, J.R., Campagnolo, D.I., and Hoeman, S. 1991. Life satisfaction of individuals with Duchenne muscular dystrophy using long-term mechanical ventilatory support. *American Journal of Physical Medicine & Rehabilitation* 70(3): 129–135.

Barnes, M.P. and Ward, A.B. 2000. *Textbook of Rehabilitation Medicine*. Oxford, U.K.: Oxford University Press.

Bethge, M., Von Groote, P., Giustini, A., and Gutenbrunner, C. 2014. The world report on disability: A challenge for rehabilitation medicine. *American Journal of Physical Medicine & Rehabilitation* 93(1): 4–11.

Bourdieu, P. 1977. *Outline of a Theory of Practice*. Cambridge, U.K.: Cambridge University Press.

Bourdieu, P. 1991. *Language and Symbolic Power.* Cambridge, U.K.: Harvard University Press.

Brock, D.W. 1993. *Life and Death*. Cambridge, U.K.: Cambridge University Press.

Brock, D.W. 2005. Preventing genetically transmitted disabilities while respecting persons with disabilities. In *Quality of Life and Human Difference*, 1st edn., eds. D. Wasserman, J. Bickenbach, and R. Wachbroit, pp. 67–100. Cambridge, U.K.: Cambridge University Press.

Centers for Disease Control and Prevention. 2000. *Measuring Healthy Days*. Atlanta, GA: Centers for Disease Control and Prevention.

Diener, E. and Suh, E. 1997. Measuring quality of life: Economic, social, and subjective indicators. *Social Indicators Research* 40(1–2): 189–216.

Dijkers, M. 2007. "What's in a name?" The indiscriminate use of the "quality of life" label, and the need to bring about clarity in conceptualizations. *International Journal of Nursing Studies* 44(1): 153–155.

Farquhar, M. 1995. Elderly people's definitions of quality of life. *Social Science & Medicine* 41(10): 1439–1446.

Finder, J.D., Birnkrant, J.D., Carl, J. et al. 2004. Respiratory care of the patient with Duchenne muscular dystrophy—ATS consensus statement. *American Journal of Respiratory and Critical Care Medicine* 170(4): 456–465.

Foucault, M. 1980. In *Power/Knowledge Selected interviews and other writings 1972-77*, ed. C. Gordon. New York: Pantheon Books.

Foucault, M. 1991. Governmentality. In *The Foucault Effect: Studies in Governmentality: With Two Lectures by and an Interview with Michel Foucault*, eds. G. Burchell, M. Foucault, C. Gordon, and P. Miller, pp. 87–104. London, U.K.: Harvester Wheatsheaf.

Gerhart, K.A., Koziol-McLain, J., Lowenstein, S.R., and Whiteneck, G.G. 1994. Quality of life following spinal cord injury: Knowledge and attitudes of emergency care providers. *Annals of Emergency Medicine* 23(4): 807–812.

Gibson, B. 2001. Long-term ventilation for patients with Duchenne muscular dystrophy: Physicians' beliefs and practices. *Chest* 119(3): 940–946.

Gill, T.M. and Feinstein, A.R. 1994. A critical appraisal of the quality of quality of life instruments. *Journal of the American Medical Association* 272: 24–31.

Gubrium, J.F. and Holstein, J.A. 2003. From the individual interview to the interview society. In *Postmodern Interviewing*, eds. J.F. Gubrium and J.A. Holstein, pp. 21–50. Thousand Oaks, CA: Sage.

Hacking, I. 2002. Inaugural lecture: Chair of philosophy and history of scientific concepts at the Collège de France. *Economy and Society* 31(1): 1–14.

Hetherington, R., Dennis, M., Barnes, M., Drake, J., and Gentili, F. 2006. Functional outcome in young adults with spina bifida and hydrocephalus. *Child's Nervous System* 22(2): 117–124.

Hunt, S.M. 1997. The problem of quality of life. *Quality of Life Research* 6(3): 205–212.

Jarvinen, M. 2000. The biographical illusion: Constructing meaning in qualitative interviews. *Qualitative Inquiry* 6(3): 370–391.

Katz, S. and Marshall, B.L. 2004. Is the functional 'normal'? Aging, sexuality and the bio-marking of successful living. *History of the Human Sciences* 17(1): 53–75.

Koch, T. 2000. Life quality vs 'quality of life': Assumptions underlying prospective quality of life instruments in health care planning. *Social Science & Medicine* 51(3): 419–427.

Koch, T. 2001. Disability and difference: Balancing social and physical constructions. *Journal of Medical Ethics* 27(6): 370–376.

Livingston, M.H., Rosenbaum, P.L., Russel, D.J., and Palisano, R.J. 2007. Quality of life among adolescents with cerebral palsy: What does the literature tell us? *Developmental Medicine and Child Neurology* 49(3): 225–231.

Metts, R.L. 2001. The fatal flaw in the disability adjusted life year. *Disability & Society* 16(3): 449–452.

Moons, P., Budts, W., and De Geest, S. 2006. Critique on the conceptualisation of quality of life: A review and evaluation of different conceptual approaches. *International Journal of Nursing Studies* 43(7): 891–901.

Parsons, J.A., Eakin, J.M., Bell, R.S., Franche, R.L., and Davis, A.M. 2008. "So, are you back to work yet?" Re-conceptualizing 'work' and 'return to work' in the context of primary bone cancer. *Social Science & Medicine* 67(11): 1826–1836.

Rapley, M. 2003. *Quality of Life Research*. London, U.K.: Sage.

Ravenscroft, A.J. and Bell, M.D.D. 2000. 'End-of-life' decision making within intensive care-objective, consistent, defensible? *Journal of Medical Ethics* 26(6): 435–440.

Robbins, R.A., Simmons, Z., Bremer, A., Walsh, S.M., and Fischer, S. 2001. Quality of life in ALS is maintained as physical function declines. *Neurology* 56(4): 442–444.

Rose, N. 1992. Governing the enterprising self. In *The Values of Enterprise Culture: The Moral Debate*, eds. P. Heelas and P. Morris, pp. 141–164. London, U.K.: Routledge.

Rose, N. 1999. *Governing the Soul: The Shaping of the Private Self*, 2nd edn. London, U.K.: Free Association Books.

Rosenbaum, P.L., Livingston, M.H., Palisano, R.J., Galuppi, B.E., and Russel D.J. 2007. Quality of life and health-related quality of life of adolescents with cerebral palsy. *Developmental Medicine and Child Neurology* 49: 516–521.

Rosengarten, M. 2005. The measure of HIV as a matter of bioethics. In *Ethics of the Body: Postconventional Challenges*, eds. M. Shildrick and R. Mykitiuk, pp. 71–90. Cambridge, MA: MIT Press.

Schneider, J.W., Gurucharri, L.M., Gutierrez, A.L., and Gaebler-Spira, D. 2001. Health-related quality of life and functional outcome measures for children with cerebral palsy. *Developmental Medicine and Child Neurology* 43: 601–608.

Schneiderman, L.J., Kaplan, R.M., Pearlman, R.A., and Teetzel, H. 1993. Do physicians' own preferences for life-sustaining treatment influence their perceptions of patients' preferences? *Journal of Clinical Ethics* 4(1): 28–33.

Scully, J.L. 2005. Admitting all variations? Postmodernism and genetic normality. In *Ethics of the Body: Postconventional Challenges*, eds. M. Shildrick and R. Mykitiuk, pp. 49–68. Cambridge, MA: MIT Press.

Sullivan, M. 2003. The new subjective medicine: Taking the patient's point of view on health care and health. *Social Science & Medicine* 56(7): 1595–1604.

Taylor, C. 1994. The politics of recognition. In *Multiculturalism*, ed. A. Gutmann, pp. 25–74. Princeton, NJ: Princeton University Press.

Tulsky, D.S. and Rosenthal, M. 2003. Measurement of quality of life in rehabilitation medicine: Emerging issues. *Archives of Physical Medicine and Rehabilitation* 84: S1–S2.

Wheatley, E.E. 2005. Disciplining bodies at risk cardiac rehabilitation and the medicalization of fitness. *Journal of Sport & Social Issues* 29(2): 198–221.

World Health Organization (WHO). 1948. *Preamble to the Constitution of the World Health Organization as adopted by the International Health Conference*, New York, June 19–22, 1946, and entered into force on April 7, 1948.

World Health Organization (WHO) 2001. International classification of functioning, disability and health. Geneva, Switzerland: World Health Organization.

World Health Organization (WHO) 2011. World report on disability. Geneva, Switzerland: World Health Organization. http://www.who.int/disabilities/world_report/2011/en/ (accessed March 11, 2015).

World Health Organization. (WHO) 2014. Health topics: Rehabilitation. http://www.who.int/topics/rehabilitation/en/ (accessed March 11, 2015).

The World Health Organization Quality of Life Group (WHOQLG). 1998. The World Health Organization quality of life assessment (WHOQOL): Development and general psychometric properties. *Social Science & Medicine* 46(12): 1569–1585.

Young, B., Rice, H., Dixon-Woods, M., Colver, A.F., and Parkinson, K.N. 2007. A qualitative study of the health-related quality of life of disabled children. *Developmental Medicine & Child Neurology* 49(9): 660–665.

Young, J.M. and McNicoll, P. 1998. Against all odds: Positive life experiences of people with advanced amyotrophic lateral sclerosis. *Health & Social Work* 23(1): 35–43.

4

Development

Barbara E. Gibson, Gail Teachman, and Yani Hamdani

In this chapter, we* question and rethink "normal development" as the primary organizing concept in children's rehabilitation. Normal development understands childhood as a predictable trajectory from infancy to adulthood characterized by a series of developmental stages that cover all aspects of personhood, including physical, intellectual, emotional, and social. This "ages and stages" framing provides the underlying rationale for a host of health and education interventions designed to maximize young people's physical and mental capacities as they "progress" toward adulthood. In the traditional rehabilitation context, therapeutic goals and treatments are designed to assist disabled children to achieve developmental milestones and approximate developmental norms and trajectories. This link between rehabilitation therapies and development is accepted almost universally as uncontroversial (Goodley and Runswick-Cole 2010) and underpins dozens of standardized scales used to assess motor, language, and social development and to guide interventions (Effgen 2005, p. 42). Pick up any text on children's rehabilitation and you will find tables, charts, and descriptions of the stages of development, accompanied by statements regarding how an understanding of developmental progression is essential for the design of treatments aimed at ameliorating disability. For example, *Pediatric Therapy* (Porr and Rainville 1999) suggests:

> Knowledge of "normal" growth and development is essential to therapy practice. Coupled with a knowledge of disease and disability, this enables the therapist to understand the impact of disability on an individual child and his or her ...capability and dysfunction. *Obviously*, this underlies any successful intervention. [p. 70, *emphasis added*]

* This chapter is modified from a previously published chapter written with my colleagues Gail Teachman and Yani Hamdani (Gibson et al. 2015).

However "obvious" it may seem, development is only one way of understanding childhood and approaching children's rehabilitation. In what follows, we situate current dominant understandings of the child and development in their historical origins, ask how well they are serving disabled children, and consider how things could be otherwise. Our project of examining "normal" development and the effects it produces aligns with the post-critical project of the book in interrogating claims to truth, how they emerged, and how they shape rehabilitation practices. We examine how biomedicine and rehabilitation divide, classify, and judge the recipients of care, and how these practices may contribute to unintentional harms. The goal is not to suggest that rehabilitation necessarily discards development, but that we remain ever vigilant in recognizing that organizing concepts are not natural but contingent human inventions that have myriad effects and are open to revision.

Developmentalism

Child development is a relatively recent idea that came to the fore in the late nineteenth and early twentieth centuries (Rose 1999, pp. 144–154). During this period, observations of young children were thought to inform evolutionary theory and help distinguish the emergence of characteristics that separate humans from animals. The development of the human embryo was seen in parallel to human physical evolution and the cultural evolution from primitive to civilized (Rose 1999, p. 145). Methods to measure, document, and influence children's physical and social development began to emerge. Key proponents of developmentalism like Piaget and Gesell constructed the standardized developmental stages and the normal development curves that are still widely used today to guide health care and education policies and practices for children and youth (James and James 2004; Rose 1999).

The emerging interest in development *as* evolution, and the systematic measurement of children's bodies and abilities, cemented a place for the science of establishing the normal child. Identifying and charting developmental milestones and age-linked performance norms provided new ways of thinking about children that were taken up by health and education professionals and the broader society—including parents. The idea of a standardized path for children's growth and development was used to underpin a wide variety of education, social, and health policies and practices that formally and informally regulated children's lives. During the late nineteenth and early twentieth centuries, children were increasingly viewed as adults-in-the-making whose progress could be tracked. The widespread measurement of markers such as height and weight were used to develop population norms against which every child could be assessed. Deviations from these norms were pathologized and thus viewed as requiring intervention. Through a series of checklists, scales, norms, and percentiles, professionals as agents of state education and health-care apparatuses could evaluate what children should be doing by a certain age, and pronounce who was normal or abnormal, advanced or slow, disabled or nondisabled. "At-risk" children could be identified and acted upon. By early twentieth century, childhood and adolescence emerged as an impermanent time of *transition*, whereby ensuring successful outcomes for children became inextricably linked with the achievement of adulthood, and more specifically a productive adulthood in the neoliberal tradition of creating *contributing* citizens (James and James 2004, pp. 143–144). Rather than subsiding, these ideas have gained further traction and are aligned with moral imperatives for life-long individual self-improvement, personal growth, change, and physical optimization that pervade contemporary life (Burman 2013).

Developmental measures are not merely aids to assess or categorize children but are in themselves, as Rose notes, "revolutions in consciousness" (Rose 1999, p. 153). They, in short, construct the ways we think about what is and is not a child in ways that are today deeply ingrained and taken for granted such that other ways of thinking about children are difficult to imagine. Discussing the monitoring of children's growth, James and James (2004, p. 145) noted:

> (A)lthough the height and weight chart claims to depict a child's unique and individual development, this uniqueness only exists in the context of a "generalised" child, derived epidemiologically from the population as a whole. Against this, the "normality" or "abnormality" of each individual child is measured and in this, "age"—that is, time passing—is critical, for it provides the context within which "successful" or "pathological" height/weight trajectories are charted. Thus the health of the child's body is "delineated not by the absolute categories of physiology and pathology, but by the characteristics of the normal population (Armstrong 1995, p. 397)," shared common characteristics that become standardized as "normality."

A critique of developmentalism has emerged from within developmental psychology (Burman 2001, 2008, 2012, 2013; Morss 1995; Motzkau 2009; Walkerdine 1993), the social studies of childhood (James and James 2004; James et al. 1998; Matthews 2007; Mayall 1996), and disability studies (Goodley and Runswick-Cole 2010, 2011, 2013; Priestley 2003). Critics note that development is not the only way or even a necessary way to understand childhood. Critical work has exposed the apparent factuality of development, which is unproblematically presented as a scientifically determined "truth." Normal development is not "natural" in these critiques but culturally produced and grounded in disparate assumptions that derive from its historical roots and misrecognized as scientific facts. As a result, development has evolved into a powerful instrument of categorization that allows value-loaded judgments regarding what is best for children and youth under the guise of putatively neutral scientific and clinical descriptions.

Within disability studies, Goodley and Runswick-Cole (2010) suggest that play has been co-opted to act as the agent of normal development. They state that the pervasive idea that "play is a child's work" takes for granted that the play is, or should be, purpose driven and always oriented to physical, social, and cognitive development and growth. Such a view of play obscures any notion of play for play's sake, or rather play (and the recreational pursuits of youth) as fun. For disabled children, Goodley and Runswick-Cole suggest that this dominant understanding of play constructs children and youth with physical or cognitive differences as "nonplaying objects" who require professional therapeutic interventions. In this way, play is a site of intervention for disabled children and pleasure in play is incidental or a means to an end, used to entice disabled children and youth to engage in therapy-driven activities. The lives of disabled children are thus pervaded with formal therapy reinforced through informal play activities geared toward normalizing their bodies and abilities. Despite therapeutic goals to the contrary, children thus risk developing a sense of their bodies and selves as problems-to-be-fixed that differentiates them from their peers and exacerbates their exclusion.

Rethinking Children's Rehabilitation

Rethinking children's rehabilitation invites us to consider the multiple effects of developmental discourses on disabled children and their families. As noted in the preceding chapters, rehabilitation and health care are rooted in dominant contemporary understandings about disability, normality, and what constitutes good quality of life. These beliefs organize programs, policies, and practices at a fundamental level and are mostly unquestioned. Rather, they operate as tacit background understandings that determine a vast range of policies and practices including programmatic funding, assessment and goal setting practices, and available treatment options (Gibson and Teachman 2012). Development is embedded in how children's rehabilitation is *structured*, organized, and delivered; institutional missions; the organization of professional teams; and referral/discharge criteria. It mediates how goals are constructed and pursued, what counts as success ("positive outcomes") or failure, and what is measured and how.

Measures of child health and development in a very real way construct how we view children as certain kinds of persons who are in transition—potentialities who can be shaped into productive, self-reliant adult citizens. As per the discussion in Chapter 3, quality of life and health status measures typically suggest better outcomes and improved quality of life the higher up on the development chain a child scores, that is, walking scores higher than wheeling. These measures, which mimic the hierarchical structuring of normal development charts, determine how children and youth are viewed as progressing, regressing, or plateauing. Yet, these scores may bear little or no relationship to young people's self-assessments (Young et al. 2013) or may not be applicable for large groups of disabled children with significant physical or cognitive impairments. Measures in the burgeoning field of "transitions" in the health and education sectors rely on the notion of childhood and youth as precursors to adulthood. Transitions "checklists" set out key social developmental milestones that signal readiness for adulthood, for example, post-secondary education, career, and independent living goals (Gall et al. 2006; Transition Developmental Checklist n.d.). Wyn and Woodman (2006, p. 497) have noted that both the concepts of development and youth transitions assume a "linear progression from one identifiable status to another" with youth reduced to a stage in transforming children into capable (working) adults. Transitions work is grounded in universal norms for a set of behaviors and abilities that are assumed to correspond with integration into adult society, and which is further conflated with good "quality of life." The assumptions built into measures of transitions are consistent with neoliberal notions that the entrance to adulthood is marked by achievement of residential and financial independence, as well as the attainment of emotional self-reliance, cognitive self-sufficiency, and behavioral self-control (Arnett and Taber 1994). Enabling children to be successful *as children* is almost unthinkable because the ideas of maximizing potential and personal development is so deeply entrenched in the collective social conscious.

Children labeled as disabled are continually exposed to assessments and normalizing interventions that shape their self-understandings. Bodies that fall outside the limits set for normal bodies and which cannot be fixed through surgery, therapy, and/or medications risk bearing the stigma of pathology. By internalizing these ideas at an early age, children may struggle to develop positive self and body images and may experience a sense of failure when they cannot achieve or maintain developmental milestones (Bottos 2003; Piggot et al. 2002). Through having their bodies singled out as in need of fixing, children learn to distinguish between normal and stigmatized bodies and internalize these negative valuations. Multiple medical, educational, and social encounters reproduce and reinforce what eventually becomes a tacit understanding of social difference, a positioning outside of an accepted norm (Priestley 1998).

We are not suggesting that the current reliance on developmentalism in rehabilitation is necessarily or uniformly "bad." What we wish to explore, however, are the potential harms that can result from misplaced applications of developmental thinking in rehabilitation practices. All conceptual commitments exert effects, which may be positive and negative, intended and unintended, and as ethical practitioners we have the responsibility to understand these effects in all their subtleties. Developmental norms always and already construct disabled children as failed children, as those who require interventions in the hopes that they can approximate the normal as closely as possible. Children with the various impairments that result in referrals to rehabilitation professionals are viewed as in need of fixing, and because most will only achieve limited successes in approximating developmental norms, they can be harmed in a number of ways. Later, we discuss research that suggests children internalize these messages to self-evaluate themselves as deficient, and describe the extraordinary efforts undertaken by parents and children to normalize children's lives and identities. As we discuss, these efforts may be accompanied by feelings of guilt, anxiety, and despair. We question if there are not other ways to support disabled children and their families, ways to help them live well with their impairments, or different narratives of disability that do not mark children as deficient.

Research with disabled children illuminates the many ways children are affected by normative ideas about disability. Walking is an example par excellence of a rehabilitation goal that is a taken-for-granted good in rehabilitation. Intense ambulation training is a major rehabilitation intervention for disabled children and is built into the system such that there may be very little individual decision-making about treatment. Notwithstanding intense therapy efforts, a number of children will not achieve functional walking and/or will use wheelchairs for some or all of their mobility needs (Bottos et al. 2001b). This approach however has been questioned within rehabilitation (Bottos et al. 2001a; Mulderij 2000; Wiart and Darrah 2002). Mulderij (2000), for example, has argued that children have a "right" to explore their worlds regardless of their disabilities and should thus be encouraged to use their own creative alternative forms of movement (crawling, rolling, carried, mobility devices).

In our research with children with cerebral palsy, we found that children held conflicting and ambivalent notions about the value of walking and walking therapies (Gibson and Teachman 2012; Gibson et al. 2012b). They weighed complex factors related to energy expenditure, the activity, the environment, and their personal preferences when making mobility choices (walk, crawl, or wheel). Moreover, they resisted negative views of disability through direct expression of pride in different aspects of their wheelchairs (speed, color, functionality) and in identification as wheelchair-users. Nevertheless, children over the age of 11 years clearly conveyed the personal importance of being identified among their peers as "someone who can walk" (see also Chapter 6). These findings help demonstrate how children are socialized to divide the world into walkers and nonwalkers and internalize which group is valorized or stigmatized. They learn a dominant message, reinforced by years of rehabilitation, that nonwalking and nonwalkers are problems to be fixed. As others have commented, by internalizing these ideas at an early age, children may struggle to develop positive self and body images and may experience a sense of failure when they cannot achieve or maintain functional walking (Bottos 2003; Piggot et al. 2002).

Similarly, parents are embedded in discourses of normal development and struggle to make sense of how these imperatives apply to their disabled children. The high value placed on having a "perfect baby" in Western cultures results in parents of disabled children grieving over the "normal" child they did not have (Piggot et al. 2002). Mothers in particular are subjected to competing responsibilities, as both advocates for care and defenders of their children's worth, thus placing a mother in a paradox of saying to her child "I love you as you are" and "I would do anything to change you" (Landsman 2003). Goodley and Runswick-Cole (2011) have noted the rise in popularity of parenting manuals and advice columns in the popular media, means that parents are fully aware of the developmental milestones set for their children and will pursue these diligently. McKeever and Miller (2004) have shown that mothers expect themselves and are expected by others to play a pivotal role in enhancing their child's future value and productivity as an adult and are socially rewarded as "good mothers" for these activities. The (in)ability of their children to reach such milestones constructs both the mother's image of her child and the image of herself as (un)successful mother.

In our interviews exploring the value of walking with parents of children with cerebral palsy (Gibson and Teachman 2012; Gibson et al. 2012b), parents were committed to doing everything possible to improve their children's abilities, but were also plagued by doubts about the wisdom of doing so. They told stories of anxiety and doubt related to their decisions to forgo, stop, or decrease the intensity of an intervention. All parents discussed the efforts needed to enable their children to "experience normal activities" and positioned their children as "normal" within the interviews (e.g., "To me, he is normal. He walks different than others, he might think a bit differently but he's normal."). Absent from their accounts was any questioning of the normal/abnormal distinction that rewards conformity to arbitrary norms of bodily forms and abilities (Thomas 2007, pp. 67–68). Rather, they reconfigured their internalized understandings to fit with their children's abilities and claim a reworked normality. By claiming that their children are "normal" or "the same" because they do the same things as other children do, parents resist negative disability discourses and work to create a positive space for their children. However, their strategies also reproduce and sustain ingrained social values that assign preferential status to nondisabled bodies—ideas that are reinforced by rehabilitation and transmitted to children.

This nascent research begins to reveal how the pursuit of normal developmental milestones may perpetrate an ongoing symbolic violence against disabled children and their parents. Bourdieu described symbolic violence as "a gentle violence, usually imperceptible and invisible even to its victims, exerted for the most part through the purely symbolic channels of communication and cognition (more precisely, misrecognition), recognition, or even feeling" (Bourdieu 2001, pp. 1–2, parentheses in the original). The visibility of bodily differences not only affects the way others perceive and act toward disabled children, it also shapes how children and their parents come to internalize these meanings. Persons come to "know their place" in the world where the meanings attached to their bodies can appear as uncontestable and "true," rather than open to revision (Edwards and Imrie 2003).

Implications for Rehabilitation Practice

Beliefs about how rehabilitation can contribute toward achievement of a good life are understood as particular to evidence and expertise in rehabilitation, yet, they map onto broader neoliberal beliefs about individuals' responsibilities to manage the work of becoming "successful" and achieving a good, happy, or productive life, for example, imperatives toward self-improvement, being the "best you can be," and reaching for your potential (Burman 2013). We need to continually ask if and how these goals "fit" rehabilitation, or if we are unreflectively imposing them because they are the "way of the world" and thus must be best for everyone. As discussed in Chapter 2, working with people labeled as disabled raises a number of questions for rehabilitation practitioners. These might also include: Is it the job of rehabilitation to help people to "fit in" and to what? How can we imagine different ways of living well? How do we balance an acceptance of diversity with the possible benefits of minimizing impairments? In the case of young people and their families questions arise regarding: How do we partner with children/youth and their parents to acknowledge their fears of the unknown and the challenges of living a trajectory that is the road not taken? In what ways are "transition" services acting to reproduce beliefs and practices about normal childhood? How could they better assist children with forging a path that fits best with their abilities and desires?

In thinking about other ways we might understand childhood and support disabled children, we can first consider the great variation in children's bodies, abilities, and rates of development, and ask if normalizing those differences is the right goal. We must also be aware that trying to approximate a typical developmental trajectory may harm some children and families in ways that are not immediately apparent. Some of the physical and social end points of child development will be unattainable for many disabled children who internalize developmental roles and expectations over time. This can have profound effects when they cannot achieve these norms, including anxiety, distress, depression, feelings of worthlessness, or "nothing to offer" (Gibson et al. 2007, 2012b, 2014). Walkerdine (1993, p. 466) has argued that the dominant narrative of development is part of a bigger "European patriarchal story," which subsumes other stories. She suggests that, "(A) move away from a universal developmentalism must be a move away from a pathologization of Otherness... (T)he way to deal with this is to produce new narratives which tell of change and transformation in the very specific conditions in which they are produced."

In rehabilitation, focusing on normal development closes off other possibilities that may better suit young people's needs and abilities. What would these alternatives look like? First of all, we would suggest exploring ways of "living well in the present" (Davies 1997) should be considered alongside development goals and the pursuit of typical adult milestones. This might include attention to achieving or maintaining relationships, personally meaningful projects, "or just plain enjoyment of life"

(Hammell 2004). These life choices do not figure in the current transitions rhetoric and we suspect many professionals working in transitions programs might struggle with supporting them. Nevertheless, we suggest that only focusing on approximating normative life trajectories closes off other possibilities that may in some cases better suit young people's needs and abilities. Recreation activities may take on a greater significance, as may hobbies, caring for others, or managing one's own care needs. These activities, because they are oriented to the present and not future development or economic contribution, may be judged as futile, trivial, or wasteful and are less likely to be supported or funded (Aitchison 2003; Gibson et al. 2009; Hammell 2004). In addition, we suggest that a move away from models that privilege normal bodies and development might open space to tap into children's own sense of their bodies, how their bodies work, and how they form connections with people, environments, and technologies to do the things they want to do (Gibson et al. 2012a).

Rethinking development creates spaces for alternate ways of living that contribute to the acceptance of differences. The centrality of work, productivity, and independence as markers of transitions and adult social status need to be balanced by *openness* to other ways of being in the world (Priestley 2003, pp. 132–142). As part of an expanded and open ethics of inclusion, rehabilitation could attend more to the nonproductive and nonmaterial contributions of individuals in society (Goodley and Runswick-Cole 2010). Moving away from thinking of development and transition as a delimited linear pathway opens up multiple other pathways that could also be explored with young people and their families. Similarly, rethinking mobility goals opens up a range of options. Early powered mobility that gives access to the world at a younger age has been advocated for a number of years (Butler 1986), but its uptake has been rather slow (Wiart and Darrah 2002). Promoting acceptance of difference also means helping families to feel comfortable with alternate modes of mobility like crawling (see Chapter 6), using assistive devices, and letting go of the pursuit of independent walking without guilt. These kinds of explorations help to create spaces for other ways of living that contribute to the acceptance of differences.

Creating space for parents and children to talk about these issues and sharing their experiences, fears, and assumptions are also important. Children's values and beliefs are forming at the same time that their parents' values and goals for their child may be shifting. Although negative views of disability and difference may be imposed on parents and disabled children, they may also resist these ideas depending on their own particular circumstances and their exposure to counter-narratives (Fisher and Goodley 2007; Landsman 2003). A challenge for rehabilitation is to determine how best to assist children in forming and maintaining positive disability identities while pursuing therapeutic interventions. Shifting away from viewing childhood as a critical period for interventions "at all costs" creates space for approaches that support disabled children to more fully enjoy and engage in the here and now of their daily lives.

Unhinging Normal and Development

In this chapter, we have suggested that a fundamental concept in children's rehabilitation, normal development, needs to be rethought and reformed on several levels. We are not suggesting that normal development be abandoned or replaced by something else. Rather, we are advocating for an opening up of possibilities for multiple ways of thinking about childhood that can collectively inform rehabilitation. Normal development became the dominant story of childhood because of a particular set of historical and cultural circumstances and beliefs that we have briefly reviewed. The point is not whether or not development is *true*, but, does it *work*? Development is not the only way to understand the lives of children, nor is it the only way of conceiving of what is best, good, or right for disabled children and youth. Once we begin to question development we open up new possibilities for working with children and families, for shared exploration of needs and hopes that will assist children and families to live well. This will sometimes involve ameliorating impairments, working on improvements of strength, speech, or walking; and it will sometimes involve advocating for acceptance of abilities, alternate ("abnormal") ways of moving or communicating, and letting go of the pursuit of normalcy.

References

Aitchison, C. 2003. From leisure and disability to disability leisure: Developing data, definitions and discourses. *Disability & Society* 18: 955–969.

Armstrong, D. 1995. The rise of surveillance medicine. *Sociology of Health & Illness* 17 (3): 393–404.

Arnett, J.J. and Taber, S. 1994. Adolescence terminable and interminable: When does adolescence end? *Journal of Youth and Adolescence* 23: 517–537.

Bottos, M. 2003. Ambulatory capacity in cerebral palsy: Prognostic criteria and consequences for intervention. *Developmental Medicine & Child Neurology* 45: 786–790.

Bottos, M., Bolcati, C., Sciuto, L., Ruggeri, C., and Feliciangeli, A. 2001a. Powered wheelchairs and independence in young children with tetraplegia. *Developmental Medicine & Child Neurology* 43: 769–777.

Bottos, M., Feliciangeli, A., Sciuto, L., Gericke, C., and Vianello, A. 2001b. Functional status of adults with cerebral palsy and implications for treatment of children. *Developmental Medicine & Child Neurology* 43: 516–528.

Bourdieu, P. 2001. *Masculine Domination*. Stanford, CA: Stanford University Press.

Burman, E. 2001. Beyond the baby and the bathwater: Post dualistic developmental psychologies for diverse childhoods. *European Early Childhood Education Research Journal* 9: 5–22.

Burman, E. 2008. *Deconstructing Developmental Psychology*. Sussex, U.K.: Routledge.

Burman, E. 2012. Deconstructing neoliberal childhood: Towards a feminist antipsychological approach. *Childhood* 19: 423–428.

Burman, E. 2013. Desiring development? Psychoanalytic contributions to antidevelopmental psychology. *International Journal of Qualitative Studies in Education* 26: 56–74.

Butler, C. 1986. Effects of powered mobility on self-initiated behaviours of very young children with locomotor disability. *Developmental Medicine & Child Neurology* 28: 325–332.

Davies, M.L. 1997. Shattered assumptions: Time and the experience of long term HIV positivity. *Social Science & Medicine* 44: 561–571.

Edwards, C. and Imrie, R. 2003. Disability and bodies as bearers of value. *Sociology* 37: 239–256.

Effgen, S.K. 2005. *Meeting the Physical Therapy Needs of Children*. Philadelphia, PA: FA Davis Company.

Fisher, P. and Goodley, D. 2007. The linear medical model of disability: Mothers of disabled babies resist with counter-narratives. *Sociology of Health & Illness* 29: 66–81.

Gall, C., Kingsnorth, S. and Healy, H. 2006. Growing up ready: A shared management approach to transition. *Physical & Occupational Therapy in Pediatrics* 38 : 47–62.

Gibson, B.E., Carnevale, F.A., and King, G. 2012a. "This is my way": Reimagining disability, in/dependence and interconnectedness of persons and assistive technologies. *Disability & Rehabilitation* 34: 1894–1899.

Gibson, B.E., Mistry, B., Smith, B., Yoshida, K.K., Abbott, D., Lindsay, S., and Hamdani, Y. 2014. Becoming men: Gender, disability, and transitioning to adulthood. *Health* 18: 93–112.

Gibson, B.E. and Teachman, G. 2012. Critical approaches in physical therapy research: Investigating the symbolic value of walking. *Physiotherapy Theory & Practice* 28: 474–484.

Gibson, B.E., Teachman, G., and Hamdani, Y. 2015. Rethinking 'normal development' in children's rehabilitation. In *Rethinking Rehabilitation: Theory and Practice*, eds. K.M. McPherson, B.E. Gibson, and A. Leplege, pp. 70–79. Boca Raton, FL: CRC Press.

Gibson, B.E., Teachman, G., Wright, V., Fehlings, D., and McKeever, P. 2012b. Children's and parents' beliefs regarding the value of walking: Rehabilitation implications for children with cerebral palsy. *Child Care Health & Development* 38: 61–69.

Gibson, B.E., Young, N.L., Upshur, R.E.G., and McKeever, P. 2007. Men on the margin: A Bourdieusian examination of living into adulthood with muscular dystrophy. *Social Science & Medicine* 65: 505–517.

Gibson, B.E., Zitzelsberger, H., and McKeever, P. 2009. 'Futureless persons': Shifting life expectancies and the vicissitudes of progressive illness. *Sociology of Health & Illness* 31: 554–568.

Goodley, D. and Runswick-Cole, K. 2010. Emancipating play: Dis/abled children, development and deconstruction. *Disabiity & Society* 25: 499–512.

Goodley, D. and Runswick-Cole, K. 2011. Problematising policy: Conceptions of 'child', 'disabled' and 'parents' in social policy in England. *International Journal of Inclusive Education* 15: 71–85.

Goodley, D. and Runswick-Cole, K. 2013. The body as disability and possibility: Theorizing the 'leaking, lacking and excessive' bodies of disabled children. *Scandinavian Journal of Disability Research* 15: 1–19.

Hammell, K.W. 2004. Dimensions of meaning in the occupations of daily life. *Canadian Journal of Occupational Therapy* 71: 296–305.

James, A. and James, A. 2004. *Constructing Childhood: Theory, Policy and Social Practice.* Hampshire, U.K.: Palgrave Macmillan.

James, A., Jenks, C., and Prout, A. 1998. *Theorising Childhood.* Cambridge, U.K.: Polity Press and Blackwell Publishers.

Landsman, G. 2003. Emplotting children's lives: Developmental delay vs. disability. *Social Science & Medicine* 56: 1947–1960.

Matthews, S. 2007. A window on the 'new' sociology of childhood. *Sociology Compass* 1: 322–334.

Mayall, B. 1996. *Children, Health and the Social Order.* Bristol, PA: Open University Press.

McKeever, P. and Miller, K.L. 2004. Mothering children who have disabilities: A Bourdieusian interpretation of maternal practices. *Social Science & Medicine* 59: 1177–1191.

Morss, J.R. 1995. *Growing Critical: Alternatives to Developmental Psychology.* New York: Routledge.

Motzkau, J.J.F. 2009. The semiotic of accusation: Thinking about deconstruction, development, the critique of practice, and the practice of critique. *Qualitative Research in Psychology* 6: 129–152.

Mulderij, K. 2000. Dualistic notions about children with motor disabilities: Hands to lean on or to reach out? *Qualitative Health Research* 10: 39–50.

Piggot, J., Paterson, J., and Hocking, C. 2002. Participation in home therapy programs for children with cerebral palsy: A compelling challenge. *Qualitative Health Research* 12: 1112–1129.

Porr, S.M. and Rainville, E.B. 1999. The special vulnerabilities of children and families. In *Pediatric Therapy: A Systems Approach*, ed. S.J. Lane. Philadelphia, PA: FA Davis.

Priestley, M. 1998. Childhood disability and disabled childhoods: Agendas for research. *Childhood* 5: 207–223.

Priestley, M. 2003. *Disability: A Life Course Approach*. Malden, MA: Polity Press.

Rose, N. 1999. *Governing the Soul: The Shaping of the Private Self*, 2nd edn. London, U.K.: Free Association Books.

Thomas, C. (2007). *Sociologies of Disability and Illness: Contested Ideas in Disability studies and medical sociology*. New York, NY: Palgrave MacMillan.

Transition Developmental Checklist. n.d. Kentucky Commission for children with special healthcare needs. Available from http://chfs.ky.gov/NR/rdonlyres/8C5EEDBE-14FC-4488-8C85-1BAC1EDE0516/0/Checklist.pdf, accessed September 26, 2015.

Walkerdine, V. 1993. Beyond developmentalism. *Theory and Psychology* 3: 451–469.

Wiart, L. and Darrah, J. 2002. Changing philosophical perspectives on the management of children with physical disabilities—Their effect on the use of powered mobility. *Disability & Rehabilitation* 24: 492–498.

Wyn, J. and Woodman, D. 2006. Generation, youth and social change in Australia. *Journal of Youth Studies* 9: 495–514.

Young, N.L., Sheridan, K., Burke, T.A., Mukherjee, S., and McCormick, A. 2013. Health outcomes among youths and adults with spina bifida. *Journal of Pediatrics* 162: 993–998.

5
In/dependence

In this chapter, I problematize independence as a taken-for-granted goal of rehabilitation and explore the idea of movements in and out of various dependencies as inherent to the human condition. Within health and disability studies, independence is conceptualized in many different ways that are often a source of debate: freedom, self-determination, sovereignty, self-sufficiency, living alone, having choice, and control. But at its most fundamental, independence relates to the modernist notion of humans as fixed individual beings, composed of separate minds that are encased in biological bodies. Questioning this foundational assumption opens up a world of possibilities for rethinking human differences. In what follows, I draw from my previous work (Gibson 2006, 2014; Gibson et al. 2012) to explore a radical notion of interdependence that decenters the individual. I consider how actions are made possible through the making and breaking of dependencies reconfigured as "assemblages" that are formed, split, reformed, and abandoned to multiple effects. In so doing, I suggest how independence goals can be re-imagined to explore various assemblages in rehabilitation practices.

Discourses of In/dependence

> *In our society dominant discourse tries never to speak its own name. Its authority is based on absence* (Ferguson 1990, cited in Graham and Slee 2008, p. 288).

Independence is a dominant discourse in rehabilitation, reflecting and reproducing broader neoliberal notions of the moral citizen. In contemporary life, we seldom question independence as a personal and social good, and see dependence as suspect and/or requiring amelioration. These ideas are not however self-evidently "true" but arise out of a particular trajectory of historical conditions, particularly in North American contexts but arguably throughout Western(ized) nations. In order to better understand the largely unchallenged valorization of independence in the West, I begin by unpacking the terms "independence" and "dependence" and the historical trajectories of their usage. To do so, I draw on Fraser and Gordon's (1994) detailed genealogy of dependency. Their substantive focus was welfare dependency in the United States, but nevertheless their comprehensive tracing of the evolution of the various meanings of dependency—from earlier largely positive connotations to the negative usages prevalent in contemporary society—illuminates the landscapes of policy, practices, and attitudes toward other forms of "dependencies" including disability.

Fraser and Gordon parse out four "registers of meaning" in current usages of dependency:

1. *Economic*: Related to an individual's need for subsistence.
2. *Socio-legal*: Referring to a lack of a separate legal or public standing, for example, children or other legal dependents.
3. *Political*: Characterized by subjection to an external ruling power and may include displaced persons or noncitizen residents.
4. *Moral/psychological*: An external judgment of individual character akin to, for example, lack of willpower, laziness, or excessive emotional neediness.

Other categories of meaning that overlap with these have been proposed in the health and social care literature, including physical, psychological, and social dependency (Fine and Glendinning 2005; Gignac and Cott 1998). For my purposes in discussing impairment and disability, I consider a *fifth register of meaning*:

5. *Functional*: Characterized by needs for various forms of physical, technological, and/or human assistance to carry out daily activities, most often discussed in relation to persons labeled as permanently or temporarily "disabled" (see below and Thomas 2007, pp. 88–90 for a discussion of how assistance needs of disabled people are devalued in comparison to other forms of need and characterized as "dependencies").

To be sure, the five registers overlap and may not encompass all meanings of dependency. Nevertheless, together they provide a frame to help unpack the concept further. These contemporary registers share in common largely negative connotations of dependency that differs from historical uses to which I now turn.

The root of the term "depends" refers to *attachment*, and more precisely, the physical relation of hanging (pendre) from something else (de). Fraser and Gordon (1994) note that in preindustrial societies, independence was not used in reference to individuals but rather to groups that were separated from other collectives, for example, independent nation states. Applications to individuals emerged into the eighteenth century, whereby an individual who owned property could be said to have an "independency," that is economic self-sufficiency ("independently wealthy") that differed from wage laborers, servants, or slaves who depended on someone else for sustenance. Dependency at the time was the usual state of affairs for most people and was not considered a negative state or personal deficiency. Rather, independency was the exceptional state. Dependence held neutral or even positive connotations in some definitions and these persist in contemporary terms like "dependable." In these formulations, to depend was linked with trusting, relying on, counting on another. Fraser and Gordon note that pejorative usages of the term did not appear in either English or American dictionaries prior to the twentieth century.

One of the most notable developments in the evolution of the meaning of dependence is the appearance of the moral/psychological register. Fraser and Gordon trace the rise of the imperative for individual independence to major social and political changes of the eighteenth and nineteenth centuries, and particularly the rise of industrial capitalism and the ideologies of Radical Protestantism. With these sociopolitical changes, formerly accepted "natural" hierarchies and subordinate relationships were increasingly challenged and rejected, underpinning major social movements of the time including abolitionism, feminism, and the organization of labor. Political and other forms of subjection came to be viewed as largely indefensible and "offenses against human dignity." Within these movements the language of individual rights loomed large and rested on the notion of the independent citizen. Independence was a linchpin of the American ideal that, as Fraser and Gordon put it, "stripped dependency of its voluntarism, emphasized its powerlessness and imbued it with stigma" (Fraser and Gordon 1994, p. 320). As part of the rhetoric of equality, freedom, and individual merit, independence became the responsibility and expectation of every citizen. These developments cemented the moral/psychological register of in/dependence and set the stage for increasing moral disapproval of those with any form of social, political, or economic dependency.

The birth of the moral/psychological register rendered all forms of dependency as deeply suspect. These meanings have persisted and arguably advanced in the contemporary Western social imaginary. Allowances may be made for those whose dependencies are viewed as unavoidable such as children or ill people, but the imperative remains for individuals to justify their dependencies and continually pursue independence in some form. The child may be dependent now, but it is allowable only as a temporary state with independence, in all its registers, as the naturalized endpoint of development (see Chapter 4). Similarly, the ill or impaired person is expected to be working toward independence in whatever forms available, including rehabilitation. Independence in self-care is a primary imperative that motivates health and rehabilitation interventions and individual "compliance" with treatment (Warren and Manderson 2008).

Fraser and Gordon (1994) suggest that the "worker" has become the "universal social subject," what I take as a standardized representation of the independent citizen who is not only economically self-sufficient, but productive, contributing, and occupied in ways that are markers of the morally good person. Those not earning a wage are expected to be otherwise contributing, usually distributed along gendered (women raising children) or generational categories, but nevertheless applicable in some form to all adults. For example, the question often asked of retired persons, "what do you do with your time?" is embedded in a context of acceptable or suspect responses. For older adults, the imperative is to "stay active" and engaged and maintain health and functional independence, so as not to be a "burden" on loved ones or a drain on public resources (Weicht 2011). These latter forms of dependence are taken for granted as social and economic problems that are expressed in individual fears of functional decline. Weicht (2011, p. 214) notes that dependence is collectively viewed as a sign of "not being healthy, of being passive, of not being self-reliant, and not being a 'proper' person in society." Independence usages and imperatives thus interweave in producing the good citizen who is active, working, and contributing rather than needy, unmotivated, idle, or lazy. Along these lines, the figure of the disabled person is engendered with multiple meanings of dependency—perceived as childlike, not working/contributing, and economically dependent (Thomas 2007, pp. 88–90). Disabled people as a class of dependent persons are thus construed as objects of pity and/or marked as social problems requiring intervention.

The moral registers of independence and dependence discourses mobilize particular practices of both institutions and individuals, which act to achieve independence and eliminate or minimize dependency in all its forms. As Fraser and Gordon (1994, p. 332) note:

> The genealogy of dependency also expresses the modern emphasis on individual personality. This is the deepest meaning of the spectacular rise of the moral/psychological register, which constructs yet another version of the independence/dependence dichotomy. In the moral/psychological version, social relations are hypostatized as properties of individuals or groups. Fear of dependency, both explicit and implicit, posits an ideal, independent personality in contrast to which those considered dependent are deviant. This contrast

> bears traces of a sexual division of labor that assigns men primary responsibility as providers or breadwinners and women primary responsibility as caretakers and nurturers and then treats the derivative personality patterns as fundamental…In this way, the opposition between the independent personality and the dependent personality maps onto a whole series of hierarchical oppositions and dichotomies that are central in modern culture: masculine/feminine, public/private, work/care, success/love, individual/ community, economy/family, and competitive/self-sacrificing.

The binaries that Fraser and Gordon list (and others such as child/adult) are imbued with positive and negative valences, for example, the hard masculine side of work and the soft feminine side of care. These ideas are prominent in the production and maintenance of the discourse of disability and the practices and projects oriented to securing independence for disabled people. I now turn to a discussion of how these ideas play out in rehabilitation and disability studies, including formulations of "interdependence" that are advanced toward remediating the dichotomy of in/dependence.

Dependence, Independence, and Interdependence in Disability Studies and Rehabilitation

Independence holds pride of place in both rehabilitation and disability studies in particular ways unique to each field. Because they share a focus on improving the lives of people with functional impairments, each field considers the relationship between individual abilities and in/dependence, albeit in very different ways that provoke debate (Reindal 1999). At the risk of oversimplifying, traditional strains of disability studies focus on sociopolitical independence as a human right and work toward operationalizing and securing this right through activism and advocacy. Rehabilitation on the other hand focuses on functional independence, traditionally viewing impairment, and dependence in a cause and effect relationship and working toward minimizing or ameliorating dependence through individualized body interventions. These very different approaches have conflicted in many ways that are highlighted throughout this book. Not the least of these is the critique of rehabilitation (and social care) as increasing the dependencies of disabled people through characterizing disability as a biomedical problem (see Chapter 2) and/or marginalizing disabled people in specialized institutions or community spaces (Thomas 2007, p. 97). Rehabilitation has responded to these critiques and others by broadening its scope and shifting emphasis away from normalizing bodily functions to enabling community participation with varying degrees of uptake in the field (Leplège et al. 2015). Developments within disability studies include a growing critique of the valorization of rights-based independence toward acknowledgment of the interconnectivity and embodied vulnerabilities that constitute the human condition (Gibson 2006; Goodley 2014; Shildrick 2000, 2002; Slater 2012).

Despite these developments and tensions, in both rehabilitation and disability studies, there remains a pervasive acceptance of independence as an essential human good that reflects broader neoliberal ideologies (Weicht 2011). Independence may include different registers of meaning, and it may be reformulated so that diverse forms of abilities and activities are caste as independence, but the basic dichotomy of independence and dependence as respectively positive and negative states remains largely unquestioned. Below I briefly review some of the registers of meaning of in/dependence in each field before discussing how the dependence/independence divide has been addressed through the intermediary concept of *interdependence*. I will suggest that, while interdependence answers many of the critiques of this divide, it also reproduces and retains the negative connotations of dependence by insisting that needing/receiving is balanced by some form of giving. Drawing on post-critical scholarship and particularly the work of Deleuze and Guattari (1987), I then break from this impulse and suggest that dependency can be reconfigured in terms of *assemblages* that all persons move in and out of with multiple effects that have implications for rehabilitation.

In/dependence in Disability Studies

At the root of the disability activism that emerged in the 1970s and 1980s was a struggle for independence, which gave birth to "the independent living movement" and continues today (Watson et al. 2004). The Independent Living Institute in Sweden currently lists 290 organizations dedicated to promoting independent living across the globe. Fundamental to the independent living philosophy is personal choice and control over everyday activities including managing one's personal life, participating in community life, and fulfilling social roles (Martinez 2003). In this formulation, independence is constructed according to notions of self-governance, self-determination, and the assertion that disabled people should have the same choices, control, and opportunities in their lives as nondisabled people:

> Independent Living is a philosophy and a movement of people with disabilities who work for self-determination, equal opportunities and self-respect. Independent Living does not mean that we want to do everything by ourselves and do not need anybody or that we want to live in isolation. Independent Living means that we demand the same choices and control in our every-day lives that our non-disabled brothers and sisters, neighbors and friends take for granted. We want to grow up in our families, go to the neighborhood school, use the same bus as our neighbors, and work in jobs that are in line with our education and interests, and start families of our own (Ratzka 2003).

The central tenets of Independent Living transform the language of needs to rights aimed at ensuring the full citizenship of disabled people. Independence here does not preclude receiving assistance, rather disabled people, as experts in their own needs, maintain control and choice over the type and delivery of assistance (Morris 2004). As Morris (1997, p. 56) notes, "Independence is not about doing everything for yourself, but about having control over how help is provided." Within disability studies, rehabilitation professionals have been charged with overemphasizing independence in self-care and entreated to shift their professional practices toward enabling decision-making (Oliver 1989).

"Care" is a key source of tension in disability studies (Watson et al. 2004). For disabled people, care as promoted and practiced by medical professionals is oriented to *taking responsibility for* "patients," that is, constructing disabled people as passive recipients of care that is bestowed and controlled by medical professionals (Gibson et al. 2009; McLaughlin 2006; Morris 1997). Disability scholars note that so-called "caring relationships" have resulted in significant harms to disabled people including physical, sexual, and emotional abuse (Saxton et al. 2001). Care is thus a loaded concept and a key site of ideological conflict between disability advocates and the health professions. The independent living philosophy more or less eliminates care talk from its lexicon and focuses instead on "consumer-directed personal assistance." Narrow interpretations of the latter construe caregivers, and particularly paid attendants, as disabled persons' "arms and legs" (Gibson et al. 2009). But a growing critique has emerged from feminist and other disability scholars who complicate the assistance/care relationship. Critics, including myself, have suggested that such an approach dehumanizes both individuals in the care relationship and ignores the mutuality inherent to successful support alliances (Fine and Glendinning 2005; Gibson et al. 2009; Kittay and Feder 2003; Watson et al. 2004; Weicht 2011). Moreover, as I elaborate later in this chapter and expand on in Chapter 6, post-critical understandings of "assistance" relationships address these tensions by obscuring the rights-bearing individual subject in favor of an examination of interdependent collectives of humans and nonhumans that can be sources of both constraints and opportunities.

In/dependence and care are central points of debate in critical disability studies that problematize rights-based approaches (Davis 2002; Goodley 2014; Hughes 2007; Reindal 1999; Shildrick 2002). These accounts share a relational approach that destabilizes dominant views of the subject as sovereign, disembodied, and disembedded and instead attend to the multiple connectivities of bodies, places, and things that shape subjectivities and characterize human experience (Reindal 1999). Disability scholars have noted that rights-based approaches tend to homogenize identities by relying on dominant neoliberal notions of the standardized person most often construed as the normalized white male subject (Davis 2002, p. 30).

An interesting example of the tension between rights-based and relational approaches comes from a paper by Jenny Slater (2012). Slater describes how through the course of her research investigating a self-advocacy program for young people with "learning difficulties," she identified her own ingrained assumptions that predisposed her to look for instances of oppressive practices. However, in her research she observed multiple exchanges of teaching and learning across students and staff, and through these encounters moved from interrogations of independence toward analysis of dynamic and embodied networks of connections. Her individual movement toward relational analyses reflects more generalized movements in the field (cf. Goodley 2011; Hughes 2007; Kuppers and Overboe 2009; McRuer 2006; Overboe 2009; Shildrick 2009).

Independence in Rehabilitation

Like rights-based approaches to disability studies, rehabilitation valorizes independence but does so in different ways. Interventions are designed to approximate normative bodies and maximize independent function, and assessment tools take for granted the goals of independence that are inherent in rehabilitation ideologies. As I discussed in Chapter 3, assessments of good or poor outcomes in rehabilitation rely on standardized measures such as the Functional Independence Measure™ (FIM), which equates greater independence (in self-care, sphincter control, transfers, locomotion, and communication/social cognition) with program success (Granger 1998). Measures of functional in/dependence not only inform individual interventions but drive programmatic practices and funding decisions. For example, in Canada, the National Rehabilitation Reporting

System (Canadian Institute for Health Information 2014) collects FIM data from adult rehabilitation providers across the country to evaluate and compare programs. Functional independence is taken for granted as the marker of successful rehabilitation across diagnostic groups, programs, and services.

Within the rehabilitation professions, independence has been characterized as "the key role of practitioners" and "the goal," "cornerstone," and "core value" of practice, while also coming under critique (Bonikowsky et al. 2012; Hammell 2009; Kirby 2013; Ramaswamy and McCandless 2013). Rehabilitation practices and individual desire for independence reinforce each other in clinical spaces. Within inpatient rehabilitation, independence in self-care is the cornerstone to returning home and is collectively pursued by clinicians, patients, and their families. Through these acts, independence as desirable is mutually reinforced and promoted within the hospital context and carried into community life. Goodwin (2008) notes that to do otherwise would be advocating dependency and viewed by professionals, care recipients, and families as failure or giving up. The moral register permeates these situations where striving for independence is valued regardless of its achievement. Trying, giving your all, working hard, and general "compliance" with treatment are the markers of the good patient and the working citizen. As Warren and Manderson (2008, p. 197) observe: "the participants of the rehabilitation program, patients, and their professional partners, in the work of doing rehabilitation and in its goals, draw on core social values of effort, cooperation and productivity." Rehabilitation practices and tools designed to identify and ameliorate dependencies thus "function to obscure and (re)secure the order of things" (Graham and Slee 2008) that is, the day to day "doing" of rehabilitation continually produces and reproduces negative meanings of dependence without any conscious intent to do so. These processes function in the background and usually are not reflected upon by practitioners until something occurs to challenge their understandings.

Conceptualizations of in/dependence in rehabilitation have shifted over time and remain slippery when viewed in different geo-temporal contexts (Bonikowsky et al. 2012). Whereas helping individuals to achieve functional independence was the primary goal of rehabilitation after World War I and arguably persists to this day, some contemporary usages align more with the Independent Living Movement and emphasize choice, control, and rights. Independence is promoted both in terms of physical function and self-determination and may be specified differently for different populations, by different professional groups, or with particular clients. Goodwin (2008) notes that dependence and independence are sometimes conceptualized along a continuum of required support, whereby rehabilitation works to move people along a predetermined path by accepting new independence challenges as they progress. The trap of this kind of thinking, as Goodwin notes, is the construction of the continuum according to a narrow range of needs and abilities that are largely defined by professionals and reproduce the in/dependence dichotomy. Moreover, independence is viewed as a property of the individual with little consideration of the relevant social and political mediators.

In an attempt to deflect professional authority in constructing in/dependence, the notion of "individually defined" independence has emerged in the rehabilitation literature. Imposed notions of functional dependence in rehabilitation practices or measures are rejected in favor of particularizing the meaning of independence for each patient according to their individual circumstances and preferences. In this vein, Struhkamp et al. (2009) suggest that clinical work differs from measurement in that it seeks to establish an independence specific to a person's situation that changes over time. Similarly, Bonikowsky et al. (2012) in a review identified nine "definition themes" of independence in the occupational therapy literature that they used to develop a definition of "personally defined" independence that consider the interplay of environmental and personal factors. This work is indicative of how rehabilitation is increasingly sensitive to the potential dangers of professionally imposed independence goals; however, there is almost no movement in the field to redress the veneration of independence. If independence is personally defined, it can mean almost anything, but the notion that it is always a *good thing* that must be diligently pursued remains largely unquestioned.

Interdependence

As a corrective to the dichotomy of in/dependence, the notion of interdependence has gained considerable traction across fields of inquiry including rehabilitation and disability studies (Gleeson 1999; Hammell 2006, 2009; Reindal 1999; Shakespeare 2000). Interdependence emphasizes mutuality and reciprocity as inherent to the human condition and conceptually functions to redress the moral registers of dependence. Dependency is seen as common to human experience, as the everyday lives of people are continually enmeshed in networks of mutual giving and receiving (Gignac and Cott 1998; Tronto 1993; Wendell 1996). Kittay (Kittay and Feder 2003; Kittay 2007) thus rejects any normative evaluations of in/dependence, arguing that dependency is a morally neutral concept. Feminists writing from the "ethics of care" have critiqued the image of the autonomous rational (male) individual and built an ethics around the relational, affective, and interconnected subject, acknowledging how carers are enmeshed in their own webs of giving and receiving (Benner and Gordon 1996; Noddings 1984; Tronto 1993). Approaches like these function to smooth away the dichotomy of givers versus receivers by suggesting that all persons do both, but in ways that are not always acknowledged. Interdependence in this approach addresses the moral uneasiness with both care and dependence by universalizing it as necessary for human flourishing (Fine and Glendinning 2005). In disability studies, Watson et al. (2004) concept of "needscapes" suggests that once needs are viewed as inherent to all social relations, the focus is switched from satisfaction of competing needs and rights to an integrated politics of needs interpretation. Across fields of practice this move requires analysis of the interrelated needs of the different embodied and embedded actors without pitting the needs of one group against another (Gibson et al. 2009; Reindal 1999).

Undoubtedly, the concept of interdependence addresses many of the untenable problems created by the figure of the neoliberal independent subject, and serves to dampen the negative moral register by exposing how dependency is a shared reality. However, I agree with Weicht (2011) that interdependence still relies heavily on a notion of *deservingness* and cannot be construed as value neutral despite some of the claims of its promoters. To my mind the emphasis on mutuality and reciprocity inherent to interdependence does not go far enough in challenging the valorization of independence.

Interdependency suggests that two or more dependencies are characteristic of the human condition that is, we are all dependent, and the corollary is that we all have others that depend on us. At least in some formulations, this reciprocal relationship seems to be forwarded to lessen the moral failures of dependency. An example is seen in the youth "transitions" literature where interdependence is promoted as "more realistic" for many young people, and is defined as "do(ing) it on my own with supports" (Stewart et al. 2009, p. 20). Instead of reciprocal dependencies common to the human condition, interdependence is presented as akin to *as independent as possible* while acknowledging the needs *of some* (i.e., disabled) people for assistance. The clear preference for independence is only mildly obscured by the language of interdependence (Hamdani et al. 2015).

Interdependence provides a vehicle for asserting the moral goodness of people who have extreme forms of dependency (economic, physical) by insisting that all persons receive help but also give help to some degree. This is of course indisputable. For example, even the comatose person provides something to her family—a focus for their love and care, a life purpose, and a point of contemplation. However, the reliance on "giving back" in these formulations reveals how interdependence contains within it the thing it purports to refute—an ongoing discomfort with dependence. Dependence is still constructed as something that needs to be softened, countered; its inherent negativity (needing) is offset by a moral good (giving). Fraser and Gordon's moral register of dependence thus persists in the idea of interdependence. With some notable exceptions (Kittay and Feder 2003; Mackenzie et al. 2014; Shildrick 2002; Weicht 2011), very little scholarship has engaged with this normative tension or worked to embrace dependency.

Escaping the moral dichotomy of in/dependence requires a theoretical shift away from the modernist sovereign subject. I have written elsewhere about how the postmodern notion of *assemblages* builds on and reformulates interdependence as an alternative to the problems of in/dependence (Gibson 2006, 2014; Gibson et al. 2012). In the remainder of this chapter, I briefly sketch out the notion of assemblages and its potential for reforming rehabilitation. I then further expand and apply these ideas to the notion of mobility in Chapter 6.

Moving Assemblages

Conceptualizing disability in terms of independence and dependence pre-empts envisioning the creative possibilities of multiple "attachments." Instead of eliminating or reducing dependencies, the project for rehabilitation becomes one of analyzing which attachments produce what effects, and sorting through how to maximize potentially fruitful attachments in keeping with an ethic of openness (Gibson 2006; Shildrick 1997, 2000, 2002). Openness is comfortable with doubt. Thus judgments about what constitutes a good or fruitful attachment are always provisional, open to revision, never settled. Openness also recognizes that every assemblage of attachments has multiple effects, some "good" and some "bad" and that the same effect can be good and bad in different ways. I use "attachments" in a particular way to recall the etymology of a dependency as something hanging from something else. Other terms further convey these ideas: assemblages, connectivities, bodies without organs, concorporations, cyborgs, becoming, and actor networks. These postmodern terms are always slippery but they collectively work to decenter the subject and admit the leaking of boundaries between subjects, bodies, technologies, and other objects or elements. Letting go of the sovereign subject frees up the inclination to declare who is dependent or independent because, as I discuss below, there is no "who" at the center but only movements of collectivities.

Postmodernism rejects the figure of the autonomous individual and reconfigure beings as becomings (Deleuze and Guattari 1987). Becoming is a process of moving in and out of various connections with heterogeneous human and nonhuman elements that produce particular effects and are then abandoned in favor of new connections. The most obvious elements of interest in rehabilitation are bodies, identities, and technologies, but assemblages can include an endless variety of elements such as physical objects, animals, events, emotions, and concepts. With becoming there is no subject engaging with other subjects but rather as Braidotti (2000, p. 159) puts it, "an assemblage of forces or passions that solidify (in space) and consolidate (in time) within the singular configuration commonly known as 'individual'." This becoming-individual does not emanate from some essential inner self, nor is s/he the product of biology, rather the assembled individual is a temporary collection of "energies" that are continually reconfigured.

The notion of "assemblages" comes from the work of Deleuze and Guattari (1987, pp. 323–350) who describe collections of heterogeneous elements that in coming together produce particular effects. Importantly, assemblages are not stable or closed systems, but rather temporary connections that continually come together and then break apart, forming different assemblages with other elements that produce different effects. Eschewing definitional closure, Deluze and Guatarri (1987, pp. 253–254) employ new terms in a variety of ways to escape the notion of bounded individual subjects and convey assemblages as unstable moving multiplicities:

> Arrive at elements that no longer have either form or function, that are abstract in this sense even though they are perfectly real. They are distinguished solely by movement and rest, slowness and speed. They are not atoms, in other words, finite elements still endowed with form. Nor are they indefinitely divisible. They are infinitely small, ultimate parts of an actual infinity, laid out on the same plane of consistency or composition. They are not defined by their number since they always come in infinites. However, depending on their degree of speed or the relation of movement and rest into which they enter, they belong to a given Individual, which may itself be part of another individual governed by another, more complex, relation, and so on to infinity... Thus each individual is an infinite multiplicity, and the whole of Nature is a multiplicity of perfectly individuated multiplicities.

Individuals in the Deleuzo-guattarian sense are multiplicities, collections of elements that may be parts of other individual multiplicities. Individuals as assemblages are never settled but change over time and space, continually *becoming*. Such a theoretical move away from stable contained bodies and subjects changes the parameters of dependence, which can be reconfigured as moments of possibility realized through multiple temporary assemblages (Gibson 2006). A space is created for appreciating and pursuing attachments. Taken-for-granted goals of independence reinforce disability as a limitation rather than possibility, reproducing and legitimizing practices that exclude particular (disabled) people. Reimagining dependencies as multiplicities opens up a theoretical space to rethink the goals of independence inherent in rehabilitation treatment, evaluation, and research practices (Gibson et al. 2012). This shift from the stable self to the fluid becoming-assemblage reconfigures interdependence in profound ways without losing its claims of shared mutualities. Mutuality and reciprocity between sovereign beings is re-imagined as the concorporation of disparate elements. Instead of giving and taking, there is becoming-together. Independence does not figure into this formulation as ideal or even possible, the project instead is to move among and between fruitful connections.

Assemblages are everywhere once you start to look. As I write this, I am aware of an assemblage formed between my ideas, typing body, and the keyboard. Words appear on a screen as together the assemblage produces a text, which is another assemblage. Each of these elements—ideas, body, keyboard, text—are part of other assemblages now and in other times and places. The assemblage contains other elements—a chair, a table, and a laptop that have positioned the body awkwardly and cause sensations of discomfort. Text and discomfort are different effects that are produced together. A switch to an audio recorder creates new assemblages that produce different texts and activate the body and in different ways. Later I can ask an assistant to transcribe the text. This dependency frees me up to do other things now and in the future, to construct different attachments.

I relate this somewhat banal example to be clear that assemblages are not limited to people labeled as disabled. Connectivity is always and everywhere. However, the analysis of different assemblages and their effects in the context of disability illuminates rehabilitation possibilities. To demonstrate, I describe various assemblages of Jessica (a pseudonym), 1 of 17 participants in an observational research study exploring place-based mediators of activity participation that included young people who use augmentative and alternative communication (AAC) (Gibson et al. 2013;

King et al. 2013). Jessica was an 18-year-old high school student who lived at home with her mother, father, younger sister, grandmother, and a paid caregiver. To make the various assemblages intelligible, I will use the convention of naming individuals according to these labels, while also highlighting the indeterminacy of each "person" and their variability as "individual multiplicities." I focus first on some "Jessica assemblages" but also consider the various configurations of "Mom," each consisting of variable bodies, technologies, identities, and other elements that together achieve particular practices and exert particular effects.

Different assemblages were implicated in Jessica's communication. Sometimes an AAC device was included to enable communication, other times it was not needed. Any assemblage that included Mom (*Jessica-Mom*) did not include the AAC device. Jessica's bodily movement and utterances were reconfigured and filtered by Mom whose body produced speech that was intelligible to others. We might describe this as "Jessica" spoke through "Mom," but this metaphor is limited as more is going on here. Jessica-Mom formed a communicating "machine" that is both singular (one machine, one communicator) and multiple (two individuals, two bodies)—what paradoxically can be called a "singular multiplicity." The Jessica-Mom machinic assemblage is temporary, it breaks apart and its elements form different assemblages in perpetual motion. *Jessica-Dad* is also a communicating machine, but it is a less efficient one. Jessica and her family explained that *Jessica-AAC* is the least efficient form of communication. It is avoided even though promoted by the rehabilitation team. Each assemblage enables communication differently but Jessica-AAC is slow, cumbersome, and tiring; emotions are harder to convey spontaneously. It also has other effects in that it is a stigmatized assemblage that marks this "Jessica" as disabled, as other.

From a rehabilitation standpoint, Jessica-AAC may be viewed as an achievement of "independent communication." This assemblage produces a better score on the FIM than Jessica-Mom, but this is not necessarily the most fruitful configuration for Jessica or her family. If independence ceases to be the goal, rehabilitation possibilities open up. How do different communication assemblages enable and disable? How can they be enhanced, reconfigured? Not only bodies and technologies but the wider possibilities outside of current contexts. How does/can the Jessica machine "plug in" to other machines (bodies, technologies, spaces, events) in the world to enable action? Independent communication with an AAC device is only one of many fruitful possibilities that can be facilitated in rehabilitation.

Jessica-Mom has other effects because "Mom" is part of other assemblages, formed and reformed with other elements. The Jessica-Mom assemblage enables communication but inhibits *becoming-mom* in other ways. The name "Mom" only describes one manifestation of becoming. Becoming-mom is also becoming-wife, becoming-daughter, becoming-worker, becoming-woman, becoming-self, and becoming-other. These classifications are limiting because they still portray a single subject with different roles and identities, but they can be put to use. Instead of closed identity categories, they can suggest potentialities and "lines of flight" (Deleuze and Guatarri 1987) that are opened and closed off in different ways with different effects. The question for rehabilitation could be how does the Jessica-Mom assemblage enable and constrain these lines of flight? What adjustments could be made and what would be the result? Asking these questions may or may not produce different interventions than those suggested by independence goals. Importantly, however, they change the philosophical parameters of assessment and treatment whereby independence no longer constrains possibilities, and dependencies are no longer necessarily construed as poor outcomes.

Letting go of independence as the "cornerstone" of practice requires a major shift in rehabilitation philosophy, but also acknowledges existing practices that may not easily fit into dominant rehabilitation ideologies. I recall presenting some of these ideas at a conference where I was daunted by the allotment of only 15 min to speak. When I was finished, a clinician in the audience proudly offered that "I'm an occupational therapist and OTs already do that" (referring to enabling assemblages). At the time, I felt like I had utterly failed to clearly elucidate my ideas. Surely OTs are not practicing according to the idea that there no subjects but only intermittent collections of heterogeneous elements! Upon reflection, however, I realized that in *the doing* of practice, clinicians facilitate the making and breaking of connections all the time, even if they would not describe what they are doing in terms of assemblages. Winance (2010) uses the terms "tinkering and adjustment" to refer to the clinical rehabilitation work whereby "care" is provided through modulating and balancing the positions of each member (technical and human) of a collective. Rehabilitation care is thus seen as a collective act of adjustment that transforms possibilities whether or not it is couched in the rhetoric of independence.

Embracing assemblages as a sensitizing concept may suggest new practices, but may also help to explain and defend existing practices that do not align with dominant rehabilitation discourses. In qualitative interviews with clinicians, I have observed how they work to describe their practices according to dominant rehabilitation principles like evidence-based practice or client-centred care (LeRoy et al. 2015). These principles do not necessarily best describe what they do, and clinicians will simultaneously resist and reproduce their tenets by remodelling the principles to support the logic of their practices. This is not necessarily a deliberate act, but rather reflects how understandings evolve through the doings of practice and discoveries of what "works." For example, clinicians labeled as "client-centred" their practices of breaking down clients' "unrealistic" goals into smaller achievable units to secure compliance and eventually help clients realize achievable outcomes. They did not share with clients that they believed the goals were unrealistic, but let them discover it on their own as therapy progressed. This description of "client-centred care" has very little overlap with expert descriptions, but better aligns with (some) clinicians' views of "good" practice that developed through experience.

As Mol (2002) has demonstrated, clinicians are motivated by a question of "what to do" for their patients, which is always a normative and practical question. What is best and how can it best be achieved? Doing good, she states "does not follow on finding out about, but is a matter of indeed doing. Of trying, tinkering, struggling, failing and trying again" (Mol 2002, p. 177). Given the many ways that rehabilitation and its aims are "enacted" in the doing (to use Mol's term), embracing dependencies as assemblages may indeed transform some practices, but may also better describe and support other existing practices. My purpose is not to replace one approach with another, but rather to resist the impulse to closure and complacency. An ethic of openness questions normative concepts that are treated as facts through the day to day doings of rehabilitation. Thus independence as the "cornerstone" of rehabilitation has to be continually questioned, doubted. Why is it the cornerstone? What effects are produced? How does it limit other creative possibilities for supporting individuals to thrive?

Assemblages have multiple effects; some are enabling, some disabling. I have, for the most part, presented the notion of facilitating assemblages as a promising avenue for rehabilitation. I do so to counter the overwhelmingly negative connotations of dependency pervasive in the Western social imagery and reflected in rehabilitation. Independence as an ideal has such a hold on contemporary practice that loosening its grip requires some doing. Nevertheless I am not suggesting that all dependencies are experienced positively. I alluded to this in the example of the Jessica-Mom assemblage that enabled communication but constrained Mom in other ways. In our work with Jessica, we noted multiple other assemblages that enabled preferred activities: playing cards, driving a boat, texting with friends. Each of these included transient attachments between particular persons, objects, and technologies embedded in different socio-material places. The "goodness of fit" between bodies, technologies, and places in each mediated actions and effects. Thus assemblage configurations are not limitless and some are more "successful" than others. The types of assemblages that are possible shape (and limit) activity choices. Jessica's human communication assemblages, for example, limit her ability to connect in different ways with peers. Similarly, wheelchair-body assemblages facilitate mobility but can constrain freedom of movement and mark the body as other (Gibson 2006; Gibson et al. 2007, 2012). The social world shapes how body-technology assemblages are interpreted, accepted, or stigmatized and how different connections can be made, sustained, or broken.

As I have suggested elsewhere (Gibson et al. 2012), thinking through the lens of assemblages, shifts rehabilitation away from a focus on enabling independence to analyzing the problems and possibilities inherent in different assemblages. This approach highlights the relational aspects of dis/ability. As Winance (2014) observes, neither abilities nor inabilities pre-exist, and nor are they attributes of an individual, but rather emerge within the contexts of heterogeneous attachments of human and nonhuman elements. With this in mind we can ask what can different configurations of people and technologies achieve in different places, and also how might they be constraining? What elements can and should be altered? For Jessica this might include any of a number of possibilities: better support for Jessica-mom, training others to form as efficient communication assemblages, research and funding for better devices, and/or education and advocacy to reduce social stigma. Interventions might (also) be aimed at increasing independent communication, but these goals need to be considered in the larger context of what avenues are most fruitful to explore for Jessica and her family. Independent communication with an AAC device is not by default the only goal worth pursuing.

Reconstructing Dependencies

In this chapter, I have traced the registers of meaning of dependency to suggest that the normative dichotomy of independence and dependence is an historical artefact that limits creative rehabilitation practices. In proposing a post-critical reading of interdependency, I have suggested that dependencies can be reconceived as assemblages of heterogeneous elements that decenter the subject and create possible avenues for a re-formed rehabilitation that embraces an ethic of openness. With this approach, independence ceases to be a driving principle of rehabilitation. I am not the first to suggest this line of flight for practice. As early as 1987, Kerr and Meyerson suggested that successful rehabilitation fostered "healthy dependency" and helping individuals to achieve the "flexibility and skill to enter comfortably into a variety of dependence relationships" (Kerr and Meyerson, 1987 p. 173).

In the next chapter, I extend the discussion of how thinking through assemblages can inform rehabilitation practices in relation to different forms of mobility. Drawing from the work of Winance (2006, 2010, 2014) and others, I offer a conception of rehabilitation practice in terms of adjustments or "collective doings" that engage humans and nonhuman elements toward the emergence of particular mobilities, abilities, and sensations that trans/form assemblages.

References

Benner, P. and Gordon, S. 1996. Caring practice. In *Caregiving: Readings in Knowledge, Practice, Ethics, and Politics*, eds. S. Gordon, P. Benner, and N. Noddings, pp. 40–55. Philadelphia, PA: University of Pennsylvania Press.

Bonikowsky, S., Musto, A., Suteu, K.A., MacKenzie, S., and Dennis, D. 2012. Independence: An analysis of a complex and core construct in occupational therapy. *The British Journal of Occupational Therapy* 75(4): 188–195.

Braidotti, R. 2000. Teratologies. In *Deleuze and Feminist Theory*, eds. C. Colebrook and I. Buchanan, pp. 156–172. Edinburgh, U.K.: Edinburgh University Press.

Canadian Institute for Health Information. National Rehabilitation Reporting System (NRS). http://www.cihi.ca/CIHI-ext-portal/internet/EN/Tabbed Content/types+of+care/hospital+care/rehabilitation/cihi010638 (accessed July 31, 2014).

Davis, L.J. 2002. *Bending over Backwards: Disability, Dismodernism, and Other Difficult Positions*. New York: NYU Press.

Deleuze, G. and Guattari, F. 1987. *A Thousand Plateaus: Capitalism and Schizophrenia*. Minneapolis, MN: University of Minnesota Press.

Ferguson, R. 1990. Introduction: Invisible centre. In *Out There: Marginalization and contemporary cultures*, ed. R. Ferguson, pp. 9–14. New York, NY: MIT Press.

Fine, M. 2005. Dependency work: A critical exploration of Kittay's perspective on care as a relationship of power. *Health Sociology Review* 14: 146–160.

Fine, M. and Glendinning, C. 2005. Dependence, independence or inter-dependence? Revisiting the concepts of 'care' and 'dependency'. *Ageing & Society* 25(04): 601–621.

Fraser, N. and Gordon, L. 1994. A genealogy of dependency: Tracing a keyword of the U.S. Welfare State. *Signs* 19(2): 309–336.

Gibson, B.E. 2006. Disability, connectivity and transgressing the autonomous body. *Journal of Medical Humanities* 27(3): 187–196.

Gibson, B.E. 2014. Parallels and problems of normalization in rehabilitation and universal design: Enabling connectivities. *Disability & Rehabilitation* 36(16): 1328–1333.

Gibson, B.E., Brooks, D., DeMatteo, D., and King, A. 2009. Consumer-directed personal assistance and 'Care': Perspectives of workers and ventilator users. *Disability & Society* 24(3): 317–330.

Gibson, B.E., Carnevale, F.A., and King, G. 2012. "This is my way": Reimagining disability, in/dependence and interconnectedness of persons and assistive technologies. *Disability & Rehabilitation* 34(22): 1894–1899.

Gibson, B.E., King G., Kushki, A., Mistry, B., Thompson, L., Teachman, G., Batorowicz, B., and McMain-Klein, M. 2013. A multi-method approach to studying activity setting participation: Integrating standardized questionnaires, qualitative methods and physiological measures. *Disability & Rehabilitation* 36(19): 1652–1660.

Gibson, B.E., Young, N.L., Upshur, R.E.G., and McKeever, P. 2007. Men on the margin: A Bourdieusian examination of living into adulthood with muscular dystrophy. *Social Science & Medicine* 65(3): 505–517.

Gignac, M.A.M. and Cott, C. 1998. A conceptual model of independence and dependence for adults with chronic physical illness and disability. *Social Science & Medicine* 47(6): 739–753.

Gleeson, B. 1999. *Geographies of Disability*. London, U.K.: Routledge.

Goodley, D. 2011. *Disability Studies: An Interdisciplinary Introduction*. London, U.K.: Sage.

Goodley, D. 2014. *Dis/Ability Studies: Theorising Disablism and Ableism*. New York: Routledge.

Goodwin, D.L. 2008. Self-regulated dependency: Ethical reflections on interdependence and help in adapted physical activity. *Sport, Ethics and Philosophy* 2(2): 172–184.

Graham, L.J. and Slee, R. 2008. An illusory interiority: Interrogating the discourse/s of inclusion. *Educational Philosophy and Theory* 40(2): 277–293.

Granger, C.V. 1998. The emerging science of functional assessment: Our tool for outcomes analysis. *Archives of Physical Medicine and Rehabilitation* 79(3): 235–240.

Hamdani, Y., Mistry, B., and Gibson, B.E. 2015. Transitioning to adulthood with a progressive condition: Best practice assumptions and individual experiences of young men with Duchenne muscular dystrophy. *Disability & Rehabilitation* 37(13): 1144–1151.

Hammell, K.W. 2006. *Perspectives on Disability and Rehabilitation*. Edinburgh, U.K.: Elsevier.

Hammell, K.W. 2009. Sacred tests: A sceptical exploration of the assumptions underpinning theories of occupation. *Canadian Journal of Occupational Therapy* 76(1): 6–13.

Hughes, B. 2007. Being disabled: Towards a critical social ontology for disability studies. *Disability & Society* 22(7): 673–684.

Kerr, N. and Meyerson, L. 1987. Independence as a goal and a value of people with physical disabilities: Some caveats. *Rehabilitation Psychology* 32(3): 173.

King, G., Gibson, B.E., Mistry, B., Pinto, M., Goh, F., Teachman, G., and Thompson, L. 2013. An integrated methods study of the experiences of youth with severe disabilities in leisure activity settings: The importance of belonging, fun, and control and choice. *Disability & Rehabilitation* 36(19): 1626–1635.

Kirby, A.V. 2015. Beyond independence: Introducing Deweyan philosophy to the dialogue on occupation and independence. *Journal of Occupational Science* 22(1): 17–25.

Kittay, E.F. 2007. Beyond autonomy and paternalism: The caring transparent self. In *Autonomy & Paternalism: Reflections on the Theory and Practice of Health Care*, eds. T. Nys, Y. Denier, and T. Vandevelde, pp. 23–70. Leuven, Belgium: Peeters Publishing.

Kittay, E.F. and Feder, E.K. 2003. *The Subject of Care: Feminist Perspectives on Dependency*. Lanham, MD: Rowman & Littlefield Publishers.

Kuppers, P. and Overboe, J. 2009. Introduction: Deleuze, disability, and difference. *Journal of Literacy & Cultural Disability Studies* 3(3): 217–220.

Leplège, A., Barral, C., and McPherson, K.M. 2015. Conceptualizing disability to inform rehabilitation: Historical and epistemological perspectives. In *Rethinking Rehabilitation Theory and Practice*, eds. K.M. McPherson, B.E. Gibson, and A. Leplège. Boca Raton, FL: CRC Press.

LeRoy, K., Boyd, K., De Asis, K., Lee, R.W., Martin, R., Teachman, G., and Gibson, B.E. 2015. Balancing hope and realism in family-centered care: Physical therapists' dilemmas in negotiating walking goals with parents of children with cerebral palsy. *Physical & Occupational Therapy in Pediatrics* 35(3): 253–264.

Mackenzie, C., Rogers, W.A., and Dodds, S. 2014. *Vulnerability: New Essays in Ethics and Feminist Philosophy*. New York: Oxford University Press.

Martinez, K. 2003. Independent living in the US & Canada. Independent Living Institute. Farsta, Sweden. http://www.independentliving.org/docs6/martinez2003.html (accessed July 31, 2014).

McLaughlin, J. 2006. Conceptualising intensive caring activities: The changing lives of families with young disabled children. *Sociological Research Online* 11(1).

McRuer, R. 2006. *Crip Theory: Cultural Signs of Queerness and Disability*. New York: NYU Press.

Mol, A. 2002. *The Body Multiple: Ontology in Medical Practice*. Durham, U.K.: Duke University Press.

Morris, J. 1997. Care or empowerment? A disability rights perspective. *Social Policy & Administration* 31(1): 54–60.

Morris, J. 2004. Independent living and community care: A disempowering framework. *Disability and Society* 19(5): 427–442.

Noddings, N. 1984. *Caring: A Relational Approach to Ethics and Moral Education*. Berkley, CA: University of California Press.

Oliver, M. 1989. Disability and dependency: A creation of industrial societies? In *Disability and Dependency*, ed. L. Barton, pp. 6–22. London, U.K.: The Falmer Press.

Overboe, J. 2009. Affirming an impersonal life: A different register for disability studies. *Journal of Literacy & Cultural Disability Studies* 3(3): 241–256.

Ramaswamy, B. and McCandless, P. 2013. Chapter 24: Physiotherapy management of Parkinson's and of older people. In *Tidy's Physiotherapy*, 15th edn., eds. S.B. Porter and N.M. Tidy, pp. 539–559. Edinburgh, U.K.: Saunders Elsevier.

Ratzka, A. 2003. The prerequisites for de-institutionalization. Cornell University ILR School, Ithaca, NY. http://digitalcommons.ilr.cornell.edu/gladnetcollect/426 (accessed July 31, 2014).

Reindal, S.M. 1999. Independence, dependence, interdependence: Some reflections on the subject and personal autonomy. *Disability & Society* 14(3): 353–367.

Saxton, M., Curry, M.A., Powers, L.E., Maley, S., Eckels, K., and Gross J. 2001. "Bring My Scooter so I can Leave You": A study of disabled women handling abuse by personal assistance providers. *Violence against Women* 7(4): 393–417.

Shakespeare, T. 2000. *Help*. Birmingham, U.K.: Venture.

Shildrick, M. 1997. *Leaky Bodies and Boundaries: Feminism, Postmodernism and (Bio)Ethics*. London, U.K.: Routledge.

Shildrick, M. 2000. Becoming vulnerable: Contagious encounters and the ethics of risk. *Journal of Medical Humanities* 21(4): 215–227.

Shildrick, M. 2002. *Embodying the Monster: Encounters with the Vulnerable Self*. London, U.K.: Sage Publications.

Shildrick, M. 2009. *Dangerous Discourses of Disability, Subjectivity and Sexuality*. Basingstoke, U.K.: Palgrave Macmillan.

Slater, J. 2012. Self-advocacy and socially just pedagogy. *Disability Studies Quarterly* 32(1).

Stewart, D., Freeman, M., Law, M., Healy, H., Burke-Gaffney, J., Forhan, M., Young, N., and Guenther, S. 2009. *"The Best Journey to Adult Life" for Youth with Disabilities: An Evidence-Based Model and Best Practice Guidelines for the Transition to Adulthood for Youth with Disabilities*. Hamilton, Ontario, Canada: CanChild.

Struhkamp, R., Mol, A., and Swierstra, T. 2009. Dealing with in/dependence: Doctoring in physical rehabilitation practice. *Science, Technology & Human Values* 34(1): 55–76.

Thomas, C. 2007. *Sociologies of Disability and Illness: Contested Ideas in Disability Studies and Medical Sociology*. New York: Palgrave MacMillan.

Tronto, J.C. 1993. *Moral Boundaries: A Political Argument for an Ethic of Care*. London, U.K.: Routledge.

Warren, N. and Manderson, L. 2008. Constructing hope dis/continuity and the narrative construction of recovery in the rehabilitation unit. *Journal of Contemporary Ethnography* 37(2): 180–201.

Watson, N., McKie, L., Hughes, B., Hopkins, D., and Gregory, S. 2004. (Inter) dependence, needs and care: The potential for disability and feminist theorists to develop an emancipatory model. *Sociology* 38(2): 331–350.

Weicht, B. 2011. Embracing dependency: Rethinking (in)dependence in the discourse of care. *The Sociological Review* 58(s2): 205–224.

Wendell, S. 1996. *The Rejected Body: Feminist Philosophical Reflections on Disability*. New York: Routledge.

Winance, M. 2006. Trying out the wheelchair: The mutual shaping of people and devices through adjustment. *Science, Technology, & Human Values* 31(1): 52–72.

Winance, M. 2010. Care and disability: Practices of experimenting, tinkering with, and arranging people and technical aids. In *Care in Practice: On Tinkering in Clinics, Homes and Farms*, eds. A. Mol, I. Moser, and J. Pols, pp. 93–117. Bielefeld, Germany: Verlag.

Winance, M. 2014. Universal design and the challenge of diversity: Reflections on the principles of UD, based on empirical research of people's mobility. *Disability & Rehabilitation* 36(16): 1334–1343.

6
Mobilities

In the previous chapter, I introduced Deleuzo-guatarrian notions of *becoming* and *assemblages* to reframe questions of independence and dependence. In this chapter, I extend this discussion by considering examples of mobility assemblages and the implications for rehabilitation research and clinical practice. Throughout the preceding chapters, I have drawn on movement as metaphor to explore rhizomatic potentialities in rehabilitation. Here I (somewhat) let go of the metaphor to explore how assembled bodies literally move through space, and how rehabilitation is oriented toward some forms of mobility over others.

Movements are everywhere in rehabilitation and act on, with, and between patients and practitioners. There are movements and connections between bodies, technologies, and places that come together and break apart. Bodies are continuously in motion and reconfiguring every day. Some reconfigurations are socially valorized ("enhancements"), others are stigmatized ("impairments"), but all are movements, changes, re-formations of the self. There are "good" and "bad" movements, for example, the normal gait cycle versus "psoatic," "equinus," or "festinate" gaits. Mobilities establish one's place in the world both in terms of material location and through the meanings assigned to different bodily movements and configurations. For example, wheelchairs and walkers allow access to the world but via often stigmatized technologies. Crawling, as I explore in the following, is largely unthinkable for anyone other than an infant. Far from being value-neutral, mobilities carry the weight of normative judgment, and rehabilitation can be a site for confirming or transforming these judgments.

My intent in this chapter is to surface the normative meanings of mobilities as an exemplar that extends and integrates the ideas discussed in the previous chapters regarding movement, normalcy, independence, development, and quality of life. I do so through drawing on the notion of assemblages outlined in Chapter 5 to consider three examples of mobilities: amputee mobilities, crawling mobilities, and wheelchair mobilities.

Mobilizing Desire

Before discussing the examples, I first consider the idea of *desire* in relation to embodied mobilities. As I discussed in Chapter 5, postmodernism questions the notion of the individual as a closed and independent entity. For Deleuze and Guattari (1983, 1987), this individuation of the subject limits *desire*, that is, flows and possibilities for making and breaking connectivities. Desiring for Deleuze and Guatarri is something very different from "wanting." A want is a compulsion to address some kind of perceived lack, instead desire (Deleuze and Guattari 1983) is conceived of as a "force of production," a fundamental flow of energy. Productive desire is a power, a passion that moves one toward something new to connect and reconnect, to move, and experiment. Wanting is repressed desire, unproductive and limiting, and is associated with fixed and individualized subjectivity:

> Desire does not lack anything; it does not lack its object. It is, rather, the subject that is missing in desire or desire that lacks a fixed subject; there is no fixed subject unless there is repression. (Deleuze and Guattari 1983, p. 26.)

Deleuze and Guattari's radicalization of desire and subjectivity requires new terms help to escape the notion of individual subjects and singular identities. "Desiring machines," "assemblages," and "becomings" are terms used to decentre the subject and point to moving networks of heterogeneous elements with kinetic boundaries that resist finalizing definitions. Desire is a free-flowing force that seeks to connect, not in order to complete itself, but to experiment and explore, to let go of the constraints of classifications and conformities, to create new hybrid machinic assemblages. Body/subjects are transitory and blend into other bodies and machines, becoming free of, and disruptive to, established systems of thought, being, and doing (Gibson 2006). A subject for Deleuze and Guattari is reconfigured as an inorganic Body without Organs (BwO), which "is desire: it is that which one desires and by which one desires" (Taguchi and Palmer 2014, p. 764).

The distinction between "wanting," a force driven by negative differences, and desire, which is driven by positive relations (Taguchi and Palmer 2014), has consequences for practice. Goals that carry the weight of conformity may never be reached, and their burdens are sustained through attempts to address a negative difference or lack and can result in anxiety, shame, guilt, and other forms of social and existential suffering. Rehabilitation and other "helping" professions are built on this notion of identifying and addressing forms of lack. Professional helping constructs a problem to be rectified, a deficiency or difference to be addressed, and envisions a future endpoint of resolution. These efforts are not "bad" or "wrong" but have multiple effects beyond the intended outcomes that are seldom explored in the bioscientific approach that dominates medicine and rehabilitation. In what follows I draw on the three mobility examples to unpack these effects and the possibilities for freeing up desire through multiple transitory connections.

Amputee Mobilities

The notion of desire provides a point of departure for considering atypical mobilities and reconfiguring the disabled body-subject. I begin with the example of amputee-mobilities to explore notions of normal walking and how rehabilitation practices both reflect and resist these notions. "Amputee rehabilitation" is a site for relearning and reinforcing typical walking patterns with the lower limb prosthesis acting as the bridge to this achievement. "Independent walking" is generally constructed as the best possible outcome in rehabilitation practice and is defined as walking "unassisted" that is, with a prosthesis but without gait aids (Hoffman 2013). Other forms of mobility (with, for example, canes, crutches, or a wheelchair) are often considered "poor outcomes" creating a moral hierarchy of assistive technologies according to the kinds of mobilities they produce. Aligned with this goal, therapy is also concerned with the quality of walking, that is, the achievement of normal walking patterns according to the standard gait cycle and its typical displacements in "swing" and "stance" phases. Hoffman (2013) notes that these efforts move beyond functional biomechanics to reflect cultural ideals of body aesthetics. Achieving typical rhythms effectively "fills in" the absent limb, neutralizing differences. Learning to walk independently with an "artificial" limb is thus a practice of normalization in body movements and styles where the ideal outcome is passing as nondisabled.

Practices of ambulation normalization have multiple effects. Efficient, pain-free mobility allows access to a world designed for walkers and makes life easier in myriad ways. By rendering the impairment invisible, stigma is minimized or avoided. The prosthesis thus enables both materially and socially. Other effects that I have discussed in earlier chapters are less immediate or transparent. Normalization practices construct the impaired body as a problem to be fixed, which reproduces negative valuations of disabled people as in needing of correction. Corrections take predictable forms of homogenization, that is, shaping the disabled body into one that looks and walks like other bodies, and erasing or narrowing differences in an impulse toward sameness, as I explored in more detail in Chapter 2. "Amputee rehabilitation" is thus both enabling and disabling in complex ways that intersect and depend on context. The prosthesis does different things in the world. This is exemplified by the experiences of Mark Mossman (2001, para 12) in his description of walking to the beach while on vacation:

> In order to get to the beach … I had to leave my limb upstairs and use crutches (salt and sand sometimes damage the hydraulic knee of my leg, so I try to avoid leaving it for long stretches on a beach). As I passed by the pool on crutches and felt the stares of roughly forty sunbathing, vacationing people, and heard the questions of several small, inquisitive children, I felt deeply disabled. I called that passage, a route I would take probably eight to ten times during the trip, the running of the gauntlet. That was what it was: a painful, bruising journey that simply had to be made. In those moments, I felt vulnerable. I felt angry. I will be honest: I felt hatred. I remember telling myself, on several occasions, that "I didn't care what they thought of me," that "I was going to do this no matter what." I remember trying hard not to look back at them, those innocent people, not to hear the questions, but instead to focus on the goal: the gateway to the beach and ultimately the sea. I knew that making eye contact meant imprisonment, displacement, perhaps even failure. I knew how the process worked: eye contact would equate deep inscription, the aggressive internalization of abnormality and disability, and I knew that too much of that would have meant a decision to just avoid the whole troublesome thing and not swim at all.

Mossman's account presents a kind of mobility trade-off. After this quotation, he goes on to describe the wonderful feeling of freedom and pleasure that he experienced once he entered the water that he says made the beach walk worth enduring the stares and whispers. We see that he gives up prosthetic walking in favor of crutch walking for practical reasons, but in doing so he exposes a difference for which he is judged and "imprisoned." The reward comes when he reaches the water, where he gets away from the inscriptive gaze of the crowd, and where the prosthesis would be a hindrance rather than a help. A new assemblage is formed with the water that provides "freedom," functionally and also ontologically. He can move more easily. He is not disabled by the stares of the crowd in this milieu, and this too is a kind of freedom.

Mobilities are political. They are assessed, categorized, and judged. Rehabilitation knows this and tries to help not just with function but with managing stigma—helping individuals to look normal, to minimize their differences, to avoid situations of "running the gauntlet." We might say that this is good in the immediate, but it also has some problematic distal effects. Normalization, or "passing," as Goffman (1963) described it, perpetuates the status quo, affirms divisions between "us and them," imprisons and spurs feelings of hatred, of failure. Mossman (2001, para 4) describes his body as a "postmodern text" that inhabits a border between two worlds that continually write and rewrite his narrative. In one place and time he is, for example, an "ill patient" in a doctor's office, and in the next moment a "healthy player" in a basketball game.

Mossman's postmodern body can be conceived of as a *desiring machine* that moves in multiple ways in and between spaces encompassing movements and stillness, connecting and releasing in ways that work, ways that enable. Categories of disability and ability no longer apply with this flexible techno-body assemblage. Troubling the categories of ill/healthy and disabled/normal acts on the stigma, deflates its power; it is no longer clear whom to point fingers at and whom to applaud. Importantly, Mossman notes that disability/ability indeterminacy has implications for all bodies. Letting go of normative bodies and abilities opens up a space for new kinds of mobilities. Doing differently, getting around in whatever way *works,* does things in the world that are positive and productive, inventing new modes and embracing discredited others.

Prosthetic bodies remind us that all bodies are imbricated in shifting networks of assemblages. More accurately, as Shildrick (2010, pp. 12–13) notes, "we are all always already prosthetic," that is caught up in a web of connections that renders indistinct boundaries "between the organic and inorganic, between the natural and artificial, or ultimately between self and other." Rather than suggesting that we are all alike, however, the point is that we are all *different.* Conventional categories of, say, disability, race or gender, are merely devices for simplifying the irreducible complexity of corporeal forms (Shildrick 2015). In this regard, disability corporealities are not unique but remind us how everyone/thing is connected. Building on this notion breaks the drive to conformity and becomes the impetus for different ways of doing in the world that inform rehabilitation. What are the possibilities inherent in the trying on of mobilities that resist the impulse to normal, that unleash desire? Or to put it more plainly, what abnormal-but-enabling mobilities emerge when we stop trying to approximate the typical?

This is not a new idea. New mobilities are invented all the time as evidenced in the history of transportation, or the evolution of the wheelchair: faster, lighter, more manoeuvrable. Sitting mobilities are evolving into upright mobilities (e.g., standing wheelchairs, the Upsee device*) for multiple reasons with multiple effects. Prosthetics too continually undergo

* The Upsee device is a harness worn by an adult that allows children with mobility impairments to walk assisted. http://www.fireflyfriends.com/upsee (accessed October 2, 2015).

design innovations. Osseo-integration allows the direct skeletal attachment of prosthesis to bone, and electrodes are implanted within residual limb muscles for myoelectric prosthetics (Pasquina et al. 2006). There is a tension in prosthetic design between form and function. For a long while, the holy grail of prosthetic design was to create something that both looked and functioned like the biological part it was designed to replace (Gutfleisch 2003, p. 139). This idea persists in some ways as more "life-like" prosthetics are designed, aided by advanced robotics and new materials that improve aesthetics. But the ideal is not yet fully realized and is not necessarily important to the people who use prosthetics (Murray 2009).

But something else is happening. Concurrent with efforts to perfect "life-like" prostheses is the emergence of the valorized bionic body; the better than normal "supercrip cyborg" (Swartz and Watermeyer 2008) that has less and less in common with typical biomorphology. Oscar Pistorius' bid to compete in the nondisabled Olympics in 2008 and 2012 became a focal point for surfacing tensions regarding new forms of enhanced techno-bodies. Concerns that his high-technology "cheetah-blades" would give him an "unfair advantage" if he were allowed to compete with nondisabled athletes revealed deeper anxieties over the need to classify his embodiment as of one kind or the other (Swartz and Watermeyer 2008). Pistorius' cyborgified body disrupts the assumption of the natural uncontaminated organic body that is reproduced in the discourse of sport and "transgresses the boundary between ability/disability, nature/machine, and so on (and) reveals the margins of ability as porous, leaky, and unstable, thereby threatening to collapse the very ontological and corporeal security of the humanist subject" (Norman and Moola 2011, p. 1273). In the debates about how to categorize Pistorius, the line between disabled and nondisabled were blurred, while at the same time reinforced. Reinforced because Pistorius was still constructed as the disabled athlete, his artificial legs were coded as a difference that materialized his disability identity, but importantly the polarities were switched, disability was seen as the advantage, nondisabled ("normal") was the disadvantage.

In reversing the polarities of disability and normality, enhanced cyborg bodies reveal both collective commitments to the construction of bodies as contained by biology, while at the same time revealing a fantasy: bodies have never been self-contained. We are all connected in one way or another (Chapter 5). Assemblic connections of desiring machines produce a range of bodily forms capable of a variety of mobilities that trouble the categories of disability and ability. All forms of prostheses whether they are artificial limbs, or the range of organic and inorganic implants, organs, or drugs, contest the shared faith in corporeal integrity even though they intend to shore it up (Shildrick 2015, p. 16). The impaired body is patched with assistive technologies in the attempt to achieve closure. A perceived lack must be effaced, made whole, but the disabled prosthetic body is still seen as poor substitute for the "real" thing. External technologies are seen as threatening to "dehumanise" the discrete, whole, unified concept of the human. This threat however can be reimagined as possibility, as positive productive force of desire.

Hybrid mobilities open up new possibilities for being and doing-in-the-world when the urge to normalize is resisted. The anxiety over enhanced techno-bodies stems from classificatory thinking, something I raised in Chapters 1 through 3. Is Pistorius disabled or not? How can he be both? Or neither? The inability to resolve indeterminacy manifests in collective anxiety, the inclination to recover and replace a lack. But if the impulse to classify is resisted, "disability" is disrupted, mobilized, and rendered meaningless—or rather meaning-*full*, which is overfull of endless possibilities. When we think of mobility and the example offered by Pistorius and other (para)athletes, new approaches to solving problems open up. Functional improvisations arise when the instinct toward sameness is resisted, when desire is free flowing, experimenting with different bodily shapes and styles. In the case of Pistorius and other "blade runners," a normal aesthetic is abandoned in favor of functional superiority, but it could have been abandoned for myriad other reasons be they functional, aesthetic, expressive, and/or political. The break from normality is extended; the need to "blend in" is forgotten because of a letting go of classificatory thinking. Previously unexplored potentials for different mobilities are enacted through a postmodern desiring BwO of replaceable parts. Categorization loses its appeal in light of the creative potentials of all bodies to be made and remade, to move in new ways that *work*. Blending-*with* instead of blending-in. Bionic limbs re-imagine mobilities that break with the appeal of the normalized body. Rather than threatening bodily integrity, the figure of the unstable cyborg-subject addresses exclusion by dispensing with identities that inhere in the so-called natural distinctions like dis/ability (Gibson et al. 2014).

My point in all of this is to say that normalization stifles creativity, and abandoning the impulse toward sameness creates possibilities for never-before imagined mobilities, and for the acceptance of previously negatively coded mobility forms. We are all always prosthetic in one way or another. For example, we are all "enwheeled" (Papadimitriou 2008) whether through wheelchairs, skateboards, scooters, cars, walkers, buses, or bicycles. We do and make do, get around and get on in ways that work. There is no reason in the world that we have to move the same way as others or according to a preset menu of options. Once we let go of the negative coding of atypical mobilities, a world of possibility opens up. We see this letting go in prosthetic design and in comments, like the following, from prosthesis-users:

> Cosmetic covers are an attempt to hide the obvious. Not needed if you've dealt with the fact that you are an amputee and don't mind being dependent on machines. In my opinion—and this it not for everyone—cosmetic covers are like sewing animal skins over your car to make it more like a "natural" mode of transport. (Murray 2009, p. 577)

The analogy here is clear: there is no "natural" mobility. The body is uncontained and normalization is no longer the aim. Instead, as Shildrick (2015) notes, disability as it is lived—with its embodied absences, displacements, and prosthetic additions—generates its own specific possibilities that both limit and extend the performativity of the self, enable and disable, opening up a "celebratory positioning of difference and transcorporeality as the very conditions of life" (Shildrick 2015, p. 14).

Assemblage thinking is rife with possibilities for a reconceived rehabilitation. Nansen (2007) suggests that such a project does not conceive of a prosthesis as a replacement for a lack, but rather as "reorganisation" that exceeds limitations. The fiction of the natural, essential, and stable body concedes to one that is continuous, permeable, and in-process. He suggests "there is no longer a 'body' but rather instantiations of bodies that rest upon a distributed and heterogenous network of relations and artifacts" (Nansen 2007, para 17). This moving body-as-desire embraces mobilities as they present themselves, always shifting. Particular dependencies are pursued when they are of use and otherwise abandoned. All bodies are caught up in these mobility networks that incorporate things as tools. In discussing assemblages of mechanical ventilation, Nansen (2007, para 17) notes:

> Traditionally, ideologies of rehabilitation emphasised separation from technological assistance as virtuous, and dependence as idleness. These ideologies are compatible with broader cultural values of independence and achievement, circumscribing the MV (mechanical ventilator) body with failure in its inability to conform to the curative goals of medicine, as well as connecting humans and technologies into similar trajectories based on usefulness, novelty, and obsolescence. The MV, adopted through necessity, imposes a range of constraints on bodily freedoms, denying notions of choice and flexibility privileged in late modernity. There is, however, an ambivalence in this reconfiguration as such attenuations are countered by the MV extending and prolonging bodies, enabling both mobility and new ways of existing outside institutions. (parentheses added)

Assemblages have effects that can both constrain and enable doing-in-the-world in material and social ways. The point is to reimagine what counts as enabling. Normal mobility? Independent mobility? What desiring machines are valorized (body-car) or disavowed (body-walker) and why? Reimagining mobilities that unleash desire by letting go of normal/disabled distinctions is better appreciated when considering those mobilities that rehabilitation practitioners most often attempt to correct, like amputee crutch walking, or as I now discuss, crawling.

Crawling Mobilities

> The room has a couch and coffee table in it. So he manoeuvres those two rooms on his belly, like, we get in the house and there isn't really room for a walker, so down he goes. But he pulls himself up on the couch, he, like, slides on and off it. He pulls himself up the coffee table, he'll pull himself up on the bookshelf on his knees and pull all the books out and then laugh at me. He's got a lot of motion going on there if you let him.
>
> Mother of five-year-old "Ray" who has cerebral palsy

Nowhere is the range of human mobility possibilities more evident than in the movements of children. Creative experimentation abounds in children's explorations of the world and how they incorporate objects, surfaces, and persons to explore their bodies and their environments. Children "try out" their bodies to see what their bodies can do, to experience new sensations, to explore their environments. Climbing, crawling, piggybacking, scrambling, galloping, rolling, wheeling are lines of flight that resist the normalizing tendency to move in adult-centric ways. Children continually become new bodies through establishing "stimulus-response circuits" where they "unhinge" themselves from habitual ways of moving, opening up "cracks in habit" and creating "zones of indeterminacy" (McLaren 2012, p. 150).

Movement experimentations are encouraged with infants but also incrementally discouraged as children age. Through immersion in their social worlds, children come to learn, as part of "growing up," what movements are permissible, valorized, or discredited and in which contexts. Movement styles embody social constructs related to age, gender, and class and are learned through a mixture of direct instruction and social cues (Bourdieu 1977). Children are taught to stand and sit up straight; running is encouraged in some places and forbidden in others; girls are admonished to keep their knees together (Bordo 1993). Movements in schools are regulated and scheduled. For example, children may be required to sit quietly in class, walk in an orderly fashion between classes, and limit dynamic movements to exercise, sport, or dance in circumscribed times and places. Mobilities are shaped by these types of overt rules as well as through the inscription of social logics that reflect aesthetic and moral orderings of good and bad bodily styles (Crossley 2005). Bourdieu (1977, p. 87) referred to this as *hexis*, a term suggesting that how we move reflects where we are from, which is achieved through the internalization of the social into the corporeal:

> Body hexis speaks directly to the motor function, in the form of a pattern of postures that is both individual and systematic, because linked to a whole system of techniques involving the body and tools, and charged with a host of social meanings and values: in all societies, children are particularly attentive to the gestures and postures which, in their eyes, express everything that goes to make an accomplished adult- a way of walking, a tilt of the head, facial expressions, ways of sitting and of using implements, always associated with a tone of voice, a style of speech and (how could it be otherwise?) a certain subjective experience.

Movement styles thus reflect and reproduce a particular social ordering internalized into a set of bodily dispositions that are acquired without being consciously learned, or deliberately practiced.

The incorporation of body techniques diminishes creative experimentation and limits desire. As they age, children's creative movements are increasingly limited to certain life spheres like sport and recreation, and are less oriented to everyday explorations of movement possibilities. Moreover mobilities that differ from the norm can be a source of teasing, scorn, or stigma for children whose movements mark them as the disabled other.

Disabled children learn early on how their ways of moving in the world may negatively "single" them out as different (Gibson and Teachman 2012). The usual response in rehabilitation is to help the child (or adult) to look and move in typical ways. The impulse, deeply ingrained in rehabilitation, is to alter the child to match the social and material order of things, to fit *in*, that is to be included in a predetermined centre (Graham and Slee 2008; Ravaud and Stiker 2001). Disability is constructed as inherent to the biological body. The alternative of course would be to "leave the child be" (leave the child do?) and change the world instead. And this is often attempted through efforts to remove material or attitudinal barriers. But these approaches oversimplify a complex set of relations. The question posed by Deleuze and Guattari (1987) of "what can a body do?" is invariably linked with the moral ordering of what *should* a body do?

The answer provided most often by professionals, parents, teachers, and disabled individuals themselves is to do what everyone else is doing, that is, to attain or approximate normative bodily styles and mobilities (see Chapter 2).

Here is the place where we could ask a different question: What could a body do if it had not learned what not to do? In other words, what are the possibilities for undiscovered creative mobilities? What is the body capable of when unconstrained by normative limits? As Deleuze and Guattari (1987) note, "we know nothing about a body until we know what it can do, in other words, what its affects are, and how they can or cannot enter into composition with other affects, with the affects of another body" (Deleuze and Guattari 1987, p. 284). Discovering what a body can do relies on unleashing desire, allowing unpredictable additions and absences that disorganize and disrupt the normative body schema (Deleuze and Guattari 1987; Shildrick 2015; Taguchi and Palmer 2014). Positive productive forces of desire enable new connections, attachments, and dependencies that are reconfigured as needed to produce assemblages that work in a given context.

Empirical research illuminates how disabled children's creative movements are promoted or discouraged and how things could be otherwise. For example, in a recent study (forthcoming) one of the parents that we interviewed spoke about her 5-year-old son's use of a walker that has since been replaced with a different model. She stated: "I think if he's in the walker, he should be putting full support on his feet and he should be using his arms to stand up into that proper position." She described how her son initially used the walker in this "proper" way before realizing he could use it like a skateboard, that is, putting weight through his arms to scoot rapidly along on the walker wheels, touching down with his feet only as needed. The parent had good intentions and I am not judging her choices; she wanted to encourage her son to use the walker therapeutically, to enhance and improve his walking potential. The boy however wanted to "let go" in the many senses of the phrase—break free of the constraints of the "proper position," play and create, experience the joy and freedom of speed, get there faster, keep up with his brother. This is the same mother that I quoted at the beginning of this section, who stated that her son has "got a lot of motion going on there *if you let him*" and who had created spaces in her home to let him move more freely. "Letting him" is a letting go of the negative forces that conspire to constrain movement. The mobility assemblage of boy-walker opens a space for multiple ways of moving that can be construed as either constraining or enabling according to different scripts of the "right" mobility aims. Becoming in the Deleuzo-guatarrian sense is not related to a future end goal such as independent walking. It's about making and breaking connections, experimenting with multiple identities, preferences, and doings in the world. Becoming mobile-walker-boy-speed.

Children actively create new bodily forms, but these possibilities are increasingly narrowed as they internalize spatial norms and rules (Stephens et al. 2015). In research with young people, Stephens et al. (2015) demonstrate how children achieve action in different ways in different environments according to tacit understandings of how movement will be perceived and acted on by others. For example, one of the youth advisors to their research suggested that disabled young people may move differently in public and private spaces, noting it was easier to get off a sofa at home because you could "stick your bum up in the air and do whatever it takes to navigate the space" (p. 14). Similarly, children distinguished different meanings associated with falling at home and at school. They described various flopping and falling movements as part of their normal repertoire of bodily styles at home, but at school, because safety concerns were paramount, they knew falling had to be avoided at all costs. Their school mobilities were thus considerably different and involved the mandatory use of aids such as wheelchairs that were not used in the home. These place-based differences re-iterate how inherent social norms of particular places are as much a part of an assemblage as the material elements of bodies and objects. The meanings attached to the material forms change, and in so doing reconfigure the assemblage.

Above I made a distinction between the appeal of high-tech athletic prostheses and the everyday marginalization experiences of amputees to make the point regarding how disability assemblages are perceived and acted on in the world. To build on this point, I now turn to a discussion of a largely disparaged form of human mobility: crawling. In the contemporary world, crawling is permitted only for the youngest humans and only in relation to their constructed roles as adults-in-the-making. The boundaries of permissible crawling are closely regulated according to developmental norms (Chapter 4). The infant is expected and encouraged to crawl sometime between 6 and 10 months after which time crawling is discouraged in favor of walking. No longer a baby, the child is assigned the new mobility-based identity of "toddler." Crawling baby progresses to walking toddler along a developmental continuum towards fully formed adult. Walking upright is more than simply a functional achievement but also an aesthetic, moral, and symbolic one. The symbolic weight of upright mobility is captured in two quotations published more than 60 years apart:

> The term "to be upright" has two connotations: to rise, to get up, and to stand on one's own feet; and the moral implication, not to stoop to anything, to be honest and just, to be true to friends in danger, to stand by one's convictions, and to act accordingly, even at the risk of one's life. We praise an upright man (sic); we admire someone who stands up for his ideas of rectitude. There are good reasons to assume that the term "upright" in its moral connotation is more than a mere allegory. (Straus 1952, pp. 530–531)

> In the famous diagram, Darwinian man unfolds himself from frightened crouch to strong surveyor of the ages, and it looks like a natural ascension: you start out bending over, knuckles dragging, timidly scouring the ground for grubs, then you slowly straighten up until there you are, staring at the skies and counting the stars and thinking up gods to rule them. (Gopnik 2014)

To walk upright is construed in Gopnik's literary musing not only as an individual achievement but the realization of human evolution that brought us out of the dirt and closer to the stars. In a different vein, Straus' phenomenological consideration of the upright body echoes Fraser and Gordon's (1994) moral/psychological register of in/dependence (Chapter 5). The straight, upright body is an achievement of moral character; it is the true body, the dependable body. In both quotations the stooped body is suspicious, dishonest, and unreliable. These persistent ideas of moral "rectitude" have implications for bodies moving closer to the ground, that is, seated mobilities, but more profoundly crawling mobilities. The positive moral and symbolic connotations associated with the descriptor "upright" are starkly juxtaposed against those surrounding the verb "to crawl." The crawler is the demeaned "groveller" who "lags behind," "makes excuses," and "cowers from danger." We see how the normativities of up or down, high or low, upright or prostrate are embedded in cultures and inscribed onto individual bodies (Bourdieu 1997). Body hexis transmits identities that are interpreted by others and suggest affinities or disconnects.

Within this minefield of meaning the functional crawler is suspect. Crawling as a form of mobility is not tolerated for anyone except the developing infant progressing toward normal bipedal gait. In medical discourse, crawling is a "milestone" that helps develop motor skills, strength, and coordination, things the baby lacks and needs. To that end, it is promoted and facilitated, but it must be temporary. Persistent crawling is a problem that requires intervention. Similarly, crawling may be used as a therapeutic device with adults (e.g., post brain injury) to decrease muscle tone, increase strength, balance, or symmetry, but no one will suggest this as a permanent form of mobility. Crawling is a means to address a lack and ultimately to enable upright walking.

Functional crawlers challenge these mobility norms. Gregor Wolbring, for example, embraces crawling as his primary mode of mobility. Born without legs he says that he "loves to crawl" and does so whenever feasible. Wolbring describes himself as a "person with a non-mainstream body function" who adapts his mobility as the situation dictates stating that there is "a situation for crawling and a situation for a wheelchair and a situation for using a car" (Swanson n.d.). This constellation of malleable assemblages constitutes "Gregor Wolbring" in different ways in different time-spaces that achieve efficient mobilities. Wolbring, like Mossman discussed earlier, embraces the nonconforming hybridity of his postmodern body while acknowledging how his mobilities are negatively coded in the dominant social orderings of disability. Thus, his preferred crawling-assemblage is inhibited in particular public spaces, a constellation of negative forces that Deleuze and Guattari might say blocks the flow of desire. Academic scholars like Wolbring and Mossman are positioned to question and resist dominant notions of right and proper mobilities, but for the child who crawls, things are both more and less complicated. More complicated because children have to learn to navigate the social rules by which normalcy is measured, and less complicated because they have more opportunities for movement experimentations.

All children and particularly disabled children learn to negotiate the multiple and sometimes conflicting imperatives of safety, independence, and normative bodily styles associated with growing *up* (Stephens et al. 2015, p. 201). Within this context, however, children resist normalizing processes and may purse creative mobilities such as crawling that build from their capacity to act and do in the world. Disabled children must negotiate the increasingly negative values assigned to crawling as they age. Stephens et al. (2015) provide examples of children preferring crawling because it is faster and more efficient. In their research, "Nick," for example, complained that he was not allowed to crawl in gym class even through his wheelchair slowed him down. He said "I could get 500 points for my team on my knees" (Stephens et al. 2015, p. 204). Interestingly, one child-participant assumed that the visiting researcher would want to see her walking even though it was not her usual or preferred way of navigating at home.

In my research examining mobility values (Gibson and Teachman 2012), children traded off opportunities and constraints according to tacit social logics of cost and reward. Choices of walking, crawling, or wheeling were not only matters of efficiency, but matters of identity. Lina (age 12) for example, shared that she preferred to crawl in people's houses but also noted the importance of being identified as "someone who can walk."

She stated that in private homes crawling allowed her to more quickly navigate among big and small obstacles, and it freed her from having to bring her walker or canes. When outside and at school, however, Lina preferred to use her walker because it was faster and more pleasurable than using her wheelchair or scooter. She said: "I always want to use my walker, because it's faster for me. And I just like using it." Lina went on to discuss more generally the importance for herself and other wheelchair users of establishing that they *can* walk (if indeed they could). In discussing a picture of a girl using a wheelchair she speculated: "She knows that she can walk, it's just that people see that she maybe can't walk. She keeps having to tell people that, like, she can walk. It's just that she doesn't."

Mobilities establish and maintain moral status. For Lina, the ability to walk conferred a preferred identity, a membership with other walkers. She made it clear that when she was using *her* walker people saw her as *a* walker (using the walker to become a walker) and they recognized that the aid was "only for support." In this case, the walker identity is both an element of the assemblage and also one of its effects. Lina had incorporated the social hierarchies of mobility assemblages into her personal schematics of body and self that were reflected in her bodily styles, mobility choices, and presentation of self to the interviewer. She formed a number of different mobility assemblages according to social and material affordances and restrictions within different milieus, but she recognized that some of these mobilities were valorized and others were suspect. She thus established an identity as someone who occupies the top of this hierarchy, that is, someone who walks. Recalling Gopnik's description of the "Darwinian man," the upright walker, occupies the highest position in the moral/mobility hierarchy and the crawler is near the bottom (has not grown "up"). The physicality of high and low mobility positions maps onto the moral orderings that are reproduced by clinicians, families, teachers, and others and transformed into the mobility aspirations of children (and adults).

The complexities of disabled children's movements in and out of assemblages of bodies, places, technologies, norms, and identities suggest that simply honoring children's choices is inadequate for helping them to thrive. Preferences for one form of mobility over another may be motivated by myriad cultural indictments that valorize upright "independent" walking over other forms (Gibson et al. 2012; Stephens et al. 2015). The radical bodily styles of crawlers like Wolbring and the children in these examples suggest that linear hierarchies do not capture or accommodate the diversity of mobilities that work for people and may limit their expression. For Stephens et al. (2015, p. 205), the legitimate focus in biomedicine on some effects such as pain or injury too often obscures other effects, the "less tangible social injuries." The latter includes risks to dignity, long term health risks, and the denial of pleasure and play for its own sake (Alexander et al. 2015, Chapter 4).

Both children and adults learn to feel shame at their nonnormative bodies and mobilities that can be addressed on a number of fronts. Dispensing with the moral ordering of right and wrong ways to move opens up desire's potential for pleasure, possibility, and opportunity. Rather than expecting disabled people to alone change the social landscape through individual acts of creativity, an ethic of openness (see Chapters 1 and 7) can be mobilized to better distinguish between the ways and means that assemblages can be potentially "oppressive" and/or "emancipatory" (Ruddick 2012). Instead of hierarchies, an open-ended web of rhizomatic connections is possible with no predetermined moral ordering. Mobility focused rehabilitation is much more than the teaching and learning of safe and efficient ways to move. It is also about forming and transforming bodies-in-society. What a body can or cannot, should or should not, do. Rehabilitated bodies are bodies that have been transformed, that fit not only particular biomedical forms but also moral forms (Papadimitriou 2007). Bodies are made and unmade in rehabilitation through the shared work of different people, technologies, processes, and encounters. Unpacking these relations, as I do in the next section, shows how they enable and constrain, free up and close down, desire.

Wheelchair Mobilities

In this section, I consider a final example, wheelchair mobilities, to focus on rehabilitation and how it works to form and shape assemblages. In each of the examples chosen for the chapter, I have deliberately focused on different elements of assemblages. The labels of "amputee," "crawling," and "wheelchair" are drawn from common classifications used to distinguish different types of people, movements, and machines, but these singular terms confound an appreciation of how elements merge, flow, and change across time and space. Said differently, "amputee mobilities" could instead be labeled "prostheses mobilities" or "walking mobilities," but none of these terms captures the shifting assemblage or its effects. As arbitrary constructions of convenience, categories provide partial, fixed, and incomplete descriptions that are focused on what a thing *is* rather than what it *does*.

To help rethink these habits of thought and the implications for rehabilitation, I draw from the work of Myriam Winance (2006, 2010, 2014), who has drawn on Actor Network Theory (Mol 2002; Moser and Law 1998) to describe the "mutual shaping" of people and wheelchairs through what she calls "processes of adjustment." Through detailed ethnographic work, Winance has described how the assemblage, or in her terms "*hybrid collectif*," of body-wheelchair is made possible through the hard work of individuals and their practitioners who engage in multiple small acts of "tinkering" to construct and maintain a "suitable arrangement" of entities (Winance 2010). "Suitable" in this instance is an arrangement that requires compromise. It creates and closes off different opportunities for doing-in-the-world. I argue that a sensitive rehabilitation is one that broadly assesses opportunities for physical, emotional, and existential possibilities afforded by assemblages.

Winance's ethnographic research illuminates the work processes of rehabilitation including the efforts of professionals, clients, and other human and nonhuman actors. In one example (Winance 2010, p. 99), she describes how a physiotherapist, Benoit, is working with Mrs. S and her husband to choose and fit a new wheelchair. Benoit notes that he would usually recommend a chair sized so that "a hand can fit between the armrest and the buttock." He knows, however, that Mrs. S wants space on the seat for her handbag so he has provided her with a chair that he would usually consider as "too wide." Benoit is told that Mrs. S will propel the chair herself at home but that her husband will push it in the community. He remarks that "it's important that the back of the chair properly supports your back, and if your husband pushes a lot, he has to be able to push without too much problem." The current chair has a back that is too high for this. Mrs. S tries the new chair and is pleased. Benoit checks with her that it is not too wide and she agrees that it is fine. He asks if she wants a strap for in front of her ankles to keep her feet in place, but Mrs. S says no. She explains that her legs need a few seconds to bend but then stay in position on their own. Through the collaborative work of these actors, an assemblage is constructed. Mrs. S shares what she feels, what she likes, how her body works, and what she does and wants to do. Benoit links these possibilities and constraints to the characteristics of the wheelchair and his notion of what is important in wheelchair fit. In this way through sharing their respective perceptions, trying it out and making compromises, a suitable body-chair assemblage emerges. One could say that one assemblage, consisting of Benoit, Mrs. S, the wheelchair, and Mr. S, produced another, a new body-chair assemblage, and that the two continue to overlap in a co-constituting relationship.

Rehabilitation involves, at least in part, defining the way that humans and nonhumans can work together, to arrange themselves to achieve action. The process of adjustment is a transfer of energies that distributes competencies to produce movement (Winance 2006, p. 59). Mobility is achieved through the collective actions and adjustments of the chair, Mrs. S, Mr. S, and Benoit. When Mrs. S is away from the clinic she will sometimes move as body-chair and sometimes as body-chair-body when her husband assists. Assembling and adjusting always involves a series of compromises. We can ask, which arrangements and adjustments achieve what actions and constrain others? To provide rehabilitation is to tinker, test, adapt, adjust; to make arrangements that are world making. This is not only the job of the practitioner, but the practitioner is part of the process. Assemblages emerge out of the possibilities presented by human and nonhuman actors. In this sense, all the actors "practice" together. The question of "what can a body do?" is focused and contextualized: What can these bodies and technologies do together in this place and time? Shaping an assemblage is shared work that is dispersed in a collective and "causes the emergence of movement sensation, possibilities and abilities for everyone" (Winance 2010, p. 95). For Winance (2006, p. 60), the "action 'to move' results from the conjunction of many small impulses coming from everywhere and passing from one actor to another."

The process of adjustment is not only mechanical, it is also emotional and embodied (Papadimitriou 2007, 2008; Winance 2006). Fitting a person with a chair is not only a technical question of biomechanics or minimizing energy expenditure. The actors explore how the person feels in and about the wheelchair, and how the chair enables or constrains particular actions. Winance (2006, p. 61) explains that wheelchair adjustment involves material and emotional adjustment through which "an extended body arises ... [and] the wheelchair becomes part of the body, that is, that through which the person acts." Assembling is an alignment of both (relatively) given and malleable characteristics of person and chair: how the body-chair will mobilize with and without Mr. S's assistance, how to adjust the seat, is a strap needed, how do legs flex and extend, how can Mrs. S's bag be accommodated? The actors share and compare their feelings and perceptions to collectively define and adjust the elements of the assemblage according to what emotions, sensations, and (in)abilities it might effect. This transformation is enacted through a therapeutic relationship where individuals connect with new assembled machines to develop new bodily styles and abilities, to do-in-the-world in new ways.

Rehabilitation after illness or injury works toward turning "I cannot do" or "I can no longer do" into "I can do (again)" (Papadimitriou 2007). As per my discussion of the shaping of children's mobilities by socio-material affordances, the chair-body assemblage involves more than its two named parts. Moreover, assemblages take some effort to construct, maintain, and adjust across time and space. Processes of adjustment within and outside of rehabilitation create a common materiality where the wheelchair is incorporated into the person, "enwheeled" as Papadimitriou (2008) puts it. Enwheelment is not immediate or automatic but requires hard work and effort. Action is made possible not only through linking elements together but through shared work to transform the body, the chair, and any other elements that enter into the assemblage. These elements may appear stable in rehabilitation, but they are continually moving and adjusting in multiple ways.

Assemblages are unstable: they move, they become. There is a mutual shaping of body and chair, the body extends beyond the skin into the metal and plastic of the machine. Heights are adjusted, parts replaced, options are added or removed (headrest, foot rest, brakes, joystick). A body-chair hexis emerges: colors are chosen, decals added, even speakers are mounted (Gibson et al. 2007). A new "ontological style" is created of increasing comfort and familiarity through which the boundary of body and chair becomes increasingly porous (Papadimitriou 2008). The chair is fitted to the body but the body also molds to the chair becomes "one with it," even though the assemblage, like all assemblages, is temporary. The body-chair is remade and unmade every day, the components age together, requiring maintenance, adjustment, intervention, and tinkering. It navigates places and spaces taking on different speeds and trajectories, plugging into to other assemblages to achieve action. This making and breaking of body-chair is incorporated into a familiar repertoire of bodily styles. The body-chair is detachable but also enduring, dispersed but connected. Psychic threads join the elements such that "my chair" is still my chair even when the body is elsewhere, that is, "otherwise occupied" (Gibson 2006). The body-chair is implicated in world making. It creates possibilities for going and doing, shaping what areas are accessible or closed off. It thus *makes the world* of the becoming assembled subject. Different assemblages will make different worlds that result in networks of possibilities and constraints.

Assemblages enable but also constrain through their relations with the affordances and injunctions of socio-material contexts. The body-chair enables mobility and freedom within a dominant culture that degrades and devalues bodies labelled as disabled wheelchair-users. Recalling Mossman's experience of "running the gauntlet" on the beach, or Lina's concern that others are aware she can walk, becoming enwheeled is a navigation between the freedom to do, and the social regulations against doing it differently. Becoming mobile involves "a constant challenge of negotiating, reorganizing and reconfiguring one's way of being, especially in public, in order to achieve the status of "active doer" (Papadimitriou 2008, p. 71). For Papadimitriou (2008, p. 71), a paradox occurs whereby "the accomplishment of becoming en-wheeled and of achieving re-embodiment by 'doing' can stigmatize users since it is this very accomplishment that brings them out in public where they are seen as unable to 'do.'"

The assemblage construction process that I outlined above is both descriptive and unapologetically prescriptive. I have drawn from a post-critical lens to describe some existing rehabilitation practices in order to illuminate *what works* or not in the broadest possible sense. It is prescriptive, not in terms of insisting on one right way of doing things but in terms of providing a new methodology that can be used for understanding what we do in rehabilitation and help better identify possibilities and problems that might otherwise be obscured. Another way of getting at this is through thought experiments regarding the goals of mobility training. What if, for example, therapy was seen as an end in itself primarily oriented to pleasures, sensations, fun, or new ways to experience the body without regard for carry over or improvement in function? In at least some rehabilitation programs this is indeed a goal, a goal that is taken seriously. For example, in some instances, "ambulation training" for individuals with spinal cord injuries is focused primarily on body sensations and learning to feel the altered body in new and different ways (Winance 2010). Such an end however does not easily align with the traditional mandates of rehabilitation, the principles of the ICF, or the domains of standardized assessment measures. It is a goal that is likely not shared too loudly with funders or proudly published in annual reports. But that does not mean it has no value. Clinicians know this. Elsewhere (Gibson and Teachman 2012) I have suggested that we should rethink ambulation training for those who have little chance of becoming functional walkers, but I admit that this conclusion only makes sense if the goal is mobility. The mobility experiences enabled through therapeutic assemblages might be ends in themselves, allowing persons to feel their bodies (physically and affectively) in new ways, or in old ways that have been lost through trauma or disease. The idea of the desiring machine when employed as a flexible principle of analysis helps to break free from assumptions of a fixed desired endpoint, to question and question again. To remain vigilant, stay open, to consider: if this, then what, and what else?

Mobility Movements

> The invention of the unknown demands new forms.
>
> Rimbaud*

* Cited in Halpern (2009).

Mobility assemblages provide a way of thinking differently about movement, circumventing the hierarchies of mobilities that permeate the social order and find expression in rehabilitation practices. In empirically presenting the range of both valorized and discredited mobilities used by disabled people, I have suggested that the moral ordering of movement impedes desire and human flourishing. For Shildrick (2015, p. 24), flourishing is expressed "in going to the limits of what is possible, embracing fluidity and radical change, dispensing with fixed identities, and affirming a becoming whose form can neither be predicted nor settled in the future." Reimagining the ontology of the body-subject creates opportunities for new contingent bodily forms and new ways of doing-in-the-world that do not rely on existing mobilities or preconceived uses of technologies and spaces.

The acceptance, promotion, and creation of new assemblages suggest a reconceived mobility ethics. This open ethic lets go of fixed standards of embodiment, programmatic goals, or rehabilitation practices and opens up transformative possibilities. Accepting that difference is the default human condition, creates opportunities for new mobility forms and new rehabilitation practices that diverge from predetermined goals such as upright or independent mobility. Rethinking mobility means attending to the social ordering of Wolbring's crawling-body below Pistorius' running-body, thinking through the conditions that perpetuate these divisions, and illuminating how things could be otherwise.

This is arguably the most "theoretical" of the topic-focused chapters in the book, but I would argue it is also the most "applied" (although I find this kind of distinction problematic). The application is this: Rehabilitation is a process of assembling bodies that has multiple physical, social, and existential effects. Assemblages enable and disable, hurt and heal, make new worlds and close off others. Doing rehabilitation then is a process of discovering what kinds of effects and possibilities result from what assemblages. This requires creativity and sensitivity about how hierarchies and social rules dampen experimentation. It requires tinkering and hard work, helping individuals become new assemblages of desiring machines that adjust in multiple ways. It requires both letting go and connecting. Assembling is what we do in rehabilitation, but deliberative and detailed analyses of these processes can provide new insights for practice that allow for exploration of new body possibilities.

References

Alexander, S. A., Frohlich, K. L. and Fusco, C. 2014. Active play may be lots of fun, but it's certainly not frivolous: The emergence of active play as a health practice in Canadian public health. *Sociology of Health & Illness* 36(8): 1188–1204.

Bordo, S. 1993. Feminism, Foucault and the politics of the body. In *Up against Foucault: Explorations of Some Tensions between Foucault and Feminism*, ed. C. Ramazanoglu, pp. 179–202. New York: Routledge.

Bourdieu, P. 1997. *Pascalian Meditations*. Stanford, CA: Stanford University Press.

Crossley, N. 2005. Mapping reflexive body techniques: On body modification and maintenance. *Body & Society* 11(1): 1–35.

Deleuze, G. and Guattari, F. 1983. *Anti-Oedipus: Capitalism and Schizophrenia*. Minneapolis, MN: University of Minnesota Press.

Deleuze, G. and Guattari, F. 1987. *A Thousand Plateaus: Capitalism and Schizophrenia*. Minneapolis, MN: University of Minnesota Press.

Fraser, N. and Gordon, L. 1994. Dependency demystified: Inscriptions of power in a keyword of the welfare state. *International Studies in Gender, State and Society* 1(1): 4–31.

Gibson, B.E. 2006. Disability, connectivity and transgressing the autonomous body. *Journal of Medical Humanities* 27(3): 187–196.

Gibson, B.E., Carnevale, F.A. and King, G. 2012. "This is my way": Reimagining disability, independence, and interconnectedness of persons and assistive technologies. *Disability and Rehabilitation* 34(22): 1894–1899.

Gibson, B.E., Mistry, B., Smith, B., Yoshida et al. 2014. Becoming men: Gender, disability, and transitioning to adulthood. *Health* 18(1): 93–112.

Gibson, B.E. and Teachman, G. 2012. Critical approaches in physical therapy research: Investigating the symbolic value of walking. *Physiotherapy Theory Practice* 28(6): 474–484.

Gibson, B.E., Young, N.L., Upshur, R.E., and McKeever, P. 2007. Men on the margin: A Bourdieusian examination of living into adulthood with muscular dystrophy. *Social Science & Medicine* 65(3): 505–517.

Goffman, E. 1963. *Stigma: Notes on the Management of Spoiled Identity*. New York: Simon & Schuster.

Gopnik, A. 2014. Heaven's gaits: What we do when we walk. *The New Yorker*. September 1, online issue. http://www.newyorker.com/magazine/2014/09/01/heavens-gaits (accessed March 10, 2015).

Graham, L.J. and Slee, R. 2008. An illusory interiority: Interrogating the discourse/s of inclusion. *Educational Philosophy and Theory* 40(2): 277.

Gutfleisch, O. 2003. Peg legs and bionic limbs: The development of lower extremity prosthetics. *Interdisciplinary Science Reviews* 28(2): 139–148.

Halpern, R. 2009. Baudelaire's "Dark Zone": The Poème en Prose as Social Hieroglyph; or the beginning and the end of commodity aesthetics. *Modernist Cultures* 4(1–2): 1–23.

Hoffman, M. 2013. Bodies completed: On the physical rehabilitation of lower limb amputees. *Health* 17(3): 229–245.

McLaren, C., Ruddick, S., Edwards, G., Zabjek, K., and McKeever, P. 2012. Children's movement in an integrated kindergarten classroom: Design, method and preliminary findings. *Children, Youth and Environments* 22(1): 145–177.

Mol, A. 2002. *The Body Multiple: Ontology in Medical Practice*. Durham, U.K.: Duke University Press.

Moser, I. and Law, J. 1998. Good passages, bad passages. *The Sociological Review* 46(S): 196–219.

Mossman, M. 2001. Acts of becoming: Autobiography, *Frankenstein*, and the postmodern body. *Postmodern Culture* 11(3). http://muse.jhu.edu/journals/postmodern_culture/v011/11.3mossman.html (accessed October 3, 2015).

Murray, C.D. 2009. Being like everybody else: The personal meanings of being a prosthesis user. *Disability Rehabilitation* 31(7): 573–581.

Nansen, B. 2007. Machine breaths: Assembling the mechanical ventilator body. *Transformations* (14). http://www.transformationsjournal.org/journal/issue_14/article_02.shtml (accessed March 10, 2015).

Norman, M.E. and Moola, F. 2011. 'Bladerunner or boundary runner?': Oscar pistorius, cyborg transgressions and strategies of containment. *Sport in Society* 14(9): 1265–1279.

Papadimitriou, C. 2007. 'It was hard but you did it': The co-production of 'work' in a clinical setting among spinal cord injured adults and their physical therapists. *Disability & Rehabilitation* 30(5): 365–374.

Papadimitriou, C. 2008. Becoming en-wheeled: The situated accomplishment of re-embodiment as a wheelchair user after spinal cord injury. *Disability & Society* 23(7): 691–704.

Pasquina, P.F., Bryant, P.R., Huang, M.E., Roberts, T.L., Nelson, V.S., and Flood, K.M. 2006. Advances in amputee care. *Archives of Physical Medicine and Rehabilitation* 87(3): 34–43.

Ravaud, J.F. and Stiker, H.J. 2001. Inclusion/exclusion: An analysis of historical and cultural meanings. In *Handbook of Disability Studies*, eds. G.L. Albrecht, K.D. Seelman, and M. Bury, pp. 490–514. London, U.K.: Sage Publications.

Ruddick, S. 2012. Power and the problem of composition. *Dialogues in Human Geography* 2(2): 207–211.

Shildrick, M. 2010. Some reflections on the socio-cultural and bioscientific limits of bodily integrity. *Body and Society* 16(3): 11–22.

Shildrick, M. 2015. "Why should our bodies end at the skin?": Embodiment, boundaries, and somatechnics. *Hypatia* 30(1): 13–29.

Stephens, L., Ruddick, S., and McKeever, P. 2015. Disability and Deleuze: An exploration of becoming and embodiment in children's everyday environments. *Body & Society* 21(2): 194–220.

Straus, E.W. 1952. The upright posture. *Psychiatric Quarterly* 26(1): 529–561.

Swanson, L. n.d. Gregor Wolbring: An ardent advocate. Abilities, Online magazine. http://abilities.ca/gregor-wolbring/ (accessed October 5, 2015).

Swartz, L. and Watermeyer, B. 2008. Cyborg anxiety: Oscar pistorius and the boundaries of what it means to be human. *Disability & Society* 23(2): 187–190.

Taguchi, H.L. and Palmer, A. July 1, 2014. Reading a Deleuzio-guattarian cartography of young girls' "School-related" ill-/well-being. *Qualitative Inquiry* 20(6): 764–771.

Winance, M. 2006. Trying out the wheelchair: The mutual shaping of people and devices through adjustment. *Science, Technology, & Human Values* 31(1): 52–72.

Winance, M. 2010. Care and disability: Practices of experimenting, tinkering with, and arranging people and technical aids. In *Care in Practice: On Tinkering in Clinics, Homes and Farms*, eds. A. Mol, I. Moser, and J. Pols, pp. 93–117. Bielefeld, Germany: Verlag.

Winance, M. 2014. Universal design and the challenge of diversity: Reflections on the principles of UD, based on empirical research of people's mobility. *Disability & Rehabilitation* 36(16): 1334–1343.

7
Re-Forming Rehabilitation

What are you doing when you are doing what you are doing? This is the question that one of my mentors, William Harvey, routinely asks of his students. When I first heard it many years ago I did not think that much of it. It was witty and seemed like a good reminder of the importance of reflexivity. But it has stuck with me ever since and comes to mind in all the instances where I have encountered practices, including my own, that have become routine and unquestioned. This deceptively simple question provides a methodology for a movement. It provides the point of departure to re-form, re-examine, and re-do practice by considering: Why are we doing this? Why this way? How does it affect people both positively and negatively? Does it need to change? How could it be done differently?

In this final chapter, I expand on the key messages of the book toward moving rehabilitation in new directions of practice, research, and scholarship. I do so by revisiting and integrating the concepts and categories discussed in each of the chapters, highlighting examples of creative practices, and signposting possibilities for change. Drawing on the post-critical lens, I summarize and further elucidate how a reflexive ethic of openness facilitates a continuous transposition of theory and practice that promotes new ways of thinking and doing rehabilitation. I conclude with some directions for disrupting the status quo, that is, for expanding post-critical rehabilitation scholarship and practice, including a call for more cross-pollination between rehabilitation and critical disability studies.

Continuities of Theory with Practice

I have argued throughout the book that questioning entrenched practices in rehabilitation (or any other system) reveals how the empirical and the theoretical are two moments of the same enterprise. Said differently, there is no practice that is free of conceptual commitments. If we continue to rely on our usual frameworks, questions of what we do and why we are bound to be answered in very narrow ways, drawing on unexamined habits of thought. For example, practices oriented to helping individuals to speak (Chapter 5) or walk (Chapter 6) in typical ways rely on a particular normative ordering of valorized or discredited bodily styles that produce limited options regarding different possible interventions. The post-critical approach that I have advocated questions the whole set of premises and assumptions that orient practices, not to say that they are necessarily wrong in every instance, but to question the assumption that they are always right. This theoretical move is not, as some might argue, questioning for its own sake. Rather, it is infinitely *practical* in that it suggests different ways, not only of thinking, but of doing practice.

Theory changes practice in profound ways, more than we might realize. It would be naive to suggest that the move away from impairment-based rehabilitation is solely, or even mostly, a response to empirical evidence—indeed, rehabilitation has rather low rates of translating research into practice (Leplège et al. 2015). Rather the move from impairment to participation is primarily a *philosophical* shift that can be traced to historical sociopolitical developments in the Western world including the emergence of the welfare state, the identification of disabled people as a group requiring state supports, and the emergence of specialty rehabilitation professionals and practices within medicine (see Leplège et al. 2015; Stiker 1999). More recently, in the 1970s and 1980s, the powerful influence of disability activists and scholars led to major reforms in how disability was defined and understood, and shaped the outcomes of interest in research. These changes are enshrined in current legislation and international policies such as the UN Convention on the Rights of Persons with Disabilities (United Nations 2006), which has specific requirements for the provision of rehabilitation services. Moreover, changes in rehabilitation practices were, and still are, directly shaped by the development of disablement models such as the Disability Creation Process (Fougeyrollas and INDCP 2010) and the ICIDH/ICF (see Chapter 2). Each of these developments progresses and constrains rehabilitation in particular ways, revealing how practices both shape and are shaped by theory, with each informing the other in the continual (r)evolution of rehabilitation.

All rehabilitation practitioners draw from particular philosophical commitments whether they do so consciously or not. Reflexive theorizing, whether at the level of individual reflection or formal analysis, provides a method for surfacing the dominant ideas that mediate practice. Theory helps us to analyze what we do and why, and how our practices might be helpful, harmful, or both. It helps us to examine deeply the effects and consequences of what we do on individuals, groups, and institutions; to consider how rehabilitation addresses or exacerbates social problems and how. A reflexive approach that critiques the dominance of bioscience is increasingly promoted in the health sciences and rehabilitation (Kinsella and Whiteford 2009; Kuper and D'Eon 2011). We might call this an expansive notion of professional or *epistemic* reflexivity (Bourdieu and Wacquant 1992) that incorporates a consideration of our individual and shared philosophical commitments.

Epistemic reflexivity speaks not only to dominant bioscientific frameworks but also to the habits of thought in post-critical and other forms of inquiry. Another maxim repeated by William Harvey (popularized by Maslow in the 1960s) comes to mind: *If all you have is a hammer, everything looks like a nail.* I have throughout this book advocated for a post-critical approach to rehabilitation through an examination of some of its most entrenched concepts and frameworks. But let me be clear that I do not intend for a post-critical approach to replace any other approach. It is not a new hammer to replace the old one. It is a method, a way of seeing that the "nails" of rehabilitation—like disability, quality of life, development, independence—may not be nails at all, and that the objects and purposes of rehabilitation should not be taken for granted as right or true. But nor should they be assumed to be false. Reflexivity thus insists that we accept ambiguity and adopt doubt as a necessary stance that should not paralyze practice but help us to remain open to other possibilities.

Instead of establishing the truth or falsity of different conceptual commitments, a post-critical approach asks "what do they *do*?" considered in the broadest sense possible. What are the apparent/immediate effects and consequences as well as the more latent or distal ones? What are the physical, psychological, social, political, cultural, and existential consequences of rehabilitation practices in teaching, research, and the clinic? In the examples provided in this book, I have examined some of the (perhaps) less apparent effects of rehabilitation's conceptual commitments and suggested some possibilities for change. What I have not done is offered any specific normative criteria for judging practice. The question of what is "good" practice remains to be determined in local contexts. It is thus left up to the reader to consider how a post-critical lens might be mobilized in different fields. For rehabilitation to grow and thrive—to move in new and varied directions that accommodate a plurality of approaches—I suggest that constant vigilance, debate, and discussion are needed. We must remain open to creative ways of rethinking, re-doing, and re-forming rehabilitation. These kinds of efforts were important in the movements away from a disease model of rehabilitation, but they continue as rehabilitation expands in new and multiple directions. Where else can they take us?

Revisiting the Ethics of Openness

The post-critical approach to rehabilitation I have outlined relies on an ethic of openness—one that blends medical, social, discursive, phenomenological, and moral perspectives while affirming that none of these perspectives are independent of the others and are inadequate when applied in isolation. The ethic of openness I promote comes from the work of Margrit Shildrick, a feminist philosopher and prominent scholar of what she terms "post conventional" critical disability studies (Shildrick 2002, 2009). Shildrick (2005) reminds us that all practice is inevitably a normative enterprise. Contra mainstream bioethics she reminds us that ethics is not outside of practice. It cannot be judged from the top-down application of principles or rules of conduct because ethics is always saturated in context and lived through our bodies. An ethics that is limited to particular problems and dilemmas that are subjected to bioethical frameworks for decision-making is thus insufficient to grapple with the intersecting psychological, social, material, historical, and discursive mediators of practice. Rehabilitation practices, like other medical practices, contribute to other societal conversations about what constitutes right and proper ways of looking, being, and doing. In the everyday doings of practice, bodies and identities are made and remade to align with common notions of the good. Nothing is neutral or objective. Whether putatively evidence-based or not, all rehabilitation practices are inescapably ethically loaded. Practices that are helpful in one way can in the same moment function to control, contain, and normalize, to produce and sustain particular modes of being and doing (Shildrick 2005). A reflexive open stance is sensitive to these multiple consequences of rehabilitation and adjusts practices accordingly.

An ethic of openness emerges from a position of doubt in which there is no predetermined right way to practice. As Shildrick (2005, pp. 14–15) outlines:

> The issue is not to "prove" the superiority of one system over another...but to take the risk of thinking otherwise. In place of certainty, determinacy, and resolution, there is a reflective awareness that outcomes are intrinsically uncertain. Real lives are not conducted singly on any neat, logical plane of abstraction, but as messy and complex constructs that are interwoven with one another in unpredictable and highly changeable ways. In the face of such a dynamic, the

> task cannot be to impose the order of answers that will prevail unchallenged over time, but to *let go* of the solid ground where certain analytical categories and concepts are fixed in advance, and to continually reopen the questions themselves. (*emphasis added*)

What does this "letting go" mean for rehabilitation practice? Firstly, a post-critical approach is a tool, not an ideology. I have included some possible implications for research and practice in each of the chapters not to prescribe a new truth, but to demonstrate possibilities, lines of flight, and creative potentials. Resisting closure, categorization, and decidability, an ethic of openness is an ethic of difference, a movement away from ossification and stasis—re-formations, perturbations, agitations, and disruptions—in the most positive and productive sense. It is about embracing uncertainty, unleashing desire (Chapter 6), changing attitudes, and assumptions not just within rehabilitation but beyond: becoming a key site for (r)evolution. The only prescriptive piece I offer is this: ask "What are you doing when you are doing what you are doing?"

What constitutes a better life for any individual cannot be known in advance. It is not equivalent with independence, or upright mobility, or normative body morphology; nor can it be reduced to a set of domains on a questionnaire. As Mol suggests (2008, pp. 75–76) "It is important to do good, to make life better than it would have otherwise been. But what it is to do good, what leads to a better life, is not given before the act. It has to be established along the way. It may differ between lives or between moments in a life." The task of health care is the task of attending to difference that is never settled but characterized by constant twists, turns, problems, frictions, and complications. It involves the hard work of doubt. Doubt is difficult for professionals who are trained to be experts, whose job it is to know things, to have answers, to educate patients (Hammell 2006, p. 199). Doubt, uncertainty, openness, and reflexivity, however, are essential to avoid stasis, to move rehabilitation in creative directions that best meet the needs of the people and communities we serve.

Implications: Mobilizing and Re-Forming

Every chapter of this book has looked at a method of categorization and/or a particular category, asked how well it is serving the recipients of rehabilitation care, and how things might be otherwise. Problematizing particular categorized objects of interest, like disability or quality of life, serves to trouble their status as natural, true, or real. Post-critical analysis reveals how objects of care are produced as categories of interest, the complex relations that sustain them, and the effects of their practical applications (Bacchi 2012). In so doing, it extends biomedicine/rehabilitation's outcomes of interest to include the social, political, and existential consequences of practice. Knowledge, the naturalized "truth" of rehabilitation, is revealed by examining what is done in and through practices (Mol 2002, pp. 1–6). With this in mind, in what follows I offer a "summary that resists closure" by revisiting Chapters 2 through 6 in terms of the effects of categorization, and the possibilities for rehabilitation in adopting a post-critical ethic of openness.

The normative ordering of disability and normalcy is likely the most profoundly influential categorization underpinning rehabilitation practices. In Chapter 2, I argued that disability is a constructed but unstable category that could be reconfigured to admit that difference is the default human condition. I suggested that an acceptance of difference is not meant to erase it, or to claim that differences do not or should not matter. Rather, acceptance requires a radical reformulation of the moral ordering of differences. This theme recurs throughout the book. An ethic of openness may not necessarily reject all forms of classification employed in biomedicine and rehabilitation, but as a responsible ethics it lays them open to scrutiny. The task is to mediate among competing interpretations of variation toward identifying the implications for individual lives (Scully 2005). "What are you doing when you are doing what you are doing?" in research and clinical practice translates into: "What are you doing *for*, *with*, and/or *to* someone and *why*?" An expansive open approach considers how practices that rely on identifying and addressing deviation from the norm always risks enabling and disabling in the same moment, if not the individual recipient of care, then the groups and groupings that it implicates.

Troubling the normal/disabled divide can facilitate creative rehabilitation practices. Bill Shannon's innovative mobilities provide a point of departure for demonstrating this point. Shannon is an artist and dancer who mobilizes with or without a skateboard using rounded tipped crutches of his own design (a video is available in Break.com [2006]). In the video Shannon uses his crutches in various fluid and seemingly effortless ways. His movements are suggestive of a dance, and indeed he is an accomplished dancer who brings in elements of hip-hop, punk, and break dancing into his celebrated performances. In his youth, as Shannon was learning to navigate material obstacles (stairs, curbs, etc.) he incorporated different movements that drew on his abilities and the tools at hand. To a rehabilitation practitioner, these movements may have been viewed as risky from a biomechanical or safety point of view. Shannon, who has a diagnosis of Legg Calvé-Perthes disease, would have been taught to mimic normal walking with elbow crutches. Instead, he developed his own adaptable methods of mobility that built on his capabilities and his aesthetic preferences. Shannon describes his flexible approach this way: "You are relating to your environment as it comes to you on an improvisational freestyle basis." His unconventional approach to mobility provides an opportunity for reflection and suggests some possible lessons for rehabilitation.

As repeatedly argued throughout the book, letting go of the moral ordering of normal/disabled and all of its expressions can produce new forms of being and doing. Shannon's hybrid mobilities defy easy categorization. His movements draw elements of more typical mobilities used by disabled and nondisabled people by incorporating crutches and skateboards as ready-to-hand tools. Rehabilitation has the opportunity to facilitate these creative solutions, not just in terms of mobility but through any practice that is open to questioning conventions by building on people's strengths in addressing their everyday challenges. Crawling as a mode of mobility (Chapter 6) is an example of an existing form that is highly discouraged in rehabilitation, as is any type of function that relies on human assistance (Chapter 5). An ethic of openness challenges these preconceived notions to develop, rather than discourage, creative solutions.

If we take Mol's assertion (quoted earlier) seriously that what leads to a better life is not known in advance, we must proceed very cautiously with judgments of quality of life. In Chapter 3, I noted some of the inherent problems and shortcomings of attempting to measure this ineffable concept that resists standardization. The value of a life is not only an intensely personal judgment, it is also a shifting one. Thus, even though it may be possible to outline "domains" of life that are implicated in life quality, the relative importance of each varies and shifts from person to person and across time and place. Measurements that reduce quality of life to a set of numbers thus risk finalizing that which is always unsettled.

From a rehabilitation perspective, we need to be especially cautious of the tendency in our research and clinical practices to equate poor function with poor quality of life. This is not to say that functional improvements do not help people. Of course they can and they do. It is the assumption that dysfunction (and/or what gets labeled as "dysfunction") is always problematic that should give us pause. In Chapter 3, I made a distinction between the concept of quality of life (life quality) and biomedicine's measurement of the construct of "QOL." I suggested that, at the very least, in every instance of QOL measurement, reflection is needed regarding what is being measured—particularly what causal links are assumed and why. If function is being measured (or symptoms, activities of daily life, etc.), there is no need to assume that low scores equate to a reduced life quality. Moreover, both formal measurement and clinical judgments of QOL perpetuate particular notions of what lives, and by extension persons, are good or bad. Measures and the normative discourses surrounding them produce particular subject positions that are difficult to subvert (Abrams and Gibson in press). The ethical implications of these practices in supporting or condemning disabled lives are too considerable to ignore.

The move in rehabilitation toward greater emphasis on quality of life and participation outcomes requires a nuanced approach to apprehending what counts as a successful intervention. Measurement scientists have increasingly grappled with how to conceptualize and measure a host of complex social outcomes including (health related) quality of life, participation, disability, and inclusion that do not fit easily within positivist frameworks. As I noted in Chapter 3, these debates continue with no signs of abatement despite the burgeoning number of measures available. I have suggested that the pursuit of the right measure, with the right constellation of domains and elements, risks perpetuating the problem even while trying to solve it. I do not dispute that it might be useful to know how much assistance a person needs with, for example, brushing their hair or eating in a restaurant. What is contentious is how that information is used in the singular or aggregate to imply the goodness of lives. Measurement practices function to categorize, produce, and sustain the normal/disabled divide. This is an example of "When all you have is a hammer, everything looks like a nail." The hammer has its uses but it is insufficient, and at times deleterious, to the task that rehabilitation has set itself—to improve the life quality of people affected by illness or injury.

Addressing the complexity of disability requires more than the decontextualized numbers supplied by objective measures. What counts to people is not easily counted but it can be interrogated both individually and collectively to inform rehabilitation practices. Listening to people's stories on their own terms, rather than structured by professionals as "cases" or "subjective histories," is a promising line of flight supported by a burgeoning corpus of qualitative research. Stories are messy, complex, full of contradictions and emotions, and shifting values that nevertheless provide insight into what matters to individuals and their sense-making practices (Frank 2000, 2010; Mattingly 1998; Smith 2013; Soundy et al. 2014; Warren and Manderson 2008). Theory and narratives can be used together to make sense of what we are doing and what care recipients are saying, and how our collective and divergent sociopolitical histories mediate what we do and think. They stimulate and ground creative, productive, movement possibilities that include, but extend beyond, dominant modes of positivist rehabilitation science.

Child development is an exemplar *par excellence* of the effects of classification in creating the seemingly stable categories we use to define people. The distinction between "child" and "adult" is a rather recent one in human history (James and James 2004) and development discourses have given rise to commonly held perceptions of the "normal" child. In Chapter 4, I cautioned against interventions aimed at approximating developmental scales that treat children solely as adults in the making. The act of categorizing people into groups is always an act of defining the characteristics of the group. The division between child and adult may start with biological age criteria, but it carries with it a host of normative expectations about how children and adults should conduct their lives and selves. Categories of dependent/independent, child/adult, and disabled/normal hold the weight of judgment in ways that conspire to mark and exclude people labeled as disabled. Bodies that fail to function according to the standards of right and proper (normal, independent) adulthood are socially marginalized and identified for rehabilitation. This is as much the case for older people as it is for children.

The normative expectations inherent in developmental discourses perpetuate idealized notions of what adults should be and do, and further reflect notions of normality/disability. Mark Priestley (2003, pp. 19–25) has termed age-based classifications "generations" and discusses generational norms in relation to other categories of oppression including race, gender, and ability. Attention to these categories, he notes, helps in the analysis of how identities intersect and are (re)produced. Generational categories are relational because they are defined only in contrast with each other. Like other identity categories there is a moral ordering that sets up power differentials between different groups such that in the child/adult hierarchy, the adult is constructed as the preferred position. This has implications not only in identifying "at-risk" children who may not fully attain proper adulthood, but also for those adults marked as "failures" of one kind or another. These are the individuals who are, for example, not working or "contributing" to society, and/or labeled as "dependent" because they need particular kinds of help with daily life. Dependency is thus equated with children and is only permissible for the very young or the very old.

While the disability/normalcy divide may be the most influential categorization in rehabilitation, the dichotomy of independence/dependence has likely been subject to the least critical scrutiny. While independence has been widely critiqued and replaced with the notion of interdependence (at least with regard to some populations), dependence remains discredited and largely unexamined, maintaining the same lowly moral positioning in a modified binary of *inter*dependence/dependence. In Chapter 5, I outlined how neoliberal notions of the independent subject pervade both rehabilitation and (traditional) disability studies, with a point of disagreement surrounding not the value of independence, but rather what forms should be pursued, for example, functional independence or self-determination. Interdependence has been introduced in both fields to acknowledge the networks of mutual giving and receiving that characterize the human condition. This move has served to expose some of the negative effects of independence discourses on those who are profoundly dependent, but perhaps most importantly, interdependence scholarship and particularly feminist studies have problematized the presumed inherent worth of independence. Nevertheless, the shift to interdependence relies on a notion of deservedness that I have suggested does not go far enough in challenging entrenched negative valuations of dependency.

In rehabilitation, interdependence is usually discussed in the context of particular populations who have ongoing functional dependencies, while independence remains the stated or implicit goal for others. Thus a curious contradiction can be observed. Interdependence is positioned as the default human condition, yet independence remains the underpinning goal for anyone who might be able to achieve it in some form or other. The result is that interdependence is often framed as a kind of consolation prize for people who will continue to require help with their activities of daily living. Rehabilitation is still firmly focused on achieving the least amount of help as needed, that is, as independent as possible. Thus interdependence in its current applications requires some significant remodeling that, I have argued, is assisted by postmodern notions of connectivity to which I now turn.

In Chapters 5 and 6, I drew on the "post" side of post-critical to suggest potential benefits of a rehabilitation that embraces dependency through the postmodern concept of assemblages. Like interdependence, assemblages insist that humans are profoundly connected. Unlike most formulations of interdependence, however, assemblage theory decenters the individual subject and instead is concerned with how human and nonhuman elements come together to enable actions. Various dependencies are enacted and abandoned in processes of becoming that create multiple ways of doing and being. Not only new ways to function, but new subject positions and identities that temporarily fuse different actors and objects into a series of connectivities that come together and break apart in continual motion. Assemblages shift the analytical gaze away from the *person* at the center (pervasively evident in visual representations of rehabilitation models) to *actions*, and to determining what configurations enable actions. Doing so creates an analytical space for escaping the moral ordering of independence and dependence that persists in common formulations of interdependence.

The implications for rehabilitation are potentially extensive. If independence is no longer an assumed goal, then a whole range of practices are open to possible reform. Certainly all the judgments and measures of function, participation, disability, and quality of life that assume independent abilities are better than those that require human or technical assistance would have to be re-examined. Moreover, clinical practices would shift from assuming that a decreased reliance on persons and devices is always worth pursuing (it is noteworthy that rehabilitation tends to order assistive devices and personal assistance, with the former positioned as preferable to the latter). Two anecdotal examples help to further demonstrate how rehabilitation might shift away from independence as a presumed endpoint.

The first example comes from a colleague, Thomas Abrams, and his personal experiences with rehabilitation. Thomas is a sociologist and disability studies scholar who has Becker's muscular dystrophy. Recently he was referred to physiotherapy because he had started to fall more frequently. He was asked about his goals to which he explained that he would like to avoid falling when walking. But the therapist suggested a reframing of his goals as "How about you want to maintain independence and falling is an obstacle there?" She then proceeded to ask him to rate his current level of independence and his goal level (Abrams and Gibson in press). Thomas rated his current level of independence at a 4 and his goal at an 8. To put these ratings in context, Thomas receives minimal or no assistance with his daily activities and his impairments are largely invisible. I would have guessed his current rating would be a 8 or 9. When I asked him why a "4," he could offer no explanation other than expressing frustration with the entire process. He did not want to be categorized according to a "level of independence" or to have his experience of illness reduced to a delimited set of goals and measures. He found the process inane and baffling.

In a more analytical vein, Thomas viewed the encounter as "enacting" his humanity in particular ways that shaped his body into a coherent object for medical intervention. He suggested that the clinical relationship required him to take up the subject position of "physiotherapy patient," which imposed a particular way of presenting his experiences and desires (Abrams and Gibson in press). I would hazard a guess that the physiotherapist had no notion of these effects, but rather felt she had helped Thomas to articulate his goals in a measurable way. The act of articulation, however, was experienced by Thomas as an act of appropriation. Constructing his desire to stop falling as a medicalized goal enacted his humanity in ways that he continues to resist, not because he does not want therapy, but because he wants a more humane form of caring that allows him to choose the ways he is "made subject to" therapeutic measures and perceived goals of independence (Abrams 2015).

A second example illustrates how reconceiving independence can change clinical practice. This comes from my collaborations with two occupational therapists (OTs) who were part of our research team exploring place-based mediators of activity participation with disabled young people who used augmentative and alternative communication (AAC). In the course of the study, which I discussed in Chapter 5 (Gibson et al. 2013; King et al. 2013), the two OTs assisted with conducting naturalistic observations, experiencing firsthand how young AAC users communicate and accomplish other tasks in their everyday environments. The OTs also contributed to our regular analysis meetings where we drew on assemblage theory to illuminate how different connectivities were enabling and/or disabling for participants. This gave the OTs the opportunity to see how contextually grounded theorizing could illuminate and inform their practices.

The OT collaborators were struck by how the experience of working on the project challenged their thinking and practices. These two women were excellent, caring practitioners with considerable experience in the field. Nevertheless, immersing themselves in the details of when, how, and why young people used AAC technologies versus communication assistants (or both) changed how they approached their work. The study revealed that AAC devices could be tremendously enabling at times, and at other times made life unnecessarily harder. Independence was often less of an issue for participants than other concerns such as the amount of effort required to use a device, but these priorities shifted with the context and over time. Drawing on the notion of enabling assemblages, the OTs modified their practices from promoting independent communication, to assessing with their clients which assemblages worked or not in what contexts. Within this framework, independent communication was still a possible outcome but not an assumed priority for every young person or in every context. Human assistance or device abandonment was viewed less as failures and more as other ways of being and doing that might work for particular AAC users and their families. This was a sometimes subtle shift that required different dialogues with families, and working together to assess, tinker, and adjust with renewed notions of what constitutes successful rehabilitation.

A post-critical lens suggests not only new practices but, as an analytical tool, helps reframe existing ones. The OTs in the example did not radically change what they did with families. They still pulled from the same toolbox of assessments and interventions in conducting their work. The transformation was instead a philosophical shift, an act of epistemic reflexivity that arose from their exposure to a new methodology for understanding rehabilitation practices that was grounded in clients' experiences. Rehabilitation practitioners are always working toward enabling individuals and are continually looking for the better ways to enhance the lives of care recipients. This may be achieved through new interventions but also through a reformed understanding of the desired endpoints. Post-critical assemblage analysis challenges the dominance of independence in rehabilitation not to discount it, but to provide a method for examining its effects and considering alternatives.

In Chapter 6, I extended the discussion of assemblages and the work of Deleuze and Guattari to examine questions of mobility and further apply the ideas explored in previous chapters. The valuing of some mobilities over others reveals and reflects the moral ordering of disability in the social world, which is extended into rehabilitation. For example, consider Bill Shannon's methods of mobilizing described earlier compared to the crawling mobilities described in Chapter 6. Shannon's skateboard symbolizes a kind of counterculture that juxtaposes often negatively marked assistive devices such as medical crutches, wheelchairs, or walkers. His creative use of a skateboard might be considered "cool," "progressive," or "enhancing," but crawling, particularly by an adult, is more likely to evoke negative reactions. Nevertheless, as I have suggested elsewhere (Gibson 2014), both raise questions about what kinds of bodies, movements, and devices are taken for granted in rehabilitation or in the design of devices and accessible spaces.

Problematizing the moral ordering of mobilities raises the question: Could functional crawling be a rehabilitation goal? Rehabilitation does not traditionally focus on supporting crawling ability, or for that matter, innovative uses of skateboards. These modes of mobility were largely discovered and developed by the individuals that employ them and not by rehabilitation professionals. One could imagine that some professionals might even actively discourage these choices. My point is that rehabilitation researchers and clinicians could have been helpful and could be highly instrumental in this regard with other clients. Leaving it up to individuals to find their own creative solutions outside of rehabilitation orthodoxy will inevitably exclude some people, including those without the time or resources, or those who have difficulty with abstract thinking, planning, or problem solving (Fadyl et al. 2015). As such, practitioners have the opportunity and, I would argue, the responsibility to challenge the status quo, to develop and support these sorts of innovations as part of their commitments to finding enabling solutions.

Rhizomatic Reforms

At the outset of this book, I claimed that my task was to foment a revolution. Perhaps at this point I can be more precise; the task is to provoke rhizomatic movements in rehabilitation. In botany, rhizomes are underground stems that connect plant life. Deleuze and Guattari (1987, pp. 3–25) have employed rhizomes to challenge traditional hierarchical modes of knowledge that resemble a tree-like structure with roots (foundations) and branches (categories and subcategories). Trees are fixed and hierarchical ("arborescent"), while rhizomes have no end or beginning. They have horizontal shoots that take off in multiple and unpredictable directions. For Deleuze and Guattari, there are "no points or positions in a rhizome, such as those found in a structure, tree, or root. There are only lines" (1987, p. 8). Rhizomes thus move continuously, making new connections, opening up potentialities for thinking differently. Nothing is fixed, sacred, or unassailable with rhizomatic modes of thinking and doing. They are exploratory, open, and ever changing.

An example of a rhizomatic approach to rehabilitation research is described by Geoffrey Edwards et al. (2014) who have developed a program of research that they call a "post-cartesian embodied perspective" that emphasizes the lived experience of the body in the world. Their aim is to open up research practices by blending traditional foci with a more expansive approach that breaks down the artificial rupture between social and biophysical research. To this end, Edwards and his colleagues are engaged in a wide array of diverse projects at different levels of intervention (micro/personal, meso/communal, and macro/societal) that intersect in their focus on the development of more inclusive cityscapes.

The team's program demonstrates rhizomatic movements in at least two ways. First it illustrates how different theoretical lenses lend themselves to different questions, different methodologies, and ultimately new interventions that address the full complexity of living with impairment for both individuals and groups—including identity, affect, design, policy, and politics, as well as more traditional foci of symptom control and function. Second they have no desire to pit social research against biophysical research or to see these as incommensurate (and, it should go without saying, no reason to pit qualitative and quantitative research against each other). Instead of replacing the dominant view with another, all perspectives are examined with regard to addressing the complexity of people's actual lives. This provides an expanded and enriched notion of rehabilitation that does not exclude or marginalize any approach. Edwards et al. (2014, p. 87) put it this way: "This (involves) an emphasis on the lived experience of the body, including issues of affect, identity, and movement but will also lead us into studying the process of worlding at scales beyond that of the individual."

Rhizomatic research and clinical practices challenge rather than reproduce the status quo. They suggest radical movement possibilities that reposition rehabilitation to partner with disabled people. What if rehabilitation, like critical disability studies, was known for challenging the taken for granted, for adopting an expansive notion of diversity, for leading a transformation in medicine and health care? This might mean that all clinicians took seriously their role to provide clients and families with opportunities to reflect on, develop, and understand different ways of understanding disability in the context of their values, values that may be shifting in response to injury or illness. Professionals would be open to changing their practices based on what they learn from clients or research participants about what gives their lives meaning, and what works or not in the contexts of their lives (Stone and Papadimitriou 2015). An important task, which I have highlighted throughout the book, would be to determine how best to assist individuals in developing and maintaining a positive disability identity while pursuing meaningful therapeutic goals. Such practices most certainly already exist, but they are overshadowed by the priorities that emanate from bioscience-based approaches.

Countering entrenched ideas about disability and the possibilities for a meaningful life do not happen quickly or easily, but require a conscious and sustained effort in multiple areas of practice. As Barnard says (cited in Ezzy 2000, p. 607), the hopeful person, rather than being defined by particular wishes, "is continually open to the possibility that reality will disclose as yet unknown sources of meaning and value." Rehabilitation practitioners can facilitate this movement, they can act as midwives for the birth of new kinds of hope by also being continually open to new sources of meaning and value. Dominant views of disability pervade society but rehabilitation should play a central role in contesting these assumptions not only in their own reasoning but in how they work with recipients of care, colleagues, funders, and policy makers. Rehabilitation has the opportunity, and perhaps the obligation, to adopt these practices pervasively.

Choices and Directions

Writing a book always involves a series of choices that have various conceptual and practical motivations. It is not surprising that the choices I made for each of the chapters reflect my ongoing research commitments, my previous clinical experience and research training, and the issues for which I am most passionate. Rather than apologize for an unavoidable partiality, I offer instead some potential future directions.

As noted, my primary purpose was to demonstrate how a post-critical approach could be employed to re-form rehabilitation, but the book necessarily provides only a partial accounting of how this might be achieved. There are some notable gaps created by the focus on physical rehabilitation and the imbalance of examples across different professional and/or patient groups. Cognitive impairment and aging are likely most noticeably absent from the discussion, and I hope others who work in these fields will expand on the discussion. There is a rich and growing corpus of critical disability studies related to intellectual and developmental disability (Anastasiou and Kauffman 2011; Goodley and Griet 2008; Goodley and Rapley 2001; Roets et al. 2008) as well in the field of critical gerontology (Kontos 2004; Warren and Manderson 2008) that have implications for rehabilitation. By this point, however, I hope readers can see how a post-critical methodology could be used to illuminate any area of practice with any population. Doing so will no doubt deepen, broaden, and reform the approach I have outlined, take it in differing rhizomatic directions, which of course is welcomed.

Without any conscious intent on my part, the successive chapters in the book, more or less with some exceptions, increasingly engage with a postmodern lens. Postmodern scholarship is often difficult to comprehend for those with little previous exposure to philosophy or social theory, and the work of Deleuze and Guattari particularly has been accused of a certain impenetrability. Rather than attempt a detailed exposition of their (or any other theorist's) ideas, I have instead endeavored to offer a more accessible text by applying the ideas to the case of rehabilitation. This does not replace an engagement with the original texts but perhaps offers a point of entry for those new to the ideas. Application is always a particular interpretation that filters knowledge from divergent sources in directions that are unique to each author. Inevitably, there is a distortion, a reframing of concepts that drifts from how they were originally conceived and presented. That is no doubt the case here. Sometimes these distortions occurred deliberately with my full knowledge, and undoubtedly there are others for which I am not fully aware. These acts of interpretation are unavoidable but also necessary. They need to be useful in moving the field, to enable tinkering, adjusting, and reforming in the spirit of avoiding the ossification of practice or theory.

The increased uptake of post-critical approaches to rehabilitation necessarily requires building capacity in theory and its applications. There is already a growing cadre of rehabilitation scholars and students who are attracted to these approaches and are applying them in their work. To that end, it is a very exciting time for rehabilitation. Delving into the rabbit hole of theory can be immensely rewarding and challenging. Nevertheless, for the work to be sufficiently nuanced, it is imperative that new scholars engage with primary sources. This book is meant to be an entry, not an end point. Graduate students who want to pursue post-critical rehabilitation research are advised to choose programs that provide the time and space to take diverse courses including those from outside one's home department, to choose supervisors who are familiar with theory and not just the substantive area of interest, and finally to read as widely as possible from diverse fields of inquiry. Movements in professional, graduate, or post-graduate rehabilitation training programs would be enhanced by inclusion of content that not only teaches the field but engages in its critique. We also need networks of researchers and practitioners to support and sustain these efforts. At time of writing there are nascent efforts to develop international PT and OT networks, a plan to launch a related rehabilitation journal, and a new multidisciplinary text devoted to *Rethinking Rehabilitation Theory and Practice* (McPherson et al. 2015). It is my hope that these efforts will continue to grow and thrive and will contribute to a more mature and nuanced field that broadly cross-pollinates with other disciplines, and partners with disabled people.

Finally, rehabilitation cannot hope to grow and transform without engaging with our colleagues in critical disability studies. In these efforts we might look to the Nordic countries who have a tradition of expansive phenomenologically informed rehabilitation research, and long established partnerships between rehabilitation professionals and disabled people advocating together to improve services and human rights. The Nordic relational model of disability (Goodley 2011, pp. 15–18) makes space for both the biophysical and the social mediators of disability by always considering each in relation to the other. This perspective allows professionals and advocates to work hand in hand to improve services in ways that are meaningful to their recipients. The approach is not without its risks (Goodley 2011, pp. 15–18), nevertheless it signals other possibilities for better alignment of rehabilitation with the diverse needs of disabled people.

The potential for rehabilitation reform is also engendered in calls for distancing rehabilitation from its affiliations with biomedicine. In disability studies, Dan Goodley has drawn on the work of Vic Finklestein to describe the Professionals Allied to the Community approach (PAC) (Goodley 2011, pp. 172–174). PAC suggests that health and welfare professionals can better serve disabled people by shifting their alliances from medicine to the communities they serve. This shift necessitates a change in emphasis toward challenging the multiple sources of disablement—social, material, political, emotional, or psychological—to facilitate human flourishing. Rather than advocating for the abandonment of impairment-based interventions, the emphasis is on revisiting care priorities reflected in the philosophical underpinnings of rehabilitation that continue to be strongly aligned with bioscience and pathology. In a similar vein, Stone and Papadimitriou (2015) have questioned the ongoing positioning of rehabilitation within biomedicine given that much of practice is oriented to helping people become "newly abled" through existential and social learning, rather than addressing medical problems. Both approaches suggest the inclination toward risk, safety, and health need to be (re)considered in relation to concerns of meaning, social inclusion, and human dignity: that deficit models be realigned to focus on maximizing abilities, that participation be broadened to the contexts of citizenship and emancipation, and that space be created for the celebration of difference and diversity.

Movement without Conclusion

Movement is a method, a philosophy, for rehabilitation. What are we doing when we are doing what we are doing? We are moving. Adjusting, tinkering, enabling, enacting, flowing, dancing, oscillating, perturbing, disrupting. Rehabilitation is not static or settled; it is a point of agitation and doubt. Movement happens whether we will it or not. Rehabilitation has its own velocity. This is not to say professionals are powerless to effect change. When movement is accepted as unavoidable, we have the collective ability and the responsibility (response-ability?) to discover where we came from, why, and ask which directions we are headed and if indeed those directions are best for the people we serve. This book has been one kind of *intermezzo* toward this analysis, part of a movement without end.

References

Abrams, T. 2015. Cartesian dualism and disabled phenomenology. *The Scandinavian Journal of Disability Research*, pp. 1–14. DOI: 10.1080/15017419.2014.995219.

Abrams T. and Gibson, B.E. (in press). Putting Gino's lesson to work: Actor-network theory, enacted humanity, and rehabilitation. *Health*.

Anastasiou, D. and Kauffman, J.M. 2011. A social constructionist approach to disability: Implications for special education. *Exceptional Children* 77(3): 367–384.

Bacchi, C. 2012. Why study problematizations? Making politics visible. *Open Journal of Political Science* 2(1): 1–8.

Bourdieu, P. and Wacquant, L.J.D. 1992. *An Invitation to Reflexive Sociology*. London, U.K.: University of Chicago Press.

Break.com. 2006. Crutch. http://www.break.com/video/bill-shannon-crutch-177786 (accessed October 3, 2015).

Deleuze, G. and Guattari, F. 1987. *A Thousand Plateaus: Capitalism and Schizophrenia*. Minneapolis, MN: University of Minnesota Press.

Edwards, G., Noreau, L., Boucher, N. et al. 2014. In *Disability, Rehabilitation Research and Post-Cartesian Embodied Ontologies—Has the Research Paradigm Changed?*, vol. 8, eds. B. Altman and S. Barnartt. pp. 73–102. Bradford, U.K.: Emerald Group Publishing Limited. http://www.emeraldinsight.com/doi/abs/10.1108/S1479-354720140000008005 (accessed October 3, 2015).

Ezzy, D. 2000. Illness narratives: Time, hope and HIV. *Social Science and Medicine* 50: 605–617.

Fadyl, J., McPherson, K., and Nicholls, D. 2015. Re/creating entrepreneurs of the self: Disclosures of worker and employee 'value' and current vocational rehabilitation practices. *Sociology of Health & Illness* 37(4): 506–521.

Fougeyrollas, P. and International Network on the Disability Creation Process (INDCP). 2000. Human development model-disability creation process. http://www.indcp.qc.ca/hdm-dcp/hdm-dcp (accessed January 29, 2015).

Frank, A. 2000. Social bioethics and the critique of autonomy. *Health* 4(3): 378–394.

Frank, A. 2010. *Letting Stories Breathe: A Socio-Narratology*. Chicago, IL: University of Chicago Press.

Gibson, B.E. 2014. Parallels and problems of normalization in rehabilitation and universal design: Enabling connectivities. *Disability & Rehabilitation* 36(16): 1328–1333.

Gibson, B.E., King, G., Kushki, A. et al. 2013. A multi-method approach to studying activity setting participation: Integrating standardized questionnaires, qualitative methods and physiological measures. *Disability & Rehabilitation* 36(19): 1652–1660.

Goodley, D. 2011. *Disability Studies: An Interdisciplinary Introduction*. London, U.K.: Sage Publications.

Goodley, D. and Griet, R. 2008. The (be)comings and goings of 'developmental disabilities': The cultural politics of 'impairment'. *Discourse: Studies in the Cultural Politics of Education* 29(2): 239–255.

Goodley, D. and Rapley, M. 2001. How do you understand "learning difficulties"? Towards a social theory of impairment. *Mental Retardation* 39(3): 229–232.

Hammell, K.W. 2006. *Perspectives on Disability and Rehabilitation*. Edinburgh, U.K.: Elsevier.

James, A. and James, A. 2004. *Constructing Childhood: Theory, Policy and Social Practice*. Hampshire, U.K.: Palgrave Macmillan.

King, G., Gibson, B.E., Mistry, B. et al. 2013. An integrated methods study of the experiences of youth with severe disabilities in leisure activity settings: The importance of belonging, fun, and control and choice. *Disability & Rehabilitation* 36(19): 1626–1635.

Kinsella, E.A. and Whiteford, G.E. August 2009. Knowledge generation and utilisation in occupational therapy: Towards epistemic reflexivity. *Australian Occupational Therapy Journal* 56(4): 249–258.

Kontos, P.C. 2004. Ethnographic reflections on selfhood, embodiment and Alzheimer's disease. *Aging & Society* 24:829–849.

Kuper, A. and D'Eon, M. 2011. Rethinking the basis of medical knowledge. *Medical Education* 45(1): 36–43.

Leplège, A., Barral, C., and McPherson, K.M. 2015. Conceptualizing disability to inform rehabilitation: Historical and epistemological perspectives. In *Rethinking Rehabilitation Theory and Practice*, eds. K.M. McPherson, B.E. Gibson, and A. Leplege. Boca Raton, FL: CRC Press.

Mattingly, C. 1998. *Healing Dramas and Clinical Plots: The Narrative Structure of Experience*. Cambridge, U.K.: Cambridge University Press.

McPherson, K.M., Gibson, B.E., and Leplège, A. 2015. Rethinking rehabilitation: Theory, practice, history—And the future. In *Rethinking Rehabilitation Theory and Practice*, eds. K.M. McPherson, B.E. Gibson, and A. Leplège. Boca Raton, FL: CRC Press.

Mol, A. 2002. *The Body Multiple: Ontology in Medical Practice*. Durham, U.K.: Duke University Press.

Mol, A. 2008. *The Logic of Care: Health and the Problem of Patient Choice*. New York: Routledge.

Priestley, M. 2003. *Disability: A Life Course Approach*. Malden, MA: Polity Press.

Roets, G., Reinaart R., Adams, M., and Hove, G.V. 2008. Looking at lived experiences of self-advocacy through gendered eyes: Becoming femme fatale with/out 'learning difficulties'. *Gender and Education* 20(1): 15–29.

Scully, J.L. 2005. Admitting all variations? postmodernism and genetic normality. In *Ethics of the Body: Postconventional Challenges*, eds. M. Shildrick and R. Mykitiuk, pp. 49–68. Cambridge, MA: MIT Press.

Shildrick, M. 2002. *Embodying the Monster: Encounters with the Vulnerable Self*. London, U.K.: Sage.

Shildrick, M. 2005. Beyond the body of bioethics: Challenging the conventions. In *Ethics of the Body: Postconventional Challenges*, eds. M. Shildrick and R. Mykitiuk, pp. 1–26. Cambridge, MA: MIT Press.

Shildrick, M. 2009. *Dangerous Discourses of Disability, Subjectivity and Sexuality*. London, U.K.: Palgrave.

Smith, B. 2013. Sporting spinal cord injuries, social relations, and rehabilitation narratives: An ethnographic creative non-fiction of becoming disabled through sport. *Sociology of Sport Journal* 30(2): 132–152.

Soundy, A., Roskell, C., Stubbs, B., Collett, J., Dawes, H., and Smith, B. 2014. Do you hear what your patient is telling you? Understanding the meaning behind the narrative. *Wayahead* 18:10–13.

Stiker, H.J. 1999. The birth of rehabilitation. In *A History of Disability*, pp. 121–189. Ann Arbor, MI: University of Michigan Press.

Stone, D.A. and Papadimitriou, C. 2015. Rehab as an existential, social learning process: A thought experiment. In *Rethinking Rehabilitation Theory and Practice*, eds. K.M. McPherson, B.E. Gibson, and A. Leplege. Boca Raton, FL: CRC Press.

United Nations. 2006. Convention on the rights of persons with disabilities. http://www.un.org/disabilities/convention/conventionfull.shtml (accessed January 29, 2015).

Warren, N. and Manderson, L. 2008. Constructing hope dis/continuity and the narrative construction of recovery in the rehabilitation unit. *Journal of Contemporary Ethnography* 37(2): 180–201.

Index

Printed in the United States
by Baker & Taylor Publisher Services

Lecture Notes in Artificial Intelligence 10604

Subseries of Lecture Notes in Computer Science

More information about this series at http://www.springer.com/series/1244

Gao Cong · Wen-Chih Peng
Wei Emma Zhang · Chengliang Li
Aixin Sun (Eds.)

Advanced Data Mining and Applications

13th International Conference, ADMA 2017
Singapore, November 5–6, 2017
Proceedings

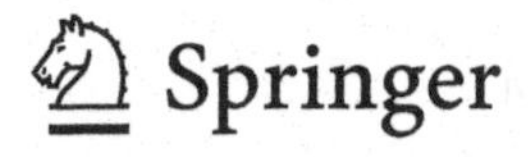
Springer

Editors
Gao Cong
Nanyang Technological University
Singapore
Singapore

Chengliang Li
Wuhan University
Wuhan
China

Wen-Chih Peng
National Chiao Tung University
Hsinchu
Taiwan

Aixin Sun
Nanyang Technological University
Singapore
Singapore

Wei Emma Zhang
Macquarie University
Sydney, NSW
Australia

ISSN 0302-9743 ISSN 1611-3349 (electronic)
Lecture Notes in Artificial Intelligence
ISBN 978-3-319-69178-7 ISBN 978-3-319-69179-4 (eBook)
https://doi.org/10.1007/978-3-319-69179-4

Library of Congress Control Number: 2017956084

LNCS Sublibrary: SL7 – Artificial Intelligence

Printed on acid-free paper

This Springer imprint is published by Springer Nature
The registered company is Springer International Publishing AG
The registered company address is: Gewerbestrasse 11, 6330 Cham, Switzerland

Preface

It is our great pleasure to introduce the proceedings of the 13th International Conference on Advanced Data Mining and Applications (ADMA). ADMA aims at bringing together data mining researchers from around the world, and also at providing a leading international forum for the dissemination of original data mining findings and practical data mining experience. Over the years, ADMA has grown to become a flagship conference in the field of data mining and applications.

There were 118 papers submitted to ADMA 2017. Each paper was assigned to at least three Program Committee members to review. All papers were rigorously reviewed and had at least three reviews. At the end, 20 papers were accepted as spotlight research papers with long presentation and 38 were accepted as regular research papers with short presentation, which include five application and case study papers. In addition, six research demonstration proposals were selected to be included in the proceedings. The conference program of ADMA 2017 was also complemented by three outstanding keynotes given by world-renowned experts, Ming-Syan Chen, Kyuseok Shim, and Anthony Tung, as well as an invited industry keynote talk session, delivered by several invited industry speakers. We would like to particularly thank the keynote speakers.

We would like to thank the Program Committee members and external reviewers for their time and comprehensive reviews and recommendations, which were crucial to the final paper selection and production of a high-quality technical program. The schedule of the reviewing process was extremely tight. The Program Committee members' tremendous efforts to complete the review reports before the deadline are greatly appreciated.

We would like to express our gratitude to all individuals, institutions, and sponsors that supported ADMA 2017. This high-quality program would not have been possible without the expertise and dedication of our Program Committee members. We are grateful to the general chairs, Aixin Sun and Hady Lauw, for their guidance and great efforts, the demonstration chairs, Zhifeng Bao and Xin Cao, for their tireless efforts, the publicity chairs, Ju Fan and Hongzhi Yin, for their work in attracting submissions, the publication chairs, Chenliang Li and Wei Emma Zhang, for their great efforts in compiling all accepted papers and working with the Springer team to produce the proceedings, the award chair, Xiaoli Li, the Web chair, Yihong Zhang, for managing the website, the special issue chairs, Michael Sheng and Xiuzhen Zhang, the local organization chairs, Zhen Hai and David Lo, for the local arrangements ensuring the conference runs smoothly, and the registration chair, Victor Chu, for handling the registration process. We would like to express our sincere thanks to Zhen Hai and Kaiqi Zhao for helping with scheduling the conference program, and to Chua Beng Lay Joanne and Boh-Nah Kiat Joo for their support in managing the conference account hosted in Nanyang Technological University. We would also like to thank the Organizing Committee of CIKM 2017 for their support. All of them helped make

ADMA 2017 a success. Furthermore, we would like to acknowledge the support of the members of the conference Steering Committee. Finally, we would like to thank all researchers, practitioners, and students who contributed with their work and participated in the conference.

We hope that participants in the conference and the readers of the proceedings will find the papers in the proceedings interesting and rewarding.

November 2017

Gao Cong
Wen-Chih Peng

Organization

General Chairs

Aixin Sun	Nanyang Technological University, Singapore
Hady Lauw	Singapore Management University, Singapore

Program Chairs

Gao Cong	Nanyang Technological University, Singapore
Wen-Chih Peng	National Chiao Tung University, Taiwan

Proceedings Chairs

Chenliang Li	Wuhan University, China
Wei Emma Zhang	Macquarie University, Australia

Publicity Chairs

Ju Fan	Renmin University of China, China
Hongzhi Yin	University of Queensland, Australia

Special Issue Chairs

Michael Sheng	Macquarie University, Australia
Xiuzhen Zhang	RMIT University, Australia

Local Arrangements Chairs

David Lo	Singapore Management University, Singapore
Zhen Hai	Institute for Infocomm Research, A*STAR, Singapore

Registration Chair

Victor Chu	Nanyang Technological University, Singapore

Demo Chairs

Zhifeng Bao	RMIT University, Australia
Xin Cao	The University of New South Wales, Australia

Awards Committee Chair

Xiaoli Li	Institute for Infocomm Research, A*STAR, Singapore

Web Chair

Yihong Zhang	Nanyang Technological University, Singapore

Steering Committee

Xue Li	University of Queensland, Australia (Chair)
Jie Cao	Nanjing University of Finance and Economics, China
Michael Sheng	Macquarie University, Australia
Jie Tang	Tsinghua University, China
Shuliang Wang	Beijing Institute of Technology, China
Kyu-Young Whang	Korea Advanced Institute of Science and Technology, Korea
Min Yao	Zhejiang University, China
Osmar Zaiane	University of Alberta, Canada
Chengqi Zhang	University of Technology Sydney, Australia
Shichao Zhang	Guangxi Normal University, China

Program Committee

Swati Agarwal	IIIT-Delhi, India
Djamal Benslimane	Lyon 1 University, France
Tossapon Boongoen	Mae Fah Luang University, Thailand
Yi-Shin Chen	National Tsing Hua University, Taiwan
Lisi Chen	Hong Kong Baptist University, SAR China
Yuan Fang	Institute for Infocomm Research, Singapore
Kaiyu Feng	Nanyang Technological University, Singapore
Philippe Fournier-Viger	Harbin Institute of Technology Shenzhen Graduate School, China
Tao Guo	Nanyang Technological University, Singapore
Jialong Han	Nanyang Technological University, Singapore
Bryan Hooi	Carnegie Mellon University, USA
Wei Hu	Nanjing University, China
Guangyan Huang	Deakin University, Australia
Chih-Chieh Hung	Tamkang University, Taiwan
Shafiq Joty	University of British Columbia, Canada
Jianxin Li	University of Western Australia, Australia
Xutao Li	Harbin Institute of Technology, China
Haiquan Li	University of Arizona, USA
Cheng-Te Li	National Cheng Kung University, Taiwan
Jinyan Li	University of Technology Sydney, Australia
Gang Li	Deakin University, Australia
Guosheng Lin	Nanyang Technological University, Singapore

Demo Program Committee

Xutao Li	Harbin Institute of Technology (Shen Zhen), China
Hua Mao	Sichuan University, China
Ryan McConville	Bristol University, UK
Ruiming Tang	Huawei Noah's Ark lab, Hong Kong, SAR China
Qingyao Wu	South China University of Technology, China
Jianqiu Xu	Nanjing University of Aeronautics and Astronautics, China
Yi Yu	National Institute of Informatics, Japan
Chao Zhang	University of Illinois at Urbana-Champaign, USA
Zhiwei Zhang	Hong Kong Baptist University, SAR China
Yuxin Zheng	Tencent, China
Jingbo Zhou	Baidu Research, China

Contents

Classification and Clustering Methods

Behavior Modeling and User Profiling

Natural Language Processing and Text Mining

Data Mining Applications

Database and Distributed Machine Learning

Querying and Mining Strings Made Easy

Majed Sahli[1(✉)], Essam Mansour[2], and Panos Kalnis[3]

[1] Saudi Aramco, Dhahran, Saudi Arabia
majed.sahli@aramco.com
[2] Qatar Computing Research Institute, HBKU, Doha, Qatar
emansour@qf.org.qa
[3] KAUST, Thuwal, Saudi Arabia
panos.kalnis@kaust.edu.sa

Abstract. With the advent of large string datasets in several scientific and business applications, there is a growing need to perform ad-hoc analysis on strings. Currently, strings are stored, managed, and queried using procedural codes. This limits users to certain operations supported by existing procedural applications and requires manual query planning with limited tuning opportunities. This paper presents StarQL, a generic and declarative query language for strings. StarQL is based on a native string data model that allows StarQL to support a large variety of string operations and provide semantic-based query optimization. String analytic queries are too intricate to be solved on one machine. Therefore, we propose a scalable and efficient data structure that allows StarQL implementations to handle large sets of strings and utilize large computing infrastructures. Our evaluation shows that StarQL is able to express workloads of application-specific tools, such as BLAST and KAT in bioinformatics, and to mine Wikipedia text for interesting patterns using declarative queries. Furthermore, the StarQL query optimizer shows an order of magnitude reduction in query execution time.

1 Introduction

Strings are sequences of symbols. Textual content on the Internet and genomic sequences are examples of important strings [16]. Textual content holds information critical for corporations to understand consumer behaviour, banking firms to identify fraudulent activities, and governmental agencies to find criminal groups. Generally, string analysis involves a single long string (e.g., the human genome or the Wikipedia text) or large collections of short strings (e.g., DNA reads or words in a Wikipedia article). More strings are being produced and propagated due to technological advances [17] and information sharing [7]. For example, the National Center for Biotechnology Information[1] (NCBI) reported that the size of the genomic sequences stored in the GenBank repository has doubled approximately every 18 months. Ambitious projects that require large string analysis include the Cancer Genome Atlas[2] and the Square Kilometre Array Telescope[3].

[1] ftp://ftp.ncbi.nih.gov/genbank/gbrel.txt.
[2] http://cancergenome.nih.gov.
[3] https://www.skatelescope.org.

G. Cong et al. (Eds.): ADMA 2017, LNAI 10604, pp. 3–17, 2017.
https://doi.org/10.1007/978-3-319-69179-4_1

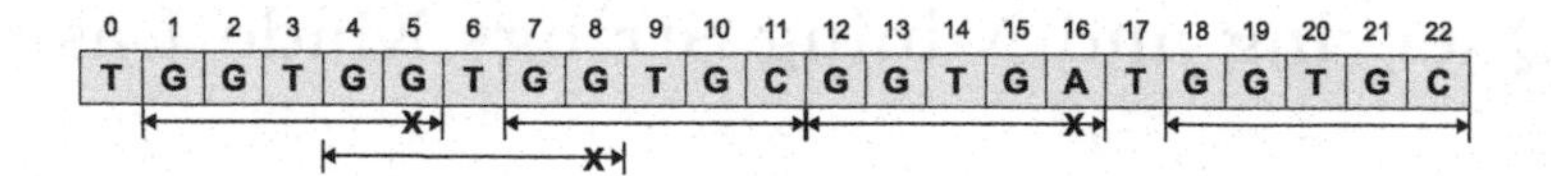

Fig. 1. Example string S over DNA alphabet $\Sigma = \{\mathtt{A}, \mathtt{C}, \mathtt{G}, \mathtt{T}\}$. Matches for `GGTGC` are indicated, allowing one mismatch and overlapping matches.

In string analysis, multiple operations are executed to extract information. One of the most basic string operations is pattern matching. It is a core operation used in most string algorithms. However, even this core and basic operation can be simple, as in the case of exact matching; or more involved, as in approximate matching. Counting pattern matches leads to the problem of identifying frequent patterns, which in turn leads to the motif extraction problem. String operations have different semantics when dealing with a single string as opposed to multiple strings. For instance, matches within a single string provide insights different from those of a single match in several strings.

One could map a string to a relation and its symbols to attributes to analyze strings using SQL. However, strings are usually large and vary in size, and the order of their symbols matters. Alternatively, considering a whole string as a single attribute is not a feasible solution because string operations require primitives not served by SQL's `LIKE` operator, such as repeated patterns and common substrings. Attempts to extend SQL with string operations do not provide native and generic string support because they are limited by their original data models [13,27].

Hence, procedural codes are currently used to analyze string datasets. For example, BLAST [1] is used for matching, where it finds regions of local similarity between biological sequences. Another example is KAT[4], a k-mer counting tool used to analyze substring frequency spectra [15]. To analyze strings, users manually move data and run different applications or use pipeline systems to automate this process.

This paper presents a declarative query language for strings, called StarQL. StarQL provides native support for string operations and generic primitives that cover users' needs in different applications. While StarQL is generic and works for any string and application, examples use DNA sequences for ease of exposition.

Example 1. *Suppose we have a DNA sequence S and we need to know if* `GGTGC` *is frequent in S or not. Assume a pattern is frequent if it appears 5 times or more in the string and that matches need not be exact as shown in Fig. 1.*

SQL can be used to count matches of a candidate pattern but matches are limited to the capabilities of the `LIKE` *operator. Using weighted scoring matrices in the case of DNA sequence similarity is not an option. Using procedural code, we can implement a string scanner and a distance function to find and count matches. However, hard-coded queries contradict with the essence of ad-hoc analysis.*

---

[4] http://www.tgac.ac.uk/KAT/.

In StarQL, finding out the number of matches for GGTGC *in S is achieved by the following query.*

```
(1) SELECT COUNT(MATCH(dna, "GGTGC", user_dist(2)));
```

Finding out if a pattern is frequent or not is a simple task. A more involved and realistic task is to extract all frequent patterns in a string. Such patterns are referred to as *motifs* and they require counting the matches for a large number of candidate motifs. SQL cannot handle candidate motifs generation so users need procedural code that implements Apriori-based or pattern-growth algorithms to extract motifs. However, extracting motifs in StarQL is equivalent to the following simple and customizable query.

```
(2) SELECT RMOTIFS(dna, freq=100, minlen=3, maxlen=9, edit(2));
```

The StarQL language is based on a simple and native string model. Considering strings as sequences of symbols and sets of related strings as collections allows the support of a large variety of string operations and is extensible to support application-specific operators. To escape the procedural code trap, StarQL supports user-defined functions. For instance, matching is a universal string operation but different applications use different matching criteria. In Example 1, `user_dist` is a user-defined distance function used when matching DNA sequences given a weighted scoring matrix. Moreover, the native string model allows StarQL queries to be smartly rewritten based on their operation semantics to reduce execution time. The paper also proposes a scalable and efficient data structure suitable for parallel query processing and handling large strings.

In summary, our contributions are the following.

- We develop StarQL, a declarative query language for strings and provide a semantic-based optimization for StarQL queries.
- We propose StarIN, a scalable and efficient data structure for implementing StarQL that avoids the limitation of traditional string indexing techniques.
- We conduct comprehensive experiments on real datasets from Wikipedia and the Human genome DNA sequence and run on a supercomputer.

The rest of this paper is organized as follows. Section 2 summarizes the related work. In Sect. 3, we introduce the syntax and semantics of StarQL, our query language. Section 4 presents our StarIN data structure. We then evaluate our language in Sect. 5 and conclude the paper in Sect. 6.

2 Related Work

Several string data models and languages are theoretically sound but impractical to implement [13]. Richardsons introduced one of the early declarative query language for strings [19]. In his model, a string starts with a symbol and the every symbol is considered the next instance of the symbol to its left. However, it is known that temporal logic modalities have limited support for recursion or iteration [28], both needed for string queries.

Currently, string analytics require running multiple standalone applications. Users need to move data between applications that use different formats and have different requirements in order to draw conclusions. This gave rise to string analysis pipeline systems (e.g., SeqWare Pipeline [18]) for users to define the steps and order of execution.

Attempts for native string support in databases exist, but most cases take an application-specific approach. SRS is an information indexing and retrieval system [8]. It targets flat files and makes use of the internal structure of their formats. SRS only allows users to draw links between different files using atomic non-sequence fields [9]. For example, SRS users can only query the description fields of FASTA-formatted and EMBL-formatted nucleotide and peptide sequences. SEQ is a string database system based on distinct domains for string elements and their underlying order type [24]. This is beneficial if users need to compute moving averages on time series. However, SEQ model limits parsing tasks, such as matching.

Relational databases deal with strings as atomic entities and queries over their internal structure are limited to the `LIKE` construct in the de facto query language, SQL. Simple extensions build on the rich and well-established data management literature and systems by introducing strings as relational domains [6]. Works of this type include extensions to the relational calculus [4,11,12,14]. Periscope/SQ [27] extended PostgreSQL with matching operations over biological sequences and reported simple matching queries over sequences of 5,000 symbols only. It is challenging to express common string queries, such as motifs and k-mers, with only matching operations.

Most relational databases support a limited number of data types. To handle strings as first-class types, researchers moved to object-oriented databases [3,13]. Nevertheless, support of string operations in object-oriented databases does not provide an ultimate solution as meta data overhead grows. Generally, extentions of existing databases are limited by their original data models and are undesired as they require the modification of mature systems [25].

3 A Declarative Strings Query Language

We consider strings as sequences of symbols from a certain alphabet, grouped into collections. A string of zero symbols is an empty string, and a collection of zero non-empty strings is an empty collection. Depending on how string collections are generated, they could consist of several long strings or many short strings. A collection of strings has a certain alphabet. For example, the DNA alphabet consists of the four characters {`A`, `C`, `G`, `T`}. Evidently, string queries have one or more strings as input and may produce one or more strings as output.

In StarQL, queries are categorized according to their applicability and results to administrative and analytic queries. Administrative queries are used to manage the string database and its string collections. Analytic queries are used to extract information. StarQL provides novel query optimizations based on the query semantics and operations.

StarQL adopts a declarative SQL-like syntax, which is easy to understand. Figure 2 shows an abstract BNF of some of the StarQL constructs. Complex string analysis can be performed by easily nesting different constructs to form queries. Next, we discuss StarQL constructs, grouped according to functionality, and give examples of their usage.

```
<query>       := <query> | <import> ; | <select> ; |
                 <delete> ; | <aggregate> ;
<identifier>  := $PATH$ | $ID$
<delete>      := DELETE <identifier>
<dist>        := HAMMING($int$) | EDIT($int$) | USER($int$)
<length>      := MINLEN $int$ MAXLEN $int$ | LEN $int$
<motif-type>  := RMOTIFS | CMOTIFS
<motif-ops>   := FREQ $int$ <length> <dist>
<slct-cls>    := <identifier> | <generator> | <extractor>
<motifs>      := <motif-type>(<slct-cls> <motif-ops>)
<kmers>       := KMERS(<slct-cls> <length>)
<generator>   := <motifs> | <kmers>
<type>        := ALL | ANY
<matches>     := EXACT(<slct-cls> <type> <slct-cls>) |
                 EXACT(<slct-cls> "$PATTERN$") |
                 REGEX(<slct-cls> <type> <slct-cls>) |
                 REGEX(<slct-cls> "$PATTERN$") |
                 APPROX(<slct-cls> <type> <slct-cls> <dist>) |
                 APPROX(<slct-cls> "$PATTERN$" <dist>)
<range>       := RANGE(<slct-cls> FROM $pos1$ TO $pos2$)
<prefixes>    := PREFIXES(<slct-cls> <length>)
<suffixes>    := SUFFIXES(<slct-cls> <length>)
<extractor>   := <prefixes> | <suffixes> | <range> | <matches>
<prefix>      := PREFIX(<slct-cls> <slct-cls> <dist>) |
                 PREFIX(<slct-cls> "$PATTERN$" <dist>) |
<suffix>      := SUFFIX(<slct-cls> <slct-cls> <dist>) |
                 SUFFIX(<slct-cls> "$PATTERN$" <dist>) |
<substring>   := SUBSTR(<slct-cls> <slct-cls> <dist>) |
                 SUBSTR(<slct-cls> "$PATTERN$" <dist>) |
<filter>      := <prefix> | <suffix> | <substring> | <matches> | <metadata>
<sort>        := ORDER BY <metadata>
<whr-cls>     := <whr-cls> | <filter> | LIMIT $int$ | <sort>
<select>      := SELECT <slct-cls> [AS <identifier>] [WHERE <whr-cls>]
<import>      := IMPORT <identifier> AS <identifier> |
                 IMPORT <select> AS <identifier>
```

Fig. 2. Abstract BNF for StarQL.

3.1 Query Constructs

Administration. The IMPORT and DELETE utilities provide simple ways for users to load, index, and purge string collections. Strings can be imported from

the file system or from query results. The newly created collection is named and given a unique ID. The number of strings and the total length of all the strings are saved as collection properties. For example, a user imports a dataset of human DNA shotgun reads from disk by running the following query.
(3) `IMPORT "/datasets/shotgun/human" AS hdna;`

Matching. The `EXACT` matching command finds exact matches of a pattern in a collection. The output is either a collection of one string, the matched pattern along with the number of exact matches, or an empty collection if no matches are found. To find matches within a certain distance threshold, the `APPROXIMATE` matching command is used. The result is a collection of as many unique substrings that match with their respective counts in the original collection. The capabilities of a regular expression matching command are vital for several string applications. The `REGEX` matching command finds substrings that match a regular expression pattern. For example, assume a user needs to find matches of the regex expression "`AC..CA`" in the previously imported collection `hdna`. The query to find and save the results is written as follows.
(4) `IMPORT (SELECT REGEX(hdna, "AC..CA")) AS re;`

Extraction. The `PREFIXES` extraction command extracts all the unique prefixes in a collection of strings. The input is a collection along with the desired prefix length range. The output is a collection of all unique prefixes within required length range. The `SUFFIXES` extraction command is similar to `PREFIXES` but for suffixes. The `RANGE` extraction command extracts all the unique substrings that exist at a specific position in a collection of strings. In our running example, a user may be interested in the different substrings of length 2 that exist between a pair of "`AC`". If `re` consisted of {`ACCCAC, ACGTAC, ACTTAC, ACATAC`}, then the output would be {`CC, GT, TT, AT`} and the query is written as follows.
(5) `SELECT RANGE(re, FROM 2 TO 3);`

Generation. The following commands generate new strings from existing collections. The `RMOTIFS` command finds all the repeated motifs supported by at least one string in the collection operated on. The input is a collection along with the desired motif properties; namely, minimum length, maximum length, and frequency threshold. The `CMOTIFS` command finds all the common motifs supported by a user specified number of strings in a certain collection. The input is a collection along with the desired motif properties. The `K-MERS` generation command finds all the unique k-mers in a collection of strings. The input is a collection along with the desired substring length k. The output is a collection of the unique k-mers from all the strings in the collection. For example, the k-mers of length 3 from the previously saved collection `re` are {`AAC, CCC, CCA, CAC, ACG, CGT, GTA, TAC, ACT, CTT, TTA, ACA, CAT, ATA`}. To generate these k-mers, the following query is used.
(6) `SELECT KMERS(er, LEN = 3);`

Filtering. Existing collections can be filtered according to matches or metadata properties. The `PREFIX` filtering command finds the strings that share a certain prefix; either exactly or approximately. The input is a collection of strings, a prefix pattern, and a distance function and threshold. The output is a collection of strings with matching prefixes. The `SUFFIX` filtering command works similarly for suffixes. The `SUBSTRING` filtering command finds the strings that share a certain substring; either exactly or approximately. The `LENGTH` filtering command finds strings of a certain length range. Continuing our running example, assume the user is interested in the k-mers of length 3 that include the 2 characters between the pair of "AC" in the regular expression matches, `r = {CC, GT, TT, AT}`. The resulting filtered k-mers are `{CCC, CCA, CGT, GTA, CTT, TTA, CAT, ATA}`. This is accomplished using the following query.

```
(7) SELECT KMERS(er, LEN=3) AS k WHERE SUBSTRING(k, r);
```

3.2 User-Defined Functions

StarQL supports user-defined functions to add new operations or introduce application-specific logic using routines executed by other functions. For example, one of the main routines used in string operations is the distance function. A distance function accepts two strings as input and outputs a scalar value indicating the dissimilarity of these strings. Biologists can augment StarQL with weighted matrices to measure distances between DNA sequences.

3.3 String Query Optimizations

It is not always straightforward to optimize string queries because the order of executing string operations could change the final results. We can optimize string queries not only based on the cost of each string operation but also based on the semantics of these operations. To start, we find an execution order that preserves the query logic while generating less intermediate data. For example, if a query involves multiple matching operations, one of which is against the longest common substring, then finding the longest common substring first reduces intermediate results and the search space for subsequent matching operations.

To ensure correctness, we use the syntax of StarQL to determine the semantics. In particular, the final output is always a subset of the operation after a `SELECT` keyword. Conditions after a `WHERE` keyword are interpreted from left to right, but not necessarily executed in this order. Using this convention, how StarQL interprets queries is clear to users. Only valid plans are compared internally to optimize efficiency. For instance, the following nested query extracts suffixes of length 3 from the repeated motifs found in Wikipedia.

```
(8) SELECT SUFFIXES(RMOTIFS(wiki, MAXLEN=20, FREQ=1000), LEN=3);
```

StarQL's query plans are based on the categories of StarQL operations, where execution plans start with operations that generate or extract strings, then apply operations that filter, limit or sort these strings. Furthermore, StarQL enables

Algorithm 1. STARQL QUERY OPTIMIZER ALGORITHM

1: **procedure** OPTIMIZE(Q)
2: $T \leftarrow$ tokenize(Q)
3: $T.initial = Q.first\_token$
4: **while** $T.initial$ NOT $collection\_id$ **do**
5: $T \leftarrow$ tokenize($T.initial$)
6: **end while**
7: $T.filters \leftarrow Q.last\_token$
8: **if** $T.filters$ in $MATCH \,||\, EXTRACT$ **then**
9: $push\_down(T.filters)$
10: **end if**
11: $S \leftarrow detect\_semantics(T)$
12: $P \leftarrow S.optimal\_plan$
13: **return** P
14: **end procedure**

semantic-based optimizations, where query operations can be rewritten using other operations. While maintaining query logic, semantic-based optimizations reduce computational complexity, intermediate results, and execution time.

Algorithm 1 describes the StarQL query optimizer. First, a query is tokenized and tokens are assigned to categories. Then, operations that can be reordered to minimize intermediate results without affecting semantics are shuffled. For instance, we do not push filter operations into generate operations to keep semantics intact. Finally, StarQL re-writes query operations based on their semantics. This is possible because some StarQL operations can be expressed in terms of other operations. The optimizer takes advantage of such cases to find an equivalent set of operations with less cost given the data and the user parameters.

Table 1. An example for a schema-based optimization in StarQL.

```
SELECT RMOTIFS(wiki, freq=500, len=9, HAMMING(1)) as m WHERE EXACT(m, "australia");
```

PLAN A (naïve)		PLAN B (optimized)	
●	OUTPUT(Y)	●	OUTPUT(Z)
Filter	Y = EXACT(X, "australia")	Filter	Z = Y >= 500
Generate	X = RMOTIFS(wiki, freq=500, len=9, \ HAMMING(1))	Aggregate	Y = COUNT(X)
		Match	X = APPROXIMATE(wiki, "australia", \ HAMMING(1))

Consider for example, a user query that checks if the string "australia" is a repeated pattern in a Wikipedia collection. A naïve plan starts by generating the repeated motifs. Then the intermediate results will be filtered by the string "australia". The StarQL optimizer will rewrite this query in terms of counting approximate matches for the pattern we filter at the end. Table 1 shows the two plans. Plan A uses more resources and generates excessive intermediate results whereas Plan B eliminates the expensive repeated motifs operator and replaces it with a count of approximate matches.

4 A Scalable Data Structure

This section introduces a scalable and efficient data structure that supports the efficient implementation and parallel execution of StarQL operations.

4.1 StarIN: A Scalable Index for Strings

It is accepted that a suffix tree is space-efficient because it is a compressed trie. Nevertheless, long common labels are less expected in large collections of strings as the probability of having different combinations from a fixed alphabet increases with string length and collection size. Consequently, the construction complexity added for compacting path labels is unjustifiable given the expected space saving. In cases where most suffix tree labels are single characters, a trie is superior in both space requirement and access time.

We argue that parallel computation should be used with more basic data structures to support scalable and efficient string operations. StarIN is a novel suffix trie index that indexes all suffixes of all strings and retains the frequency of every path label. Because we are targeting large collections of strings; each node stores a single character, avoiding the need to reference strings to retrieve path labels. The path label frequency is used to answer and optimize many string operations without the need to access strings. StarIN is constructed in linear time by traversing the trie from the root using the suffixes. When a suffix exists, node counts are incremented. Otherwise, new nodes are created for the newly added suffix with initial count of 1. StarIN also eliminates the need for different terminating symbols or maintaining string identifiers and compacting path labels. Some information that would have been readily available in a GST requires extra computation in StarIN. However, such information is efficiently generated when needed in a distributed fashion.

Figure 3 shows an example StarIN index. When exact positions or counts within each string are required, we utilize well-known string algorithms to efficiently extract this information in parallel. StarIN balances preprocessing time, index size, and execution efficiency. For instance, Boyer-Moore search algorithm is run in parallel to find original strings that satisfy a certain filter query after pruning the search space using the suffix trie and an External R-Way merge sort algorithm is used to eliminate duplicate results after a pattern extraction query is executed.

4.2 Parallel Support for StarQL Operations

StarIN supports StarQL primitives, which include complex operations that require parallelization in order to finish in reasonable time. Tuning problem

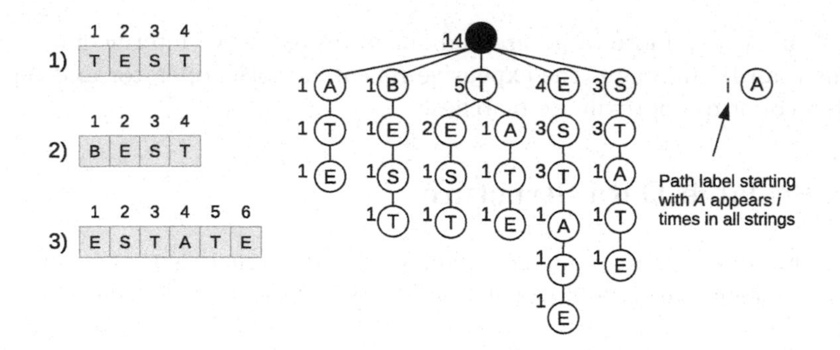

Fig. 3. Example proposed index as opposed to the generalized suffix tree.

decomposition depends on the number of available workers and the load of the query. Given our StarIN data structure, a collection is decomposed into sub-collections and assigned to workers. The StarIN footprint of each sub-collection fits in memory. Complex query operators are solved in parallel by utilizing the underlying infrastructure and the decomposed data structure. Next we show by example how we utilize parallel computation to extract information that is not stored in our StarIN data structure.

Assume a user was interested in finding the positions where "EST" appears in S. Using StarIN, we would know from traversing the trie that "EST" appears three times. To find the exact positions, a parallel search is executed where the strings in S are distributed among workers to search for the three occurrences. This search is feasible because it is a bounded exact search and the cost is distributed between workers.

To extract the longest common substring in S, we run `LCS(S)` which first extracts the longest substrings that appear at least $|S| = 3$ times then verify that they exist in every string at least once. In the first step, the candidate solutions are ordered according to their length, {EST, ST, E, T}. In order to stop short, if possible, verification starts from the longest candidate. An exact parallel search is used to verify that "EST" appears in every string, which is the case in this example and the result is {EST}. Finally, to generate 3-mers of S, `KMERS(S, LEN=3)`, the suffix trie branches of length three are simply spelled out {ATE, BES, TES, TAT, EST, STA}.

Example 2. *Consider a user needs to find text that appears frequently in Wikipedia. The user has to work around spelling mistake and simple differences such as noun plurals and verb tenses. First, the Wikipedia archive is imported into the string database using the* `IMPORT` *StarQL construct. The database indexes the dataset using StarIN and may partition or replicate indexes depending on size and available resources.*

To find all frequent patterns, a query to generate motifs is used. Motifs are patterns that appear frequently but not necessarily exactly [21, 22]. StarQL supports different distance functions for approximate matching. Running on 480 cores, the motifs search space (a combinatorial tree over the English alphabet) is partitioned to thousands of tasks. The workload is balanced by dynamically assigning tasks and the results are gathered and returned to the user.

The user may decide to filter out motifs of length 4 or less as they correspond to common short words, such as articles and prepositions. The user allows an edit distance of 2 characters so words like "fishes" and "fishy" count as occurrences for the motif "fish". The length and approximate matching parameters are readily available in StarQL. The user in our example may form and submit the following StarQL query.

(9)
```
SELECT RMOTIFS(wiki, FREQ=1000, MINLEN=4, MAXLEN=10, \
  EDIT(3)) AS wikipats;
```

We indexed the Wikipedia archive using StarIN. Our system executes first the repeated motifs operation in parallel. Since the motifs search space is a combinatorial tree, it is logically partitioned into many sub-trees. In analytics workload, the number of sub-trees affects the utilization of the computing resources [20]. On a supercomputer, the StarQL optimizer estimates the query workload using a sampling technique and determines that 2,048 cores can be fully utilized. The original archive is not accessed because StarIN is annotated with counts. The resulting repeated motifs are also in the form of a suffix trie. Therefore, further operations to extract the common suffixes, for example, are quickly executed on the resulting collection, `wikipats`.

5 Experimental Evaluation

This section presents different aspects of evaluating our StarQL language: the expressiveness power, the StarQL query optimizer, the scalability of StarIN, and the overall performance of using StarQL. We implemented StarQL in a strings database system using C/C++ and MPI based on StarQL and StarIN. The system was demonstrated using large datasets and different varieties of queries [23]. The implementation uses a master/worker architecture. As an MPI-based system, it can be used in workstations, clusters, or supercomputers. Our large-scale string database system is available for download[5].

5.1 StarQL Expressiveness

StarQL expresses queries in a natural and readable way. Consider the simple query of finding exact matches of `EEK` in a collection of protein sequences `R`. Table 2 shows this query in PiQL and StarQL. While StarQL is more readable, PiQL [26] is also limited to matching biological sequences. For instance, PiQL cannot express a simple query over a text archive like the following StarQL query, which returns the unique words of lengths 5 to 7 from Wikipedia prefixes.

```
SELECT PREFIXES(Wiki, minlen=5, maxlen=7);
```

BLAST is the widely used bioinformatics tool. We can express a BLAST script in StarQL to efficiently execute in our implementation. The BLAST

[5] http://cloud.kaust.edu.sa/Pages/stardb.aspx.

Table 2. Expressing the same simple query using PiQL and StarQL syntax.

Language	Query
PiQL	`SELECT * FROM MATCH(R, p, "EEK", EXACT, 3)`
StarQL	`SELECT EXACT(R, "EEK");`

workload was generated using the human and mouse immunoglobulin variable region dataset from NCBI[6]. This dataset is composed of 141,465 DNA sequences of lengths that range between 97 and 3,177,340. We invoked BLAST version 2.0 with the default parameters for the tool *blastn* and the query string `ACCGTTCAGTT`. To our surprise, BLAST returns one match that represents a sufficiently high-scoring ungapped alignment. However, its heuristics imply that the same BLAST command could yield different results between different runs.

We imported the dataset in our implementation and issued the following StarQL query. Since we implemented exact algorithms, our StarQL query finds all results. Firstly, we find two exact matches of the query string. Moreover, we find 35 approximately matching substrings that appear in the dataset 451 times. From here, using StarQL we can further process these results to analyze the dataset by running other operators without the need to move data between systems and without running other procedural tools.

(10) `SELECT APPROX(igSeqNt, "ACCGTTCAGTT", USER(1));`

Furthermore, we compare our implementation capabilities against the following state-of-the-art procedural repeated motif extractors: PSMILE [5], FLAME [10], and VARUN [2]. Although the procedural codes are specialized, our implementation generates the same output up to 3 orders of magnitude faster. For example, for a certain exact-length motif query, FLAME runs for 4 h while our implementation finishes serially in 1 h and using 12 cores in 7 min. our implementation is able to handle 3 order of magnitude larger strings and scaled efficiently on a supercomputer whereas the only parallel motif extractor [5] reported scaling to 4 cores.

5.2 The StarQL Query Optimizer

In this experiment, we show the benefit of our semantic-based query optimization. In StarQL, string operators could result in large string collections so query plans with small intermediate results and less complex operations are favoured. Figure 4 shows the size of intermediate results and execution times for the query plans discussed in Table 1 of Sect. 3.3. The gain in memory footprint and execution time from semantic-based optimization is significant. Note that the optimized query executes more operations but (i) they are lightweight as the aggregate and filter operations answers are readily available in the data structure of StarQL model, and (ii) they result in less data access and intermediate results. Fewer intermediate results consumes less memory and requires less instructions to build and use in further steps.

[6] ftp://ftp.ncbi.nih.gov/blast/db/FASTA/igSeqNt.gz.

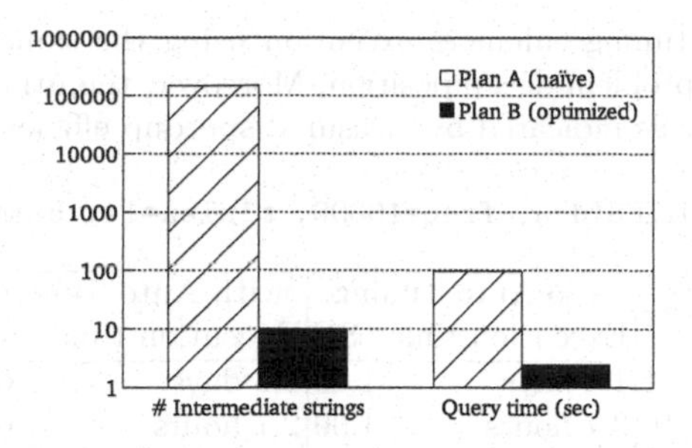

Fig. 4. Semantic-based optimizations of StarQL queries dramatically decreases intermediate results and reduce serial execution time by replacing operations while maintaining semantics. Plan A and Plan B are shown in Table 1.

5.3 Scalability and Parallel Support

For time-consuming string queries, scaling out to finish in reasonable time is essential for online analysis of strings. The parallelization of string operations supported by StarQL's data model and proposed data structures effectively achieves this goal. For a StarQL query that involves generating all motifs, the efficient representation of StarIN reduced the serial execution time from 4 h to less than an hour and a half on the same hardware. This query is executed by our implementation in less than a minute when scaling out to 256 cores. Table 3 shows our implementation using a supercomputer to execute a more complex query in seconds instead of hours.

Due to the flexibility of StarIN, we are able to find the best problem decomposition and determine the degree of parallelism to highly utilize resources with minimal overhead. Therefore, our implementation automatically tunes the execution parameters (i.e., problem decomposition and number of cores to use) to achieve the near optimal resource utilization. Because we can generate many small tasks, we utilize our automatic tuning framework [20] to find the best decomposition (i.e., maximum number of tasks with minimal parallel overhead)

Table 3. StarQL implementation scalability on a Blue Gene/P supercomputer. Query load is increased by increasing the allowed hamming distance to 4. The serial execution time of the query is 5.2 h. Speedup efficiency is the ratio of speedup to number of cores with an optimal value of 1.

```
SELECT RMOTIFS(dna, freq=10000, len=12, hamming(4));
```

Cores	Time (sec)	Speedup Efficiency
512	38	0.97
1024	19	0.97
2048	10	0.97
4096	5	0.92
8192	3	0.76

Table 4. Automatic tuning enhances execution using the same number of cores by determining the best problem decomposition. Moreover, the utilization of resources is enhanced dramatically as indicated by measured speedup efficiency (SE).

```
SELECT RMOTIFS(dna, freq=10000, minlen=12, hamming(3));
```

Cores	w/o Auto Tuning		with Auto Tuning	
	Execution time	SE	Execution time	SE
1	1.6 days	1.00	1.6 days	1.00
16	2.7 hours	1.00	2.7 hours	1.00
1,024	2.5 minutes	0.96	2.4 minutes	0.99
2,048	1.5 minutes	0.79	1.2 minutes	0.98
4,096	53 seconds	0.67	39 seconds	0.91

and estimate the serial and parallel runtimes to predict utilization. Table 4 shows the gain in time and utilization by automatically tuning the execution of the same query on the supercomputer.

6 Conclusion

We need to deal with large strings that may not fit on a single machine. Similarly, some string queries are computationally demanding and require parallel execution to finish in reasonable times. This paper proposed StarQL, a declarative query language for strings; and StarIN, a scalable and efficient data structure. We demonstrated the expressiveness of StarQL and the scalability of StarIN by utilizing a supercomputer to process string queries on large real datasets.

References

1. Altschul, S.F., Gish, W., Miller, W., Myers, E.W., Lipman, D.J.: Basic local alignment search tool. J. Mol. Biol. **215**(3), 403–410 (1990)
2. Apostolico, A., Comin, M., Parida, L.: VARUN: discovering extensible motifs under saturation constraints. IEEE/ACM Trans. Comput. Biol. Bioinform. **7**(4), 752–762 (2010)
3. Balkir, N., Sukan, E., Ozsoyoglu, G., Ozsoyoglu, G.: Visual: a graphical icon-based query language. In: Proceedings of International Conference on Data Engineering (ICDE) (1996)
4. Benedikt, M., Libkin, L., Schwentick, T., Segoufin, L.: String operations in query languages. In: Proceedings of PODS (2001)
5. Carvalho, A.M., Oliveira, A.L., Freitas, A.T., Sagot, M.F.: A parallel algorithm for the extraction of structured motifs. In: Proceedings of the ACM Symposium on Applied Computing (SAC) (2004)
6. Date, C.: An Introduction to Database Systems, 8th edn. Pearson/Addison-Wesley, Boston (2003)
7. Dube, K., Mansour, E., Wu, B.: Supporting collaboration and information sharing in computer-based clinical guideline management. In: 18th IEEE Symposium on Computer-Based Medical Systems (CBMS), Dublin, Ireland (2005)

8. Etzold, T., Argos, P.: SRS - an indexing and retrieval tool for flat file data libraries. Comput. Appl. Biosci. **9**(1), 49–57 (1993)
9. Etzold, T., Argos, P.: Transforming a set of biological flat file libraries to a fast access network. Comput. Appl. Biosci. **9**(1), 49–57 (1993)
10. Floratou, A., Tata, S., Patel, J.M.: Efficient and accurate discovery of patterns in sequence data sets. TKDE **23**(8), 1154–1168 (2011)
11. Ginsburg, S., Wang, X.S.: Regular sequence operations and their use in database queries. J. Comput. Syst. Sci. **56**(1), 1–26 (1998)
12. Ginsburg, S., Wang, X.: Pattern matching by RS-operations: towards a unified approach to querying sequenced data. In: Proceedings of PODS (1992)
13. Grahne, G., Hakli, R., Nykänen, M., Tamm, H., Ukkonen, E.: Design and implementation of a string database query language. Inf. Syst. **28**(4), 311–337 (2003)
14. Grahne, G., Nykänen, M., Ukkonen, E.: Reasoning about strings in databases. In: Proceedings of the Thirteenth ACM SIGACT-SIGMOD-SIGART Symposium on Principles of Database Systems, PODS 1994 (1994)
15. Mapleson, D., Garcia Accinelli, G., Kettleborough, G., Wright, J., Clavijo, B.J.: KAT: a K-mer analysis toolkit to quality control NGS datasets and genome assemblies. Bioinformatics **33**(4), 574–576 (2017)
16. Mathur, A., Sihag, A., Bagaria, E., Rajawat, S., et al.: A new perspective to data processing: Big data. In: Proceedings of INDIACom, pp. 110–114 (2014)
17. Niedringhaus, T.P., Milanova, D., Kerby, M.B., Snyder, M.P., Barron, A.E.: Landscape of next-generation sequencing technologies. Anal. Chem. **83**(12), 4327–4341 (2011)
18. O'Connor, B.D., Merriman, B., Nelson, S.F.: Seqware query engine: storing and searching sequence data in the cloud. BMC Bioinf. **11**(12), S2 (2010)
19. Richardson, J.: Supporting lists in a data model (a timely approach). In: Proceedings of the 18th International Confernce on Very Large Data Bases, VLDB 1992 (1992)
20. Sahli, M., Mansour, E., Alturkestani, T., Kalnis, P.: Automatic tuning of bag-of-tasks application. In: International Conference on Data Engineering (ICDE) (2015)
21. Sahli, M., Mansour, E., Kalnis, P.: Parallel motif extraction from very long sequences. In: Proceedings of the ACM International Conference on Information and Knowledge Management (CIKM) (2013)
22. Sahli, M., Mansour, E., Kalnis, P.: ACME: a scalable parallel system for extracting frequent patterns from a very long sequence. VLDB J. **23**(6), 871–873 (2014)
23. Sahli, M., Mansour, E., Kalnis, P.: StarDB: a large-scale DBMS for strings. Proc. VLDB **8**, 1844–1847 (2015)
24. Seshadri, P., Livny, M., Ramakrishnan, R.: The design and implementation of a sequence database system. In: Proceedings of the International Conference on Very Large Data Bases, VLDB 1996 (1996)
25. Stonebraker, M., Cetintemel, U.: "One size fits all": an idea whose time has come and gone. In: Proceedings of International Conference on Data Engineering (ICDE) (2005)
26. Tata, S., Friedman, J., Swaroop, A.: Declarative querying for biological sequences. In: Proceedings of International Conference on Data Engineering (ICDE), pp. 87–87, April 2006
27. Tata, S., Lang, W., Patel, J.M.: Periscope/SQ: interactive exploration of biological sequence databases. In: Proceedings of VLDB (2007)
28. Wolper, P.: Temporal logic can be more expressive. In: 22nd Annual Symposium on Foundations of Computer Science, SFCS 1981, pp. 340–348, October 1981

Distributed Training Large-Scale Deep Architectures

Shang-Xuan Zou, Chun-Yen Chen, Jui-Lin Wu, Chun-Nan Chou, Chia-Chin Tsao, Kuan-Chieh Tung, Ting-Wei Lin, Cheng-Lung Sung, and Edward Y. Chang(✉)

HTC Research,Taipei, Taiwan
edward_chang@htc.com

Abstract. Scale of data and scale of computation infrastructures together enable the current deep learning renaissance. However, training large-scale deep architectures demands both algorithmic improvement and careful system configuration. In this paper, we focus on employing the system approach to speed up large-scale training. Taking both the algorithmic and system aspects into consideration, we develop a procedure for setting mini-batch size and choosing computation algorithms. We also derive lemmas for determining the quantity of key components such as the number of GPUs and parameter servers. Experiments and examples show that these guidelines help effectively speed up large-scale deep learning training.

Keywords: Deep learning · Neural network · Convolutional neural networks · Distributed learning · Speedup · Performance tuning

1 Introduction

In the last five years, neural networks and deep architectures have been proven very effective in application areas such as computer vision, speech recognition, and machine translation. The convincing factor that makes deep learning shine is *scale*, in both data volume and computation resources. Large network and large scale of training data demands scalable computation. However, scaling up computation is not merely throwing in an infinite number of CPUs and GPUs. As Amdahl's law [2] states, the non-parallelizable portion of a computation task may cap computation speedup. Non-parallelizable overheads in deep learning frameworks should be carefully mitigated to speed up training process.

Several open-source projects (e.g., Caffe [25], MXNet [7], TensorFlow [1], and Torch [9]) have been devoted to speeding up training deep networks. They can be summarized into two approaches: deep-learning algorithm optimization and algorithm parallelization. The former includes using faster convolution algorithms, improving stochastic gradient decent with faster methods, employing compression/quantization, and tuning the learning rate with advanced optimization techniques. Indeed, most open-source libraries have quickly adopted available state-of-the-art optimizations. However, most users in academia and industry do not

G. Cong et al. (Eds.): ADMA 2017, LNAI 10604, pp. 18–32, 2017.
https://doi.org/10.1007/978-3-319-69179-4_2

know how to set parameters, algorithmic and system, to conduct cost-effective training. Researchers and professionals face at least the following questions in three levels, which are intra-GPU, inter-GPU, and inter-machine:

1. With X amount of data, what is the size of each mini-batch (X_{mini}) and how to maximize GPU utilization?
2. How many GPUs (G) should be employed, and how should such a system be configured?
3. How many parameter servers (N_{ps}) should be deployed when building a distributed system?

In this work, we identify computation bottlenecks of representative frameworks and aim to answer the above questions by providing system configuration guidelines given the characteristics of the training data and hardware parameters.

1.1 Related Work

Since deep-learning training is time-consuming, many previous studies devoted to improve the training performance. These prior contributions can be divided into two approaches: algorithmic and system. The algorithmic approach accelerates the training algorithm, whereas the system approach focuses on employing improved resources to achieve parallel training. To ensure scalability, the system approach may require enhancing the training algorithm to take full advantage of the increased resources.

Algorithmic Approach. Stochastic gradient descent (SGD) is the de facto optimization algorithm for training a deep architecture. Many SGD techniques have been developed for achieving faster convergence to the global minimum. The settings of hyper-parameters such as learning rate and mini-batch size are crucial to the training performance. Hinton and Bengio [4,21] provide recommendations on setting hyper-parameters commonly used in gradient-based training. Batch renormalization can be an effective strategy to train a network with small or non-i.i.d mini-batches [23].

More efficient algorithms can improve speed. Some FFT-based convolution schemes were proposed [31] to achieve speedup. Additionally, Firas et al. proposed three matrix layout schemes using lowering operations [19]. *Caffe con Troll* implemented a CPU-GPU hybrid system that contains several lowering operations, and at the same time, employs a simple automatic optimizer to select the best lowering. Some compression algorithms [15] were developed for both good compression ratios and fast decompression speed to enable block-wise uncompressed operations, such as matrix multiplication are executed directly on the compressed representations.

System Approach. Convolution and matrix multiplication are two common arithmetic operations used in a deep learning computation task. A GPU is well-suited for speeding up such operations since these operations are parallelizable. To achieve further speedup, the next logical step is to employ multiple GPUs, and to configure a distributed clusters of CPUs and GPUs. The computation time can be largely reduced via data parallelism and/or model parallelism. Many projects have proven parallelism to be helpful [8,13,22,26,34,38].

According to Amdahl's law, the peak performance of a parallel architecture is capped by the overhead portion of the computation task. In the context of deep learning, its training overhead includes synchronization between distributed threads, disk I/O, communication I/O, and memory access. To reduce synchronization delay, Zinkevich et al. [40] proposed an asynchronous distributed SGD algorithm to guarantee parallel acceleration without tight latency constraints. Chen et al. [6] proposed adding backup workers in synchronous SGD algorithm to mitigate the bottleneck. To reduce the impact of I/O on the overall speedup, most open-source frameworks attempt to conceal I/O behind computation via the pipeline approach proposed in [30]. Such approach requires a computation unit to be sufficiently long so as to hide I/O overheads as much as possible. The pipeline approach, however, demands carefully setting up the unit size of computation (or mini-batch size) and the number of parameter servers. We will propose how to best estimate these configuration parameters in Sect. 3.

Computation Frameworks. There have been several deep learning open-source efforts. Representative frameworks are CNTK [12], Theano [24], Caffe [25], MXNet [7], TensorFlow [1], and Torch [9]. Among these frameworks, MXNet and TensorFlow are built-in distributed training frameworks. Users can easily develop algorithms running on computing clusters with thousands of CPUs or GPUs. Several works are proposed to give users a glimpse on the factors that they must take into consideration. Bahrampour et al. [3] provided a comparative study on different frameworks with respect to extensibility, hardware utilization, and performance. Shi et al. [35] conducted studies on performance of selected frameworks. These works offer practitioners a high-level guideline to select an appropriate framework. Given a selected framework, our work aims to provide further configuration guidelines to make training both fast and cost-effective.

1.2 Contribution Summary

In summary, this work makes the following contributions:

1. Identifying computation bottlenecks and devising their remedies.
2. Quantifying remedies into an optimization model. We formulate our remedies into an optimization model to determine the optimal mini-batch size and carefully balance memory and speed trade-offs so as to employ the fastest algorithms given the memory constraint.
3. Recommending distributed configuration involving multiple GPUs and parameter servers.

2 Training Process and Setup

Figure 1 depicts a general architecture of deep-learning training and data flow. A worker is basically a commodity computer equipped with G GPUs. When aiming to improve parallelism via a distributed architecture, a worker and a parameter server can be replicated into multiple copies connected by a network. The training samples are divided into mini-batches. The mini-batch processing pipeline in the training process consists of seven steps. After the model parameters W and the data processing pipeline is initialized, the training process repeats until an approximate minimum is obtained.

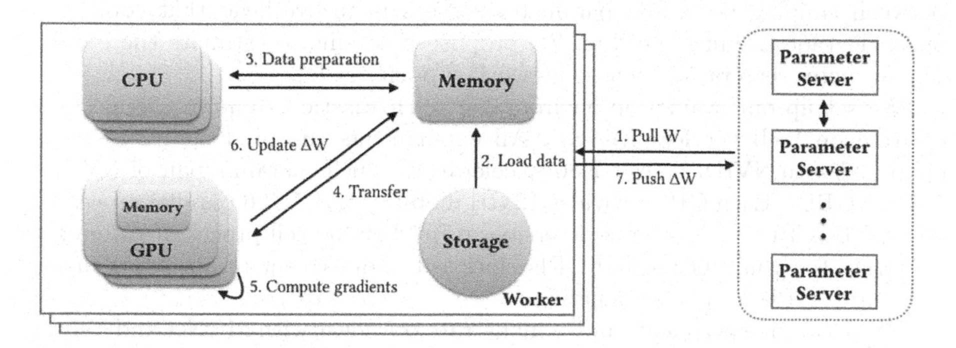

Fig. 1. Deep learning system architecture. The batch processing pipeline in the general training process can be divided into seven steps.

1. *Parameter refresh.* In distributed training, the latest copy of model parameters W is pulled from parameter servers at the beginning of each mini-batch processing. W is then loaded onto GPU memory. A distributed environment consists of N_w workers and N_{ps} parameter servers for managing shared parameters.
2. *Data loading.* A subset of the X training instances called *mini-batch* of size X_{mini} is loaded from the persistent storage to the main memory.
3. *Data preparation.* X_{mini} instances are transformed into the required input format. These instances may be augmented to mitigate the over-fitting problem and enrich sample diversity.
4. *Host to GPU transfer.* The mini-batch is loaded onto the memory of a GPU. If G GPUs are employed, G different mini-batches are loaded onto G GPUs.
5. *GPU processing.* Required computations including matrix multiplication and convolution are performed on G GPUs for the gradients against the given mini-batch.
6. *Parameter update.* The delta ΔW is derived from the gradients and applied to the previous version of W in main or GPU memory.
7. *Distributed update.* The parameter updates are sent to parameter servers when distributed machines are configured.

Among the seven steps, step 5 performs computation, and the other steps that cannot be hidden behind step 5 are considered as overheads. The larger fraction of the time which those overhead steps take, the less effective parallelism can achieve. Therefore, our tasks are minimizing overhead time and hiding overheads via pipelining as much as possible. The remainder of this paper is to demonstrate how the following parameters can be carefully tuned to achieve such goals, organized into three sections. In Sect. 3.1, we provide a procedure to recommend a mini-batch size that leads to maximum training performance. Section 3.2 provides an in-depth analysis on training in a multi-GPU environment. We provide a lemma to estimate the number of GPUs G for a desired factor of speedup. In Sect. 3.3, we address issues involving distributed workers. The communication between training hosts and parameter servers is an overhead that could seriously degrade training speedup. We propose a scheme to estimate the number of parameter servers N_{ps}, whose network capacity is B_{ps}.

We set up our evaluation environment with Elastic Compute Cloud (EC2) of Amazon Web Services (AWS)[1]. All experiments run on EC2 P2 instances equipped with NVIDIA Tesla K80 Accelerators which contain a pair of NVIDIA GK210 GPUs. Each GPU provides 12 GB memory and 2,496 parallel processing cores. The CPU is a customized version of Intel Broadwell processor running at 2.7 GHz. To avoid unexpected GPU clock rate adjustment in our experiments, we disable GPU autoboost function.

We perform experiments and demonstrate our ideas with MXNet and TensorFlow. Virtual machines are launched from Amazon deep learning AMI (Amazon Machine Image) $v2.1$ preloaded with NVIDIA CUDA toolkit $v7.5$ and cuDNN $v5.1$. We conduct experiments on the ILSVRC-2012 dataset, the subset of ImageNet [14] containing 1,000 categories and 1.2 million images on SSD. The other set containing 50,000 labeled images is used as validation data.

3 Configuration of High Performance Training System

We study configurations in three incremental steps, starting from a single GPU (Sect. 3.1), then expanding our benchmarking to multiple GPUs (Sect. 3.2), and finally to distributed nodes where each node consists of multi-GPUs (Sect. 3.3). Each of these three steps focuses on analyzing one system configuration.

3.1 Training on Single GPU Instance

In this section, we first point out the common performance pitfalls in developing neural networks. We illustrate that the setting of mini-batch size is the primary factor that determines training speed. We then formulate selecting the mini-batch size X_{mini} as an optimization problem and provide a procedure to solve for X_{mini} that can achieve fastest training speed.

[1] GPU instances on Google Compute Engine (GCE) do not support GPU peer-to-peer access, and hence we will defer our GCE experiments till such support is available.

Identifying System Issues. Most neural networks are initially designed according to some heuristics. Researchers may not have the full picture about their model's feasibility, convergence quality, and prediction quality unless they conducted some experiments. During the experimental process, various hyper-parameter values may be tested exhaustively by a trial-and-error process. According to our own experience, it is typically unknown at the beginning to know how long it would take to run a round of training job, let alone configure a cost-effective system that can maximize training speed. A suboptimal system configuration can lead to excessive execution time because of encountering the following issues:

- *Shortage of GPU memory space.* A GPU cannot start computation without the data and metadata being loaded into GPU memory. A neural network designed without system knowledge may require more memory capacity than available memory. This excessive memory use may cause unnecessary thrashing and prolong training time.
- *Ineffective trade-off between speed and memory.* Deep learning frameworks may execute operations of a training task in different algorithms, which have different speed and memory-use trade-offs. The selection of using which algorithm is a layer-dependent decision. The selection factors include input data size, layer parameters, mini-batch size, and available GPU memory space. Consider the convolution operation as an example. An FFT-based implementation runs faster than a GEMM-based one but it requires more memory. The training speed may be degraded when a large X_{mini} exhausts memory capacity in order to run a faster FFT-based algorithm. Thus, when tuning factors mentioned above, we should consider the impact on memory consumption because the memory budget affects the selection of algorithm.

Selecting a good mini-batch size, one must examine from both the algorithmic and system aspects. From the algorithmic aspect, the mini-batch size is suggested to be larger than the number of output classes and a mini-batch contains at least one sample from each class [21]. The diversified training data leads to more stable convergence. From the system aspect, a proper mini-batch size helps to improve the parallelism inside GPU and enables the faster implementation of an operator. Based on the suggested mini-batch size considering the algorithmic aspect, we introduce the system aspect into deciding X_{mini}.

Choosing Convolution Algorithms. Speeding up convolution involves GPU memory and computation speed trade-off. There are different algorithms for implementing the convolution operation. GEMM-based implementations converts convolution to a matrix multiplication, which can be slow but the up side is that it requires less memory space. FFT-based implementations run faster than the GEMM-based by using efficient matrix multiplication and reducing the number of floating point operations. However, FFT-based implementations demand substantially more memory as the filters are padded to be the same size as the input. In addition, FFT-based implementations require extra memory space for feature mapping on domain transformation. Take AlexNet as an example, the memory space required by the first layer with FFT is 11.6 times of that with GEMM given mini-batch size 128.

To further understand the impact of X_{mini}, we experimented with MXNet and TensorFlow, and plot system throughput (y-$axis$) versus X_{mini} (x-$axis$) in Fig. 2(a). Although different frameworks may yield different throughputs, the trend remains the same, that is, the system throughput degrades once after X_{mini} reaches a threshold. The reason why the throughput drops is that MXNet and TensorFlow run a slower version of convolution due to the constrained free memory caused by the increased X_{mini}. How to determine the optimal X_{mini}? We next formulate the problem of determining X_{mini} as an optimization problem.

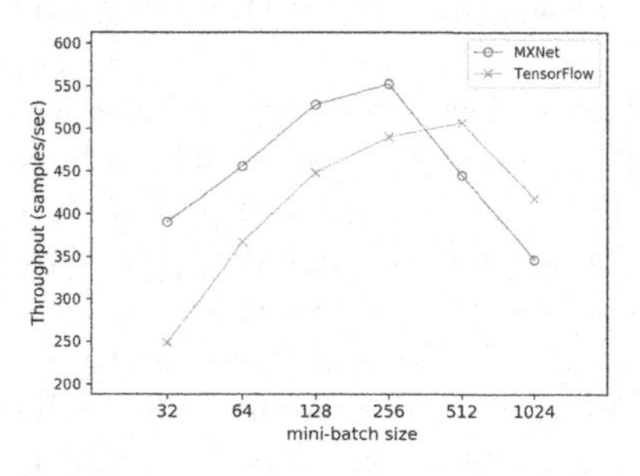

(a) Throughts vs. mini-batch sizes.

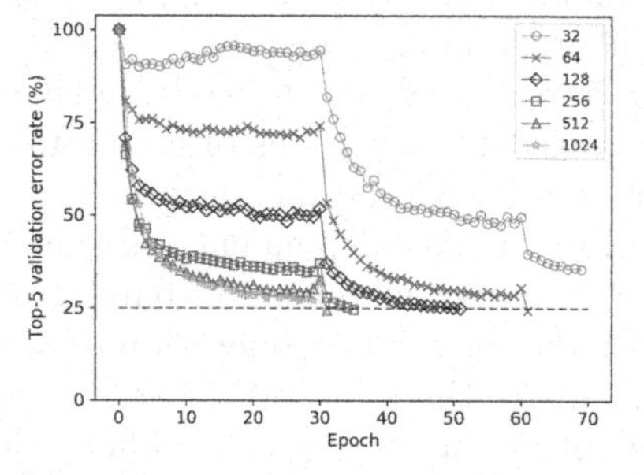

(b) Learning curves vs. mini-batch sizes.

Fig. 2. Dual impact of mini-batch size

Optimizing Mini-batch Size. In order to formulate the problem of determining X_{mini}, we first define a memory constraint M_{bound}, which is built into the later optimization formulas for X_{mini}. During our formulation, most of the symbols follow in the same fashion of [11].

Deriving M_{bound}.

We assume that a CNN such as AlexNet [27] consists of two major components: feature extraction and classification. Further, we assume that the feature extraction part comprises of n layers where stacked convolution layers are optionally followed by pooling layers, and the classification part consists of m fully-connected layers. We use $B_i \times H_i \times D_i$ and $B_{i+1} \times H_{i+1} \times D_{i+1}$ where $i \in \{0, 1, \ldots, n\}$ to represent the sizes of inputs and outputs of convolution layers (or pooling layers), respectively. In particular, the size $B_0 \times H_0 \times D_0$ represents the size of input data. If we take training AlexNet on the ImageNet [14] as the example, $B_0 \times H_0 \times D_0$ is equal to $224 \times 224 \times 3$. For the ith layer of convolution and pooling layers, we denote its spatial extent (i.e. the size of filters) as F_i, its stride as S_i, its amount of padding as P_i, and its number of filters as K_i. Please note that if the ith layer is a pooling layer, its K_i is equal to zero, i.e.

$K_i = 0$. Thus, the inputs and outputs in the feature extraction part have the following relations:

$$\begin{aligned} B_{i+1} &= (B_i - F_{i+1} + 2P_{i+1})/S_{i+1} + 1, \\ H_{i+1} &= (H_i - F_{i+1} + 2P_{i+1})/S_{i+1} + 1, and \\ D_{i+1} &= \begin{cases} K_{i+1}, & \text{if } (i+1)^{th} \text{ layer is convolution layer} \\ D_i, & \text{if } (i+1)^{th} \text{ layer is pooling layer} \end{cases}. \end{aligned} \tag{1}$$

The memory allocated for the feature extraction part of CNNs includes the input data, outputs (i.e. feature maps) of all the layers, model parameters, and gradients. We assume that all the values are stored by using single precision floating point (32 bits). Based on the aforementioned notations and Eq. (1), the memory usage for the input data and outputs of all layers in the feature extraction part can be calculated as follows:

$$M_{FM} = \sum_{i=0}^{n} B_i \times H_i \times D_i \times X_{mini} \times 32. \tag{2}$$

Regarding the model parameters, there are two kinds of parameters: weights and biases. Though the biases are often omitted for simplicity in the literature, we take them into account here in order to estimate the memory usage precisely. Besides, we assume that the size of the gradients is twice as the size of the model parameters[2]. Thus, we can derive the memory usage for the model parameters and their related gradients by the following equation:

$$\begin{aligned} M_{MP} = &\sum_{i=1}^{n} F_i \times F_i \times D_{i-1} \times K_i \times 3 \times 32 \quad (weights) \\ &+ \sum_{i=1}^{n} K_i \times 3 \times 32 \quad (biases). \end{aligned} \tag{3}$$

Furthermore, the memory allocated for the classification part of CNNs contains the outputs of all neurons and model parameters. We use L_j where $j \in \{1, \ldots, m\}$ to denote the number of neurons at j^{th} layer. Again, we make the same assumption that the size of the gradients is twice as the size of the model parameters. Therefore, the memory usage for the classification part of CNNs is as follows:

$$\begin{aligned} M_C = &\sum_{j=1}^{m} L_j \times 32 \quad (outputs) \\ &+ \sum_{j=1}^{m-1} L_j \times L_{j+1} \times 3 \times 32 \quad (weights) \\ &+ (m-1) \times 3 \times 32 \quad (biases). \end{aligned} \tag{4}$$

[2] For each training instance, we need to store the gradients of all model parameters. The aggregated gradients of all model parameters are also required for a specific batch.

According to Eqs. (2) to (4), the memory constraint M_{bound} can be approximately determined by the following equation:

$$M_{bound} = M_{GPU} - M_{FM} - M_{MP} - M_C, \quad (5)$$

where M_{GPU} is the total memory of a GPU in terms of bits.

Deriving X_{mini}.

Assuming that there are p kinds of convolution algorithms, and q layers in the CNN. (In the case that we have illustrated so far, $p = 2$. Other choices of convolution algorithms can be Winograd minimal convolution algorithm [28], Strassen algorithm [10], fbfft [37], etc.) The parameter $x_{k,l} \in \{0, 1\}$ represents whether the kth layer uses the lth convolution algorithm or not. When $x_{k,l}$ is evaluated to 1, it means that the kth layer uses the lth algorithm to compute convolution. The value $T_{k,l}$ is the time consumption at the kth layer for the lth algorithm. The value $M_{k,l}$ is the memory consumption at the kth layer for the lth algorithm. Thus, the problem of determining X_{mini} can be formulated an optimization problem as follows:

$$\begin{aligned} & min \sum_{k=1}^{q} \sum_{l=1}^{p} x_{k,l} \times T_{k,l} \\ & s.t. \sum_{k=1}^{q} \sum_{l=1}^{p} x_{k,l} \times M_{k,l} \leq M_{bound} \quad \& \quad \forall k \sum_{l=1}^{p} x_{k,l} = 1, \end{aligned} \quad (6)$$

where the M_{bound} is derived from Equation (mem:bound).

Obviously, Eq. (6) is an integer linear programming (ILP) problem [32], which is NP-hard. However, there are several off-the-shelf heuristic methods and libraries (e.g. GLPK [17]) for solving ILP problems. Given a range of mini-batch sizes that can attain good accuracy, we can derive the estimated training time for each mini-batch size by solving Eq. (6). The mini-batch size which leads to the minimal training time is then the suggested X_{mini}.

This far, we assume that a CNN model is given to determine X_{mini} and layer-dependent convolution algorithms to maximize training speed. We can make two further adjustments:

- *Permit X_{mini} reduction.* The researchers may need to compromise on smaller mini-batch size if the target one is not feasible or does not deliver acceptable performance under the constraint of GPU memory size. Ghadimi et al. [16] shows that the convergence rate of SGD on a non-convex function is bounded by $O(1/\sqrt{K})$, where K is the number of samples seen, i.e., mini-batch size. It can be interpreted that a range of mini-batch sizes can deliver similar convergence quality. In Fig. 2(b), the x-axis depicts the epoch number and the y-axis depicts the top-5 validation error rate[3]. The figure shows that indeed

[3] AlexNet achieved 18.2% top-5 error rate in in the ILSVRC-2012 competition, whereas we obtained 21% in our experiments. This is because we did not perform all the tricks for data augmentation and fine-tuning. We choose 25% as the termination criterion to demonstrate convergence behavior when mini-batch sizes are different.

a range of mini-batch sizes enjoy similar convergence quality. Therefore, we could reduce X_{mini} to increase M_{bound} to permit more memory space to run a faster convolution execution to achieve overall speedup.

- *Permit model adjustment.* Suppose that the constrained space of memory prevents us from running a faster algorithm. We could adjust the CNN model to free up some memory. For instance, if the ith layer can be sped up ten times and the jth only twice. To accommodate running a faster algorithm for the ith layer, we could adjust both layers to e.g., use a larger stride or memory-efficient filters.

3.2 Scale with Multiple GPUs

When one GPU cannot handle the training task timely, employing multiple GPUs is the next logical step to share the workload and achieve speedup. When G GPUs are used and the maximal 100% efficiency is achieved, the speedup is G times. Let α denote the system efficiency between 0% and 100%. Lemma 1 provides the estimated efficiency given G GPUs.

Lemma 1. *Let T denote the total training time, where T can be divided into computation time T_C and overhead T_O. Let R_O denote the ratio of overhead or $R_O = T_O/T_C$. Suppose the desired efficiency of the system is α, where $\alpha \leq 100\%$. The efficiency can be estimated as*

$$\alpha = \frac{1 + R_O}{1 + GR_O}.$$

Proof. Details of the proof is documented in the extended version of this paper [41].

Lemma 1 can be used to estimate system efficiency given R_O and G, and also can be used to estimate the acceptable R_O given α and G. For example, given four GPUs and target efficiency $\alpha = 80\%$, the ratio of overhead that cannot be hidden behind computation must not exceed 9%.

To estimate R_O, a practitioner can quickly profile the training program for a couple of epochs. Some frameworks such as MXNet and TensorFlow provide the capability to visualize the execution of a training task, which can be used to derive R_O. If a computation framework is not equipped with a profiling tool, one can visualize program execution using **nvprof**[4]. Suppose a practitioner is asked to make $3x$ speedup of a training task, and she measures $R_O = 10\%$. According to the lemma, she can configure a 4 GPU system to achieve the performance objective.

To evaluate Lemma 1, we conduct the training on four neural networks to compare the estimated speedup with actual speedup. Though the estimated R_O is a constant and in real-time overheads could be stochastic, Fig. 3 shows that in all cases the estimated speedup matches the the actual speedup. Therefore,

[4] **nvprof** only profiles GPU activities, so the CPU activities cannot be analyzed.

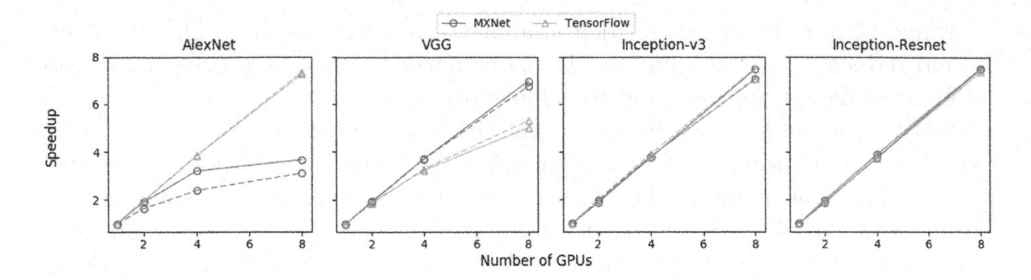

Fig. 3. Comparison of speedup (dotted-line: estimated, solid-line: actual)

the lemma can be used to estimate the performance gain of using G GPUs and devise a cost-effective training plan including system configuration and parameter settings.

The overall speedup can be improved by reducing computation overheads. We conclude this subsection by providing two overhead reduction suggestions.

- *Data transfer pipelining.* Low throughput of feeding training data is a major bottleneck that degrades the multi-GPU training performance as the demand for bus bandwidth for loading data grows with the number of GPUs. Pipelining data loading (I/O) with computation is the effective way to reduce the overhead brought by data preparation. The impact of disk I/O can be further alleviated by using better disk or reducing expensive file operations like seek. Modern frameworks such as TensorFlow and MXNet provide the way to rearrange training samples so that the data can be read in sequentially. The load for decoding and augmenting training data may cause extreme high CPU usage and drags the performance of data provision. The computation intensive jobs should be avoided on CPUs.
- *Peer-to-peer parameter updates.* Synchronizing parameter updates among GPUs, as indicated in step 6 in Fig. 1, is another common bottleneck in multi-GPU training environment. A naive implementation is to keep the latest model at main memory, transfer the latest copy to GPUs at the beginning of batch processing, and aggregate updates from all GPUs. It leads to bus contention and huge data load between main memory and GPUs under CUDA programming model. To alleviate the hot spot issue, the weight updates can be completed via GPU high-speed DMA if GPU supports peer-to-peer transfer.

If multiple GPUs with low computing overhead still cannot meet the desired performance, distributed training is the option you can consider. We'll discuss the topic in the next section.

3.3 Distributed Training

Distributed training has become increasingly important because of the growth of dataset size and model complexity. To effectively orchestrate multiple machines for a training task, the system must provide a way to manage the globally shared model parameters. The parameter server architecture, i.e., a cluster of machines to manage parameters, is widely-used to reduce I/O latency for handling parameter updates [29,30]. As shown in Fig. 1, parameter servers maintain latest parameter values and serve all workers. The workers retrieve updated parameters from the cluster, complete computation, and then push updates back to the cluster of parameter servers.

Parameter updates can be performed either synchronously or asynchronously. Employing synchronous updates ensures consistency but suffers from the performance dragger issue. Updating parameters asynchronously gains training speed and may not significantly affect training accuracy according to prior studies [13]. When I/Os can be performed asynchronously, fetching and updating parameters can be hidden behind computation and hence computation overhead can be mitigated. We assume that an asynchronous update policy is employed.

Let N_{ps} denote the number of parameter servers. How many parameter servers should be configured to hide the computation overhead? We select N_{ps} when $N_{ps} + 1$ can no longer speed up the training task. Before we prove our lemma that derives the most effective N_{ps}, we enumerate two desired subgoals or conditions.

The first subgoal is that the computation duration of a worker should be longer than its communication time with the parameter cluster. In other words, the I/O time between a worker thread and its designated parameter servers is shorter than the computation time of that worker. This condition allows parameters being pre-fetched before a new round of computation commences. Therefore, the I/O overhead can be hidden behind computation. The second subgoal is to distribute parameter-update workload evenly among parameter servers. We assume a dynamic load-balancing policy (e.g., [5]) can be employed to distribute parameter retrieval and update workload almost evenly among N_{ps} servers.

Lemma 2. *Given a round of GPU computation time T_C on a worker, number of workers N_w, and parameter size S_p, the minimum number of parameter servers N_{ps}, whose network capacity is B_{ps}, required to mask communication I/Os is*

$$N_{ps} \simeq \left\lceil \frac{2S_P Nw}{B_{ps}T_C} \right\rceil.$$

Proof. Details of the proof is documented in the extended version of this paper [41].

Lemma 2 suggests a back-of-the-envelop estimate on N_{ps} given two ideal conditions. When the conditions do not hold, more parameter servers should be employed to be able to mask I/O overhead. Three measures are recommended:

1. *Increase T_C.* When workload cannot be evenly distributed, the computation time should be longer to mask most I/Os. Therefore, a good strategy is to maintain a large T_C. In other words, having a larger mini-batch size when the memory capacity permits is helpful. Goyal et al. [18] proposed a scheme to use

a larger mini-batch size without loss of accuracy. Besides, a larger mini-batch leads to less number of parameter updates and improves overall performance.
2. *Improve B_ps.* Increasing channel bandwidth can reduce time for pushing/pulling parameters. Insufficient bandwidth of the communication channel may throttle the training performance. Thus, high speed networking is highly recommended when applying distributed training.
3. *Balance workload.* Prior works [5,30] propose effective data placement methods to balance dynamic workload. Such load balancing schemes can avoid I/O bottlenecks, and lead to overall overhead reduction.

4 Concluding Remarks

AlphaGo showed that more training data can only be helpful towards improving machine intelligence and competitiveness. Recently, Residual Neural Networks [20,36] shows that in both theory and practice, more layers of neural networks correlates to a higher achieved accuracy by a trained classifier. At a 2016 machine learning workshop [33], Andrew Ng presented that the traditional biases and variance trade-off have not appeared in training large-scale deep architectures. In other words, the larger the scale, the better suited the architecture is for improving the intelligence of a "machine".

This "larger the better" conjecture certainly demands that database and machine learning communities devise data management and data mining systems that can handle an ever increasing workload. We foresee that not only will algorithmic research continue flourishing, but system research and development will as well. Already we have seen that GPU vendors are enhancing distributed GPU implementations. Advances in interconnected technology and implementation will help reduce both I/O overhead in data loading and in parameter updates.

In this work, we provided practical guidelines to facilitate practitioners the configuration of a system to speed up training performance. Our future work will focus on effectively managing such large-scale training systems to achieve both high accuracy and cost-effectiveness in three specific areas:

- *Flexibility.* Prior work [39] provided a flexibility to work with any compatible open-source frameworks. For example, we expect to simultaneously work with multiple frameworks such as MXNet and TensorFlow to complete a large-scale training task running on Azure, AWS, GCE, and other available commercial clouds.
- *Scalability and elasticity.* In addition to the parameter estimation performed in this work, we will research dynamic schemes to adjust allocation and scheduling parameters according to the dynamic workload nature of distributed systems.
- *Ease of management.* We plan to devise tools with the good user experience for monitoring and managing the training system.

References

1. Abadi, M. et al.: TensorFlow: large-scale machine learning on heterogeneous systems, 2015. Software available from tensorflow.org (2015).
2. Amdahl, G.M.: Validity of the single processor approach to achieving large scale computing capabilities. In: Proceedings of the Spring Joint Computer Conference, 18–20 April 1967, pp. 483–485. ACM (1967)
3. Bahrampour, S. et al.: Comparative study of deep learning software frameworks. In: arXiv.org. arxiv: 1511.06435v3 [cs.LG], November 2015
4. Bengio, Y.: Practical recommendations for gradient-based training of deep architectures. In: Montavon, G., Orr, G.B., Müller, K.-R. (eds.) Neural Networks: Tricks of the Trade. LNCS, vol. 7700, pp. 437–478. Springer, Heidelberg (2012). doi:10.1007/978-3-642-35289-8_26
5. Chang, E., Garcia-Molina, H., Li, C.: 2D BubbleUp: managing parallel disks for media servers. Technical report, Stanford InfoLab (1998)
6. Chen, J. et al.: Revisiting distributed synchronous SGD. arXiv preprint arXiv:1604.00981 (2016)
7. Chen, T. et al.: MXNet: a flexible and efficient machine learning library for heterogeneous distributed systems. arXiv preprint arXiv:1512.01274 (2015)
8. Chilimbi, T.M. et al.: Project adam: building an efficient and scalable deep learning training system. In: OSDI, vol. 14, pp. 571–582 (2014)
9. Collobert, R., Kavukcuoglu, K., Farabet, C.: Torch7: a matlab-like environment for machine learning. In: EPFL-CONF-192376 (2011)
10. Cong, J., Xiao, B.: Minimizing computation in convolutional neural networks. In: Wermter, S., Weber, C., Duch, W., Honkela, T., Koprinkova-Hristova, P., Magg, S., Palm, G., Villa, A.E.P. (eds.) ICANN 2014. LNCS, vol. 8681, pp. 281–290. Springer, Cham (2014). doi:10.1007/978-3-319-11179-7_36
11. CS231n Convolutional neural network for visual recognition (2017). http://cs231n.github.io/
12. Dally, W.J.: CNTK: an embedded language for circuit description. Department of Computer Science, California Institute of Technology, Display File
13. Dean, J. et al.: Large scale distributed deep networks, pp. 1223–1231 (2012)
14. Deng, J. et al.: ImageNet: a large-scale hierarchical image database. In: CVPR 2009 (2009)
15. Elgohary, A., et al.: Compressed linear algebra for large-scale machine learning. Proc. VLDB Endow. **9**(12), 960–971 (2016)
16. Ghadimi, S., Lan, G.: Stochastic first-and zeroth-order methods for nonconvex stochastic programming. SIAM J. Optim. **23**(4), 2341–2368 (2013)
17. GNU linear programming kit (2012). https://www.gnu.org/software/glpk/
18. Goyal, P. et al.: Accurate, large Minibatch SGD: training ImageNet in 1 h. arXiv preprint arXiv:1706.02677 (2017)
19. Hadjis, S., et al.: Caffe con troll: shallow ideas to speed up deep learning, April 2015. arXiv.org. arXiv: 1504.04343v2 [cs.LG]
20. He, K. et al.: Deep residual learning for image recognition, pp. 770–778 (2016)
21. Hinton, G.: A practical guide to training restricted Boltzmann machines. Momentum **9**(1), 926 (2010)
22. Iandola, F.N. et al.: FireCaffe - near-linear acceleration of deep neural network training on compute clusters. In: CVPR, pp. 2592–2600 (2016)
23. Ioffe, S.: Batch renormalization: towards reducing Minibatch dependence in batch-normalized models, February 2017. arXiv.org. arXiv: 1702.03275v1 [cs.LG]

24. Bergstra, J. et al.: Theano: a CPU and GPU math expression compiler (2010)
25. Jia, Y. et al.: Caffe: convolutional architecture for fast feature embedding. In: Proceedings of the 22nd ACM International Conference on Multimedia, pp. 675–678 (2014)
26. Krizhevsky, A.: One weird trick for parallelizing convolutional neural networks. arXiv preprint arXiv:1404.5997 (2014)
27. Krizhevsky, A., Sutskever, I., Hinton, G.E.: ImageNet classification with deep convolutional neural networks. In: Pereira, F. et al. (eds.) Advances in Neural Information Processing Systems, vol. 25, pp. 1097–1105. Curran Associates Inc. (2012)
28. Lavin, A., Gray, S.: Fast algorithms for convolutional neural networks. In: Proceedings of the IEEE Conference on Computer Vision and Pattern Recognition, pp. 4013–4021 (2016)
29. Li, M. et al.: Scaling distributed machine learning with the parameter server. In: OSDI (2014)
30. Liu, Z. et al.: PLDA+: parallel latent Dirichlet allocation with data placement and pipeline processing. ACM Trans. Intell. Syst. Technol. **2**(3), 26:1–26:18 (2011). ISSN, pp. 2157–6904, doi:10.1145/1961189.1961198. http://doi.acm.org/10.1145/1961189.1961198
31. Mathieu, M., Henaff, M., LeCun, Y.: Fast training of convolutional networks through FFTs. In: CoRR abs/1312.5851 cs.CV (2013)
32. Nemhauser, G.L., Wolsey, L.A.: Integer programming and combinatorial optimization. In: Nemhauser, G.L., Savelsbergh, M.W.P., Sigismondi, G.S. (eds.) Constraint Classification for Mixed Integer Programming Formulations. Wiley, Chichester (1992). COAL Bull. **20**, 8–12 (1988)
33. Ng, A.Y.: The nuts and bolts of machine learning. In: NIPS Workshop on Deep Learning and Unsupervised Feature Learning (2016)
34. Niu, F. et al.: A lock-free approach to parallelizing stochastic gradient descent. arXiv preprint arXiv:1106.5730 (2011)
35. Shi, S. et al.: Benchmarking state-of-the-art deep learning software tools, August 2016. arXiv.org. arXiv:1608.07249v5 [cs.DC]
36. Szegedy, C., Ioffe, S., Vanhoucke, V.: Inception-v4, Inception-ResNet and the impact of residual connections on learning. In: CoRR abs/1602.07261 (2016). http://arxiv.org/abs/1602.07261
37. Vasilache, N. et al.: Fast convolutional nets with fbfft: a GPU performance evaluation. arXiv preprint arXiv:1412.7580 (2014)
38. Zhang, H. et al.: Poseidon: a system architecture for effcient GPU-based deep learning on multiple machines. arXiv preprint arXiv:1512.06216 (2015)
39. Zheng, Z. et al.: SpeeDO: parallelizing stochastic gradient descent for deep convolutional neural network. In: NIPS Workshop on Learning Systems (2015)
40. Zinkevich, M. et al.: Parallelized stochastic gradient descent, pp. 2595–2603 (2010)
41. Zou, S.-X. et al.: Distributed training large-scale deep architectures. HTC technical report (2017). https://research.htc.com/publications-and-talks

Fault Detection and Localization in Distributed Systems Using Recurrent Convolutional Neural Networks

Guangyang Qi[1(✉)], Lina Yao[1(✉)], and Anton V. Uzunov[2(✉)]

[1] University of New South Wales, Sydney, Australia
qiguangyang@gmail.com, lina.yao@unsw.edu.au
[2] Defence Science and Technology Group, Adelaide, Australia
anton.uzunov@dst.defence.gov.au

Abstract. Early detection of faults is essential to maintaining the reliability of a distributed system. While there are many solutions for detecting faults, handling high dimensionality and uncertainty of system observations to make an accurate detection still remains a challenge. In this paper, we address this challenge with a two-dimensional convolutional neural network in the form of a denoising autoencoder with recurrent neural networks that performs simultaneous fault detection and diagnosis based on real-time system metrics from a given distributed system (e.g. CPU usage, memory consumption, etc.). The model provides a unified way to automatically learn useful features and make adaptive inferences regarding the onset of faults without hand-crafted feature extraction and human diagnostic expertise. In addition, we develop a Bayesian change-point detection approach for fault localization, in order to support the fault recovery process. We conducted extensive experiments in a real distributed environment over Amazon EC2 and the results demonstrate our proposal outperforms a variety of state-of-the-art machine learning algorithms that are used for fault detection and diagnosis in distributed systems.

1 Introduction

Advancements in the Internet of Things and sensor technologies have fostered the realization of new distributed systems for homeland security, environmental monitoring, health-care and smart spaces. These systems also have demonstrable applicability to a wide range of Defence scenarios, from supporting the mental health of soldiers in the field via continuous real-time monitoring and information processing, to the autonomous protection of enterprise networks from cyber security attacks. One of the most important quality attributes of such distributed systems is reliability, which can be seen as the ability to detect and remedy a variety of faults occurring in single or multiple components in order to maintain functionality. Ensuring distributed systems reliability in turns requires examining the reliability of each individual component before predicting or assessing the reliability of the whole system. One of the key prerequisites for this is to

G. Cong et al. (Eds.): ADMA 2017, LNAI 10604, pp. 33–48, 2017.
https://doi.org/10.1007/978-3-319-69179-4_3

effectively detect faults at an early stage and to determine effective diagnosis techniques so that a recovery scheme can be activated accordingly by isolating faults and making repairs.

Fault detection based on machine learning (ML) has been extensively studied in the past few years, with researchers working on extracting fault patterns from the historical data of past system operations, which can be further utilized to predict fault occurrences [3,4,7]. However, three major open issues remain. (i) Many information processing tasks can be very easy or very difficult depending on how the collected information is represented, which directly has an impact on performance. The complexity of distributed systems makes suitable metrics hard to model and many existing approaches depend on hand-crafted features like mean/variation and human diagnosis expertise, which are usually noise-prone and biased by different feature extraction and selection schemes. (ii) Existing approaches usually combine two distinct functions into one: feature extraction and classification. Using fixed and hand-crafted features in this single function may be a suboptimal choice, however, and would require significant computational cost that, in general, would prevent their usage in real-time applications. (iii) It is very difficult to measure a large number of inter-correlated variables in a distributed system for conducting fault diagnosis. Most existing approaches, such as those based on Bayesian networks or conditional random fields, are unable to address this challenge very well, since they cannot model both the spatial and temporal dependencies between the system metrics of a component or a node to discriminate between various types of faults.

In recent years, deep learning's revolutionary advances in image processing [9] and speech recognition [6] have gained significant attention [5,10]. Deep learning attempts to model high level representations hidden in raw data and classify patterns by stacking multiple layers of information processing modules in hierarchical architectures. It has been demonstrated that this approach enables the codification of more complex abstractions as data representations in the higher layers, while capturing complex relationships within the data itself. Deep learning enables the development of a unified ML framework integrating feature extraction and inference for the early and accurate detection of faults.

In this paper, we aim to address the three aforementioned challenges by developing a two-dimensional convolutional neural network based fault detection and diagnosis model for distributed systems, along with a fault localization algorithm for supporting recovery. In our model, 2D convolution and pooling operations are applied to multivariate system metrics, in order to capture local dependencies along both temporal and spatial dimensions; an autoencoder layer is used for learning robust representations; and a recurrent neural network layer is used to capture the correlations between continuous streams of unprocessed system metrics, thereby improving efficacy. The proposed approach automatically learns spatiotemporal features from raw distributed system metrics, and does not require any form of transformation, manual feature extraction, or pre- and post-processing; the model and change-point algorithm can work directly over raw system run-time metrics for fault detection and diagnosis. The paper thus makes the following contributions:

- We present an automated fault detection and diagnosis model for general distributed systems based on a hybrid recurrent convolutional neural network with denoising auto-encoders (RCNN-A).
- We present a Bayesian change-point detection approach for localizing faults to the granularity of a distributed node, thus providing useful guidance for robust fault recovery.
- We have implemented our proposed model in a real-world distributed system on top of the Amazon EC2 cloud computing platform, and inject a range of common faults to evaluate efficacy. The experimental results show that our method outperforms a series of state-of-the-art ML algorithms, which are used in the literature for fault detection and diagnosis. Access to a live demonstration of the whole experimental system will be made availableon Insdata[1].

The remainder of this paper is organized as follows. Section 2 provides an overview of related work. Our proposed approaches and their associated details are presented in Sect. 2. Experimental details and results together with two use cases are discussed in Sect. 4. Finally, we draw conclusions in Sect. 5.

2 Related Work

Fault management refers to a class of related approaches aiming to strengthen the reliability of distributed systems [15], and can be categorised into two areas: fault detection and fault diagnosis. For fault detection, there are three main methods: invariant checking, reference implementation and model checking. Invariant checking and reference implementation methods can only detect faults that are obviously abnormal in currently running executions, whereas model checking can achieve more comprehensive detection via an exhaustive search. Unlike a random-check walk-through, model checking is a high confidence fault checking method [15]. For fault diagnosis, log-based causality analysis is the most comprehensive method, which is used in [4]. The latter reference proposes the use of different approaches for automated fault identification, including a signature-based method. Signature-based methods perform well with respect to scalability and simplicity; however, these and other inference methods cannot provide high confidence in the results of detection [15]. Cook et al. also implement FixSym, which is based on ML algorithms and which can automate the detection of system faults. The three ML algorithms in FixSym are Nearest neighbour, K-means clustering and Adaboost [14]. From the experiments conducted by Cook et al., FixSym can detect 95.2% of the faults in a test generating 50 faults within 90 s. The ML algorithms clearly helped the fault diagnosis to achieve a decent level of accuracy; however, the authors did not discuss how to improve the performance

[1] http://insdata.org/opensource/faultpredition.

and accuracy of the classification methodology. In addition, their paper does not clarify the overall efficacy of the method compared to other fault detection methods. In [3], Cid-fuentes et al. present BARCA (Behaviour Identification Architecture), which employs a similar method to Cook et al. to diagnose faults in order to identify the online behaviour in distributed systems, using Support Vector Machines (SVM) [2] for the classification process. BARCA consists of a two layer classification from the extracted features on system usages. The first layer is a one-class classifier which identifies the normal state and any other unexpected behaviour. The second layer is a multi-class classifier that can distinguish the different types of behaviours in a distributed system. The results of BARCA indicate an over 90% accuracy for behaviour detection and modelling. However, the two layer classification would also result in very high performance overheads, and the error rate in the first layer could be enlarged in the second layer.

3 Fault Detection and Diagnosis Approach

In this section, we describe the workflow and implementation of our end-to-end fault detection and localization approaches for distributed systems.

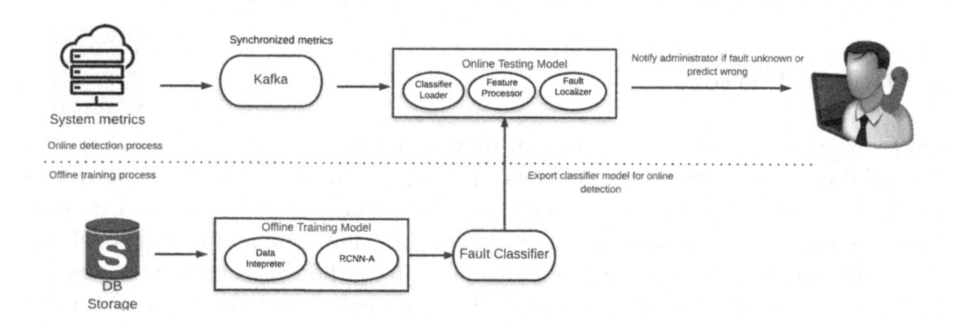

Fig. 1. Workflow of fault detection and localization

The overall workflow can be outlined briefly as follows (see Fig. 1). First of all, raw system metrics such as CPU usage, network usage, etc. are collected during system execution. A data pre-processing component combines and "resizes" these metrics so that the resulting data set can be correctly ingested by our RCNN-based model. A data interpreter normalizes and transforms the same dataset into 2-D vectors (vectorization process). Given such normalized 2-D vectors, a fault predictor (classifier) – which consists of several components for loading a saved classifier – can calculate the class of a fault and its probability. If the probability is higher than a presupposed threshold value, the implementation will send out a notification to an administrator or an external system and add the labeled data to a database for future classifier updating. A fault-healing module will reboot the tier service to resume the system back to a normal state.

3.1 Fault Detection

The diagram of our proposed fault detection approach is shown in Fig. 2. The system usage metrics data is mapped into a 2-D grid of measurements (feature matrix), and first processed by a convolutional neural network to produce feature maps representing a specific system status (e.g. normal, or abnormal for a certain fault type). These maps are subsequently processed by a denoising autoencoder layer, and the information is finally allowed to flow into a recurrent neural network to further capture sequential dependencies along a temporal dimension.

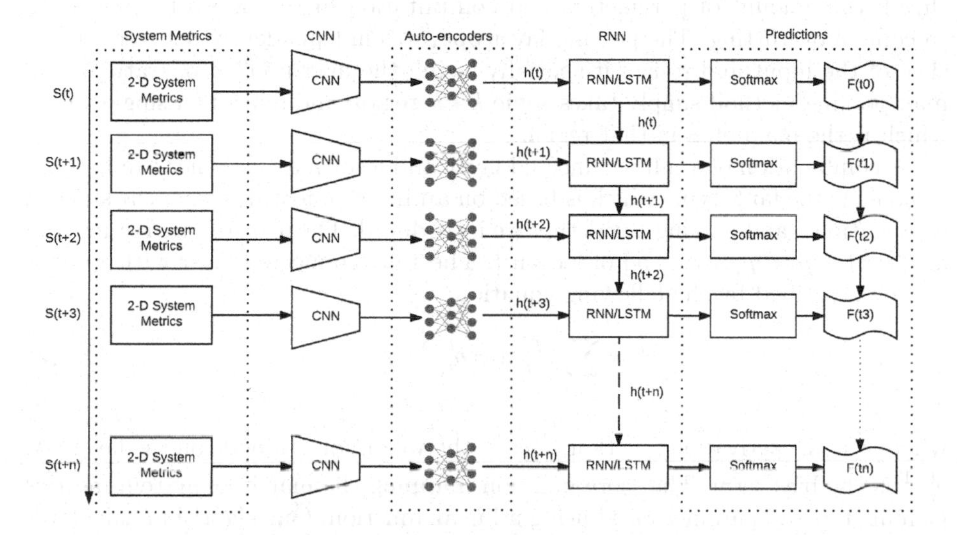

Fig. 2. Fault detection: System status is represented as a sequence of metrics $s(t)$ (e.g. CPU usage, memory consumption, network activity, etc.) from each node, which form 2D convoluational features. These features are input to an autoencoder layer, then temporal dependencies are aggregated across the sequences by a recurrent neural network layer, where the hidden state $h(t-1)$ is calculated from the previous system metrics. The updated hidden state for the current sequence $h(t)$ is used as an input to predict the fault category $F(t)$ with given conditional probabilities.

Convolutional Network Layer. Convolutional neural networks (CNNs) are feed-forward, constrained neural networks comprised of convolutional and subsampling layers, together with one or multiple fully connected multilayer neural networks. A CNN is formed by a stack of distinct layers that transform the input volume into an output volume through a differentiable function. We define the CNN process of the input sequence as a 2-D vector D_t for representing a system's fault status. The convolution kernel size is $a \times b$, with stride size of $i \times j$. For an input sequence I_w of window size w, the output of the ith layer is a matrix of 2-D vector values. The convolutional layer is the core function of CNN, hence we design a convolution layer ℓ with an $m \times m$ filter ω. The output of convolution is defined as follows:

$$x_{ij}^{\ell} = \sum_{a=0}^{m-1} \sum_{b=0}^{m-1} \omega_{ab} y_{(i+a)(j+b)}^{\ell-1}. \tag{1}$$

Our model for fault diagnosis consists of two convolutional layers, two pooling layers, one fully connected layer, one autoencoder layer and an output layer with a recurrent neural layer, as shown in Fig. 2. It is common to periodically insert a pooling layer in-between successive convolutional layers in a CNN architecture. Its function is to progressively reduce the spatial size of the representation to shrink the amount of parameters and computation in the network, and hence to control overfitting. The pooling layer operates independently on every depth slice of the input and resizes it spatially, using the max pooling operation. The max pooling method simply takes some $k * k$ region and outputs a single value, which is the maximum in that region.

A combination of a fully-connected layer and a softmax classifier can be used to analyze the fault type, which is based on an input of features from the stacked convolutional and pooling layers that we introduced. The features are regularized as a vector $p = [p_1, p_2, ..., p_l]$ of length l. The fully-connected layer with l nodes can be described by the following equation:

$$h_i^l = \sum_j \omega_{ij}^{l-1} (\sigma(p_i^{l-1}) + b_i^{l-1}) \tag{2}$$

where σ is the activation function, ω_{ij}^{l-1} is the weight of i-th node on the layer l-1. b_i^{l-1} is the bias term. The score function mapping the matrix of system metrics to fault types is parameterized using a linear function. Our algorithm calculates the scores in each iteration until convergence. The output of the softmax layer is defined as:

$$P(f|p) = argmax \frac{exp(p^{L-1} w^L + b^L)}{\sum_{k=1}^{N_f} exp(p^{L-1} w_k)} \tag{3}$$

where f is the fault type, L is the last layer index, and N_c is the total number of fault classes.

Denoising Autoencoder Layer. A classical autoencoder is a neural network trained to produce outputs equal to the inputs. It is a three-layer network, and its typical structure is comprised of one hidden layer, while the input and the output layers have the same size. The Denoising Autoencoder (DA) is an extension of a classical autoencoder, wherein the initial inputs are corrupted by means of additive isotropic Gaussian noise, and was introduced as a building block for deep networks in [13]. DA has proved to be a robust algorithm that can make unsupervised representations in a feature pattern become more clear. In DA, the linear encoding and decoding processes have the same value weight matrices, which are the vectors of biases of the input and output layers. A regularization function is used to adjust the extremely large or extremely small weights in a specific dataset. Using a DA, one hidden neural layer can be trained with noisy data as input and clean pattern data as output. We add a DA stage after the CNN processing to extract the useful intermediate representations of system metrics X.

Recurrent Neural Network Layer. Recurrent neural networks (RNN) aim to tackle the problem of processing an arbitrarily long time-series sequence of data using a neural network. RNN is able to learn dependencies over time with feedback connections. RNN takes a new sequence of data and generates the output by aggregating the information of the current time-stamp and previous time-steps. In this work, system metrics may have a relation to forward and backward contexts, so it is essential to design a process of carrying memory forward mathematically. We apply Recurrent Neural Networks with Long Short-Term Memory Units (LSTMs) to keep a short memory of the state forward spread into the next learning process. The basic formula of an RNN is $h_t = \phi(W_{x_t} + Uh_{t-1})$, where the hidden state at time step t is h_t. This is a function of the input at the same time step x_t, modified by a weight matrix W. The general formula of an RNN is $h_t = \phi(W_{x_t} + Uh_{t-1} + b)$, where the hidden state at time step t is h_t. U and b are the parameter matrices and vectors, respectively. An improved LSTM in our fault detection is implemented as follows:

$$\begin{aligned} f_t &= \phi(W_f x_t + U_f h_{t-1} + b_f) \\ i_t &= \phi(W_i x_t + U_i h_{t-1} + b_i) \\ o_t &= \phi(W_o x_t + U_o h_{t-1} + b_o) \\ h(t) &= o_t \circ \sigma_h(f_t + i_t \circ o_t) \end{aligned} \tag{4}$$

where f_t is the forget gate for the weight of remembering old information. i_t is the input gate vector. The weight of acquiring new information o_t is the output gate vector W. $h(t)$ is the final output function of state candidate vectors. A temporal pooling layer is then applied for integrating the information across the system metrics along the temporal dimension, in order to capture the long-term dependency of the system metrics time-series. This layer aggregates combined features generated by the CNN and RNN to produce a single feature representation for each sequence. The detailed process of fault detection and diagnosis is expressed in Algorithm 1. The whole system is implemented in Java, and the code will be publicly available on Insdata[2].

3.2 Fault Localization

Once a fault is positively identified to have occurred, fault localization is utilized to trace back across numerous components in the distributed system in order to position the onset of possible to-be faulty component/components. We have developed a fault localization algorithm based on Bayesian change-points [1] – which have been successfully used for the modelling and prediction of time series

[2] http://insdata.org/opensource/faultpredition.

Algorithm 1. Fault Detection and Localization

```
   Data: Matrix of system metrics (2-D vector) D_i
   Result: Predicted fault class C
 1 initialization of the program;
 2 load classifier M;
 3 set window size w;
 4 while Real-time monitoring process is running do
 5 |    read current matrix of system metrics D_i;
 6 |    detect change-point C_n^T using Bayesian model;
 7 |    if size of D_i greater than w then
 8 |    |    ND_i = normalize(D_i);
 9 |    |    F_i = vec(ND_i);
10 |    |    F, θ = classify(F_i);
11 |    |    if θ ≥ threshold then
12 |    |    |    output F;
13 |    |    |    store labelled matrix D_t;
14 |    |    |    while D_t ≥ sizeK do
15 |    |    |    |    train CNN-based model;
16 |    |    |    |    start updating M;
17 |    |    |    end
18 |    |    |    loc(C_n^T, F);
19 |    |    else
20 |    |    |    notify();
21 |    |    end
22 |    else
23 |    |    collect(D);
24 |    end
25 end
```

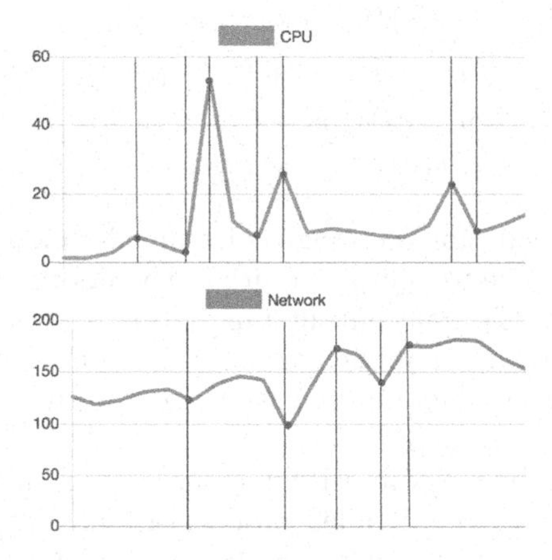

Fig. 3. Bayesian online changepoint detection for system metrics.

in various application areas – to pinpoint where the fault happens for more efficient fault recovery. The change-point model is expressed in terms of run lengths, where run length will drop to zero when a change-point occurs. The predictive distribution is computed on the posterior distribution based on the current run-length, as follows:

Note that the predictive distribution $P(x_{t+1}|x_{1:t})$ depends only on the recent data x_t^r. In our distributed system, the change-point will be detected for four types of metrics: CPU usage, Memory usage, Disk read bytes and Network received bytes. The fault localization module will monitor the four different types of data series every second and export the change-point into a database. Faults in a distributed system can be injected for many reasons and perform fluctuations of workload. An abnormal change-point is possibly related to a fault injection in the system. Therefore, when a fault happens to the system, we assume that the node which has an abnormal change-point closest to the time of fault detection is the source of the fault.

$$P(x_{t+1}|x_{1:t}) = \sum_{r_t} P(x_{t+1}|r_t, x_t^r)P(r_t|x_{1:t}) \tag{5}$$

4 Experiments

4.1 Experimental Settings

Hardware and Software. Our testbed for the (offline) model training phase consists of a nine-node virtual network on Amazon Web Services EC2 cloud, where each node runs Ubuntu Linux, and one node runs an Apache web server. A collection of Bash shell scripts are used to simulate different activities (running processes, etc.) and behaviours which periodically happen in the system. In accord with our fault model, six types of fault injection tools have been developed, which are used to generate the different types of faults. Our tests run on c4.4xlarge type of compute optimized AWS nodes, with the server being a c4.2xlarge node with a 16-core CPU and 30 GB memory. All system metrics data is collected by our distributed log system, the design of which is based on Kafka[3] - an open source library written in Scala and Java developed by the Apache Software Foundation. A local NoSQL database (MongoDB) is deployed for data storage and processing. The six types of faults are periodically injected. It is noted that we assume faults only occur on one node at a time in our experiments. We use the Sigar library[4] to collect the CPU, Memory, Disk and Network real time data twice per second on each node of the system. In data collection session, we simulate the fault into distributed system and collect the system metrics of each type for total 14 h. Over 350000 frames of system metrics were used for our training experiments.

Fault Categorization. Faults in a distributed system can be broadly categorized into system crash faults, timing faults and hardware faults [8,12]. In this paper, we consider a restricted set of 6 faults, which we nevertheless consider to be representative of the different fault categories in a distributed system, and use these as the basis of our fault model. Table 1 summarizes these faults and describes the corresponding software-fault-injection methods used in this work (Fig. 4).

[3] https://kafka.apache.org/.
[4] https://github.com/hyperic/sigar.

Table 1. Fault categories

Fault type	Fault description	Injection method
Node crash	One computer node in the network within which the distributed system operates ceases to work – for example, as a result of the node's power being switched off, or due to an irrecoverable operating system execution error	Periodically shutdown one network node in the AWS EC2 testbed
Application server crash	An application server ceases to work, e.g., as a result of an overload or an execution error	Randomly shutdown the Apache server running on a given node. Use Siege to simulate 20 users continuously making requests to the server
Component crash	The processes underlying one or more system components are killed	Kill a database component periodically while an application is fetching data from the database
Network congestion	The network links connecting two or more nodes in the distributed system become saturated with traffic	Use netem to simulate network latency and packet loss. Simulate 1000 users visiting the Apache server continuously (flooding)
CPU overload	A thread, application or component consumes an abnormally high amount of CPU time continuously. This fault could also lead to a Node Crash	Run an emulation program which periodically utilizes over 99% of CPU time for a sufficiently long time
Memory leak	A process continually consumes an increasing amount of memory that is not released	Run an emulation program which starts hundreds of threads that individually allocate and consume a high amount of memory

4.2 Overall Comparison

We have compared our CNN-based model with a series of algorithms used for fault detection in related literature, including Support Vector Machine (SVM) [3], Naive Bayes (NB) [7], Multilayer Perceptron (MLP), K-nearest neighbors (KNN) [11], AdaBoost [4], Conditional Random Fields (CRFs), Hidden Markov Model (HMM), and Decision Tree (DT). The results are shown in Table 2. As can be seen from the table, some algorithms perform better when

Table 2. Comparison with different models

Model/Training ratio	0.1	0.3	0.5	0.7	0.9
MLP	0.2771	0.3638	0.4267	0.5223	0.79
SVM	0.3406	0.4017	0.4018	0.6873	0.6985
KNN	0.3815	0.4156	0.4108	0.566	0.8081
NB	0.4379	0.4971	0.5128	0.5826	0.6267
CRF	0.3341	0.5127	0.5121	0.732	0.6735
HMM	0.1287	0.1483	0.1561	0.245	0.3854
Decision Tree	0.4421	0.433	0.6137	0.6465	0.6878
AdaBoost	0.1815	0.3601	0.3484	0.3667	0.4171
RCNN-A	0.3633	0.4626	0.5184	0.7006	**0.8712**

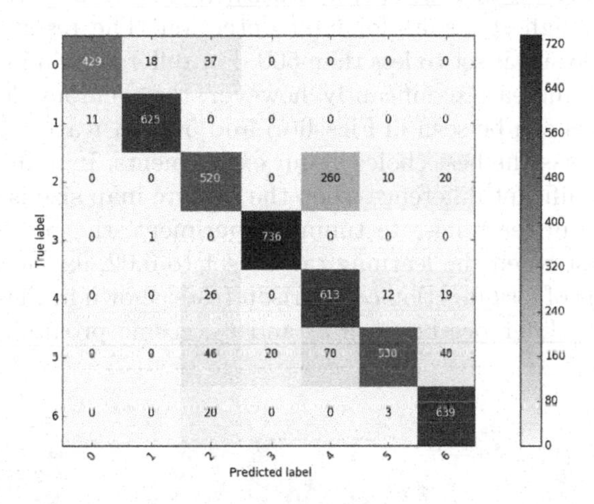

Fig. 4. Confusion matrix over 6 Fault categories, 0: Memory leak, 1: CPU overload, 2: Node crash, 3: Database component crash, 4: Application server crash, 5: Network congestion, 6: Normal

the training process has a different dataset size. CRF is the only algorithm to perform similarly to our model when the training set is less than 90% of the whole dataset. KNN can achieve more than 80% accuracy when the training dataset ratio is 90%. All the other algorithms are comparatively lower than 70% no matter how one changes the training dataset ratio. Our model achieves the highest accuracy when the training dataset is larger in size, e.g., 90% training data, which converts to approximately $\sim 310,000$ system metric records. It should be noted that in these experiments all algorithms were used with raw system metrics (i.e. without feature extraction) to ensure consistency; and we used 5-fold cross-validation.

4.3 Parameter Tuning

In this section, we conduct a series of empirical studies for analyzing the impact of different hyperparameters for the proposed approach. In order to study the best configuration (set of hyperparameters) for our model, we extensively explored: (1) Impact of different configurations of the recurrent convolutional neural network; (2) Impact of a set of key (neural) network parameters such as portion of the training set, learning rate, size of convolutional filter, polling size, and activation function parameter.

Figures 6(a) and 5(a) shows the performance tends to be similar since batch size increases to 50. With larger batch size, the performance will consume more memory while have less iterations per epoch. Balancing the batch size between 50 – 1000 is a challenge when we ran the training algorithm on our server node. Thus, 1000 is the best choice because it saves the overall running time instead of using more memory. In Figs. 6(b) and 5(b), it is obvious that a node size of 1000 reaches the highest results for fault detection. The results are extremely low when the node size is set to less than 500. For different window sizes, the feature map size will increase significantly, however, the accuracy does not increase proportionately, as can be seen in Figs. 6(c) and 5(c). A feature map size of 400 (window size 16) was the best choice in our experiments. In addition, the results do not show a significant difference when the feature map size is varied between 200 and 800. In our learning-rate tuning experiment, the precision and recall reach their highest when the learning rate is set to 0.02, as shown in Figs. 6(d) and 5(d). In terms of loss-function comparison tests, shown in Figs. 6(e) and 5(e), there is a notable difference between ℓ_1 and ℓ_2, cosine proximity and negative

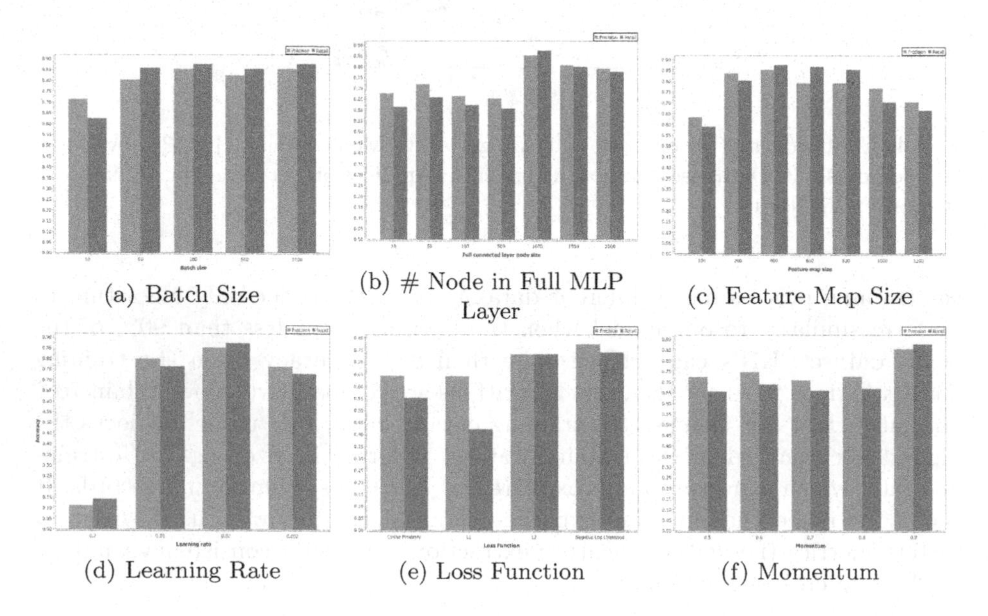

(a) Batch Size (b) # Node in Full MLP Layer (c) Feature Map Size

(d) Learning Rate (e) Loss Function (f) Momentum

Fig. 5. Precision and recall comparison with different parameter settings

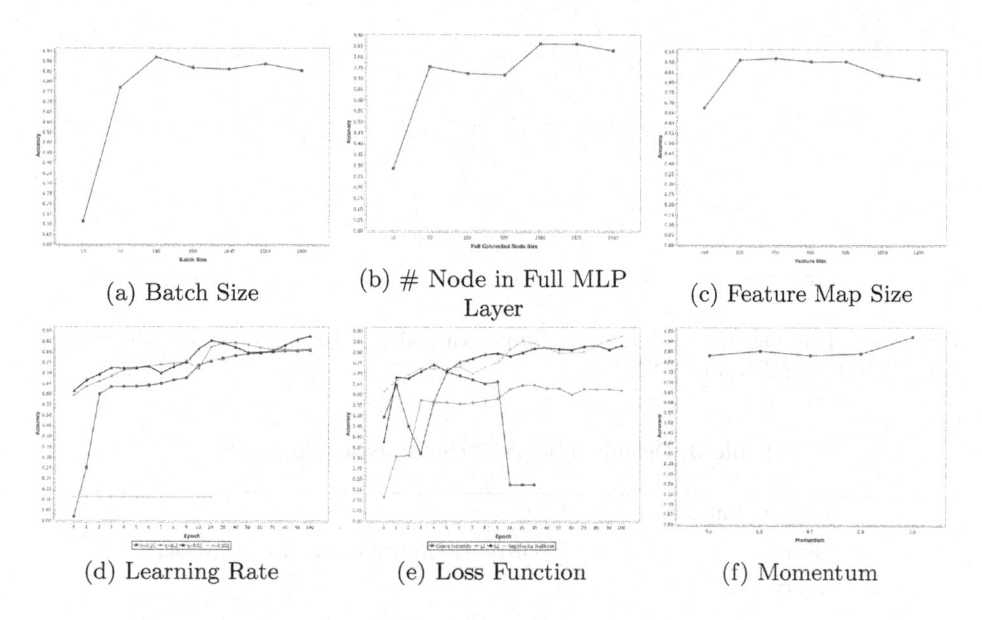

(a) Batch Size (b) # Node in Full MLP Layer (c) Feature Map Size

(d) Learning Rate (e) Loss Function (f) Momentum

Fig. 6. Accuracy comparison with different parameter settings

log likelihood. In particular, ℓ_1 and cosine proximity perform very poorly on our dataset, while negative log likelihood appears to be the best choice. Momentum does not appear to be strongly related to the performance of our CNN for fault detection. Figures 6(f) and 5(f) show that a momentum of 0.9 is the best choice; other values of this parameter lead to similar results.

Finally, based on different ratios of training datasets and evaluation datasets, the accuracy decreases truly linearly, as shown in Fig. 6. The accuracy shown in the comparison tests (Fig. 6) follows a similar trend to that described previously for precision and recall. In those experiments, the fault classification accuracy is higher than precision and recall. In order to further investigate the efficacy of our proposal, we plot the accuracy evolution process when training occurs after each epoch, as shown in Fig. 6. From this we can observe that the patterns in the raw metric data collected for each fault type become increasingly distinguished layer by layer. The cosine proximity loss function degrades significantly after ten epochs, which is due to the optimization algorithm dropping into a local minimum solution. Cosine proximity is not useful with respect to our fault detection algorithm, as the achievable accuracy in the first five epochs is only 65%. For the learning rate comparison test, the accuracy stays around 10% while the learning rate set to 0.2, which is too large for the dataset, as shown in Fig. 6. We conducted additional experiments to determine the balance ratio of training dataset size and time. These results (Figs. 3 and 6(a and b)) show that the training time linearly grows with the dataset size growth, and that the accuracy is also related to the dataset's size. The optimal setting of our proposed hybrid model is summarized in Table 3.

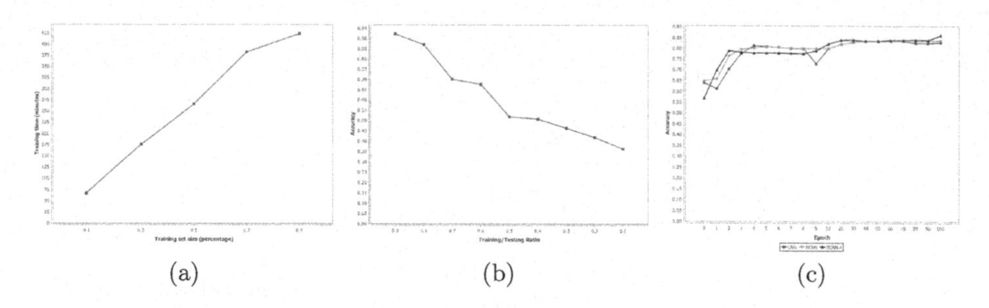

(a) (b) (c)

Fig. 7. (a) Training time variation (b) Impact of training/testing ratio (c) Comparison with RCNN-A, CNN and RNN

Table 3. Default settings of the proposed approach

Hyper parameter	Value
Layer	Recurrent, Convolution, Auto-encoder
Iteration	2
Epoch	100, Early stopping
Learning rate	0.2–0.002
Kernel size	2, 1
Stride	1, 1
Pooling size	2, 1
Pooling method	MAX
Momentum	0.9
Batch size	100–2000
Auto-encoder layer size	100–1000
Full connected node	10–1000
Optimization Algorithm	Stochastic gradient descent

Table 2 shows a confusion matrix of fault (class) prediction. It is obvious that the accuracy of class "node crash" and "application server crash" are confused in our fault classifier, which is the most significant case that decreases the overall accuracy. Network congestion is also predicted incorrectly the most times by our model. We also compare our approach with other deep neural network architectures such as (pure) convolutional neural networks and recurrent neural networks. Figure 7(c) shows that our model outperforms both (pure) CNN and RNN when the epoch is greater than 90.

We have developed a web-based user interface which provides access to monitoring the system metrics of all active (system) nodes on a network, simulation of fault injection to a given node, analysis and a view the detection history of our proposed algorithm. The web-based user interface is used for our fault detection system demonstration and can be accessed with a browser on any platform. The demonstration can be found at Insdata[5].

5 Conclusion

In this paper, we outlined our work towards an automated fault management solution for distributed systems using a recurrent convolutional neural network model for fault detection, along with a Bayesian change-point algorithm for pinpointing nodes from which the fault originated. With respect to this model and from our studies so far, our explorations presented in this paper have shown a promising proof of deep learning's capability to accurately support fault-related inferences by directly analyzing raw system data. Our proposed model outperforms a series of state-of-the-art algorithms used for fault detection and diagnosis in distributed systems.

Acknowledgements. The research of Lina Yao and Guangyang Qi was funded by the Defence Science Institute (DSI), an initiative of the State Government of Victoria, as part of a collaborative project between DST Group and UNSW Sydney under the DSI CERA program.

References

1. Adams, R.P., MacKay, D.J.: Bayesian online changepoint detection. arXiv preprint arXiv:0710.3742 (2007)
2. Byun, H., Lee, S.W.: Applications of support vector machines for pattern recognition: a survey. In: Lee, S.W., Verri, A. (eds.) SVM 2002. LNCS, vol. 2388, pp. 213–236. Springer, Heidelberg (2002). doi:10.1007/3-540-45665-1_17
3. Cid-Fuentes, J.A., Szabo, C., Falkner, K.: Online behavior identification in distributed systems. In: 2015 IEEE 34th Symposium on Reliable Distributed Systems (SRDS), pp. 202–211. IEEE (2015)
4. Cook, B., Babu, S., Candea, G., Duan, S.: Toward self-healing multitier services. In: 2007 IEEE 23rd International Conference on Data Engineering Workshop, pp. 424–432. IEEE (2007)
5. Goodfellow, I., Bengio, Y., Courville, A.: Deep learning. MIT Press, Cambridge (2016)
6. Hinton, G., Deng, L., Yu, D., Dahl, G.E., Mohamed, A.R., Jaitly, N., Senior, A., Vanhoucke, V., Nguyen, P., Sainath, T.N., et al.: Deep neural networks for acoustic modeling in speech recognition: the shared views of four research groups. IEEE Signal Process. Mag. **29**(6), 82–97 (2012)
7. Jia, R., Abdelwahed, S., Erradi, A.: Towards proactive fault management of enterprise systems. In: 2015 International Conference on Cloud and Autonomic Computing (ICCAC), pp. 21–32. IEEE (2015)
8. Kola, G., Kosar, T., Livny, M.: Faults in large distributed systems and what we can do about them. In: Cunha, J.C., Medeiros, P.D. (eds.) Euro-Par 2005. LNCS, vol. 3648, pp. 442–453. Springer, Heidelberg (2005). doi:10.1007/11549468_51

[5] http://insdata.org/opensource/faultpredition.

9. Krizhevsky, A., Sutskever, I., Hinton, G.E.: Imagenet classification with deep convolutional neural networks. In: Advances in Neural Information Processing Systems, pp. 1097–1105 (2012)
10. LeCun, Y., Bengio, Y., Hinton, G.: Deep learning. Nature **521**(7553), 436–444 (2015)
11. Nandi, A., Mandal, A., Atreja, S., Dasgupta, G.B., Bhattacharya, S.: Anomaly detection using program control flow graph mining from execution logs. In: Proceedings of the 22nd ACM SIGKDD International Conference on Knowledge Discovery and Data Mining, pp. 215–224. ACM (2016)
12. Tanenbaum, A.S., Van Steen, M.: Distributed Systems. Prentice-Hall, Upper Saddle River (2007)
13. Vincent, P., Larochelle, H., Bengio, Y., Manzagol, P.A.: Extracting and composing robust features with denoising autoencoders. In: Proceedings of the 25th International Conference on Machine Learning, pp. 1096–1103. ACM (2008)
14. Witten, I.H., Frank, E.: Data Mining: Practical Machine Learning Tools and Techniques. Morgan Kaufmann, San Francisco (2005)
15. Zhou, W.: Fault management in distributed systems. Technical report MS-CIS-10-03, University of Pennsylvania, Department of Computer and Information Science (2010)

Discovering Group Skylines with Constraints by Early Candidate Pruning

Ming-Yen Lin[1], Yueh-Lin Lin[1], and Sue-Chen Hsueh[2(✉)]

[1] Feng Chia University, Taichung 40724, Taiwan
[2] Chaoyang University of Technology, Taichung 41349, Taiwan
schsueh@cyut.edu.tw

Abstract. Skyline query has been an important issue in the database community. Many applications nowadays request the skyline after grouping tuples, such as fantasy sports, so that the group skyline problem becomes the research focus. Most previous algorithms intended to quickly sift through the numerous combinations but fail to address the problem of constraints. In practice, nearly all groupings are specified with constrains, which demand solutions of constrained group skyline. In this paper, we propose an algorithm called CGSky to efficiently solve the problem. CGSky utilizes a pre-processing method to exclude the unnecessary tuples and generate candidate groups incrementally. A pruning mechanism is devised in the algorithm to prevent non-qualifying candidates from the skyline computation. Our experimental results show that CGSky improves an order of magnitude over previous algorithms in average. It also shows that CGSky has good scale-up capability on different data distributions.

Keywords: Skyline query · Group skyline · Constraint · Constrained skyline

1 Introduction

Skyline is a query operator that helps users to retrieve interesting tuples from databases [5, 8, 9]. These tuples are not dominated by any other tuples. A typical example is that in a hotel relation having price and distance-to-beach attributes. A user is likely to ask for hotels that are both cheap and close to the beach. If the price of a hotel h is higher than that of a hotel h′ and the distance-to-beach of h is not shorter than that of h′, h is *dominated* by h′, written as $h' \succ h$, and h can be excluded from the query result. Skyline queries return the sets of tuples that are not *dominated* by any other tuples. Typically, a user may specify some constraints on certain attributes, such as price, so that constrained skyline [2, 13, 15, 21] might be more common in practice. For example, the skyline query for best web-portal advertising plan might be constrained by 'cost $\leq$ 6000'. Skyline query and constrained skyline query thus are used in many multi-criteria decision support applications.

Although (constrained) skyline query may retrieve non-dominated tuples, interesting groups generated from combinations of single tuples can be more desirable in some applications. For example, to increase visibility of new products, a company may advertise on more than one web portal so that the skyline result contains combinations of portals, which combinations are not dominated by other ones, considering the total

G. Cong et al. (Eds.): ADMA 2017, LNAI 10604, pp. 49–62, 2017.
https://doi.org/10.1007/978-3-319-69179-4_4

'cost' and the total 'number-of-visitors' (#visitors) attributes. Given a number of portals, a user may specify that a group is composed of 2 portals. The problem of group skyline [17] is to find the groups, considering all the combinations of 2 portals, which are not dominated by other groups. The attribute-values of the group thus are aggregate-values (e.g. sum) of the 2 portals. Applications querying the skylines of groups are commonplace, such as baseball teams of 9 persons as a group, fantasy basketball of 5 persons as a group, Hackathon of 3 persons as a group, etc. The cardinality of a group (9 in baseball, 5 in basketball, etc.) is specified by users, which is called the group cardinality, denoted by k. In addition, the aggregate-function is also specified by users, which can be sum(), min(), max(), and so on. Because group skyline has to consider all the combinations of certain cardinality, the problem is more complicated than traditional skyline problems.

Nevertheless, no previous studies have discussed group skylines with constraints. A common scenario is that not all combinations are acceptable due to certain constraints. For example, advertising web-portals may subject to a limited total budget, which means the total cost (by summing cost of the portals in the combination) cannot exceed certain amount. Given a query of investment portfolios for stocks, the investors may have a budget limit of 10000 for the non-dominated portfolio of 3 stocks ($k = 3$). Also, NBA league rules that every NBA team cannot exceed a certain amount of team salary, which means the total salary is constrained. The result of the group skyline would be groups of players having good (aggregated) scoring/defense capability while satisfying the total salary constraint.

Table 1. An example of web portals datasets.

Tuple	Web Portal	Cost	#Visitors	Skyline
t_1	Facebook	3	4	V
t_2	Google	10	4	
t_3	Yahoo	5	1	
t_4	Apple Daily	7	10	V
t_5	Mobile01	8	6	
t_6	PChome	6	7	V

However, finding group skylines with constraints is complicated. In Table 1, tuples t_1, t_4, and t_6 are skyline tuples since $t_1 \succ t_2$, $t_1 \succ t_3$, and $t_6 \succ t_5$, when smaller 'cost' and larger '#visitors' are preferred in web-portal advertising plans. Using the 6 tuples for groups of cardinality $k = 3$, there are total 20 groups as listed in Table 2. Although t_3 is not a skyline tuple in Table 1, group G_5 having t_1, t_3 and t_4 is a group skyline tuple. Similarly, tuple t_5, dominated by t_6 in Table 1, becomes the member of the group skyline tuple G_{20}. That is, both combinations of skyline tuples and that of non-skyline tuples have to be considered in the group skyline finding process. The number of combinations can be very huge. For example, assume that a dataset contains 500 tuples and group cardinality $k = 5$, about C(500, 5) = 2.6×10^{11} candidate groups will be generated in total. To compute such a huge amount of combinations is a serious challenge. Furthermore, the constraint can only be considered after groups are formed because the constraint is specified against the aggregated attribute-value. This restricts effective pruning of candidate groups and is more time-consuming, comparing to specifying constraint on single tuples of a typical skyline query. Constrained skyline may exclude tuples that do not satisfy the constraint a priori to reduce the computation but constrained group skyline needs to generate all candidate groups to exclude the groups unsatisfying the constraint. Therefore, the discovery of the group skyline with constraints is much more difficult than that of both skyline with constraints and group skyline without constraints.

Table 2. Enumerated groups of cardinality 3 for the dataset in Table 1.

Group	Members	Cost	#Visitors	Skyline
G_1	t_1, t_2, t_3	18	9	
G_2	t_1, t_2, t_4	20	18	
G_3	t_1, t_2, t_5	21	14	
G_4	t_1, t_2, t_6	19	15	
G_5	t_1, t_3, t_4	15	15	V
G_6	t_1, t_3, t_5	16	11	
G_7	t_1, t_3, t_6	14	12	V
G_8	t_1, t_4, t_5	18	20	
G_9	t_1, t_4, t_6	16	21	V
G_{10}	t_1, t_5, t_6	17	17	
G_{11}	t_2, t_3, t_4	22	15	
G_{12}	t_2, t_3, t_5	23	11	
G_{13}	t_2, t_3, t_6	21	12	
G_{14}	t_2, t_4, t_5	25	20	
G_{15}	t_2, t_4, t_6	23	21	
G_{16}	t_2, t_5, t_6	24	17	
G_{17}	t_3, t_4, t_5	20	17	
G_{18}	t_3, t_4, t_6	18	18	
G_{19}	t_3, t_5, t_6	19	14	
G_{20}	t_4, t_5, t_6	21	23	V

The problem of finding group skyline with constraint is defined as follows. Given a database of n tuples $D = \{t_1, t_2, \ldots, t_n\}$ of m numeric attributes, user-specified group cardinality k ($k > 1$), and a constraint c, the objective is to find the set of group skyline tuples satisfying c. A tuple t_i is represented as $(t_i[A_1], t_i[A_2], \ldots, t_i[A_m])$. Tuple t_x *dominates* tuple t_y, denoted by $t_x \succ t_y$, if $\forall\, i\ (1 \leq i \leq m)$, $t_x[A_i] \geq t_y[A_i]$, and $\exists\, j\ (1 \leq j \leq m)$, $t_x[A_j] > t_y[A_j]$. The operators '>' and '$\geq$' can be replaced by '<' and '$\leq$' when smaller values are preferred, such as the smaller 'cost' and the larger 'number-of-visitors' the example of Table 1. A group tuple $Gx = \{t_1', t_2', \ldots, t_k'\}$ is a combination of k distinct tuples in D, where $t_p' \in D\ \forall 1 \leq p \leq k$. Gx also has m attributes and the attribute value of $Gx[A_i] = \sum_{p=1}^{k} t_p'[A_i]$ $(1 \leq i \leq m)$ if sum() is the preferred aggregate-function. The *Gx* is also called a *k-tuple* group since it has *k* tuples. A group tuple *Gx* satisfying constraint *c* is denoted by G_x^c. A group G_x^c is said to dominate group G_y^c, denoted by $G_x^c \succ_G G_y^c$, if and only if $\forall\, i\ (1 \leq i \leq m)$, $G_x^c[A_i] \geq G_y^c[A_i]$, and $\exists\, j\ (1 \leq j \leq m)$, $G_x^c[A_j] > G_y^c[A_j]$. G_x^c is a group skyline tuple satisfying *c* if there exists no G_y^c such that $G_y^c \succ_G G_x^c$. The objective is to find the set of all the group skyline tuples satisfying *c*.

For example, given dataset D in Table 1, group cardinality k = 3, and constraint c = 'Cost < 19', all the 20 combinations are listed in Table 2. When constraint c is not considered, the group skyline tuples are G5, G7, G9, and G20. The group skyline tuples satisfying c are G_5^c, G_7^c, and G_9^c because G20 does not satisfy 'Cost < 19' constraint. Alternatively, we said that the three group tuples are constrained group skyline tuples.

In this paper, we present a novel algorithm called CGSky (*Constrained Group Skyline*), for solving troblem of computing group skyline with constraints. In the following context, the group skyline tuples satisfying the constraint are simply called the group skyline tuples, or collectively named the group skyline.

The rest of the paper is as follows. Section 2 briefly reviews the related work. The proposed CGSky algorithm is presented in Sect. 3. Section 4 describes the experimental results. Finally, Sect. 5 concludes the paper.

2 Related Work

The skyline operator was first introduced in [1] and many algorithms have been proposed. These algorithms can be categorized into generic and index-based types. Generic skyline algorithms do not need pre-computation, such as BNL [1], D&C [1], SFS [4], SSPL [10], etc. Index-based skyline algorithms utilize the pre-processing data structures to avoid scanning the entire dataset, such as NN [12], BBS [18], Bitmap [20], etc. Generic skyline algorithms usually incur high I/O cost, while the efficiency of index-based ones will decrease as the number of attributes increases.

Constrained skyline was proposed on the extension of the BBS algorithm [6]. The main idea of constrained skyline is to compute the results satisfying user preferences. Two types of constraint problems were described. The constrained skyline problem [2] uses the constraint to filter out tuples first, then computes the results using the remaining tuples. The skyline with constraints problem is to computing the skyline first, then using the constraint to filter out the results dis-qualifying the constraint.

Computing the group skyline is a complicated task. GDynamic [11] algorithm utilizes an incremental method to overcome the bottleneck, which is the number of candidate groups. There are $\binom{n}{c}$ possible combinations for n tuples and group cardinality of c. The Improved Decomposition Algorithm (IDA) [6] is a combinatorial skyline algorithm. The dynamic programing algorithm based on order-specific property (OSM) [22] is also a group skyline algorithm. While the G-Skyline [14] is a group skyline algorithm without using aggregate function as the foundation of group dominance relation. Among these algorithms, the IDA algorithm utilizes a pre-processing method to compute the number of dominating numbers for each tuple. Moreover, the pre-processing result will output a dominance table for speeding up the formation of groups. However, all these algorithms ignore that the group skyline might incorporate the need of certain constrains. The focus of the study is to push constraints into the computation process so that the skyline finding process can be greatly accelerated. As indicated in the experimental results, the proposed algorithm successfully improve the discovering process.

3 Proposed Algorithm

The proposed CGSky algorithm, inspired by the IDA algorithm [6], computes the constrained group skyline in three phases: early tuple-pruning, candidate-group generation, and group-dominance checking. Figure 1 is an overview of the CGSky algorithm. The dominance relationships among tuples are computed and tuples cannot become members of group skyline tuples are pruned in the phase of early tuple-pruning. The remaining tuples are sorted in ascending order of the constraint attribute in this phase. The sorted tuples are used to generate candidate groups recursively in the phase of candidate-group generation. Finally, the resulting group skyline tuples satisfying the constraint are found by applying any (single-tuple) skyline algorithm, such as SFS [4], on the candidate groups in the phase of group-dominance checking.

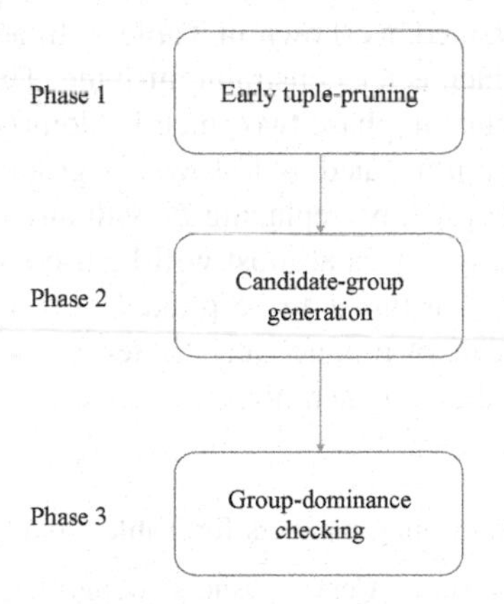

Fig. 1. An overview of the CGSky algorithm.

3.1 Phase One: Dominance-Table Computation

First, Phase one of the CGSky algorithm reduces the number of candidate groups by pruning tuples that cannot become members of the final group skyline tuples. In this phase, the CGSky algorithm first computes the dominance relationships among tuples in D. For each tuple t, the number of tuples dominating t is accumulated. The number is referred to as the *dominating number* of t, denoted by *dom*(t). Once a tuple's dominating number is larger than the group cardinality *k*, the tuple is pruned and no candidate group will include this tuple as a member. Any group formed by these eliminated tuples is impossible to be a skyline group tuple, as proved in Theorem 1. That is, if *dom*(t) $\geq k$, then tuple t is eliminated from the generation of candidate groups of cardinality k. For convenience, we use '$t \oplus^{k-1} G_x$' to represent the group tuple formed by a (k-1)-tuple group G_x and tuple t. CGSky then sorts tuples by ascending order of the constraint attribute. Sorting tuples by the constraint attribute is beneficial to the generation of candidate groups, as presented in Sect. 3.2

Theorem 1. Tuple t with *dom*(t) $\geq k$ cannot form a skyline group tuple for group cardinality of k.

Proof. Tuple t is dominated by at least k tuples in dataset D since *dom*(t) $\geq k$. Assume t is included in a group tuple $G = t \oplus^{k-1} G_x$, we will show that there exists a group tuple G', which is formed by $t' \oplus^{k-1} G_x$ and $G' \succ_G G$. (i) Let the set of tuples dominating t be $H = \{t_1', t_2', \ldots, t_k'\}$ if *dom*(t) = k. When $H \cap {}^{k-1}G_x = \phi$, there exists $t' \in H$, $G' = t' \oplus^{k-1} G_x \succ_G G = t \oplus^{k-1} G_x$ since $t' \succ t$. Let $H \cap {}^{k-1}G_x = {}^{p}G_y$ $(1 \leq p \leq k\text{-}1)$ and $H' = H - {}^{p}G_y$, thus there are (k-p) tuples in H' dominating t. Then there exists $t' \in H'$, $G' = t' \oplus ({}^{p}G_y \oplus^{k-p-1} G_z) \succ_G t \oplus ({}^{p}G_y \oplus^{k-p-1} G_z)$ since $t' \succ t$. (ii) If *dom*(t) > k then we just pick k tuples from the set dominating t to constitute $H = \{t_1', t_2', \ldots, t_k'\}$, the rest of the proof is the same as (i). Thus, any group having t must be dominated by some other group. Tuple t with *dom*(t) $\geq k$ cannot form a skyline group tuple and can be safely eliminated from the generation of candidate groups. □

For example, tuples in Table 1 are processed in this phase and the dominating number of each tuple is obtained, as shown in Table 3. In addition, tuples are sorted in ascending order of Cost, which is the constraint attribute. Tuple t_2 is not engaged in the generation of candidate groups in phase two since its dom(t_2) > k for group cardinality k = 3. The exclusion can be illustrated as follows. A group G formed by including t_2 will be dominated by a group G′, by replacing t_2 with any one of the four dominating tuples $\{t_1, t_6, t_4, t_5\}$. Only two tuples at most will be used to form G for k = 3 so that there are always two remaining tuples to be picked to form G′. Obviously, G′ dominates G. Consequently, t_2 cannot produce any 'potential' group skyline tuple and can be eliminated from the candidate generation.

Table 3. Dominating numbers for Table 1 (sorted by Cost).

Tuple	Cost	#Visitors	dom(t_i)
t_1	3	4	0
t_3	5	1	1
t_6	6	7	0
t_4	7	10	0
t_5	8	6	2
t_2	10	4	4

3.2 Phase Two: Candidate-Group Generation

Figure 2 presents the pseudo-code of the candidate-group generation. The CGSky algorithm invokes GenCandidate with parameters (D[1, n], k, limit), where D[1, n] is the dataset after the early pruning in phase one, k is the group cardinality, and limit is the upper bound of the constraint value. The subroutine generates all the candidate groups of cardinality k satisfying the constraint (limit). The principle of this phase is as follows.

```
Subroutine GenCandidate
Input: D[p,q] – list of tuples t_p, t_p+1, …, t_q
       k – group cardinality
       limit – constraint limit // constraint attribute A_c
Output: A = set of candidate group tuples
1. A = ϕ ;
2. if (k=1)
3.    for i = p to q do
4.      if (t_i[Ac] ≥ limit) break ;
5.      add {t_i} to A ;
6.    endfor
7.    return A ;
8. endif
9. for i = p to q-(k-1)
10.  if (t_i[A_c] ≥ limit) break ;
11.  A' = GenCandidate(D[i+1,q], k-1, limit-t_i[A_c]) ;
12.  if (A'= ϕ) break ;
13.  for each set S in A'
14.    Add t_i to S ;
15.    Add S to A ;
16.  endfor
17. endfor
18. return A;
```

Fig. 2. Pseudo-code of the candidate-group generation.

Given the sorted list of tuples $[t_p, t_{p+1},\dots, t_i, t_{i+1},\dots, t_q]$, if tuple t_i with constraint-attribute value t_i[Ac] will constitute a k-tuple group with a (k-1)-tuple group Gx, then the aggregate-value of Gx[Ac] must be less than (limit′ = limit-t_i[Ac]). In addition, the Gx is constructed from potential combinations of (k-1) tuples from list $[t_{i+1},\dots, t_q]$. Recursively, if tuple t_{i+1} with constraint-attribute value t_{i+1}[Ac] will constitute a (k-1)-tuple group with a (k-2)-tuple group Gx′, then the aggregate-value of Gx′ [Ac] must be less than (limit′-t_{i+1}[Ac]). The Gx′ is constructed from potential combinations of (k-2) tuples from list $[t_{i+2},\dots, t_q]$. The recursion eventually would reach the formation of 1-tuple group from list $[t_p', t_p'_{+1},\dots, t_q]$, constrained by certain upper bound $limit^z$. When some tuple t_s in the list having $t_s[Ac] \geq limit^z$ is unqualified, all the rest of tuples are impossible to satisfy the bound since tuples are sorted in ascending order of constraint value (lines 2–8). Therefore, we may prevent a large number of "unqualified" candidate groups from generation. Furthermore, when no combination is generated during the construction of certain group tuple, assume that such combinations are to be used with t_h, then no tuples after t_h in the list may generate a qualified group (lines 9–17).

For example, let the CGSky algorithm invoke GenCandidate(D[$\boldsymbol{t_1}$, t_3, t_6, t_4, t_5], k = 3, limit = **19**) in Table 3. Tuple t_1 can only form qualified candidates with 2-tuple groups, generated from D[t_3, t_6, t_4, t_5] and constrained by (2-tuple group) limit of 19-t_1[Cost] = 16. This will invoke GenCandidate(D[$\boldsymbol{t_3}$, t_6, t_4, t_5], k = 2, limit = **16**). The call with t_3 can only form qualified candidates with 1-tuple groups, generated from D [t_6, t_4, t_5] and constrained by limit of 16-t_3[Cost] = 11. GenCandidate(D[t_6, t_4, t_5], k = 1, limit = **11**) returns {t_6}, {t_4} and {t_5} so that {t_3, t_6}, {t_3, t_4} and {t_3, t_5} are returned. The three will be collected for t_1 to form 3-tuple groups {t_1, t_3, t_6}, {t_1, t_3, t_4} and {t_1, t_3, t_5} later. The GenCandidate(D[t_3, $\boldsymbol{t_6}$, t_4, t_5], k = 2, limit = **16**) continues with t_6. This call with t_6 can only form qualified candidates with 1-tuple groups, generated from D[t_4, t_5] and constrained by limit of 16-t_6[Cost] = 10. GenCandidate (D[t_4, t_5], k = 1, limit = **10**) returns {t_4} and {t_5} so that {t_6, t_4} and {t_6, t_5} are returned. The two will be collected for t_1 to form 3-tuple groups {t_1, t_6, t_4} and {t_1, t_6, t_5} later. The GenCandidate(D[t_3, t_6, $\boldsymbol{t_4}$, t_5], k = 2, limit = **16**) continues with t_4. This call with t_4 can only form qualified candidates with 1-tuple groups, generated from D [t_5] and constrained by limit of 16-t_4[Cost] = 9. GenCandidate(D[t_5], k = 1, limit = **9**) returns {t_5} so that {t_4, t_5} is returned. This one will be collected for t_1 to form a 3-tuple group {t_1, t_4, t_5} later. The call with t_1 now stops.

Next, GenCandidate(D[t_1, $\boldsymbol{t_3}$, t_6, t_4, t_5], k = 3, limit = **19**) continues with tuple t_3. Tuple t_3 can only form qualified candidates with 2-tuple groups, generated from D[t_6, t_4, t_5] and constrained by (2-tuple group) limit of 19-t_3[Cost] = 14. This will invoke GenCandidate(D[$\boldsymbol{t_6}$, t_4, t_5], k = 2, limit = **14**). The call with t_6 can only form qualified candidates with 1-tuple groups, generated from D[t_4, t_5] and constrained by limit of 14-t_6[Cost] = 8. GenCandidate(D[t_4, t_5], k = 1, limit = **8**) returns {t_4} so that {t_6, t_4} is returned. The {t_6, t_4} will be used with t_3 to form 3-tuple groups {t_3, t_6, t_4} later.

Subsequently, GenCandidate(D[t_1, t_3, $\boldsymbol{t_6}$, t_4, t_5], k = 3, limit = **19**) continues with tuple t_6. Tuple t_6 can only form qualified candidates with 2-tuple groups, generated from D[t_4, t_5] and constrained by (2-tuple group) limit of 19-t_6[Cost] = 13. This will invoke GenCandidate(D[t_4, t_5], k = 2, limit = **13**). The call with t_4 can only form qualified candidates with 1-tuple groups, generated from D[t_5] and constrained by limit of 13-t_4[Cost] = 6. GenCandidate(D[t_5], k = 1, limit = **6**) returns empty so that the call with t_4, invoked by the call with t_6 are stopped. Any invocation after t_6 cannot generate valid 3-tuple groups so the recursion ends. The candidate 3-tuple groups are {t_1, t_3, t_6}, {t_1, t_3, t_4}, {t_1, t_3, t_5}, {t_1, t_6, t_4}, {t_1, t_6, t_5}, {t_1, t_4, t_5}, and {t_3, t_6, t_4}.

3.3 Phase Three: Group-Dominance Checking

The resulting group skyline tuples satisfying the constraint are found by applying any common skyline algorithm, such as the BNL algorithm [1], on the candidate groups. The final group skyline with constraints includes {t_1, t_3, t_6}, {t_1, t_3, t_4}, and {t_1, t_6, t_4}.

Note that only 8 candidates, rather than 20 candidates, are generated by the CGSky algorithm. The number of candidates required for dominance checking using common skyline algorithms is greatly reduced.

4 Experimental Results

Comprehensive experiments were executed to assess the performance of the proposed algorithm. All the algorithms were executed on a Windows 7 PC, with Intel(R) Core (TM) i5-4460 3.2 GHz, 16 GB RAM and 1 TB hard disk. A modified IDA algorithm [6], called IDA*, and CGSKY were compared in the experiments. Both were implemented in Java. The IDA algorithm [6] is one of the representative group skyline algorithms up-to-date. The IDA* algorithm extends IDA with an additional phase of selecting the groups satisfying the constraints. Both synthetic datasets and a real dataset were used in the experiments. Here, we report the results on anti-correlated datasets, the results on independent and correlated datasets were similar.

Similar to most skyline algorithms, the synthetic datasets include distributions of correlated, anti-correlated and independent data. Distinct datasets were generated using different parameters including data size n, group cardinality k, number of attributes m, and constraint (limit) c. The used parameters are summarized in Table 4. The default setting was $n = 500$, $k = 3$, $m = 3$, and $c < 120$. The range of values for each attribute was uniformly distributed from 0 to 100. All the attribute values were independently generated in the independent dataset. For a correlated dataset, if the value of the first attribute is x, the values of the rest attributes range from x*0.95 to x*1.05. For an anti-correlated dataset, if the value of the first attribute is x, the values of the rest attributes range from 100-x*0.95 to 100-x*1.05.

Table 4. Parameter values used in the synthetic datasets.

Parameter	Used value	Default
Data Size n	100, 300, 500, 700, 900	500
Group cardinality k	2, 3, 4, 5	3
Attribute m	2, 3, 4, 5	3
Constraint c	80, 120, 160, 200, 240	120

Figure 3 shows the results of executions on anti-correlated datasets of $k = 3$, $m = 3$, and $c < 120$, by varying the data size n from 100 to 900. The results on independent datasets and correlated datasets were similar. As the data size increases, both the number of candidate groups and the number of constrained group skyline tuples increase. In average, CGSky runs four times faster than IDA*. Table 5 lists the number of candidate tuples, that of candidate groups, and that of group skyline tuples with respect to the algorithms. For example, in Table 5 with $n = 100$, both algorithms eliminated 60 tuples having dominating number larger than the group cardinality. This leaves C(40, 3) = 4980 candidate groups generated for IDA* while CGS generated only 2013 candidates by incorporating the constraint during candidate generation. The number of (constrained) group skyline tuples was the same for both algorithms.

Figure 4 shows the results of executions on anti-correlated datasets of n = 500, k = 3, and c < 120, by varying the number of attributes m from 2 to 5. In average, CGSky runs 11.1 times faster than IDA*. IDA* spent 1400 s to compute the answer when m = 5. As listed in Table 6, the number of candidate groups for IDA* is 5.6 times for CGSky when m = 4. The increase in the number of attributes has a great impact on the total execution time since the number of "incomparable" tuples increases exponentially.

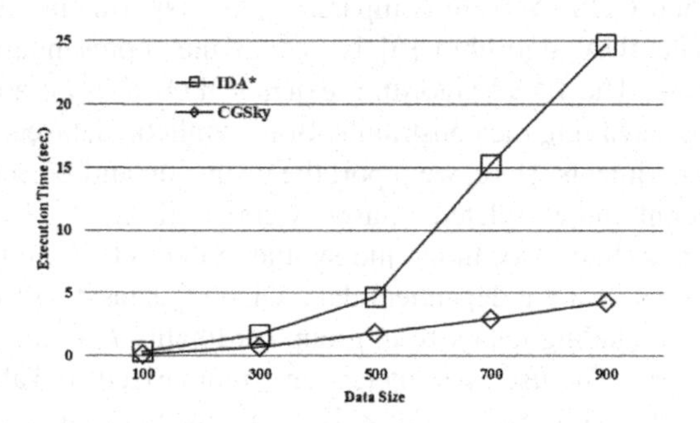

Fig. 3. Results on varying data size *n*.

Table 5. Number of candidate tuples and candidate-groups w.r.t. *n*.

n	Candidate tuples	IDA*	CGSky
100	40	9880	2013
300	66	45760	15693
500	90	117480	41971
700	119	273819	94130
900	133	383306	124480

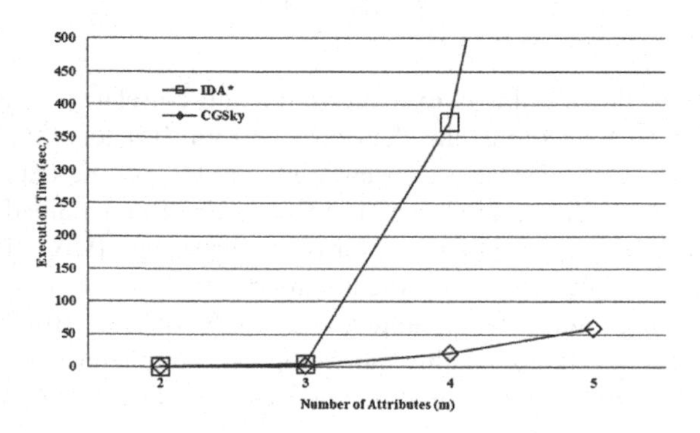

Fig. 4. Results on varying number of attributes *m*.

Table 6. Number of candidates, candidate-groups, and group-skyline tuples w.r.t. *m*.

m	Candidate tuples	IDA*	CGSky
2	31	4495	3121
3	90	117480	41971
4	182	988260	174493
5	272	3317040	421015

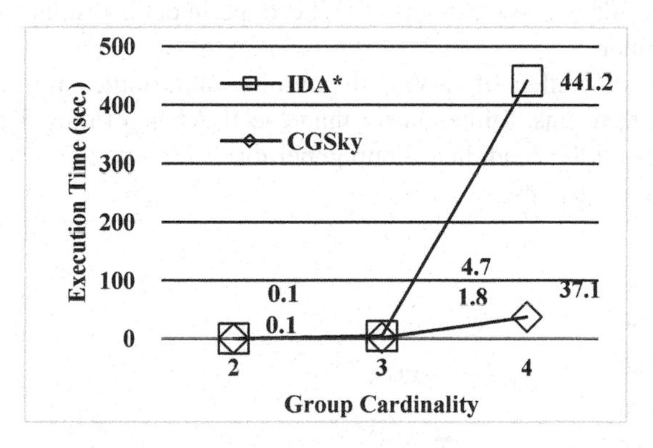

Fig. 5. Results of varying group cardinality *k*.

Table 7. Number of candidates, candidate-groups, and group-skyline tuples w.r.t. *k*.

k	Candidate tuples	IDA*	CGSky
2	71	2485	1452
3	91	121485	30918
4	111	5989005	1675519
5	127	254231775	21450113

Next, we investigated the results of varying group cardinality, which was varied from 2 to 5, with n = 500, m = 3, and c < 120. In average, CGSky runs 5.2 times faster than IDA*, as shown in Fig. 5. When k = 5, IDA* spent 8000 s and CGSky spent 3196 s for the computation. Table 7 indicates that CGSky effectively eliminated a large number of candidate groups. IDA* had to process 3.6 times of candidate groups than CGSky did. That is why CGSky outperforms IDA* for about 11 faster with group cardinality k = 4.

The next experiment was varying constraint c from 80 to 240 on anti-correlated datasets, with n = 500, m = 3, and k = 3. The execution time of the IDA* algorithm stayed nearly constant of 4.7 s since the time-consuming process of finding group skyline tuples took the same time, and the constraint is used only to retrieve groups passing the threshold. The execution time of the CGSky algorithm increased as the constraint value increased, because the number of candidates increased. The CGSky algorithm finished less than 1 s for 'c < 80', increased to 1.7 s for 'c < 120', but kept less than 4 s for 'c < 240'. Note that the constraint can be useless when the constraint value is close to 300 for k = 3.

The experiments continued with the read-world dataset, from http://tw.global.nba.com/statistics/ with the NBA 2015-2016 regular season data. This data contains 412 players with five attributes: salary, points, rebounds, assists, and steals. The salary attribute is the constraint attribute. The salary constraint of 70 million is set for 12 players by NBA league so the default salary constraint used in the experiment was about 30 million for group cardinality k = 5. The number of attributes was varied from 2 to 5 and the result is shown in Fig. 6. The experimental results of varying k and varying c are similar.

Figure 6 shows the effect of varying the number of attributes m from 2 to 5. Again, the CGSky algorithm runs 3 times faster than the IDA* algorithm. This confirms that the early pruning and the candidate group generation are very effective in reducing the number of candidate groups.

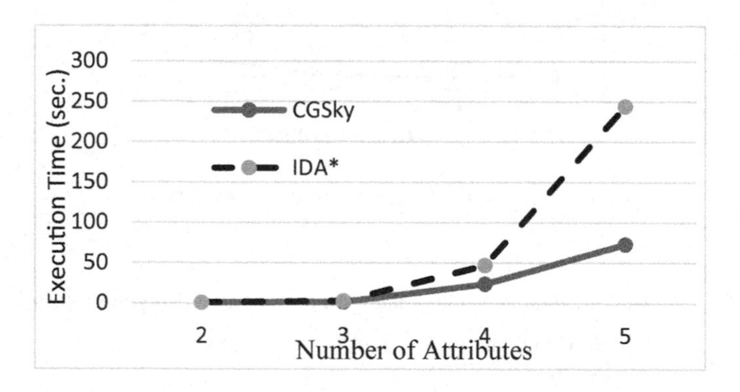

Fig. 6. Results on NBA real-datasets by varying *m*.

5 Conclusion

In this paper, we propose the CGSky algorithm for discovering constrained group skylines. The CGSky algorithm features in the reduction of candidate groups and pruning impossible candidate combinations from applying the constraints. The comprehensive experiments comprising synthetic and real datasets confirm that the CGSky algorithm outperform the well-known IDA algorithm by an order of magnitude faster in average. Future extension of the study could be finding the group skyline where group members are formed with specified characteristics, or finding group skylines with constraints in distributed computing platforms [3, 7, 16, 19].

Acknowledgements. The authors appreciate the valuable comments from the reviewers. This research was supported partly by the Ministry of Science and Technology, R.O.C. under grant MOST 105-2634-E-004-001.

References

1. Borzsonyi, S., Kossmann, D., Stocker, K.: The skyline operator. In: Proceedings of the 17th International Conference on Data Engineering, pp. 421–430 (2001)
2. Chen, L., Cui, B., Lu, H.: Constrained skyline query processing against distributed data sites. IEEE Trans. Knowl. Data Eng. (TKDE) **23**(2), 204–217 (2011)
3. Chen, L., Hwang, K., Wu, J.: MapReduce skyline query processing with a new angular partitioning approach. In: 26th IEEE International Parallel and Distributed Processing Symposium Workshops & PhD Forum, pp. 2262–2270 (2012)
4. Chomicki, J., Godfrey, P., Gryz, J., Liang, D.: Skyline with presorting. In: Proceedings of the 19th International Conference on Data Engineering, pp. 717–719 (2003)
5. Chomicki, J., Ciaccia, P., Meneghetti, N.: Skyline queries, front and back. SIGMOD Rec. **42**(3), 6–18 (2013)
6. Chung, Y.C., Su, I.F., Lee, C.: Efficient computation of combinatorial skyline queries. Inf. Syst. **38**(3), 369–387 (2013)
7. Dean, J., Ghemawat, S.: MapReduce: simplified data processing on large clusters. In: 6th Symposium on Operating System Design and Implementation (OSDI), pp. 137–150 (2004)
8. Dellis, E., Seeger, B.: Efficient computation of reverse skyline queries. In: Proceedings of the 33rd International Conference on Very Large Data Bases, pp. 291–302 (2007)
9. Endres, M., Roocks, P., Kießling, W.: Scalagon: An Efficient Skyline Algorithm for All Seasons. In: Renz, M., Shahabi, C., Zhou, X., Cheema, M.A. (eds.) DASFAA 2015. LNCS, vol. 9050, pp. 292–308. Springer, Cham (2015). doi:10.1007/978-3-319-18123-3_18
10. Han, X., Li, J., Yang, D., Wang, J.: Efficient skyline computation on big data. IEEE Trans. Knowl. Data Eng. (TKDE) **25**(11), 2521–2535 (2013)
11. Im, H., Park, S.: Group skyline computation. Inf. Syst. **188**, 151–169 (2012)
12. Kossmann, D., Ramsak, F., Rost, S.: Shooting stars in the sky: an online algorithm for skyline queries. In: Proceedings of 28th International Conference on Very Large Data Bases, pp. 275–286 (2002)
13. Lee, J., Hwang, S.W.: Toward efficient multidimensional subspace skyline computation. VLDB J. **23**(1), 129–145 (2014)
14. Liu, J., Xiong, L., Pei, J., Luo, J., Zhang, H.: Finding pareto optimal groups: group-based skyline. Proc. VLDB Endowment **8**(13), 2086–2097 (2015)
15. Mortensen, M.L., Chester, S., Assent, I., Magnani, M.: Efficient caching for constrained skyline queries. In: Proceedings of the 18th International Conference on Extending Database Technology (EDBT), pp. 337–348 (2015)
16. Mullesgaard, K., Pedersen, J.L., Lu, H., Zhou, Y.: Efficient skyline computation in MapReduce. In: Proceedings of the 17th International Conference on Extending Database Technology (EDBT), pp. 37–48 (2014)
17. Magnani, M., Assent, I.: From stars to galaxies: skyline queries on aggregate data. In: Proceedings of the 16th International Conference on Extending Database Technology (EDBT), pp. 477–488 (2013)
18. Papadias, D., Tao, Y., Fu, G., Seeger, B.: An optimal and progressive algorithm for skyline queries. In: Proceedings of the 2003 ACM SIGMOD International Conference on Management of Data, pp. 467–478 (2003)
19. Park, Y., Min, J.K., Shim, K.: Parallel computation of skyline and reverse skyline queries using MapReduce. Proceedings of the VLDB Endowment **6**(14), 2002–2013 (2013)

20. Tan, K.L., Eng, P.K., Ooi, B.C.: Efficient progressive skyline computation. In: Proceedings of 27th International Conference on Very Large Data Bases, pp. 301–310 (2001)
21. Zhang, M., Alhajj, R.: Skyline queries with constraints: integrating skyline and traditional query operators. Data Knowl. Eng. **69**(1), 153–168 (2010)
22. Zhang, N., Li, C., Hassan, N., Rajasekaran, S., Das, G.: On skyline groups. IEEE Trans. Knowl. Data Eng. (TKDE) **26**(4), 942–956 (2014)

Comparing MapReduce-Based k-NN Similarity Joins on Hadoop for High-Dimensional Data

Přemysl Čech[1(✉)], Jakub Maroušek[1], Jakub Lokoč[1], Yasin N. Silva[2], and Jeremy Starks[2]

[1] SIRET Research Group, Department of Software Engineering, Faculty of Mathematics and Physics, Charles University, Prague, Czech Republic
{cech,lokoc}@ksi.mff.cuni.cz, marousej@artax.karlin.mff.cuni.cz

[2] Arizona State University, Tempe, USA
{ysilva,Jeremy.Starks}@asu.edu

Abstract. Similarity joins represent a useful operator for data mining, data analysis and data exploration applications. With the exponential growth of data to be analyzed, distributed approaches like MapReduce are required. So far, the state-of-the-art similarity join approaches based on MapReduce mainly focused on the processing of vector data with less than one hundred dimensions. In this paper, we revisit and investigate the performance of different MapReduce-based approximate k-NN similarity join approaches on Apache Hadoop for large volumes of high-dimensional vector data.

Keywords: Hadoop · MapReduce · k-NN · Approximate similarity join · HTTPS data

1 Introduction

The k-NN similarity joins serve as a powerful tool in many domains. In the data mining and machine learning context, k-NN joins can be employed as a preprocessing step for classification or cluster analysis. In data exploration and information retrieval, similarity joins provide a similarity graph with the most relevant entities for each object in the database. Their applications can be found for example in the image and video retrieval domain [6,7], and in network communication analysis and malware detection frameworks [2,10]. Because data volumes are often too large to be processed on a single machine (especially for high-dimensional data), we study the use of the distributed MapReduce environment [5] on Hadoop[1]. Hadoop MapReduce is a widely adopted technology and considered an efficient and scalable solution for distributed big data processing.

Related papers [8,14,15] have deeply analyzed advantages, disadvantages and bottlenecks of distributed MapReduce systems Hadoop and Spark[2]. [21]. In this

[1] http://hadoop.apache.org/.

[2] http://spark.apache.org/.

G. Cong et al. (Eds.): ADMA 2017, LNAI 10604, pp. 63–75, 2017.
https://doi.org/10.1007/978-3-319-69179-4_5

paper, we study similarity join algorithms that were designed and implemented on Apache Hadoop. The comparison considers methods employing data organization/replication strategies initialized randomly as they enable convenient application and usage on different domains. Although a study tackling similarity joins have been previously published for Hadoop [18], the study focused just on two-dimensional data. The need of effective and efficient high-dimensional-data k-NN similarity joins led us to revise available MapReduce algorithms and integrate further adaptations. In the paper, we study three different approaches which offer diverse ways of approximate query processing with a promising trade-off between error and computation time (when compared to exact k-NN similarity joins).

The main contribution of this paper is a revision of similarity join algorithms and their comparison. Particularly, we report findings for high-dimensional data (200, 512 and 1000 dimensions) and show the benefits of the pivot-based approach.

The paper is structured in the following order. In Sect. 2, all essential definitions are presented. Section 3 summarizes all investigated k-NN similarity join algorithms with revisions. In Sect. 4, we examine the presented approaches in multiples experimental evaluations and discuss the results, and finally, in Sect. 5, we conclude the paper.

2 Preliminaries

In this section, we present fundamental concepts and basic definitions related to approximate k-NN similarity joins. All the definitions use the standard notations [18,22].

2.1 Similarity Model and k-NN Joins

In this paper we address the efficiency of k-NN similarity joins of objects o_i modeled by high-dimensional vectors $v_{o_i} \in \mathbb{R}^n$. In the following text, a shorter notation v_i will be used instead of v_{o_i}. In connection with a metric distance function $\delta : \mathbb{R}^n \times \mathbb{R}^n \rightarrow \mathbb{R}_0^+$, the tuple $M = (\mathbb{R}^n, \delta)$ forms a metric space that serves as a similarity model for retrieval (low distance means high similarity and vice versa)[3].

Let us suppose two sets of objects in a metric space M: database (train) objects $S \subseteq \mathbb{R}^n$ and query (test) objects $R \subseteq \mathbb{R}^n$. The similarity join task is to find the k nearest neighbors for each query object $q \in R$ from the set S employing a metric function δ. Usually, the Euclidean (L_2) metric is employed. Formally:

$$kNN(q, S) = \{X \subset S; |X| = k \wedge \forall x_i \in X, \forall y \in S - X : \delta(q, x_i) \leq \delta(q, y)\}$$

[3] Note that the effectiveness of the distance function and feature extraction mapping from o_i to v_i is the subject of similarity modeling.

The k-NN similarity join is defined as:

$$R \bowtie S = \{(q,s) | q \in R, s \in kNN(q,S)\}.$$

Because of the high computational complexity of similarity joins, we focus on approximations of joins which can significantly reduce computation costs while keeping reasonable precision. Formally an approximate k-NN query for an object $q \in R$ is labeled as $kNN_a(q)$ and defined as ϵ-approximation of exact k-NN:

$$kNN_a(q,S) = \{X \subset S; |X| = k \wedge \max_{x_i \in kNN(q,S)} \delta(q,x_i) \leq \max_{x_i \in X} \delta(q,x_i) \leq \epsilon \cdot \max_{x_i \in kNN(q,S)} \delta(q,x_i)\}$$

where $\epsilon \geq 1$ is an approximation constant. The corresponding approximate k-NN similarity join is defined as:

$$R \bowtie_a S = \{(q,s) | q \in R, s \in kNN_a(q,S)\},$$

For high-dimensional vector representations, all the pairwise distances between dataset vectors tend to be similar and high with respect to the maximal distance (the effect of high intrinsic dimensionality [22]). The ϵ constant for such datasets and given k would have to be small to guarantee a meaningful precision with respect to exact search. At the same time, filtering methods considering small ϵ would often result in inefficient (i.e., too expensive) approximate kNN query processing. Therefore, in this work we do not consider such guarantees for the compared methods (theoretical limitations of the guarantees are out of the scope of this paper). In the experiments, we focus just on the error of the similarity join approximation. The k-NN query approximation precision (or recall with respect to the exact k-NN search) is defined as:

$$precision(k,q,S) = \frac{|kNN(q,S) \cap kNN_a(q,S)|}{k}$$

2.2 MapReduce Environment

Since data volumes are significantly increasing every day, centralized solutions are often intractable for large data processing. Therefore, the need for effective distributed data processing is emerging. In this paper, we have adopted the MapReduce [5] paradigm that is often used for parallel processing of big datasets. The algorithms described in Sect. 3 are implemented in the Hadoop MapReduce environment which consists of several components. Datasets are stored in the Hadoop distributed file system (HDFS), which is designed to form a big virtual file space to contain data in one place. Data files are physically stored on different data nodes across the cluster and are replicated in multiple copies (protection against a hardware failure or a data node disconnection). Name nodes manage access to data according to the distance from a request source to a data node (it finds the closest data node to a request).

In Hadoop, every program is composed of one or more MapReduce jobs. Each job consists of three main phases: a map phase, a shuffle phase and a reduce phase. In the map phase, data are loaded from the HDFS file system, split into fractions and sent to mappers where a fraction of data is parsed, transformed and prepared for further processing. The output of the map phase are `<key, value>` pairs. In the shuffle phase, all `<key, value>` pairs are grouped and sorted by the key attribute and all values for a specific key are sent to a target reducer. Ideally, each reducer receives the same (or similar) number of groups to equally balance a workload of the job. In the reduce phase all reducers process values for an obtained key (or multiple keys) and usually perform the main execution part of the whole job. Finally, all computed results from the reduce phase are written back to the HDFS.

3 Related k-NN Similarity Joins

In this paper we study a pivot-based approach for general metric spaces and two vector space approaches - space-filling Z-curve and locality sensitive hashing.

3.1 Pivot-Based Approach

The original version of this approximate k-NN join algorithm [2] utilizes pivot space partitioning based on a set of preselected global pivots $p_i \in P \subset S$. This approach was inspired by the Lu et al. work [11], which focused on exact similarity joins. The algorithm is composed of two main phases: the preprocessing phase and the actual k-NN join computation phase.

In the preprocessing phase, both sets of database and query objects (S and R) are distributed into Voronoi cells C_i using the Voronoi space partitioning algorithm according to the preselected pivots P (a cell C_i is determined by the pivot $p_i \in P$). The set of all created cells is denoted as C. Next, all distances d_{j_i} from objects $o_j \in S \cup R$ to all pivots p_i ($d_{j_i} = \delta(o_j, p_i)$) have to be computed, and for every object o_j the nearest pivot p_n with the distance d_{j_n} is stored within the o_j data record. Also, global statistics are evaluated for every Voronoi cell C_i such as the covering radius, number of objects o_j and total size of all objects o_j in the particular cell C_i. At the end of the preprocessing phase, the Voronoi cells C_i are clustered into bigger groups G_l. Every group G_l should contain objects of a similar total size to properly balance further parallel k-NN join workload.

The second phase performs k-NN join of two sets S and R in a parallel MapReduce environment (one MapReduce job). Every computing unit (one reducer red_l) receives a subset $S_l \subset S$ of database objects and $R_l \subset R$ of query objects corresponding to a group G_l precomputed in the previous phase. Because not all nearest neighbors for query objects $q_l \in R_l$ may be present in a group G_l (especially for query objects near G_l space boundaries), a replication heuristic is employed. Specifically, every database object located in each cell $C_j \in C$ is replicated to groups $G^m \subset G$ (and corresponding nearest cells) containing pivots p_i that are within *ReplicationThreshold* nearest pivots to pivot p_j.

At each reducer, metric filtering rules and additional approximate filtering (only the closest cells to the query are considered) are employed to speed up the query processing. Additional details of this algorithm can be found in the original paper [2]. The output of a reducer red_l is a set of the k nearest neighbors for every query object $q_l \in R_l$. An overview of the space partitioning and replication algorithm is depicted in Fig. 1a.

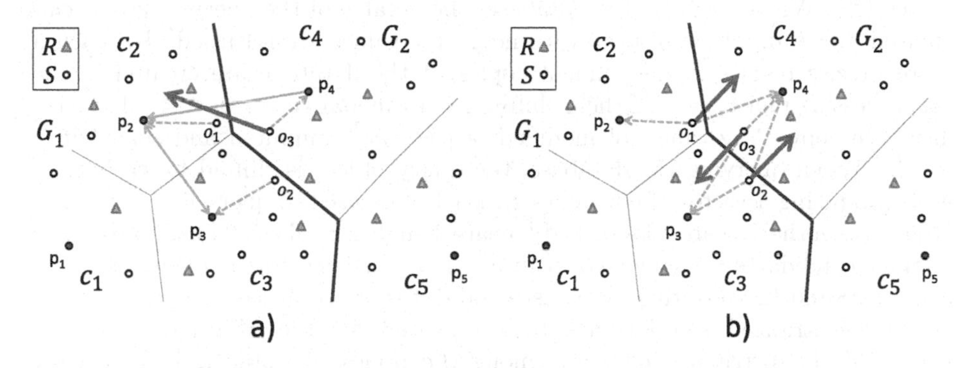

Fig. 1. An example of the Voronoi space partitioning and replication of database objects $o_n \in S$. The first part (a) depicts the replication based on distances between pivots p_i. For the *ReplicationThreshold* = 2 only the object o_3 is replicated to the other group G_1, whereas o_1 and o_2 have the closest pivot to the corresponding pivot p_i (in the cell c_i) in the same group. In the (b) scenario, for the $MaxRecDepth = 2$ all three objects o_n near groups boundaries are replicated to the other group because the second closest pivot to the objects o_n lies in the other group.

Algorithm Revision. In this paper, we use a slightly modified version of the previously described algorithm. The main difference is the utilization of a repetitive (recursive) Voronoi partitioning inspired by indexing techniques in metric spaces such as M-Index [16]. Basically, every object o_j is identified by a pivot permutation [3] determined by a set of closest pivots instead of a single closest pivot. The modification influences mainly the preprocessing phase and also the database objects replication heuristic. An example of the use of the revised algorithm is represented in Fig. 1b.

We define a new parameter $MaxRecDepth$ which sets a threshold for the maximum depth of the Voronoi space partitioning. In the preprocessing phase, for every object o_j ($o_j \in S \cup R$) the distances to all pivots are evaluated and the ordered list of the $MaxRecDepth$ nearest pivots $P_j \subset P$ is stored (in the form of pivot IDs) with object o_j.

The replication heuristic in the beginning of the second phase utilizes directly the stored lists of nearest pivots. Specifically, every database object o_j located in a cell $C_j \in C$ is replicated to groups $G_i \subset G$ that contain cells determined by pivots from P_j.

3.2 Space-Filling Curve Approach

A space-filling curve is a bijection which maps an object from an n-dimensional space to a one-dimensional value, trying to preserve the locality of objects with high probability. For example, the z-order curve creates values (referenced as *z-values*) that can be computed easily by interleaving the binary representation of coordinate values. Z-curves can be used to efficiently approximate kNN search [20]. When querying the database, the z-value of the query object is calculated and k database objects with nearest z-values are returned. To reach a more precise results, c independent copies of the database are created in the preprocessing phase, each of them shifted by a random vector $v_i \in \mathbb{R}^n$. For each database copy C_i, z-values of modified objects are computed and sorted in a list L_i. When querying the database, the query object is shifted by each v_i as well, producing a vector of c z-values z_i. Each z_i is used to query list L_i for $2 \cdot k$ objects with the k nearest lower and k nearest higher z-values. Thus, up to $2 \cdot c \cdot k$ distinct candidates are collected in total, their distance to the query object is computed and the resulting k nearest candidates are returned.

The centralized solution has been adapted for the MapReduce framework [23]. To distribute the work among the nodes, the objects in each copy C_i are split in n partitions, depending on their z-value. Inside each partition, each present query object is used to find $2 \cdot k$ nearest database object candidates using z-values[4] and also the distances to the candidates are evaluated. Each partition is processed by a separate reducer. Using a suitable number of partitions and having data equally distributed, the portion of data for each reducer is small enough to be stored in a node memory. Finally, the nearest objects for each query are detected by merging the candidate results obtained from all copies C_i. We have modified the original source code [23] to keep the partition objects in memory and to optimize the serialization of z-values.

3.3 Locality Sensitive Hashing Approach

Locality Sensitive Hashing (LSH) [4] is another technique that can be used in the context of k-NN Similarity Join algorithms. Specifically, Stupar et al. proposed RankReduce [19], a MapReduce-based approximate algorithm to simultaneously process a small number of k-NN search queries in a single MapReduce job using LSH. The key idea behind RankReduce is to use hashing to build an index that assigns similar records to the same hash table buckets. Unlike the original RankReduce method, our implementation compares only database and query objects from the same bucket. Our method is composed of two MapReduce jobs: a hashing job including k-NN evaluation and a merging job. During the map phase of the hashing job, both database S and query objects R are hashed using a set of l hash tables each containing j hash functions of the form $h_{a,B}(v) = \lfloor (a \cdot v + B)/W \rfloor$, where W is a parameter. For every input record $v \in S \cup R$ a set

[4] The presence of k lower and k higher z-values of database objects is ensured during the partitioning phase by replication.

of output keys (buckets) key_l is evaluated. One key_l represents a unique string formed from j hash functions corresponding to the hash table l. The map phase emits pairs of the form (key_l, v). In the reduce phase of the hashing job, local k-NN candidates are computed for a subset of queries and database objects in every bucket identified by the key key_l. In the second MapReduce job, all partial results are loaded, grouped by the query object IDs and global k-NN results for all queries are produced.

3.4 Exact k-NN Similarity Join Approach

In order to be able to evaluate the performance of approximate methods, an exact k-NN similarity join was also implemented. We used the pivot space approach (Subsect. 3.1) with *ReplicationThreshold* parameter set to the number of pivots (thus, all database objects were replicated to all reducers) and the *filter* parameter explained in the original paper [2] was set to the value 1 (meaning all Voronoi cells C_i are processed on each reducer).

4 Experimental Evaluation

In this section, we experimentally evaluate and compare the presented MapReduce k-NN similarity join algorithms. Main emphasis is put on scalability, precision and the overall similarity join time of all solutions for high-dimensional data. First, we describe the test datasets and the evaluation platform, then we investigate parameters for all the methods and, finally, we compare the performance of all the approaches in multiple testing scenarios.

4.1 Description of Datasets and Test Platform

In the experiments, we perform k-NN similarity joins on three vector datasets with various number of dimensions: 200, 512 and 1000. The 200 and 1000-dimensional datasets contain histogram vectors which were formed from a few key features located in HTTPS proxy logs collected by the Cisco cloud. Features were transformed into vectors using two techniques. The dataset with 200 dimensions was created by uniform feature mapping into a 4-dimensional hypercube [9]. In the dataset with 1000 dimensions, each HTTPS communication feature was assigned to the closest pre-trained Gaussian utilizing a well known density estimation technique called Gaussian Mixture Model (GMM) [12]. The resulting vectors are histograms of occurrences of each Gaussian. These feature extraction algorithms are also implemented in the MapReduce framework. Our implementation is inspired by works [2,9,13]. The algorithm processes all HTTPS communication features in parallel, groups them by a given key and applies a specific feature transformation strategy to produce final descriptors (vectors).

The last dataset consists of 335944 officially provided key frames from the TRECVid IACC.3 video dataset [1]. The descriptors for each key frame were extracted from the last fully connected layer of the pretrained VGG deep neural network [17] and further reduced to 512 dimensions using PCA.

All datasets are divided into the database S and query points R. The number of database objects ranges from about $|S|$ =150 000 to 450 000 objects. The size of the query part ranges from about $|R|$ =180 000 to 320 000 objects in every dataset. Every object contains an ID and a vector of values stored in the space saving format presented in the paper [2]. The size of datasets vary according to the number of dimensions from 0.5GB to 3GB of data in the sparse text format. We employ the Euclidean (L_2) distance metric as the similarity measure.

The experiments ran on a virtualized Hadoop 2.6.0 cluster with 20 worker nodes, each having 6 GB RAM and 2 core CPU (Intel(R) Xeon(R) running at 2.20 GHz) and were implemented in Java 1.7.

4.2 Fine Tuning of Experimental Methods

In this subsection, we investigate parameters for every tested algorithm. Note that all time values include not only the running time of the k-NN similarity join but also the preprocessing time. The parameter tuning tests ran on the 1000-dimensional dataset and the k value was set to 5.

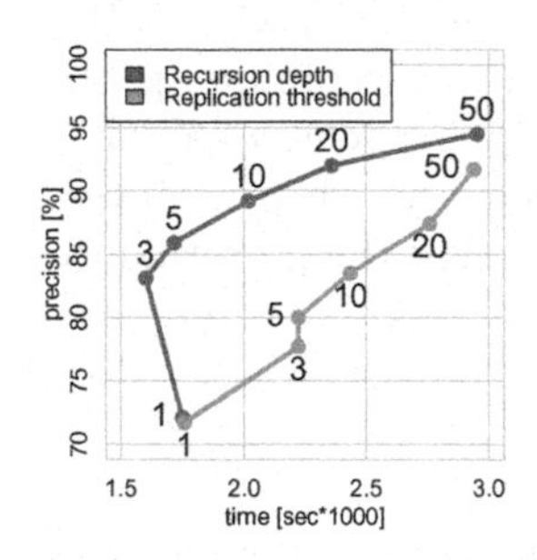

Fig. 2. Pivot-based approach parameters tuning

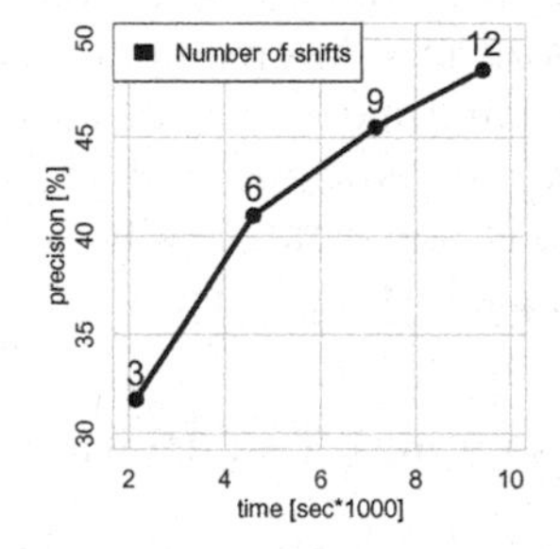

Fig. 3. Z-curve approach number of shifts tuning

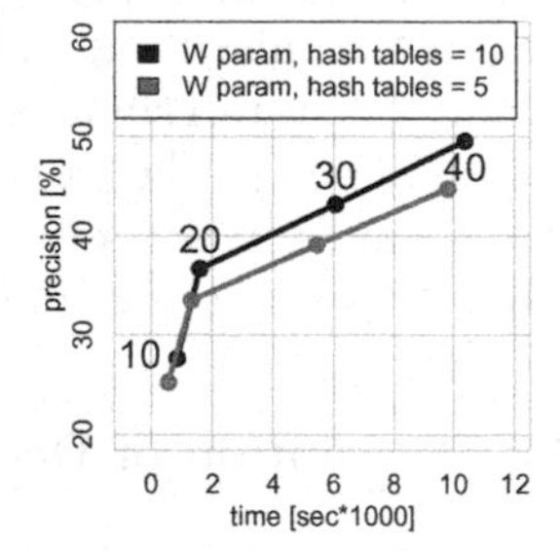

Fig. 4. LSH approach W parameter tuning

In Fig. 2, we compare the *ReplicationThreshold* and *MaxRecDepth* parameters for related and revised pivot-based (Voronoi) approaches described in Sect. 3.1. Although lower parameter values run faster, they do not achieve convincing accuracy. For the rest of the experiments, we fixed *MaxRecDepth* parameter to the value 10 which promises a competitive precision and running time trade off. In the following experiments, we do not consider the original version with *ReplicationThreshold*. In general, the Voronoi space partitioning approach used 2000 randomly preselected pivots, Voronoi cells C_i were grouped into 18 distinct groups G_l and the *filter* parameter explained in the original paper [2] was set to the value 0.05.

You may notice that the total running time for some lower parameter values is longer than for following higher values, e.g. *ReplicationThreshold* = 3 and 5 or $MaxRecDepth = 1$ and 3. Despite more replications, a shorter k-NN evaluation time is caused by the efficient candidate processing in the actual algorithm evaluation on each reducer where parent filtering and lower bound filtering techniques in a metric space are utilized [2,22]. Note that closer k objects to many queries appear in their group and so the ranges of k-NN queries get tighter. Hence, more candidates are filtered out by the triangle inequality and the total number of actual distance computations is lower.

Figure 3 displays the precision and overall time for the Z-curve approach for growing number of random vector shifts presented in Sect. 3.2. We may observe that more shifts slightly increases approximation precision, but running time is prolonged significantly. In other experiments, we fixed the number of shifts to value 5. We used 40 partitions, in order to fit the number of reducers. The Z-curve parameter ϵ was set to 0.128 which provided reasonably balanced size of partitions while keeping shorter pre-processing time. Notice that in the paper [23], different ϵ values did not affect the precision.

In Fig. 4, we examine the influence of the parameter W on the performance of the LSH method described in Sect. 3.3. With growing W, both precision and time increase substantially. Longer running time for higher W values is mainly caused by hashing objects into bigger buckets (more objects fall into the same bucket). However, this parameter heavily depends on the specific dataset. For other experiments, we fixed $W = 1$ for the 200-dimensional dataset, $W = 100$ for the 512-dimensional TrecVid dataset and $W = 20$ for the 1000-dimensional dataset. Generally, we used 10 hash tables each containing 20 hash functions.

4.3 Comparison of Methods

We propose multiple testing scenarios designed to test the main aspects of each k-NN approximate similarity join algorithm.

Size-Dependent Computation. Each of the datasets, both train and test vectors, were sampled in order to create subsets containing $\frac{1}{4}$, $\frac{1}{2}$, $\frac{3}{4}$ and all of the original data. The methods were tested on each sample. The graphs 5, 6 and 7 show that the running time generally increases with higher dimensionality and dataset size. Surprisingly, the Z-curve method is sometimes slower than the exact algorithm, due to the high index initialization costs. The revised pivot space method shows to have the best approximation precision/speed tradeoff across all datasets.

As we can see in the Figs. 8, 9 and 10, the approximation precision of the methods does not significantly change with the size when each dataset is considered separately. In all cases, the precision of the pivot space method is clearly the highest, ranging from 73% for the 200-dimensional dataset up to 88% for the 1000-dimensional dataset.

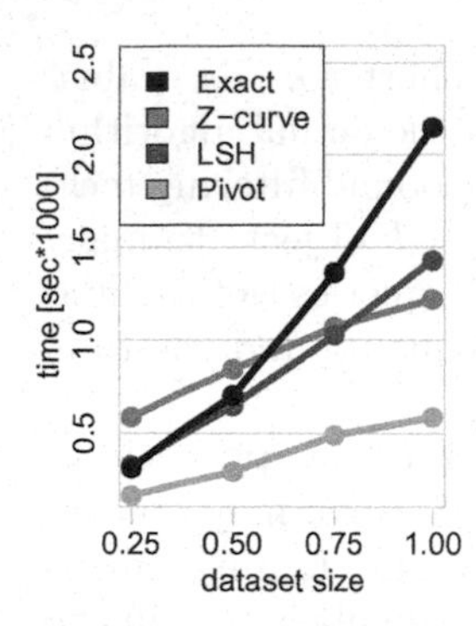

Fig. 5. 200-dimensional dataset: computation time

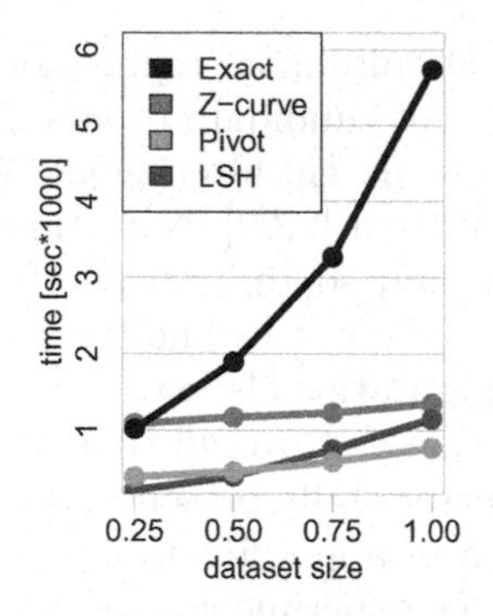

Fig. 6. 512-dimensional dataset: computation time

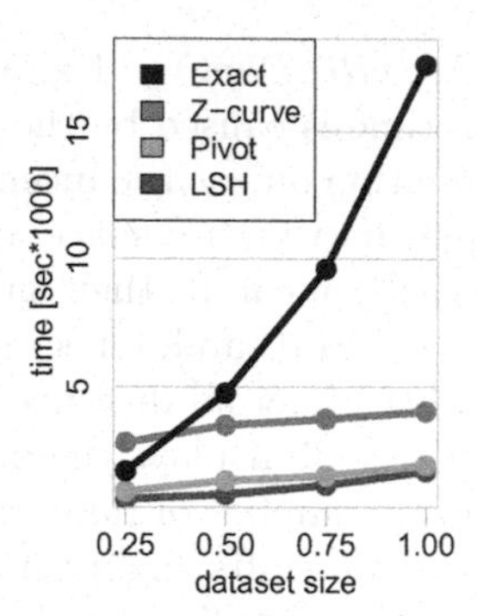

Fig. 7. 1000-dimensional dataset: computation time

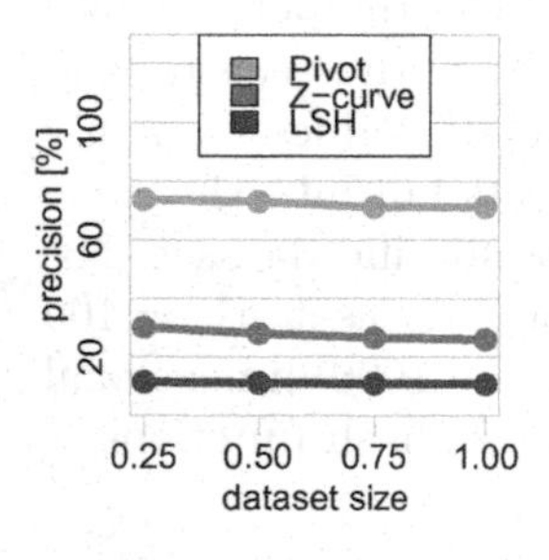

Fig. 8. 200-dimensional dataset: precision

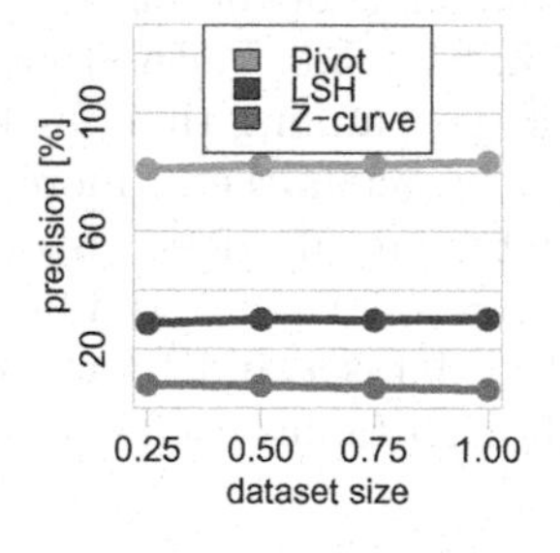

Fig. 9. 512-dimensional dataset: precision

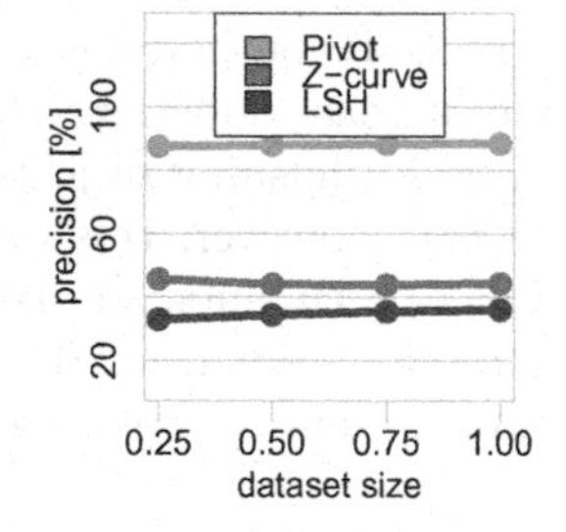

Fig. 10. 1000-dimensional dataset: precision

K-Dependent Computation. In the graphs 11 and 12, we investigate the influence of increasing the parameter k (from the k nearest neighbors) on the precision and total similarity join time. All the presented experiments were performed on the 1000-dimensional dataset. The precision stays the same or slowly decreases for the pivot space and LSH methods, whereas time complexity is gradually increasing, but the difference is only marginal. On the other hand, the growing k increases the precision and time complexity for the Z-curve approach. This observation could be explained by more database objects replications to neighboring partitions caused by higher k (this property comes from the original distributed Z-curve design described in the paper [23]). The results of all the methods follow trends identified in the previous graphs. The pivot space approach outperforms other algorithms in the precision/speed tradeoff.

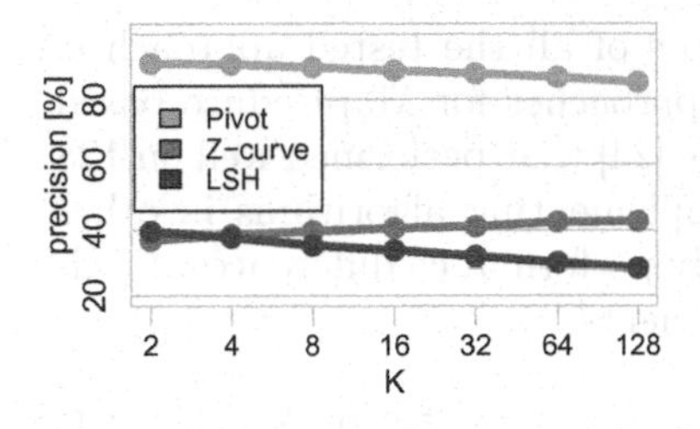

Fig. 11. k-dependent computation: precision

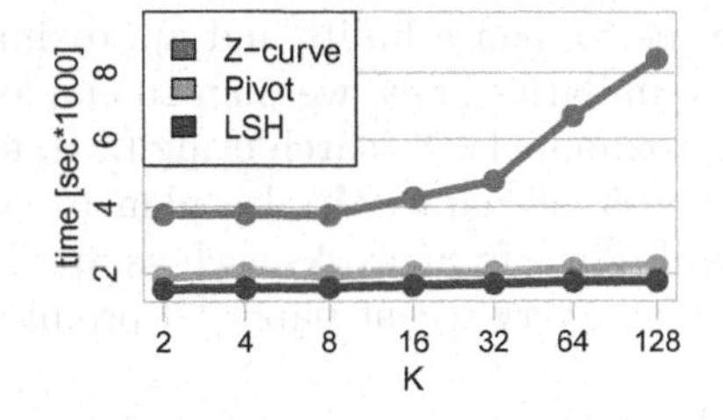

Fig. 12. k-dependent computation: time

4.4 Discussion

In the experiments, three related approximate MapReduce-based k-NN similarity joins on Hadoop were investigated using settings recommended in the original papers. Note that the Z-curve and LSH (RankReduce) related methods used primarily low-dimensional datasets during the design of the approaches (30 dimensions in [23], 32 an 64 dimensions in [19]). In the experiments, the pivot-based approach using the repetitive Voronoi partitioning significantly outperformed the other two methods in the precision/efficiency tradeoff. Our hypothesis is that for high-dimensional data the Z-curve and LSH methods suffer from the random shifts and hash functions that do not reflect data distributions. We verified this hypothesis on our synthetic 10-dimensional dataset in which all three methods provided expected behavior, as presented in the original papers. Note that specific subsets of the dataset could potentially reside in low-dimensional manifolds. Hence, finetuning specific parameters of the two methods (number of shifts in Fig. 3 and W in Fig. 4) do not provide a significant performance boost.

On the other hand, the pivot-based approach uses representatives from the data distribution and employs pairwise distances to determine data replication strategies. As demonstrated also by metric access methods for k-NN search [16,22], it seems that the distance-based approach can be also directly used as a robust and intuitive method for approximate k-NN similarity joins in high-dimensional spaces.

5 Conclusions

In this paper, we focused on approximate k-NN similarity joins in the MapReduce environment on Hadoop. Although comparative studies have been proposed for the considered approaches, the studies focused mainly on data with less than one hundred dimensions. According to our findings, the dimensionality affects the conclusions about the compared approaches. Two out of three methods previously tested for low-dimensional data did not perform well under their original recommended design and settings.

In the future, we plan to thoroughly analyze and track the bottlenecks of all the methods and try to provide a theoretically sound explanation about the performance limits and approximation errors of all the tested approaches. For similarity joins, we plan to employ other approaches for MapReduce based approximate kNN search using LSH, for example [24] that performed well on 128 dimensional data. We also plan to consider implementing algorithms in other MapReduce frameworks such as Spark and study performance differences. Findings in a very recent paper [8] promise improvements.

Acknowledgments. This project was supported by the GAČR 15-08916S and GAUK 201515 grants.

References

1. Awad, G., Fiscus, J., Michel, M., Joy, D., Kraaij, W., Smeaton, A.F., Quénot, G., Eskevich, M., Aly, R., Jones, G.J.F., Ordelman, R., Huet, B., Larson, M.: TRECVID 2016: evaluating video search, video event detection, localization, and hyperlinking. In: Proceedings of TRECVID 2016. NIST, USA (2016)
2. Čech, P., Kohout, J., Lokoč, J., Komárek, T., Maroušek, J., Pevný, T.: Feature extraction and malware detection on large HTTPS data using MapReduce. In: Amsaleg, L., Houle, M.E., Schubert, E. (eds.) SISAP 2016. LNCS, vol. 9939, pp. 311–324. Springer, Cham (2016). doi:10.1007/978-3-319-46759-7_24
3. Chavez Gonzalez, E., Figueroa, K., Navarro, G.: Effective proximity retrieval by ordering permutations. IEEE Trans. Pattern Anal. Mach. Intell. **30**(9), 1647–1658 (2008)
4. Datar, M., Immorlica, N., Indyk, P., Mirrokni, V.S.: Locality-sensitive hashing scheme based on p-stable distributions. In: Proceedings of the Twentieth Annual Symposium on Computational Geometry, SCG 2004, NY, USA, pp. 253–262. ACM, New York (2004)
5. Dean, J., Ghemawat, S.: MapReduce: simplified data processing on large clusters. Commun. ACM **51**(1), 107–113 (2008)
6. Ferhatosmanoglu, H., Tuncel, E., Agrawal, D., Abbadi, A.E.: Approximate nearest neighbor searching in multimedia databases. In: Proceedings 17th International Conference on Data Engineering, pp. 503–511 (2001)
7. Giacinto, G.: A nearest-neighbor approach to relevance feedback in content based image retrieval. In: Proceedings of the 6th ACM International Conference on Image and Video Retrieval, CIVR 2007, NY, USA, pp. 456–463. ACM, New York (2007)
8. Gu mundsson, G. ., Amsaleg, L., Jónsson, B. ., Franklin, M.J.: Towards engineering a web-scale multimedia service: a case study using spark. In: Proceedings of the 8th ACM on Multimedia Systems Conference, MMSys 2017, Taipei, Taiwan, pp. 1–12, 20–23 June 2017 (2017)
9. Kohout, J., Pevny, T.: Unsupervised detection of malware in persistent web traffic. In: 2015 IEEE International Conference on Acoustics, Speech and Signal Processing (ICASSP) (2015)
10. Lokoč, J., Kohout, J., Čech, P., Skopal, T., Pevný, T.: k-NN classification of malware in HTTPS traffic using the metric space approach. In: Chau, M., Wang, G.A., Chen, H. (eds.) PAISI 2016. LNCS, vol. 9650, pp. 131–145. Springer, Cham (2016). doi:10.1007/978-3-319-31863-9_10
11. Lu, W., Shen, Y., Chen, S., Ooi, B.C.: Efficient processing of k nearest neighbor joins using mapreduce. Proc. VLDB Endow. **5**(10), 1016–1027 (2012)

12. Marin, J.M., Mengersen, K., Robert, C.P.: Bayesian modelling and inference on mixtures of distributions. In: Dey, D., Rao, C. (eds.) Bayesian Thinking: Modeling and Computation, Handbook of Statistics, vol. 25, pp. 459–507. Elsevier, Amsterdam (2005)
13. Mera, D., Batko, M., Zezula, P.: Towards fast multimedia feature extraction: Hadoop or storm. In: 2014 IEEE International Symposium on Multimedia, pp. 106–109, December 2014
14. Moise, D., Shestakov, D., Gudmundsson, G., Amsaleg, L.: Indexing and searching 100m images with Map-Reduce. In: International Conference on Multimedia Retrieval, ICMR 2013, Dallas, TX, USA, 16–19 April 2013, pp. 17–24 (2013)
15. Moise, D., Shestakov, D., Gudmundsson, G., Amsaleg, L.: Terabyte-scale image similarity search: experience and best practice. In: Proceedings of the 2013 IEEE International Conference on Big Data, 6–9 October 2013, Santa Clara, CA, USA, pp. 674–682 (2013)
16. Novak, D., Batko, M.: Metric index: an efficient and scalable solution for similarity search. In: Proceedings of the 2009 Second International Workshop on Similarity Search and Applications, pp. 65–73. IEEE, Washington, DC (2009)
17. Simonyan, K., Zisserman, A.: Very deep convolutional networks for large-scale image recognition. CoRR abs/1409.1556 (2014)
18. Song, G., Rochas, J., Huet, F., Magoulès, F.: Solutions for processing k nearest neighbor joins for massive data on MapReduce. In: 2015 23rd Euromicro International Conference on Parallel, Distributed, and Network-Based Processing, pp. 279–287, March 2015
19. Stupar, A., Michel, S., Schenkel, R.: RankReduce - processing k-nearest neighbor queries on top of MapReduce. In: LSDS-IR (2010)
20. Yao, B., Li, F., Kumar, P.: K nearest neighbor queries and kNN-joins in large relational databases (almost) for free. In: ICDE (2010)
21. Zaharia, M., Xin, R.S., Wendell, P., Das, T., Armbrust, M., Dave, A., Meng, X., Rosen, J., Venkataraman, S., Franklin, M.J., Ghodsi, A., Gonzalez, J., Shenker, S., Stoica, I.: Apache spark: a unified engine for big data processing. Commun. ACM **59**(11), 56–65 (2016)
22. Zezula, P., Amato, G., Dohnal, V., Batko, M.: Similarity Search: The Metric Space Approach. Advances in Database Systems. Springer, Boston (2006). doi:10.1007/0-387-29151-2
23. Zhang, C., Li, F., Jestes, J.: Efficient parallel kNN joins for large data in MapReduce. In: Proceedings of the 15th International Conference on Extending Database Technology, EDBT 2012, NY, USA, pp. 38–49. ACM, New York (2012)
24. Zhu, P., Zhan, X., Qiu, W.: Efficient k-nearest neighbors search in high dimensions using MapReduce. In: 2015 IEEE Fifth International Conference on Big Data and Cloud Computing, pp. 23–30, August 2015

A Higher-Fidelity Frugal Quantile Estimator

Anis Yazidi[1(✉)], Hugo Lewi Hammer[1], and B. John Oommen[2]

[1] Department of Computer Science, Oslo and Akershus University College of Applied Sciences, Oslo, Norway
anis.yazidi@hiao.no

[2] School of Computer Science, Carleton University, Ottawa, Canada

Abstract. The estimation of the quantiles is pertinent when one is mining data streams. However, the complexity of quantile estimation is much higher than the corresponding estimation of the mean and variance, and this increased complexity is more relevant as the size of the data increases. Clearly, in the context of "infinite" data streams, a computational and space complexity that is linear in the size of the data is definitely not affordable. In order to alleviate the problem complexity, recently, a very limited number of studies have devised *incremental* quantile estimators [7,12]. Estimators within this class resort to updating the quantile estimates based on the most recent observation(s), and this yields updating schemes with a very small computational footprint – a constant-time (i.e., $O(1)$) complexity. In this article, we pursue this research direction and present an estimator that we refer to as a Higher-Fidelity Frugal [7] quantile estimator. Firstly, it guarantees a substantial advancement of the family of Frugal estimators introduced in [7]. The highlight of the present scheme is that it works in the discretized space, and it is thus a pioneering algorithm within the theory of discretized algorithms (The fact that discretized Learning Automata schemes are superior to their continuous counterparts has been clearly demonstrated in the literature. This is the first paper, to our knowledge, that proves the advantages of discretization within the domain of quantile estimation). Comprehensive simulation results show that our estimator outperforms the original Frugal algorithm in terms of accuracy.

Keywords: Quantile estimation · Stochastic Point Location · Discretized estimation

1 Introduction

Estimation is probably the most fundamental and central problem in many areas of engineering and computer science. The entire training phase of classification deals with estimation in one way or the other. While solutions to estimating

B. John Oommen—*Chancellor's Professor*; *Fellow: IEEE* and *Fellow: IAPR*. This author is also an *Adjunct Professor* with the University of Agder in Grimstad, Norway.

G. Cong et al. (Eds.): ADMA 2017, LNAI 10604, pp. 76–86, 2017.
https://doi.org/10.1007/978-3-319-69179-4_6

the mean (and central or non-central moments) of a distribution have been well established for centuries, we consider the problem of estimating the quantiles of a distribution with minimal time and space requirements.

Apart from the phenomenon of estimation, there are three rather distinct computational paradigms that have emerged within the general area of computational intelligence listed below:

1. The first of these involves the Stochastic Point Location SPL problem [8] where the Learning Mechanism (LM) attempts to learn a point on the "line" when all that it receives are signals from a random environment, i.e., whether *it* is to the "Left" or "Right" of the unknown point. This point that the LM attempts to learn may be, for example, a parameter of a control system.
2. The second of these involves the concept of discretization. Unlike learning in a continuous probability space, it has been shown that in the field of Learning Automata (LA), it is advantageous to discretize the probability space. Discretized LA are, generally speaking, both faster and more accurate than their corresponding continuous counterparts.
3. The third of these are the unique issues encountered when one seeks to estimate the quantiles of a distribution rather than the mean or central/non-central moments of a distribution in an *incremental* manner.

Conceptually, the fundamental contribution of this paper is to present a single solution that represents the confluence of these three distinct paradigms.

2 On Enhancing the Frugal Estimator

Since our contribution falls into the family of *Incremental* Quantile Estimators, we now present an overview of this class of estimators.

2.1 Incremental Quantile Estimators

An incremental estimator, by definition, resorts to the last observation(s) in order to update its estimate. The research on developing incremental quantile estimators is sparse. Probably, one of the outstanding early and unique examples of incremental quantile estimators is due to Tierney, proposed in 1983 [10], and which resorted to the theory of stochastic approximation. Applications of Tierney's algorithm to network monitoring can be found in [4]. The shortcoming of Tierney estimator [10] is that it requires the incremental constructions of local approximations of the distribution function in the neighborhood of the quantiles, and this increases the complexity of the algorithm. Our goal is to present an algorithm that does not involve any local approximations of the distribution function. Recently, a generalization of the Tierney's [10] algorithm was proposed by the authors of [5], where the authors proposed a batch update of the quantile, where the quantile is updated every $M \geq 1$ observations.

In the same context of incremental estimators, Ma, Muthukrishnan and Sandler [7] recently devised an innovative incremental quantile estimator[1] called the Frugal scheme, that follows randomized rules of updates. The first algorithm presented in the manuscript of Ma, Muthukrishnan and Sandler [7] is a Frugal approach for estimating the median. The procedure for estimating the median is simple but also "surprising": One increments the estimate of the median by a fixed amount Δ ($\Delta > 0$) whenever the observation from the data stream is larger than the median, and decrements the estimate of the median by Δ whenever the observation is smaller than the corresponding estimate. Nevertheless, the Frugal algorithm presented later in the same manuscript in order to tackle any quantile estimate (apart from the median), is not a generalization of the median case. In fact, according to the general update equations, if we are attempting to find the 50% quantile (median) of the data stream, we need to increment up randomly with 50% probability (for observations larger than the median estimate) and decrement down randomly with 50% probability (for observations smaller than the median estimate). Thus, intuitively, the Frugal [7] algorithm fails to generalize the median case as we observe that the randomization is unnecessary for estimating the median. Moreover, we can intuitively infer that the Frugal algorithm will suffer also from the "unnecessary" randomization for quantile estimates that fall in neighborhood of 50%.

In [12], Yazidi and Hammer devised a truly multiplicative incremental quantile estimation algorithm. The main difference between that and the current work is that the latter algorithm operates on a continuous space, while this present work is in a discretized space.

When it comes to memory efficient methods that require a small storage footprint, histogram based methods form an important class. Viewed from this perspective, a representative work is due to Schmeiser and Deutsch [9] who proposed the use of equidistant bins, where the boundaries are adjusted online. Arandjelovic et al. [1] used a different idea than equidistant bins by attempting to maintain bins in a manner that maximizes the entropy of the corresponding estimate of the historical data distribution, and where the bin boundaries were adjusted in an online manner.

In [6], Jain et al. resorted to five markers so as to track the quantile, where the markers corresponded to different quantiles and the min and max of the observations. Their concept was similar to the notion of histograms, where each marker had two measurements, its height and its position. By definition, each marker had some ideal position, and some adjustments were made so as to keep it in its ideal position by counting the number of samples that exceeded the marker. Thus, for example, if the marker corresponded to the 80% quantile, its ideal position would be around the point corresponding to the 80% of the data points below the marker. Subsequently, based on the positions of the markers, the quantiles were computed by modeling it such that the curve passing through

[1] With some insight, one sees that this elegant median estimation procedure is similar to the Boyer and Moore algorithm [2] for computing the majority item in a stream, using only a single pass.

three adjacent markers was parabolic, and by using piecewise parabolic prediction functions[2].

Finally, it is worth mentioning that an important research direction that has received little attention in the literature revolves around updating the quantile estimates under the assumption that portions of the data are deleted. Such an assumption is realistic in many real-life settings where data needs to be deleted due to the occurrence of errors, or because they are out-of-date and thus should be replaced. The deletion triggered a re-computation of the quantile [3], which is considered a complex operation. The case of deleted data is more challenging than the case of insertion of new data, because data insertion can be handled easily using either sequential or batch updates, while quantile update upon deletion requires more complex update operations.

2.2 The Higher-Fidelity Frugal Estimator

To motivate our work, we concur with Arandjelovic et al. [1] who remark that most quantile estimation algorithms are not single-pass algorithms and are, thus, not applicable for streaming data. On the other hand, the single pass algorithms are concerned with the exact computation of the quantile and thus require a storage space of the order of the size of the data which is clearly an unfeasible condition in the context of "Big Data" streams. Thus, the work on quantile estimation using more than one pass, or storage of the same order of the size of the observations seen so far, is not relevant in the context of this paper. We also affirm the need for storage-constrained and single-pass algorithms.

In this article, we extend the results from Frugal [7] and present a Higher-Fidelity Frugal (H-FF) scheme where the median can be seen as an instantiation of our algorithm and not as exceptional case that requires a different set of rules. In addition, our H-FF scheme is shown to be faster and more accurate than the original Frugal scheme [7]. For the rest of the paper, in order to avoid confusion, we will refer to the original Frugal algorithm due to Ma, Muthukrishnan and Sandler [7], as the Original Frugal (OF). As mentioned earlier, our H-FF algorithm is based on the theory of Stochastic Point Location [8], and although the latter theory has found applications within discretized binomial and multinomial estimation in [13], as we shall see, its application here is unique. In addition, one can observe that the binomial/multinomial discretized estimators proposed by Yazidi et al. in [11,14] and Frugal [7] are similar. In fact, if we use the same update equations as in [11,14] with the "binary" observation being whether the current estimate sample is larger than the current estimate, then, interestingly, we obtain the OF scheme [7]!

[2] Clearly, though, such an approach would not be able to handle the case of non-stationary quantile estimation as the positions of the markers would be affected by stale data points.

Let $Q_i = a + i.\frac{(b-a)}{N}$ and suppose that we are estimating the quantile in the interval[3] $[a, b]$. Note $Q_0 = a$ and $Q_N = b$. Let Δ be $\frac{(b-a)}{N}$. Further, we suppose that the estimate at each time instant $\widehat{Q}(n)$ takes values from the $N+1$ possible values, i.e., $Q_i = a + i.\Delta$, where $0 \le i \le N$.

For the sake of completeness, we will give the update equations for the OF algorithm introduced in [7]. Please note that the equations are slightly modified so as to obtain estimates within $[a, b]$. In addition, the step size Δ has a general form and is not limited to unity as done in [7].

$$\widehat{Q}(n+1) \leftarrow Min(\widehat{Q}(n) + \Delta, b), \text{ If } \widehat{Q}(n) \le x(n) \text{ and } rand() \le q, \tag{1}$$

$$\widehat{Q}(n+1) \leftarrow Max(\widehat{Q}(n) - \Delta, a), \text{ If } \widehat{Q}(n) > x(n) \text{ and } rand() \le 1-q, \tag{2}$$

$$\widehat{Q}(n+1) \leftarrow \widehat{Q}(n), \text{ Otherwise}, \tag{3}$$

where $Max(.,.)$ and $Min(.,.)$ denote the max and min operator of two real numbers while $rand()$ is a random number generated in $[0, 1]$.

Our H-FF algorithm has two different update equations depending on whether the quantile we are estimating is larger or smaller than the median.

Update equation for $q \le 0.5$:

$$\widehat{Q}(n+1) \leftarrow Min(\widehat{Q}(n) + \Delta, b), \text{ If } \widehat{Q}(n) \le x(n) \text{ and } rand() \le \frac{q}{1-q}, \tag{4}$$

$$\widehat{Q}(n+1) \leftarrow Max(\widehat{Q}(n) - \Delta, a), \text{ If } \widehat{Q}(n) > x(n), \tag{5}$$

$$\widehat{Q}(n+1) \leftarrow \widehat{Q}(n), \text{ Otherwise}. \tag{6}$$

Update equations for $q > 0.5$:

$$\widehat{Q}(n+1) \leftarrow Min(\widehat{Q}(n) + \Delta, b), \text{ If } \widehat{Q}(n) \le x(n), \tag{7}$$

$$\widehat{Q}(n+1) \leftarrow Max(\widehat{Q}(n) - \Delta, a), \text{ If } \widehat{Q}(n) > x(n) \text{ and } rand() \le \frac{1-q}{q}, \tag{8}$$

$$\widehat{Q}(n+1) \leftarrow \widehat{Q}(n), \text{ Otherwise}. \tag{9}$$

Theorem 1. *Let us assume that we are estimating the q-th quantile of the distribution, i.e., $Q^* = {F_X}^{-1}(q)$. Then, applying the updating rules given by Eqs. (4)–(6) for the case when $q \le 0.5$, and Eqs. (7)–(9) when $q > 0.5$ yields:* $\lim_{N\to\infty} \lim_{n\to\infty} E(\widehat{Q}(n)) = Q^*$.

The proof of theorem is quite involved and is omitted here for the sake of brevity. The proof can be found in a unabridged version of this article [15].

---

[3] Throughout this paper, there is an implicit assumption that the true quantile lies in $[a, b]$. However, this is not a limitation of our scheme; the proof is valid for any bounded and probably non-bounded function.

2.3 Salient Differences Between the H-FF, SPL and OF

It is pertinent to mention that there are some fundamental differences between the H-FF and the SPL, both with regard to their *computational paradigms* and with regard to their respective *analyses*. There are also some fundamental differences between the H-FF and the OF schemes. We state them briefly below.

2.3.1 Differences Between the *Paradigms* of the H-FF and SPL

The following are the differences between the *paradigms* of the H-FF and SPL:

- Although the rationale for updating in the H-FF is *apparently* similar to that of the SPL algorithm [8], there are some fundamental differences. First, we emphasize that the SPL has a significant advantage. Indeed, the SPL assumes the existence of an "Oracle", the presence of which is, unarguably, a "bonus". In our case, since there is no "Oracle", the H-FF scheme has to simulate such an entity. Or more precisely, it has to infer the behavior of a fictitious "Oracle" from the incoming samples.
- Further, unlike the SPL, the H-FF has no specific LM either. The learning properties of the LM must now be encapsulated into the estimation procedure.

2.3.2 Differences Between the *Analyses* of the H-FF and SPL

The following are the differences between the *analyses* of the H-FF and SPL:

- From a cursory perspective, it could *appear* as if the Markov Chain that we have presented, and its analysis, are rather identical to those presented in [8]. However, although the similarities are few, the differences are more vital. The main differences are the following:
  1. First of all, unlike the original SPL, there is a non zero probability that in our present updating scheme, the estimate remains unchanged at the next time instant.
  2. As opposed to original SPL, in our case, the scheme never stays at the same state at the next time instant, except at the end states. Rather, the environment (our simulated "Oracle") directs the simulated LM to move to the right or to the left, or to stay at the same position.
- Unlike the work of [8], the probability that the "Oracle" suggests the move in the correct direction, is not constant over the states of the estimator's state space. This is quite a significant difference, since it renders our model to be characterized by a Markov Chain with state-*dependent* transition probabilities.
- A major advantage of this estimator and SPL-based estimators, in general, is that they are, by design, adequate to dynamic environments. In fact, the estimator is memory-less, and this is a consequence of the Markovian property. Thus, whenever a change takes place in the unknown underlying value of the target quantile to be tracked, our H-FF will *instantly* change its search direction since the properties of transition probabilities of the underlying random walk, change too.

2.3.3 Other Salient Differences Between the H-FF and OF

- Our H-FF is "semi-randomized" in the sense that only one direction of the updates is randomized and not both directions as in the case of the OF algorithm. In fact, whenever $q \leq 0.5$, we observe that the randomization is only applied for moving to the left (decrementing the estimate with probability $\frac{q}{1-q}$ which is less than unity). Similarly, when estimating a quantile q such that $q > 0.5$, the randomization is only applied for moving to the right (incrementing the estimate with probability $\frac{1-q}{q}$, which is again strictly less than unity).
- A fundamental observation is that for the median case, i.e., when $q = 05$, we obtain the Frugal update proposed as a exceptional case that deviates from the main scheme in [7] since $\frac{q}{1-q} = 1$. Formally, the median is estimated as follows:

$$\widehat{Q}(n+1) \leftarrow Min(\widehat{Q}(n) + \Delta, b) \text{ if } \widehat{Q}(n) \leq x(n), \tag{10}$$

$$\widehat{Q}(n+1) \leftarrow Max(\widehat{Q}(n) - \Delta, a) \text{ if } \widehat{Q}(n) > x(n). \tag{11}$$

3 Experimental Results

In order to demonstrate the strength of our scheme (denoted as H-FF), we have rigorously tested it and compared it to the OF estimator proposed in [7] for different distributions, under different resolution parameters, and in both dynamic and stationary environments. The results we have obtained are conclusive and demonstrate that the convergence of the algorithms conforms to the theoretical results, and proves the superiority of our design to the OF algorithm [7]. To do this, we have used data originating from different distributions, namely:

- Uniform in $[0, 1]$,
- Normal $N(0, 1)$,
- Exponential distribution with mean 1 and variance 1, and
- Chi-square distribution with mean 1 and variance 2.

In all the experiments, we chose a to be -8 and b to 8. Note that whenever the resolution was N, the estimate was moving with either an additive or subtractive step size equal to $\frac{b-a}{N}$. Thus, a larger value of the resolution parameter, N, implied a smaller step size, while a lower value of the resolution parameter, N, led to smaller step sizes. Initially, at time 0, the estimates were set to the value $Q_{\lfloor * \rfloor \frac{N}{2}}$. The reader should also note that an additional aim of the experiments was to demonstrate the H-FF's salient properties as a novel quantile estimator using only *finite* memory.

In this set of experiments, we examined various stationary environments. We used different resolutions, and as mentioned previously, we set $[a, b] = [-8, 8]$. In each case, we ran an ensemble of 1,000 experiments, each consisting of 500 iterations.

In Tables 1, 2, 3 and 4, we report the estimation error for the OF and H-FF for different values of the resolutions, N, for the Uniform, Normal, Exponential and Chi-squared distributions respectively. We catalogue the results for different values of the quantile being estimated, namely, q: 0.1, 0.3, 0.499, 0.7 and 0.9. From these tables we observe that the H-FF outperformed the OF in almost all the cases, i.e., for different distributions and for different resolutions. A general observation is that the error for both schemes diminished as we increased the resolution. For example, from Table 1, we see that the error for $q = 0.1$ decreased from 0.144 to 0.044 as the resolution increased from 50 to 500.

Table 1. The estimation error for the OF and H-FF algorithms for the Uniform distribution and for different values of the resolutions N and target quantiles.

q	0.1		0.3		0.499		0.7		0.9	
N	H-FF	OF	H-FF	OF	H-FF	F	H-FF	OF	H-FF	OF
50	0,144	0,144	0,197	0,198	0,245	0,246	0,220	0,220	0,176	0,175
100	0,104	0,103	0,146	0,146	0,160	0,161	0,157	0,159	0,122	0,122
150	0,074	0,075	0,121	0,122	0,135	0,137	0,128	0,131	0,100	0,101
200	0,069	0,068	0,106	0,107	0,117	0,120	0,113	0,115	0,088	0,089
250	0,063	0,063	0,096	0,097	0,106	0,109	0,102	0,106	0,081	0,083
300	0,055	0,056	0,089	0,090	0,098	0,104	0,096	0,102	0,080	0,082
350	0,051	0,052	0,083	0,085	0,091	0,097	0,094	0,099	0,081	0,084
400	0,050	0,050	0,078	0,081	0,088	0,095	0,091	0,098	0,082	0,086
450	0,046	0,047	0,075	0,077	0,083	0,091	0,089	0,098	0,083	0,087
500	0,044	0,044	0,072	0,075	0,082	0,091	0,088	0,097	0,084	0,089

A very intriguing characteristic of our estimator is that as the resolution increased, the estimation error diminished (asymptotically). In fact, the limited memory of the estimator did not permit us to achieve zero error, i.e., 100% accuracy. As noted in the theoretical results, the convergence centred around the smallest interval $[z\Delta, (z+1)\Delta]$ containing the true quantile. Informally speaking, a higher resolution increased the accuracy while a low resolution decreased the accuracy.

Another interesting remark is that both the OF and H-FF seemed to perform almost equally well for extreme quantiles, i.e., quantiles that are close to 0 or close to 1. However, as the true value of the quantile to be estimated became closer to 0.5, i.e., median, the H-FF had a markedly clearer superiority when compared to the OF.

The reader should note that the choice of 0.499 instead of 0.5 was deliberate in order to "avoid" using the exceptional rules presented with regard to the OF in [7], and that coincide with the rules of H-FF for the median. Thus, the estimation of the quantile for the value 0.499 was performed using the OF rules

Table 2. The estimation error for the OF and H-FF algorithms for the Normal distribution and for different values of the resolutions N and target quantiles.

q	0.1		0.3		0.499		0.7		0.9	
N	H-FF	OF	H-FF	OF	H-FF	F	H-FF	OF	H-FF	OF
50	0,341	0,339	0,376	0,377	0,361	0,358	0,377	0,376	0,956	0,956
100	0,259	0,259	0,258	0,260	0,251	0,250	0,259	0,258	1,030	1,042
150	0,235	0,239	0,210	0,213	0,205	0,203	0,212	0,212	1,082	1,096
200	0,229	0,236	0,188	0,192	0,176	0,175	0,190	0,191	1,122	1,133
250	0,233	0,244	0,171	0,175	0,157	0,156	0,170	0,175	1,154	1,170
300	0,242	0,258	0,161	0,165	0,144	0,142	0,160	0,168	1,187	1,204
350	0,254	0,272	0,152	0,162	0,133	0,129	0,152	0,159	1,216	1,237
400	0,273	0,293	0,148	0,155	0,124	0,120	0,148	0,158	1,245	1,273
450	0,290	0,310	0,143	0,155	0,116	0,113	0,144	0,154	1,277	1,302
500	0,305	0,329	0,142	0,154	0,112	0,109	0,142	0,152	1,303	1,332

Table 3. The estimation error for the OF and H-FF algorithms for the Exponential distribution and for different values of the resolutions N and target quantiles.

q	0.1		0.3		0.499		0.7		0.9	
N	H-FF	OF	H-FF	OF	H-FF	F	H-FF	OF	H-FF	OF
50	0,159	0,158	0,253	0,254	0,335	0,332	0,399	0,401	0,473	0,464
100	0,109	0,109	0,181	0,182	0,235	0,237	0,285	0,290	0,378	0,385
150	0,078	0,078	0,149	0,148	0,193	0,198	0,237	0,247	0,370	0,381
200	0,074	0,073	0,129	0,130	0,169	0,174	0,215	0,227	0,386	0,404
250	0,066	0,066	0,116	0,117	0,153	0,160	0,204	0,219	0,416	0,442
300	0,057	0,058	0,107	0,109	0,141	0,152	0,200	0,218	0,459	0,489
350	0,056	0,056	0,099	0,102	0,134	0,147	0,195	0,219	0,501	0,540
400	0,053	0,053	0,095	0,097	0,130	0,144	0,197	0,223	0,544	0,587
450	0,048	0,048	0,090	0,094	0,125	0,142	0,199	0,228	0,598	0,639
500	0,047	0,048	0,088	0,091	0,122	0,142	0,203	0,237	0,638	0,687

as per Eqs. (1)–(3) to avoid the unnecessary randomization of the OF around the median that could lead to higher errors, which was the earlier-mentioned shortcoming of the OF scheme.

Please note too that for the target values of the quantiles that were close to the initial point 0, the error was smaller than for those that are far away from initial point. Thus, for example, in Table 1, the error was lowest for the 10% quantile which is 0.1, which in this case, is closer to 0 than any other quantile in the the table, namely, 0.3 0.499, 0.7 and 0.9.

Table 4. The estimation error for the OF and H-FF algorithms for the Chi-squared distribution and for different values of the resolutions N and target quantiles.

q	0.1		0.3		0.499		0.7		0.9	
N	H-FF	OF	H-FF	OF	H-FF	F	H-FF	OF	H-FF	OF
50	0,088	0,088	0,254	0,254	0,348	0,345	0,453	0,454	0,600	0,606
100	0,063	0,063	0,149	0,149	0,234	0,231	0,322	0,326	0,519	0,525
150	0,051	0,052	0,126	0,125	0,192	0,192	0,270	0,272	0,535	0,567
200	0,045	0,045	0,105	0,104	0,167	0,170	0,245	0,253	0,597	0,638
250	0,040	0,040	0,094	0,095	0,150	0,153	0,227	0,243	0,686	0,731
300	0,037	0,036	0,085	0,085	0,139	0,142	0,220	0,238	0,765	0,822
350	0,033	0,033	0,079	0,079	0,129	0,136	0,218	0,239	0,842	0,915
400	0,031	0,031	0,074	0,075	0,122	0,128	0,220	0,244	0,933	0,987
450	0,029	0,029	0,070	0,070	0,118	0,125	0,218	0,254	1,003	1,062
500	0,027	0,027	0,067	0,068	0,113	0,121	0,222	0,258	1,073	1,134

4 Conclusion

This paper describes a scheme which is a confluence of three paradigms, namely, working with the foundations of Stochastic Point Location (SPL), the discretized world, and estimation of the quantiles in an incremental manner. We present a new quantile estimator which merges all these three concepts, and which we refer to as a Higher-Fidelity Frugal [7] (H-FF) quantile estimator. We have shown that the H-FF represents a substantial advancement of the family of Frugal estimators introduced in [7], and in particular to the so-called Original Frugal (OF) estimator.

Simulation results show that our estimator outperforms the OF algorithm in terms of accuracy.

References

1. Arandjelovic, O., Pham, D.S., Venkatesh, S.: Two maximum entropy-based algorithms for running quantile estimation in nonstationary data streams. IEEE Trans. Circuits Syst. Video Technol. **25**(9), 1469–1479 (2015)
2. Boyer, R.S., Moore, J.S.: MJRTY-a fast majority vote algorithm. In: Boyer, R.S. (ed.) Automated Reasoning: Essays in Honor of Woody Bledsoe, pp. 105–117. Springer, Netherlands (1991). doi:10.1007/978-94-011-3488-0_5
3. Cao, J., Li, L.E., Chen, A., Bu, T.: Incremental tracking of multiple quantiles for network monitoring in cellular networks. In: Proceedings of the 1st ACM Workshop on Mobile Internet Through Cellular Networks, pp. 7–12. ACM (2009)
4. Chambers, J.M., James, D.A., Lambert, D., Wiel, S.V.: Monitoring networked applications with incremental quantile estimation. Stat. Sci. **21**(4), 463–475 (2006)
5. Chen, F., Lambert, D., Pinheiro, J.C.: Incremental quantile estimation for massive tracking. In: Proceedings of the Sixth ACM SIGKDD International Conference on Knowledge Discovery and Data Mining, pp. 516–522. ACM (2000)

6. Jain, R., Chlamtac, I.: The P2 algorithm for dynamic calculation of quantiles and histograms without storing observations. Commun. ACM **28**(10), 1076–1085 (1985)
7. Ma, Q., Muthukrishnan, S., Sandler, M.: Frugal streaming for estimating quantiles. In: Brodnik, A., López-Ortiz, A., Raman, V., Viola, A. (eds.) Space-Efficient Data Structures, Streams, and Algorithms. LNCS, vol. 8066, pp. 77–96. Springer, Heidelberg (2013). doi:10.1007/978-3-642-40273-9_7
8. Oommen, B.J.: Stochastic searching on the line and its applications to parameter learning in nonlinear optimization. IEEE Trans. Syst. Man Cybern. Part B **27**(4), 733–739 (1997)
9. Schmeiser, B.W., Deutsch, S.J.: Quantile estimation from grouped data: the cell midpoint. Commun. Stat. Simul. Comput. **6**(3), 221–234 (1977)
10. Tierney, L.: A space-efficient recursive procedure for estimating a quantile of an unknown distribution. SIAM J. Sci. Stat. Comput. **4**(4), 706–711 (1983)
11. Yazidi, A., Granmo, O.-C., Oommen, B.J.: A stochastic search on the line-based solution to discretized estimation. In: Jiang, H., Ding, W., Ali, M., Wu, X. (eds.) IEA/AIE 2012. LNCS, vol. 7345, pp. 764–773. Springer, Heidelberg (2012). doi:10.1007/978-3-642-31087-4_77
12. Yazidi, A., Hammer, H.: Quantile estimation using the theory of stochastic learning. In: Proceedings of the 2015 Conference on Research in Adaptive and Convergent Systems, pp. 7–14. ACM (2015)
13. Yazidi, A., Oommen, B.J.: Novel discretized weak estimators based on the principles of the stochastic search on the line problem. IEEE Trans. Cybern. **46**(12), 2732–2744 (2016)
14. Yazidi, A., Oommen, B.J., Horn, G., Granmo, O.C.: Stochastic discretized learning-based weak estimation: a novel estimation method for non-stationary environments. Pattern Recognit. **60**(C), 430–443 (2016)
15. Yazidi, Anis Hammer L., H., Oommen, B.J.: Higher-fidelity frugal and accurate quantile estimation using a novel incremental (2017, to be submitted for publication). Journal version

Recommender System

Fair Recommendations Through Diversity Promotion

Pierre-René Lhérisson[1,2](✉), Fabrice Muhlenbach[1], and Pierre Maret[1]

[1] Université de Lyon, UJM-Saint-Etienne, CNRS,
Laboratoire Hubert Curien UMR 5516, 42023 Saint Etienne, France
{pr.lherisson,fabrice.muhlenbach,pierre.maret}@univ-st-etienne.fr
[2] 1D Lab, 5 rue Javelin Pagnon, 42000 Saint Etienne, France

Abstract. We address the problem of overspecialization in streaming platform recommender systems. The personalization of web pages by delivering content to users is a challenging task in data mining. But it has been proved that beside optimizing the relevance accuracy such systems should also rely on other factors like diversity or novelty. In this paper we focus on modeling users' boundary area of interest by selecting the most diverse items they liked in the past. We apply diversification while building the top-N list of recommendations. We select the items we want to recommend from an area where we consider a user will find item different from what she or he likes in the past. We evaluate our approach in offline analysis on two datasets, showing that our approach brings diversity and is competitive against implicit state-of-the-art method.

Keywords: Recommender systems · Diversity · Accuracy · Content-based · Multimedia streaming

1 Introduction

Recommender systems are a means of matching existing goods and services and users of these products by applying some data mining techniques. When it comes to cultural products offered by streaming platforms, it can be assumed that these tools are essential for filtering the immensity of the product catalogs of these platforms in order to give to all users the items that best meet their expectations, in a personalized way. The most popular items are the most purchased, they are a very small minority of the catalog, the rest following a long tail distribution. Thanks to the digital revolution, one can thus imagine that through the diversity of user tastes, it is now possible that cultural creators find more easily people interested in their creations. Unfortunately this is not the case... The "death of the long tail" is a phenomenon that gets amplified with the digital era [10]. With the arrival of digital market and streaming platforms, some people predicted that the superstar artists would be overthrow by the artists in the long tail (e.g., indie music artists) [3]. But we have seen the contrary happening: the superstars get more incomes [19]. If one can argue that the long tail effect does

G. Cong et al. (Eds.): ADMA 2017, LNAI 10604, pp. 89–103, 2017.
https://doi.org/10.1007/978-3-319-69179-4_7

not have the same impact in others markets like book, movie, and video game, we can also say that some companies still rely on blockbusters to make money, following the Pareto effect. This superstar economy can also have bad effect on the creation because non-superstars can less and less live from their creation. So, for sustainability reasons, it is becoming more and more important to find ways to drift away from the current system. This can be done by helping users to filter in a fairly way the information. Even if we are no longer in the brick and mortar world where the choices were very limited, we still observe a concentration of the active catalog. This can be explained by the policy of most of the recommender systems: recommend popular items, or similar items to those that have already been appreciated in the past [9]. However popular items tend to bias the recommendation: they bias the system because, although if they are very few in the catalog, they attract the overwhelming majority of recommendations. In addition, most often the most popular items are only popular for a limited time, even if some work has focused on items that remain popular over time [35].

To counter this effect, it is necessary to filter the information in a way that users can be aware of the existing diversity and can make informed choices. By adopting such strategy we assume that users will get a chance to extend their profile and avoid the "filter bubble" [23]. Let's consider a streaming platform that promotes diversity and novelty through its catalog, and that remunerates the artists through a fair trade. The noble objective of such streaming platform would be that every artist get his/her part of the cake. By bypassing popularity and focusing on diversity and novelty in the recommendation list we only focus on adding value to the user [15]. Users can explore and understand the space of options. The underlying assumption is that, by favoring exploration, the system will make the set of users interact at least once with all the items. Some experiments show that many items are not reachable by browsing through the top-N list of recommendations, unless it is designed specifically for this purpose [27].

Our main insight is that, instead of focusing on providing value to the users, our system should try to embrace the provider's viewpoint. Each item should have a chance to appear in a recommendation list. We believe that it is the task of the system to ensure a good coverage of the catalog while adding novelty and diversity to the users list. Indeed, even with nearly unlimited choice, customers agglomerate around popular items and do not spend their time browsing on niche items [29]. But the task of presenting novel and diverse list to user is not an easy one [11]: novelty can have a bad impact on user; too unfamiliar items can frustrate users; and users respond better to diverse list of recommendations. However each item in a diverse list of recommendations can be seen as a novel item with respect to the rest of the list [30].

The problem of finding diverse items to propose to a user is usually solved by finding a trade-off between accuracy and diversity. In our paper we try to follow this approach by emphasizing diversity. Instead of proposing only valuable recommendations –i.e., recommendations that will be directly consumable by the users and that will not last in time–, we offer multiple diverse items by applying a recommendation model that will extend the spectrum of users' interests. We make the hypothesis that such recommendation will contribute to a cultural enrichment. Diverse recommendations will make a lasting impression to the users.

After mentioning the diversity in recommender systems in Sect. 2, we present a recommendation model that promotes the diversity in Sect. 3. The experiments and results are discussed in Sects. 4 and 5. Finally, we propose future research and possible extensions of this research in Sect. 6.

2 Related Work

In recommender system, it has been shown that we can not rely only on accuracy, popularity and similarity to guide the users on their choices [18,36]. We have to rely on other factors if we want to navigate through the long tail [9]. Many criteria have been introduced to validate recommender systems, like diversity [8], novelty, and all related concepts such as serendipity [12], or usefulness [2]. According to the user's needs and desires, some approaches try dynamically to adjust the compromise between accuracy, diversity and novelty [24].

In the following, we will focus more on diversity in recommender systems. To propose diverse items, most of the time the system has to balance between similarity and diversity [28], preference and diversity [36], or popularity and accuracy [9]. Selecting diverse items has been proven to be an NP-hard problem. A common approach to solve this problem is to apply a greedy approach and maximize a modular/submodular objective function [4,7]. The gain we get from adding a diverse item in the list can be computed in an implicit way [7] or in an explicit way [33].

Some work prior to the recommendation step is to model the user profile to know his/her short and long point of interest [34] or to know the propensity of the user to appreciate a diversified recommendations list. The user is put on clusters based on the length of the set of items he or she interacted with and his or her propensity to diversity [21]. The goal is to take into account the various ranges of interest of individuals. In the same context, it is possible to identify the diversity within the user profiles and generate partial recommendations based on homogeneous subsets of user preferences which they combine afterwards to produce a final list of recommendations [32]. The user profile partitioning was addressed also in [37], but the goal there was to bring novelty to top-N list of recommendations. Most of those techniques for user ranges of interest were done on a collaborative filtering recommender system scenario. The user profile understanding was used in the "Outside-The-Box" method [1], which takes some risks to help users make fresh discoveries by creating clusters of items and identifying clusters that are underexposed to users.

3 Diversity Promotion Model

3.1 Introduction to the Mexican-Hat Diversity Model (MHDM)

To tackle the overspecialization problem encountered in recommender systems, we introduce in our approach a new objective function for diversity and a model called "Mexican-Hat Diversity Model" (MHDM). We also propose a method for identifying the diversity of each user. The solutions for those two methods can be found greedily. To explain how these algorithms work, it is necessary to introduce some elements of notation beforehand.

We have a finite set of users $\mathcal{U} = u_1, ..., u_m$ and a set of finite items $\mathcal{I} = i_1, ..., i_n$. The items are more or less close the ones to the others depending on a dissimilarity function $\mathcal{D}$ based on the content describing these items.

We want to present to each user u_α of $\mathcal{U}$ a set $\mathcal{R}_\alpha$ of r_α recommended items based on the previous consumed items ($\mathcal{P}_\alpha$). Each user u_α has appreciated and/or consumed a set $\mathcal{P}_\alpha$ of p_α preferred items, with $\mathcal{P}_\alpha \subset \mathcal{I}$. Our objective is to provide a set of recommended items $\mathcal{R}_\alpha$ having the most interesting diversity for the user u_α. To this end, we can follow the process described in Algorithm 1.

3.2 Identifying the Diversity of a User Profile

The first step is to identify the most diverse user profile by selecting a limited but diverse number of items that are considered to be the "seed items." We consider a set $\mathcal{S}_\alpha$ of s_α seed items extracted from the set $\mathcal{P}_\alpha$ of preferred items. These s_α seed items are chosen for having the most important diversity between them. For this, we initialize the list with the items having the most important difference, then we add to the list in an iterative process another item fp (the farthest point) having the maximal global difference with the selected items, which means that the minimal distance between this item fp and all the selected items is greater than the other items not yet selected.

3.3 Promoting Diversity from the User Profile

From the time a diverse user profile has been identified with seed items, it is necessary to grow these seeds in a diversity space. The seed items $\mathcal{S}_\alpha$ are used to define a set of recommended items $\mathcal{R}_\alpha$ by following the steps described in Algorithm 1. Each seed item of the list $\mathcal{S}_\alpha$ is used to find another item to recommend, and all of them constitute a list $\mathcal{R}_\alpha$. For finding the corresponding items, we propose to use a "Mexican hat" shape function having interesting properties, as it will be explained below.

3.4 Diversity Search Function: The Mexican Hat

To find an area of interest from a dissimilarity value, we propose a "Mexican hat" shaped model which enables to delimit the boundaries of fairly diversified cultural items proposed by an online streaming platform.

To promote the presence of diversity in cultural services (e.g., music, literature, video games, videos), we hypothesize that a given cultural service allows an interesting exploration of diversity insofar as this recommended cultural service is sufficiently dissimilar from a reference one, i.e., in the case of music recommendation, if the recommended music is sufficiently different from the music usually

Algorithm 1. GrowTheDiversitySeed

Data: list of diverse seed items $\mathcal{S}_\alpha$.
Result: list of diverse items recommended $\mathcal{R}_\alpha$.
begin
  $\mathcal{R}_\alpha = \{\}$
  for $i_a \in \mathcal{S}_\alpha$ **do**
    $i^* = \arg\max_{i \in \mathcal{I}} MHDM(i_a, sd(I))$
    $\mathcal{R}_\alpha = \mathcal{R}_\alpha \cup \{i^*\}$
    $\mathcal{I} = \mathcal{I}/\{i^*\}$

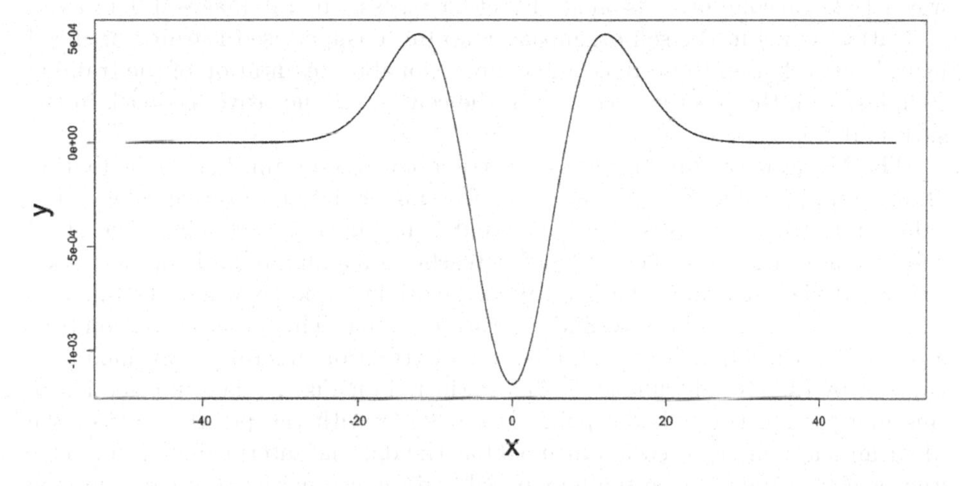

Fig. 1. Mexican hat wavelet.

listened and liked by a given listener. Therefore, we need to find a function to define criteria for establishing an area of interest with the following properties: (i) the function must return a minimum (or negative) value when the dissimilarity is zero, (ii) the function must grow as the dissimilarity increases to a maximum value, (iii) the function must decrease after this optimum until tending towards zero when dissimilarity tends towards infinity, and (iv) the function must depend on few parameters, such as the average or the standard deviation of the dissimilarity values calculated on the set of available content for describing the cultural services.

The Mexican hat function, as shown on Fig. 1, seems to hold these four desired properties. The Mexican hat is the (negative) normalized second derivative of the normal distribution function $\mathcal{N}(\mu, \sigma)$. The normal distribution is a very common continuous probability distribution characterized by the mean of the distribution μ and the standard deviation σ. Knowing the mean μ and the standard deviation σ, the probability density of the normal distribution is given by:

$$f(x) = \frac{1}{\sigma\sqrt{2\pi}}\ \mathrm{e}^{-\frac{1}{2}\left(\frac{x-\mu}{\sigma}\right)^2}$$

When $\mu = 0$, the second derivative is given by this formula:

$$f''(x) = \mathrm{e}^{-\frac{1}{2}\left(\frac{x}{\sigma}\right)^2}\ \left(\frac{-\sigma^2 + x^2}{\sigma^5\sqrt{2\pi}}\right)$$

This function (shown on Fig. 2) looks like an upside-down sombrero (a "Mexican hat") and has been used for a wide range of applications, e.g., as a model seismic wavelet [25], in computer vision for detecting edges in digital images [17], or as an activation kernel in the self-organizing map (an unsupervised learning artificial neural network used to produce a low-dimensional representation of the training samples) with the positive feedback in the center, and negative feedback in the surround [16].

The Mexican hat function is symmetric about the origin. For a distribution of dissimilarity value $X = x_1, x_2, \ldots, x_n$ (dissimilarities are positive values), the value of f'' will be negative for $x \simeq 0$ and minimal for $x = 0$. The value of f'' will increase with the value of x until it reaches a maximum, and will decreased towards 0 when the value of x is far from the origin. To know where the function starts to decrease, we have to find the turning point. This point corresponds to a zero of the third derivative of the normal distribution function. This maximum is given by the straight line $o = \sqrt{3} \times \sigma$ (in red on Fig. 2). The intersection of this line passing through the point $o = \sqrt{3} \times \sigma$ with the positive side of the Mexican hat is interpreted in our model as the optimal intermediate item. This item is considered to have the best possible diversity: neither too close nor too far from the compared item. We consider this turning point as the center of the intermediate area. To find the boundaries of this area, we took $o \pm \gamma$ with the intervals $\gamma = (\sqrt{3} - 1) \times \sigma$ (limits in green on Fig. 2). Indeed, $b_{\text{inf}} = (\sqrt{3} \times \sigma) - \gamma$ is the moment when the value of the function becomes positive. Therefore, we can define two boundaries: the lower bound $b_{\text{inf}} = (\sqrt{3} \times \sigma) - \gamma$ and the upper bound $b_{\text{sup}} = (\sqrt{3} \times \sigma) + \gamma$.

This Mexican hat-based model relies on parameters such as the standard deviation and the mean of a distribution of dissimilarity values with respect to a given item. Once we have the dissimilarity values, the other parameters are easy to obtain. On a recommender scenario, this method allows us to eliminate close and distant items and focus on the intermediate items that have features slightly different from the ones the user usually consumes. This method is all the more interesting because the more diversity we have in our items, the greater the scope of the function.

For searching the optimal item for each seed item, as shown on Fig. 2, the Algorithm 1 will tend to look for candidate items that have more difference to the optimal diverse item (right part of the interval) than less difference (left part of the interval). If there is no item at the optimum, the search for a candidate item can be done on the left of the optimum (with less difference with the seed item)

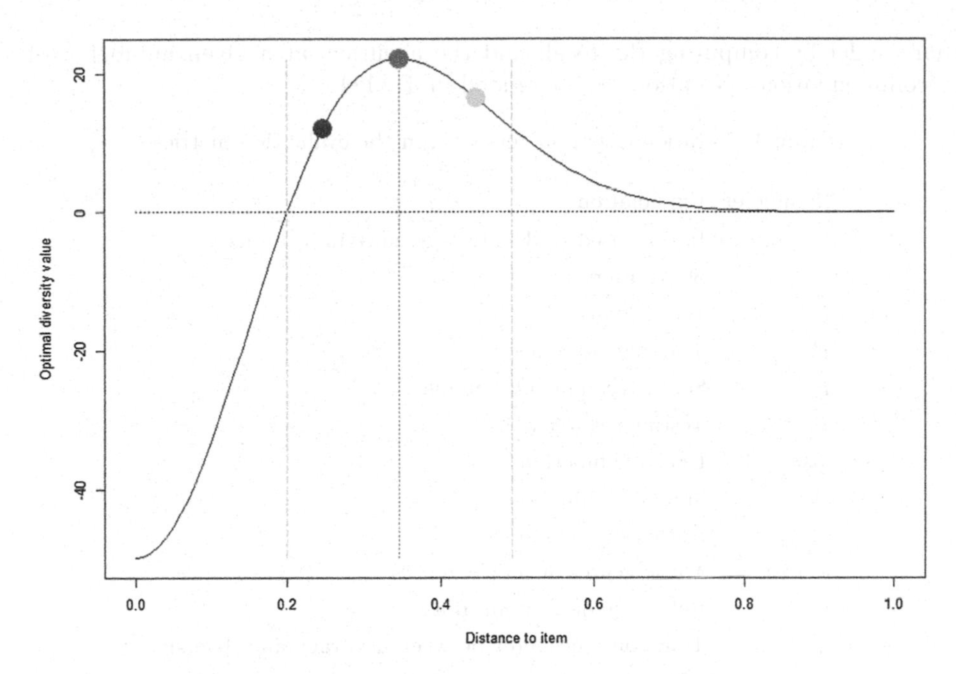

Fig. 2. Area of diversity interest resulting from the Mexican hat function: The distance to a reference (seed) item is represented on X-axis and the diversity interest on Y-axis. The optimal diversity zone is located between the two green limits. The maximal optimal diversity is obtained for the red dot. (Color figure online)

or on the right of the optimum (more difference). However, for the same distance to the optimum, the function will favor an item located on the right side, i.e., having more distance with the seed item (green dot on the Fig. 2) than on the left side, e.g., the blue dot on Fig. 2 have a smaller value compared to the green one even if its distance with the optimum is identical.

4 Experiments

In this section, we present a comparative analysis of the Mexican-Hat Diversity Model (MHDM) and two state-of-the-art diversity re-ranking algorithms. We evaluate our approach in offline top-N movie recommender system and music recommender system.

4.1 Evaluation Metrics

First we present different state-of-this-art diversity measures proposed to evaluate the diversity component of recommendations made in automated systems. For this task, we used metrics from the literature capturing individual diversity, coverage (i.e., aggregate diversity), and novelty. As it is mentioned, gaining diversity is done by losing accuracy. Therefore we also measure the accuracy of our model by computing the recall and the accuracy at a given number k of recommendations. Notations are reminded in Table 1.

Table 1. Notation of parameters used in the evaluation metrics.

Parameter	Explanation
i, j, k, u	Indices used to denote a given item or an user
U	Set of users
I	Set of items
P	Training set items
R	Set of recommended items
T	Testing set items
$dist$	Distance function
sim	Similarity function
rat	Rating of an item
$genres$	Music genres or movie genres
rel	Relevance of an item in a list
λ	Trade-off parameter between accuracy and diversity

Intra-List Diversity (ILD). The intra-list diversity measures the individual diversity of a list of recommendations. It has been proposed in [36] and it computes the average distance between all pairs of items in the list of recommended items. In our experiment we use a mixed distance based on the content of the item and the users items interactions:

$$\frac{1}{|U|}\sum_{u \in U}\frac{1}{k(k-1)}\sum_{(i,j)\in R_u} dist(i,j)$$

Genre Coverage. The genre coverage helps us measure the diversity of topics in the recommendations. It helps to measure if all the user interests are covered in the list. We use the formula proposed by [22]:

$$\frac{1}{|U|}\sum_{u \in U}\frac{\left|\bigcup_{i \in R_u} genres(i) \bigcap \bigcup_{i \in P_u^+} genres(i)\right|}{\left|\bigcup_{i \in P_u^+} genres(i)\right|}$$

Catalog Coverage. The catalog coverage is an important measure for the streaming platform point of view. It evaluates the percentage of items in the catalog that are recommended at least once. Thus this can help to improve the distribution of items across the users.

$$\frac{\left|\bigcup_{u \in U} R_u\right|}{|I|}$$

Precision@k. This precision is the fraction of retrieved items that are relevant in the list of k recommended items with T_u the set of item in the test for the ith user.

$$\frac{1}{|U|} \sum_{u \in U} \frac{1}{k} |R_u \cap T_u|$$

Recall@k. It is the fraction of relevant items that are in the list of k recommended items.

$$\frac{1}{|U|} \sum_{u \in U} \frac{|R_u \cap T_u|}{T_u}$$

Normalized Distributed Cumulative Gain@k (nDCG). Normalized discounted cumulative gain@k takes into account the relevance of recommendations with respect to the test set for a user, giving more weight to the items higher on the ranking list. The $nDCG@k$ metric is computed as follows, with rel_i denoting the relevance of item i on the similarity list:

$$\frac{1}{|U|} \cdot \sum_{u \in U} \frac{1}{iDCG@N} \sum_{i=1}^{k} \frac{2^{rel_i} - 1}{log_2(1+i)}$$

with $iDCG@k$ denoting the best possible (recommendation list exactly the same as test set) $DCG@k$ score. The possible values of rel_i are 0 and 1, 0 if the artist is not in the test set, and 1 if the artist is in the test.

Expected Popularity Complement. It computes the percentage of items in the long-tail that are present in the recommendation list [31]. We use the formula in [20]. We define $|rat(i)|$ as the number of users who rated the item i and $|\arg\max(rat)|$, as the number of ratings of the most rated item in the item set.

$$\frac{1}{|U|} \sum_{u \in U} \frac{1}{k} \sum_{i \in R_u} 1 - \frac{|rat(i)|}{|\arg\max(rat)|}$$

In brief, Intra-List Diversity, Catalog Coverage, and Genre Coverage measure diversity; nDCG@k, Recall@k and Precision@k evaluate the accuracy; and the Expected Popularity Complement is used to measure the novelty.

4.2 Baselines

We choose two baseline diversification algorithms to compare our method: the Maximal Marginal Relevance (MMR) [7] and an extension of MMR, the Max-Sum Diversification (MSD) [5].

Maximal Marginal Relevance (MMR). It is a linear combination of the user's profile item similarity and the maximum similarity of the item to the selected item set.

$$\arg \max_{i \in I/P \cup R} \lambda sim_1(u,i) - (1-\lambda) \max_{j \in R} sim_2(i,j)$$

Max-Sum Diversification (MSD). Like in MMR, the objective function of MSD is a linear combination of a function that measures the relevance of an item for a user and a function that measures the diversification between the items.

$$\arg \max_{R \subseteq I/P} \lambda r(i) + (1-\lambda) \sum_{i \in R} \sum_{j \in R-i} dist(i,j) \mid |R| \leq k$$

For the two baseline diversification algorithms, the purpose is to maximize an objective function with a trade-off parameter $\lambda \in [0,1]$.

4.3 Experiments on Public Datasets

We use two datasets for our offline experiments, a *MovieLens* dataset [14] and a *Last.fm* dataset [6]. The results are presented on Table 2 for MovieLens dataset and Table 3 for Last.fm dataset: the results are scaled between 0 and 100, the best results are in bold font, and the second best results are in italic font. For each user on the two datasets, we hold 80% of the ratings for the training part and the 20% left for testing. For the *Last.fm* dataset, we convert the users' listenings to a 1-to-5 rating value. We use the genres (*MovieLens*) and the tags (*Last.fm*) to create the item distance matrix. For the *Last.fm* dataset we reduce the item tag matrix using Latent Semantic Analysis (LSA) prior computing the distance matrix. For the implementation of the *MSD* algorithm, we use a state-of-the-art item-based collaborative filtering implemented in R *recommenderlab* package [13] to predict the ratings. We consider these predicted ratings as the relevance part in *MSD*. We consider the normalized sum of the item features in the train part as the profile of a user for the *MMR* algorithm. We use a cosine similarity to compute the similarity between the user and an item. For *MMR* and *MSD*, we use $\lambda = 0.1, 0.5$, and 0.8. We show also the results we obtained for the item-based collaborative filtering (*IBCF*). For our method, we use the value in the train set to create the seed items for the user profile. We use the *IBCF* ratings for our algorithm by doing a linear combination of the rating for an item and the value given by the Mexican hat function. We present then two versions of our Mexican-hat diversity model: $MHDM_S$, a "Simple" version

Table 2. Experimental results on top-k recommendations for MovieLens dataset with $k = 10$.

	IBCF	MSD			MMR			$MHDM_R$	$MHDM_S$
		$\lambda = 0.1$	$\lambda = 0.5$	$\lambda = 0.8$	$\lambda = 0.1$	$\lambda = 0.5$	$\lambda = 0.8$		
ILD	51.00	**76.97**	*69.70*	68.41	61.00	53.54	50.89	64.54	64.77
Genre cov.	51.26	**95.26**	*85.00*	72.45	54.69	54.01	51.30	87.68	88.40
Catalog cov.	70.96	46.33	70.18	71.66	33.56	*72.00*	**79.00**	58.22	51.10
Precision@k	0.76	**10.39**	2.67	1.47	2.87	2.89	2.62	5.39	*5.72*
Recall@k	0.40	**3.66**	1.10	0.89	1.15	1.18	1.09	2.47	*2.64*
nDCG@k	0.79	**12.31**	3.70	1.53	4.97	4.81	4.51	0.95	*5.93*
EPC	**90.83**	75.74	85.14	86.09	39.48	43.05	44.00	88.00	*88.44*

Table 3. Experimental results on top-k recommendations for Last.fm dataset with $k = 10$.

	IBCF	MSD			MMR			$MHDM_R$	$MHDM_S$
		$\lambda = 0.1$	$\lambda = 0.5$	$\lambda = 0.8$	$\lambda = 0.1$	$\lambda = 0.5$	$\lambda = 0.8$		
ILD	17.00	35.00	26.00	24.00	60.00	**67.00**	**67.00**	22.00	*53.00*
Catalog cov.	45.00	42.00	44.00	44.00	**47.00**	39.00	39.00	**47.00**	18.00
Precision@k	0.37	1.71	0.57	0.40	*1.92*	1.37	1.39	0.49	**3.55**
Recall@k	0.44	1.91	0.69	0.47	*2.07*	1.44	1.44	0.58	**3.82**
nDCG@k	0.45	3.93	0.95	0.51	*3.08*	1.56	1.44	0.57	**3.34**
EPC	88.95	97.04	*98.20*	**98.37**	91.90	91.92	92.00	97.60	95.16

without taking into account the ratings, and $MHDM_R$, a version of the model taking into account the *Ratings*. We do not use a trade-off coefficient for this implementation. Our codes, datasets and experiments are available online[1].

5 Results and Discussions

We compare our method to two diversification methods (*MSD* and *MMR*) and the *IBCF* method with common metrics used for k recommended items. At first, we observe that all the diversification methods obtain better accuracy scores (*Precision@k*, *Recall@k*, *nDCG@k*) compared to the *IBCF* algorithm on the two datasets. We expect the accuracy to increase and the diversity to decrease with the increase of λ, but we observe this only for the diversification but not for the accuracy (*MSD* and *MHDM*). This is explained by the low precision, recall, and *nDCG* scores of the *IBCF*, as the higher λ gives more weight to the initial ranking of the *IBCF*. This does not happen to *MMR* because its relevance score does not depend on the ratings. For *MovieLens* dataset, *MSD* obtained the overall best results. For the *Last.fm*, no method produces the best scores for each metrics.

[1] https://www.dropbox.com/sh/uwcp1xfz6afckif/AAAJiBeGUEhs0HEH4E-_-n-ca?dl=0.

Ours $MHDM_S$ and $MHDM_R$ methods do not overcome all algorithms in terms of diversification but are always one of the top performers. We explain this by the fact that *MHDM* does not maximize the intra-list diversity *ILD* like *MSD*. The diversification is done by retrieving items in an intermediate zone that is neither too similar nor too different than what the user preferred in the past. This leads also to the good results observed in the recall, precision and $nDCG$, especially on the *Last.fm* dataset. We see that by adding the ratings on $MHDM_R$: our results on *MovieLens* are not affected, but we cannot say that for *Last.fm*. One of the advantages of this technique is that we do not have to rely on the ratings, and we do not need a hyperparameter such as λ.

6 Conclusion and Future Work

We present in this paper a method that brings diversity in recommendation list. We build a recommendation model and we conduct offline experiments on two public datasets. The results show that our method competes well against the existing diversification algorithms. We believe that a recommender list should not only be a shortlist chosen by the system which is the reflection of the past behavior of the user. We believe that in those shortlist we can put "boldness" by going further than the boundary of the user profile. Indeed, given less choice people are more satisfied even when the quality is not as good [26]. But we have to be careful, because we do not want to frustrate the users with recommendations too bold and too far from their interests. This is why our Mexican-Hat Diversity Model seek to promote diversity, without looking to maximize this criteria. For an online streaming platform, a MHDM recommender system will have the advantage of covering all the cultural content it offers to users, reaching the long tail as expected with the arrival of the digital revolution [3].

The essential element to remember from this proposal is that the Mexican-Hat Diversity Model (MHDM) seems to fulfill three main characteristics sought in the recommendations of cultural services on streaming platforms:

1. A MHDM recommender system that is seeking to promote diversity has a pedagogical virtue in order to reach the full spectrum of the user's interest and even to seek to enlarge it. The system will not play the easy game of recommending the most popular items that will easily appeal to everyone directly, but do not satisfy it in the long run. Conversely, the system will not perform too much customization on items already appreciated by each user, which will induce a history he or she will be doomed to repeat, an endless-loop and narrowing version of him- or herself [23].
2. For the online streaming platform, a MHDM recommender system will have the advantage of covering more easily all the cultural content it offers to users, reaching the long tail as expected with the arrival of the digital revolution [3].
3. For the artists and other cultural content producers distributed by the platform, a MHDM recommender system will be more likely to recommend each of them in a fair mode, without privileging the superstars, giving everyone the opportunity to contribute to the cultural diversity of the world.

In a world where artificial systems will increasingly play the role of intermediary between us and existing goods and services through choice-making, it seems that our MHDM proposal is both an original and sustainable answer by the diversity promotion.

References

1. Abbassi, Z., Amer-Yahia, S., Lakshmanan, L.V.S., Vassilvitskii, S., Yu, C.: Getting recommender systems to think outside the box. In: Bergman, L.D., Tuzhilin, A., Burke, R.D., Felfernig, A., Schmidt-Thieme, L. (eds.) Proceedings of the 2009 ACM Conference on Recommender Systems, RecSys 2009, New York, NY, USA, 23–25 October 2009, pp. 285–288. ACM (2009)
2. Adamopoulos, P., Tuzhilin, A.: On unexpectedness in recommender systems: or how to better expect the unexpected. ACM Trans. Intell. Syst. Technol. (TIST) **5**(4), 54:1–54:32 (2014)
3. Anderson, C.: The Longer Long Tail: How Endless Choice is Creating Unlimited Demand. Random House Business, New York (2009)
4. Ashkan, A., Kveton, B., Berkovsky, S., Wen, Z.: Optimal greedy diversity for recommendation. In: Yang, Q., Wooldridge, M. (eds.) Proceedings of the Twenty-Fourth International Joint Conference on Artificial Intelligence, IJCAI 2015, Buenos Aires, Argentina, 25–31 July 2015, pp. 1742–1748. AAAI Press (2015)
5. Borodin, A., Lee, H.C., Ye, Y.: Max-sum diversification, monotone submodular functions and dynamic updates. CoRR abs/1203.6397 (2012)
6. Cantador, I., Brusilovsky, P., Kuflik, T.: Second workshop on information heterogeneity and fusion in recommender systems (HetRec 2011). In: Proceedings of the 5th ACM conference on Recommender systems, RecSys 2011, NY, USA. ACM, New York (2011)
7. Carbonell, J.G., Goldstein, J.: The use of MMR, diversity-based reranking for reordering documents and producing summaries. In: Croft, W.B., Moffat, A., van Rijsbergen, C.J., Wilkinson, R., Zobel, J. (eds.) Proceedings of the 21st Annual International ACM SIGIR Conference on Research and Development in Information Retrieval, SIGIR 1998, Melbourne, Australia, 24–28 August 1998, pp. 335–336. ACM (1998)
8. Castells, P., Hurley, N.J., Vargas, S.: Novelty and Diversity in Recommender Systems. In: Ricci, F., Rokach, L., Shapira, B. (eds.) Recommender Systems Handbook, pp. 881–918. Springer, Boston (2015). doi:10.1007/978-1-4899-7637-6_26
9. Celma, Ò.: Music recommendation and discovery in the long tail. Ph.D. thesis, Universitat Pompeu Fabra, Barcelona, Catalonia, Spain (2008)
10. Celma, Ò.: Music Recommendation and Discovery – The Long Tail, Long Fail, and Long Play in the Digital Music Space. Springer, Heidelberg (2010)
11. Ekstrand, M.D., Harper, F.M., Willemsen, M.C., Konstan, J.A.: User perception of differences in recommender algorithms. In: Eighth ACM Conference on Recommender Systems, RecSys 2014, Foster City, Silicon Valley, CA, USA, 6–10 October 2014, pp. 161–168 (2014)
12. Ge, M., Delgado-Battenfeld, C., Jannach, D.: Beyond accuracy: evaluating recommender systems by coverage and serendipity. In: Amatriain, X., Torrens, M., Resnick, P., Zanker, M. (eds.) Proceedings of the 2010 ACM Conference on Recommender Systems, RecSys 2010, Barcelona, Spain, 26–30 September 2010, pp. 257–260. ACM (2010)

13. Hahsler, M.: recommenderlab: Lab for Developing and Testing Recommender Algorithms (2017). Rpackageversion0.2-2. http://lyle.smu.edu/IDA/recommenderlab/
14. Harper, F.M., Konstan, J.A.: The movielens datasets: history and context. ACM Trans. Interact. Intell. Syst. (TiiS) **5**(4), 19:1–19:19 (2016)
15. Jannach, D., Adomavicius, G.: Recommendations with a purpose. In: Sen, S., Geyer, W., Freyne, J., Castells, P. (eds.) Proceedings of the 10th ACM Conference on Recommender Systems, Boston, MA, USA, 15–19 September 2016, pp. 7–10. ACM (2016)
16. Kohonen, T.: Self-organizing Maps. Springer Series in Information Sciences, 3rd edn. Springer, Heidelberg (2001)
17. Marr, D., Hildreth, E.C.: Theory of edge detection. Proc. R. Soc. Lond. B, Biol. Sci. **207**(1167), 187–217 (1980)
18. McNee, S.M., Riedl, J., Konstan, J.A.: Being accurate is not enough: how accuracy metrics have hurt recommender systems. In: Olson, G.M., Jeffries, R. (eds.) Extended Abstracts Proceedings of the 2006 Conference on Human Factors in Computing Systems, CHI 2006, Montréal, Québec, Canada, 22–27 April 2006, pp. 1097–1101. ACM (2006)
19. Mulligan, M.: The death of the long tail: the superstar music economy, mIDiA Consulting internal report. https://musicindustryblog.wordpress.com/2014/03/04/the-death-of-the-long-tail/
20. Niemann, K., Wolpers, M.: A new collaborative filtering approach for increasing the aggregate diversity of recommender systems. In: The 19th ACM SIGKDD International Conference on Knowledge Discovery and Data Mining, KDD 2013, Chicago, IL, USA, 11–14 August 2013, pp. 955–963 (2013)
21. Noia, T.D., Rosati, J., Tomeo, P., Sciascio, E.D.: Adaptive multi-attribute diversity for recommender systems. Inf. Sci. **382–383**, 234–253 (2017)
22. Parambath, S.P., Usunier, N., Grandvalet, Y.: A coverage-based approach to recommendation diversity on similarity graph. In: Sen, S., Geyer, W., Freyne, J., Castells, P. (eds.) Proceedings of the 10th ACM Conference on Recommender Systems, Boston, MA, USA, 11–14 September 2016, pp. 15–22. ACM (2016)
23. Pariser, E.: The Filter Bubble: What The Internet Is Hiding From You. Penguin Press, New York (2011)
24. Ribeiro, M.T., Lacerda, A., Veloso, A., Ziviani, N.: Pareto-efficient hybridization for multi-objective recommender systems. In: Sixth ACM Conference on Recommender Systems, RecSys 2012, Dublin, Ireland, 9–13 September 2012, pp. 19–26 (2012)
25. Ricker, N.: Wavelet functions and their polynomials. Geophysics **9**(3), 314–323 (1944)
26. Schwartz, B.: The Paradox of Choice - Why More Is Less. Harper Perennial, New York (2004)
27. Seyerlehner, K., Flexer, A., Widmer, G.: On the limitations of browsing top-N recommender systems. In: Bergman, L.D., Tuzhilin, A., Burke, R.D., Felfernig, A., Schmidt-Thieme, L. (eds.) Proceedings of the 2009 ACM Conference on Recommender Systems, RecSys 2009, New York, NY, USA, 23–25 October 2009, pp. 321–324. ACM (2009)
28. Smyth, B., McClave, P.: Similarity vs. diversity. In: Aha, D.W., Watson, I. (eds.) ICCBR 2001. LNCS, vol. 2080, pp. 347–361. Springer, Heidelberg (2001). doi:10.1007/3-540-44593-5_25

29. Steck, H.: Item popularity and recommendation accuracy. In: Mobasher, B., Burke, R.D., Jannach, D., Adomavicius, G. (eds.) Proceedings of the 2011 ACM Conference on Recommender Systems, RecSys 2011, Chicago, IL, USA, 23–27 October 2011, pp. 125–132. ACM (2011)
30. Vargas, S.: Novelty and diversity evaluation and enhancement in recommender systems. Ph.D. thesis, Universidad Autonoma de Madrid, Spain, February 2015
31. Vargas, S., Castells, P.: Rank and relevance in novelty and diversity metrics for recommender systems. In: Proceedings of the 2011 ACM Conference on Recommender Systems, RecSys 2011, Chicago, IL, USA, 23–27 October 2011, pp. 109–116 (2011)
32. Vargas, S., Castells, P.: Exploiting the diversity of user preferences for recommendation. In: Ferreira, J., Magalhães, J., Calado, P. (eds.) Open research Areas in Information Retrieval, OAIR 2013, Lisbon, Portugal, 15–17 May 2013, pp. 129–136. ACM (2013)
33. Wasilewski, J., Hurley, N.: Intent-aware diversification using a constrained PLSA. In: Proceedings of the 10th ACM Conference on Recommender Systems, Boston, MA, USA, 15–19 September 2016, pp. 39–42 (2016)
34. Yang, M.-H., Gu, Z.-M.: Personalized recommendation based on partial similarity of interests. In: Li, X., Zaïane, O.R., Li, Z. (eds.) ADMA 2006. LNCS (LNAI), vol. 4093, pp. 509–516. Springer, Heidelberg (2006). doi:10.1007/11811305_56
35. Zhang, J., Zhu, X., Li, X., Zhang, S.: Mining item popularity for recommender systems. In: Motoda, H., Wu, Z., Cao, L., Zaiane, O., Yao, M., Wang, W. (eds.) ADMA 2013. LNCS (LNAI), vol. 8347, pp. 372–383. Springer, Heidelberg (2013). doi:10.1007/978-3-642-53917-6_33
36. Zhang, M., Hurley, N.: Avoiding monotony: improving the diversity of recommendation lists. In: Pu, P., Bridge, D.G., Mobasher, B., Ricci, F. (eds.) Proceedings of the 2008 ACM Conference on Recommender Systems, RecSys 2008, Lausanne, Switzerland, 23–25 October 2008, pp. 123–130. ACM (2008)
37. Zhang, M., Hurley, N.: Novel item recommendation by user profile partitioning. In: 2009 IEEE/WIC/ACM International Conference on Web Intelligence, WI 2009, Milan, Italy, 15–18 September 2009, Main Conference Proceedings. pp. 508–515. IEEE Computer Society (2009)

A Hierarchical Bayesian Factorization Model for Implicit and Explicit Feedback Data

ThaiBinh Nguyen[1(✉)] and Atsuhiro Takasu[1,2]

[1] Department of Informatics, SOKENDAI (The Graduate University for Advanced Studies), Tokyo, Japan
{binh,takasu}@nii.ac.jp
[2] National Institute of Informatics, Tokyo, Japan

Abstract. Matrix factorization (MF) is one of the most efficient methods for performing collaborative filtering. An MF-based method represents users and items by latent feature vectors that are obtained by decomposing the rating matrix of users to items. However, MF-based methods suffer from the cold-start problem: if no rating data are available for an item, the model cannot find a latent feature vector for that item, and thus cannot make a recommendation for it. In this paper, we present a hierarchical Bayesian model that can infer the latent feature vectors of items directly from the *implicit feedback* (e.g., clicks, views, purchases) when they cannot be obtained from the rating data. We infer the full posterior distributions of these parameters using a Gibbs sampling method. We show that the proposed method is strong with overfitting even if the model is very complex or the data are very sparse. Our experiments on real-world datasets demonstrate that our proposed method significantly outperforms competing methods on rating prediction tasks, especially for very sparse datasets.

Keywords: Collaborative filtering · Item embedding · Implicit feedback · Explicit feedback · Matrix factorization

1 Introduction

With the emergence of big data, recommender systems have become a core part of online services. The goal of a recommender system is to model user preferences by analyzing their history data and providing them with personalized recommendations. Collaborative filtering (CF) is an efficient approach for recommender systems that aims at predicting the rating of a user for an item given the past rating history of the users. Among various CF-based methods, matrix factorization (MF) is one of the most powerful approaches [2,11].

MF-based algorithms represent user preferences and item attributes by latent feature vectors in a shared latent space. Typically, an MF-based algorithm finds the latent feature vectors of users and items by fitting the model with the observed ratings given in the user–item rating matrix [2,11,12,15]. However, because each user can only rate a limited number of items, the rating

G. Cong et al. (Eds.): ADMA 2017, LNAI 10604, pp. 104–118, 2017.
https://doi.org/10.1007/978-3-319-69179-4_8

matrix is usually extremely sparse. Therefore, the performance of rating prediction declines if an item has too few ratings; or in an extreme case, if an item has no prior ratings, the system cannot learn its latent feature vector, and thus cannot recommend it to any user. This problem is referred to as the *cold-start* problem.

To address this problem, a common approach is to exploit other information about users and items, known as *side information* or *auxiliary information.* There are various types of side information, depending on the item being recommended (e.g., the genres of movies or text content of books). Such side information is successfully combined with traditional CF-based algorithms to alleviate the cold-start problem. For instance, in [1,14,16], text content was exploited for article recommendations; music content for song recommendations [9], or text content and category information for movie recommendations [10]. One limitation of these models is that such side information is not always available, or, in many cases, that information is available, but less informative for describing items (e.g., some items are described by a few keywords or very short texts).

This work focuses on exploiting another kind of feedback known as *implicit feedback* (e.g., clicks, views, purchases) as the auxiliary data. The advantage of using implicit feedback is that it is abundant and easily collected during the interactions of users with the system without requiring users to provide further interactions.

Related Work. In [2], the authors proposed SVD++ which exploits implicit feedback to boost the performance of the original probabilistic matrix factorization (PMF) model [11]. However, in SVD++, implicit feedback is a binary matrix that indicates "who rates what", obtained by binarizing the rating data, an item has implicit feedback if and only if it has rating data; therefore, this model cannot model an item if it has no ratings.

Co-rating [5] combines explicit and implicit feedback in a unified framework. In the model, the explicit feedback are normalized into the range [0, 1] and added to the implicit feedback matrix to form a unique matrix. This matrix is then factorized to obtain the latent feature vectors of users and items. In this way, the feature vector of an item can be inferred even if it does not have any rating data. The limitation of this method is that, after forming the final matrix, implicit and explicit feedback cannot be distinguished; therefore, this model cannot take into account the uncertainty of the implicit feedback.

In [13], the authors proposed a method for combining implicit and explicit feedback using expectation maximization (EM). To predict ratings for an item for which rating data are not available, the rating is inferred from ratings of its neighbors in terms of click data. However, the algorithm is based on an iterative EM-based algorithm in which the E-phase is a matrix factorization model. In other words, matrix factorization is performed multiple times and is therefore computationally expensive.

In [8], the authors proposed a probabilistic model for combining explicit and implicit feedback for making recommendations. In this model, the latent feature vector of an item for which rating data are not available can be learned directly from the implicit feedback data. This is a combination of PMF [11] and an item embedding model; the model learns latent feature vectors for an item from the implicit feedback. In detail, the model consists of simultaneously factorizing the rating matrix and the positive point-wise mutual information (PPMI) matrix that is constructed from the click data. The item vectors are obtained by the factorization of the PPMI matrix and are then adjusted by the rating matrix. Although this model successfully combines implicit feedback data in learning latent feature vectors of items, it is prone to overfitting if the hyperparameters (i.e., the regularization parameters) are not tuned carefully. Usually, the hyperparameter tuning is very costly, especially when there are many hyperparameters, or when the data are large.

Present Work. In this paper, we propose a fully hierarchical Bayesian treatment for the model proposed by Nguyen et al. [8]. In this model, instead of finding a point estimate for the model parameters, our method infers the full posterior distribution of these model parameters to capture their uncertainty. The missing ratings are predicted by integrating out the latent feature vectors of users and items. To this end, we place the Gaussian inverse Wishart priors on the mean vectors and covariance matrices of the latent feature vectors for the rating matrix and PPMI matrix [8]. We develop a Markov chain Monte Carlo (MCMC)-based method for inferring the full posterior distribution.

2 Preliminary

Suppose we have N users and M items. For each user–item pair (u, i), there can be two types of feedback: *explicit feedback* (also known as *rating data*) and *implicit feedback* (also known as *click data*). The rating data are represented by matrix $\mathbf{R} \in \mathbb{R}^{N \times M}$, in which element r_{ui} is the rating of user u for item i. r_{ui} can be a real number or a binary value (e.g., like/dislike). The click data are represented by a binary matrix $\mathbf{P} \in \{0, 1\}^{N \times M}$, where $p_{ui} = 1$ indicates that user u has clicked i at least once, and $p_{ui} = 0$ otherwise.

Generally, the rating matrix $\mathbf{R}$ is extremely sparse with many missing values (i.e., r_{ui} is not observed). We are interested in predicting these missing ratings.

2.1 Item Embedding Model According to Implicit Feedback Data

Word embedding techniques have shown their success in many natural language processing tasks [3,6]. By viewing each item in a recommender system as a word, the same assumptions that underlie word embedding models can be applied to modeling items. In [8], the authors proposed a method for an item embedding model based on implicit feedback data, i.e., a model that captures the relationship between items that are clicked by the same users.

In this item embedding model, item i is represented by two vectors: an *item vector* $\mathbf{w}_i$ and a *context vector* $\mathbf{z}_i$. The vectors have different roles: the item vector describes the distribution of the item, and the context vector describes the distribution of the co-occurrence of an item with other items in its context.

In [8], the authors proposed an item-embedding scheme in which the *item vector* and the *context vector* are obtained by factorizing the PPMI matrix corresponding to the click data [8]:

$$PPMI(i, j) = \mathbf{w}_i^\top \mathbf{z}_i \tag{1}$$

The PPMI matrix is obtained by replacing the negative values by zeros in the point-wise mutual information (PMI) matrix. The elements of the PMI matrix are correlation measures for the co-occurrence of two items. Empirically, the PMI of items i and j can be approximated using the observed data:

$$PMI(i, j) = \log \frac{\#(i, j)|\mathcal{D}|}{\#(i)\#(j)}, \tag{2}$$

where $\#(i)$ and $\#(j)$ are the numbers of times items i and j are clicked, respectively. $\mathcal{D}$ is the set of item pairs that appear in the combined click history of all users. $\#(i, j)$ is the number of users who clicked both i and j.

2.2 Probabilistic Model for Implicit and Explicit Feedback Data

After producing the item embedding model according to implicit feedback, Nguyen et al. [8] proposed a model that combines implicit and explicit feedback in a unified framework (PIE). PIE is a combination of the item-embedding model (described in Sect. 2.1) and the matrix factorization for rating data. In PIE, the latent feature vector $\mathbf{y}_i$ of item i is obtained by adding a small deviation $\mathbf{t}_i$ to the item vector $\mathbf{z}_i$. The graphical model of PIE is shown in Fig. 1a.

The main drawback of this model is that the parameter learning is a point estimation (MAP estimate), which is prone to overfitting when applying the trained model to unseen data. To avoid overfitting, we must tune the hyperparameters carefully. One approach is grid-search: we form a set of appropriate configurations of hyperparameters and train the model with these configurations. The configuration that produces the best performance on the validation set will be selected. However, in general, grid search is very costly, especially for large-scale data, or when the number of hyperparameters is large.

A straightforward way to avoid hyperparameter tuning is to introduce priors to the hyperparameters and optimize the log-posterior over both model parameters and hyperparameters. In this way, the hyperparameters will be learned from the data instead of tuned manually. However, this solution does not significantly improve the generalization of the model because it is still a point estimation and cannot capture the uncertainty of the model parameters.

3 Proposed Method

To address drawbacks described above, we propose a hierarchical, fully Bayesian model (HBFM) that can capture the uncertainty of the model parameters. Instead of approximating the posterior by its mode (the MAP estimate), we approximate the full posterior distributions of model parameters.

3.1 The Model

We place the Gaussian inverse Wishart priors on the mean vectors and covariance matrices of the latent feature vectors. The graphical model is shown in Fig. 1b.

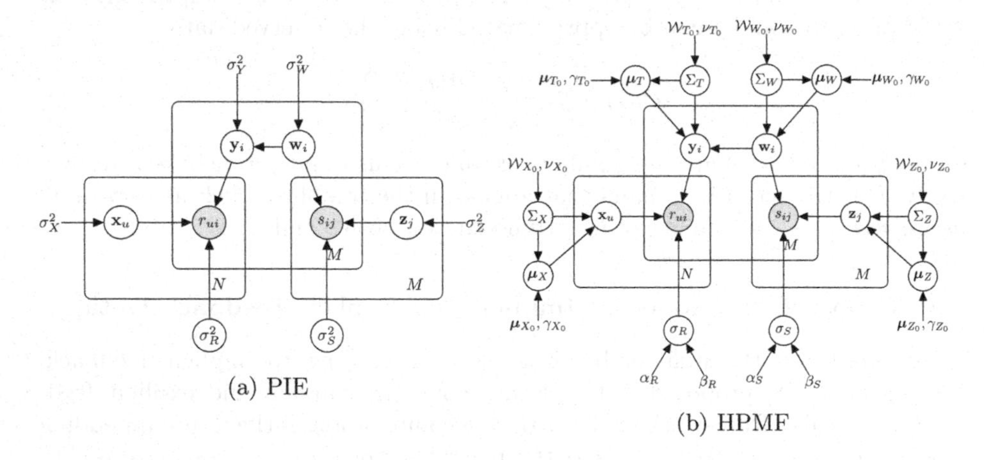

(a) PIE

(b) HPMF

Fig. 1. Graphical models of PIE [8] and HPMF (this paper). Because of space limitations, we omit the bias terms.

We assume that r_{ui} and s_{ij} are Gaussian distributions as follows:

$$p(r_{ui}|\mathbf{x}_u, \mathbf{y}_i, \theta_u, \rho_i, \sigma_R^2) = \mathcal{N}(r_{ui}|\mathbf{x}_u^\top \mathbf{y}_i + \eta_{ui}, \sigma_R^2) \tag{3}$$

$$p(s_{ui}|\mathbf{w}_i, \mathbf{z}_j, \sigma_S^2) = \mathcal{N}(s_{ij}|\mathbf{w}_i^\top \mathbf{z}_j, \sigma_S^2), \tag{4}$$

where θ_u and ρ_i are the biases of user u and item i, respectively; $\mathbf{y}_i = \mathbf{t}_i + \mathbf{w}_i$; $\eta_{ui} = \mu + \theta_u + \rho_i$; and μ is the global mean of the ratings.

The prior distributions of the latent feature vectors are assumed to be multivariate Gaussian distributions:

$$\begin{aligned} p(\mathbf{X}|\boldsymbol{\Theta}_X) &= \prod_{u=1}^{N} \mathcal{N}(\mathbf{x}_u|\boldsymbol{\mu}_X, \boldsymbol{\Sigma}_X), \quad p(\mathbf{T}|\boldsymbol{\Theta}_T) = \prod_{i=1}^{M} \mathcal{N}(\mathbf{t}_i|\boldsymbol{\mu}_T, \boldsymbol{\Sigma}_T) \\ p(\mathbf{W}|\boldsymbol{\Theta}_W) &= \prod_{i=1}^{M} \mathcal{N}(\mathbf{w}_i|\boldsymbol{\mu}_W, \boldsymbol{\Sigma}_W), \quad p(\mathbf{Z}|\boldsymbol{\Theta}_Z) = \prod_{j=1}^{M} \mathcal{N}(\mathbf{z}_u|\boldsymbol{\mu}_Z, \boldsymbol{\Sigma}_Z) \end{aligned} \tag{5}$$

where $\boldsymbol{\mu}_X$, $\boldsymbol{\mu}_T$, $\boldsymbol{\mu}_W$, and $\boldsymbol{\mu}_Z$ are the mean vectors and $\boldsymbol{\Sigma}_X$, $\boldsymbol{\Sigma}_Y$, $\boldsymbol{\Sigma}_W$, and $\boldsymbol{\Sigma}_Z$ are the covariance matrices of $\mathbf{x}_u$, $\mathbf{y}_i$, $\mathbf{w}_i$, and $\mathbf{z}_j$, respectively; $\boldsymbol{\Theta}_X = \{\boldsymbol{\mu}_X, \Sigma_X\}$, $\boldsymbol{\Theta}_T = \{\boldsymbol{\mu}_T, \Sigma_T\}$, $\boldsymbol{\Theta}_W = \{\boldsymbol{\mu}_W, \Sigma_W\}$, and $\boldsymbol{\Theta}_Z = \{\boldsymbol{\mu}_Z, \Sigma_Z\}$.

To model the uncertainty of the latent feature vectors, we do not treat them as distributions of fixed hyperparameters. Instead, we further place Gaussian-inverse Wishart priors on $\boldsymbol{\Theta}_X$, $\boldsymbol{\Theta}_T$, $\boldsymbol{\Theta}_W$, and $\boldsymbol{\Theta}_Z$:

$$p(\boldsymbol{\Theta}_X|\boldsymbol{\Phi}_{X_0}) = \mathcal{N}(\boldsymbol{\mu}_X|\boldsymbol{\mu}_{X_0}, \boldsymbol{\Sigma}_X/\gamma_{X_0})\mathcal{W}^{-1}(\boldsymbol{\Sigma}_X|\mathcal{W}_{X_0}, \nu_{X_0}) \tag{6}$$

$$p(\boldsymbol{\Theta}_T|\boldsymbol{\Phi}_{T_0}) = \mathcal{N}(\boldsymbol{\mu}_T|\boldsymbol{\mu}_{T_0}, \boldsymbol{\Sigma}_T/\gamma_{T_0})\mathcal{W}^{-1}(\boldsymbol{\Sigma}_T|\mathcal{W}_{T_0}, \nu_{T_0}) \tag{7}$$

$$p(\boldsymbol{\Theta}_W|\boldsymbol{\Phi}_{W_0}) = \mathcal{N}(\boldsymbol{\mu}_W|\boldsymbol{\mu}_{W_0}, \boldsymbol{\Sigma}_W/\gamma_{W_0})\mathcal{W}^{-1}(\boldsymbol{\Sigma}_W|\mathcal{W}_{W_0}, \nu_{W_0}) \tag{8}$$

$$p(\boldsymbol{\Theta}_Z|\boldsymbol{\Phi}_{Z_0}) = \mathcal{N}(\boldsymbol{\mu}_Z|\boldsymbol{\mu}_{Z_0}, \boldsymbol{\Sigma}_Z/\gamma_{Z_0})\mathcal{W}^{-1}(\boldsymbol{\Sigma}_Z|\mathcal{W}_{Z_0}, \nu_{Z_0}), \tag{9}$$

where: $\boldsymbol{\Phi}_{X_0} = \{\boldsymbol{\mu}_{X_0}, \gamma_{X_0}, \mathcal{W}_{X_0}, \nu_{X_0}\}$, $\boldsymbol{\Phi}_{T_0} = \{\boldsymbol{\mu}_{T_0}, \gamma_{T_0}, \mathcal{W}_{T_0}, \nu_{T_0}\}$, $\boldsymbol{\Phi}_{W_0} = \{\boldsymbol{\mu}_{W_0}, \gamma_{W_0}, \mathcal{W}_{W_0}, \nu_{W_0}\}$, and $\boldsymbol{\Phi}_{Z_0} = \{\boldsymbol{\mu}_{Z_0}, \gamma_{Z_0}, \mathcal{W}_{Z_0}, \nu_{Z_0}\}$.

Here, $\mathcal{W}^{-1}$ is the inverse Wishart distribution with ν_0 degrees of freedom and a $d \times d$ scaling matrix $\mathcal{W}_0$:

$$\mathcal{W}^{-1}(\boldsymbol{\Sigma}|\mathcal{W}_0, \nu_0) = \frac{1}{C}|\boldsymbol{\Sigma}|^{-(\nu_0-d-1)/2}\exp(-\frac{1}{2}Tr(\mathcal{W}_0\boldsymbol{\Sigma}^{-1})), \tag{10}$$

where C is a normalizing constant and $Tr(.)$ is the trace of a matrix.

The Gaussian inverse Wishart prior is adopted because it is the conjugate prior of the multivariate Gaussian distribution. This selection of the prior allows the conditional distributions derived from the posterior distributions to be sampled easily. Similarly, we place inverse Gamma priors [17] on the variance σ_R^2:

$$p(\sigma_R^2|\alpha_R, \beta_R) \quad = \quad IG(\sigma_R^2|\alpha_R, \beta_R), \tag{11}$$

where $IG(.)$ is the inverse Gamma distribution [17]:

$$IG(x|\alpha, \beta) = \frac{\beta^\alpha}{\Gamma(\alpha)}x^{-\alpha-1}exp(-\frac{\beta}{x}) \tag{12}$$

Choosing the inverse Gamma distribution, which is the conjugate prior of the variance of a Gaussian distribution, makes it easy to sample from the posterior distribution. Indeed, this distribution has also been proven to model the unknown variance of a Gaussian distribution effectively [17].

We place Gaussian priors over the bias terms as follows.

$$p(\theta_u|\sigma_\theta^2) = \mathcal{N}(\theta_u|0, \sigma_\theta^2), \quad p(\rho_i|\sigma_\rho^2) = \mathcal{N}(\rho_i|0, \sigma_\rho^2), \tag{13}$$

where, σ_θ^2 and σ_ρ^2 are inverse Gamma distributions [17]:

$$p(\sigma_\theta^2|\alpha_\theta, \beta_\theta) = IG(\sigma_\theta^2|\alpha_\theta, \beta_\theta), \quad p(\sigma_\rho^2|\alpha_\rho, \beta_\rho) = IG(\sigma_\rho^2|\alpha_\rho, \beta_\rho) \tag{14}$$

We place an inverse Gamma [17] prior on the variance of σ_S^2 of r_{ij}:

$$p(\sigma_S^2|\alpha_S, \beta_S) \quad = \quad IG(\sigma_S^2|\alpha_S, \beta_S) \tag{15}$$

3.2 Posterior Inference

Our goal is to find the posterior distribution of the model parameters. The posterior distribution is analytically intractable, so we employ MCMC-based methods, which are widely used for approximating distributions [7]. The key idea of these methods is to construct a Markov chain that converges to the posterior distribution of the model. Each state of the Markov chain is a set of model parameters. The posterior distribution is characterized by the samples from that Markov chain. In this paper, we use Gibbs sampling [7], a kind of MCMC that alternatively samples each variable conditioned on the remaining variables.

Sampling $\mathbf{x}_u$, $\mathbf{t}_i$ $\mathbf{w}_i$, and $\mathbf{z}_j$. The conditional distribution over the user latent feature vector $\mathbf{x}_u$, conditioned on the observed ratings, the latent feature vectors of items, and the hyperparameters, is Gaussian:

$$\begin{aligned} p(\mathbf{x}_u|\mathbf{R}, \mathbf{Y}, \boldsymbol{\mu}_X, \boldsymbol{\theta}, \boldsymbol{\rho}, \boldsymbol{\Sigma}_X) &= \mathcal{N}(\mathbf{x}_u|\boldsymbol{\mu}^*_{X_u}, \boldsymbol{\Sigma}^*_{X_u}) \\ &\propto p(\mathbf{x}_u|\boldsymbol{\mu}_X, \boldsymbol{\Sigma}_X) \prod_{i \in \mathcal{R}_u} \mathcal{N}(r_{ui}|\mathbf{x}_u^\top \mathbf{y}_i + \eta_{ui}, \sigma_R^2), \end{aligned} \tag{16}$$

where $\eta_{ui} = \theta_u + \rho_i + \mu$, $\boldsymbol{\theta} = \{\theta_u\}_{u=1}^N$, $\boldsymbol{\rho} = \{\rho_i\}_{i=1}^M$, and

$$\boldsymbol{\Sigma}^*_{X_u} = \left(\boldsymbol{\Sigma}_X^{-1} + \frac{1}{\sigma_R^2} \sum_{i \in \mathcal{R}_u} \mathbf{y}_i \mathbf{y}_i^\top\right)^{-1} \tag{17}$$

$$\boldsymbol{\mu}^*_{X_u} = \boldsymbol{\Sigma}^*_{X_u} \left[\boldsymbol{\Sigma}_X^{-1} \boldsymbol{\mu}_X + \frac{1}{\sigma_R^2} \sum_{i \in \mathcal{R}_u} (r_{ui} - \eta_{ui}) \mathbf{y}_i\right]. \tag{18}$$

Similarly, we can obtain the posterior distribution of $\mathbf{t}_i$, $\mathbf{w}_i$ and $\mathbf{z}_j$.

Sampling $\boldsymbol{\Theta}_X = \{\boldsymbol{\mu}_X, \boldsymbol{\Sigma}_X\}$, $\boldsymbol{\Theta}_T = \{\boldsymbol{\mu}_T, \boldsymbol{\Sigma}_T\}$, $\boldsymbol{\Theta}_W = \{\boldsymbol{\mu}_W, \boldsymbol{\Sigma}_W\}$, and $\boldsymbol{\Theta}_Z = \{\boldsymbol{\mu}_Z, \boldsymbol{\Sigma}_Z\}$. The posterior distribution over $\boldsymbol{\Theta}_X = \{\boldsymbol{\mu}_X, \boldsymbol{\Sigma}_X\}$ conditioned on user latent feature vectors and $\boldsymbol{\Phi}_{X_0} = \{\boldsymbol{\mu}_{X_0}, \gamma_{X_0}, \mathcal{W}_{X_0}, \nu_{X_0}\}$ is a Gaussian inverse Wishart distribution:

$$p(\boldsymbol{\mu}_X, \boldsymbol{\Sigma}_X|\mathbf{X}, \boldsymbol{\Phi}_{X_0}) = \mathcal{N}(\boldsymbol{\mu}_X|\boldsymbol{\mu}^*_{X_0}, \boldsymbol{\Sigma}_X/\gamma^*_{X_0})\mathcal{W}^{-1}(\boldsymbol{\Sigma}_X|\mathcal{W}^*_{X_0}, \nu^*_{X_0}) \tag{19}$$

$$\propto p(\mathbf{X}|\boldsymbol{\mu}_X, \boldsymbol{\Sigma}_X) p(\boldsymbol{\mu}_X, \boldsymbol{\Sigma}_X|\boldsymbol{\Phi}_{X_0}), \tag{20}$$

where:

$$\boldsymbol{\mu}^*_{X_0} = \frac{\gamma_{X_0}\boldsymbol{\mu}_{X_0} + N\bar{\mathbf{x}}}{\gamma_{X_0} + N}, \quad \gamma^*_{X_0} = \gamma_{X_0} + N, \nu^*_{X_0} = \nu_{X_0} + N \tag{21}$$

$$\mathcal{W}^*_{X_0} = \mathcal{W}_{X_0} + N\bar{\mathbf{S}} + \frac{\gamma_{X_0} N}{\gamma_{X_0} + N}(\boldsymbol{\mu}_{X_0} - \bar{\mathbf{x}})(\boldsymbol{\mu}_{X_0} - \bar{\mathbf{x}})^\top \tag{22}$$

$$\bar{\mathbf{x}} = \frac{1}{N}\sum_{u=1}^{N} \mathbf{x}_u, \quad \bar{\mathbf{S}} = \frac{1}{N}\sum_{u=1}^{N} \mathbf{x}_u \mathbf{x}_u^\top \tag{23}$$

Similarly, we can obtain the posterior distributions over $\boldsymbol{\Theta}_T$, $\boldsymbol{\Theta}_W$, and $\boldsymbol{\Theta}_Z$ using exactly the same form.

Sampling bias terms $\boldsymbol{\theta_u}$ and $\boldsymbol{\rho_i}$. The posterior distribution over the user bias term θ_u is Gaussian:

$$\begin{aligned} p(\theta_u|\mathbf{R},\mathbf{X},\mathbf{Y},\boldsymbol{\rho},\sigma_R^2) &= \mathcal{N}(\theta_u|\xi_u^*,(\sigma_{\theta_u}^*)^2 \\ &\propto p(\mathbf{R}|\mathbf{X},\mathbf{Y},\boldsymbol{\rho},\sigma_R^2)p(\theta_u|\sigma_\theta^2), \end{aligned} \tag{24}$$

where:

$$(\sigma_{\theta_u}^*)^2 = \left(\frac{1}{\sigma_\theta^2}+\frac{|\mathcal{R}_u|}{\sigma_R^2}\right)^{-1}, \quad \xi_u^* = \left(\frac{\sigma_{\theta_u}^*}{\sigma_R}\right)^2 \sum_{i\in\mathcal{R}_u}\left[r_{ui}-(\mu+\rho_i+\mathbf{x}_u^\top\mathbf{y}_i)\right] \tag{25}$$

The posterior distribution over the ρ_i can be obtained using the same form.

Sampling $\boldsymbol{\sigma_R^2}$ and $\boldsymbol{\sigma_S^2}$. The posterior distribution over σ_R^2, conditioned on the rating data, user latent factor matrix $\mathbf{X}$, item latent factor matrix $\mathbf{Y}$, and bias matrices $\boldsymbol{\theta}$, $\boldsymbol{\rho}$, is given as:

$$\begin{aligned} p(\sigma_R^2|\mathbf{R},\mathbf{X},\mathbf{Y},\alpha_R,\beta_R) &= IG(\sigma_R^2|\alpha_R^*,\beta_R^*) \\ &\propto p(\mathbf{R}|\mathbf{X},\mathbf{Y},\boldsymbol{\theta},\boldsymbol{\rho},\sigma_R^2)p(\sigma_R^2|\alpha_R,\beta_R) \end{aligned} \tag{26}$$

where:

$$\alpha_R^* = \alpha_R + \frac{|\mathcal{R}|}{2}, \quad \beta_R^* = \beta_R + \frac{1}{2}\sum_{(i,j)\in\mathcal{R}}\left[r_{ui}-(\mathbf{x}_u^\top\mathbf{y}_i+\eta_{ui})\right]^2 \tag{27}$$

The conditional distribution over σ_S^2 can be obtained using the same form.

Sampling $\boldsymbol{\sigma_\theta^2}$ and $\boldsymbol{\sigma_\rho^2}$. The conditional distribution over σ_θ^2 conditioned on the bias terms of users is an inverse Gamma distribution:

$$p(\sigma_\theta^2|\boldsymbol{\theta},\alpha_\theta,\beta_\theta) = IG(\sigma_\theta^2|\alpha_\theta^*,\beta_\theta^*) \quad \propto \quad p(\boldsymbol{\theta}|\sigma_\theta^2)p(\sigma_\theta^2|\alpha_\theta,\beta_\theta), \tag{28}$$

where:

$$\alpha_\theta^* = \alpha_\theta + \frac{N}{2}, \quad \beta_\theta^* = \beta_\theta + \frac{1}{2}\sum_{u=1}^{N}\theta_u^2 \tag{29}$$

The conditional distribution over σ_ρ^2 conditioned on the bias terms of items can be obtained using the same form.

Computational Complexity. From the formulas for posterior distribution sampling, we can observe that the most expensive computations lie in the sampling of the latent feature vectors ($\mathbf{x}_u$, $\mathbf{t}_i$, $\mathbf{w}_i$ and $\mathbf{z}_j$), which require computing the inverses of matrices. It is easy to show that in each iteration, the complexity for sampling the latent feature vectors of N users (matrix $\mathbf{X}$) is $\mathcal{O}(d^2|\mathcal{R}|+d^3N)$. Similarly, the complexities for sampling matrix $\mathbf{T}$, $\mathbf{W}$, and $\mathbf{Z}$ are $\mathcal{O}(d^2|\mathcal{R}|+d^3N)$, $\mathcal{O}(d^2|\mathcal{S}|+d^3M)$, and $\mathcal{O}(d^2|\mathcal{S}|+d^3M)$, respectively, where $|\mathcal{R}|$ and $|\mathcal{S}|$ are the numbers of observed ratings and observed clicks, respectively. However, note that the posterior distribution of $\mathbf{x}_u$ does not depend on other users; therefore, the sampling of matrix $\mathbf{X}$ can be performed efficiently in parallel. Similarly, sampling $\mathbf{T}$, $\mathbf{W}$, and $\mathbf{Z}$ can also be sped up by performing them in parallel.

3.3 Rating Prediction

The posterior predictive distribution of the unseen rating value $\hat{r}_{ui}$ of item i by user u is obtained by integrating out the model parameters and hyperparameters:

$$p(\hat{r}_{ui}|\mathcal{O}) = \int \dots \int p(\hat{r}_{ui}|\boldsymbol{\Omega})p(\boldsymbol{\Omega})d\{\boldsymbol{\Omega}\}, \quad (30)$$

where $\mathcal{O}$ is the observed data and $\boldsymbol{\Omega}$ is the set of all parameters.

The above posterior predictive distribution is analytically intractable, so we approximate it by sampling the parameters using the Gibbs sampling described in Sect. 3.2. The predicted rating value can be approximated as follows:

$$\begin{aligned} p(\hat{r}_{ui}|\mathcal{O}) &\approx \frac{1}{K}\sum_{k=1}^{K} p(\hat{r}_{ui}|\mathbf{x}_u^{(k)}, \mathbf{y}_i^{(k)}, \theta_u^{(k)}, \rho_i^{(k)}, (\sigma_R^2)^{(k)}) \\ &= \frac{1}{K}\sum_{k=1}^{K} \mathcal{N}\left(\hat{r}_{ui}|\eta_{ui}^{(k)} + \mathbf{x}_u^{(k)\top}\mathbf{y}_i^{(k)}, (\sigma_R^2)^{(k)}\right), \end{aligned} \quad (31)$$

where K is the number of samples taken from the posterior distribution, $(.)^{(k)}$ is the kth sample, and $\eta_{ui}^{(k)} = \mu + \theta_u^{(k)} + \rho_i^{(k)}$.

We consider two rating prediction tasks: (i) **in-matrix** prediction: predict the rating by user u of item i, where i has not been rated by u but has been rated by at least one other user (i.e., i appears at least once in the training set of the rating data); and (ii) **out-matrix** prediction: predict the rating by user u of item i, where i has not been rated by any user (i.e., i does not appear in the training set of the rating data).

In Eq. 31, $\mathbf{y}_i^{(k)} = \mathbf{w}_i^{(k)} + \mathbf{t}_i^{(k)}$ for the *in-matrix* prediction task; $\mathbf{y}_i^{(k)} = \mathbf{w}_i^{(k)}$ and $\eta_{ui}^{(k)} = \mu + \theta_u^{(k)}$ for the *out-matrix* prediction task.

4 Empirical Study

4.1 Datasets

Data Description. We used three public datasets of different domains with varying sizes. (1) **MovieLens 1M** (ML-1m): a dataset of user-movie ratings collected from MovieLens, an online film service. It contains 1 million ratings in the range 1–5 of 4000 movies by 6000 users. This dataset is available at GroupLens[1]. (2) **MovieLens 20M** (ML-20m): another dataset of user-movie ratings collected from MovieLens. It contains 20 million ratings in the range 1–5 of 27,000 movies by 138,000 users. This dataset is available at GroupLens[2]. (3) **Bookcrossing**: A dataset collected in August and September 2004 from the

[1] https://grouplens.org/datasets/movielens/1m/.
[2] https://grouplens.org/datasets/movielens/20m/.

Book-Crossing website[3]. This dataset contains 278,858 users (anonymized but with demographic information) providing 1,149,780 ratings (explicit/implicit) of 271,379 books. We removed users and items that had no explicit feedback.

The MovieLens datasets contain only rating data, so we employed a preprocess phase to obtain the click data. We binarized the original rating data and interpreted it as click data. Furthermore, because rating data are only a small part of the click data, we randomly selected from original ratings with different percentages, assuming that only these amounts of ratings were available. Details of these datasets after preprocessing are shown in Table 1.

Table 1. Datasets obtained by selecting ratings from the original ratings of MovieLens datasets with different percentages

Picked from ML1-20			Picked from ML20-20		
Dataset	% rating picked	Density of rating matrix (%)	Dataset	% rating picked	Density of rating matrix (%)
ML1-10	10	0.3561	ML20-10	10	0.0836
ML1-20	20	0.6675	ML20-20	20	0.1001
ML1-50	50	1.6022	ML20-50	50	0.2108

4.2 Experimental Protocol

We used the click data and 80% of the rating data to train the model; the remaining 20% of the rating data was used as the test data to evaluate the model. In evaluating the *in-matrix* prediction task, when splitting data, we made sure that every item in the test set appeared at least once in the training set. In evaluating the *out-matrix* prediction task, we made sure that none of the items in the test set appeared in the training set (to ensure that none of the items in the test set had any previous ratings).

Evaluation Metric. We used Root Mean Square Error (RMSE) as the metric to measure the performance of the models. RMSE measures the deviation between the rating predicted by the model and the true rating (given by the test set), and is defined as follows.

$$RMSE = \sqrt{\frac{1}{|Test|} \sum_{(u,i) \in Test} (r_{ui} - \hat{r}_{ui})^2}, \quad (32)$$

where $|Test|$ is the size of the test set.

[3] http://www.bookcrossing.com/.

Competing Methods. For the **in-matrix** prediction task, we compared our method with the following baseline methods:

1. *PMF* [11]: a state-of-the-art method for rating predictions
2. *BPMF* [12]: the Bayesian treatment of PMF [11]
3. *NMF* (non-negative matrix factorization) [4]: a matrix factorization method which requires the components of user and item factors to be non-negative
4. *PIE* [8]: the model described in Sect. 2.2
5. *SVD++* [2]: a factor model that exploits both explicit and implicit feedback in rating predictions

For the **out-matrix** prediction task, we compared our proposed method with PIE [8], which is described in Sect. 2.2.

Parameter Settings. We varied the dimension of the latent space ($d = 20, 30, 50, 100$) to study the performance of the models with respect to the dimensionality of the latent feature vectors.

For PMF, NMF and SVD++, we used grid search to find the optimal values of the hyperparameters that produced the best performance on a validation set. For the PIE model [8], we fixed $\lambda = 1$ and used grid search to find the optimal values of the remaining parameters that gave good performance on the validation set. For BPMF [12], hyperparameters were set following the original paper.

Regarding our proposed method, HBFM, for simplicity, we set the parameters as follows: $\mathcal{W}_{\mathcal{F}} = \mathbf{I}_d$, $\nu_{\mathcal{F}_0} = d$, $\gamma_{\mathcal{F}_0} = 1$, and $\mu_{\mathcal{F}_0} = \mathbf{0}$ ($\mathcal{F} = \{X, T, W, Z\}$). We adopted uninformative priors for the noise variances; therefore, we set the hyperparameters for the inverse Gamma distributions as follows: $\alpha_R = \alpha_S = \alpha_\theta = \alpha_\rho = 0$ and $\beta_R = \beta_S = \beta_\theta = \beta_\rho = 0$. For the Gibbs sampling process, we ignored the first 1000 samples as "burn-in". The following 100 samples were selected to approximate the posterior distributions.

4.3 Results

We report the RMSEs on the test datasets for the *in-matrix* and *out-matrix* prediction tasks in Tables 2 and 3, respectively. We can see that HBFM outperformed the competing methods for all values of d.

For small values of d (e.g., $d = 20, 50$), PIE and HP-PIE perform better than the other methods, indicating the effectiveness of exploiting click data in boosting the performance of rating predictions. When d exceeds 150, the test RMSEs for PMF, NMF, SVD++, and PIE tend to increase, whereas those for BPMF and HBFM continue to decrease. This is because when d increases, the number of parameters increases and the models become more complex. PMF, NMF, SVD++, and PIE do not handle the complexity of the model well; therefore, they tend to overfit. By contrast, BPMF and HBFM, which can manage the complexity of the models well, continue improving the test RMSEs. This shows that the full Bayesian model that can manage the uncertainty of the model parameters is an effective approach for avoiding overfitting.

Table 2. Test RMSEs for different numbers of latent features

(a) ML1-20 dataset

Methods	# of latent features d				
	20	50	100	150	200
PMF	1.0053	0.9941	0.9574	0.9628	0.9715
NMF	0.9971	0.9734	0.9571	0.9605	0.9711
SVD++	0.9464	0.9342	0.9023	0.9148	0.9235
BPMF	0.9339	0.9191	0.8971	0.8824	0.8731
PIE	0.9218	0.9021	0.8911	0.9013	0.9125
HBFM	**0.9012**	**0.8834**	**0.8617**	**0.8594**	**0.8512**

(b) ML20-20 dataset

Methods	# of latent features d				
	20	50	100	150	200
PMF	0.9627	0.9098	0.8832	0.8901	0.9015
NMF	0.8988	0.8927	0.8856	0.8942	0.9031
SVD++	0.8947	0.8655	0.8532	0.8598	0.8641
BPMF	0.8804	0.8576	0.8462	0.8397	0.8301
PIE	0.8788	0.8532	0.8474	0.8501	0.8602
HBFM	**0.8521**	**0.8401**	**0.8325**	**0.8245**	**0.8189**

(c) Bookcrossing dataset

Methods	# of latent features d				
	20	50	100	150	200
PMF	2.0231	2.0105	1.9834	1.9921	1.9989
NMF	1.9477	1.9132	1.9092	1.9132	1.9198
SVD++	1.8090	1.7968	1.7729	1.7823	1.7891
BPMF	1.7941	1.7873	1.7728	1.7693	1.7601
PIE	1.6704	1.6501	1.6341	1.6401	1.6487
HBFM	**1.6623**	**1.6431**	**1.6028**	**1.5931**	**1.5867**

Table 3. Test RMSEs for the out-matrix prediction task

# of features	ML1-20		ML20-20		Bookcrossing	
	PIE	HBFM	PIE	HBFM	PIE	HBFM
20	1.0066	**0.9902**	0.9686	**0.9523**	1.7257	**1.7028**
50	1.0062	**0.9811**	0.9436	**0.9357**	1.6484	**1.6245**
100	1.0044	**0.9801**	0.9374	**0.9211**	1.6398	**1.6201**
150	1.0089	**0.9758**	0.9403	**0.9188**	1.6405	**1.6178**
200	1.0132	**0.9695**	0.9489	**0.9101**	1.6497	**1.6102**

Impact of the Sparsity of the Dataset on the Methods. We studied the effectiveness of the proposed method for datasets with different levels of sparsity by training models with the ML1-10, ML1-20, ML1-50, ML20-10, ML20-20 and ML20-50 datasets. The test RMSEs are shown in Table 4.

Table 4. Test RMSEs for datasets with different levels of sparsity. The dimensionality of feature vectors is fixed: $d = 20$

(a) In-matrix prediction

Method	ML1m			ML20m		
	ML1-10	ML1-20	ML1-50	ML20-10	ML20-20	ML20-50
PMF	1.0471	0.9941	0.9574	0.9627	0.9098	0.8532
NMF	1.0179	0.9734	0.9571	0.8988	0.8927	0.8856
SVD++	0.9757	0.9342	0.9023	0.8947	0.8655	0.8489
BPMF	0.9364	0.9191	0.8971	0.8804	0.8576	0.8362
PIE	0.9318	0.9021	0.8801	0.8788	0.8532	0.8474
HBFM	**0.9012**	**0.8834**	**0.8617**	**0.8521**	**0.8401**	**0.8325**

(b) Out-matrix prediction

Method	ML1m			ML20m		
	ML1-10	ML1-20	ML1-50	ML20-10	ML20-20	ML20-50
PIE	1.0376	1.0066	0.9961	0.9762	0.9686	0.9601
HBFM	**1.0231**	**0.9913**	**0.9728**	**0.9634**	**0.9521**	**0.9489**

We can observe that denser rating data improved test RMSE values for all methods. This is reasonable because when more rating data are available for training, the prediction is more accurate. When the data are extremely sparse (e.g., ML1-10 or ML20-10), although managing the complexity of the model for sparse data is a challenging task, PIE and HBFM perform better than the other methods because they leverage the sparsity of rating data by the click data. For all settings, HBFM outperforms the competing methods. These results clearly show the effectiveness of exploiting click data and managing the complexity of sparse datasets.

Performance for Different Segmentations of Users. We further test the effectiveness of our method with different segments of users. We divided users into three segments based on the number of items for which they had provided ratings, and compared the performances of the methods for each group. These segments are: (i) *low*: users who provide fewer than 20 ratings; (ii) *medium*: users who provide fewer than 50 and more than 20 ratings; and (iii) *high*: users who provide 50 or more ratings.

The test RMSEs in Fig. 2 show that our method (HBFM) outperforms all competing methods for all user segments for the three datasets. From the results,

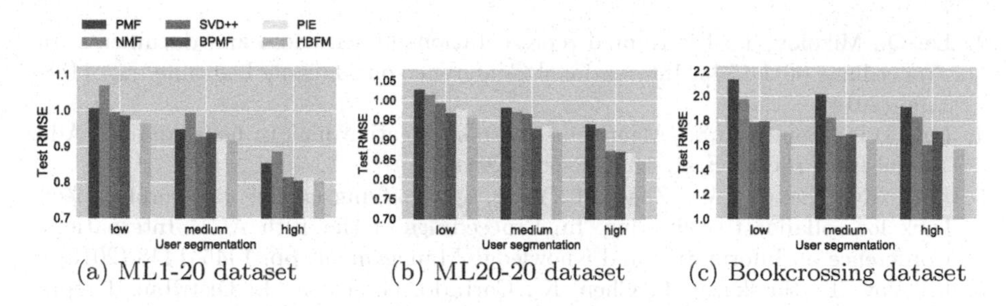

(a) ML1-20 dataset (b) ML20-20 dataset (c) Bookcrossing dataset

Fig. 2. Test RMSEs for different segmentations of users

we can also see that all the methods perform better when more explicit feedback is provided. This is reasonable because explicit feedback is much more reliable than implicit feedback for inferring users' preferences.

5 Discussion and Future Work

In this paper, we have proposed HBFM, a fully Bayesian model that combines explicit and implicit feedback to address the cold-start problem in collaborative filtering. This is a Bayesian treatment of the PIE model [8], in which priors are placed on the hyperparameters such as the covariance matrix of latent feature vectors or the variance of rating data. We developed a Gibbs sampling-based method to approximate the posterior distributions over latent feature vectors of users and items. The experiments show that HBFM provides good control over the capacity, and can be applied to models with large numbers of parameters and very sparse data.

Several future directions are possible. One is to make the model more flexible by developing a nonparametric algorithm that can efficiently find the appropriate dimensionality of latent feature vectors instead of empirically tuning the method. Another direction is to generalize the model to adopt different types of explicit feedback. In the present model, we assumed that the rating data were random variables with Gaussian distributions. This model may not work well when the data are binary feedback (e.g., like/dislike, purchase/not purchase); in that case, a Bernoulli distribution model may be more suitable.

Acknowledgments. This work was supported by a JSPS Grant-in-Aid for Scientific Research (B) (15H02789, 15H02703).

References

1. Gopalan, P.K., Charlin, L., Blei, D.: Content-based recommendations with poisson factorization. Adv. Neural Inf. Process. Syst. **27**, 3176–3184 (2014)
2. Koren, Y.: Factorization meets the neighborhood: a multifaceted collaborative filtering model. In: Proceedings of the 14th ACM SIGKDD International Conference on Knowledge Discovery and Data Mining, pp. 426–434 (2008)

3. Le, Q., Mikolov, T.: Distributed representations of sentences and documents. In: Proceedings of the 31st International Conference on Machine Learning, pp. 1188–1196 (2014)
4. Lee, D.D., Seung, H.S.: Algorithms for non-negative matrix factorization. Adv. Neural Inf. Process. Syst. **13**, 556–562 (2001)
5. Liu, N.N., Xiang, E.W., Zhao, M., Yang, Q.: Unifying explicit and implicit feedback for collaborative filtering. In: Proceedings of the 19th ACM International Conference on Information and Knowledge Management, pp. 1445–1448 (2010)
6. Mikolov, T., Sutskever, I., Chen, K., Corrado, G., Dean, J.: Distributed representations of words and phrases and their compositionality. In: Proceedings of the 26th International Conference on Neural Information Processing Systems, pp. 3111–3119 (2013)
7. Neal, R.M.: Probabilistic inference using Markov chain Monte Carlo methods. Technical report CRG-TR-93-1, Department of Computer Science, University of Toronto (1993)
8. Nguyen, T., Aihara, K., Takasu, A.: A probabilistic model for collaborative filtering with implicit and explicit feedback data. CoRR abs/1705.02085 (2017). http://arxiv.org/abs/1705.02085
9. van deb Oord, A., Dieleman, S., Schrauwen, B.: Deep content-based music recommendation. In: Proceedings of the 26th International Conference on Neural Information Processing Systems, pp. 2643–2651 (2013)
10. Park, S., Kim, Y.D., Choi, S.: Hierarchical bayesian matrix factorization with side information. In: Proceedings of the Twenty-Third International Joint Conference on Artificial Intelligence, pp. 1593–1599 (2013)
11. Salakhutdinov, R., Mnih, A.: Probabilistic matrix factorization. In: Proceedings of the 20th International Conference on Neural Information Processing Systems, pp. 1257–1264 (2007)
12. Salakhutdinov, R., Mnih, A.: Bayesian probabilistic matrix factorization using Markov chain Monte Carlo. In: Proceedings of the 25th International Conference on Machine Learning, pp. 880–887 (2008)
13. Wang, B., Rahimi, M., Zhou, D., Wang, X.: Expectation-maximization collaborative filtering with explicit and implicit feedback. In: Tan, P.-N., Chawla, S., Ho, C.K., Bailey, J. (eds.) PAKDD 2012. LNCS, vol. 7301, pp. 604–616. Springer, Heidelberg (2012). doi:10.1007/978-3-642-30217-6_50
14. Wang, C., Blei, D.M.: Collaborative topic modeling for recommending scientific articles. In: Proceedings of the 17th ACM SIGKDD International Conference on Knowledge Discovery and Data Mining, pp. 448–456 (2011)
15. Wang, H., Shi, X., Yeung, D.Y.: Collaborative recurrent autoencoder: recommend while learning to fill in the blanks. In: Advances in Neural Information Processing Systems, vol. 29, pp. 415–423 (2016)
16. Wang, H., Wang, N., Yeung, D.Y.: Collaborative deep learning for recommender systems. In: Proceedings of the 21th ACM SIGKDD International Conference on Knowledge Discovery and Data Mining, pp. 1235–1244 (2015)
17. Witkovsky, V.: Computing the distribution of a linear combination of inverted gamma variables. Kybernetika **37**(1), 79–90 (2001)

Empirical Analysis of Factors Influencing Twitter Hashtag Recommendation on Detected Communities

Areej Alsini(✉), Amitava Datta, Jianxin Li, and Du Huynh

School of Computer Science and Software Engineering,
University of Western Australia, Crawley, WA 6009, Australia
areej.alsini@research.uwa.edu.au,
{amitava.datta,jianxin.li,du.huynh}@uwa.edu.au

Abstract. Due to the limited length of tweets, hashtags are often used by users in their tweets. Thus, hashtag recommendation is highly desirable for users in Twitter to find useful hashtags when they type in tweets. However, there are many factors that may affect the effectiveness of hashtag recommendation, which includes social relationships, textual information and user profiling based on hashtag preference. In this paper, we aim to analyse the effect of these factors in hashtag recommendation on the detected communities in Twitter. In details, we seek answers to the two questions: What is the most significant factor in recommending hashtags in the context of detected communities? How the different community detection algorithms and the size of the communities affect the performance of hashtag recommendation?

To answer these questions, we detect the communities using two algorithms: Breadth First Search (BFS) and Clique Percolation Method (CPM). On the randomly detected communities, we investigate the quality and the behaviour of the recommended hashtags people consumed. From the extensive experimental results, we have the following conclusions. First, social factor is the most significant factor along with the textual factor for hashtag recommendation. Second, we find that the quality of the hashtag recommendation in the community detected using CPM clearly outperforms that using BFS. Third, incorporating user profiling increases the quality of the recommended hashtags.

Keywords: Social networks · Twitter · Hashtag recommendation · Community detection · User profiling

1 Introduction

In Twitter, choosing the right hashtag automatically for the user enables him/her to quickly join a discussion and read tweets written by other users. Currently, Twitter recommends only *trends*, the most popular contemporary hashtags among all users. Hashtag recommendation has become an active area of research. Most hashtag recommendation systems suggest the most relevant

G. Cong et al. (Eds.): ADMA 2017, LNAI 10604, pp. 119–131, 2017.
https://doi.org/10.1007/978-3-319-69179-4_9

top-k hashtags to the user's query [2,4,7,8,11,12,19]. Hashtag recommendation algorithms can be broadly classified into two categories: personalised [7,8] and non-personalised [2,4,11,12,19] systems. Personalized recommendation systems [14] address the user preferences, activities and constraints while the non-personalized recommendation systems address data of all users. The outputs of hashtag recommendation systems benefit two parties: the user and Twitter. Not only that the user will save time and effort when personalized hashtags are recommended automatically, but the quality of the Twitter's discussions will be enhanced when the used hashtags are more accurate. They also help Twitter eliminate the insignificant and noisy hashtags.

Twitter is composed of three main components which are: user, hashtag and tweet content. There are connections between users that reflect their relationship (e.g., family members) or their similarity in profession or interest. By analysing these connections in a network, *communities* can be detected. Individual users have their preferred hashtags when they tweet. *Hashtag preference* is the set of all previous hashtags used by a user [8]. Users also have *Topics preference* [20]. *Textual features* are collection of words extracted from tweets; they are therefore related to the content of tweets. Hashtags related features are *popularity*, *relevance*, *recency* and *number of authors* who are adopting a certain hashtag. Some hashtag features are used as ranking methods in hashtag recommendation systems. Previous research in hashtag recommendation used different combination of previously mentioned components or their related features to design their models. Some of these research clustered similar users [20], set of mentioned users [10] or set of followee [7] to find candidate hashtags. None of these research studied the effect of these factors on communities detected from *real-world* networks in the context of hashtag recommendation. As community detection algorithms explores densely interconnected users, it is worthwhile investigating how network communities affect the performance of hashtag recommendation.

The focus of this paper is to investigate the impact of the social factors when they are incorporated with tweet texts in hashtag recommendation on detected communities. The effect of user profiling based on hashtag preference is also investigated. Our research questions are: What is the most influencing factor on detected communities in the context of hashtag recommendation? Does the algorithm used in community detection and the size of the community affect the hashtag recommendation performance later on? To the best of our knowledge this is the first piece of research work that studies hashtag recommendation on detected communities. The Breadth-First Search algorithm (BFS) and Clique Percolation Method (CPM) algorithms are adopted in our study to detect communities. *Hit rate* is used as a measure of evaluation to compare the performance of these factors. In addition, the performance of some ranking methods that are related to popularity and relevance used in hashtag recommendation are compared.

Structure of the Paper: This paper is organized as follows: Sect. 2 discusses previous works that directly relevant to our research. Section 3 describes the dataset and methodologies used in this research. Section 4 explains the conducted experiments. Section 5 reports the results of experiments and extensive discussion on the results. Section 6 concludes the paper and outlines our future work.

2 Related Work

Our analysis is built on two lines of research: Community detection from the Twitter *real-world* network and Twitter hashtag recommendation.

Community Detection from the Twitter Real-World Network. Algorithms for detecting communities from real-world social networks focus mainly on the connections between users and the strength of these connections [1,13,16]. These algorithms gather users from the network to form communities using either Breadth-First Search (BFS) or the Clique Percolation Method (CPM). BFS works as a traversal method through a graph of users. It finds a root users and then the next level followee and so on. CPM finds overlapped communities of highly connected users [1]. CPM explores all possible k-cliques which are k number of nodes with complete connections. When two k-cliques share $k - 1$ nodes, they are considered adjacent. The union of the two adjacent k-cliques forms a community. Wagenseller et al. [6] used the size of the community, coverage, modularity, participation ratio and user interests to compare different community detection algorithms. They also studied how *good* the detected communities were, based on the similarity score between users interests. In their method, the user's interest was expressed as the top-10 most frequent hashtags. They reported that the relationships between users were poor when this method was used.

Twitter Hashtag Recommendation. The textual factor has been studied in the literature and proven to be a significant factor in hashtag recommendation. Mazzia et al. [11] used the Naive Bayes algorithm to recommend hashtags. Dovgopol et al. [2] built a hybrid hashtag recommendation model based on the K-Nearest Neighbour and Naive Bayes. Zangerle et al. [19] built their hashtag recommendation model by studying the textual similarity between tweet contents. They weighted the words in tweets using TF-IDF and computed the similarity distance using *Cosine similarity*, *Jaccard coefficient*, *Dice coefficient* and *Levenshtein distance*. They found that the *Cosine similarity* performed the best over the others.

User profiling [14] infers the user's interests, activities, preferences and behaviours. User profiling or *user based recommendation* is used to find similar users. In an early study, the biography of users has been analysed for user classification [15]. However, it is difficult to rely completely on this information as not all users provide correct biography about themselves. Some research incorporated user profiling in hashtag recommendation. Zhao et al. [20] have entrenched the user's topics preference and Kywe et al. [8] have implanted the user's hashtag preference to find similar users. From the set of similar users, candidate hashtags are extracted, ranked and recommended.

In hashtag recommendation systems, candidate hashtags can be ranked based on their popularity, relevance or recency. The definition of these ranking methods are listed below:

Tweet Hashtag Popularity. Yang et al. [18] defined *popularity* as the number of times a hashtag has been adopted in previous tweets.

User Hashtag Popularity. This means that the popularity of a hashtag is measured based on the number of authors (users) who have adopted the hashtag at least once [8,18].

Global Hashtag Popularity. For this type of hashtag popularity, the hashtag frequency is calculated over the whole dataset [19].

Tweet Hashtag Relevance. The closeness of a hashtag to the user or to the tweet content [19]. Hashtags placed in the tweet with the highest similarity score to the user's query are considered the most relevant hashtags to the user's query tweet [19].

Recency of the Hashtag. This measures the age (in days) of the hashtag that has recently been used by the user [5].

From the above definitions, we can see that some of them are general while the others are personalized. Ranking based on hashtag popularity is sometimes called ranking by frequency [8,19].

3 Methods

In this section, we compare the quality of the recommended hashtags to study the effect of the textual, social and user profiling factors on detected communities. The baseline methods, dataset, experimental settings and evaluation metrics are explained. In the previous section we have introduced different ranking methods. In this section, we focus on analysing the performance of Tweet Hashtag Relevance (THR), Tweet Hashtag Popularity (THP), User Hashtag Popularity (UHP) and Global Hashtag Popularity (GHP).

3.1 Baseline Approaches

Two baseline methods are chosen to perform our experiments. The first one is hashtag recommendation based on textual factor and the other one is hashtag recommendation based on user profiling.

Hashtag Recommendation Based on Textual Factor. In Zangerle et al.'s [19] model, the feature vectors of tweets are created using TF-IDF. The Cosine similarity is used to retrieve the top-500 similar tweets to the query tweet. Candidate hashtags are extracted from the set of similar tweets, ranked and the top-5 and top-10 hashtags are recommended. Table 1 reviews Zangerle et al.'s results. These results show the contribution of the textual factor in the application of hashtag recommendation.

Table 1. Previous research results from [19]

Ranking method	Top-5		Top-10	
	Precision	Recall	Precision	Recall
THR	7	22	5.5	26
THP	-	19	-	26.5
GHP	-	12	-	17

Hashtag Recommendation Based on User Profiling. Kywe et al.'s [8] model is our second baseline method. The feature vector of a user is his/her historical hashtags considering the duplication. TF-IDF is used to weight all the extracted hashtags. Then, the Cosine similarity is used to find the distance between users. From the tweets of the similar users, all hashtags are extracted. In Kywe et al.'s model, when the hashtags extracted from similar users and the ones extracted from similar tweets are combined, their hit rate performance is 31.56% when the top-5 hashtags are recommended and 37.19% when the top-10 hashtags are recommended.

3.2 Datasets and Pre-processing

The dataset we use is the *Dataset-UDI-TwitterCrawl-Aug2012* [9] collected by Li et al. during the period from 2011 to 2012. However, the user's personal timeline includes tweets issued from 2008 to 2012. In this dataset, there are 200 million user following relationships, 3 million user profiles and 50 million tweets for 140,000 users. Every tweet is attached with its author name, the issue date of the tweet and other data. Each user's personal timeline has at most 500 tweets. Due to hardware constraints, our sub-network consists of 745,262 users and 2 million user relationships which our machine with 32 GB RAM could just handle when the number of adjacent nodes k is set to 2. In order to study the impact of the community detection algorithm on hashtag recommendation, we adopted the Breadth-First Search algorithm (BFS) and Clique Percolation Method (CPM) to detect communities. In BFS, the first user was chosen randomly to be the root node followed by its immediate followee, then followed by the next level followee.

As a proof of concept, a straightforward exploratory analysis is conducted regarding the network we are using. Using CPM, the maximal number of k-cliques in our sub-network is 1,881,550. The number of communities and the size of the largest community are shown in Table 2. To validate our results, we tested various number of detected communities. Table 3 shows an overview of two random communities detected using BFS and CPM.

By studying these communities, some of our observations were consistent with earlier research which incorporated millions of users in the following points: Few hashtags have very high tweet hashtag popularity and the majority of hashtags have a very low tweet hashtag popularity, mostly equal to 1. These data

Table 2. Number of communities and largest community size

k	Number of communities with CPM	Size of the largest community
3	510	84,353
5	134	1,970
7	15	71

Table 3. Overview of the two random communities detected using BFS and CPM

Characteristic	BFS	CPM
Total number of users	105	100
Total number of tweets no duplication	200,588	174,965
Total number of tweets with hashtags	41,929	35,437
The rate of tweets with hashtags to the overall number of tweets	20%	20%
The total number of hashtags usage	11,632	10,443
The total number of distinct hashtags	4,355	2,655
Hashtags occurring only once	3,139	1,762

follow the long tail distribution. The top-5 most popular hashtags in the BFS-generated community are: ‘fb’: 419, ‘news’: 384, ‘ff’: 195, ‘pr20chat’: 122, ‘sxsw’: 114. The top-5 most popular hashtags in the CPM-generated community are: ‘ff’: 324, ‘alliegentry’: 255, ‘tcot’: 251, ‘cdnpoli’: 249, ‘teaparty’: 197.

We have chosen 10 communities randomly, 5 of these communities are generated using BFS and 5 are generated using CPM (when $k = 3$). Each of these communities is a separate dataset. We split each dataset into training and testing datasets since it is useful for evaluation. Essentially, we shuffled the dataset and 20% of the dataset was used in the testing. The hashtags placed in the testing dataset were removed from the original tweets and used to build the set of ground truth hashtags.

We adopted various pre-processing strategies to reduce noise in tweets content. As the performance of the ranked search results depends heavily on the pre-processing of the corpus [2], we removed duplicates in tweets, punctuation, stop words and links. All texts transformed into lower case. We used the contraction map built by Sarkar [17] that converts 122 shortened words into proper English words such as ‘won’t’ to ‘will not’. We also used the *WordNetLemmatizer* [3] algorithm to group different forms of words into one word such as ‘drive’,‘drove’, ‘driven’ and ‘driving’ into ‘drive’. The open source Python Libraries are used.

3.3 Experimental Setting

There are *general* parameters and *personalized* parameters involved in the experiments. As for the general parameters, let $D = \{d_1, d_2, \ldots, d_n\}$ be the set of tweets in the training dataset and $Q = \{q_1, q_2, \ldots, q_l\}$ be the set of tweets in the testing dataset. Let $U = \{u_1, u_2, \ldots, u_m\}$ be the set of users, and let $H = \{h_1, h_2, \ldots, h_p\}$ be the global hashtag space from D. Personalized parameters are modified parameters which differ from user to user. So, D_{u_i} is the tweets issued by the user u_i and H_{u_i} is the u_i's hashtags preference. In the training and testing datasets, every tweet is attached with its author ID. Top-n is the set of similar tweets and top-m is the set of similar users. Top-k is the set of highly ranked hashtags to be recommended to the user where we set k to 5 and 10.

3.4 Evaluation Metrics

Measuring the quality of the automatically recommended hashtags is essential to compare the results. To evaluate methods of this research, *hit rate* is adopted. The *hit rate* measure [8] gives the ratio of the number of hits to a number of attempts. A *hit* to an active tweet is considered in the counting when there is at least one matching ground truth hashtag in the tweet.

4 Experiments

In this section, two experiments are performed.

Experiment 1: Hashtag Recommendation Based on Social and Textual Factors. The aim of this experiment is to assess the contribution of the social factor when it is incorporated with tweet contents on hashtag recommendation. This experiment is performed on the ten randomly selected communities (5 are generated using BFS and 5 are generated using CPM). The reported results of the experiments are the average score of testing these communities. In this experiment, we notice that the similarity score of some of the retrieved tweets are very low or equal to zero. This motivates us to set a threshold τ to work as a dividing line between the highly similar and less similar tweets. To improve the recommendation quality, we disregard tweets that are marginally similar to the user's query q. There are two parts in this experiment. The first part records the hit rate when retrieving various number of similar tweets n to the user's query q, top-n = 10, 50, 100, 150 and 200. The second part investigates the impact of the size of the community on hashtag recommendation by increasing the number of users m. The number of users is set to 100, 200, 300 and 400 and we fix the value of the top-n to be 50. In both parts, we compare the performance of the four ranking methods: UHP, THP, THR and GHP.

Experiment 2: Hashtag Recommendation Based on Social and User Profiling Factors. The aim of this experiment is to asses the contribution of the social factor when it is incorporated with the user profiling factor based on the user's hashtag preference. This experiment is performed on the BFS and CPM generated communities. For the ten communities, top-5 and top-10 hashtags are recommended. There are two parts in this experiment. The first part records the hit rate when the hashtags extracted from the top-m similar users are considered in the recommendation. The second part records the hit rate when the hashtags extracted from the top-m similar users and the hashtags extracted from the top-n similar tweets are combined in the recommendation. In both parts, top-m is set to $1, 3, 5$ and 10 similar users and top-n equals 50 is fixed.

5 Results and Discussions

Results of Experiment 1. Figures 1 and 2 show the average hit rate (in percentage) on the BFS-generated communities when top-5 and top-10 hashtags are recommended, respectively. Figures 3 and 4 show the average hit rate when top-5 and top-10 hashtags are recommended on the CPM-generated communities. In general, there is a slight improvement when τ is used in all ranking methods but it is more clear in the UHP. When $\tau > 0.1$, more accurate results are obtained but many queries retrieve none similar tweets which reduces the overall performance.

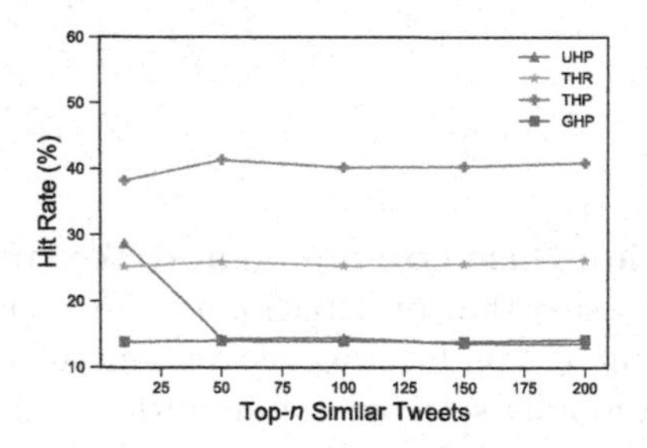

Fig. 1. Top-5 recommended hashtags average hit rates of the BFS-generated communities

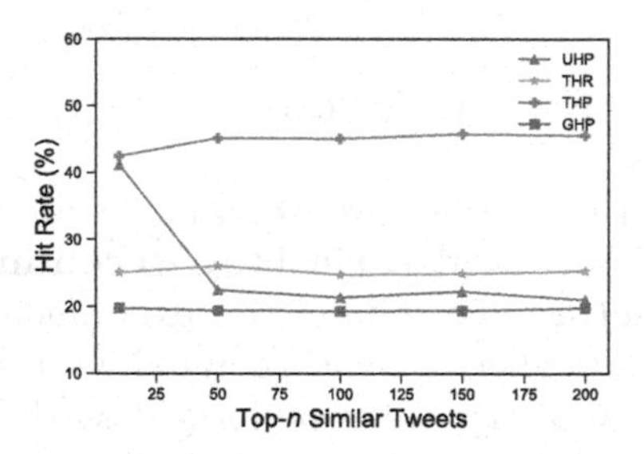

Fig. 2. Top-10 recommended hashtags average hit rates of the BFS-generated communities

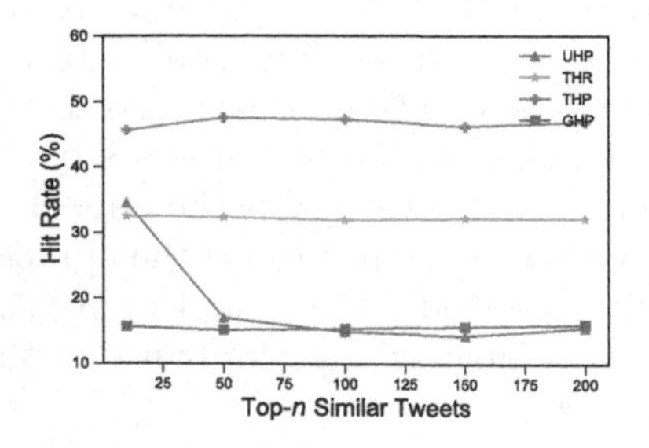

Fig. 3. Top-5 recommended hashtags average hit rates of the CPM-generated communities

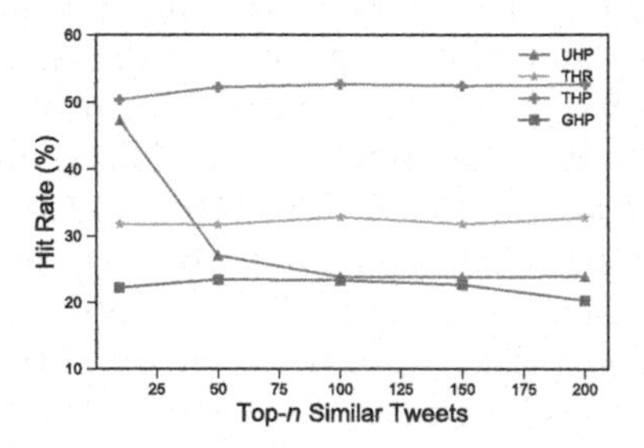

Fig. 4. Top-10 recommended hashtags average hit rates of the CPM-generated communities

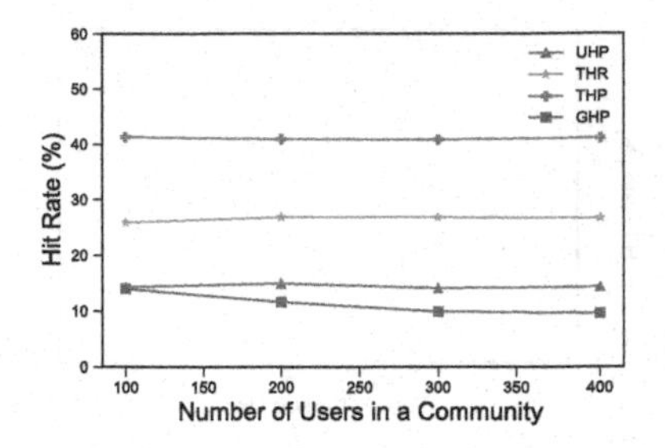

Fig. 5. Top-5 recommended hashtags on different sizes of BFS-generated communities

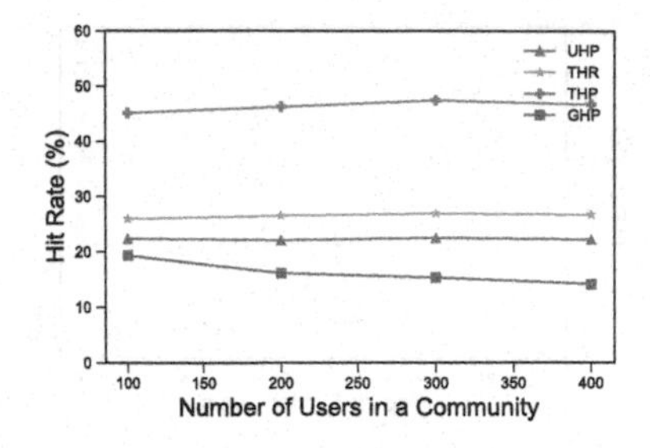

Fig. 6. Top-10 recommended hashtags on different sizes of BFS-generated communities

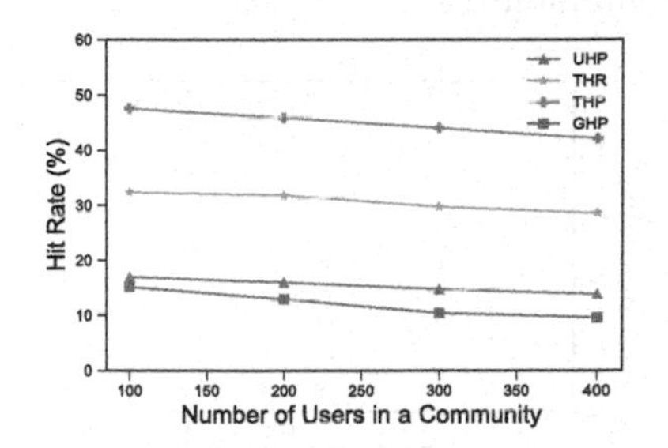

Fig. 7. Top-5 recommended hashtags on different sizes of CPM-generated communities

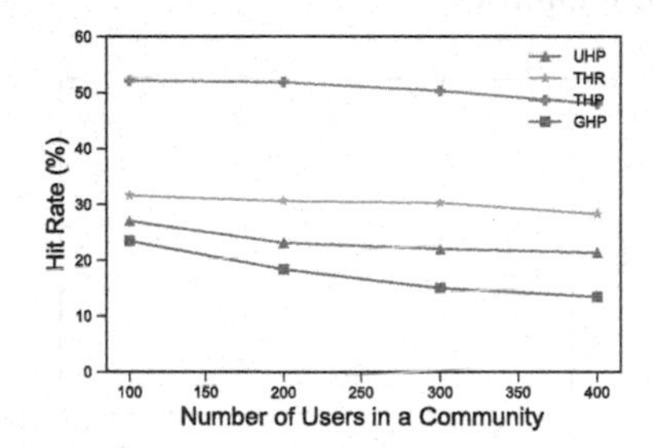

Fig. 8. Top-10 recommended hashtags on different sizes of CPM-generated communities

As a whole, the Tweet Hashtag Popularity ranking method (THP) performs better than all the other ranking methods. In the BFS-generated communities, the highest average hit rate is 41.34% when top-5 hashtags are recommended and 45.78% when the top-10 hashtags are recommended. In the CPM-generated communities, the highest average hit rate is 47.58% when the top-5 hashtags are recommended and 52.67% when the top-10 hashtag are recommended. It can be noticed that there is no significant improvement in the performance when $n > 50$ since τ is used as a filter. In general, the performance on the CPM-generated communities outperforms the BFS-generated communities. The performance on the BFS and CPM-generated communities are higher than the Zangerle's et al. paper by approximately more than 20% and 30%, respectively.

As for the results of the second part of the experiment, Figs. 5 and 6 show the average hit rate of the top-5 and top-10 recommended hashtags on the BFS-generated communities when the sizes of the communities (number of users) are increased. The highest average hit rate in the top-5 hashtag recommendation is 41.34% and 47.46% in the top-10 hashtag recommendation. It can be seen that there are no significant improvements in the performance when the sizes of the BFS-generated communities are increased to the second or to the third level. Figures 7 and 8 show the average hit rate of the top-5 and top-10 recommended

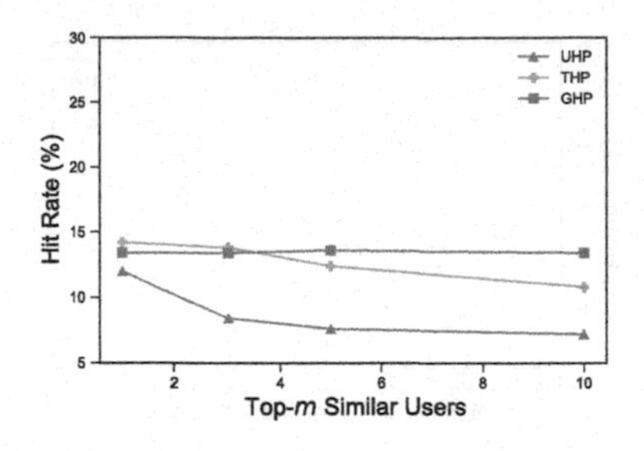

Fig. 9. Top-5 recommended hashtags average hit rates when the top-m users are considered of the BFS-generated communities

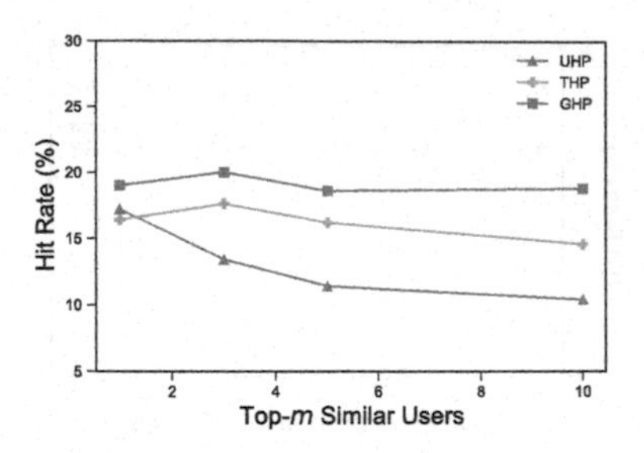

Fig. 10. Top-10 recommended hashtags average hit rates when the top-m users are considered of the BFS-generated communities

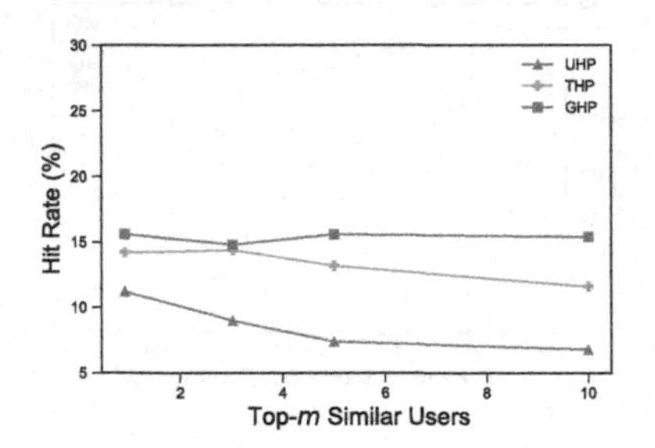

Fig. 11. Top-5 recommended hashtags average hit rates when the top-m users are considered of the CPM-generated communities

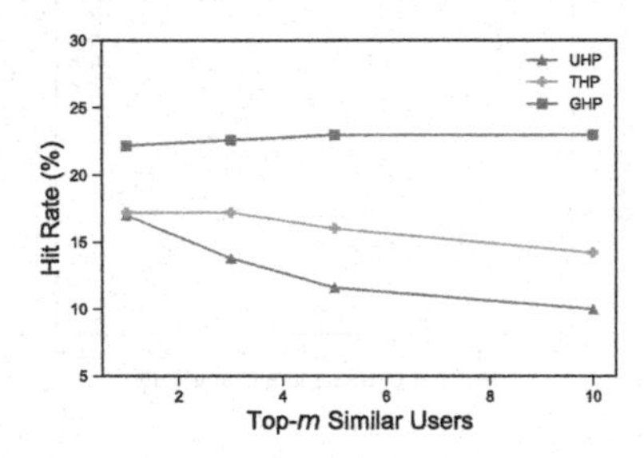

Fig. 12. Top-10 recommended hashtags average hit rates when the top-m users are considered of the CPM-generated communities

hashtags on the CPM-generated communities when the sizes of the communities (number of users) are increased. The highest average hit rate when the top-5 hashtags are recommended is 47.58% and 52.20% when the top-10 hashtags are recommended. In CPM-generated communities, it can be noticed that the performance is decreasing with the increase of the communities sizes. The overall performance on the CPM-generated communities is higher than that of the BFS communities.

Results of Experiment 2. Figures 9, 10, 11 and 12 show results of the first part of the experiment which measures the average hit rates when top-m users are considered. In this part of the experiment, the THR is not used because the tweets content are not incorporated. We notice that GHP performs the best over THP and UHP. The best results in BFS-generated communities are when the top-1 similar users are taken into account. The average hit rates of THP and UHP decrease as m increases. This means when hashtags of more than one user are considered the performance of the hashtag recommendation is decreased. This finding is consistent with Kywe's et al. finding. In THP, the best average hit rates is 14.2% when the top-5 hashtags are recommended and 17.6% when

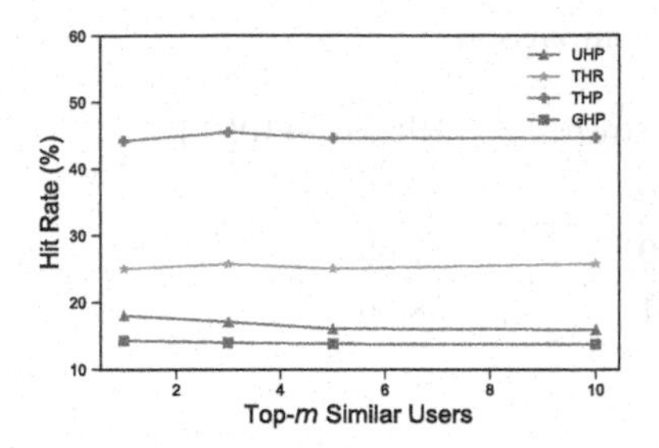

Fig. 13. Top-5 recommended hashtags average hit rates when hashtags from top-m users and top-50 tweets are considered of the BFS-generated communities

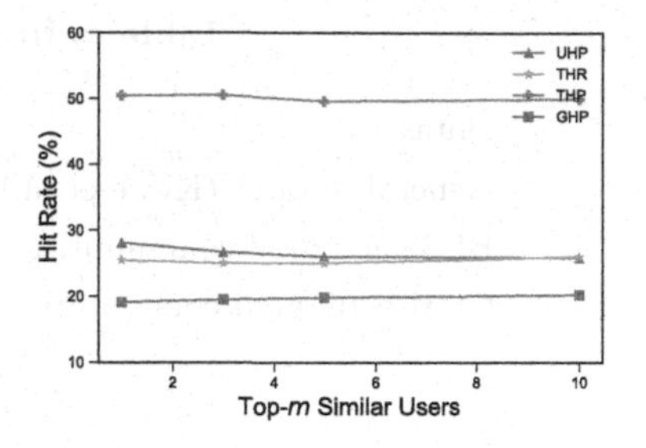

Fig. 14. Top-10 recommended hashtags average hit rates when hashtags from top-m users and top-50 tweets are considered of the BFS-generated communities

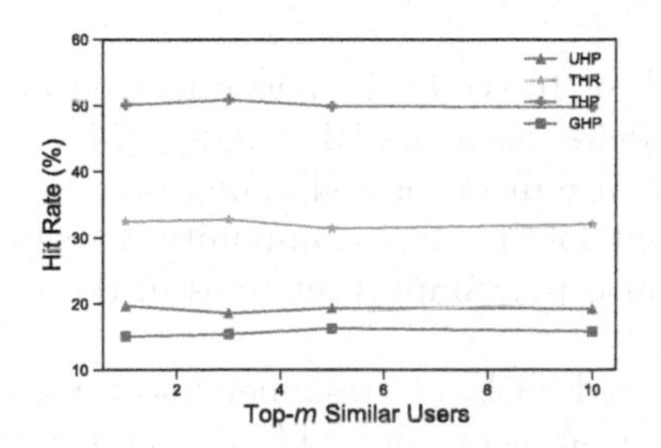

Fig. 15. Top-5 recommended hashtags average hit rates when hashtags from top-m users and top-50 tweets are considered of the CPM-generated communities

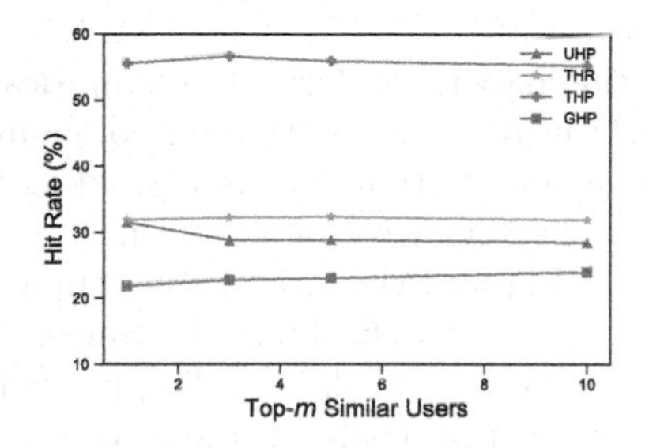

Fig. 16. Top-10 recommended hashtags average hit rates when hashtags from top-m users and top-50 tweets are considered of the CPM-generated communities

the top-10 hashtags are recommended. In the CPM-generated communities, the average hit rates of the THP in the top-5 and top-10 recommended hashtags are 14.2% and 17.21%, respectively. UHP shows the best performance when the top-1 user is considered with average hit rates equals to 11.2% and 17% to the top-5 and top-10 recommended hashtags. Therefore, the contribution of the user profiling based on the user's hashtags preference is less than the contribution of the textual factor when each of them is considered separately.

Figures 13, 14, 15 and 16 show results of the second part of the experiment. In general, the performance of the hashtag recommendation on both communities are higher than the results reported in the first part of the experiment 1 which does not incorporate user profiling. This indicates that the user profiling factor has a significant impact on enhancing the performance. These results also are higher than the results reported by Kywe et al.'s. which indicates that the social factor has a great impact on the hashtag recommendation. Table 4 shows the results compared with the results reported by Kywe's et al.'s. model. In BFS-generated communities, the best average hit rate is 45.48% in the top-5 hashtag

Table 4. Hit rates comparison

Datast	Hit rate@5(%)	Hit rate@10(%)
General dataset (Kywe et al.)	31.56	37.19
BFS-generated communities	41.89	47.63
CPM-generated communities	54.01	58.46

recommendation and 50.53% in the top-10 hashtag recommendation. In CPM-generated communities, the highest results is 50.89% when the top-5 hashtags are recommended and 56.61% when the top-10 hashtags are recommended.

6 Conclusion and Future Work

In this paper, we derived an empirical analysis to study the performance of the hashtag recommendation on communities detected using BFS and CPM when the social, textual and user profiling factors are incorporated. The results show that the social factor is the most significant factor. The community detection algorithm and the size of the community also play important roles in the performance of the hashtag recommendation.

Our future work is to design a personalized hashtag recommendation model based on the results of our investigation. In addition, we will have additional restrictions on which neighbours we are adding into the community. For example, if a node is not influential, then we should not include that node into the community.

Acknowledgements. This work is partially supported by the ARC Discovery Project under grant No. DP160102114 and UWA startup grant.

References

1. Bollobas, B., Kozma, R., Miklos, D.: Handbook of Large-Scale Random Networks. Bolyai Society Mathematical Studies, 1st edn. Springer, Heidelberg (2009)
2. Dovgopol, R., Nohelty, M.: Twitter Hash Tag Recommendation. CoRR abs/1502.00094 (2015)
3. Fellbaum, C. (ed.): WordNet: An Electronic Lexical Database. Language, Speech, and Communication. MIT Press, Cambridge (1998)
4. Ferragina, P., Piccinno, F., Santoro, R.: On analyzing hashtags in Twitter. In: Ninth International AAAI Conference on Web and Social Media (2015)
5. Harvey, M., Crestani, F.: Long Time, No Tweets! Time-aware Personalised Hashtag Suggestion, pp. 581–592. Springer, Cham (2015)
6. Wagenseller III, P., Wang, F.: Community Detection Algorithm Evaluation using Size and Hashtags. CoRR abs/1612.03362 (2016)
7. Kowald, D., Pujari, S., Lex, E.: Temporal effects on hashtag reuse in twitter: a cognitive-inspired hashtag recommendation approach (2017). arXiv:1701.01276v1

8. Kywe, S.M., Hoang, T.A., Lim, E.P., Zhu, F.: On Recommending Hashtags in Twitter Networks, pp. 337–350. Springer, Heidelberg (2012)
9. Li, R., Wang, S., Deng, H., Wang, R., Chang, K.: Towards social user profiling: unified and discriminative influence model for inferring home locations. In: KDD, pp. 1023–1031 (2012)
10. Ma, Z., Sun, A., Yuan, Q., Cong, G.: Tagging your tweets: a probabilistic modeling of hashtag annotation in Twitter. In: Proceedings of the 23rd ACM International Conference on Conference on Information and Knowledge Management, CIKM 2014, NY, USA, pp. 999–1008. ACM, New York (2014)
11. Mazzia, A., Juett, J.: Suggesting hashtags on Twitter. In: EECS 545 Project, Winter Term (2011)
12. Otsuka, E., Wallace, S.A., Chiu, D.: A hashtag recommendation system for Twitter data streams. Comput. Soc. Netw. **3**(1), 3 (2016). https://doi.org/10.1186/s40649-016-0028-9
13. Palla, G., lászló Barabási, A., Vicsek, T.: Quantifying social group evolution. Nature **446**, 664–667 (2007)
14. Peñas, P., del Hoyo, R., Vea-Murguía, J., González, C., Mayo, S.: Collective knowledge ontology user profiling for Twitter automatic user profiling. In: Proceedings of the 2013 IEEE/WIC/ACM International Joint Conferences on Web Intelligence (WI) and Intelligent Agent Technologies (IAT), WI-IAT 2013, vol. 1, pp. 439–444. IEEE Computer Society, Washington, DC (2013)
15. Pennacchiotti, M., Popescu, A.M.: A machine learning approach to Twitter user classification. In: ICWSM (2011)
16. Saramäki, J., Pekka Onnela, J., Kertész, J., Kaski, K.: Characterizing motifs in weighted complex networks (2005)
17. Sarkar, D. (ed.): Text Analytics with Python. Apress, Bangalore (2016)
18. Yang, L., Sun, T., Zhang, M., Mei, Q.: We Know What @You #Tag: does the dual role affect hashtag adoption? In: Proceedings of the 21st International Conference on World Wide Web, WWW 2012, pp. 261–270. ACM, New York (2012)
19. Zangerle, E., Gassler, W., Specht, G.: On the impact of text similarity functions on hashtag recommendations in microblogging environments. Soc. Netw. Anal. Min. **3**(4), 889–898 (2013)
20. Zhao, F., Zhu, Y., Jin, H., Yang, L.T.: A personalized hashtag recommendation approach using LDA-based topic model in microblog environment. Fut. Gener. Comput. Syst. **65**(C), 196–206 (2016)

Group Recommender Model Based on Preference Interaction

Wei Zheng[1], Bohan Li[1,2,4](✉), Yanan Wang[1], Hongzhi Yin[3], Xue Li[3], Donghai Guan[1], and Xiaolin Qin[1]

[1] College of Computer Science and Technology, Nanjing University of Aeronautics and Astronautics, Nanjing, China
{jive, bhli}@nuaa.edu.cn

[2] Collaborative Innovation Center of Novel Software Technology and Industrialization, Nanjing, China

[3] School of Information Technology and Electrical Engineering, University of Queensland, St Lucia, Australia

[4] Jiangsu Easymap Geographic Information Technology Corp., Ltd., Yangzhou, China

Abstract. With the application of recommender system increasing, the research and application of group recommender have been paid more attention. In the course of group activities, the unknown preferences of users are often affected by other members of the group. However, in the existing group recommender system, this effect is not taken into account. In this paper, we propose a novel recommender model that incorporates the preference interaction in the group recommender into rating predicting process. The model is divided into two parts: self-prediction and preference-interaction, the preference-interaction will be systematically analyzed and illustrated. For every user in the group, we use group activity history information and recommender post-rating feedback mechanism to generate personalized interactive parameters. Thus, it can improve the group's recommender accuracy. Finally, the model is combined with the collaborative filtering algorithm and compared with the algorithm without the model on the MovieLens dataset. The experiment results show that the model proposed in this paper can improve the accuracy of the group recommender results obviously.

Keywords: Recommender systems · Group recommender · Preference interaction · Collaborative filtering

This work is supported by the National Natural Science Foundation of China (61672284, 61373015, 41301407), the Funding of Security Ability Construction of Civil Aviation Administration of China (AS-SA2015/21), the Innovation Funding of Nanjing University of Aeronautics and Astronautics (NJ20160028), the Project Funded by the Priority Academic Program Development of Jiangsu Higher Education Institutions, the Australian Research Council Discover Project (DP140100104), Linkage Project (LP160100630).

G. Cong et al. (Eds.): ADMA 2017, LNAI 10604, pp. 132–147, 2017.
https://doi.org/10.1007/978-3-319-69179-4_10

1 Introduction

In informational era, the e-commerce is developing rapidly. With the enormous growth of web, the information overload problem is becoming increasingly serious, while the recommender system can effectively alleviate the problem [1]. At present most of the areas of the recommended system is only for a single user. However, in daily life, many of consuming behavior of user is in the form of group participation, such as multiple users to dinner, travel, movies, order takeout and so on [7]. In response to this situation, the recommender system needs to consider the collaboration among users within the group, so the algorithm design and model implementation process is more complicated than the single-user recommender system, the recommender system in which multiple users are involved is referred to group recommender. The main difference in the process of group recommender and single-user recommender is that the group recommender requires an aggregation of group membership preferences, and through various forms of aggregation strategies, the recommender results in the overall satisfaction, fairness, comprehensibility to reach the corresponding demand [2, 8].

In the group recommended process, group members are going to participate a series of consumer activities, so there will be some interactions among the group members in the general case, such as the exchange of their previous consumption situation or their preferences and so on, while these interactions often have effects on the unknown preferences of members in the group, such as the following example:

Example 1: A, B, C three users are going to watch movies. User A has ever watched the movie I and rated it, while user B and C haven't watched the movie I, that's to say, for the movie I, the preference of user A is known and the preferences of user B and C are unknown. Therefore, if there are interactions among the three users regarding the movie I, then user A's preference (rating) will influence the unknown preference of user B and C for the movie I during the interaction.

Example 2: A, B, C three users are going to eat dinner together. Users A and B have been to the restaurant I and rated it, while user C hasn't been to the restaurant I, so for the restaurant I, the preferences of user A and B is known and the preference of user C is unknown. Therefore, if there are interactions among the three users regarding the restaurant I, then user A and B's preferences (ratings) will influence the unknown preference of user C for the restaurant I during the interaction.

As can be seen from the above examples, for each item in the group, which can divide the group users into two categories, one is the preference known users for the item, the other is the preference unknown users for the item. In Example 1, A is the preference known user, and B and C are preferences unknown users. In Example 2, A and B are preferences known users, and C is preference unknown user. If there are interactions in the group, the preference of the preference known users will, to a certain extent, affect the preferences of users who are the preferences unknown users. In addition to the movies and restaurants, most of the group consume activities are related to the impact above.

Currently, most of the group recommender algorithms do not take into account this kind of interaction relations, but the impact of this interaction is often particularly important in group recommender, which is one of the main characteristics of group recommender that are different from single-user recommender. There are some group recommender studies that take into account the impact of the interaction, but these studies only focus on the process of preference aggregation within the group member, the main idea is based on the characteristics, roles, influences and other factors of group users to assign a different weight for them, and then aggregate preference base on these weights, through the user weight to reflect the interaction between users, nevertheless, these methods can't reflect the effect of the known preferences influence on the unknown preferences.

The preference interaction model proposed in this paper is different from the preference interaction in previous group recommender. The model focuses on the effect of preference interaction on the unrated items in group members. That is, if a group user's rating is unknown for a specific item, it means that the user is completely unaware of the item, therefore base on emotional contagion and conformity phenomena [3], the member's preference for the item will naturally be influenced by other users in the group who rated the item. The interact effect of this type is different from the related literature's interaction which using the way of user's weight, because for the unknown items of ourselves, we tend to be more dependent on others, so that the potential preference is not limited to the influence of other users in the group.

2 Related Work

2.1 Multiple Recommenders

At present, there is no unity standard to classify the recommender system. From the point of view of models, the basic models for recommender systems work with two kinds of data [4, 12], which are the user-item interactions, such as ratings or buying behavior, and the attribute information about the users and items such as textual profiles or relevant keywords. Methods that use the former are referred to as collaborative filtering methods, whereas methods that use the latter are referred to as content-based recommender methods. In addition, the demographic filtering recommenders, utility-based recommenders, association rule-based filtering recommenders are also frequently-used [16, 18].

As the rapid development of LBS and social media, the context-award and social networks recommender system are very popular, Yin et al. [5, 9, 10] think that users' behaviors in social media systems are generally influenced by intrinsic interest as well as the temporal context, so they proposed a latent class statistical mixture model

TCAM. Besides they proposed a spatial context-aware recommender LCARS [5, 11] to deal with the sparse matrix problem when people travel to a new city where they have no activity history.

Nevertheless, the recommenders above are all designed for severing single user, if there are situations that the target use becomes group, the methods can not fit well. So the group recommenders appear to recommend for group users.

2.2 Group Recommender

MusicFX [15] is one of the earliest group recommender studies, its processing method is analyze the user's personal preferences, and find an appropriate music for group users in the fitness center to play. PolyLens [17] is an extension of the single-user recommender system MovieLens, which aims to recommend appropriate movies for group users by using collaborative filtering to predict individual unrated items and using least misery strategies to aggregate personal preferences. Furthermore, Chen et al. [6] proposed a method of considering user's interaction in group recommender aggregation. They suggested that different user in the group had different group influences during recommender aggregation, and using genetic algorithm to get the weight of group members, to a certain extent, it can improve the fairness of the preference aggregation process. Campos et al. [19] used the Bayesian network to represent the interactions and the group decision process among group members. Bayesian network learning method and user history rating were used to obtain the relationship between group members. There are more and more researches about getting different users' weight in group recommender through various methods.

After the survey we found, some of the algorithms have referred the preference interaction among users, but its interaction process are different from our model, there is no conflict, the main difference is as follows: The key to the interaction of existing literature is the weight, that is, different users has different influence, its interaction works on the recommender aggregation process. The key to the interaction of our algorithm is the influence of unknown preference, its interaction works on the preference prediction process. In summary, the interaction in this paper as a supplement to the traditional group recommender still has some research significance.

2.3 Preference Prediction

Recommender system for user preference prediction commonly apply collaborative filtering, the method predict the recommender items by similarity calculation. There are two main types of collaborative filtering: user-based collaborative filtering (UBCF) and item-based collaborative filtering (IBCF) based on different similarity. When we get the user-item rating matrix, we need to calculate the similarity between users or items at first, and the Pearson similarity is usually used to calculate the similarity in recommend system. In the case of UBCF, the Pearson similarity between user u and v is calculated as follows:

$$sim(u,v) = \frac{\sum_{i \in I}(r_{u,i} - \overline{r_u})(r_{v,i} - \overline{r_v})}{\sqrt{\sum_{i \in I}(r_{u,i} - \overline{r_u})^2}\sqrt{\sum_{i \in I}(r_{v,i} - \overline{r_v})^2}} \tag{1}$$

Where $r_{u,i}$ represents the rating of item u for item i, If $\Sigma_{i \in I}$ is replaced by $\Sigma_{i \in I_u \cap I_v}$ in the calculation process, the formula is changed to only consider the user's common rating items, the resulting sim(u, v) is a number between –1 and 1, the higher the value, the higher the similarity.

After obtaining the similarity between users, we can get a set of user S similar to the target user u, so the prediction rating of user u for item i can be expressed as:

$$p_{u,i} = \overline{r_u} + \frac{\sum_{v \in S} Sim(u,v)\left(r_{v,i} - \overline{r_v}\right)}{\sum_{v \in S}|Sim(u,v)|} \tag{2}$$

The similarity calculation and rating prediction formula of IBCF can also be obtained similarly, no longer list in this paper.

2.4 Recommender Aggregation

The traditional recommender system is recommended for a single user, so after predicting users' unrated items, we can give recommenders base on the user-item rating matrix. However, as for group recommender, the recommended results need to satisfy all of the group member's need, so it is also necessary to take into account the synergies problem between group members, and then aggregating group members' preferences through some strategies is needed.

According to the stage of preference aggregation in group recommender, the content of recommender aggregation is different, mainly divided into two categories: aggregating recommenders [14] and aggregating ratings [13]. Aggregating recommenders refers to generating a personal recommender list according to the personal preferences of the users in the group, and then combining the individual recommender list of all the users in the group according to the aggregation strategy to obtain the recommender list of the group. Aggregating ratings refers to aggregate all the group members' ratings into one overall rating as the group rating at first, and then based on the group rating for further recommenders. As the preference aggregation process will involve every group users' rating about the candidate items, the user's unrated items need to be firstly predicted, and then aggregate group members' preferences. So the process usually combines with collaborative filtering to generate recommended results for group recommenders.

3 Group Recommender Based on Preference Interaction

3.1 Preference Interaction Among Group Members

In group recommender, the participants is a group of users, there must be some association among the users, they might be relatives or friends, which will inevitably occur some interactive activities, some of group users' unknown items will be affected by the other members during the procedure, thus it will influence the preferences of group members, for example, expand the example 1 in the introduction section, because the group G consists of user A, B, C is going to watch a movie together, their ratings record about the films Titanic and Star Wars are given in Fig. 1, where "?" represents the film that the user has not rated, it means that the user has not watched the film. In group G, for the film Titanic only user A has rated it, and for Star Wars, its rating users are A and B, so if there is interaction within the group, then the users B and C's unknown rating for Titanic's will be affected by user A's rating of 5, user C's unknown rating for Star War will be affected by user A's rating of 3 and user C's score of 4, as shown in Fig. 1.

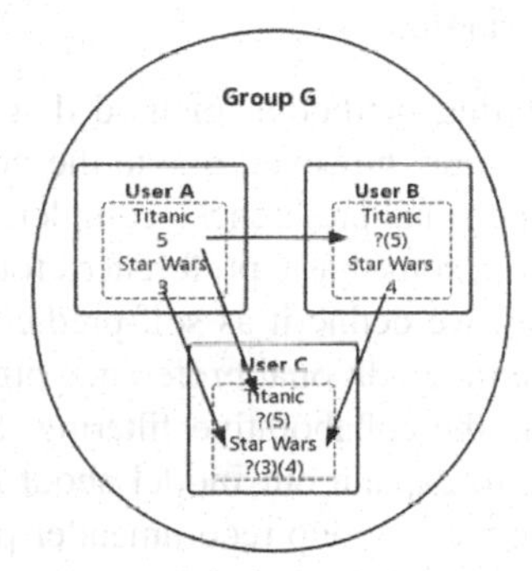

Fig. 1. The sketch map of unrated item influenced by interaction in the group

Therefore, based on the above-mentioned influence relationship, the following rating prediction method is proposed, which is affected by the interaction of members' preference in the group, it is defined as follows:

$$R(I)_{u,i} = \overline{r_u} + \frac{\sum_{v \in U_{g,i}} w_{u,v}\left(r_{v,i} - \overline{r_v}\right)}{\sum_{v \in U_{g,i}} w_{u,v}}, u \in g \tag{3}$$

Where $R(I)_{u,i}$ represents the unknown rating's predict rating for item i of user u in group g that is influenced by the preference interaction of the other members in the group. $U_{g,i}$ represents the set of users in group g that have rated the item i. $w_{u,v}$ denotes the impact weight of the user v on the user u. In reality, the degree of influences among the users within the group may not be the same, so we should take into account the different impact of different users when we generate $R(I)_{u,i}$, the following gives an implicit method to access $w_{u,v}$.

In the real life, the closer the relationship between people tends to be more frequent activities with each other, which means more interaction. Therefore, $w_{u,v}$ can also be used to express the intimacy between people, we can use the degree of intimacy between users to approximate the value of $w_{u,v}$. The value of $w_{u,v}$ may be based on the following idea if there is no data source for intimacy between users: The more the number of common activities between users, the more intimate between users, the higher the value of $w_{u,v}$ is. Therefore, $w_{u,v}$ is defined as follows:

$$w_{u,v} = 1 + \lg(s_{u,v} + 1) \quad (4)$$

Where $s_{u,v}$ represents the number of times that the user u and v are in common activities, $w_{u,v}$ increases linearly with the increase of $s_{u,v}$, obviously it is unreasonable for practical application, so we calculate the logarithm of $s_{u,v}$ to limit its growth rate. As the model is used continuously, the value of $w_{u,v}$ tends to be stable, the difference between users' intimacy is more obvious, and the rating prediction results will be more accurate.

3.2 Preference Prediction for Group Recommender Based on the Preference Interaction

Formula (3) has obtained a rating prediction method that is influenced by the interaction of members within the group, however, due to the different personality of users, the user will not abandon his personal preferences completely for his unrated item, and therefore, the user will still retain some basic preferences for the item. For the impact of this factor on prediction rating, we define it as self-predicting part R(S). For the self-predicting part, we usually use the traditional preference prediction algorithm based on rating, the most typical one is the collaborative filtering. So we will use UBCF and IBCF algorithms as examples to explain our model about R(S) in the following.

Based on the basic idea above, a group recommender preference predicting model based on preference interaction is proposed. The model combines the influence of preference interaction and the self-prediction of users in group activity. For this prediction model, the basic formula as follow:

$$R_{u,i} = e_u R(I)_{u,i} + (1 - e_u) R(S)_{u,i} \quad (5)$$

Where $R_{u,i}$ denotes the predicting rating of the item i by user u, e_u denotes the influence of the preference interaction-part of group user u, $1 - e_u$ denotes the influence of the self-predicting part of user u. The whole process of rating prediction is shown in Algorithm 1, the algorithm is illustrated by combining the model and UBCF algorithm. The reason why applying the parameter e_u is considering the differences degree of users being affected, some users self-awareness is relatively strong, for their unknown items are also less susceptible to others, the value of such users' e_u is low, and some users are just the opposite, their preferences for unknown items more susceptible to others, and their e_u is high.

For the acquisition of e_u, we propose an implicit method based on feedback mechanism, that is, after each group recommender activity, if the user u rate his original unrated item i as $r_{u,i}$, $r_{u,i}$ can be a feedback parameter to adjusted e_u, that is, each feedback $r_{u,i}$ can be used to obtain the once value of e_u : $e_u^{(s)}$ according to formula (5), that is:

$$e_u^{(s)} = \frac{r_{u,i} - R(S)_{u,i}}{R(I)_{u,i} - R(S)_{u,i}}, R(I)_{u,i} \neq R(S)_{u,i} \tag{6}$$

When $e_u^{(s)} < 0$, the value of $e_u^{(s)}$ is 0, or if $e_u^{(s)} > 1$, the value of $e_u^{(s)}$ is 1, if $R(I)_{u,i} = R(S)_{u,i}$, indicating preference-interaction part and self-predicting part have same rating, the value of e_u feedback this time is meaningless, then discard it.

Algorithm 1 UBCF Algorithm Based on Preference Interaction: I-UBCF

Input: The user u and item i to which the unrated item belongs, and the group g to which u belongs
Output: Unrated item's predictive rating $R_{u,i}$

```
1.  RatedGroup ← getRatedUsers(g,u,i);   //Get all the group users that rated the item i except u
2.  if rateGroup == null then
3.      R_{u,i} ← UBCF(u,i);   //When the set of rated users is null, apply the UBCF predict the r_{u,i}
4.  else
5.      influencedRating ← 0;
6.      weightAmount ← 0;
7.      for every RatedUser in RatedGroup do   //For every user in the set that consist of rated users
8.          influencedRating ← influencedRating + w_{u,ratedUser}(r_{ratedUser,i} − ave(r_{ratedUser}));
            // Aggregate the influenced ratings of all users in the group
9.          weightAmount ← weightAmount + w_{u,ratedUser};
            // Aggregate the weight of all users in the group
10.     end for
11.     RI_{u,i} ← ave(r_u) + influencedRating / weightAmount;
        //Calculate the ratings of preference-interaction part
12.     RS_{u,i} ← UBCF(u,i);   //Calculate the ratings of self-predicting part
13.     R_{u,i} ← e_u * RI_{u,i} + (1 − e_u) * RS_{u,i};
        //Calculate the predicting rating by I-UBCF
14. end if
15. return R_{u,i};   // Returns the predict rating for unrated item
```

Taking into account the degree of dependence of each user will change gradually as the changing of user's mentality, personality or status, therefore, every time for the value of e_u can be obtained by calculating the latest 10 values of, that is:

$$e_u = \frac{\sum_{e_u^{(s)} \in E_u} e_u^{(s)}}{|E_u|} \tag{7}$$

Where E_u represents the set of feedback values of $e_u^{(s)}$ for the latest ten times of user u. The whole process of obtaining feedback e_u as shown in Algorithm 2.

Algorithm 2 The obtain algorithm of e_u: CalculateInteraction

Input: The self-predicting part $RS_{u,i}$ and preference-interaction part $RI_{u,I}$ of I-UBCF, and the true rating $r_{u,I}$ of the user after recommender

Output: The obtained Once value of e_u

```
1.  if RI_u,i != RS_u,i then
2.      e_us ← (r_u,i – RS_u,i) / (RI_u,i – RS_u,i);   //Calculate once feedback value e_us
3.      if e_us < 0 then
4.          e_us ← 0;   // Assign 0,if the value is less than 0
5.      else if e_us > 1 then
6.          e_us ← 1;   // Assign 1,if the value is greater than 1
7.      end if
8.      if E_u.length == 10 then
9.          removeOldestElement(E_u);   //Delete the oldest element when Eu contains more than 10 elements
10.     end if
11.     addElement(E_u, e_us);   //Add the newest element e_us
12. end if
13. e_u ← sum(E_u) / E_u.length;   //Calculate the average of E_u and assign to e_u
14. return e_u;   //Return the value of e_u
```

3.3 Algorithm Application

Take the movie recommender as an example. The data in Table 1 are intercepted from the MovieLens dataset, which contains five users' rating record for four movies. The five users are represented by User1–5. Assume they are in the same group, just recommend movies for them. The red marked ratings are predicted by UBCF, they are originally the items that the user unrated, the user's interaction parameter e_u and average rating $\overline{r_u}$ is also available in the table. The user's history group information in group g as shown in Table 2, the number represents the number of common activities between two users. The purpose of the algorithm is to consider preference interaction in the process of rating prediction. That is to say, we need to modify the marked red ratings in Table 1 by the proposed preference interaction algorithm to make it more suitable for the actual recommender.

Table 1. The user information table of group g

		Lion King (1)	Forrest Gump (2)	Brave Heart (3)	Twelve Monkeys (4)	e_u	$\overline{r_u}$
g	User1	3	4	**2.2**	**2.4**	0.3	3.1
	User2	3	5	4	**4.1**	0.5	3.9
	User3	**4.2**	**3.1**	5	**4.2**	0.7	4.2
	User4	2	**2.8**	3	**1.6**	0.2	2.2
	User5	4	5	**3.3**	**4.2**	0.3	4.1

Table 2. The grouped record in group g

	User1	User2	User3	User4	User5
User1	-	20	0	3	1
User2	20	-	12	5	0
User3	0	12	-	0	15
User4	3	5	0	-	1
User5	1	0	15	1	-

First of all, according to the data in Table 3, calculate the users intimacy between users $w_{u,v}$ in the group applying formula (4), such as $w_{1,2} = 1 + \lg 21$, therefore $w_{1,2} = 2.32$, $w_{1,3} = 1 + \lg 1$, so $w_{1,3} = 1$. The intimacy between other members in the group can also be calculated similarly.

After calculating the intimacy between users, we can calculate the ratings of preference-interaction part. Take the calculation of User1's preference interaction rating for Brave Heart as an example. Firstly we need to get all the users in the group that rated Brave Heart, they are User2, User3, and User4, so User1's preference for Brave Heart will be affected by them, and then we need to get the intimacy of the User1, $w_{1,2} = 2.32$, $w_{1,3} = 1$, $w_{1,4} = 1.6$. According to formula (3), the preference-interaction part of the predicted rating of User1 for Brave Heart can be calculated as $R(I)_{1,3} = 3.3$. In the following, aggregate the ratings of self-prediction and preferences interaction parts, by Table 2, User1's interaction parameter $e_1 = 0.3$, the rating of self-predicting part $R(S)_{1,3} = 2.2$. Therefore, the rating of Brave Heart of User1 can be calculated by formula (5), $R_{1,3} = 2.5$. For the prediction of User1's rating about Twelve Monkeys, there is no user in the group who has rated Twelve Monkeys, that is, all users in the group is not familiar with Twelve Monkeys, so there is no preference interaction about the prediction of Twelve Monkeys. The rest of prediction about the unrated in the table can also be similar. The user information of the group g adjusted by the above process is shown in Table 3, where the blue rating items indicate the adjusted ratings by preference interaction. Then you can do the next step of the recommender using the table.

Table 3. The grouped record in group g

		Lion King (1)	Forrest Gump (2)	Brave Heart (3)	Twelve Monkeys (4)	e_u	$\overline{r_u}$
g	User1	3	4	**2.5**	**2.4**	0.3	3.1
	User2	3	5	4	**4.1**	0.2	3.9
	User3	**4.1**	**3.4**	5	**4.2**	0.7	4.2
	User4	2	**2.7**	3	**1.6**	0.5	2.2
	User5	4	5	**3.6**	**4.2**	0.3	4.1

3.4 The Framework of Preference Interactive Group Recommender System

The life cycle of the traditional group recommender system can be divided into four stages: collecting the data of group member, obtaining the preference information of group member, generating group recommender, recommender evaluation and feedback. In [16], a four-layer group recommender framework based on the above four phases is presented. On the basis of the framework, we propose a group recommender algorithm model based on preference interaction. The framework is changed into a five-layer structure, and the contents of each layer are shown in Fig. 2.

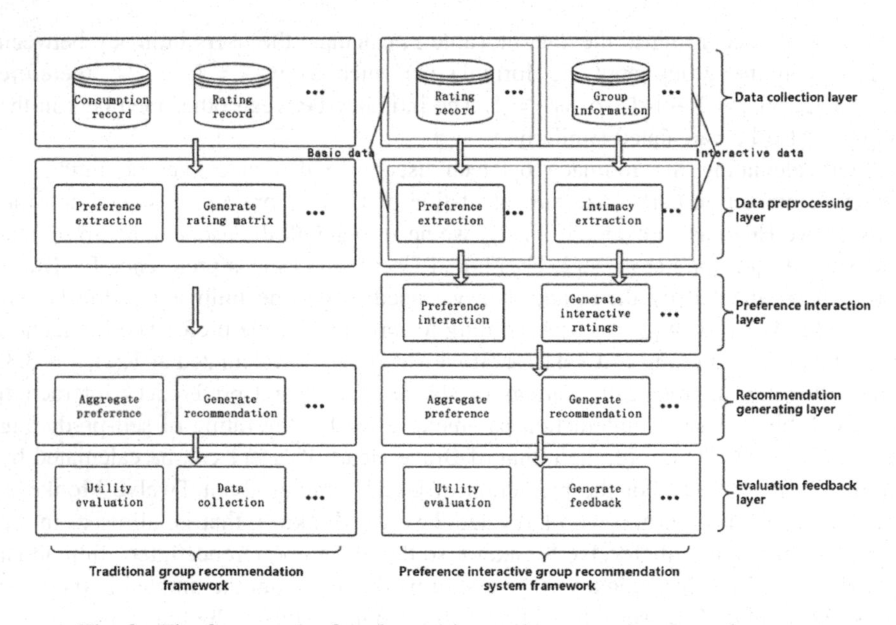

Fig. 2. The framework of preference interactive group recommender system

4 Experiment and Analysis

4.1 Dataset

The dataset used in this experiment is the MovieLens 100 K dataset, which was collected by GroupLens Laboratories on a large number of users' movie ratings on the movielens website, it includes 943 users for a total of 100000 five-point ratings for 1682 movies (1–5 points), and each user has already rated at least 20 movies.

There is currently no dataset related to the group recommender, including the dataset selected for this experiment, which only contains the recommender data related to the user's individual information and does not include any group information. Therefore, the dataset is need to be pretreated, refer to the processing method in [14], firstly group the users into the specific group size, then, simulate $w_{u,v}$ according to the normal distribution of intimacy between users, and compare the different algorithms under different interaction parameter e_u at the same time. In order to measure the algorithm, the experiment applies the standard method to divide the dataset into two parts, that is, randomly select 60% of the data as the training set, 40% as the test set, the algorithm recommends items using the data of training set, and then according to the data of test set to verify the recommended results.

Since the source of the dataset is the personal rating for the movies preferences, and there is no information related to group, obviously there is no interaction between the users in the dataset. Therefore, on the basis of the original dataset, we simulate a dataset with interaction factors, that is collect 30 people of our lab's common consumer activities and personal character so that to extract the e_u between them, and then approximate its Gaussian distribution, further simulates the interaction parameters between users in the dataset based on the distribution. Using the interaction parameters adjusts the test set, and then the adjusted dataset is regarded as the simulated dataset with users' preference interaction.

The main purpose of the experiment is to compare the group recommender algorithm based on preference interaction with the algorithm without preference interaction, besides the experiments are evaluated in two datasets, the original dataset and the dataset with preference interaction, in order to prove the importance of preference interaction during the process of preference prediction.

4.2 Evaluation System

RMSE [6] and nDCG [20] are used to evaluate the algorithm model. RMSE can be used to evaluate the quality of the rating prediction, and it represents the root mean square errors of the predicted ratings and actual ratings:

$$RSME = \sqrt{\frac{\sum_{i=1}^{M}\left(R_{u,i} - r_{u,i}\right)}{M}} \tag{8}$$

Where M denotes the number of predicted ratings in the dataset, $R_{u,i}$ denotes the predicted rating of item i by user u, and $r_{u,i}$ is the actual rating. RSME is a non-negative value, the lower the value is, the higher precision of the predicted value.

nDCG is a standard information retrieval evaluation index, which can be used to evaluate the accuracy of the recommended list, the formula is as follows:

$$\begin{aligned} DCG_n &= rel_1 + \sum_{i=2}^{n} \frac{rel_i}{\log_2 i} \\ nDCG_n &= \frac{DCG_n}{maxDCG_n} \end{aligned} \tag{9}$$

Where rel_i represents the actual rating of the i-th item in the recommended list, $maxDCG_n$ represents the max possibility value of DCG_n, that is the optimal order of the n items about the value of DCG_n, n represents the number of recommended results, n = 5 in this experiment, it is closer to the actual recommender list length.

In order to compute nDCG, we need to know the true ratings of all the items in the recommended list. However, only a small number of items in the recommended list have ratings in the test set, so we apply the method of [14] to calculate nDCG, that is calculate the nDCGs of the projection of recommended list in the test set, For example, suppose the ordered recommended list of users u rec = [1, 4, 5, 8, 3, 7, 6, 2, 9], but the user's rating in the test set only 7 items test = [1, 4, 7, 8, 9, 12, 14, 20], so we only need to calculate the nDCG of the projection $rec_{projection}$ = [1, 4, 8, 7, 9], and the average value of all users' nDCGs is the experimental result. The value of nDCG is between 0 and 1, the greater the value, the higher the recommended accuracy.

4.3 Experimental Results

Experiments compare the group recommender algorithm based on preference interaction with the algorithm without preference interaction under different group size and e_u. Where I-UBCF represents the UBCF algorithm based on the preference interaction and I-IBCF represents the IBCF algorithm based on the preference interaction.

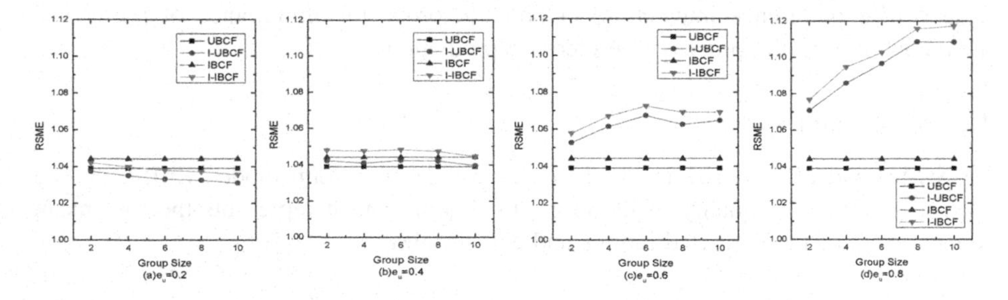

Fig. 3. The comparison of RSME in original dataset

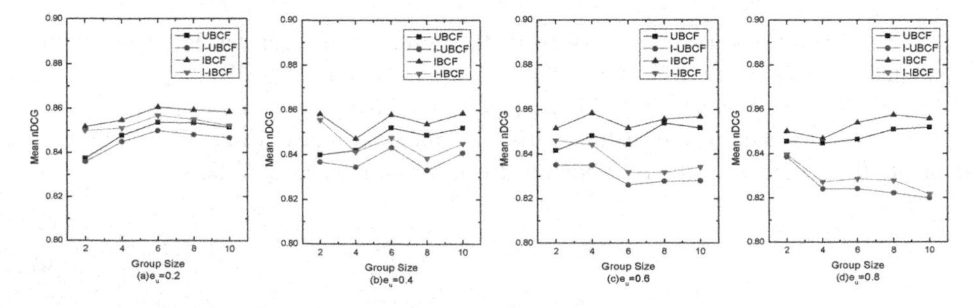

Fig. 4. The comparison of nDCG in original dataset

It can be concluded from Fig. 3 under the original dataset, that the RSME value is not affected by the change of the group size, because the RSME value of traditional collaborative filtering is not associated with group. Figure 4 shows that the accuracy of the recommender list given by the traditional group recommender algorithm is better than that of the interactive algorithm in the original dataset, and the gap becomes larger as the group size becomes larger. Therefore, it can be conclude that the proposed group recommender algorithm is not suitable for the recommender systems without group interaction. However, since the interaction parameters proposed by the model are obtained by means of feedback, the value of e_u becomes moderately low with the use of the model and will not affect the efficiency of the whole group recommender system.

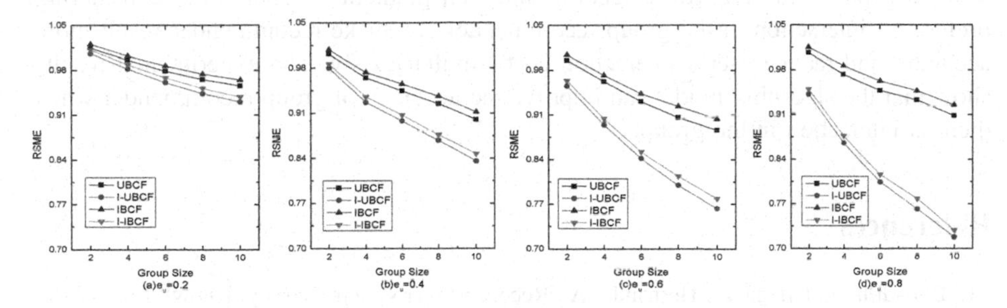

Fig. 5. The comparison of RSME in adjusted dataset

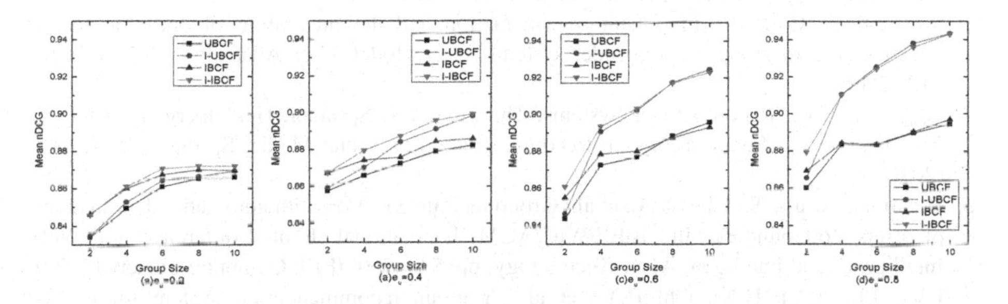

Fig. 6. The comparison of nDCG in adjusted dataset

From Fig. 5 we can see that group recommender with preference interaction has a smaller prediction error, especially in larger groups. As for Fig. 6, the performance of the proposed algorithm is improved obviously when the interactive parameter e_u and the group size are larger. It can be concluded that the algorithm presented in this paper has more advantages in the group with preference interaction.

According to the experimental results, we can draw a conclusion that the preference interactive group recommender algorithm outperforms the traditional group recommender algorithm when there is a preference interaction among the groups. In practical application of group recommender, the recommended target is often some groups of social relations, which involves the interaction between users. And in the model of the recommended algorithm, the users' interaction parameters e_u and $w_{u,v}$ are obtained through adaptive way, so in the recommended group, regardless how much of the number of interactions it involves, the algorithm model will gradually adjusted to the best effect as the using of the model, therefore the algorithm model proposed in this paper has some practical significance in the group recommender scenario involving user interaction.

5 Conclusions

In the group recommender, the unknown preferences of the users are easier influenced by the members in the group. According to this idea, this paper proposes a group recommender algorithm model based on preference interaction. The model is an optimization for the preference prediction process. The prediction process is divided into two parts: preference-interaction and self-prediction. Therefore, considering preference interaction in the group recommender can make recommender result more accurate, and reduce user's interaction cost simultaneously. The experimental results show that the algorithm model can improve the accuracy of group recommender when there is interaction in the group.

References

1. Bobadilla, J., Ortega, F., Hernando, A.: Recommender systems survey. Knowl. Based Syst. **46**(1), 109–132 (2013)
2. Garcia, I., Pajares, S., Sebastia, L., Onaindia, E.: Preference elicitation techniques for group recommender systems. Inf. Sci. **189**(8), 155–175 (2012)
3. Masthoff, J., Gatt, A.: In pursuit of satisfaction and the prevention of embarrassment: affective state in group recommender systems. User Model. User Adap. Inter. **16**(3), 281–319 (2006)
4. Aggarwal, C.C.: Recommender Systems: The Textbook. Springer, Heidelberg (2016)
5. Yin, H., Cui, B.: Spatio-Temporal Recommendation in Social Media. Springer, Singapore (2016)
6. Boratto, L., Carta, S., Chessa A., et al.: Group recommendation with automatic identification of users communities. In: IEEE/WIC/ACM International Joint Conference on Web Intelligence and Intelligent Agent Technology, pp. 547–550. IEEE Computer Society (2009)
7. Kim, J.K., Kim, H.K., Oh, H.Y., et al.: A group recommendation system for online communities. Int. J. Inf. Manage. **30**(3), 212–219 (2010)
8. Crossen, A., Budzik, J., Hammond, K.J.: Flytrap: intelligent group music recommendation. In: Proceedings of the 7th International Conference on Intelligent User Interfaces, San Francisco, USA, pp. 184–185 (2002)
9. Yin, H., Cui, B., Chen, L., et al.: A temporal context-aware model for user behavior modeling in social media systems. In: International Conference Proceedings on Management of Data, pp. 1543–1554. Association for Computing Machinery (2014). Special Interest Group on Management of Data
10. Yin, H., Cui, B., Chen, L., et al.: Dynamic user modeling in social media system. ACM Trans. Inf. Syst. **33**(3), 10 (2015)
11. Yin, H., Cui, B., Chen, L., et al.: Modeling location-based user rating profiles for personalized recommendation. ACM Trans. Knowl. Discov. Data **9**(3), 1–41 (2015)
12. Ricci, F., Rokach, L., Shapira, B., et al.: Introduction to Recommender Systems Handbook. Springer, Boston (2011)
13. Garcia, I., Sebastia, L., Onaindia, E.: On the design of individual and group recommender systems for tourism. Exp. Syst. Appl. **38**(6), 7683–7692 (2011)
14. Baltrunas, L., Makcinskas, T., Ricci, F.: Group recommendations with rank aggregation and collaborative filtering. In: ACM Conference on Recommender Systems, pp. 119–126. ACM (2010)

15. Mccarthy, J.F., Anagnost, T.D.: MusicFX: an arbiter of group preferences for computer supported collaborative workouts. In: ACM Conference on Computer Supported Cooperative Work, pp. 363–372. ACM (2000)
16. Boratto, L.: Group recommender systems: state of the art, emerging aspects and techniques, and research challenges. In: Ferro, N., Crestani, F., Moens, M.-F., Mothe, J., Silvestri, F., Di Nunzio, G.M., Hauff, C., Silvello, G. (eds.) ECIR 2016. LNCS, vol. 9626, pp. 889–892. Springer, Cham (2016). doi:10.1007/978-3-319-30671-1_87
17. O'Connor, M., Cosley, D., Konstan, J.A., et al.: PolyLens: a recommender system for groups of users. In: Proceedings of the seventh Conference on European Conference on Computer Supported Cooperative Work, pp. 199–218. Kluwer Academic Publishers (2001)
18. Gartrell, M., Xing, X., Lv, Q., et al.: Enhancing group recommendation by incorporating social relationship interactions. In: International ACM SIGGROUP Conference on Supporting Group Work, Group 2010, Sanibel Island, Florida, USA, November, pp. 97–106 (2010)
19. Campos, L.M.D., Fernández-Luna, J.M., Huete, J.F., et al.: Managing uncertainty in group recommending processes. User Model. User Adap. Inter. **19**(3), 207–242 (2009)
20. Pessemier, T.D., Dooms, S., Martens, L.: Comparison of group recommendation algorithms. Multimedia Tools Appl. **72**(3), 2497–2541 (2014)

Identification of Grey Sheep Users by Histogram Intersection in Recommender Systems

Yong Zheng(✉), Mayur Agnani, and Mili Singh

School of Applied Technology, Illinois Institute of Technology, Chicago, IL 60616, USA
yzheng66@iit.edu, {magnani,msingh32}@hawk.iit.edu

Abstract. Collaborative filtering, as one of the most popular recommendation algorithms, has been well developed in the area of recommender systems. However, one of the classical challenges in collaborative filtering, the problem of "Grey Sheep" user, is still under investigation. "Grey Sheep" users is a group of the users who may neither agree nor disagree with the majority of the users. They may introduce difficulties to produce accurate collaborative recommendations. In this paper, discuss the drawbacks in the approach that can identify the Grey Sheep users by reusing the outlier detection techniques based on the distribution of user-user similarities. We propose to alleviate these drawbacks and improve the identification of Grey Sheep users by using histogram intersection to better produce the user-user similarities. Our experimental results based on the MovieLens 100 K rating data demonstrate the ease and effectiveness of our proposed approach in comparison with existing approaches to identify grey sheep users.

Keywords: Recommender system · Collaborative filtering · Grey sheep

1 Introduction

Recommender system is well-known to assist user's decision making by recommending a list of appropriate items to the end users tailored to their preferences. Several recommender systems have been developed to provide accurate item recommendations. There are three types of these algorithms: collaborative filtering approaches, content-based recommendation algorithms and the hybrid recommendation models [4]. Collaborative filtering (CF) is one of the most popular algorithms since it is effective and it does not rely on any content information.

Most of the efforts on the development of CF algorithms focus on the effectiveness of the recommendations, while far too little attention has been paid to the problem of "Grey Sheep" users which is one of the classical challenges in collaborative filtering. "Grey Sheep" (GS) users [6,11] is a group of the users who may neither agree nor disagree with the majority of the users. They may introduce difficulties to produce accurate collaborative recommendations. Therefore, it has been pointed out that GS users must be identified from the data and treated individually for these reasons:

G. Cong et al. (Eds.): ADMA 2017, LNAI 10604, pp. 148–161, 2017.
https://doi.org/10.1007/978-3-319-69179-4_11

- They may leave negative impact on the quality of recommendations for the users [6–9,11,13,14] in the collaborative filtering algorithms.
- Collaborative filtering approaches do not work well for GS users [6–9,13]. GS users should be treated separately with another type of the recommendation models, such as content-based approaches.
- Due to the presence of GS users, the poor recommendations may result in critical consequences [6,9,11]: unsatisfied users, user defection, failure among learners, inaccurate marketing or advertising strategies, etc.

Most recently, we propose a novel approach to identify the GS users by the distribution of user-user similarities in the collaborative filtering approach [15]. However, one of the drawbacks in this approach is that the user-user similarity cannot be measured if two users did not rate the same items. Also, the user-user similarities may not be reliable if the number of co-rated items by two users is limited. In this paper, we propose an improved approach to alleviate this problem. More specifically, we propose to utilize histogram intersection to re-produce the distribution of user-user similarities.

Our contributions in this paper can be listed as follows:

- Our proposed approach improves the identification of GS users by the distribution of user-user similarities.
- It is the first time to compare different methods of identifying the GS users. The proposed approach in this paper was demonstrated as the best performing one based on the MovieLens 100 K rating data set.

2 Related Work

In this section, we introduce collaborative filtering first, discuss the characteristics of GS users, and finally introduce the corresponding progress of identifying the GS users.

2.1 Collaborative Filtering

Rating prediction is a common task in the recommender systems. Take the movie rating data shown in Table 1 for example, there are four users and four movies. The values in the data matrix represent users' rating on corresponding movies. We have the knowledge about how the four users rate these movies. And we'd like to learn from the knowledge and predict how the user U_4 will rate the movie "Harry Potter 7".

Collaborative filtering [11,14] is one of the most popular and classical recommendation algorithms. There are memory-based collaborative filtering, such as the user-based collaborative filtering (UBCF) [12], and model-based collaborative filtering, such as matrix factorization. In this paper, we focus on the UBCF since it suffers from the problem of GS users seriously.

The assumption in UBCF is that a user's rating on one movie is similar to the preferences on the same movie by a group of K users. This group of the

Table 1. Example of a movie rating data

	Pirates of the Caribbean 4	Kung Fu Panda 2	Harry Potter 6	Harry Potter 7
U_1	4	4	1	2
U_2	3	4	2	1
U_3	2	2	4	4
U_4	4	4	1	2

users is well known as K nearest neighbors (KNN). Namely, they are the top-K users who have similar tastes with a given user. Take Table 1 for example, to find the KNN for user U_4, we observe the ratings given by the four users on the given movies except "Harry Potter 7". We can see that U_1 and U_2 actually give similar ratings as U_4 – high ratings (3 or 4-star) on the first two movies and low rating on the movie "Harry Potter 6". Therefore, we infer that U_4 may rate the movie "Harry Potter 7" similarly as how the U_1 and U_2 rate the same movie.

To identify the KNN, we can use similarity measures to calculate user-user similarities or correlations, such as the cosine similarity shown by Eq. 1.

$$sim(U_i, U_j) = \frac{\overrightarrow{R_{U_i}} \bullet \overrightarrow{R_{U_j}}}{\|\overrightarrow{R_{U_i}}\|_2 \times \|\overrightarrow{R_{U_j}}\|_2} \tag{1}$$

We use a rating matrix similar to Table 1 to represent our data. $\overrightarrow{R_{U_i}}$ and $\overrightarrow{R_{U_j}}$ are the row vectors for user U_i and U_j respectively, where the rating is set as zero if a user did not rate the item. The size of these rating vectors is the same as the number of movies. In Eq. 1, the numerator represents the dot product of the two user vectors, while the denominator is the multiplication of two Euclidean norms (i.e., L2 norms). The value of K in KNN refers to the number of the top similar neighbors we need in the rating prediction functions. We need to tune up the performance by varying different numbers for K.

Once the KNN are identified, we can predict how a user rates one item by the rating function described by Eq. 2.

$$P_{a,t} = \bar{r}_a + \frac{\sum\limits_{u \in N} (r_{u,t} - \bar{r}_u) \times sim(a, u)}{\sum\limits_{u \in N} sim(a, u)} \tag{2}$$

where $P_{a,t}$ represents the predicted rating for user a on the item t. N is the top-K nearest neighborhood of users a, and u is one of the users in this neighborhood. The sim function is a similarity measure to calculate user-user similarities or correlations, while we use cosine similarity in our experiments. Accordingly, $r_{u,t}$ is neighbor u's rating on item t, $\bar{r}_a$ is user a's average rating over all items, and $\bar{r}_u$ is u's average rating.

This prediction function tries to aggregate KNN's ratings on the item t to estimate how user a rates t. However, the predicted ratings may be not accurate if user a is a GS user, since the user similarities or correlations between a and his or her neighbors may be very low. From another perspective, if a GS user is selected as one of the neighbors for a common user, it may result in odd recommendations or predictions since GS users may have unusual tastes on the items.

2.2 Grey Sheep Users

Due to the fact that UBCF takes advantage of the user-user similarities to produce the recommendations, the user characteristics in the collaborative filtering techniques become one of the key factors that can affect the quality of recommendations. McCrae et al. categorize the users in the recommender systems into three classes [11]: "the majority of the users fall into the class of *White Sheep* users, where these users have high rating correlations with several other users. The *Black Sheep* users usually have very few or even no correlating users, and the case of black sheep users is an acceptable failure[1]. The bigger problem exists in the group of *Grey Sheep* users, where these users have different opinions or unusual tastes which result in low correlations with many users; and they also cause odd recommendations for their correlated users". Therefore, Grey Sheep (GS) user usually refers to "a small number of individuals who would not benefit from pure collaborative filtering systems because their opinions do not consistently agree or disagree with any group of people [6]".

There are two significant characteristics of GS users indicated by the related research: On one hand, *GS users do not agree or disagree with other users* [7,11]. Researchers believe GS users may fall on the boundary of the user groups. Ghazanfar et al. [7,8] introduces a clustering technique to identify the GS users, while Gras et al. [9] reuses the outlier detection based on the user's rating distributions. On the other hand, *GS users may have low correlations with many other users, and they have very few highly correlated neighbors* [6].

2.3 Identification of Grey Sheep Users

There are several research [6,11,13,14] that point out the problem of GS user, define or summarize the characteristics of GS users, but very few of the existing work were made to figure out the solutions to identify GS users.

By paying attention to the first characteristics of GS users mentioned in Sect. 2.2, researchers believe GS users may fall on the boundary of the user groups. Ghazanfar et al. [7,8] proposes a clustering technique to identify the GS users, while they define improved centroid selection methods and isolates the GS users from the user community by setting different user similarity thresholds. The main drawback in their approach is the difficulty to find the optimal number

[1] The problem of black sheep users is caused by the situation that we do not have rich or even no rating profiles for these users. It is acceptable failure since the problem can be alleviated or solved if these users will continue to leave more ratings on the items.

of clusters, as well as the high computation cost to end up convergence in the clustering process, not to mention the unpredictable varieties by initial settings and other parameters in the technique. In their experiments, they demonstrate that content-based recommendation algorithms can be applied to improve the recommendation performance for the GS users. By contrast, Gras et al. [9] reuses the outlier detection based on the distribution of user ratings. They additionally take the imprecision of ratings (i.e., prediction errors) into account. However, the rating prediction error can only be used to evaluate whether a user is a GS user, it may not be appropriate to utilize it to identify GS users. It is because GS user is not the only reason that leads to large prediction errors. In other words, a user associated with large prediction errors is not necessary to be a GS user.

Another characteristics is that *GS users may have low correlations with many other users, and they have very few highly correlated neighbors* [6]. Most recently, we made the first attempt to take advantage of this characteristics to identify the GS users by the distribution of user-user similarities in the collaborative filtering approach [15]. More specifically, we statistically analyze a user's correlations with all of the other users, figure out bad and good examples, and reuse the outlier detections to identify potential GS users. Note that our work is different from the Gras et al. [9]'s work, since they stay to work on the distribution of user ratings, while we exploit the distribution of user similarities.

However, one of the drawbacks in the approach [15] is that the user-user similarity cannot be measured if two users did not rate the same items. Also, the user-user similarities may not be reliable if the number of co-rated items by two users is limited. In this paper, we propose an improved approach to alleviate this problem.

3 Methodologies

We first briefly introduce the basic solution proposed in [15]. Afterwards, we introduce and discuss the proposed approach to improve the basic solution in this section.

3.1 Basic Solution by the Distribution of User Similarities

As mentioned in [6], White Sheep users are the common users that have high correlations with other users. Namely, we can find a set of good KNN for White Sheep users. By contrast, GS users have correlations with other users but most of the correlations are relatively low. The basic solution in [15] relies on the following assumptions: A White Sheep user usually has higher correlations with other users, therefore its distribution of user similarities is expected to be left-skewed and the frequency at higher similarities should be significantly larger. In terms of the GS users, we do not have many high correlations with other users, and most of the user similarities are low. In short, the distribution of user similarities for GS users may have the following characteristics:

- It is usually a right-skewed distribution.
- The descriptive statistics of the user similarities, such as the first, second and third quartiles (q1, q2, q3), as well as the mean of the correlations, may be relatively smaller, since GS users have low correlations with other users.

Therefore, the basic solution in [15] can be summarized by the following four steps: distribution representations, example selection, outlier detection and examination of GS users.

Distribution Representations. The first step is to obtain user-user similarities and represent the distribution of user similarities for each user in the data set. We use the cosine similarity described by Eq. 1 to calculate the user-user similarity between every pair of the users. Note that the similarity of two users may be zero if there are no co-rated items by them. We remove the zero similarities from the distribution, since we only focus on the known user-user similarities in our data.

Table 2. Example of distribution representations

User	q1	q2	q3	Mean	STD	Skewness
40459	0.051	0.089	0.133	0.098	0.060	0.964
7266	0.028	0.056	0.091	0.064	0.045	1.245
34975	0.128	0.181	0.243	0.193	0.093	0.671
34974	0.093	0.149	0.209	0.156	0.084	0.568
34977	0.047	0.077	0.121	0.112	0.115	2.516
...	...	...	...	...	...	...

As a result, we are able to obtain a list of non-zero user-user similarities for each user. We further represent each user by the descriptive statistics of his or her distribution of the user similarities, including, q1, q2, q3, mean, standard deviation (STD) and skewness, as shown by Table 2.

Example Selection. Outlier detection [5,10] refers to the process of the identification of observations which do not conform to an expected pattern or other items in a data set. Thus it has been selected to distinguish GS users from other users in our approach. Gras et al. [9]'s work also points out that the identification of GS users is closely related to the outlier detection problem in data mining.

To apply the outlier detection, we need to select *good* (i.e., White Sheep users) and *bad* (i.e., potential GS users) examples in order to construct a user matrix similar to Table 2. This step is necessary especially when there are large scale of the users in the matrix. We suggest to filter the users by the descriptive statistics of their similarity distributions, such as the first quartile (q1), the second quartile (q2), the third quartile (q3), as well as mean of the similarity values, etc. More specifically, the bad examples could be selected by the following constraints:

- **Low similarity statistics**: In this case, q1, q2, q3 and mean may be much smaller than other users. We can select a lower-bound as the threshold. For example, if a user's mean similarity is smaller than *the first quartile* of mean similarities (i.e., the list of mean values over all of the users), this user is selected as one of the bad examples. The constraints could be flexible. They can be applied to the mean similarity only, or they could be applied to any subsets of {q1, q2, q3, mean} at the same time.
- **The degree of skewness**: This time, we apply a constraint on the skewness. For example, if a user's skewness value in his or her similarity distribution is larger than *the third quartile* of skewness values over all of the users, this user may be selected as one of the bad examples. It is because GS users may have very few highly correlated neighbors, and most of their user correlations are pretty low, which results in a heavily right-skewed similarity distribution.

Note that the constraints could be flexible or strict. The best choice may vary from data to data.

Outlier Detection. There are several outlier detection [5,10] techniques, such as the probabilistic likelihood approach, the clustering based or the density based methods, etc. We adopt a density based method which relies on the local outlier factor (LOF) [3]. LOF is based on the notion of local density, where locality is given by the $\mathbb{k}$ nearest neighbors[2] whose distance is used to estimate the density. The nearest neighbor, in our case, can be produced by using distance metrics on the feature matrix, while the feature matrix is the distribution representation matrix as shown in Table 2. By comparing the local density of a user to the local densities of his or her neighbors, one can identify regions of similar density, and the users that have a substantially lower density than their neighbors can be viewed as the outliers (i.e., the GS users) finally. Due to that the distances among the users are required to be calculated, we apply a normalization to the matrix in Table 2 in order to make sure all of the columns are in the same scale.

A user will be viewed as a common user if his or her LOF score is close to the value of 1.0. By contrast, it can be an outlier (i.e., potential GS user) if the LOF score is significantly larger or smaller than 1.0. We set a threshold for the LOF score, and tune up the results by varying the values of $\mathbb{k}$ and the LOF threshold in our experiments in order to find qualified GS users as many as possible. Note that, not all of the identified outliers are GS users, since it is possible to discover the outliers from the good examples too. We only consider the outliers from the bad examples as GS users in our experiments.

[2] We use $\mathbb{k}$ to distinguish it from the K in KNN based UBCF algorithm.

Examinations. With different values of $\mathbb{k}$ and the LOF threshold, we are able to collect different sets of the users as the GS users. We use the following approaches to examine the quality of the GS users:

- The recommendation performance for the group of GS users by collaborative filtering must be significantly worse than the performance for the White Sheep users. More specifically, the average rating prediction errors (see Sect. 4.1) based on the rating profiles associated with these GS users must be significantly higher than the errors that are associated with non-GS users. If the prediction errors for GS users and the remaining group of the users are close, we will perform two-independent sample statistical test to examine the degree of significance.
- We additionally visualize the distribution of similarities for GS users, in comparison with the one by non-GS users. The distribution of user similarities for GS and White sheep users are right and left-skewed respectively.

We tune up the values of $\mathbb{k}$ and the LOF threshold to find GS users as many as possible. But note that GS users are always a small proportion of the users in the data.

3.2 Improved Approach by Histogram Intersection

The basic solution by the distribution of user similarities is highly dependent with the user-user similarities and the distribution of these similarity values. However, there is a well-known drawback in the similarity calculations (such as the cosine similarity or the Pearson correlations) – the similarity between two users can be obtained only when they have co-rated items. Also, the similarity value may be not that reliable if the number of co-rated items is limited.

Therefore, we seek solutions to improve the quality of user-user similarities. One of the approaches is to generate user-user similarities by the histogram intersections [2] based on the distribution of cosine similarities. More specifically, we use cosine similarity to calculate the user-user similarity values first. As a result, each user can be represented by the distribution of similarities between other users and him or her. We can represent this distribution by a histogram which is constructed by N bins. Each bin can be viewed as a bar in the histogram. In our experiment, we use 40 bins with distance of 0.025 (i.e., the range is [0, 1] which represents the similarity). Furthermore, the similarity between two users can be re-calculate by the similarity between two histograms. Histogram intersection becomes one of the ways to measure the similarity between two histograms.

An example can be shown by Fig. 1. The blue and orange regions represent two histograms, while the pink areas stand for the histogram intersections. Larger the pink area is, more similar two histograms will be.

Assume there are two users u_1 and u_2. We use I and M to represent the histogram representation of u_1 and u_2's distribution of user-user similarities. These similarity values are obtained by the cosine similarity in UBCF.

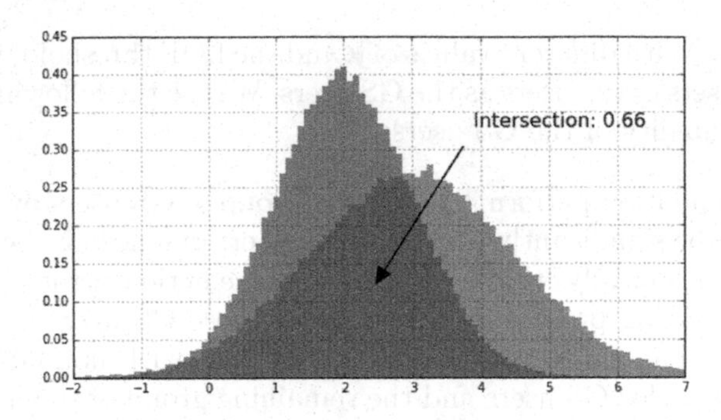

Fig. 1. Example of histogram intersections

The similarity between u_1 and u_2 by the histogram intersection can be simply re-calculated by:

$$sim(u_1, u_2) = \frac{\sum_{j=1}^{N} Min(I_j, M_j)}{\sum_{j=1}^{N} M_j} \tag{3}$$

where N represents the number of bars or bins in the histogram. I_j and M_j indicate the frequency value in the jth bar or bin in histogram I and M respectively. The function Min is used to get the minimal value between I_j and M_j. By this way, we can still calculate the similarity between two users, even if they do not have co-rated items.

4 Experiments and Results

4.1 Experimental Settings

We use the MovieLens 100 K rating data set[3] which is a movie rating data available for research. In this data, we have around 100,000 ratings given by 1,000 users on 1,700 movies. We simply split the data into training and testing set, where the training set is 80% of the whole data. Each user has rated at least 20 movies. We believe these users have rich rating profiles, and black sheep users are not included in this data.

We apply our proposed methodologies on the training set to identify GS users, and examine them by the recommendation performance over the test set. To obtain the prediction errors, we apply UBCF described by Eq. 2 as the collaborative filtering recommendation algorithm. In UBCF, we adopt the cosine similarity to measure the user-user similarities, and vary different value of K ($K = 100$ is the besting setting in our experiments) in order to find the best KNN. The recommendation performance is measured by mean absolute error

[3] https://grouplens.org/datasets/movielens/100k/.

(MAE) which can be depicted by Eq. 4. T represents the test set, where $|T|$ denotes the total number of ratings in the test set. $R_{a,t}$ is the actual rating given by user a on item t. (a, t) is the <user, item> tuple in the test set. $P_{a,t}$ is the predicted rating by the function in Eq. 2. The "abs" function is able to return the absolute value of the prediction error.

$$MAE = \frac{1}{|T|} \sum_{(a,t) \epsilon T} abs(P_{a,t} - R_{a,t}) \tag{4}$$

4.2 Results and Findings

We follow the four steps in Sect. 3 to identify the GS users from the training set. As mentioned in the Sect. 3.1, it is flexible to set different constraints to select good and bad examples. In our experiments, we tried both strict and loose constraints. The strict constraints can be described as follows: we go through the distribution representation matrix, and select the bad examples (i.e., potential GS users) if his or her q1, q2 and mean similarity value is smaller than the first quartile of the q1, q2 and mean distribution of all the users. According, the loose constraints will seek the bad examples by using the filtering rule that q1, q2 and mean similarity value is smaller than the second or the third quartile of the q1, q2 and mean distribution of all the users. However, there is not clear pattern to say which constraint is better. In our experiments, the loose constraints can help find more GS users if we use the basic solution in Sect. 3.1, while the strict constraint is the better one if we use the improved approach discussed in Sect. 3.2. In the following paragraphs, we only present the optimal results based on the corresponding constraints. The group of bad examples is further filtered by the

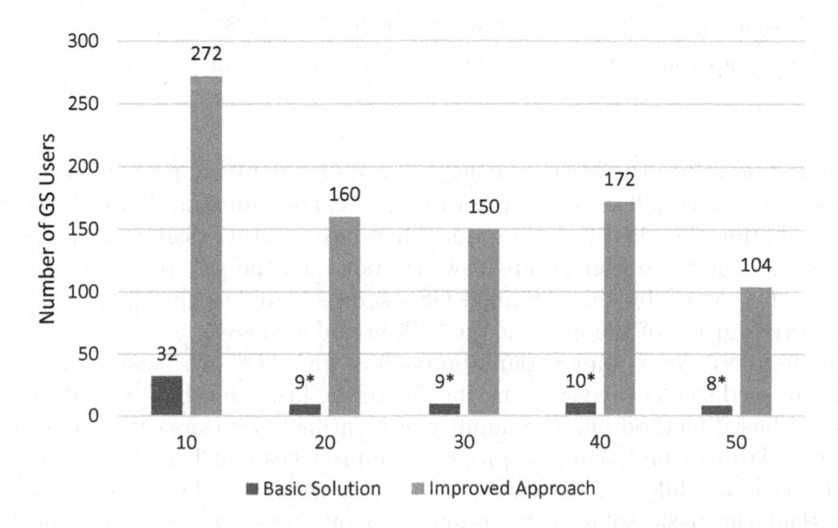

Fig. 2. The number of GS Users identified by different k values. Note that (*) tells that the two-independent sample statistical test was failed in that setting.

skewness – the users with skewness value smaller than the third quartile of the skewness distribution over all the users will be removed.

Afterwards, we blend the good and bad examples, and apply the LOF technique to identify the GS users. We tried different values of $\mathbb{k}$ and LOF thresholds in our experiments. The number of GS users identified can be shown by Fig. 2, while the x-axis represents $\mathbb{k}$ value. Note that the GS users are only the outliers from the bad examples. In addition, the group of GS users can only be considered as effective ones if the MAE of the rating profiles associated with these users is significantly larger than the MAE based on the non-GS users. We use 95% as confidence level, and apply the two-independent sample statistical test to examine whether they meet this requirement.

Based on the Fig. 2, we can observe that more GS users can be identified if we use the improved approach which utilizes the histogram intersection to produce user-user similarities. More specifically, by varying different value of $\mathbb{k}$ and LOF thresholds, we can only find qualified GS users by setting $\mathbb{k}$ as 10 in the basic solution. The results based on other $\mathbb{k}$ values failed the statistical tests, which tells that the MAE value by these GS users in UBCF is not significantly larger than the MAE obtained from non-GS users.

In addition, the statistical tests are all passed when we vary the $\mathbb{k}$ value in the improved approach discussed in Sect. 4. However, the difference between the MAE values by the GS users and non-GS users could be very small. Therefore, we decide to choose the result by using $\mathbb{k}$ as 50 as the optimal result, while the MAE by GS users is 0.810 and it is 0.760 for the non-GS users.

Table 3. MAE results

	All users	Good examples	Bad examples	Remaining users	GreySheep
Basic solution	0.765	0.766	0.763	0.762	0.844
Improved approach	0.765	0.766	0.777	0.760	0.810

Table 3 describes the MAE evaluated based on the rating profiles in the test set associated with different groups of the users. The "remaining users" refer to users excluding the identified GS users. There are no statistically differences on MAE values for these user groups if we do not take the group of GS uses into account. The MAE by the identified GS users is significantly higher than the one by other group of the users at the 95% confidence level.

Furthermore, we compare our approaches with the two existing methods which are used to identify GS users: the clustering based method [8] and the distribution based method [9]. The number of identified GS users can be described by Fig. 3. We can find that our proposed approaches can beat the clustering-based method, while the distribution-based method is able to find more GS users than the basic solution we propose in our previous research. The best performing solution is still the one that we utilize the histogram intersection

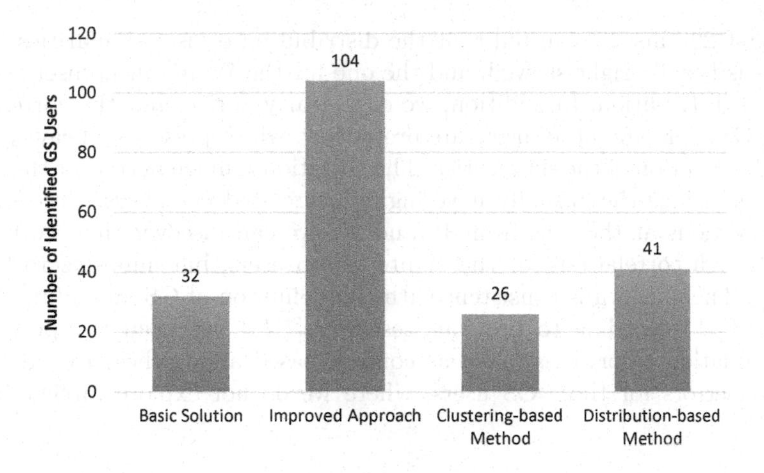

Fig. 3. Comparison between our approaches and existing methods

to calculate the user-user similarities. Keep in mind that the complexity of our proposed approach is much lower than these two existing methods, since we only need to apply the outlier detection techniques after the example selections.

We look into the characteristics of identified GS and White Sheep users. We select two GS users and two White Sheep users as the representatives, visualize the distribution of user similarities, as shown in Fig. 4. The bars in slate blue and coral present the histograms for two users, while the bars in plum capture the overlaps between two histograms. The x-axis is the bins of the similarities, while we put the similarity values (in range [0, 1]) into 40 bins with each bin size as 0.025. The y-axis can tell how many similarity or correlation values that fall in corresponding bins. These distributions of user similarities are produced by the histogram intersection – that's the reason why the similarity values are not that close to 1.0.

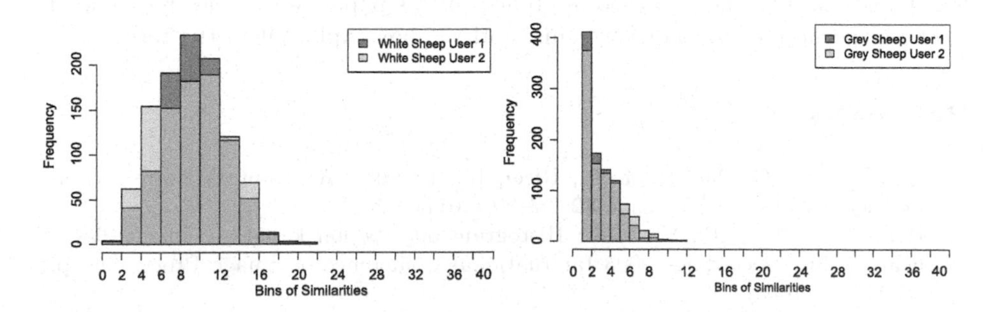

Fig. 4. Visualization of the similarity distributions

We can observe that the distributions for both GS and White Sheep users are right-skewed, if we take all of the 40 bins into consideration. While focusing on the first 20 bins, we can tell that the distribution of user similarities by the GS users is heavily right-skewed, and the one for the White Sheep users is close to normal distribution. In addition, we can clearly notice that the correlations between GS users and other users are pretty low, which presents a heavily right-skewed distribution of the similarities. The situation is much better for the White Sheep users, since they usually have highly correlated neighbors. According to the observations at the bins from 12 and 20, we can discover that we have at least 300 high correlations for the White Sheep users, but almost zero for the GS users. This pattern is consistent with the definition of GS and White Sheep users in [11]. According to previous research [7,11], we need to apply other recommendation algorithms (such as content-based approaches) to reduce the prediction errors for these GS users, where we do not explore further in this paper.

5 Conclusions

In this paper, we improve the approach of identifying Grey Sheep users based on the distribution of user similarities by utilizing the histogram intersection to better produce user-user similarities. The proposed approach in this paper is much easier than the previous methods [7,9,11] in terms of the complexity. The improved approach that utilizes the histogram intersection is demonstrated as the best performing solution in comparison with the existing methods to identify Grey Sheep users in the MovieLens 100 K data.

In our future work, we will apply the proposed approach to other data sets rather than the data in the movie domain. Also, we believe the same approach can also be used to identify *Grey Sheep items* in addition to the Grey Sheep users. The problem of Grey Sheep users may not only happen in the traditional recommender systems, but also exist in other types of the recommender systems. For example, in the context-aware recommender systems [1,16,17], the definition of Grey Sheep users could be the users who have unusual tastes in specific contextual situations. The proposed approach in this paper can be easily extended to these special recommender systems, and we may explore it in the future.

References

1. Adomavicius, G., Mobasher, B., Ricci, F., Tuzhilin, A.: Context-aware recommender systems. AI Magazine **32**, 67–80 (2011)
2. Barla, A., Odone, F., Verri, A.: Histogram intersection kernel for image classification. In: Proceedings 2003 International Conference on Image Processing, p. III-513-16 (2003)
3. Breunig, M.M., Kriegel, H.P., Ng, R.T., Sander, J.: LOF: identifying density-based local outliers. In: ACM Sigmod Record, vol. 29, pp. 93–104. ACM (2000)
4. Burke, R.: Hybrid recommender systems: survey and experiments. User Modeling User-adapted Interact. **12**(4), 331–370 (2002)
5. Chandola, V., Banerjee, A., Kumar, V.: Anomaly detection: a survey. ACM Comput. Surv. (CSUR) **41**(3), 15 (2009)

6. Claypool, M., Gokhale, A., Miranda, T., Murnikov, P., Netes, D., Sartin, M.: Combining content-based and collaborative filters in an online newspaper. In: Proceedings of ACM SIGIR Workshop on Recommender Systems, vol. 60 (1999)
7. Ghazanfar, M., Prugel-Bennett, A.: Fulfilling the needs of gray-sheep users in recommender systems, a clustering solution. In Proceedings of the 2011 International Conference on Information Systems and Computational Intelligence, pp. 18–20 (2011)
8. Ghazanfar, M.A., Prügel-Bennett, A.: Leveraging clustering approaches to solve the gray-sheep users problem in recommender systems. Expert Syst. Appl. **41**(7), 3261–3275 (2014)
9. Gras, B., Brun, A., Boyer, A.: Identifying grey sheep users in collaborative filtering: a distribution-based technique. In: Proceedings of the 2016 Conference on User Modeling Adaptation and Personalization, pp. 17–26. ACM (2016)
10. Hodge, V., Austin, J.: A survey of outlier detection methodologies. Artificial Intell. Rev. **22**(2), 85–126 (2004)
11. McCrae, J., Piatek, A., Langley, A.: Collaborative filtering. http://www.imperialviolet.org (2004)
12. Resnick, P., Iacovou, N., Suchak, M., Bergstrom, P., Riedl, J.: Grouplens: an open architecture for collaborative filtering of netnews. In: Proceedings of the 1994 ACM Conference on Computer Supported Cooperative Work, pp. 175–186. ACM (1994)
13. Ruiz-Montiel, M., Aldana-Montes, J.F.: Semantically enhanced recommender systems. In: Meersman, R., Herrero, P., Dillon, T. (eds.) OTM 2009. LNCS, vol. 5872, pp. 604–609. Springer, Heidelberg (2009). doi:10.1007/978-3-642-05290-3_74
14. Su, X., Khoshgoftaar, T.M.: A survey of collaborative filtering techniques. Adv. Artificial Intell. **2009**, 4 (2009)
15. Zheng, Y., Agnani, M., Singh, M.: Identifying grey sheep users by the distribution of user similarities in collaborative filtering. In: Proceedings of The 6th ACM Conference on Research in Information Technology. ACM (2017)
16. Zheng, Y., Burke, R., Mobasher, B.: Splitting approaches for context-aware recommendation: an empirical study. In: Proceedings of the 29th Annual ACM Symposium on Applied Computing, pp. 274–279. ACM (2014)
17. Zheng, Y., Mobasher, B., Burke, R.: CSLIM: contextual SLIM recommendation algorithms. In: Proceedings of the 8th ACM Conference on Recommender Systems, pp. 301–304. ACM (2014)

Social Network and Social Media

A Feature-Based Approach for the Redefined Link Prediction Problem in Signed Networks

Xiaoming Li[1], Hui Fang[2(✉)], and Jie Zhang[1]

[1] School of Computer Science and Engineering, Nanyang Technological University, Singapore, Singapore
{lixiaoming,zhangj}@ntu.edu.sg

[2] Shanghai University of Finance and Economics, Shanghai, China
fang.hui@mail.shufe.edu.cn

Abstract. Link prediction is an important research issue in social networks, which can be applied in many areas, such as trust-aware business applications and viral marketing campaigns. With the rise of signed networks, the link prediction problem becomes more complex and challenging as it introduces negative relations among users. Instead of predicting future relation for a pair of users, however, the current research focuses on distinguishing whether a certain link is positive or negative, on the premise of the link existence. The situation that two users do not have relation (i.e., no-relation) is also not considered, which actually is the most common case in reality. In this paper, we redefine the link prediction problem in signed social networks by also considering "no-relation" as a future status of a node pair. To understand the underlying mechanism of link formation in signed networks, we propose a feature framework on the basis of a thorough exploration of potential features for the newly identified problem. We find that features derived from social theories can well distinguish these three social statuses. Grounded on the feature framework, we adopt a multiclass classification model to leverage all the features, and experiments show that our method outperforms the state-of-the-art methods.

Keywords: Signed social network · Link prediction · No-relation

1 Introduction

Signed network, literally denotes the network which contains both positive and negative links among nodes. Under this network structure, the relationship between online users can be 'friend' or 'foe', and 'trust' or 'distrust', etc. The rise of this new type of user relationship networks has broad implications for real businesses nowadays, and more and more online systems such as Slashdot (friend or foe, www.slashdot.org), Epinions (trust or distrust, www.epinions.com) and even Facebook have adopted signed network structure and features. For example, Facebook introduced a handful of new reaction buttons, besides 'like' option, to show different attitudes such as 'angry' and 'sad' to other users. In other words,

G. Cong et al. (Eds.): ADMA 2017, LNAI 10604, pp. 165–179, 2017.
https://doi.org/10.1007/978-3-319-69179-4_12

relationship between online users are not only limited to positive (e.g. friend and trust) anymore, but try to add more alternatives to be consistent with the human relationship in real life.

The increasing interest in signed social networks has brought great impact on many traditional research topics, one of which is link prediction. Link prediction, which aims to infer the formation of a possible link in the near future, is well studied in the last few years as its significant contributions to improve and enhance online experiences [11,14], in the form of further facilitating applications such as recommenders for products or friends [22] and social networks [23]. Link prediction in unsigned networks aims to predict the future connection status between two nodes, or a dyad, either linked or not. On the contrary, connection status of two nodes in signed networks could be positive, negative and no-relation, which increases the difficulty of link prediction.

On the other hand, link sign prediction in signed networks focuses on predicting signs of existing links [4,7,9,18], which is a binary classification problem. In other words, this kind of research basically ignores the no-relation status. The rationale behind this assumption might be two parts: (1) if no-relation is considered as a link status, positive or negative ones will be highly imbalanced and sparse contrasted with no-relation, and thus most of the machine learning methods incline to predict the dyad status to be no-relation for the sake of maximum accuracy; (2) for some traditional applications (e.g. spam email detection), the assumption of link existence is inherently satisfied.

However, most link prediction applications in signed networks cannot be simply treated as the sign prediction problem as aforementioned. For example, in voting prediction, a user might vote a candidate entity as positive or negative, but in most cases, the user will choose not to vote the entity. Therefore, the existing methods cannot be directly adopted to address these kinds of applications. To conclude, the previous approaches mainly suffer from two issues: (1) they ignore the no-relation status, which accounts for the majority of the real relationship in signed social networks; (2) instead of predicting the future relationship status of any two nodes, these approaches actually consider a static network as they assume the existence of links with uncertain signs.

In this paper, we design a link prediction approach for signed social networks, to predict future link status, which could be positive, negative or no-relation. We take no-relation and future status into consideration, which are the two major differences compared with the previous studies in the literature. To address the problem, we first thoroughly explore features which may potentially affect future link status of any two nodes, especially to investigate the related features which can well distinguish no-relation from the other two statuses. On the basis of the thorough feature exploration, we propose a feature framework, where features of different categories try to distinguish the three link statuses, for link prediction in signed networks, and design a simple but effective feature selection mechanism to show how to apply the feature framework in real applications. With the feature framework, we establish a feature based link prediction model in signed networks. Experiments verify the effectiveness of the proposed feature framework, and demonstrate that our model outperforms the state-of-the-art approaches for both the measurements of Positive AUC and Generalized AUC [18].

To summarize, the main contributions of our work are two-folds:

1. We redefine the link prediction problem by taking an initial step to consider 'no-relation' as a future dyad status for link prediction in signed networks. Besides, we focus on predicting the future relationship status of any two nodes, rather than distinguishing the sign of a certain link in a static network, which is the common setting of the current approaches [4,7,9,18].
2. We propose a structured feature framework for the redefined problem on the basis of a thorough feature analysis to reveal the underlying mechanism regarding link formation in signed networks. The feature framework, grounded on both well-known theories and sound observations, can serve as a guidance for research on the new problem.

2 Related Work

We summarize the literature into two parts: (1) link prediction in unsigned networks; and (2) link prediction in signed networks.

Link prediction in unsigned networks has been well studied during the past decade. Existing methods can be divided into two classes: unsupervised and supervised ones. Unsupervised methods consist of neighbor-based metrics and path-based metrics [11]. They calculate a "link formation score" for each pair of nodes to indicate their possibility to be linked or not in the near future. Popular neighbor-based metrics include: the number of common neighbors [1], Adamic/Adar Index [1], Jaccard Coefficient [11], Preferential attachment [16] and Resource Allocation Index [24]. These ranking metrics are derived from neighborhood structure. Meanwhile, the features related to the path between two nodes in a network structure are also used to compute the similarities of node pairs, like Katz [8], Vertex Collocation Profile [12] and ProfFlow [13]. Popular supervised methods include: feature-based classification models [2], and latent feature models [15]. However, link prediction in unsigned networks considers only two possible future connection statuses of two nodes, i.e., linked or not-linked, while in signed networks, three connection statuses are possible: positive, negative, and no-relation. Therefore, all the features and metrics need to be re-investigated in the signed network scenario, because neighbors and paths can be negative in signed networks.

Existing attempts for signed link prediction mainly focus on how to distinguish positive and negative links, and topology feature-based approaches are dominant in the literature. For example, based on balance theory and status theory, Leskovec et al. [9] identify triangle-based features of each two users and their common neighbours to predict the sign (i.e., positive or negative) between each two users. Besides, k-cycle-based features are proposed in [4] where triangle-based features ($k = 3$) are specially explored. It also shows that longer cycles

($k = 5$) significantly benefit sign prediction, while the performance gain is not significant beyond $k = 5$. Papaoikonomou et al. [17] leverage the pattern of frequent subgraph among node pairs, to predict link status. Another type of popular methods is the low-rank models. For example, Hsieh et al. [7] verify that signed networks naturally present a low-rank structure, and a matrix factorization model is proposed to infer link signs. However, all the aforementioned methods assume the existence of links with uncertain signs. Song and Meyer [18] also adopt a low-rank model to infer link signs, which learns the latent features by minimizing the generalized AUC loss. Although it takes the no-relation into consideration, the major purpose of the work is to distinguish positive and negative link status, and the no-relation information is only used in the training period of the model.

We can see that the no-relation status is ignored in the existing studies, while no-relations actually account for the majority of the real relationship in signed social networks. Besides, we need to re-investigate the features adopted in the literature for link prediction. We then can design more specific approaches for the newly redefined problem (i.e., link prediction in signed network) on the basis of a better feature design and problem analysis.

3 Redefined Link Prediction Problem

Here we first formalize our redefined link prediction problem in signed social networks. Specifically, let $G = (V, E^P, E^N, X)$ denote a signed social network, where V is the node set; E^P is the set of positive links and E^N is the set of negative links; X refers to the set of no-relation. $G_t = (V, E_t^P, E_t^N, X_t)$ denotes the snapshot of the network at time t. Our research question is: *given a series of network snapshots G_0, G_1, ..., G_t, and any node pair (i, j) (i.e. dyad) where $x_{ij} \in X_t$, to predict the connection status of x_{ij} at time $t+1$, which can belong to E_{t+1}^P, E_{t+1}^N or X_{t+1}.*

To be more specific, in this paper, we aim to solve three questions as below:

1. What has been changed with the introduction of no-relation?
2. What is the link formation mechanism behind signed network evolution? or which specific features influence link formation in signed networks?
3. How to evaluate link prediction performance involving no-relation?

To address these questions, we propose a link prediction approach in signed networks, including a feature framework of six categories, a feature-based link prediction model, and a feature selection mechanism.[1] We also introduce two techniques to address the data imbalance issue for link prediction in signed networks.

[1] The preliminary version [10] of our work has been published at AAAI 2017 as a student abstract.

4 Feature Framework

4.1 Data Description

We first introduce the datasets used in this work. We obtain two publicly available datasets[2] with the signed structure, i.e., Epinions and Slashdot. In both social networks, users can establish trust and distrust relationship, i.e., positive or negative links with other users. Table 1 provides descriptive statistics for these datasets.

Table 1. Dataset statistics

	Epinions	Slashdot
Users	131, 828	82, 140
Users with degree ≥ 10	17, 664	17, 794
Users with degree ≥ 25	9, 134	8, 325
User pairs with positive links	717, 667	425, 072
User pairs with negative links	123, 705	124, 130
User pairs with no-relations	$1.7 * 10^{10}$	$6.7 * 10^{9}$

From Table 1, we can quickly summarize two general data patterns that occur in signed networks: (1) sparsity: a signed network is quite sparse, as there are no more than 10.2% users with degree ≥ 25 in both real social networks; and (2) imbalance: the number of linked pairs is smaller than pairs of no-relation by four orders of magnitude. Meanwhile, the number of positive and negative links are also imbalanced.

4.2 Feature Design Principles

The design of a feature set is always the keystone of a feature-based prediction method. Link prediction in unsigned networks adopts features, such as the number of common friends, to distinguish linked and not-linked status corresponding to those with the value of 1 and 0 in unsigned networks. On the contrary, previous link prediction in signed networks designs features to discriminate positive links and negative links, with the value of 1 and -1 respectively. In our newly identified link prediction problem in signed networks, as three link statuses (with the value of 1, 0 and -1) are involved, the feature set should be re-considered.

An ideal feature is expected to well distinguish the three link statuses, however, as indicated before, there is no previous feature study considering the three statuses together. To fill this gap, we propose a feature framework for the new research problem, aiming to serve as a guidance and elicit more related research. We not only adopt existing features in previous studies [9,20] on both unsigned and signed network scenarios, but also derive new features based on our analysis

[2] https://snap.stanford.edu.

and observations. We then combine and summarize these features into six major categories, and then explore the influence of each category on link formation in signed networks. We also indicate how our features have addressed our problem uniquely. All features are discussed in the following section.

4.3 Feature Definition

Balance Theory [3] can be simply explained as "my friend's friend is my friend", or "my enemy's enemy is my friend". In other words, two users will more likely become friends if they have many common friends. Thus, we define **pp** and **pp_ratio** to represent the number and the fraction of the common 'positive' neighbors (friends) between two users, and **nn** and **nn_ratio** to represent the number and the fraction of the 'negative' neighbors (enemies). Besides, given two users, we also check the number of their neighbors which are one's friends but the other's enemies, denoted by **pn**. Based on balance theory, a large **pn** represents a high chance for a negative link establishment. Then we define a feature **bal_diff** to check the contradiction within the balance theory. When user i and j have largely the same number of 'friends' and 'enemies', a positive or negative sign will eventually make the network unbalanced, on the basis of social balance theory. In this research, balance theory is extended such that the no-relation status can make the graph more balanced.

Status Theory [5,9] refers to that, a positive link $i \rightarrow j$ indicates the node status of j is higher than i. Therefore, given a common neighbor w, if link $i \rightarrow w$ and $w \rightarrow j$ are both positive, link $i \rightarrow j$ is more likely to be positive since the status of j is higher than i. Thus, given two users i and j, we define **sta_diff_p** (**sta_diff_n**) as the number of their neighbors which indicate j's status is higher (lower) than i. Then **sta_diff** is used to represent the status difference between these two users, while **sta_diff_ratio** takes into account the fraction of the status difference. Status theory is extended in this research, as two users tend to have no-relation if they have nearly equal status.

Reciprocity [6] is the tendency that two nodes with bidirectional links between each other always have the same sign. In Epinions dataset, 83.5% of user pairs with bidirectional links have the same sign. Therefore, we can infer the status of the link $i \rightarrow j$ by the sign of the backward link $j \rightarrow i$, named as **reciprocity**. This feature will be useful if there exist many bidirectional links in the network.

Rich-get-richer [21] indicate two active or popular users will more likely get linked. Thus, we derive 10 features to capture this phenomenon. Given two user i and j, we define **out_p** and **out_p_ratio** to represent the number and the fraction of positive links coming from i. Similarly, **out_n** takes into account the negative links. Meanwhile, two features **in_p** and **in_p_ratio** are the number and the fraction of the positive links pointed to j. Besides, if i's out_p_ratio and j's in_p_ratio are both high, there will be more likely a positive link between i and j. However, if i's out_p_ratio (or out_n_ratio) is large and the j's in_n_ratio (or in_p_ratio) is large, which indicates that i is active and tends to trust others, but j is not trustworthy and distrusted by others, there will be no-relation between i and j. Therefore, we adopt 4 features **prprs**, **prnrs**, **nrprs**, **prnrs** to capture those observations and check whether those features can indicate no-relation status.

Clustering [11] adopts the similar insight with link prediction in unsigned networks. It measures per-dyad side features like the number of common neighbors. The underlying assumption is that two users likely get connected if they have many common neighbors. In this work, we use 5 features **CN** [11], **Katz** [8], **JC** [11], **PA** [16], **Status Similarity** [19]. In signed network, a smaller feature in this category indicates a higher chance to have no-relation.

Frequent Subgraph [4,9] considers triads constructed by users i, j and their common neighbors. Each link between a user and its neighbor may have two directions, i.e., forward and backward, meanwhile it can be positive or negative. Therefore, based on the combination of the directions and signs, there will be 16 types of triads. We use p and n to represent the positive and negative signs, and f and b denote the link direction, so these triads represent as $ppff$, $pnfb$, etc., as shown in Fig. 1.

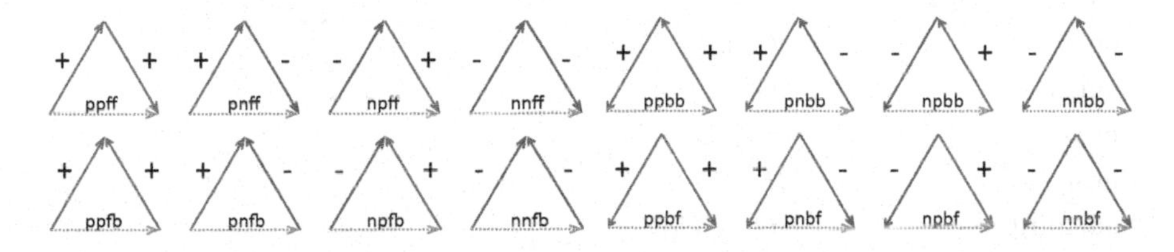

Fig. 1. The sixteen triads are fundamental and crucial units for network topology analysis [4,9].

In summary, balance theory, status theory and reciprocity mainly capture the signed network characteristics; rich-get-richer considers per-node side features meanwhile clustering captures per-dyad side features; and frequent subgraph captures relatively larger scale topological features.

We adopt the following notation: let $1, 2, \cdots, N$ be N users; Let S_{ij} be the link sign from user i toward user j; Let O_i, I_i be user i's outgoing and incoming link sets, respectively. Specifically, O_i^+, I_i^+ represent the positive link sets, and O_i^-, I_i^- the negative link sets; Let C_{ij} be the set of the common neighbors between users i and j; ppff, pnff, ... are basic triad units. Table 2 summarizes the full list of the features we derived from social theories.

Table 2. Features derived from social theories

Feature	Notation
Balance theory	
pp	ppff + ppfb + ppbf + ppbb
nn	nnff + nnfb + nnbf + nnbb
pn	$\|C\|$− pp − nn
pp_ratio	pp/$\|C\|$
nn_ratio	nn/$\|C\|$
bal_diff	pp + nn − pn
Status theory	
sta_diff	sta_diff_p − sta_diff_n
sta_diff_p	ppff + nnbb + pnfb + npbf
sta_diff_n	nnff + ppbb + npfb + pnfb
sta_diff_ratio	sta_diff_p/(sta_diff_p + sta_diff_n)
Reciprocity	
Reciprocity	S_{ji}
Rich-get-richer	
out_p	$\|O_i^+\|$
out_n	$\|O_i^-\|$
in_p	$\|I_j^+\|$
in_n	$\|I_j^-\|$
out_p_ratio	$\|O_i^+\|/\|O_i\|$
in_p_ratio	$\|I_j^+\|/\|I_j\|$
prprs	$(\|O_i^+\|/\|O_i\|) * (\|I_j^+\|/\|I_j\|)$
prnrs	$(\|O_i^+\|/\|O_i\|) * (\|I_j^-\|/\|I_j\|)$
nrnrs	$(\|O_i^-\|/\|O_i\|) * (\|I_j^-\|/\|I_j\|)$
nrprs	$(\|O_i^-\|/\|O_i\|) * (\|I_j^+\|/\|I_j\|)$
Clustering	
cn	$\|C\|$
Katz	ppff + pnff + npff + nnff
Jaccard coefficient	$\|C_{ij}\|/(\|O_i\| + \|O_j\| + \|I_i\| + \|I_j\|)$
Preferential attachment	$(\|O_i\| + \|I_i\|) * (\|O_j\| + \|I_j\|)$
Status similarity	$1/(\delta(i) + \delta(j) - 1)$, $\delta(i) = \|I_i^+\| + \|O_i^-\| - \|O_i^+\| - \|I_i^-\|$

5 Signed Link Prediction

The proposed feature-based model can be stated as:

$$\min_{\alpha,\beta} \sum l(S_{ij}, L(\alpha f(u_i, u_j) + \beta u_{ij})) + \frac{\lambda_1}{2}\|\alpha\|_2^2 + \frac{\lambda_2}{2}\|\beta\|_2^2 \qquad (1)$$

where S_{ij} is the ground truth of link status; L(·) is the link prediction function; $l(\cdot,\cdot)$ is the loss function; u_{ij}, u_i and u_j are corresponding features; $\frac{\lambda_1}{2}\|\alpha\|_2^2$ and $\frac{\lambda_2}{2}\|\beta\|_2^2$ are regularizers.

Link prediction function L(·) is a function with a value of 1, −1 or 0, which represents positive, negative or no-relation respectively. Under this setting, a multiclass classification algorithm should be adopted, such as SVM and decision trees. In this paper, we adopt the multinomial logistic regression model.

Loss function $l(\cdot,\cdot)$ is user-specified and application-depended. For example, in recommendation systems, loss for an incorrectly predicted −1 or 0 can be relatively low, while the loss for a mistakenly identified 1 should be set high, as the prediction performance on 1 is of the most importance.

Features mainly consist of two parts: per-dyad side, u_{ij} is the feature set of dyad (i,j), such as **sta_diff**, **pp**, **pp_ratio**; per-node side, $f(u_i, u_j)$ is the function to leverage the node-side features of u_i and u_j, like **prprs**, which is the multiplication of i's **out_p_ratio** and j's **in_p_ratio**.

5.1 Feature Selection Mechanism

Before using these potential predictive features, we need to investigate whether these features can distinguish different classes, or have different influences on each class. As aforementioned, an ideal feature is expected to well distinguish the three link statuses. For each specific application, to effectively adopt the feature framework, we should firstly investigate whether each theoretically sound feature is suitable for the real application.

To do this, we statistically check the mean of each feature for each class (i.e. positive, negative or no-relation), taking Epinions dataset as an example. We conduct One-Way ANOVA test on $M_1(f_i)$, $M_0(f_i)$ and $M_{-1}(f_i)$, where f_i denotes a feature and $M(\cdot)$ denotes its average value. The corresponding null hypothesis is: $H_0 : M_1(f_i) = M_0(f_i) = M_{-1}(f_i)$. If a feature is rejected at the significance level of $\alpha = 0.01$ with p-value < 0.001, the feature is dropped in this application. We choose a smaller significance level and p-value here in order to strongly support the alternate hypothesis, i.e., try to select the features which can better distinguish those three classes. Figure 2 shows the kernel smoothed density distribution of some selected features. As shown in Fig. 2, we can easily understand why these features work. For example, in the figure, "prprs", the multiplication of node i's outgoing positive link ratio and node j's incoming positive link ratio, shows totally different distributions for different link status.

5.2 Handling Imbalance Issue

The imbalance issue is one of the most serious problems for link prediction in signed networks, where the number of no-relation pairs $\gg$ the number of positive links $\gg$ the number of negative links, as shown in Table 1. Therefore, if we conduct experiments based on the full dataset, positive and negative links will be almost ignored as there are overwhelmingly no-relation pairs. Meanwhile,

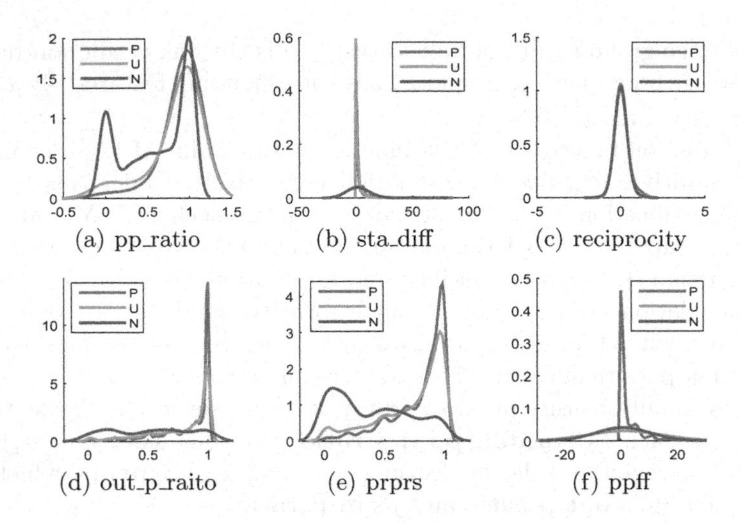

Fig. 2. Kernel smoothed density distribution of selected features. Details of features are given in Table 2. P, U and N in legends represent positive, no-relation and negative link respectively. [Figures are best viewed in color]

the accuracy performance can reach to almost 100% since the learning model can predict all pairs as no-relation.

Thus, the first technique is under sampling, where we randomly draw a set of links including an equal amount of samples for each link status. Specifically, since the negative link is the smallest in quantity, for every negative link, we randomly draw a positive link and a no-relation pair.

Another technique is to use the measurements of ranking rather than the accuracy metric, to evaluate the prediction performance of different methods. As we have three statuses in signed networks, we aim to rank user pairs based on the predicted link scores, and make positive links be ranked higher at the top, and negative links lower in the bottom of the list. That is, the ranking order comes as positive, no-relation, negative ones in the list. In this work, we adopt GAUC (Generalized AUC) [18], an extension of AUC, as a metric which can measure the ranking performance for three statuses. A score of 1.0 indicates a perfect classifier while 0.5 represents a random classifier. This metric is insensitive to the imbalanced data.

6 Experiments

In this section, we conduct experiments using Epinions and Slashdot datasets to demonstrate the effectiveness of our feature framework, and the superiority of our link prediction approach compared to the state-of-the-art methods.

6.1 Experimental Setting

First, we aim to design an experimental environment which can well represent the link prediction scenario in reality. One realistic scenario is that, given a certain number of user pairs which currently are not linked, we predict which user pair will form a positive link or a negative link, or still have no-relation in the future. Since Epinions dataset contains a timestamp for each generated link, we can use it to test the performance of our method on future link prediction. We divide the dataset into three parts by timestamps: $T1$, $T2$ and $T3$, which represent the past, current and future respectively. Because there are 578,996 links marked with the timestamp 1/10/2001, we treat this timestamp as "past" and use those links to derive training features. And we split the rest into two parts: training set consists of the links (or user pairs) formed during $T2$ (till 4/30/2002); and the testing set includes the links formed in the period of $T3$ (till 8/12/2003) but the features are measured in both periods of $T1$ and $T2$. Although there is an overlap between the feature sets of the training and testing data, this experiment setting is exactly consistent with the training and prediction process in the real-world scenarios. Based on the undersampling method discussed in Sect. 5.2, we sample a positive link and a no-relation dyad for every negative link, to ensure the training and testing data are balanced. Specifically, the number of samples in $T2$ and $T3$ are 18489 and 15741 respectively.

Since there is no timestamp information in the Slashdot dataset, we adopt the traditional training/testing setting [7,9], i.e., by randomly drawing a sample of user dyads including positive, negative and no-relation ones with the equal amount as training and testing set respectively. We adopt 10-fold cross validation for this dataset. Besides, to measure the effectiveness and robustness of our approach, we test our approach under different settings. We filter user pairs by different number of common neighbors, i.e., minimum as 1, 10 and 25. In the following experiments, if not stated otherwise, we show the result on user pairs with at least 1 neighbor since this is a more general setting.

Evaluation Metrics. As discussed in Sect. 5.2, we will use measurements of ranking rather than of accuracy. We adopt the generalized AUC (i.e., GAUC) metric [18], which is defined as:

$$GAUC = \frac{1}{|P|+|N|}(\frac{1}{|U|+|N|}\sum_{a_i \in P}\sum_{a_s \in U \cup N} I(L(a_i) > L(a_s))$$
$$+\frac{1}{|P|+|N|}(\frac{1}{|U|+|P|}\sum_{a_j \in N}\sum_{a_t \in U \cup P} I(L(a_j) < L(a_t))$$

where $|P|$, $|N|$, $|U|$ represent the number of positive links, negative links, and no-relations, respectively; a represents a link; and L$(\cdot)$ is the link score function. GAUC is an extension of AUC, and provides a ranking metric considering the three link statuses.

The other metric is PAUC (positive AUC), which measures the classification performance over positive links and non-positive links. We do not show NAUC (negative AUC) results here since NAUC results can be derived from GAUC and AUC, where GAUC can be treated as the weighted sum of PAUC and NAUC.

Benchmark Approaches. We compare our approach with the following methods:
• Common Neighbors (CN) [11], ranks user pairs by the number of their common neighbors, including both the positive and negative common neighbors.
• Katz [8], ranks user pairs by the number of directional routes. CN and Katz are always used as the baselines for link prediction.
• Triad and Degree feature-based method(All23) [9], adopts total 23 features based on topolgy triads and user degree, and use regression as the learning model.
• Matrix Factorization (MF) [7], learns latent features from the social matrix with non-zero elements, and rank user pairs by the multiplication of latent features. This is a point-wise approach for sign prediction.
• Optimizing GAUC (OptGAUC) [18], optimizes the GAUC metric through matrix factorization with the ranking order of the positive, no-relation, and negative links. It is a pair-wise approach for sign prediction.

6.2 Prediction Performance

As shown in Table 3, we can see that our approach outperforms others on both GAUC and PAUC metrics, under different dataset settings.

Table 3. Performance comparison

	Epinions						Slashdot					
Method	cn ≥ 1		cn ≥ 10		cn ≥ 25		cn ≥ 1		cn ≥ 10		cn ≥ 25	
	GAUC	PAUC	GAUC	PAUC	GAUC	PAUC	GAUC	PAUC	GAUC	PAUC	GAUC	PAUC
CN	0.576	0.587	0.566	0.57	0.545	0.556	0.625	0.649	0.643	0.697	0.645	0.699
Katz	0.591	0.592	0.602	0.571	0.549	0.55	0.661	0.665	0.697	0.752	0.712	0.758
MF	0.654	0.645	0.657	0.651	0.662	0.658	0.552	0.545	0.565	0.558	0.561	0.559
OptGAUC	0.715	0.72	0.709	0.702	0.719	0.712	0.603	0.599	0.613	0.601	0.619	0.605
Triads + Degree	0.742	0.736	0.825	0.777	0.838	0.798	0.878	0.853	0.887	0.862	0.892	0.865
Ours	**0.827**	**0.799**	**0.834**	**0.791**	**0.840**	**0.807**	**0.923**	**0.904**	**0.924**	**0.897**	**0.926**	**0.898**

CN and Katz do not perform well because they do not differentiate the signs of neighbors and links. Thus we conclude that traditional link prediction methods cannot directly be applied for link prediction in signed networks. OptGAUC outperforms MF, indicating that no-relation information used in OptGAUC helps improve its link prediction. As the PAUC measurement can be treated as an extended version of AUC in traditional unsigned networks, we can thus conclude that negative links as new information for link prediction can improve the performance of predicting positive links in signed networks.

6.3 Feature Framework Analysis

In order to check the effectiveness of each feature category and the robustness of the feature framework, we first check the prediction performance of each feature category. As shown in Table 4, the learning model with any feature category outperforms random guessing (GAUC = 0.5). Specifically, the best performance in terms of both GAUC and PAUC is given by balance theory and frequent subgraph for Epinions dataset, meanwhile, cluster and frequent subgraph outperform others in Slashdot dataset. The full model which adopts all features shows the best performance, demonstrating the effectiveness of feature combinations.

Table 4. The effectiveness of each feature category

Feature category	Epinions		Slashdot	
	GAUC	PAUC	GAUC	PAUC
Balance theory	0.733	0.734	0.808	0.794
Status theory	0.72	0.703	0.647	0.639
Reciprocity	0.538	0.549	0.622	0.645
Rich-get-richer	0.738	0.715	0.691	0.682
Cluster	0.617	0.638	0.820	0.807
Frequent subgraph	0.799	0.776	0.843	0.825
Full model	**0.827**	**0.799**	**0.924**	**0.904**

Furthermore, we evaluate the performance of our approach by removing the features of a certain category each time. The experimental results are shown in Table 5, where each row represents the prediction results in terms of GAUC and PAUC after dropping features of the corresponding category. We can see that the performance of each incomplete framework is worse than the complete one involving the features of all the six categories.

Table 5. The effectiveness of the framework by removing one feature category

Feature category	Epinions		Slashdot	
	GAUC	PAUC	GAUC	PAUC
Balance theory	0.801	0.774	0.921	0.902
Status theory	0.818	0.789	0.902	0.872
Reciprocity	0.822	0.791	0.905	0.874
Rich-get-richer	0.816	0.795	0.921	0.903
Cluster	0.823	0.798	0.875	0.867
Frequent subgraph	0.824	0.796	0.916	0.895
Full model	**0.827**	**0.799**	**0.924**	**0.904**

6.4 Link Prediction Model Comparison

We also examine the performance of different multiclass classifiers for the link prediction function in our feature-based approach. This test is conducted within the WEKA framework, and each model adopts the default parameter setting. Experimental results in Table 6 indicate that our approach with the multinomial logistic regression model achieves the best performance in term of GAUC.

Table 6. GAUC performance on different multiclass classification models

Classifier	Epinions	Slashdot
SVM	0.497	0.583
Decision tree	0.679	0.865
Adaboost	0.684	0.794
Naïve Bayes	0.796	0.866
Random forest	0.81	0.798
Multinomial logistic regression	**0.827**	**0.924**

7 Conclusions and Future Work

In this paper, we redefine the link prediction problem in signed networks, by considering no-relation as a future status of a user pair. For this problem, we further propose a feature framework grounded on thorough theoretical analysis, and design a feature selection mechanism and feature-based prediction model to apply the framework in real applications. We also indicate two techniques to handle the imbalance issue for link prediction in signed networks. Experiments in Epinions and Slashdot dataset show that our model outperforms existing methods in terms of GAUC and PAUC, and also demonstrate that each category of our feature framework and our choice of the multinomial logistic regression model are effective.

This work takes an initial step to consider 'no-relation' as a future status for link prediction in signed networks, and our proposed feature framework can serve as a leading guidance for research on the new problem. For future work, firstly, we will investigate more real-world datasets to further evaluate the significance of the new problem and the effectiveness of our approach. Secondly, we will explore more features and design an advanced model specifically for link prediction in signed networks.

Acknowledgement. This work was supported by the National Natural Science Foundation of China (Grant No. 71601104).

References

1. Adamic, L.A., Adar, E.: Friends and neighbors on the web. Soc. Netw. **25**(3), 211–230 (2003)
2. Al Hasan, M., Chaoji, V., Salem, S., Zaki, M.: Link prediction using supervised learning. In: SDM (2006)
3. Antal, T., Krapivsky, P.L., Redner, S.: Social balance on networks: the dynamics of friendship and enmity. Phys. D Nonlinear Phenom. **224**(1), 130–136 (2006)
4. Chiang, K.Y., Natarajan, N., Tewari, A., Dhillon, I.S.: Exploiting longer cycles for link prediction in signed networks. In: CIKM, pp. 1157–1162. ACM (2011)
5. Davis, J.A., Leinhardt, S.: The structure of positive interpersonal relations in small groups (1967)
6. Falk, A., Fischbacher, U.: A theory of reciprocity. Games Econ. Behav. **54**(2), 293–315 (2006)
7. Hsieh, C.J., Chiang, K.Y., Dhillon, I.S.: Low rank modeling of signed networks. In: SIGKDD, pp. 507–515. ACM (2012)
8. Katz, L.: A new status index derived from sociometric analysis. Psychometrika **18**(1), 39–43 (1953)
9. Leskovec, J., Huttenlocher, D., Kleinberg, J.: Predicting positive and negative links in online social networks. In: WWW, pp. 641–650. ACM (2010)
10. Li, X., Fang, H., Zhang, J.: Rethinking the link prediction problem in signed social networks. In: AAAI (2017)
11. Liben-Nowell, D., Kleinberg, J.: The link-prediction problem for social networks. JAIST **58**(7), 1019–1031 (2007)
12. Lichtenwalter, R.N., Chawla, N.V.: Vertex collocation profiles: subgraph counting for link analysis and prediction. In: WWW, pp. 1019–1028. ACM (2012)
13. Lichtenwalter, R.N., Lussier, J.T., Chawla, N.V.: New perspectives and methods in link prediction. In: SIGKDD, pp. 243–252. ACM (2010)
14. Lü, L., Zhou, T.: Link prediction in complex networks: a survey. Phys. A Stat. Mech. Appl. **390**(6), 1150–1170 (2011)
15. Menon, A.K., Elkan, C.: Link Prediction via Matrix Factorization. In: Gunopulos, D., Hofmann, T., Malerba, D., Vazirgiannis, M. (eds.) ECML PKDD 2011. LNCS, vol. 6912, pp. 437–452. Springer, Heidelberg (2011). doi:10.1007/978-3-642-23783-6_28
16. Newman, M.E.: Clustering and preferential attachment in growing networks. Phys. Rev. E **64**(2), 025102 (2001)
17. Papaoikonomou, A., Kardara, M., Tserpes, K., Varvarigou, T.A.: Predicting edge signs in social networks using frequent subgraph discovery. IEEE Internet Comput. **18**(5), 36–43 (2014)
18. Song, D., Meyer, D.A.: Recommending positive links in signed social networks by optimizing a generalized auc. In: AAAI, pp. 290–296 (2015)
19. Symeonidis, P., Tiakas, E.: Transitive node similarity: predicting and recommending links in signed social networks. WWW **17**(4), 743–776 (2014)
20. Tang, J., Chang, Y., Liu, H.: Mining social media with social theories: a survey. ACM SIGKDD Explor. Newsl. **15**(2), 20–29 (2014)
21. Tufekci, Z.: Who acquires friends through social media and why? "rich get richer" versus "seek and ye shall find". In: ICWSM (2010)
22. Zhang, J., Lv, Y., Yu, P.: Enterprise social link recommendation. In: CIKM, pp. 841–850. ACM (2015)
23. Zhao, T., Zhao, H.V., King, I.: Exploiting game theoretic analysis for link recommendation in social networks. In: CIKM, pp. 851–860. ACM (2015)
24. Zhou, T., Lü, L., Zhang, Y.C.: Predicting missing links via local information. EPLB-Condens. Matter Complex Syst. **71**(4), 623–630 (2009)

From Mutual Friends to Overlapping Community Detection: A Non-negative Matrix Factorization Approach

Xingyu Niu, Hongyi Zhang(✉), Micheal R. Lyu, and Irwin King

Department of Computer Science and Engineering,
The Chinese University of Hong Kong, Shatin, Hong Kong
neoxyniu@gmail.com, {hyzhang,lyu,king}@cse.cuhk.edu.hk

Abstract. Community detection provides a way to unravel complicated structures in complex networks. Overlapping community detection allows nodes to be associated with multiple communities. *Matrix Factorization (MF)* is one of the standard tools to solve overlapping community detection problems from a global view. Existing MF-based methods only exploit link information revealed by the adjacency matrix, but ignore other critical information. In fact, compared with the existence of a link, the number of mutual friends between two nodes can better reflect their similarity regarding community membership. In this paper, based on the concept of mutual friend, we incorporate *Mutual Density* as a new indicator to infer the similarity of community membership between two nodes in the MF framework for overlapping community detection. We conduct data observation on real-world networks with ground-truth communities to validate an intuition that mutual density between two nodes is correlated with their community membership cosine similarity. According to this observation, we propose a *Mutual Density based Non-negative Matrix Factorization (MD-NMF)* model by maximizing the likelihood that node pairs with larger mutual density are more similar in community memberships. Our model employs stochastic gradient descent with sampling as the learning algorithm. We conduct experiments on various real-world networks and compare our model with other baseline methods. The results show that our MD-NMF model outperforms the other state-of-the-art models on multiple metrics in these benchmark datasets.

Keywords: Complex networks · Overlapping community detection · Matrix factorization

1 Introduction

In complex networks, there usually exist groups inside which nodes are connected more densely with one another than with the nodes outside. These groups of nodes are called *communities* [13]. In reality, these groups usually have physical meanings such as members of the same organization, scientists with publications in the same area, or proteins sharing the same function. Thus, uncovering

G. Cong et al. (Eds.): ADMA 2017, LNAI 10604, pp. 180–194, 2017.
https://doi.org/10.1007/978-3-319-69179-4_13

such latent communities in complex networks has attracted great research interests in the past decade [11]. Classic methods assume communities are mutually exclusive, i.e., each node of a network belongs to one and only one community. However, in real-world complex networks like social networks and biological networks, such community membership restriction does not apply because a node may have multiple characteristics and thus belongs to multiple communities. As a result, a more challenging problem named *overlapping community detection* has been introduced in recent years [31].

Matrix Factorization (MF), as one of the standard framework to solve the problem of overlapping community detection, detects communities from a global view [31]. Taking the adjacency matrix G of the given network as input, MF-based models assign the number of communities in advance, and seek out a node-community weight matrix F, which matches the information revealed by the input as accurately as possible. Early work [23,29] simply aims to approximate G entry by entry with FF^T, which only makes use of the mathematical representation of adjacency matrix, but ignores its physical meaning. The most obvious information an adjacency matrix provides is the link information. Thus, recent work [32,35] assumes that nodes sharing more communities have a higher probability to be linked and formulates the problem with a generative objective function. In other words, a link can be regarded as an indicator to reflect the similarity of community membership between two nodes.

However, a link is not a perfect indicator for two major reasons. First, it is common that two nodes sharing several communities do not have a link between them, or two nodes with no common community are connected. A survey conducted on Facebook [9] shows that edges between two individuals from different communities outnumber edges connecting users in the same community. For example, a salesperson may make connections with many strangers to sell his products, and the establishment of links between salespeople and customers does not indicate any similarity between their community memberships. In cases like these, links become noise instead of evidence. Second, a link is a binary indicator in an unweighted network. Given two linked node pairs with no other information at all, it is impossible to distinguish which one is more similar.

Inspired by the definition of tie strength [12], we incorporate a more powerful indicator, which is the number of mutual friends between two nodes, to reflect their community membership similarity. The definition of tie strength reveals that the stronger tie the two nodes own, the larger overlap in their friendship circles they will have. This idea can be incorporated into our matrix factorization framework for overlapping community detection, which meets the common sense that the more communities two nodes share, the more mutual friends they will have. For example, if two individuals attended the same class in high school, joined the same basketball team, and work in the same company now, they should know many mutual friends in different communities, i.e., their ego-networks (friend circles) are densely overlapped. Compared to a link, the number of mutual friends is no longer a binary indicator and it provides more confidence to predict the similarity of community membership between two nodes. However, it still suffers from several issues: the lack of friends of two nodes may limit the number of mutual friends between them, and communities with different sizes may contribute different numbers of mutual friends to each node pair. To handle these limitations, we incorporate *Mutual Density* as a more consistent indicator, which is defined as the Jaccard similarity of two nodes' ego-networks. Under the general description of "neighborhood similarity", the concept of mutual density has been applied in community detection under different assumptions [1,3,21,26,28]. However, none of these methods are based on matrix factorization and none of them use mutual density to measure the similarity of community membership between two nodes.

In this paper, we introduce mutual density and the number of mutual friends as the new indicators instead of links themselves for inferring community membership similarity in the matrix factorization framework. We conduct data observation on real-world networks with ground-truth communities to validate that mutual density is more consistent with community memberships similarity than the other two indicators. Thus, we formulate our *Mutual Density based Non-negative Matrix Factorization (MD-NMF)* model, which incorporates mutual density as the community similarity indicator and employs a novel objective function to ensure that a node pair with higher mutual density is more likely to have a higher community membership similarity. From a node's perspective, we ensure that it is more likely to join the same communities with its acquaintances than with its strangers. To solve the optimization problem, we apply projected stochastic gradient descent with sampling. By applying our model to real-world and open-source network datasets, we find that our new MD-NMF model outperforms several state-of-the-art methods on either modularity or F_1 score.

The main contributions of this paper are:

1. We incorporate *Mutual Density* as a new indicator to reflect the community membership similarity between two nodes in substitution for a link within the matrix factorization framework for overlapping community detection.
2. We find that there is consistency between the mutual density of two nodes and their community memberships similarity by empirically studying real-world networks with ground-truth communities.
3. We propose a novel *Mutual Density based Non-negative Matrix Factorization (MD-NMF)* model for overlapping community detection by formulating mutual density properly in the matrix factorization framework. Our model outperforms state-of-the-art baselines.

2 Definition and Data Observation

2.1 Problem Definition

Definition 1 (Community Detection). *Given an unweighted and undirected graph $G(V, E)$, community detection aims to find a communities set $S = \{C_i | C_i \neq \emptyset, C_i \neq C_j, 1 \leq i, j \leq p\}$ where C_i represents a community consisting a set of nodes, to maximizes a particular objective function f, i.e.,*

$$\max f(G, S), \tag{1}$$

where p is the number of communities.

Different from the traditional community detection problem, an overlapping community detection problem allows communities to overlap with each other. This relaxation enables the *Matrix Factorization* approach to be employed. In MF-based methods, the graph is represented by its adjacency matrix $G \in \{0,1\}^{n \times n}$, whose (i,j) entry indicates whether node i and node j are connected or not. The goal is to find a node-community weight matrix F, with its entry $F_{u,c}$ representing the weight of node u in community c, and apply F to approximate the adjacency matrix.

2.2 Indicator Definitions

To infer the community membership similarity between two nodes, we have mentioned three indicators in Introduction. They are link existence $l(u,v)$, the number of mutual friends $m(u,v)$ and mutual density $d(u,v)$, where u and v are both nodes in V. We formally define each of them as follows.

Definition 2 (Link Existence). *Given a graph $G(V,E)$ and two nodes $u, v \in V$, the link existence between u and v is*

$$l(u,v) = \begin{cases} 1 & if\ G_{uv} = 1, \\ 0 & else \end{cases}. \tag{2}$$

Definition 3 (The Number of Mutual Friends). *Given a graph $G(V,E)$ and two nodes $u, v \in V$, the number of mutual friends between u and v is*

$$m(u,v) = \mid \{i \mid (u,i) \in E\ and\ (v,i) \in E\} \mid . \tag{3}$$

Definition 4 (Mutual Density). *Given a graph $G(V,E)$ and two nodes $u, v \in V$, the mutual density between u and v is*

$$d(u,v) = \frac{\mid \{i \mid (u,i) \in E\ and\ (v,i) \in E\} \mid}{\mid \{j \mid (u,j) \in E\ or\ (v,j) \in E\} \mid}. \tag{4}$$

2.3 Data Observation

To validate (1) the number of mutual friends is better than a link in inferring community membership similarity, and (2) mutual density is more stable compared with the number of mutual friends, we conduct two experiments on two

Table 1. Dataset statistics. $|V|$: number of nodes, $|E|$: number of edges, $|C|$: number of ground-truth communities, D: average degree of nodes, M: average number of nodes per community, A average number of joined communities per node.

Dataset	|V|	|E|	|C|	D	M	A
Amazon	335k	926k	49k	3.38	100.0	14.83
DBLP	317k	1.0M	2.5k	4.93	429.8	2.57

large real-world networks with ground-truth communities [33]. Table 1 shows the statistics of these two networks, which are **Amazon** and **DBLP**.[1]

To quantify the community membership similarity between two nodes, we use *cosine similarity* as our measurement, which is defined as follows.

Definition 5 (Cosine Similarity of Community Membership). *Given a graph with p ground-truth communities $\{C_i|i = 1, 2, \cdots, p\}$, the cosine similarity of community membership $s(u, v)$ between u and v is*

$$s(u, v) = \frac{\boldsymbol{u} \cdot \boldsymbol{v}^T}{\|\boldsymbol{u}\|_2 \|\boldsymbol{v}\|_2}, \quad (5)$$

where $\boldsymbol{u} \in \mathcal{R}^p$ is the community membership vector of node u and u_i represents the weight u belongs to community C_i.

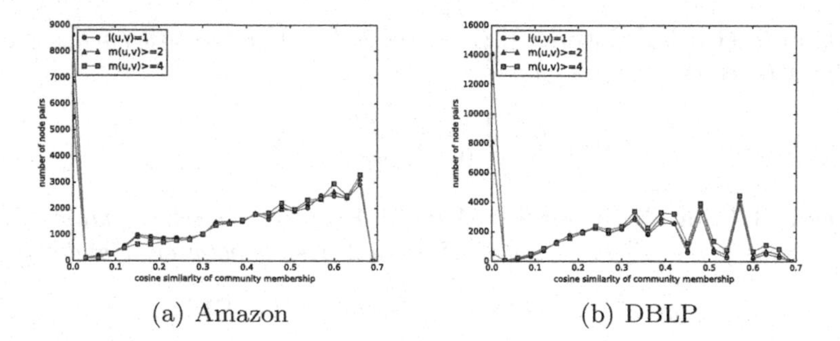

(a) Amazon (b) DBLP

Fig. 1. The number of sampled node pairs having a same value of cosine similarity

First, we randomly sample 100,000 node pairs with links as well as 100,000 node pairs with at least two or four mutual friends and compute the cosine similarity of community membership for each node pair. Figure 1 plots the number of 3 different types of node pairs with the same value of cosine similarity. We expect all three types of node pairs to share at least one community and thus to have non-zero cosine similarity. However, nearly 14,000 node pairs with links do not share any communities. The error rate is about 14%. On the other side, less than 8% of the node pairs with at least two mutual friends and only about 1% of the node pairs with at least four mutual friends are out of our expectation. When the value of cosine similarity is non-zero, all three types are pretty similar, and the number of node pairs with four mutual friends is slightly greater than the other types. Thus, the number of mutual friends is a more accurate and more flexible indicator compared to the existence of links.

Second, we compare the stability of indicator between the number of mutual friends and mutual density. A stable indicator is expected to be monotonic while community membership similarity increases. We sample 10,000 node pairs each

[1] http://snap.stanford.edu/data/.

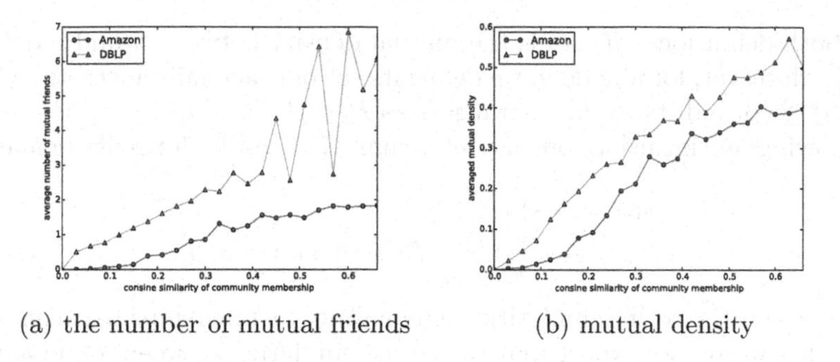

(a) the number of mutual friends (b) mutual density

Fig. 2. Averaged value of each indicator as a function of cosine similarity in community membership

time with a certain value of cosine similarity and calculate the average number of mutual friends and average mutual density of these node pairs. The result is shown in Fig. 2. We can see that on the DBLP data, the average number of mutual friends vibrates up and down while average mutual density is almost monotonic as cosine similarity increases. Thus, mutual density is a more stable indicator than the number of mutual friends to infer community membership similarity.

In summary, mutual density is the best indicator among all three indicators we mentioned with highest accuracy and stability.

3 Mutual Density Based NMF Model

3.1 Model Assumption

From the data observation, we can see that the cosine similarity of community membership between two nodes is correlated with their mutual density. It leads to the intuition of our model that two nodes with larger mutual density are more likely to have higher cosine similarity of community membership.

To formally illustrate our model assumption, we need to define two relationships between two nodes in the first place: α-acquaintance and β-stranger.

Definition 6 (α-acquaintance). *Given $\alpha \in [0,1]$, for two nodes $u, v \in V$, v is u's α-acquaintance if and only if*

$$d(u,v) \geq \alpha.$$

By the symmetry of $d(u,v)$, u is also v's α-acquaintance.

Definition 7 (β-stranger). *Given $\beta \in [0,1]$, for two nodes $u, v \in V$, v is u's β-stranger if and only if*

$$d(u,v) \leq \beta.$$

By the symmetry of $d(u,v)$, u is also v's β-stranger.

In both definitions, $d(u,v)$ is the mutual density between u and v defined in Eq. (4). Moreover, for a node u, we define its set of α-acquaintances as $A(u,\alpha) = \{i|d(u,i) \geq \alpha\}$ and its set of β-strangers as $B(u,\beta) = \{j|d(u,j) \leq \beta\}$.

Following our intuition, our model assumption can be formally defined as

$$\begin{aligned} &s(u,i) > s(u,j), \\ &\text{if } i \in A(u,\alpha),\ j \in B(u,\beta), \text{and } \alpha > \beta, \end{aligned} \tag{6}$$

where $s(u,i)$ is the cosine similarity of community memberships between u and i.

In other words, we expect that the cosine similarity between u and any of its α-acquaintances should be greater than the cosine similarity between u and any of its β-strangers. Adjusting α and β for different graphs enables us to make sure that the difference of cosine similarity is significant. If α is only slightly greater than β, we are not confident enough to make such assumption.

3.2 Model Formulation

In the MD-NMF model, we aim to find the node-community weight matrix F which maximizes the likelihood that every node in the graph has higher cosine similarity in community membership with all its α-acquaintances than with all its β-strangers. For each node u, we want to maximize

$$\mathcal{P}(\underset{u}{>}|F,\alpha,\beta) = \prod_{i \in A(u,\alpha)} \prod_{j \in B(u,\beta)} \mathcal{P}(s(u,i) > s(u,j)|F). \tag{7}$$

Given any two nodes $u, v \in V$, we can obtain their node-community weight vectors F_u, F_v from F. From the observation that the higher cosine similarity of community membership vectors between two nodes, the greater mutual density they will have, we define the probability that $s(u,i) > s(u,j)$ given the node-community membership matrix as

$$\mathcal{P}(s(u,i) > s(u,j)|F) = \sigma\left(\frac{F_u F_i^T}{\|F_u\|_2 \|F_i\|_2} - \frac{F_u F_j^T}{\|F_u\|_2 \|F_j\|_2}\right), \tag{8}$$

where σ is the sigmoid function $\sigma(x) = \frac{1}{1+e^{-x}}$. For simplicity, we define $\phi(i,j) = \frac{F_i F_j^T}{\|F_i\| \|F_j\|}$, so we have

$$\mathcal{P}(s(u,i) > s(u,j)|F) = \sigma(\phi(u,i) - \phi(u,j)). \tag{9}$$

Since the sigmoid function maps any real value into $(0,1)$, this probability approaches to 1 when $\phi(u,i) \gg \phi(u,j)$ and approaches to 0 when $\phi(u,i) \ll \phi(u,j)$.

By multiplying Eq. (7) for each node and combining Eqs. (8) and (9), we can derive the final learning objective of the MD-NMF model, which is

$$
\begin{aligned}
l(F) &= \max_{F \in R_+^{n \times p}} \log \prod_{u \in V} \mathcal{P}(\underset{u}{>} | F, \alpha, \beta) - \lambda \cdot reg(F) \\
&= \max_{F \in R_+^{n \times p}} \sum_{u \in V} \sum_{i \in A(u,\alpha)} \sum_{j \in B(u,\beta)} \log \mathcal{P}(s(u,i) > s(u,j) | F) \\
&\quad - \lambda \cdot reg(F) \\
&= \max_{F \in R_+^{n \times p}} \sum_{u \in V} \sum_{i \in A(u,\alpha)} \sum_{j \in B(u,\beta)} \log \sigma(\phi(u,i) - \phi(u,j)) \\
&\quad - \lambda \cdot reg(F),
\end{aligned}
\tag{10}
$$

where $reg(F)$ is a regularization term in order to prevent overfitting of F, and λ is the regularization parameter. For the simplicity of differentiation, we set $reg(F) = \|F\|_F^2$, which is the Frobenius norm of F.

3.3 Parameter Learning

To make our model scalable to large datasets, we employ the widely used paradigm of *Stochastic Gradient Descent (SGD)* as our learning algorithm. Also considering the non-negativity constraint, we apply a projected gradient method [18] which maps the vector with negative parameters back to the nearest point in the projected space. Following the learning objective l, we update the matrix F by

$$
\Theta_{t+1} = \max\{\Theta_t + \delta \frac{\partial l}{\partial \Theta}, 0\} , \tag{11}
$$

where δ is the learning rate and Θ can be any entry of matrix F.

Algorithm 1 describes the whole iterative process of parameter learning. In each iteration, the time complexity is $O(|E|p)$, where $|E|$ is the number of edges and p the number of communities. Because we need to save the whole node-community weight matrix F in memory, the space complexity of the algorithm is $O(|V|p)$, where V is the number of nodes. When V becomes too large, the algorithm needs huge memory to store the whole matrix F, which is the limitation of the algorithm. To scale this algorithm to billions of nodes, distributed storage and update of F should be considered.

Choosing the Number of Communities. Before running Algorithm 1, we need to set the number of communities p in advance. After conducting some experiments on small datasets, we find that if we set p to be larger than the intended p and learn the parameters accordingly, our detected communities contain the results we obtain with the intended p as well as some duplicated communities or trivial communities with few nodes. Thus, our strategy is to pick a relatively large p based on the number of nodes and edges in the network and further refine our results via merging or deletion.

Algorithm 1. Overlapping community detection using *MD-NMF*

Require: G, the adjacency matrix of original graph; α, the acquaintance threshold; β, the stranger threshold
Ensure: F, the node-community weight matrix
1: initialize F
2: compute initial loss
3: **repeat**
4: **for** $num\_samples = 1$ to $|E|$ **do**
5: sample node u from V uniformly at random
6: sample node i from u's α-acquaintances set $A(u, \alpha)$ uniformly at random
7: sample node j from u's β-strangers set $B(u, \beta)$ uniformly at random
8: **for** each entry Θ in F_i, F_j and F_k **do**
9: update Θ according to Equation (11)
10: **end for**
11: **end for**
12: compute loss
13: **until** convergence or *max_iter* is reached

Acquaintances and Strangers Sampling. For node $u \in V$ and any of its α-acquaintances i, if $\alpha > 0$, it is guaranteed that u and i have mutual friends. To find i, we first do a breadth-first search and group all u's neighbors as well as friends of these neighbors into a set. Then we filter out any node k with $d(u, k) < \alpha$ in this set and sample i from the remaining nodes uniformly at random. If u does not have any α-acquaintance, we sample another u and repeat the above process until we get a valid u. To sample the β-stranger of u, we simply sample a random node from graph until we get the β-stranger. From Table 1 we can see that in each graph, the average degree of nodes is much smaller than the number of edges. Thus the time complexity sampling acquaintances and strangers of a node remains constant.

Setting Membership Threshold. For each node, to determine whether it belongs to a particular community, our strategy is to set a membership threshold t for the node-community membership matrix, i.e., if $F_{u,k} \geq t$, we say that node u is associated with community k. t is a hyper-parameter which is tuned via experimental results.

4 Experiments

4.1 Dataset

The real-world datasets we use include the two large networks we have described in the data observation section, as well as six benchmark networks collected by Newman[2]. Table 2 lists the basic information of the six benchmark datasets. They are relatively small compared to the two large networks and have no ground-truth communities.

[2] http://www-personal.umich.edu/mejn/netdata.

Table 2. Statistics of six Newman's datasets. $|V|$: number of nodes, $|E|$: number of edges.

Dataset	|V|	|E|
Dolphins	62	159
Books about US politics (Books)	105	441
American college football (Football)	115	613
Network science	1,589	2742
Power grid	4,941	6,594
High-energy theory (High-energy)	8,361	15,751

4.2 Comparison Methods

For comparison, we select the following six baseline approaches, namely *Sequential Clique Percolation (SCP)* [16], *Demon* [8], *Bayesian Non-negative Matrix Factorization (BNMF)* [23], *Bounded Non-negative Matrix Tri-Factorization (BNMTF)* [36], *BigCLAM* [34], and *Preference-based Non-negative Matrix Factorization (PNMF)* [35]. Notice that the latter four approaches are also based on matrix factorization.

4.3 Evaluation Metrics

We use modularity as the evaluation metric for small datasets without ground-truth communities and F_1 score for large datasets with ground truth communities.

Modularity. The classic modularity is defined as

$$Q = \frac{1}{2|E|} \sum_{u,v \in V} (G_{u,v} - \frac{d(u)d(v)}{2|E|}) I_{u,v},$$

where $d(u)$ is the degree of node u, $G_{u,v}$ is the (u, v) entry of the adjacency matrix G, and $I_{u,v} = 1$ if u, v are in the same community otherwise 0 [20].

In the overlapping scenario, since a node pair may share more than one communities, a minor modification has been made by replacing $I_{u,v}$ with $|C_u \cap C_v|$, i.e., the number of overlapped community between u and v:

$$\hat{Q} = \frac{1}{2|E|} \sum_{u,v \in V} (G_{u,v} - \frac{d(u)d(v)}{2|E|}) |C_u \cap C_v|.$$

From the definition, we can see that greater value of modularity reveals denser connectivity within the detected communities because only linked node pairs sharing common communities contribute positively to the value. This metric has also been frequently used in previous MF-based works [34,35].

F_1 Score. The F_1 score of a detected community S_i is defined as the harmonic mean of

$$precision(S_i) = \max_j \frac{S_j^{'} \cap S_i}{|S_i|}$$

and

$$recall(S_i) = \max_j \frac{S_j^{'} \cap S_i}{|S_j^{'}|},$$

i.e.,

$$F_1 = \frac{precision(S_i) \cdot recall(S_i)}{precision(S_i) + recall(S_i)},$$

where $S_j^{'}$ is one of the given ground-truth communities. The overall F_1 score of the result of detected communities is the average F_1 score of all communities in the detected communities set.

4.4 Results

For the small networks, we set the learning rate θ as 0.5 and p ranging from 10 to 50. We assume each node joins at most 3 to 10 communities and set the threshold based on this assumption. For the large network datasets, we set θ much greater because the normalized term in cosine similarity limits the altered amount of weight in each gradient descent iteration. We set p ranging from 1,000 to 5,000 and assume that each node joins at most 100 communities. The maximum number of iteration is set to be 100, while in most cases F converges before reaching the iteration limit.

Table 3. Comparison of experiment results in terms of modularity.

Dataset	SCP	Demon	BNMF	BNMTF	BigCLAM	PNMF	MD-NMF
Dolphins	0.305	0.680	0.507	0.507	0.423	0.979	**1.019**
Books	0.496	0.432	0.461	0.492	0.592	0.864	**0.987**
Football	0.605	0.540	0.558	0.573	0.518	1.049	**1.163**
Network science	0.729	0.642	0.661	0.741	0.503	1.657	**1.695**
Power grid	0.044	0.195	0.342	0.368	1.010	1.105	**1.228**
High-energy	0.543	0.962	0.565	0.600	0.964	0.973	**1.031**

Table 3 shows the results in terms of modularity on six small benchmark networks without ground-truth communities. We can see that our MD-NMF model outperforms all baseline methods on all datasets on modularity, including *LC* that leverages the general concept of "neighborhood similarity" as well and *PNMF* that is also based on a pairwise objective function but employs links as the indicator.

Table 4. Comparison of experiment results in terms of F_1 score.

Dataset	SCP	BigCLAM	PNMF	MD-NMF
Amazon	0.0315	0.0441	0.0419	**0.0961**
DBLP	0.0967	0.0390	0.0985	**0.1013**

Table 4 shows the results on two large benchmark networks with ground-truth communities. We can see that only three of our comparison methods are able to scale to networks of such size. On both Amazon and DBLP dataset, our MD-NMF model prevails on the metric F_1 score.

5 Related Work

5.1 Community Detection

Community detection has been an important line of research in physics and computer science for a long period, and many different classes of approaches are proposed to solve this problem [11]. Apart from tradition graph partitioning/clustering approaches [15], modularity-based methods are particularly designed for community detection tasks [20]. As the most well-known quality function by far, modularity can be directly optimized. Since optimizing modularity has been proven to be an NP-complete problem [6], many heuristics are proposed to solve it in polynomial time [7,10,19]. However, these classic community detection algorithms have a severe limitation that a node belongs to one and only one community.

Until recently, major attention has been focused on the case where communities are allowed to be overlapped [31]. According to the general strategy, overlapping community detection methods can be classified into local methods and global methods. Local methods adopt divide-and-conquer which discovers communities in small subgraphs before merging small communities into larger ones based on some criteria [8,17,30]. Global methods employ stochastic block models [2,14] or community affiliation models [32] which aim to figure out the relationship between nodes and communities in a macro view. As one of the major frameworks, *Matrix Factorization (MF)* introduces a node-community membership matrix to match the adjacency matrix according to some optimization function [23,29,34,36].

5.2 Mutual Friends

Mutual friend as a strong factor to indicate the closeness between two nodes has been investigated in many social-related tasks. Friend recommender systems provide the potential friends list through discovering the latent information behind network topology and friends in common [4,25]. Link prediction models in complex networks use common neighbors to evaluate the probabilities of link establishments [5]. Online social rating networks make use of the co-commenting and co-rating behaviors of users to recommend products and predict new rating [27]. In community detection problem, mutual friends have also been employed to measure the strength of connections between nodes. Newman defines connection strength as the normalized term of mutual friends and uses it to cluster nodes [21]. Tang and Liu directly interpret Jaccard similarity as node similarity to fit into K-means algorithm for community detection [28]. Steinhaeuser and Chawla exam Jaccard coefficient as an edge weighting method and employ it in community detection. However, this algorithm fails to detect any community structure without the addition of node attribute [26]. Alvari et al. regard neighborhood similarity, i.e., the number of common neighbors, as a similarity measure and incorporate it into a game theory framework [3]. Ahn et al. explicitly give the definition of link similarity and hierarchically cluster links accordingly [1].

In this paper, mutual density has the same mathematical form as Jaccard similarity or link similarity but is used for measuring the community membership similarity. Thus, we can still calculate mutual density between two nodes even if they are not linked. Also, our model is built on the matrix factorization framework instead of link clustering.

5.3 Bayesian Personalized Ranking

The pairwise objective function of our model is based on the Bayesian Personalized Ranking [24]. This method and its extensions are originally proposed to solve the ranking problem in recommender systems [22,37]. Zhang et al. employ this model on the overlapping community detection problem [35]. They focus on the link indicator and assume that each node shares more common communities with its neighbors than its non-neighbors, which is more realistic both conceptually and experimentally.

6 Conclusion

In this paper, we propose a *Mutual Density based Non-negative Matrix Factorization* model for overlapping community detection. We introduce mutual density as a more consistent indicator of community membership similarity than links in traditional methods. The formulation of our model is based on empirical findings that mutual density correlates with the cosine similarity of community membership. Our learning objective maximizes the likelihood that each node has a more similar community membership with its acquaintances than its strangers. Experiment results show that our new model outperforms the other baseline methods as well as the link-based *PNMF* model in real-world datasets.

References

1. Ahn, Y.Y., Bagrow, J.P., Lehmann, S.: Link communities reveal multiscale complexity in networks. Nature **466**(7307), 761–764 (2010)
2. Airoldi, E.M., Blei, D.M., Fienberg, S.E., Xing, E.P.: Mixed membership stochastic blockmodels. J. Mach. Learn. Res. **9**(1981–2014), 3 (2008)
3. Alvari, H., Hashemi, S., Hamzeh, A.: Detecting overlapping communities in social networks by game theory and structural equivalence concept. In: Deng, H., Miao, D., Lei, J., Wang, F.L. (eds.) AICI 2011. LNCS, vol. 7003, pp. 620–630. Springer, Heidelberg (2011). doi:10.1007/978-3-642-23887-1_79
4. Armentano, M.G., Godoy, D.L., Amandi, A.A.: A topology-based approach for followees recommendation in twitter. In: Workshop Chairs, p. 22 (2011)
5. Backstrom, L., Leskovec, J.: Supervised random walks: predicting and recommending links in social networks. In: Proceedings of the Fourth ACM International Conference on Web Search and Data Mining, pp. 635–644. ACM (2011)
6. Brandes, U., Delling, D., Gaertler, M., Görke, R., Hoefer, M., Nikoloski, Z., Wagner, D.: On Modularity-np-completeness and Beyond. Univ., Fak. für Informatik, Bibliothek (2006)
7. Clauset, A., Newman, M.E., Moore, C.: Finding community structure in very large networks. Phys. Rev. E **70**(6), 066111 (2004)
8. Coscia, M., Rossetti, G., Giannotti, F., Pedreschi, D.: Demon: a local-first discovery method for overlapping communities. In: Proceedings of the 18th ACM SIGKDD International Conference on Knowledge Discovery and Data Mining, pp. 615–623. ACM (2012)
9. De Meo, P., Ferrara, E., Fiumara, G., Provetti, A.: On facebook, most ties are weak. Commun. ACM **57**(11), 78–84 (2014)
10. Duch, J., Arenas, A.: Community detection in complex networks using extremal optimization. Phys. Rev. E **72**(2), 027104 (2005)
11. Fortunato, S.: Community detection in graphs. Phys. Rep. **486**(3), 75–174 (2010)
12. Gilbert, E., Karahalios, K.: Predicting tie strength with social media. In: Proceedings of the SIGCHI Conference on Human Factors in Computing Systems, pp. 211–220. ACM (2009)
13. Girvan, M., Newman, M.E.: Community structure in social and biological networks. Proc. Natl. Acad. Sci. **99**(12), 7821–7826 (2002)
14. Karrer, B., Newman, M.E.: Stochastic blockmodels and community structure in networks. Phys. Rev. E **83**(1), 016107 (2011)
15. Kernighan, B.W., Lin, S.: An efficient heuristic procedure for partitioning graphs. Bell Syst. Tech. J. **49**(2), 291–307 (1970)
16. Kumpula, J.M., Kivelä, M., Kaski, K., Saramäki, J.: Sequential algorithm for fast clique percolation. Phys. Rev. E **78**(2), 026109 (2008)
17. Li, Y., He, K., Bindel, D., Hopcroft, J.E.: Uncovering the small community structure in large networks: a local spectral approach. In: Proceedings of the 24th International Conference on World Wide Web, pp. 658–668. ACM (2015)
18. Lin, C.J.: Projected gradient methods for nonnegative matrix factorization. Neural Comput. **19**(10), 2756–2779 (2007)
19. Newman, M.E.: Fast algorithm for detecting community structure in networks. Phys. Rev. E **69**(6), 066133 (2004)
20. Newman, M.E.: Modularity and community structure in networks. Proc. Natl. Acad. Sci. **103**(23), 8577–8582 (2006)

21. Newman, M.: Communities, modules and large-scale structure in networks. Nat. Phys. **8**(1), 25–31 (2012)
22. Pan, W., Chen, L.: Gbpr: group preference based bayesian personalized ranking for one-class collaborative filtering. IJCAI **13**, 2691–2697 (2013)
23. Psorakis, I., Roberts, S., Ebden, M., Sheldon, B.: Overlapping community detection using bayesian non-negative matrix factorization. Phys. Rev. E **83**(6), 066114 (2011)
24. Rendle, S., Freudenthaler, C., Gantner, Z., Schmidt-Thieme, L.: Bpr: Bayesian personalized ranking from implicit feedback. In: Proceedings of the Twenty-Fifth Conference on Uncertainty in Artificial Intelligence, pp. 452–461. AUAI Press (2009)
25. Silva, N.B., Tsang, R., Cavalcanti, G.D., Tsang, J.: A graph-based friend recommendation system using genetic algorithm. In: IEEE Congress on Evolutionary Computation, pp. 1–7. IEEE (2010)
26. Steinhaeuser, K., Chawla, N.V.: Community detection in a large real-world social network. In: Social Computing, Behavioral Modeling, and Prediction, pp. 168–175. Springer, Boston (2008)
27. Symeonidis, P., Tiakas, E., Manolopoulos, Y.: Product recommendation and rating prediction based on multi-modal social networks. In: Proceedings of the Fifth ACM Conference on Recommender Systems, pp. 61–68. ACM (2011)
28. Tang, L., Liu, H.: Community detection and mining in social media. Synth. Lect. Data Min. Knowl. Discov. **2**(1), 1–137 (2010)
29. Wang, F., Li, T., Wang, X., Zhu, S., Ding, C.: Community discovery using nonnegative matrix factorization. Data Min. Knowl. Discov. **22**(3), 493–521 (2011)
30. Whang, J.J., Gleich, D.F., Dhillon, I.S.: Overlapping community detection using seed set expansion. In: Proceedings of the 22nd ACM International Conference on Conference on Information and Knowledge Management, pp. 2099–2108. ACM (2013)
31. Xie, J., Kelley, S., Szymanski, B.K.: Overlapping community detection in networks: the state-of-the-art and comparative study. ACM Comput. Surv. (CSUR) **45**(4), 43 (2013)
32. Yang, J., Leskovec, J.: Community-affiliation graph model for overlapping network community detection. In: 2012 IEEE 12th International Conference on Data Mining (ICDM), pp. 1170–1175. IEEE (2012)
33. Yang, J., Leskovec, J.: Defining and evaluating network communities based on ground-truth. In: Proceedings of the ACM SIGKDD Workshop on Mining Data Semantics, p. 3. ACM (2012)
34. Yang, J., Leskovec, J.: Overlapping community detection at scale: a nonnegative matrix factorization approach. In: Proceedings of the Sixth ACM International Conference on Web Search and Data Mining, pp. 587–596. ACM (2013)
35. Zhang, H., King, I., R., L.M.: Incorporating implicit link preference into overlapping community detection. In: Proceedings of the Twenty-Ninth AAAI Conference on Artificial Intelligence. ACM (2015)
36. Zhang, Y., Yeung, D.Y.: Overlapping community detection via bounded nonnegative matrix tri-factorization. In: Proceedings of the 18th ACM SIGKDD International Conference on Knowledge Discovery and Data Mining, pp. 606–614. ACM (2012)
37. Zhao, T., McAuley, J., King, I.: Leveraging social connections to improve personalized ranking for collaborative filtering. In: Proceedings of the 23rd ACM International Conference on Conference on Information and Knowledge Management, pp. 261–270. ACM (2014)

Calling for Response: Automatically Distinguishing Situation-Aware Tweets During Crises

Xiaodong Ning(✉), Lina Yao(✉), Xianzhi Wang, and Boualem Benatallah(✉)

University of New South Wales, Sydney, NSW, Australia
{z5122770,xiaodong.ning}@student.unsw.edu.au, lina.yao@unsw.edu.au,
sandyawang@gmail.com, boualem.benatallah@unsw.edu.au

Abstract. Recent years have witnessed the prevalence and use of social media during crises, such as Twitter, which has been becoming a valuable information source for offering better responses to crisis and emergency situations by the authorities. However, the sheer amount of information of tweets can't be directly used. In such context, distinguishing the most important and informative tweets is crucial to enhance emergency situation awareness. In this paper, we design a convolutional neural network based model to automatically detect crisis-related tweets. We explore the twitter-specific linguistic, sentimental and emotional analysis along with statistical topic modeling to identify a set of quality features. We then incorporate them to into a convolutional neural network model to identify crisis-related tweets. Experiments on real-world Twitter dataset demonstrate the effectiveness of our proposed model.

Keywords: Convolutional neural network · Situational awareness

1 Introduction

With the arrival of the information age, Twitter has become a popular platform for people to post situations, exchange information, seek and offer advice during crises [2]. Such tweets has great significance for both the people affected by crises and those who plan to help the affected people. First, rich and useful situation-aware tweets are an important information source for decision-making agencies like governments to make a reasonable emergency plan for allocating rescuers and relief materials. Second, tweets have the advantage of timeliness, which can reflect the situations and circumstances at real time. According to the expert experience, there is a 72 h 'golden window' for post-crisis relief, and as the time passes, rescue efficiency degrades significantly. Therefore, quick acquisition of tweets about crises can improve the response speed of government, and further reduce the casualties and property damage. For the above reasons, it is essential to design an efficient information extraction technique that can capture the valuable tweets about an crisis as soon as it happens [3].

G. Cong et al. (Eds.): ADMA 2017, LNAI 10604, pp. 195–208, 2017.
https://doi.org/10.1007/978-3-319-69179-4_14

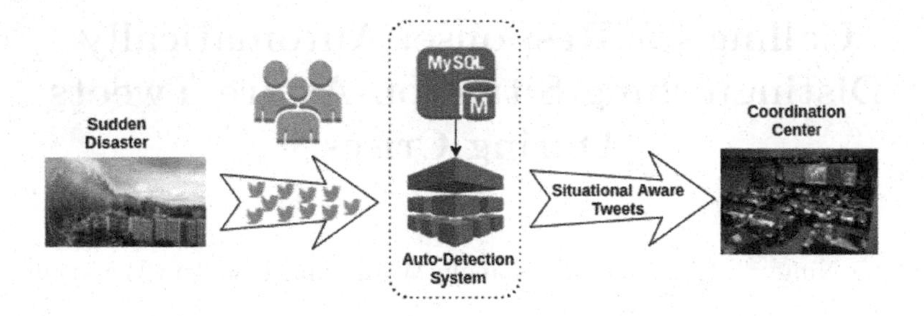

Fig. 1. Overall flow chart of detecting situation-aware tweets

Generally, tweets can be collected by event-related keywords using Twitter's public API during crisis. However, the collected tweets are generally in huge number, a significant fraction of which is noise (or irrelevant information). Consequently, facing with the overwhelming amount of information, it is unfeasible to select the situation-aware tweets manually. Therefore, it is essential to design an automatic, efficient model to detect the situation-aware valuable ones from online tweets. In fact, situation-awareness is a focused field of study aimed at understanding the environment and is critical to the decision-making as response to mass emergencies. Although there are several previous research efforts on situation awareness, most of them [6,7,9] train and validate their models for each individual event. These models do not show the capability of handling cross-crisis task. Some other researchers [1,8] train cross-crisis model from dataset of previous events and validate it for a new event which are partly annotated by humans. For this reason, they require data annotated by humans to train the model before it can start working while annotation can be highly time-consuming whereas time is precious in crises.

Based on the above discussion, we propose an automatic model to discriminate the situation awareness tweets for a *new* crisis event without human-participation.

- We present an automatic approach to capturing the critical crisis-related information conveyed on social media to enhance public responses to crisis situation in the real world.
- We design a set of quality features based on text-based measures such as emotions, linguistics, topics and entities to characterize various aspects of situation-aware tweets.
- We learn an effective one dimensional CNN-based predictive model for detecting crisis-related situation-aware tweets from a *new* crisis event, and deploy the model on a real-world twitter dataset including 6 categories of crisis events. Our model yields an increase of multiple evaluation metrics compared with a series of baseline and the state-of-the-arts methods. It also provides us a thorough understanding of the predictive results.

2 Approach Overview

As we mentioned above, only a fraction of tweets filtered by the crisis related key words and locations are 'Situation-awareness'. For example, we show two tweets about 'Boston Bombing' which are collected by key words in Fig. 2.

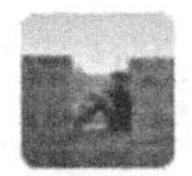

Ramsay Jalal 램지 @RamsayJalal · 19 Apr 2013
Suspect was THROWING explosives from car! Plus there may be two active bombs near Arsenal mall! #Boston #Watertown

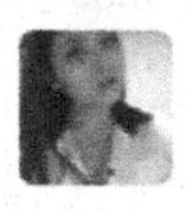

Noeliaa @Nellyy_95 · 15 Apr 2013
Disasters like this make you realize that your problems aren't too bad:\ #PrayForBoston

Fig. 2. Two tweets about the 'Boston Bombing' crisis

We can find that both of the two tweets are collected by the keyword 'Boston Bomb' using Twitter's API, yet the first one is situation-aware to the crisis while the second one is not situation-aware (the first one describes the details of the crisis while the second one just talks irrelevant things). By analyzing the content carefully, we find that the language styles are different between the two tweets. The emotional index is higher in the first one while the subjectivity is stronger in the second one. Therefore, we distinguish between the situation-aware and the other tweets according to their language attributes. For this reason, our approach involves two main steps: feature extraction and model learning (the overall structure of our methodology is shown on Fig. 1.

2.1 Feature Extraction

In this section, we extract several types of content-based features from each tweet to detect whether it is situation-aware or not.

Linguistic Features. According to the research in the sociology and psychology, linguistic features can reflect the mental activities and behavioral intention of posters. We extract four kinds of linguistic attributes: subjectivity, part-of-speech, tenses and lexical density. Specifically, we use Textblob[1] to calculate the subjectivity scores of tweets. Each subjectivity score ranges within $(0, 1)$ and higher score indicates stronger subjectivity of tweet. We analyze the tense of tweets by measuring the different verb tenses: 'past tense', 'present participle', 'base form' and 'past participle' using the Stanford's Part-of-speech (POS) tool.[2] The values of verb tenses are calculated by counting the occurrences of corresponding words in the content. Lexical density is measured by keywords such as 'verb', 'adverb', 'symbol' and 'number' (also done by POS). Finally, the linguistic features add up to a 43-dimensional vector.

[1] https://textblob.readthedocs.io/en/dev/.
[2] https://nlp.stanford.edu/software/tagger.shtml.

Table 1. Mn (Mean), Std (Standard deviation) of the linguistic representative attributes across the Situation-Awareness (SA) and Non-Situational Awareness (Non-SA) tweets. PRP = personal pronoun, SYM = symbol, VBD = verb past tense, RBS = superlative adverb, SUB = subjectivity; JJ = adjective; NN = nourns; CD = cardinal number.

Feature types		Linguistic features							
Subtypes		PRP	SYM	VBD	RBS	SUB	JJ	NN	CD
Situational awareness	Mn	0.45	0.01	0.86	0.46	0.01	1.05	3.69	0.35
	Std	0.78	0.12	0.99	0.79	0.15	1.03	2.47	0.69
Non-situational awareness	Mn	1.01	0.005	1.01	0.72	0.03	0.94	1.90	0.20
	Std	1.12	0.01	1.17	0.68	0.09	1.03	1.72	0.57

Emotional Features. In order to estimate the emotional features in tweets, we analyze three aspects: emotional states, emotional intensity and content polarity. The emotional states are measured by 10 emotional terms in tweets such as 'joy', 'sadness', 'anger', 'nervousness', 'fear', 'disgust', etc. The score of each term is estimated using the Empath API [5].[3] We analyze the emotional intensity of each tweet by averaging the arousal scores of its words given in ANEW dictionary (Affective Norms for English Words).[4] Polarity is measured in a score between $(0, 1)$ by analyzing the whole tweet using the Textblob API. Finally, we get a 17-dimensional vector for this part.

Table 2. Mn (Mean), Std (Standard deviation) of the emotional representative attributes across the Situation-Awareness (SA) and Non-Situational Awareness (Non-SA) tweets.

Feature types		Emotional features						
Subtypes		Arousal	Polarity	Sad	Nervous	Angry	Joy	Disgust
Situational awareness	Mn	5.26	0.03	0.03	0.15	0.20	0.003	0.009
	Std	0.85	0.08	0.08	0.26	0.31	0.07	0.097
Non-situational awareness	Mn	4.40	0.07	0.01	0.06	0.04	0.005	0.002
	Std	1.26	0.04	0.07	0.13	0.12	0.06	0.049

Entity-Based Features. Besides the former two types of features, we also take the entity-based features into consideration. Typically, some entities are associated closely with the relevant tweets during mass emergencies, e.g., 'government', 'journalism', and 'Medical Emergency'. We choose up to 17 entity-topics (each topic contains several entity words which are related to that topic) and measure the corresponding scores in each tweet using the Empath API.

[3] http://empath.stanford.edu/.
[4] https://tomlee.wtf/2010/06/16/anew/.

Table 3. Mn (Mean), Std (Standard deviation) of the entity-based representative attributes across the Situation-Awareness (SA) and Non-Situational Awareness (Non-SA) tweets.

Feature types		Entity features					
Subtypes		Journalism	Government	Medical	Injury	Sympathy	Weak
Situational awareness	Mn	0.015	0.02	0.015	0.03	0.023	0.07
	Std	0.09	0.13	0.128	0.18	0.15	0.28
Non-situational awareness	Mn	0.008	0.004	0.008	0.01	0.015	0.03
	Std	0.015	0.07	0.015	0.12	0.13	0.19

Topical Features. Although the specific locations and events can be different in various crises, the core content of tweets posted fall into several common topics such as relief, blessing, seeking for help, news report, etc. Previous research [22–24] has already shown topical features can be a strong complement for the handcrafted attributes due to its ability of capturing the latent semantic features in social media. Then we apply latent Dirichlet allocation (LDA) model to extract the topics in tweets. With the empirical evaluations, the optimal number of topics is set as 7 in our work. We show the several top frequent words for each clustered topic in Table 4. From the table, we can observe that the clustered words in each topic are significantly different. Topic 2 is closely related to relief (e.g. support, redcross, donate, etc.) while the topic 3 contains many news report related words such as: http, bbc, hit, news, etc. To demonstrate the effectiveness of word clustering from LDA, we choose topic 2 as example (as it is related to relief) and show the top-10 most relevant term frequencies within it compared to the overall frequencies in Fig. 3(a). From the figure, we can observe that topic 2 accounts for the overwhelming proportion of the overall ten term frequencies meaning that extracted topics are separated well.

In order to give an intuitive insight, we select some representative terms from the former three kinds of features by calculating the means and standard deviations of them in 'SA' and 'Non-SA' Tweets in Tables 1, 2 and 3. We can clearly observe that there exists distinguishable feature distribution patterns between 'SA' and 'Non-SA' tweets. Figure 3(b) shows the significant difference of topic distributions between the 'SA' and 'Non-SA' tweets. We further characterize the distribution differences in tweets based on the categories as following:

Feature Analysis. *Linguistic Feature*: We can observe that 'SA' tweets show significantly higher mean value than 'Non-SA' ones in nouns(+94%) and cardinal numbers(+75%) while the latter shows 200% and 124% higher values in subjectivity and personal pronoun respectively. Presumably, the different distributions of linguistic features conform to the common sense as situation-aware tweets always provide more objective content with nouns and cardinal numbers during crisis.

Table 4. LDA vocabulary distribution

LDA topic	Vocabulary
Topic1	*need,volunteer, share, tweet, http, evacuation, safe, affect...*
Topic2	*help, victim, donate, need, redcross, find, relief, support...*
Topic3	*http, video, photo, facebook, bbc, hit, news, youtube, ...*
Topic4	*day, trend, hours, weather, tonight, place, night, update...*
Topic5	*suspect, caught, police, attack, arrest, rip, tragedy, fire, kill...*
Topic6	*thank, love, good, better, happy, well, final, tomorrow, hope...*
Topic7	*lol, joke, want, sigh, really even, guy, more, extremely...*

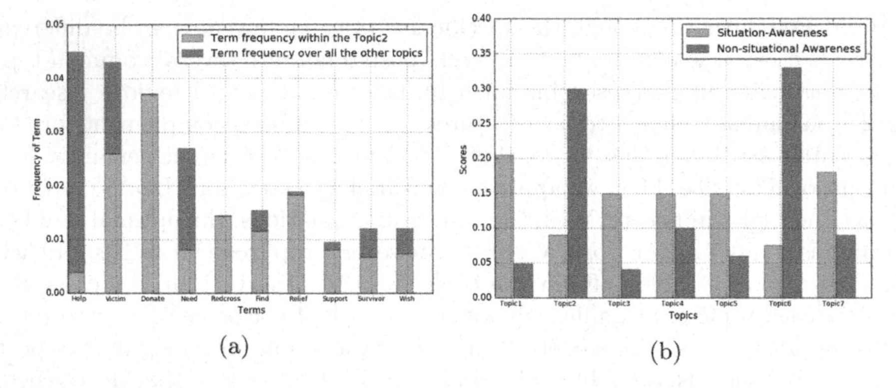

Fig. 3. (a) Top-10 most relevant term frequencies within topic 2 compared to the term frequencies over all the other topics; (b) Topic distributions between 'Situation-awareness' and 'Non-Situational Awareness' tweets;

Emotional Feature: From the chosen emotional features, it is notable that 'SA' tweets show higher mean value in all of the negative emotions (e.g. sad(+200%), angry(+400%), nervous(+150%).etc) than 'Non-SA' ones while the values of joy and polarity are higher in the latter. We can infer that 'SA' tweets tend to associate with strong negative emotions due to distress caused by crisis while 'Non-SA' tweets generally talk about irrelevant topics.

Entity Feature: As for entity features, the mean values of 'SA' tweets are consistently higher than 'Non-SA' tweets in all the chose entity topics, which confirms assumption in the previous feature extraction part. It is reasonable that situation-aware contains more crisis-related entities.

Topical Feature: By analyzing the topic distributions among two categories, we can find that the mean value are much higher in 'Non-SA' tweets in topic 2 and topic 6 while 'SA' tweets get higher values in other topics. The words appearing in the topic 2 and 6 can be regarded as 'support and blessing' related terms while the other topics contain many detail-related terms which can transmit situation-aware information.

2.2 Situation-Awareness Identification

To identify the situation-aware tweets in each crisis. we propose a 1D-CNN model in an empirical data-driven manner. Deep learning has been proven to achieve promising performance in various domains such as image processing [10] and speech recognition [11], as a result of its ability to model high-level representations and capture complex relationships of data via a stacking multiple layered architecture. Recently, it is also adapted to the field of social media content analysis [12,13]. We show the overall structure of our model in Fig. 4.

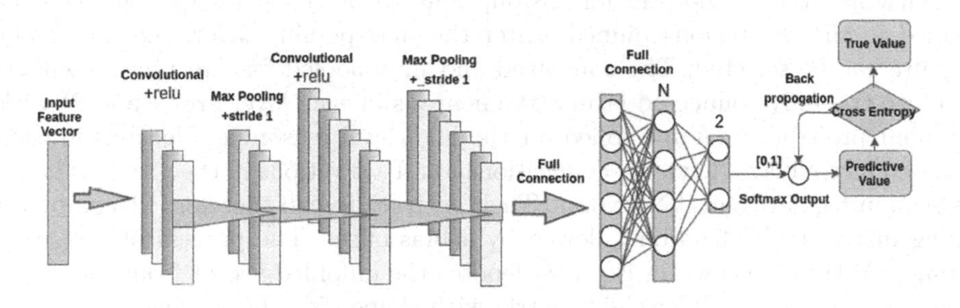

Fig. 4. 1DCNN architecture

We will explain the details of our model in the following part. The list of quality features above are used in a form of vectors as input of our model. The specific structure of our model is as follows: The first and third layers are convolutional layers, the second and forth are max-pooling layers, and the fifth and sixth are two fully-connected layers. The first and third convolutional layers in our model take a set of $F1$ and $F2$ independent filters respectively and slide them over the whole feature vector with stride size Fs and filter length Fl. Along the way, dot product is taken between the filters and chunks of the input feature. Filters are used to generate the feature vectors in each filter length. In this way, the original feature vector is projected into a stack of feature maps (vector maps in our work). Additionally, we apply the rectified linear unit (ReLU) activation function on the dot product from filters. We take the first convolutional layer as example to show the details of convolutional operation and RELU function in Eqs. 1 and 2: $Conv_i(j)$ denotes the j_{th} convolutional output from the i_{th} filter and input vector I (84 dimensional vector in our work); F_i denotes the i_{th} filter vector; $Convrelu_i(j)$ denotes the relu function result of the $Conv_i(j)$;

$$Conv_{ij} = I[j * Fs, (j * Fs + Fl)] * F_i \tag{1}$$

$$Convrelu_{ij)} = Max(0, Conv_{ij}) \tag{2}$$

After the convolutional layers, the hidden relationships between features can be combined by the dot product from each filter. The captured features can play an important role in the final performance in our model.

The multiple filters in convolutional layers can be updated automatically via the evolution of network. Followed by each convolutional layer, we add one max-pooling layer with max-filter length Pl and stride size Ps. Similar to previous part, we show the details of first max-pooling layer in Eq. 3: $Max(i,j)$ denotes the j_{th} max-pooling output from the i_{th} convolutional layer output with Relu $Convrelu_i$;

$$Maxoutput(i,j) = Max(Convrelu_i[j * Ps, (j * Ps + Pl)]) \tag{3}$$

The max-pooling layer can down-sample the feature representation, reducing its dimensionality and allowing for assumptions to be made about features contained in the sub-regions binned. After the max-pooling layer, the important feature can be selected. The convolved and max-pooled feature vectors will be fed into two fully-connected layers (the neurons in each layer are N and 2) with dropout probability (Kp) applied for the high-level reasoning. Neurons in each fully-connected layer have full connections to all activations in the previous layer, as seen in regular Neural Networks. Their activations can therefore be computed using matrix multiplication followed by a bias offset. The process of first fully connected layer is shown in Eq. 4: L denotes the unfolded vector from the previous layer; W denotes the weight matrix with shape $(N \times L)$; B denotes the bias vector with N length; $Output(N)$ denotes the output vector of this layer;

$$Output(N) = W \times L + B \tag{4}$$

Finally, we use the softmax as the output layer of the last fully-connected layer. Each node in the softmax layer produces the probabilities of two classes including 'situation-aware' and 'non-situational aware'. The class with higher probability will be output as the prediction.

3 Experiments

3.1 Settings

Dataset. We use the tweets dataset provided by [4], which contains six crises that occurred in English-speaking countries between October 2012 and July 2013. This dataset was collected using Twitter's API by event-related keywords and geolocations. All the tweets in this dataset have been manually classified into 'Situation-Aware' and 'Non-situational Aware'. Table 5 presents the details of our dataset, where we observe that the numbers of 'SA' and 'Non-SA' Tweets are approximately equal.

Baseline Methods. We choose the following baseline methods (the parameters of all method are tuned for optimal performance), including *Random Forrest* (the number estimators as 300, max depth as 5) [6], *Xgboosting* (learning rate as 0.05, max depth as 4 and minimum descending value of cost function as 0.1) [14], *Logistic Regression*, *Decision Tree* (max depth as 3), *Support Vector Machine* (kernel as 'poly' and C parameter as 1), *AdaBoosting* (number of estimators as

Table 5. Statistics of dataset

Crisis	# of SA Tweets	# of Non-SA Tweets
Sandy hurricane	6138	3870
Alberta flood	5189	4842
Boston bombing	5638	4364
Oklahoma tornado	4827	5165
Queensland floods	5414	4619
West texas explosion	5246	4760

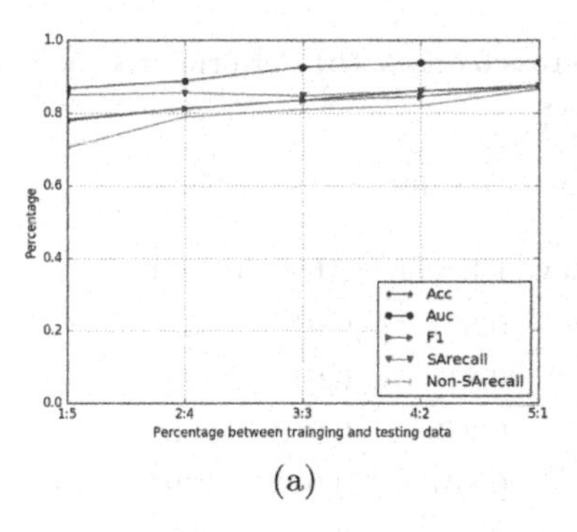

(a)

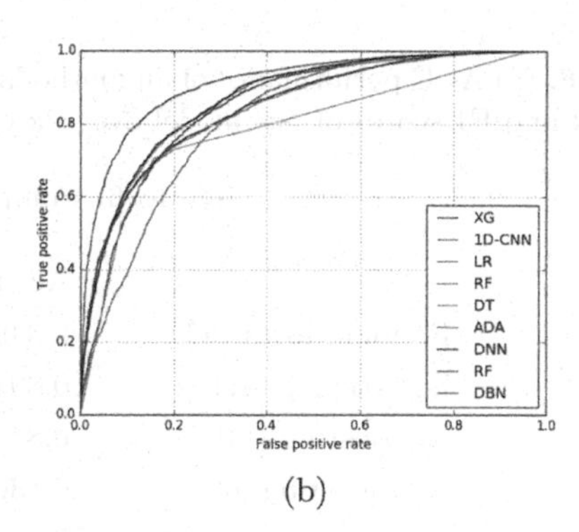

(b)

Fig. 5. (a) Cross-crisis performance comparison with varied training/testing ratio. The X-axis indicates the number of crisis topic used for training, and the rest of crisis topics used for testing; (b) ROC performance over crisis topic *'Sandy Hurricane'*;

200 and learning rate as 0.3) [6]. Besides the above methods, we also choose two deep learning based methods as our baseline: *Deep Belief Network* (four hidden layers (with 110,200,400,300 units in each layer), learning rate as 0.001,activation function as relu, number of epochs as 200) and *Deep Neural Network* (four hidden layers (with 500, 600, 400, 200 in each layer), learning rate as 0.0001, training epochs as 1000).

3.2 Results

Parameter Tuning. We conducted extensive experiments to determine the optimal configuration of parameters for the 1D-CNN. There are two types of parameters in our model: the first type includes weights and biases in the model layers, which can be initiated randomly and learned afterwards from each iteration; the second type includes the parameters that should be configured manually. In particular, we select nine most common hyper-parameters for our 1D-CNN model, namely the learning rate lr, the dropout probability Kp (used to prevent overfitting), convolutional filters length Fl, number of filters in the first convolutional layer $F1$, number of filters in the third convolutional layer $F2$, stride size

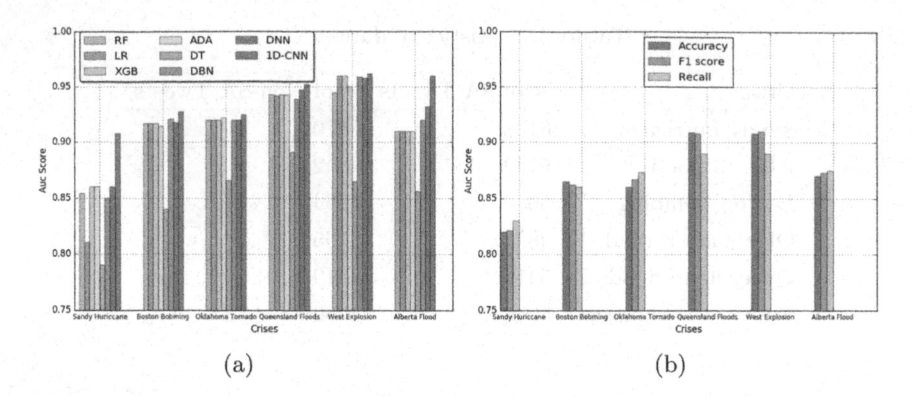

Fig. 6. (a) AUC performance of all methods across 6 crises. (b) Performance (accuracy, recall and F1 score) of our model over six crises

Table 6. Comparison results

	Accuracy	F1 score	AUC	Recall
Random forest [6]	0.849	0.851	0.914	0.852
Logistic regression	0.808	0.81	0.91	0.825
Xgboosting [14]	0.845	0.843	0.918	0.855
Adaboosting [6]	0.836	0.837	0.916	0.839
Decision tree	0.79	0.80	0.851	0.797
Support vector machine	0.816	0.814	0.91	0.823
Deep belief network	0.822	0.825	0.919	0.83
Deep neural network	0.847	0.848	0.92	0.846
Ours	**0.871**	**0.872**	**0.94**	**0.87**

in convolutional layers Fs, max-filter length Pl, stride size Ps in max-pooling layers and number of neurons in first connection layer N. Since the weight W and bias b in each neural layer can be learned automatically via the evolution of model network, we focus on tuning the hyper-parameters lr, Kp, Fl, $F1$, $F2$, Fs, Pl, Ps and N. In particular, we fix the number of iterations as 1000 for each experiment and try different combinations of parameters by changing the value of one parameter and keep the other eight parameters. Finally, we set $lr = 0.0001$, $Kp = 0.05$, $Fl = 3$, $F1 = 2$, $F2 = 2$, $Fs = 1$, $Pl = 2$, $Ps = 1$, $N = 1200$ as default setting of our method.

Performance Study. The aim of our work is to effectively and automatically discriminate the 'SA' tweets for a totally new crisis, hence we design our experiments by choosing five events as training data and leave the sixth event as testing data iteratively (similar to six-fold validation where validation dataset comes from a new crisis). We evaluate the performance of each classifier by four metrics: Accuracy, Recall, AUC, and F1 score. Table 6 shows the overall

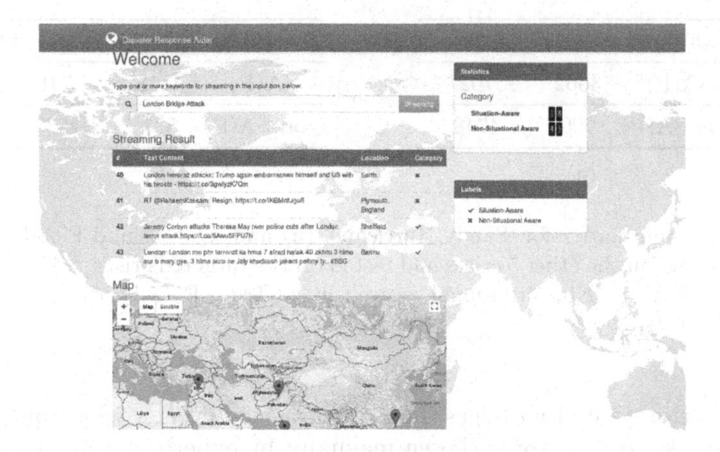

Fig. 7. Website interface

comparison results. From the table, we can observe that our method outperforms the baseline methods consistently in all the four metrics. It is notable that all of the baseline models (except decision tree) achieve more than 80% in accuracy, f1 score, recall and 90% in auc score, which confirms the high effectiveness of our feature engineering. Random forest provides best performance among the non-deep learning methods while deep neural network presents a similar performance. As for another deep learning model, deep belief network does not show better performance than other baseline methods. In particular, our model achieves improvement in recall, F1 score and accuracy by 2%, and 2.6% in AUC compared to the high baseline, which confirms convolutional layer can indeed capture some hidden but important relationships among features. In addition, we also evaluate the cross-crisis performance comparison with varied training/testing ratio, ROC performance over crisis topic 'Sandy Hurricane', AUC performance of all methods across 6 crises and details of 1D-CNN performance over six crises in Figs. 5 and 6. In the end, we choose 'Sandy Hurricane' and 'Queensland Floods' as examples and show their confusion matrix in Fig. 8.

Additionally, we build a website for interaction with our system and show web-interface in Fig. 7. We provide an input box for user to enter a crisis-related keyword or geo-location and then return the classified tweets with their location in the rolling box. We also display the geo-location of each tweet in the global map to give an insight for user. And we also provide a demo[5] based on the real crisis 'London Bridge Attack' to show our system.

4 Related Work

There are many previous work on managing social media information during disaster. Olteanu et al. [4] proposed a crisis lexicon to efficiently query twitter

[5] https://youtu.be/J1GbLppA50c.

N=10012	SA(T)	Non-SA(T)
SA(P)	3662	702
Non-SA(P)	900	4748

(a)

N=10033	SA(T)	Non-SA(T)
SA(P)	4118	501
Non-SA(P)	577	4837

(b)

Fig. 8. Confusion matrix for 'Sandy Hurricane' (a) and 'Queensland Floods' (b). The model is trained on the other 5 crises and tested on the targeted crisis. 'SA'='Situation-aware'; 'Non-SA' = 'Non-situational aware'; T = True; P = Predicted; N = total number of tweets;

to extract crisis-related messages during emergency events, which outperforms using only a set of key words chosen manually by experts. Imran et al. [7] utilized naive bayes classifier (NB) to classify the tweets into four categories and [8] implemented the conditional random field (CRF) to extract valuable information from the classified tweets. Imran et al. [15] utilized an unsupervised algorithm to capture the dynamic crisis-related topics from social media. Stowe et al. [16] presented a system for classifying disaster-related tweets with support vector machine classifier. In 2014, Imran et al. [1] proposed an artificial intelligence disaster response platform for detecting the situation-aware tweets during disaster by combining the human intelligence and machine intelligence, and they [17] study two challenges in their design: identifying which elements should be labeled and determining when to ask for annotations to be done. Similarly, Popoola [18] developed an online platform that involves citizens participation for timely information verification during natural disasters. Verma et al. [9] utilized two classifiers(naive bayes and max entropy) to detect whether a tweet is situation-aware or not. Ashktorab et al. [19] proposed a method to detect whether the tweet is damage or causality related. MacEachren [20] proposed a web-enabled geo-visual analytics approach to leveraging Twitter in support of crisis management and displaying the tweets content based on place, time and concept characteristics. Morstatter [25] developed a system for analysts with little information about an disaster to gain knowledge through the use of effective visualization techniques. This system connects human intelligence with rich data so that human clues can inform search and guide a users query to form better understanding about the disaster. Horita [21] proposed a framework which utilizes an extended model $oDMN^+$ for improving the understanding of how to leverage big data in the organizations decision-making.

Among the previous works, [1,7,9,16–19] are most related to our work. However, some of them [1,19] focus only on the application area instead of the model and feature extraction. Among the other works, [18] requires a lot of human participation to verify a disaster information and cannot automatically distinguish informative messages during disaster. [7,9,16] train and validate their models for each individual event. Those models do not show capability of handling cross-event task. [7,17] try to train cross-event model from dataset of previous events and validate it for a new event which are partly annotated by humans. In other words, the methods proposed in the previous work require data annotated by humans to train the model before it can start working. Annotation can be highly time-consuming whereas time is precious in crises. Compared to previous work, our model can automatically distinguish the situation-aware tweets during a new crisis without human participation and experimental results over real dataset show that our model can excellently handle the inter-event identification task.

5 Conclusions

In this paper, we present a convolutional neural network based model for automatic extraction of situation-aware tweets posted during crises. Our model extracts a set of text-based features of tweets: emotional, linguistic, topical and entity-based attributes, and utilizes an one-dimensional CNN to capture the hidden relationships between those features. Experimental results on a real dataset demonstrate that our model can excellently handle the cross-crisis classification task (AUC 94%, recall 87%, accuracy 87.1% and F1 score 87.2%) and perform better than a series of baseline methods. In future work, we will investigate multi-modal features of tweets and embed our current model into a multi-view learning framework. We also plan to further fuse the model into a dynamic crisis tracking system through social media streams.

References

1. Muhammad, I., et al.: AIDR: Artificial intelligence for disaster response. In: Proceedings of the 23rd International Conference on World Wide Web. ACM (2014)
2. Takeshi, S., Okazaki, M., Matsuo, Y.: Earthquake shakes Twitter users: real-time event detection by social sensors. In: Proceedings of the 19th International Conference on World wide web. ACM (2010)
3. Jie, Y., et al.: Using social media to enhance emergency situation awareness. IEEE Intell. Syst. **27**(6), 52–59 (2012). APA
4. Alexandra, O., et al.: CrisisLex: a lexicon for collecting and filtering microblogged communications in crises. In: ICWSM (2014)
5. Ethan, F., Chen, B., Bernstein, M.S.: Empath: understanding topic signals in large-scale text. In: Proceedings of the 2016 CHI Conference on Human Factors in Computing Systems. ACM (2016)
6. Niharika, S., Kumaraguru, P.: Call for service: character- izing and modeling police response to serviceable requests on Facebook. In: CSCW (2017)
7. Muhammad, I., et al.: Extracting information nuggets from disaster-related messages in social media. In: ISCRAM (2013)
8. Muhammad, I., et al.: Practical extraction of disaster-relevant information from social media. In: Proceedings of the 22nd International Conference on World Wide Web. ACM (2013)
9. Sudha, V., et al.: Natural language processing to the rescue? extracting "situational awareness" tweets during mass emergency. In: ICWSM (2011)
10. Alex, K., Sutskever, I., Hinton, G.E.: Imagenet classification with deep convolutional neural networks. In: Advances in Neural Information Processing Systems (2012)

11. Souvik, K., et al.: Joint acoustic factor learning for robust deep neural network based automatic speech recognition. In: 2016 IEEE International Conference on Acoustics, Speech and Signal Processing (ICASSP). IEEE (2016)
12. Tingmin, W., et al.: Twitter spam detection based on deep learning. In: Proceedings of the Australasian Computer Science Week Multiconference. ACM (2017)
13. Duyu, T., et al.: Coooolll: a deep learning system for twitter sentiment classification. In: SemEval@ COLING (2014)
14. Tianqi, C., Guestrin, C.: Xgboost: a scalable tree boosting system. In: Proceedings of the 22nd ACM sigkdd International Conference on Knowledge Discovery and Data Mining. ACM (2016)
15. Muhammad, I., Castillo, C.: Towards a data-driven approach to identify crisis-related topics in social media streams. In: Proceedings of the 24th International Conference on World Wide Web. ACM (2015)
16. Kevin, S., et al.: Identifying and categorizing disaster-related tweets. In: Conference on Empirical Methods in Natural Language Processing (2016)
17. Muhammad, I., et al.: Coordinating human and machine intelligence to classify microblog communications in crises. In: ISCRAM (2014)
18. Abdulfatai, P., et al.: Information verification during natural disasters. In: Proceedings of the 22nd International Conference on World Wide Web. ACM (2013)
19. Zahra, A., et al.: Tweedr: mining twitter to inform disaster response. In: ISCRAM (2014)
20. Alan M, M., et al.: Geo-twitter analytics: Applications in crisis management. In; 25th International Cartographic Conference (2011)
21. Flvio EA, H., et al.: Bridging the gap between decision-making and emerging big data sources: an application of a model-based framework to disaster management in Brazil. Decis. Support Syst. **97**, 12–22 (2017)
22. Matthew S, G.: Predicting crime using Twitter and kernel density estimation. Decis. Support Syst. **61**, 115–125 (2014)
23. Thapen, N., Simmie, D., Hankin, C.: The early bird catches the term: combining twitter and news data for event detection and situational awareness. J. Biomed. Semant. **7**(1), 61 (2016)
24. Kar Wai, L., Buntine, W.: Twitter opinion topic model: Extracting product opinions from tweets by leveraging hashtags and sentiment lexicon. In: Proceedings of the 23rd ACM International Conference on Conference on Information and Knowledge Management. ACM (2014)
25. Fred, M., et al.: Understanding twitter data with tweetxplorer. In: Proceedings of the 19th ACM SIGKDD International Conference on Knowledge Discovery and Data Mining. ACM (2013)

Efficient Revenue Maximization for Viral Marketing in Social Networks

Yuan Su[1(✉)], Xi Zhang[1], Sihong Xie[2], Philip S. Yu[3,4], and Binxing Fang[1]

[1] Beijing University of Posts and Telecommunications, Beijing, China
{timsu,zhangx,fangbx}@bupt.edu.cn
[2] Lehigh University, Bethlehem, PA, USA
sxie@cse.lehigh.edu
[3] University of Illinois at Chicago, Chicago, IL, USA
psyu@cs.uic.edu
[4] Institute for Data Science, Tsinghua University, Beijing, China

Abstract. In social networks, the problem of revenue maximization aims at maximizing the overall revenue from the purchasing behaviors of users under the influence propagations. Previous studies use a number of simulations on influence cascades to obtain the maximum revenue. However, these simulation-based methods are time-consuming and can't be applied to large-scale networks. Instead, we propose calculation-based algorithms for revenue maximization, which gains the maximum revenue through fast approximate calculations within local acyclic graphs instead of the slow simulations across the global network. Furthermore, a max-Heap updating scheme is proposed to prune unnecessary calculations. These algorithms are designed for both the scenarios of unlimited and constrained commodity supply. Experiments on both the synthetic and real-world datasets demonstrate the efficiency and effectiveness of our proposals, that is, our algorithms run in orders of magnitude faster than the state-of-art baselines, and meanwhile, the maximum revenue achieved is nearly not affected.

Keywords: Revenue maximization · Social networks · Viral marketing

1 Introduction

Revenue maximization [1,10,14,20,23,25] is the problem of devising the marketing strategy to obtain the optimal revenue in social networks, by determining the price of a commodity and identifying a small set of influential vertices to give out commodities for free. In contrast to influence maximization [5–8,13,18,19], revenue maximization takes into account the impact of prices on adopting commodities, and quantifies the revenue obtained from the adoption after the information diffusion process.

In networks, one user's valuation towards a commodity often exhibits positive network externalities [2,4,12,17,21,23,24], i.e., a user's valuation will be positively influenced by other users who have already purchased the commodity.

G. Cong et al. (Eds.): ADMA 2017, LNAI 10604, pp. 209–224, 2017.
https://doi.org/10.1007/978-3-319-69179-4_15

Hoping to increase the future revenue, in networks, a seller can give out some commodities for free to some individuals to drive up the demands of the commodities. We study the seller's marketing strategy as follows: the seller selects a set S of consumers and gives each of them a commodity for free, and then sets a unified price λ for the other consumers to buy the commodity, such that the expected revenue is maximized. Different from the influence maximization problem, there exists a challenge in revenue maximization when optimizing the price λ. Specifically, lowering the price λ increases the number of purchasers but may not improve the total revenue, while raising the price loses potential purchases and may not improve the total revenue as well. Such a complex relationship is an inherent and challenging problem in revenue maximization.

We consider two scenarios of commodity supply, the unlimited supply and the constrained supply. The unlimited supply means that a commodity is with nearly zero marginal cost of manufacturing and the seller supply is unrestricted [23], e.g., the number of SIM cards released by a telecommunication company can be considered to be unlimited. The constrained supply suits that a seller has limited production or service capacity, e.g., the tickets of a cinema are restricted. For the scenario of unlimited supply, a randomized algorithm using a large number of simulations on influence cascades for revenue estimation is proposed in [23], which is time-consuming and can't be applied to large-scale networks. Moreover, it does not consider the "awareness" of a commodity in the dynamic process of commodity adoptions. In the dynamic process, a user won't be "aware" of a commodity until one of her in-degree neighbors adopted it. Thus, awareness should be the premise of the purchasing behavior and need to be incorporated into the dynamic process. For the scenario of constrained supply, a heuristic algorithm is proposed in [25], which, however, is only suitable to the situation that each user's inherent valuation of a commodity is known. This is a strong assumption that commonly does not hold in the real-world viral marketing, where a consumer's inherent estimation is usually unknown to the sellers.

To address the aforementioned problems, we consider the awareness of a commodity as the premise of a user's purchase, and generalize the revenue maximization problem by setting each user's inherent valuation as unknown. We then propose efficient and effective algorithms for both the scenarios of the unlimited supply and the constrained supply. Firstly, a fast method of approximate revenue calculation using local acyclic graphs is proposed to replace the time-consuming simulations on influence cascades. The intuition is to restrict the influence spreading to a vertex within its local acyclic graph, and the activation probability of this vertex can be calculated approximately in its local acyclic graph instead of the original large network. Based on this method, for the scenario of unlimited supply, we propose an efficient algorithm, i.e., the Calculation-based Randomized (CR) algorithm, in which the revenues are approximately calculated based on local acyclic graphs. For the scenario of constrained supply, we develop an efficient algorithm called the Calculation-based max-Heap updating Greedy (CHG) algorithm. The main idea of this algorithm contains two crucial parts: (1) fast approximate revenue calculation based on the local acyclic graphs;

(2) max-Heap updating scheme, which relies on the submodularity of the objective function of the revenue maximization problem. We conduct extensive experiments on both the synthetic and real-world networks. The results indicate that the proposed algorithms can achieve almost the same revenue while running in orders of magnitude faster than the baselines.

The contributions of this paper are summarized as below:

- We address the problem of revenue maximization for both the cases that the commodity supply is unlimited and constrained, and propose a fast and general method to approximately calculate the revenue.
- For unlimited commodity supply, an efficient algorithm CR is proposed based on the approximate revenue calculations; for constrained commodity supply, an efficient algorithm CHG is proposed based both on the approximate revenue calculations and max-Heap updating scheme.
- The results of experiments demonstrate the efficiency and effectiveness of CR algorithm and CHG algorithm, which can run orders of magnitude faster than the state-of-art baselines while gaining almost the same revenue.

2 Revenue Maximization Problem

In this section, we first describe the price-sensitive dynamic process in social networks, and then formally present the problem of revenue maximization.

The social network. Given a commodity, a social network is represented as a weighted graph $G = (V, E)$, where V is the set of potential consumers, and E is the set of edges. For each vertex $v \in V$, her inherent valuation of the commodity $\chi_v \in [0, 1]$ is selected uniformly at random in $[0, 1]$, under the assumption that her inherent valuation is unknown. If the purchase by one vertex u will directly encourage the desire of another vertex v for the commodity, there exists an edge $e_{u,v} \in E$ from u to v, and the influence weight on edge $e_{u,v}$ is represented by $w_{u,v} > 0$. If there is no edge between vertices u and v, then $w_{u,v} = 0$. The non-negative and non-decreasing function $F : \mathbb{R}^+ \rightarrow \mathbb{R}^+$ transforms the edge weight into the valuation increment. Given a set of vertices S which can directly influence the purchase decision of v, then v's valuation will be $\chi_v + F(\Sigma_{u \in S} w_{u,v})$.

The price-sensitive dynamic process. The activation of a vertex by a commodity has two important factors [16,20]: awareness and purchase. For the awareness, if one vertex is activated by the commodity, she makes her out-degree neighbors aware of the commodity, which means that these neighbors are exposed to the commodity and know about it. In other words, a vertex is aware of the commodity in condition that at least one of her in-degree neighbors is activated by the commodity. For the purchase, if some vertices are activated by the commodity in the network, they will exert influences on their out-degree neighbors, while the influence strength is denoted by the edge weights. Then the valuations of the out-degree neighbors towards the commodity will be incremented. A vertex who is aware of the commodity will purchase it if her valuation outweighs the price. A vertex is activated by a commodity if it is aware of the commodity and purchase that commodity.

The diffusion proceeds in discrete steps. Initially at step $t = 0$, all the vertices in seed set S_0 are activated, and the seller sets a fixed price $\lambda \in \Lambda$ for the commodity. Here Λ is the price set. At each step $t \geq 1$, for each vertex v, if some of v's in-degree neighbors are activated by the commodity, v becomes aware of the commodity, and then v's valuation will be updated by $\chi_v^t = \chi_v + F(\Sigma_{i\in S_{t-1}} w_{i,v})$, where $S_{t-1} \subseteq V$ is the set of vertices activated after time $t-1$. In this paper, we set $F(x) = x$ for convenience, following the same setting as in [23,25]. If $\chi_v^t \geq \lambda$, then v will purchase the commodity. This process continues and the dynamic process propagates until no more vertices are activated. If the commodity supply is constrained, when the activated number achieved is larger than the quantity Q of the commodity, the dynamic process terminates. For any vertex, if it has purchased the commodity, it will stay activated. Different from Linear Threshold Model [18] adopted in influence maximization problem where the commodity price is not considered, in revenue maximization problem, it is obvious that λ will affect the number of infected nodes: the higher the price, the fewer vertices will be activated; while the lower the price, the more vertices will be activated.

In our setting, a vertex is activated by the commodity in the propagation of social influence if and only if (1) the vertex is in the seed set, or (2) at least one of v's in-degree neighbors are activated by the commodity, i.e., v is aware of the commodity, and v's current valuation is no less than the price of the commodity.

In this paper, we set $\Sigma_u w_{u,v} \leq \lambda$, specifically, $\Sigma_u w_{u,v} \in [0, \alpha]$ and $\lambda \in [\alpha, 1]$ where $\alpha \in [0, 1]$. Please note that if all the in-degree neighbors of vertex v are activated, as $\chi_v \in [0, 1]$ is selected uniformly at random, v's valuation $\chi_v + \Sigma_u w_{u,v}$ ($u \in v$'s in-degree neighbors) will be selected in $[\Sigma_u w_{u,v}, 1 + \Sigma_u w_{u,v}]$ uniformly at random. Then the activation probability that $\chi_v + \Sigma_u w_{u,v} \geq \lambda$ is $1 - \lambda + \Sigma_u w_{u,v}$. This probability is exactly guaranteed in [0, 1] as $\Sigma_u w_{u,v} \in [0, \alpha]$ and $\lambda \in [\alpha, 1]$. Besides, in the case that not all the in-degree neighbors are activated, we can get the same conclusion. These settings can make price-sensitive dynamic process have better probability characteristics for mathematical calculations.

Revenue maximization problem. The seller selects a set of vertices S as seeds and gives them the commodity for free. After the diffusion process, the number of activated vertices $\sigma(S, \lambda)$ is obtained, while the revenue comes from the number of activated vertices except the seeds, that is, $\sigma(S, \lambda) - |S|$. We define the revenue function as $\pi : 2^V \times \Lambda \rightarrow \mathbb{R}$. Then $\pi(S, \lambda) = \lambda(\sigma(S, \lambda) - |S|)$.

Formally, we define *Revenue Maximization Problem* as follows: given a commodity and a graph $G = (V, E)$, the problem is to determine the optimal price λ for this commodity and identify a seed set S to be the initial consumers, such that the expected revenue $\pi(S, \lambda)$ is maximized.

3 Approximate Revenue Calculation

In order to solve the revenue maximization problem efficiently, we provide a method for approximate revenue calculation based on local acyclic graph constructions, which is the basis for the proposed heuristic algorithms.

Activation Probability Calculation. In general directed graphs, there exists loops, and the expected social influence spread from the seed set is difficult to compute. But if the directed graphs are acyclic, the computation of the expected social influence can be conducted. For an acyclic graph G_A, given a seed set $S \subseteq V$ and the price λ, let $ap_\lambda(S, v)$ be the activation probability of vertex v.

We first topologically sort [15] all the vertices into a linear order $\{v_1, v_2, ...v_n\}$, where n is the number of vertices, with the seeds at the beginning of this order, and then compute $ap_\lambda(S, v_i)$ $(1 \leq i \leq n)$ for all v_i following this order. The influence on a vertex v_i comes from the vertices in front of v_i in this topological order, but not comes from the vertices behind, with the reason that the graph G_A is acyclic. In other words, the valuation of v_i is influenced by the vertices in front of it in the order. Suppose the number of seed set S is k. The first k vertices in this topological order $\{v_1, v_2, ...v_k\}$ are the seeds, so that $ap_\lambda(S, v_i) = 1(i \leq k)$ as they have already been activated. For the vertex v_{k+1}, the influence of her valuation comes from the set $\{v_1, v_2, ...v_k\}$. If some of her in-degree neighbors are from the seed set, v_{k+1}'s valuation will increase to $\chi_{v_{k+1}} + \sum_{v_i \in S} w_{v_i,v_{k+1}}$. Because $\chi_{v_{k+1}} \in [0, 1]$ is selected uniformly at random, $\chi_{v_{k+1}} + \sum_{v_i \in S} w_{v_i,v_{k+1}}$ will be selected in $[\sum_{v_i \in S} w_{v_i,v_{k+1}}, 1 + \sum_{v_i \in S} w_{v_i,v_{k+1}}]$ uniformly at random. If $\chi_{v_{k+1}} + \sum_{v_i \in S} w_{i,v_{k+1}} \geq \lambda$, then v_{k+1} will adopt the commodity. Thus, the probability of v_{k+1}'s adoption is $ap_\lambda(S, v_{k+1}) = 1 - \lambda + \sum_{v_i \in S} w_{v_i,v_{k+1}}$. As $S = \{v_1, v_2, ...v_k\}$ and $ap_\lambda(S, v_i) = 1(i \leq k)$, then we got $ap_\lambda(S, v_{k+1}) = 1 - \lambda + \sum_{v_i \in \{v_1,v_2,...v_k\}} ap_\lambda(S, v_i) w_{v_i,v_{k+1}}$. Similarly, for the vertex v_{k+2}, the influence on her valuation comes from $\{v_1, v_2, ...v_{k+1}\}$. Her valuation will become $\chi_{v_{k+2}} + \sum_{i \in \{v_1,v_2,...v_{k+1}\}} ap_\lambda(S, v_i) w_{v_i,v_{k+2}}$. Then the probability of v_{k+2}'s adoption is $ap_\lambda(S, v_{k+2}) = 1 - \lambda + \sum_{v_i \in \{v_1,v_2,...v_{k+1}\}} ap_\lambda(S, v_i) w_{v_i,v_{k+2}}$. For vertex $v_i(i > k+2)$, the probability of adoption can be computed in the similar way. Suppose the set of vertices in front of vertex v_i in the topological order is C_{v_i}. In general, for each vertex $v_i(i > k)$, it can be derived that the activation probability is

$$ap_\lambda(S, v_i) = 1 - \lambda + \sum_{u \in C_{v_i}} ap_\lambda(S, u) w_{u,v_i} \quad (1)$$

The activation probability of vertex v_i is computed according to that of the vertices in front of v_i in the topological order. When computing the activation probability of v_i, all the activation probability of v_i's in-neighbors have been computed. Equation (1) shows that the activation probability of all the vertices can be calculated linear to the number of edges of an acyclic graph.

However, real-world social networks are not acyclic, so we cannot use Eq. (1) directly. To address this problem, we construct a local acyclic graph for every vertex v, and then use the activation probability of v in its local acyclic graph to approximate that in the original network. For each price λ, vertex v is associated

Algorithm 1. $LA_\lambda(v)$ construction

1: Initialize $LA_\lambda(v) \leftarrow v$, set v newly added and $inf_{LA_\lambda(v)}(v,v) = 1$
2: **for** every added vertex $x \in LA_\lambda(v)$ **do**
3:   **for** every in-neighbor u ($u \notin LA_\lambda(v)$) of x **do**
4:     **if** u is first check **then**
5:       $inf_{LA_\lambda(v)}(u,v) = w_{u,x} \times inf_{LA_\lambda(v)}(x,v)$
6:     **else**
7:       $inf_{LA_\lambda(v)}(u,v) += w_{u,x} \times inf_{LA_\lambda(v)}(x,v)$
8:     **if** $inf_{LA_\lambda(v)}(u,v) \geq \theta$ **then**
9:       Add u into $LA_\lambda(v)$
10:       Add all $e_{u,y}$ (y in $LA_\lambda(v)$) into $LA_\lambda(v)$
11: **Output** $LA_\lambda(v)$

with a local acyclic graph $LA_\lambda(v)$, which denotes a subgraph of G rooted at v. We need to find $LA_\lambda(v)$ that covers a significant portion of influence from other vertices to v and ignores the others. Given a seed set S, we assume that the influence from S to v is only propagated within $LA_\lambda(v)$.

Influence Calculation. The influence to v propagated from u in an acyclic graph G_A, defined as $inf_{G_A}(u,v)$, is v's incremental activation probability, in the case that u is activated relative to that u is not activated. We topologically sort [15] all the vertices that can reach v in G_A into a sequence, and then reverse this sequence into a new order. Initially, $inf_{G_A}(v,v) = 1$. Then for each node $u \neq v$ according to the order

$$inf_{G_A}(u,v) = \sum_{x \in V \setminus \{v\}} w_{u,x} inf_{G_A}(x,v) \tag{2}$$

In an acyclic graph G_A, supposing that the item price is λ and the seed set is S, the incremental activation probability of v contributed from u is $(1 - ap_\lambda(S,u)) inf_{G_A}(u,v)$, which can be derived by repeatedly expanding $ap_\lambda(S,v)$ using Eq. (1), where $inf_{G_A}(u,v)$ is calculated according to Eq. (2).

Local Acyclic Graph Construction. According to Eq. (2), the influence $inf_{LA_\lambda(v)}(u,v)$ from u to v can be calculated in constructing an acyclic graph $LA_\lambda(v)$. Algorithm 1 shows how to construct the local acyclic graph of each vertex v and calculate the influences from other vertices to v. Let $\theta \in [0,1]$ be a threshold, and we need to make sure that $inf_{LA_\lambda(v)}(u,v) \geq \theta$ for each vertex u in $LA_\lambda(v)$. The intuition behind is that we need to find $LA_\lambda(v)$ that covers a significant portion of influences from other vertices to v and ignores the vertices that have only little influence to v. Initially vertex v is added into $LA_\lambda(v)$. Then in each iteration, for every newly added vertex $x \in LA_\lambda(v)$, for every in-neighbor u of x, we calculate $inf_{LA_\lambda(v)}(u,v)$ and select every vertex u satisfying $inf_{LA_\lambda(v)}(u,v) \geq \theta$, and then add these vertices into $LA_\lambda(v)$ together with all the corresponding edges. The process continues until there is a vertex u with $inf_{LA_\lambda(v)}(u,v) < \theta$. The runtime of constructing each $LA_\lambda(v)$ is linear to $|E|$.

Total Revenue Calculation. For each price λ, vertex v is associated with a local acyclic graph $LA_\lambda(v)$. We use the activation probability of v in its local acyclic graph to approximate that in the original network. Given a seed set S, we assume that the influence from S to v is only propagated within $LA_\lambda(v)$. The activated number $\sigma(S,\lambda)$ is $\sum_v ap_\lambda(S,v)$, then the expected revenue $\pi(S,\lambda)$ is

$$\pi(S,\lambda) = \lambda(\sum_{v\in V} ap_\lambda(S,v) - |S|) \tag{3}$$

Marginal Revenue Calculation. Suppose the current seed set is S, if a vertex u is selected as a seed, the incremental influence that u imposes on the activation probability of v, i.e., $ap_\lambda(S\cup\{u\},v) - ap_\lambda(S,v)$, is $(1-ap_\lambda(S,u))inf_{LA_\lambda(v)}(u,v)$. We define the incremental marginal revenue from u as $\pi(u|S,\lambda)$. Applying Eq. (3),

Algorithm 2. CR Algorithm

1: **for** every price λ **do**
2: **for** each vertex $v \in V$ **do**
3: $LA_\lambda(v)$ construction
4: Initialize $X_0 \leftarrow \emptyset$, $Y_0 \leftarrow V$, $n \leftarrow |V|$
5: **for** $i = 1$ to n **do**
6: $a_i \leftarrow \pi(u_i|X_{i-1},\lambda)$ according to Eq. (4)
7: $b_i \leftarrow \pi(u_i^-|Y_{i-1},\lambda)$ according to Eq. (5)
8: $a'_i \leftarrow max\{a_i, 0\}$, $b'_i \leftarrow max\{b_i, 0\}$
9: **with probability** $a'_i/(a'_i + b'_i)$ **do**:
10: $X_i \leftarrow X_{i-1} \cup \{u_i\}$, $Y_i \leftarrow Y_{i-1}$
11: **else** (with probability $b'_i/(a'_i + b'_i)$) **do**:
12: $X_i \leftarrow X_{i-1}$, $Y_i \leftarrow Y_{i-1}\backslash\{u_i\}$
13: $S \leftarrow X_n$ (or equivalently Y_n)
14: Calculate $\pi(S,\lambda)$ according to Eq. (3)
15: **Output** λ and S with the maximum $\pi(S,\lambda)$
16: * If $a'_i = b'_i = 0$, we assume $a'_i/(a'_i + b'_i) = 1$

Algorithm 3. CG Algorithm

1: **for** every price λ **do**
2: **for** each vertex $v \in V$ **do**
3: $LA_\lambda(v)$ construction
4: Initialize $S_0 \leftarrow \emptyset$
5: **for** $i = 1$ to Q **do**
6: **if** $(\sigma(S_{i-1},\lambda) = \sum_v ap_\lambda(S_{i-1},v)) \geq Q$ **then**
7: **break**
8: **for** each vertex $v \in V\backslash S_{i-1}$ **do**
9: Calculate $\pi(v|S_{i-1},\lambda)$ according to Eq. (4)
10: $u = argmax_{v\in V\backslash S_{i-1}} \pi(v|S_{i-1},\lambda)$
11: **if** $\pi(u|S_{i-1},\lambda) \leq 0$ **then**
12: **break**
13: $S_i \leftarrow S_{i-1} \cup \{u\}$
14: For price λ, the seed set is S_i
15: Calculate $\pi(S_i,\lambda)$ according to Eq. (3)
16: **Output** λ and S_i with the maximum $\pi(S_i,\lambda)$

$$\pi(u|S,\lambda) = \pi(S\cup\{u\},\lambda) - \pi(S,\lambda) = \lambda(-1 + (1-ap_\lambda(S,u))\sum_{v\in V} inf_{LA_\lambda(v)}(u,v)) \tag{4}$$

Similarly, if $u \in S$ is removed from S, the decreased marginal revenue is

$$\pi(u^-|S,\lambda) = \lambda(1 + (ap_\lambda(S\backslash\{u\},u) - 1)\sum_{v\in V} inf_{LA_\lambda(v)}(u,v)) \tag{5}$$

The local acyclic graph constructions as well as the total and marginal revenue calculations are the basis for the proposed heuristic algorithms.

4 The Proposed Algorithms

We propose two efficient algorithms: (1) the Calculation-based Randomized (CR) algorithm for unlimited commodity supply; (2) the Calculation-based max-Heap updating Greedy (CHG) algorithm for constrained commodity supply.

4.1 CR Algorithm

For unlimited commodity supply, instead of time-consuming simulations in [23], we calculate the approximate marginal and total revenue.

Algorithm 2 shows CR. In the main loop of lines 1–14, we pick a price in each round and identify the corresponding seed set. Lines 2–3 are the preparation phase for each price, in which each $LA_\lambda(v)$ is generated, and $inf_{LA_\lambda(v)}(u,v)$ for all $u \in LA_\lambda(v)$ are gained as well. Lines 5–12 identify whether a vertex is selected as a seed. Instead of using a large number of simulations to get the marginal revenue, line 6 calculates the incremental marginal revenue from vertex u_i when the seed set is X_{i-1}, and line 7 calculates the decreased marginal revenue from vertex u_i when the seed set is Y_{i-1}. Lines 9–12 give the probability of vertex u_i being selected as a seed or the probability being not selected as a seed. Line 13 gives the seed set at the predetermined price, and line 14 calculates the total revenue of this seed set and the predetermined price. Finally, in line 15, we choose the price and the corresponding seed set achieving the maximum revenue. The time complexity of CR is $O(|\Lambda||V||E|)$.

4.2 CHG Algorithm

For the scenario of constrained commodity supply, we propose CG and CHG. A vertex with greater influence should be regarded as more important, so that greedily selecting the individuals with greatest influence as seeds can lead to a feasible solution. To make the algorithm more efficient, in CG and CHG, we approximately calculate the revenue within the local acyclic graphs. Compared with CG, CHG uses a max-Heap updating scheme to reduce unnecessary calculations to achieve better efficiency.

Algorithm 3 shows CG. In the main loop of lines 1–15, we select a price λ in each round and identify the seed set at λ. Lines 2–3 are the preparation phase for each price, in which each $LA_\lambda(v)$ is generated, and $inf_{LA_\lambda(v)}(u,v)$ for all $u \in LA_\lambda(v)$ are obtained as well. In the seed selecting process for price λ, we iteratively select a seed with the maximum marginal revenue (lines 5–13), where the marginal revenue can be calculated as Eq. 4. The iteration process can be terminated in two cases: (1) the number of the activated vertices exceeds the quantity of the commodity Q (lines 6–7); (2) the examined seed's marginal revenue is negative (lines 11–12). The seed set at each price λ is obtained in line 14. Finally, we choose the price and the corresponding seed set achieving the maximum revenue (line 16). In CG, the marginal revenue from one vertex (line 9), the activated number of a seed set (line 6), the total revenue by setting a price and a seed set (line 15) are all calculated based on the local acyclic graphs. The time complexity of CG is $O(Q|\Lambda||V||E|)$.

However, there is still a limitation of CG. To identify the seed with the maximum marginal revenue, given the current seed set S_{i-1}, we have to enumerate all candidate vertices to obtain the one with the maximum marginal revenue. Actually, for some of the vertices, the computations for their marginal revenue

Algorithm 4. CHG Algorithm

```
1: for every price λ do
2:     for each vertex v ∈ V do
3:         LA_λ(v) construction
4:     Initialize S_0 ← ∅, and initialize a hash map M_λ
5:     Build max-Heap H_λ with π({v}|∅, λ) of all v ∈ V
6:     for i = 1 to Q do
7:         if (σ(S_{i-1}.λ) = Σ_v ap_λ(S_{i-1}, v)) ≥ Q then
8:             break
9:         Clear hash map M_λ
10:        while the i'th seed not obtained do
11:            v = H_λ.pop()
12:            if v ∉ M_λ (unchecked) then
13:                Calculate π({v}|S_{i-1}, λ) based on Eq. (4)
14:                Add ⟨v, π({v}|S_{i-1}, λ)⟩ into H_λ
15:                Put ⟨v, calculated⟩ into M_λ (set checked)
16:                continue
17:            if v ∈ M_λ (checked) then
18:                S_i ← S_{i-1} ∪ {v}
19:        if π({v}|S_{i-1}, λ) ≤ 0 then
20:            Remove v from S_i
21:            break
22:     For price λ, the seed set is S_i
23:     Calculate π(S_i, λ) according to Eq. (3)
24: Output λ and S_i with the maximum π(S_i, λ)
```

can be avoided. The intuition behind is that revenue functions follow the submodular property, i.e., the marginal revenue from a vertex decreases as the seed set grows. It has been proved that the revenue function $\pi(S, \lambda)$ is non-negative submodular [3,9,23] if the commodity supply is unlimited, and it is obvious that the property also holds when the commodity supply is constrained, for the quantity constraint will not break this property. Then we propose the CHG algorithm using a max-Heap updating scheme to prune unnecessary calculations.

In CHG algorithm, the process to identify seeds at price λ is as follows. Firstly we calculate the marginal revenue $\pi(v|\emptyset, \lambda)$ for each vertex $v \in V$, and build a max-Heap H_λ with the initial marginal revenue $\pi(v|\emptyset, \lambda)$ of every vertex. Obviously, the top vertex on the max-Heap is the first seed selected for price λ, denoted by u. We pop u, add u into S_0, adjust the heap, and set all the vertices in the max-Heap unchecked. Then we keep updating this heap to select the rest seeds. Specifically, in the following iterations, we pop the top vertex v in the max-Heap, and deal with v in two cases: (1) if v's marginal revenue $\pi(v|S_{i-1}, \lambda)$ is unchecked, we calculate $\pi(v|S_{i-1}, \lambda)$, add $\langle v, \pi(v|S_{i-1}, \lambda)\rangle$ into the max-Heap H_λ, and set it checked; (2) if v's marginal revenue is already checked, v will be chosen as a seed, and thus the current iteration will be terminated and all the vertices in the max-Heap is set unchecked. A hash map M_λ is used to maintain whether a vertex is checked or not. According to the submodular property, if the marginal revenues of some vertices obtained in previous iterations is less than the marginal revenue from another vertex in the current iteration, it's not possible for those vertices to be selected as seeds in the current iteration. Consequently, unnecessary computations can be pruned. Algorithm 4 shows CHG. The marginal revenue from one vertex (line 13), the activated number of a seed set (line 7), and the total revenue by setting a price and a seed set (line 23) are all calculated based on the local acyclic graphs. In the seed selecting process for price λ, we first build a max-Heap (line 5), and then iteratively select a seed with the maximum marginal revenue from the heap (lines 6–21). The time complexity of CHG algorithm is $O(Q|\Lambda||V||E|)$. With regard to the effectiveness, the maximum revenue obtained by CHG is the same as that of CG.

5 Evaluation

In this section, we conduct experiments on both synthetic networks and real-world networks to demonstrate the efficiency and effectiveness of the proposed algorithms CR and CHG. All the algorithms are implemented in JAVA, and performed on Intel(R) Xeon(R) CPU E5-2620 v3 @ 2.40 GHz.

5.1 Experimental Setup

Datasets. We do experiments in synthetic networks and real-world networks. Synthetic networks are power-law graphs generated by NetworkX [1] with various sizes, which will be introduced in details in Sect. 5.2. We use four real-world networks: (a) Residence Hall Friendship (RHF) network [11] with 217 vertices and 2,672 edges; (b) Ego-Facebook (EgoFB) network [22] with 4,039 vertices and 88,234 edges; (c) NetHEPT network [5] with 15,233 vertices and 58,891 edges; and (d) NetPHY network [5] with 37,154 vertices and 231,584 edges.

For each network, we need to generate the weights on all edges with a random method, that is, the weight of each edge is firstly generated uniformly at random in the range $[0, \alpha]$. To meet $\Sigma_u w_{u,v} \leq \alpha$, the weights of all in-neighbor edges of a vertex v are divided by the number of v's in-neighbor edges. Here we set $\alpha = 0.5$ in the experiment. For each network, we repeated this process for 10 times, and the results (including the running time, the maximum revenue and the corresponding price) for evaluations are the mean value of the results obtained each time. When constructing acyclic graphs, the threshold θ is set to 0.01. In the experiments, we set the prices of a commodity as a set Λ of input parameters [0.50, 0.52, 0.54, ..., 0.70], and $\lambda \in \Lambda$.

Baselines. We compare our algorithms with three baselines described as follows.

Randomized Algorithm. It is the algorithm proposed in [23], and we compare CR with it for unlimited supply of commodities.

Greedy Algorithm. It is the variant of CG, in which the marginal and the total revenue are gained by simulations but bot by calculations. It is compared with CG and CHG for constrained supply of commodities.

PRUB+IF Algorithm. It is proposed in [25] for constrained supply of commodities, which is compared with CG and CHG. Please note that this algorithm

[1] https://networkx.github.io/.

only suites the cases that each user's inherent valuation is known by the seller, which is a strong assumption that does not hold in real-world scenarios. To address this issue, we generalize this algorithm by setting each user's inherent valuation as random variables. Specifically, in the process of obtaining the upper bound of the maximum revenue, each user's valuation is set as the average of 1,000 random values in the range [0, 1].

All the baselines and proposed algorithms are run in the price-sensitive dynamics process described in Sect. 2. For the baselines, 2000 simulations are executed to estimate the revenue for each candidate price and seed set. In each simulation, the valuation of each user is generated at random. This number of simulations is chosen to make the estimates accurate while considering the poor efficiency of the baselines. As the running time of the baselines are linear to the number of simulations, if our proposed algorithms are much faster than the baselines with 2000 simulations, then we can conclude that they would be more efficient than the baselines conducting a larger number of simulations. For the evaluations of effectiveness, in each algorithm of CR, CG, CHG and the baselines,

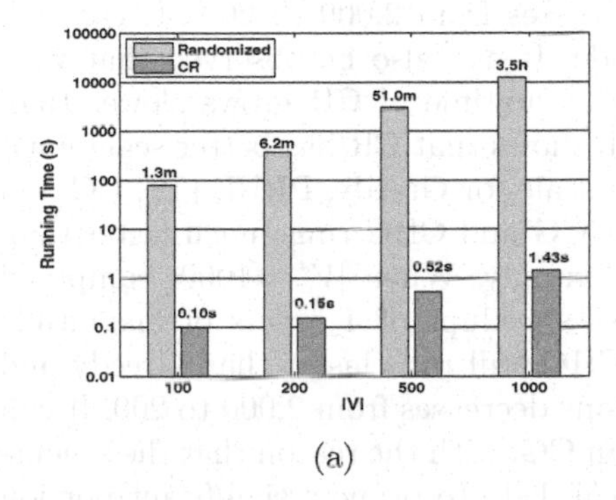

(a)

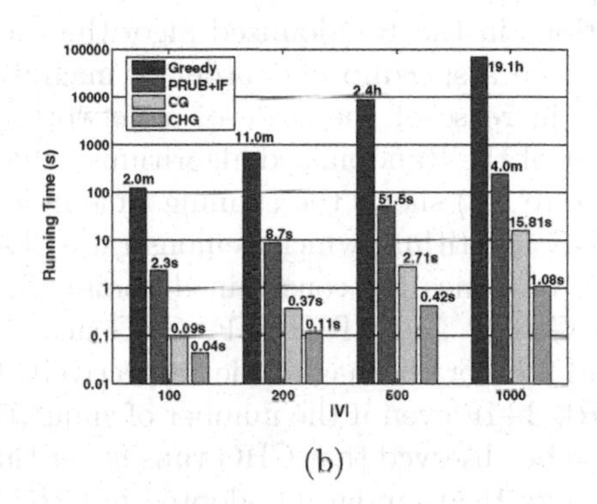

(b)

Fig. 1. The running time (in log scale) on synthetic networks for: (a) unlimited commodity supply; (b) constrained commodity supply where $Q/|V| = 60\%$.

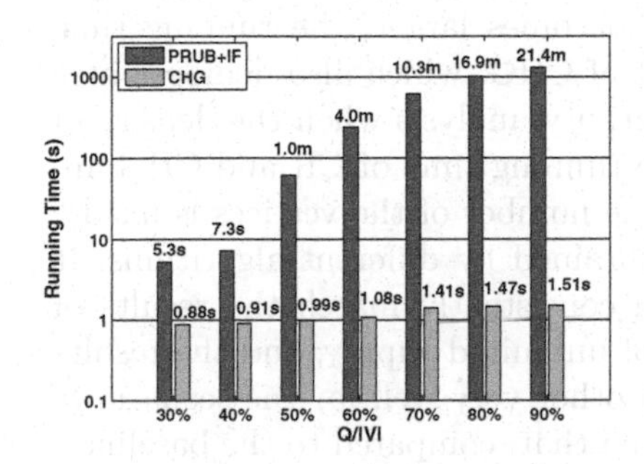

Fig. 2. The running time (in log scale) in a network (1,000 vertices, 3,000 edges) as the quantity of the commodity varies.

Table 1. The running time of CR and CHG ($Q/|V| = 60\%$) on a network (500 vertices) when the density varies.

$\|E\|$	1500	3000	4500	6000	7500
CR	0.52 s	0.62 s	0.65 s	1.03 s	1.26 s
CHG	0.42 s	0.55 s	0.88 s	1.30 s	1.49 s

after selecting λ and S, we use the average revenue by 2000 simulations as the result to compare. To make fair comparisons, we use the same settings in the baselines as our work.

5.2 Results on Synthetic Networks

We generate different scales of synthetic power-law graphs with 100, 200, 500 and 1,000 vertices, each with 300, 600, 1,500 and 3,000 edges respectively to evaluate the algorithms. Please note that as the baseline algorithms are not scalable, we can only use small datasets to conduct the comparisons. Later we will evaluate our methods on large-scale real-world networks to show the scalability.

Figure 1(a) shows the running time in log scale for the Randomized algorithm and CR algorithm, which demonstrates that, when the quantity of the commodities is unlimited, the Randomized algorithm runs much slower than CR. For example, when $|V|$ is 1000, CR achieves a speedup of 3 orders of magnitude against the Randomized algorithm. Note that as the runtime of the Randomized algorithm is linear to the number of simulations, even if the number of simulations in the Randomized algorithm decreases from 2,000 to 20, CR can still achieve a speedup of 1 order of magnitude. It can also be observed that with the increase of the scale of a network, the runtime of CR grows slower than that of the Randomized algorithms, which shows that CR has better scalability. Figure 1(b) shows the running time in log scale for Greedy, PRUB+IF, CG and CHG algorithm, which demonstrates that CG and CHG runs much faster than the baselines for constrained commodity supply. When $|V|$ =1000, compared to Greedy and PRUB+IF, CHG achieves speedups of 4 orders of magnitude and 2 orders of magnitude respectively. CHG still runs faster than Greedy and PRUB+IF even if the number of simulations decreases from 2,000 to 200. It can also be observed that CHG runs faster than CG, with the reason that the scheme of max-Heap updating adopted in CHG can help to prune a significant portion of the calculations. Figure 2 shows the running time in log scale of PRUB+IF and CHG on a network with 1,000 vertices and 3,000 edges, as the quantity of the commodities varies. As the quantity becomes larger, the running time of PRUB+IF increases much more than that of CHG, which also demonstrates the efficiency of CHG. In Table 1 we do sensitivity analysis when the density of the graph varies. It can be observed that the running time of CR and CHG are almost linear to the number of edges when the number of the vertices is fixed.

Figure 3 shows the maximum revenues obtained by different algorithms. It can be observed that the results of CR can consistently match the results of the Randomized algorithm for the scenario of unlimited supply, and the results of CHG and other baselines also match each other very well for the scenario of constrained supply. Thus it can be summarized that, compared to the baselines, the maximum revenues obtained by CR and CHG are almost not impacted, with a much better efficiency.

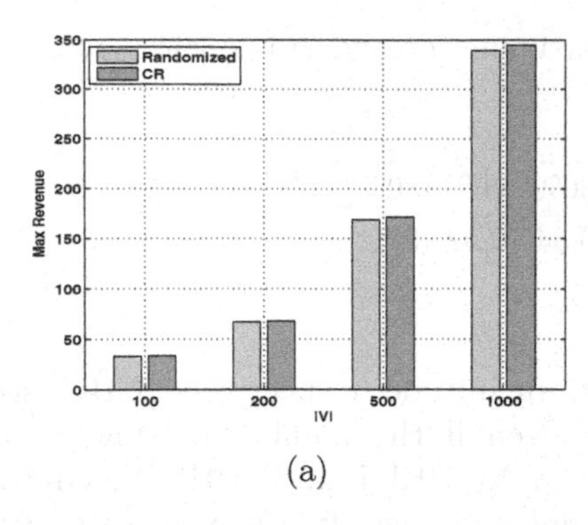

(a)

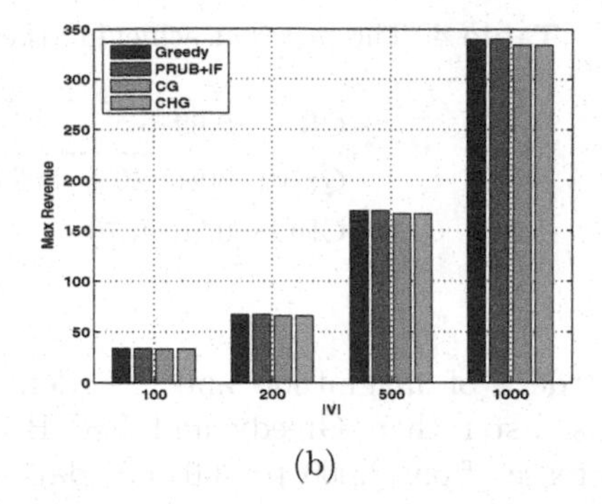

(b)

Fig. 3. The maximum revenues on synthetic networks for: (a) unlimited commodity supply; (b) constrained commodity supply where $Q/|V| = 60\%$.

Table 2. The running time on real-world networks.

Datasets	RHF	EgoFB	NetHEPT	NetPHY
Unlimited commodity supply				
Randomized	1359.8 s	N/A	N/A	N/A
CR	0.7 s	31.7 s	161.3 s	2790.3 s
Constrained commodity supply				
Greedy	584.3 s	N/A	N/A	N/A
PRUB+IF	35.5 s	18123.9 s	N/A	N/A
CG	0.6 s	363.1 s	43633.9 s	N/A
CHG	0.5 s	24.3 s	363.3 s	13640.2 s

Table 3. The maximum revenues on real-world networks.

Datasets	RHF	EgoFB	NetHEPT	NetPHY
Unlimited commodity supply				
Randomized	71.8	N/A	N/A	N/A
CR	71.5	1392.2	4636.2	11557.5
Constrained commodity supply				
Greedy	70.6	N/A	N/A	N/A
PRUB+IF	70.6	1376.3	N/A	N/A
CG	70.2	1296.5	4631.6	N/A
CHG	70.2	1296.5	4631.6	11448.3

5.3 Results on Real-World Networks

In this section, we conduct experiments on real-world networks. Please note that in these experiments, if the running time of an algorithm exceeds 24 h, we just stop running this algorithm and discard its results of the running time and the maximum revenue, and mark them as "N/A" in the corresponding table.

Table 2 shows the runtime of the baselines and the proposed algorithms. For unlimited commodity supply, it can be observed that CR algorithm runs much faster than the Randomized algorithm. For the residence hall friendship dataset, CR achieves a speedup of 4 orders of magnitude against the Randomized algorithm. As the runtime of the Randomized algorithm is linear to the number of simulations, even if the number of simulations in the Randomized algorithm decreases from 2,000 to 20, CR can still achieve a speedup of 2 orders of magnitude. For the other three datasets which have larger size than the residence hall friendship dataset, the Randomized algorithm runs over 24 h, but CR is quite efficient. For the dataset NetPHY that has the largest size, CR runs less than an hour. For the scenario of constrained commodity supply, it is shown that CG and CHG runs much faster than the baselines. For the residence hall friendship dataset, compared to Greedy and PRUB+IF, CHG achieves speedups of

Table 4. The prices at achieving the maximum revenue on Ego-Facebook.

CR	0.52						
$Q/\|V\|$	30%	40%	50%	60%	70%	80%	90%
CHG	0.70	0.70	0.62	0.54	0.52	0.52	0.52

3 orders of magnitude and 2 orders of magnitude respectively. CHG still runs faster than Greedy and PRUB+IF even if the number of simulations decreases from 2,000 to 200. For datasets of NetHEPT and NetPHY, Greedy and PRUB+IF run over 24 h, while CHG runs quite fast. It can also be observed that CHG runs faster than CG, with the reason that the scheme of max-Heap updating adopted in CHG works well, which can help to prune a significant portion of the calculations. According to Table 2, it can be concluded that the baselines are constrained in efficiency, while the proposed algorithms show good scalability and would be feasible solutions for real-world scenarios.

Table 3 shows the maximum revenues. It can be observed that the results of CR match those of the Randomized algorithm, and the results of CHG and other baselines also match each other very well. Thus it can be summarized that, compared with the baselines, CR and CHG can successfully obtain almost the same maximum revenue with superiority in efficiency.

We also study the chosen price at the maximum revenue from CR and CHG. It is shown in Table 4 that in Ego-Facebook network, for unlimited commodity supply, the selected price is a lower value within the range, 0.52 in our case, which reveals a good strategy should focus on the number of activated vertices when the differences among the candidate prices are not large. For constrained commodity supply, when the quantity of the commodity is small, the selected price should be high. The possible reason is that both the higher and lower price can result in a significant number of activated vertices relative to the small quantity of the commodities, and thus the higher price can bring in more revenue. We can also see that the chosen price decreases as the amount of the commodity grows larger. The possible reason is that as the quantity of the commodity grows, the higher price can no longer make the number of the activated vertices approach to the quantity of the commodity. As a result, we have to lower the price to increase the number of the activated vertices. It is consistent with the marketing strategies in real-world applications.

6 Conclusion

In this paper, two efficient revenue maximization algorithms CR and CHG are proposed for both the scenarios of unlimited and constrained commodity supply respectively. In these algorithms, local acyclic graphs are constructed which help to gain the revenue through fast calculation. Furthermore, a max-Heap updating scheme is proposed to prune unnecessary calculations in CHG. Experiments on both the synthetic networks and real-world networks demonstrate the efficiency and effectiveness of the proposed algorithms.

Acknowledgments. This work is supported in part by the State Key Development Program of Basic Research of China (No. 2013CB329605), the National Key Research and Development Program of China (No. 2016QY03D0605), the Natural Science Foundation of China (No. 61300014, 61372191, 61672313), NSF through grants IIS-1526499, and CNS-1626432.

References

1. Akhlaghpour, H., Ghodsi, M., Haghpanah, N., Mirrokni, V.S., Mahini, H., Nikzad, A.: Optimal iterative pricing over social networks (Extended abstract). In: Saberi, A. (ed.) WINE 2010. LNCS, vol. 6484, pp. 415–423. Springer, Heidelberg (2010). doi:10.1007/978-3-642-17572-5_34
2. Bensaid, B., Lesne, J.P.: Dynamic monopoly pricing with network externalities. Int. J. Ind. Organ. **14**(6), 837–855 (1996)
3. Buchbinder, N., Feldman, M., Naor, J., Schwartz, R.: A tight linear time (1/2)-approximation for unconstrained submodular maximization. SIAM J. Comput. **44**(5), 1384–1402 (2015)
4. Cabral, L.M.B., Salant, D.J., Woroch, G.A.: Monopoly pricing with network externalities. Int. J. Ind. Organ. **17**(2), 199–214 (1999)
5. Chen, W., Wang, Y., Yang, S.: Efficient influence maximization in social networks. In: KDD, pp. 199–208 (2009)
6. Chen, W., Yuan, Y., Zhang, L.: Scalable influence maximization in social networks under the linear threshold model. In: ICDM, pp. 88–97 (2010)
7. Cohen, E., Delling, D., Pajor, T., Werneck, R.F.: Sketch-based influence maximization and computation: Scaling up with guarantees. In: CIKM, pp. 629–638 (2014)
8. Domingos, P., Richardson, M.: Mining the network value of customers. In: KDD, pp. 57–66 (2001)
9. Feige, U., Mirrokni, V.S., Vondrak, J.: Maximizing non-monotone submodular functions. SIAM J. Comput. **40**(4), 1133–1153 (2011)
10. Fotakis, D., Siminelakis, P.: On the efficiency of influence-and-exploit strategies for revenue maximization under positive externalities. Theor. Comput. Sci. **539**, 68–86 (2014)
11. Freeman, L., Webster, C., Kirke, D.: Exploring social structure using dynamic three-dimensional color images. Soc. Netw. **20**(2), 109–118 (1998)
12. Fromlet, H.: Predictability of financial crises: lessons from Sweden for other countries. Bus. Econ. **47**(4), 262–272 (2012)
13. Goyal, A., Lu, W., Lakshmanan, L.V.S.: SIMPATH: an efficient algorithm for influence maximization under the linear threshold model. In: ICDM, pp. 211–220 (2011)
14. Hartline, J., Mirrokni, V., Sundararajan, M.: Optimal marketing strategies over social networks. In: WWW, pp. 189–198 (2008)
15. Kahn, A.B.: Topological sorting of large networks. Commun. ACM **5**(11), 558–562 (1962)
16. Kalish, S.: A new product adoption model with price, advertising, and uncertainty. Manag. Sci. **31**(12), 1569–1585 (1985)

17. Katz, M., Shapiro, C.: Network externalities, competition, and compatibility. Am. Econ. Rev. **75**(3), 424–440 (1985)
18. Kempe, D., Kleinberg, J., Tardos, E.: Maximizing the spread of influence through a social network. In: KDD, pp. 137–146 (2003)
19. Leskovec, J., Krause, A., Guestrin, C., Faloutsos, C., VanBriesen, J., Glance, N.: Cost-effective outbreak detection in networks. In: KDD, pp. 420–429 (2007)
20. Lu, W., Lakshmanan, L.V.S.: Profit maximization over social networks. In: ICDM, pp. 479–488 (2012)
21. Mason, R.: Network externalities and the coase conjecture. Eur. Econ. Rev. **44**(10), 1981–1992 (2000)
22. McAuley, J., Leskovec, J.: Learning to discover social circles in ego networks. In: NIPS, pp. 539–547 (2012)
23. Mirrokni, V.S., Roch, S., Sundararajan, M.: On fixed-price marketing for goods with positive network externalities. In: Goldberg, P.W. (ed.) WINE 2012. LNCS, vol. 7695, pp. 532–538. Springer, Heidelberg (2012). doi:10.1007/978-3-642-35311-6_43
24. Sundararajan, A.: Local network effects and complex network structure. BE J. Theor. Econ. **7**(1) (2007)
25. Teng, Y., Tai, C., Yu, P.S., Chen, M.: An effective marketing strategy for revenue maximization with a quantity constraint. In: KDD, pp. 1175–1184 (2015)

Generating Life Course Trajectory Sequences with Recurrent Neural Networks and Application to Early Detection of Social Disadvantage

Lin Wu[1,2](✉), Michele Haynes[1], Andrew Smith[1], Tong Chen[2], and Xue Li[2]

[1] Australian Research Council Centre of Excellence in Children and Families over the Life Course, Institute for Social Science Research, The University of Queensland, Indooroopilly 4068, Australia
{lin.wu,m.haynes,a.smith7}@uq.edu.au

[2] Information Technology and Electrical Engineering, The University of Queensland, St Lucia 4072, Australia
tong.chen@uq.edu.au, xueli@itee.uq.edu.au

Abstract. Using long-running panel data from the Household, Income and Labour Dynamics in Australia (HILDA) survey collected annually between 2001 and 2015, we aim to generate a sequence of events for individuals by processing real life trajectories one step at a time and predict what comes next. This is motivated by the need for understanding and predicting forthcoming patterns from these disadvantage dynamics which are represented by multiple life-course trajectories evolutions over time. In this paper, given longitudinal trajectories created from HILDA survey waves, we develop a model with Long Short-term Memory recurrent neural networks to generate complex trajectory sequences with long-range structure. Our method uses a multi-layered Long Short-Term Memory (LSTM) approach to map the input sequence to a vector of a fixed dimensionality, and then another deep LSTM to decode the target sequence from the vector. The generated sequences over time use the social exclusion monitor (SEM) indicator to determine the level of social disadvantage for each individual. The sequences are encoded by predefined social exclusion factors, which are binary values to indicate the occurrence of corresponding factors. To model the correlations among social exclusion domains, we use the Mixture Density Networks which are parameterized by the outputs of LSTM. Our main result is the high prediction accuracy on personal life course trajectories created from real HILDA data. Moreover, the proposed model can synthesize, and impute some missing trajectories given partial observations from respondent individuals. More importantly, we examine the relative roles of different advantage dimensions in explaining changes in life trajectories in Australia, and find that the domains of employment, education, community and personal safety are highly correlated to the decreased disadvantage measurement. While, domains regarding material resources, health and social support are of direct relevance to increase social disadvantage with varied contribution extent.

G. Cong et al. (Eds.): ADMA 2017, LNAI 10604, pp. 225–242, 2017.
https://doi.org/10.1007/978-3-319-69179-4_16

Keywords: Recurrent neural networks · Mixture density model · Social disadvantage · Life course data trajectory

1 Introduction

Social disadvantage monitoring is essential for policy planning and understanding the drivers of disadvantage is important for reducing the disparity between the advantaged and disadvantaged groups. Australia provides an important case study in gaining insights into the drivers and dynamics of disadvantage. For example, in 2014, Australia ranked 1st in the World in terms of average wealth [20]. However, the proportion of the population that is relatively poor, which is one in eight, and is increasing. And the share of the population that is deeply and persistently disadvantaged has not decreased in the last decade, and income inequality is on the rise [2,35]. Thus, it is critical to provide tools for strategic planning and policymaking to devise policy interventions that maximize economic growth and reduce socio-economic deprivation in cost-effective ways.

A main challenge in understanding the level of social exclusion and disadvantage in the Australian context is how to model the various factors contributing to the changes in the level of disadvantage, and how to predict their future trajectories regarding individuals. All approaches to measuring social exclusion/disadvantage confront, either explicitly or implicitly, the issue of how to identify individual dimension of exclusion that are driving factors to the level of disadvantage. In [13], Martinez Jr. and colleagues examine the trends in multidimensional disadvantage in Australian between 2001 and 2013, and find that this has been relatively stable, with some evidence of upwards trend following from the 2008 Global Financial Crisis. Their further examination on the relative roles of different exclusion domains suggests that recent year-to-year changes in multi-dimensional disadvantage are mainly driven by fluctuations in social support, health and material resources. They explain the changes in disadvantage dynamics by using a decomposition methodology, and specifically, they adopt the Shapley-based decomposition method proposed by Shorrocks et al. [19]. Unlike a straightforward Oaxaca-Blinder decomposition method that only entails fitting a linear regression model and perusing the estimated regression coefficients [8], the Shapley-based alternative is able to explain average differences in characteristics and their underlying distribution. However, the Shapley-based decomposition algorithm has an inherent limitation where the estimated contribution factor may differ when the specific ordering of factors varies. This is because the Shapley-based decomposition constructs a counter-factual distribution for sum-score based disadvantage score by changing the value of each factor from the observed value at the initial time period to the observed value at the succeeding time period, one at a time, by holding the values of all other factors constant. As a consequence, to estimate the contribution of each factor, this method has to average across all possible permutations. This methodology is unable to capture the temporal dependency among life course trajectories measuring potential disadvantage. Also, the decomposition methodology does not estimate the correlations among driving factors of social disadvantage.

In this paper, we investigate individual trajectories of social exclusion in Australia, employing a deep recurrent model that generates life course sequences with long range structure. To encode people's life course trajectories, we apply the multidimensional measures that identify seven domains of exclusion: material resources; employment; education and skills; health and disability; social; community; and personal safety [17]. Additionally, to describe the trajectories more realistically, we include demographic characteristics which include gender, age, country of birth, housing situation, education attainment, marital status, and number of children (please refer to Tables 1 and 2). Our approach is premised on Recurrent Neural Networks (RNNs) [18] which have recently become a popular choice for modeling variable-length sequences. The rationale is that, the RNNs can be trained to condition their predictions on real data sequences one step at a time and predict what comes next. The predictions in our approach are assumed to be probabilistic, so that novel sequences can be generated from RNNs by iteratively sampling from the network's output, and then feeding in the sample as input at the next step. However, RNNs are using internal representations to perform their predictive distributions, in which the output variables cannot be modeled faithfully. To this end, we combine the recurrent model with a mixture density network [5,6] to allow more accurate prediction on the future trajectories. We apply the proposed approach to a nationally representative house panel survey: the Household, Income and Labour Dynamics in Australia (HILDA) survey, which provides longitudinal over 15 years and is rich in covariates.

Our key contributions are fourfold. First, to the best of our knowledge, we are the first study that models the sequences of life course trajectories using a deep recurrent model, which allows us to synthesize multi-variate data and generate sequences in future setting. Second, the longitudinal structure of the HILDA survey data allows us to examine the persistence of social disadvantage over a wide range of economic, social and health related dimensions. Third, we perform simulations to evaluate the accuracy of our model in its prediction ability.

2 Data and Definitions

The data used for this study comprise the 15 waves of the HILDA survey, an ongoing Australian household panel survey, providing rich information collected annually over the period 2001 to 2015 [21,34]. Wave 1 of the panel contained 14,000 individuals living in 7,682 households across Australia and was largely representative of the Australian population. The HILDA survey is very well suited to the early detection on social disadvantage since it collects yearly information from respondents on a wide variety of subjects relating to economic, health, and social wellbeing. Subjects include labor market and education activity, family circumstances, income, expenditure, disability, health, significant life events, satisfaction with various aspects of life and experience of financial hardship. Thus, this richness of data, combined with its longitudinal structure and its nationally representative design, is extremely valuable for the study of social disadvantage. We restrict our analytical sample to the working-age population (aged 25–60 years) so that any observed changes in disadvantage are not artificially affected by changes experienced by people who enter the labor for the first time or exit it permanently. Also, this is the conventional approach in the literature (OECD2009) [15] and makes it possible to compare with comparative study in [13]. A preprocessing step is to keep records from individuals who provide their answers in all 15 waves, and we ignore those who having their responses partially missing in any wave. As a result, we have 6,347 persons and for each person his/her trajectory is encoded by a mixture of variables: demographic characteristics, namely, sex, location of residence, household type, country of birth, Indigenous status, housing situation, and education attainment [16], and 21 indicators across seven life domains [17] to measure social exclusion.

We include demographic indicators into the life course trajectories for the sake of describing the real life trajectory at individual level more accurately from which RNN would be working well by feeding more variables as inputs. On the other hand, demographic incidence of social disadvantage provides more meaningful understanding on the generated life trajectories in regards to a specific community group. For example, consider the case of a woman aged 30s, lone parent with dependent children, we can artificially change the status of her household type to see how her trajectory pattern would be involving over time and if the indicator of household type would be the driving factor for her to move into or out of social disadvantage. Moreover, there are commonalities in the demographic composition of the socially excluded group from which representative patterns on life course trajectories can be mined out. The demographic characteristics are listed in Table 1. We investigate the social disadvantage by employing a multi-dimensional measure that can produce a single aggregate measure of the level of exclusion experienced by the individuals. Developed through consultations held in 2008 and 2009 [16] with a wide

Table 1. Demographic characteristics.

Gender	Male
	Female
Age	15–24 years
	25–34 years
	35–44 years
	45–54 years
	55–64 years
	65 years plus
Country of birth	Australian born
	Immigrant-English speaking country
	Immigrant-Non-English speaking country
	Indigenous
Housing situation	Home-owner (outright)
	Home-owner with mortgage
	Private renter
	Public housing
	Other housing situation
Education attainment	Bachelor degree or higher
	Diploma
	Cert III or IV
	Year 12
	Cert I or II or Cert not defined
	Year 11 and below
Marital status	Single, never married
	Cohabitation
	Married
	Separated/divorced
Number of children	No children
	under 5 years
	6–18 years
	≥18 years

Table 2. Indicator of social disadvantage dimensions in HILDA.

Domain	Indicator	Description
Material resources	Household income	1 if income ≤ 60% of median income
Employment	Long-term unemployment	1 if currently unemployed, looked for work for the past 4 weeks, and was employed for the preceding 12 months
	Unemployment	1 if unemployed
	Marginal attachment to labor force	1 if not employed but looking for work or not employed and not looking for work due to the belief of being unlikely to find work
	Underemployment	1 if working less 35 hours per week
	Living in a jobless household	1 if no household member is employed and at least one household member is aged 15 to 64
Education and skills	Pool English proficiency	1 if speaks a language other then English at home, and reports not speaking English well
	Low level of education	1 if does not study full-time and his highest qualification is less than high school completion
	Limited work experience	1 if has spent fewer than 3 years in paid employment
Health and disability	Poor general health	1 if has poor general health (0–50 on a 0–100 scale)
	Poor physical health	1 if has poor physical health (0–50 on a 0–100 scale)
	Poor mental health	1 if has poor mental health (0–50 on a 0–100 scale)
	Long-term health condition	1 if has long-term health condition, disability or impairment
	Disabled member in the household	1 if lives in a household that has a disabled member
Social support	Little social support	1 if receives little social support (0–30 on a 0 70 scale)
	Low social activities	1 if gets together socially with friends/relatives at most once or twice every 3 months
Communication participation	Low neighborhood satisfaction	1 if the satisfaction with neighborhood is low (0–5 on a 0–10 scale)
	Low community connection	1 if the satisfaction with feeling part of local community is low (0–5 on a 0–10 scale)
	Non-participation in community activities	1 if not currently a member of a sporting, hobby or community-based club/association
	Non-participation in voluntary work	1 if not engaged in any voluntary work activity in a typical week
Personal safety	Poor received personal safety	1 if the satisfaction with safety is low (0–5 on a 0–10 scale)

range of social researchers, community groups and government agencies, the measure identifies seven domains of social disadvantage: (1) material resources; (2) employment; (3) education and skills; (4) health and disability; (5) social; (6) community; and (7) personal safety. Within each domain are selected indicator, which are listed in Table 2.

2.1 Social Disadvantage Measurement

The panel data from the HILDA survey contain annual measurements of individual level factors involving over time that are known or suspected to contribute to social exclusion and disadvantage. Moreover, some variables are correlated in some way to lead to the formation of disadvantage. For example, a lower household income might be closely related to disabled member in the household. This makes the dataset fit for examining trends in multi-variate life course trajectories at individual and or household level. To capture the level of disadvantage, we use the Social Exclusion Monitor (SEM), a multidimensional social exclusion index created by the MIAESR in liaise with the Brotherhood of St Laurence [17]. This enables comparability with earlier studies. Our analysis involves integrating information from 21 indicators available on an annual basis in the survey data into a single exclusion index, decomposable into 7 life domains. The design of the SEM framework take into account issues of measurability, objectivity, parsimony and correspondence to community notions of social exclusion [14,16]. To gauge the reliability of the SEM in this sample, Martinez Jr. and colleagues [13] calculated Cronbach's α for all the 21 indicators and estimated it to be 0.51. This can be explained by the weak correlation between some of the indicators, for instance, some indicators in the social support and community participation dimensions are weakly correlated with those in other dimensions. However, when Cronbach's α is calculated across the scores for the seven domains, its value is 0.68. Thus, to augment the selected indicators, we use a number of indicators describing the demographic characteristics, which have somewhat correlation and render the SEM more robust in this study. Please see [14] for detailed discussion of the statistical properties of the SEM.

A sum-score approach is employed to combine the 21 indicators into 7 domain indices, which are then added up to create the final multi-dimensional exclusion index. Let S^j denote the a person's score on the j-th domain of social exclusion. Each domain consists of n_j component indicators, denoted by s^c, which are binary variables whose value is either 0 (not disadvantaged) or 1 (disadvantaged). The term S^j is calculated by taking the arithmetic mean of the component indicators included in the j-th domain, as formulated in Eq. 1.

$$S^j = \frac{\sum_{c=1}^{n_j} s^c}{n_j}. \tag{1}$$

Let S denote the SEM index, which is the sum of S^j ($j = 1, \ldots, 7$) and can be defined as $S = \sum_{j=1}^{7} S^j$. Apparently, the values of the resulting index range between 0 and 7, in which higher values correspond to higher levels of social-economic disadvantage. As done by many earlier studies [13,16,17], equal weights are assigned to each dimension and indicator within each domain. This simplifies algebraic manipulation substantially, and most importantly, prevents subjective judgments to permeate disadvantage definitions [1]. The multi-dimensional disadvantage HILDA can be quantized using three headcount measures: "marginal", "deep", and "very deep". Following [13], we adopt the thresholds used by the Brotherhood of St Laurence and MIAESR: "marginally disadvantaged" individuals are those individuals who score more than 1 but less than 2 in the multi-dimensional disadvantage index described above, "deeply disadvantaged" individuals are those whose score between 2 to 3, and "very deeply disadvantaged" individuals are those who score 3 or more [3].

3 The Prediction Network on Life Course Trajectory

3.1 Preliminary: Recurrent Neural Networks

Recurrent Neural Networks (RNNs) are a rich class of dynamic models that can be used to generate sequences in music [7], text, and motion capture data. A common problem to all conditional generative models is that if the networks' predictions are only based on the last few inputs, and these inputs were themselves predicted by the network, it has little opportunity to recover from past mistakes. In most RNNs, $\mathcal{H}$ (in Eq. 2) is an element-wise sigmoid function, which is unable to store information about past inputs for very long and not robust to "mistakes".

3.2 Predicting Life Course Trajectory on HILDA

Given an input trajectory sequence $\mathbf{x} = [x_1, \ldots, x_T]$ where each $x_t, 1 \leq t \leq T$ is a life course trajectory vector, we pass the sequence through weighted connections to a stack of N recurrently connected hidden layers to compute the first hidden trajectory sequences $\mathbf{h}^n = [h_1^n, \ldots, h_T^n]$, and then the output trajectory sequence $\mathbf{y} = [y_1, \ldots, y_T]$. Each output vector y_t is used to parameterize a predictive distribution $Pr(x_{x+1}|y_t)$ over the possible next output x_{t+1}. The first element x_1 of every input sequence is always a null vector whose entries are zeros, and the network emits a prediction for x_2, the first real input, with no prior information. The network is deep in both space and time in the sense that every piece of information passing either vertically or horizontally through the computation graph will be acted on by multiple successive weight matrices and nonlinearities. We remark that we have skip connections from the inputs to all hidden layers, and from all hidden layers to the outputs. This operation is to ease the training of deep networks, by reducing the number of processing steps between the bottom of the network and the top, and thereby mitigating the vanishing gradient problem [4]. Figure 1(a) illustrates the basic recurrent neural network prediction architecture used in this paper. Note that when $N = 1$, the architecture reduces to an ordinary single layer next step prediction RNN.

The hidden layer activations are computed by iterating the following equations from $t = 1$ to T and from $n = 2$ to N:

$$h_t^1 = \mathcal{H}(W_{ih^1}x_t + W_{h^1h^1}h_{t-1}^1 + b_h^1), h_t^n = \mathcal{H}(W_{ih^n}x_t + W_{h^{n-1}h^n}h_t^{n-1} + W_{h^nh^n}h_{t-1}^n + b_h^n), \quad (2)$$

where W terms denote weight matrices, *e.g.*, W_{ih^n} is the weight matrix connecting the inputs to the n-th hidden layer, and $W_{h^{n-1}h^n}$ is the recurrent connection

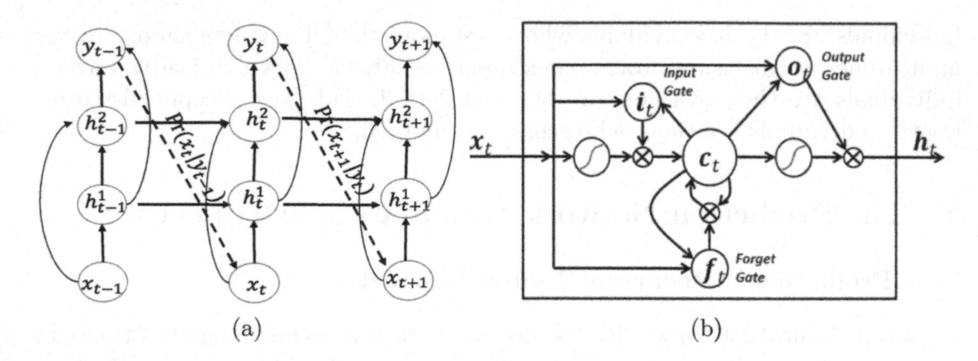

Fig. 1. (a) Deep recurrent neural network prediction architecture. The circles represent network layers, the solid lines represent weighted connections and the dashed lines denote predictions. The network is deep both space (vertically) and time (horizontally). Generating sequences is repeatedly prediction what will happen next by treating past predictions as if they were real. (b) Long Short-term Memory Cell. The idea of LSTM is to use linear memory cells surrounded by multiplicative gate units to store read, write and reset information. Input gate (i_t): scales input to cell (write). Output gate (o_t): scales output from cell (read). Forget gate (f_t): scales old cell value (reset).

between hidden states, the b terms denote bias vectors, and $\mathcal{H}$ is the hidden layer function. Given the hidden sequences, the output sequence can be computed as:

$$\hat{y}_t = b_y + \sum_{n=1}^{N} W_{h^n y} h_t^n, y_t = \mathcal{Y}(\hat{y}_t), \tag{3}$$

where $\mathcal{Y}$ is the output layer function. The complete network therefore defines a function, parameterized by the weight matrices, from input trajectory histories $x_{1:t}$ to output vector y_t. The output vector y_t can be used to parameterize the predictive distribution for the next input via the form of $Pr(x_{t+1}|y_t)$. This corresponds to sampling from the conditional model $Pr(x) = \Pi_t Pr(x_t|x_{1:t-1})$. In practice, the form of $Pr(x_{t+1}|y_t)$ must be chose carefully in order to match the input data. In particular, finding a good predictive distribution for multivariate, real-valued HILDA time series data, which is usually referred to be *density modeling* in this paper, could be very challenging.

The probability provided by the network to the input sequence $\mathbf{x}$ is $Pr(\mathbf{x}) = \Pi_{t=1}^{T} Pr(x_{t+1}|y_t)$, and the sequence loss $\mathcal{L}(\mathbf{x})$ used to train the network is the negative logarithm of $Pr(\mathbf{x})$:

$$\mathcal{L}(\mathbf{x}) = -\sum_{t=1}^{T} \log Pr(x_{t+1}|y_t). \tag{4}$$

The partial derivatives of the loss with respect to the network weights can be efficiently calculated with back-propagation through time [36], and the whole network can be trained with gradient descent.

3.3 Long Short-Term Memory (LSTM)

The RNN can easily map sequences to sequences whenever the alignment between the inputs and the outputs is known ahead of time. Apparently, it is more clear to apply RNN to personal trajectory problems whose input and output sequences have fixed lengths without complicated relationships. A simple strategy for general sequence learning is to map the input sequence into a fixed-sized vector using one RNN, and then to map the vector to the target sequence with another RNN [9,11,22]. While it could work since the RNN is provided with all the relevant information, it would be difficult to train the RNNs due to the resulting long term dependencies [4]. However, the Long Short-Term Memory (LSTM) [12] is known to learn problems with long range temporal dependencies, so an LSTM may succeed in this setting. LSTM architecture uses a purpose-built memory cells to store information, is better at finding and exploiting long range dependencies in the data. Figure 1(b) illustrates a single LSTM memory cell. In LSTM, the hidden layer function $\mathcal{H}$ is implemented by the following composite function:

$$\begin{aligned} i_t &= \sigma(W_{xi}x_t + W_{hi}h_{t-1} + W_{ci}c_{t-1} + b_i) \\ f_t &= \sigma(W_{xf}x_t + W_{hf}h_{t-1} + W_{cf}c_{t-1} + b_f) \\ c_t &= f_t c_{t-1} + i_t tanh(W_{xc}x_t + W_{hc}h_{t-1} + b_c) \\ o_t &= \sigma(W_{xo}x_t + W_{ho}h_{t-1} + W_{co}c_t + b_o) \\ h_t &= o_t tanh(c_t), \end{aligned} \tag{5}$$

where σ is the logistic sigmoid function, and i, f, o and c are the input gate, forget gate, output gate, cell, and cell input activation vectors, respectively. Note all these parameters are the same size as the hidden vector h. W denotes weight matrix for which we use subscripts to distinguish their function, *e.g.*, W_{hi} is the hidden-input gate matrix, W_{xo} is the input-output gate matrix. The weight matrices from the cell to gate vectors (*e.g.*, W_{ci}) are diagonal, so element m in each gate vector only receives input from element m of he cell vector. $b_\star$ ($\star = i, f, c, o$) are bias terms corresponding to gates.

3.4 Mixture Density Outputs on Life Course Trajectory

In real-world application, such as life course trajectory time series data, the variance of the data is not constant while exhibits complex stochastic process. For problems involving the prediction of continuous variables, the average value of $Pr(x_{t+1}|y_t)$ provides only a very limited description of the properties of the future input's variables. This is particularly true for problems in which the mapping to be learned is multi-valued, as often arises in the solution of HILDA survey data since the average of several correct next values is not necessarily itself a correct value. In order to attain a complete description of the data, for the purposes of predicting the outputs corresponding to the new input vectors, we need to model the conditional probability distribution of the output variables, again conditioned on the input life course sequence. In this section, we present an improved network model obtained by combining a LSTM with a mixture density network [5,6] which is to use the outputs of LSTM to parameterize a mixture distribution.

In mixture density networks, a subset of the outputs are used to define the mixture weights, while the remaining outputs are used to parameterized the individual mixture components. The mixture weight outputs are normalized with a soft-max function to ensure they from a valid discrete distribution, and the other outputs are passed through suitable functions to keep their values within meaningful ranges[1]. Mixture density networks are trained by maximizing the log probability density of the targets under the induced distributions. Note that the densities are normalized (up to a fixed constant), and are therefore straightforward to differentiate and pick unbiased sample from. In our scenario, mixture density outputs is combined with LSTM, in which the output distribution is conditioned not only on the current input, but also on the history of the previous inputs. Given the input trajectory at individual level across 15 waves $x_t = [x_{tk}]_{k=1}^{21}$, $(t = 1, \ldots, 15)$, which consists of 21 real values elements that defines the his social exclusion status. Then a mixture of multi-variate Gaussians was used to predict $[x_{tk}]$, and each output vector y_t consists of the a set of means μ^j, standard deviations σ^j, correlations ρ^j, and mixture weight π^j for the M mixture components. That is

$$x_t \in \mathbb{R} \times \ldots \times \mathbb{R}; y_t = \left([\pi_t^j, \mu_t^j, \sigma_t^j, \rho_t^j]_{j=1}^M \right). \tag{6}$$

Note that the mean and standard deviation are 21-dimensional vectors and correlation is encoded into a 210-dimensional vector, whereas the component weight is scalar. The vectors y_t are obtained from the LSTM outputs $\hat{y}_t$, where $\hat{y}_t = \left([\hat{\pi}_t^j, \hat{\mu}_t^j, \hat{\sigma}_t^j, \hat{\rho}_t^j]_{j=1}^M \right) = b_y + \sum_{n=1}^N W_{h^n y} h_t^n$ and $\mathcal{Y}$ maps $\hat{y}_t$ to y_t:

$$\begin{aligned} \pi_t^j &= \frac{\exp(\hat{\pi}_t^j)}{\sum_{j'=1}^M \exp(\hat{\pi}_t^{j'})} \rightarrow \pi_t^j \in (0,1), \sum_j \pi_t^j = 1 \\ \mu_t^j &= \hat{\mu}_t^j \rightarrow \mu_t^j \in \mathbb{R}; \sigma_t^j = \exp(\hat{\sigma}_t^j) \rightarrow \sigma_t^j > 0; \rho_t^j = \tanh(\hat{\rho}_t^j) \rightarrow \rho_t^j \in (-1,1) \end{aligned} \tag{7}$$

The probability density $Pr(x_{t+1}|y_t)$ of the next input x_{t+1} given the output vector y_t is defined as follows:

$$Pr(x_{t+1}|y_t) = \sum_{j=1}^M \pi_t^j \mathcal{N}(x_{t+1}|\mu_t^j, \sigma_t^j, \rho_t^j) \tag{8}$$

where

$$\mathcal{N}(x|\mu, \sigma, \rho) = \frac{1}{2\pi \prod_k^{21} \sigma_k \sqrt{1-\rho^2}} \exp\left[\frac{-Z}{2(1-\rho^2)} \right] \tag{9}$$

with

$$Z = \sum_{k=1}^{21} \frac{(x_k - \mu_k)^2}{\sigma_k^2} - \sum_{k \neq l}^{21} \sum_{l=1}^{21} \frac{2\rho_{kl}(x_k - \mu_k)(x_l - \mu_l)}{\sigma_k \sigma_l}. \tag{10}$$

[1] For instance, the exponential function is typically applied to outputs used as scale parameters, which are required to be positive.

Thus, the sequence loss of Eq. 4 can reformulated to be as follows

$$\mathcal{L}(\mathbf{x}) = -\sum_{t=1}^{T} \log \left(\sum_{j=1} \pi_t^j \mathcal{N}(x_{t+1}|\mu_t^j, \sigma_t^j, \rho_t^j) \right). \tag{11}$$

The derivatives with respect to the mixture density outputs can be found by first defining the component responsibilities γ_t^j:

$$\hat{\gamma}_t^j = \pi_t^j \mathcal{N}(x_{t+1}|\mu_t^j, \sigma_t^j, \rho_t^j); \gamma_t^j = \frac{\hat{\gamma}_t^j}{\sum_{j'=1}^{M} \hat{\gamma}_t^{j'}}. \tag{12}$$

Then observing that

$$\frac{\partial \mathcal{L}(\mathbf{x})}{\partial \hat{\pi}_t^j} = \pi_t^j - \gamma_t^j; \frac{\partial \mathcal{L}(\mathbf{x})}{\partial (\hat{\mu}_t^j, \hat{\sigma}_t^j, \hat{\rho}_t^j)} = \gamma_t^j \frac{\partial \log \mathcal{N}(x_{t+1}|\mu_t^j, \sigma_t^j, \rho_t^j)}{\partial (\hat{\mu}_t^j, \hat{\sigma}_t^j, \hat{\rho}_t^j)} \tag{13}$$

where

$$\begin{aligned} \frac{\partial \log \mathcal{N}(x|\mu,\sigma,\rho)}{\partial \hat{\mu}_k} &= \frac{C}{\sigma_k} \sum_{k,l}^{21} \left(\frac{x_k - \mu_k}{\sigma_k} - \frac{\rho_{kl}(x_l - \mu_l)}{\sigma_l} \right); \\ \frac{\partial \log \mathcal{N}(x|\mu,\sigma,\rho)}{\partial \hat{\sigma}_k} &= \frac{C(x_k - \mu_k)}{\sigma_k} \sum_{k,l}^{21} \left(\frac{x_k - \mu_k}{\sigma_k} - \frac{\rho_{kl}(x_l - \mu_l)}{\sigma_l} \right) - 1; \\ \frac{\partial \log \mathcal{N}(x|\mu,\sigma,\rho_{kl})}{\partial \hat{\rho}_{kl}} &= \frac{(x_k - \mu_k)(x_l - \mu_l)}{\sigma_k \sigma_l} + \rho_{kl}(1 - CZ) \end{aligned} \tag{14}$$

where $C = \frac{1}{1-\rho^2}$.

4 Case Study: Life Course Trajectory Generation in Australia 2001–2015

4.1 Training Details

Our hardware platform is based on a single Nvidia GPU of GTX 980. The network architecture consists of three hidden layers with 1000, 500, and 500 LSTM units, respectively. We divide training dataset into mini-batches where less computation is used to update the weights, and gradient computation for many cases is to simultaneously use matrix-matrix multiplies which are very efficient, especially on GPUs. The whole HILDA sample dataset is divided into 5347 and 100 to be training set and test set, respectively. RMSProp [23] divides the learning rate for a weight by running average of the magnitudes of recent gradients for that weight. This is because the magnitude of the gradient can be very different for different weights and can change during learning, and thus it is hard to choose a single global learning rate. In essence, RMSprop is to keep a moving average of the squared gradient for each weight:

$$MeanSquare(w,t) = 0.9MeanSquare(w,t-1) + 0.1\left(\frac{\partial \mathcal{L}}{\partial w(t)}\right)^2 \tag{15}$$

It is empirically shown that dividing the gradient by $\sqrt{MeanSquare(w,t)}$ makes the learning work much better. To avoid over-fitting on the training data, we use the regularization: weight noise with a standard deviation of 0.075 applied to the network weights at the start of each training sequence. We have found that retraining with iteratively increased regularization is considerably faster than training from random weights with regularization.

4.2 Results

In the first experiment, we perform self-evaluations to examine the performance of our method with respect to varied network architectures. Specifically, we evaluate the prediction accuracy against different combinations of network structures and gradient computations, which include RNN + Stochastic Gradient Descent (SGD), LSTM + SGD, LSTM + RMSProp. The accuracy of prediction results are reported in Table 3. Note that the accuracy is computed as the counting difference between the predicted values and the ground truth ones. We can see that the LSTM with RMSProp is able to achieve higher prediction accuracy compared with RNN/(LSTM) + SGD. The main reason is RMSProp is more suitable for the training on sequences in which the gradients can be maintained over time. It can also be observed that the network of LSTM performs better as the number of hidden layers increases. However, to balance the training efficiency, we keep three hidden layers of LSTM units. Moreover, we examine the effect of additional demographic dimensions by adding the features of demographic, marital status, and number of children into training sequences. And Table 3 shows that the inclusion of these dimensions are helpful in improving the prediction accuracy. Also, Table 4 reports the accuracy on each disadvantage dimension.

Furthermore, we discover year-on-year variation in each dimension in the aspect of persistence over time. To visualize the results, we use the Recurrence

Table 3. Evaluation on real HILDA. The demographic variables include gender, age, country of birth, housing situation, and education attainment.

Dataset: HILDA	Prediction accuracy		
Train/test: 5347/1000			
RNN + SGD	29.6% (2 layers)	35.7% (3 layers)	36.4% (4 layers)
LSTM + SGD	33.4% (2 layers)	40.4% (3 layers)	42.0% (4 layers)
LSTM + RMSProp	34.9% (2 layers)	46.6% (3 layers)	47.1% (4 layers)
LSTM + RMSProp + Demographic	35.3% (2 layers)	47.2% (3 layers)	47.5% (4 layers)
LSTM + RMSProp + Demographic + Marital status + Number of children	35.3% (2 layers)	47.3% (3 layers)	47.5% (4 layers)

Table 4. The prediction accuracy on each disadvantage variable.

	Prediction accuracy		
Household income	33.6% (2 layers)	45.3% (3 layers)	45.7% (4 layers)
Long-term unemployment	37.6% (2 layers)	49.3% (3 layers)	49.8% (4 layers)
Unemployment	33.8% (2 layers)	45.5% (3 layers)	46.0% (4 layers)
Marginal attachment to labor force	33.9% (2 layers)	45.6% (3 layers)	46.1% (4 layers)
Underemployment	34.5% (2 layers)	46.2% (3 layers)	46.7% (4 layers)
Living in a jobless household	34.8% (2 layers)	46.0% (3 layers)	46.5% (4 layers)
Pool english proficiency	36.7% (2 layers)	48.4% (3 layers)	48.9% (4 layers)
Low level of education	35.1% (2 layers)	45.8% (3 layers)	46.3% (4 layers)
Limited work experience	34.4% (2 layers)	46.1% (3 layers)	46.6% (4 layers)
Pool general health	33.3% (2 layers)	45.0% (3 layers)	45.5% (4 layers)
Pool physical health	34.5% (2 layers)	46.2% (3 layers)	46.7% (4 layers)
Poor mental health	34.6% (2 layers)	46.3% (3 layers)	46.7% (4 layers)
Long-term health condition	33.2% (2 layers)	44.9% (3 layers)	45.4% (4 layers)
Disabled member in the household	35.7% (2 layers)	46.7% (3 layers)	47.7% (4 layers)
Little social support	32.8% (2 layers)	44.5% (3 layers)	45.0% (4 layers)
Low social activities	34.5% (2 layers)	46.2% (3 layers)	46.7% (4 layers)
Low neighborhood satisfaction	36.6% (2 layers)	48.3% (3 layers)	48.9% (4 layers)
Low community connection	34.2% (2 layers)	45.9% (3 layers)	46.4% (4 layers)
Non-participation in community activities	33.8% (2 layers)	45.5% (3 layers)	46.0% (4 layers)
Non-participation in voluntary work	33.4% (2 layers)	45.1% (3 layers)	45.6% (4 layers)
Poor received personal safety	34.0% (2 layers)	45.7% (3 layers)	46.2% (4 layers)
Material resources	33.6% (2 layers)	45.3% (3 layers)	45.7% (4 layers)
Employment	33.9% (2 layers)	46.5% (3 layers)	47.0% (4 layers)
Education and skills	35.4% (2 layers)	46.7% (3 layers)	47.2% (4 layers)
Health and disability	34.2% (2 layers)	45.8% (3 layers)	46.4% (4 layers)
Social support	33.6% (2 layers)	45.3% (3 layers)	45.8% (4 layers)
Communication participation	34.5% (2 layers)	46.2% (3 layers)	46.7% (4 layers)
Personal safety	34.0% (2 layers)	45.7% (3 layers)	46.2% (4 layers)

Plot [10] to illustrate the repetition of persistence in each dimension. A recurrence plot is a plot showing, for a given moment in time, the times at which the phase space trajectory visits roughly the same area in the phase space. In other words, a recurrence is a time the trajectory returns to a location it has visited before. The recurrence plot depicts the collection of pairs of times at which the trajectory is at the same place, i.e. the set of (i, j) with $\boldsymbol{x}(i) = \boldsymbol{x}(j)$. This can show many things, for instance, if the trajectory is strictly periodic at the period T, then all such pairs of times will be separated by a multiple of T and visible as diagonal lines. To make the plot, continuous time and continuous phase space are discretized, taking e.g. $\boldsymbol{x}(i)$ as the location of the trajectory at time i, and counting as a recurrence any time the trajectory gets sufficiently close (say, within ϵ) to a point it has been previously. Concretely then, recurrence/non-

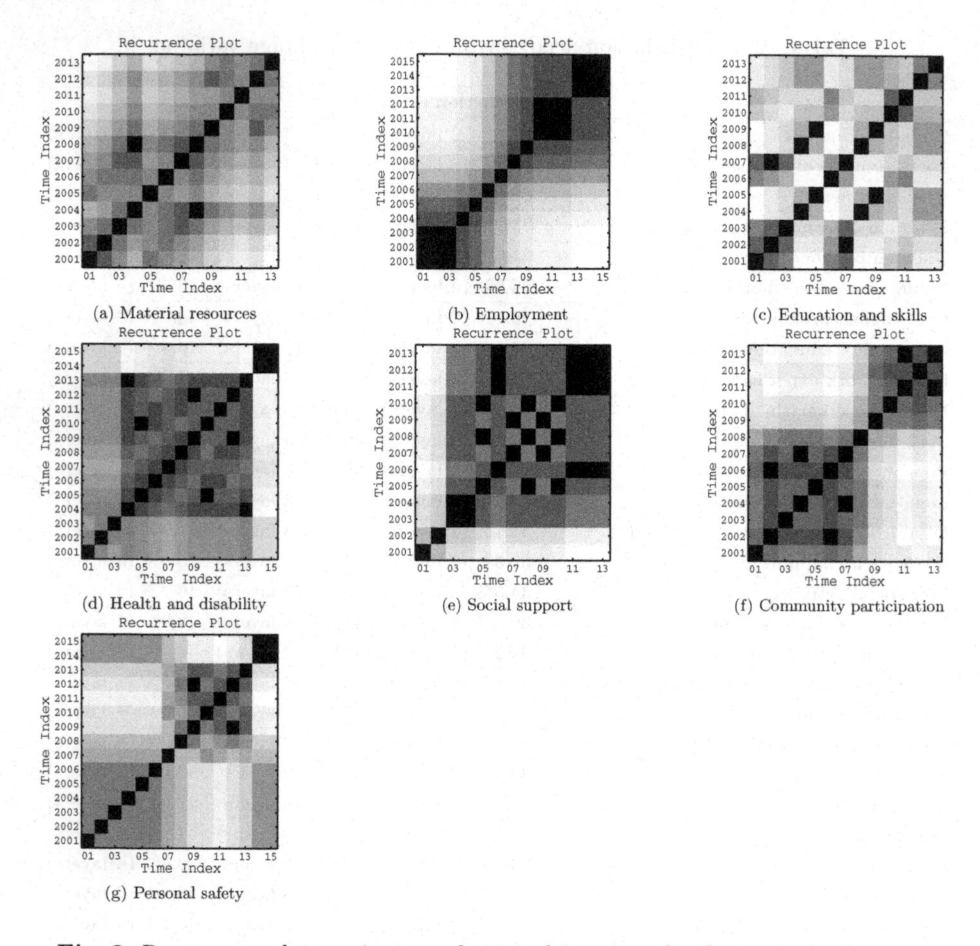

(a) Material resources (b) Employment (c) Education and skills

(d) Health and disability (e) Social support (f) Community participation

(g) Personal safety

Fig. 2. Recurrence plot on time trends in multi-variate disadvantage dimensions.

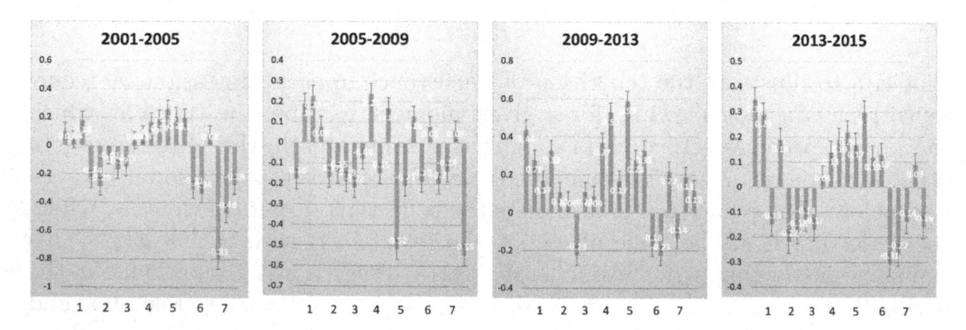

Fig. 3. 1-Material resources (↑); 2-Employment (↓); 3-Education and skills (↓); 4-Health and disability (↑); 5-Social support (↑); 6-Community participation (↓); 7-Personal safety (↓).

recurrence can be recorded by the binary function:

$$R(i,j) = \begin{cases} 1 & if ||\boldsymbol{x}(i) - \boldsymbol{x}(j)|| \leq \epsilon \\ 0 & otherwise, \end{cases} \tag{16}$$

and the recurrence plot puts a (black) point at coordinates (i, j) if $R(i, j) = 1$. Figure 2 illustrate the over-time trajectories of disadvantages with respect to the seven domains. There sorts of recurrence observations can be seen: (1) For employment and community participation, the trajectories exhibit very similar in the period of 2001–2007, and the period of 2009–2015, while trajectories are quite divergent from those in 2001–2007. This is because of the onset of Global Financial Crisis (at around 2008), which seems to have reversed long-running trends towards disadvantage reductions in employment and community participation; This discovery is consistent with the results revealed by Martinez Jr and his colleagues [13]. The GFC seems to have the same effect on the personal safety. (2) For the dimensions of health and disability and social support, the trajectories exhibit more frequent yet persistent recurrent visit over-time; This can some extent reflect the trend towards somewhat trap in disadvantage, e.g., a person has been suffering long-term poor health condition would get stuck into this disadvantage profoundly. (3) For the two dimensions of education and skills and material resource, trajectories are more or less similar to each other because they are relative stable over-time whilst there are some divergence in education and skills because some people finish off or terminate their educations.

To investigate the contributing effect to the increasing or decreasing poverty rates, we decompose the annual changes in SEM. The results are shown in Fig. 3. A bar which has a self-contained value is associated with a given factor and the above over the value 0 indicates that factor contributed to the increased poverty rates. Conversely, when the bar is below the value 0, it means the corresponding factor contributed to decreasing poverty rates. And the self-contained particular value inside the bar means how much that factor contribute the change of rates. We can see that: (1) in the period of 2001–2005 in Australia, changes in personal safety, employment, community participation contributed to the decreasing poverty; on the other hand, changes in material resources, health and social support contributed to increasing poverty rates; (2) in the 2005–2009 period, changes in almost all domains contributed to decreasing poverty and extent of reduction is equitably; nonetheless, changes in material resources and health contributed to the increasing poverty; (3) in the 2009–2013 period during GFC, all factors contributed to increasing poverty; (4) in the 2013–2015 period, changes in most of domains contributed to increasing poverty with an exception in education and community participation which lead to decreasing poverty rates.

5 Conclusion

In this paper, we present a novel approach of studying social disadvantage by using a deep recurrent model. The proposed method processes the sequences of life course trajectories at individual levels over time, and outputs the future sequence with moderate prediction accuracy. The showcase of HILDA survey data has demonstrated the ability of Long Short-Term Memory recurrent neural networks to generate real-valued sequences with complex, long-range structure using next-step prediction. The significance of this paper is to gain a better insight into the internal representation of life course data, and to use this to manipulate the data distribution directly. Therefore, the proposed model is able to foresee the social deprivation and exclusion progressively. Future work will investigate more thoroughly the driving factors of changes in social disadvantage for individual and subgroups. Also, we would leverage multi-dimensional data study [24–33,38,41,42] and recent deep learning methods [37,39,40] into an improved prediction system.

Acknowledgement. Lin Wu's research was funded by the Australian Research Council Centre of Excellence in Children and Families over the Life Course and supported by a Life Course Centre Staff Exchange Scheme 2017. We acknowledge the use of HILDA survey funded by Australian Government Department of Social Services and support from The Melbourne Institute.

References

1. Alkire, S., Foster, J.: Counting and multidimensional poverty measurement. J. Public Econ. **95**(7–8), 476–487 (2011)
2. Azpitarte, F.: Has economic growth in Australia been good for the income-poor? And for the multidimensionally poor? Soc. Indic. Res. **113**(1), 1–37 (2014)
3. Azpitarte, F.: Social exclusion monitor bulletin (2013). http://library.bsl.org.au/jspui/bitstream/1/6083/1/AzpitarteBowman_Social_exclusion_monitor_bulletin_Jun2015.pdf
4. Bengio, Y., Simard, P., Frasconi, P.: Learning long-term dependencies with gradient decent is difficult. IEEE Trans. Neural Netw. **5**(2), 157–166 (1994)
5. Bishop, C.M.: Mixture density networks. Technical report (1994)
6. Bishop, C.M.: Neural Networks for Pattern Recognition. Oxford University Press, New York (1995)
7. Boulanger-Lewandowski, N., Bengio, Y., Vincent, P.: Modeling temporal dependencies in high-dimensional sequences: application to polyphonic music generation and transcription. In: International Conference on Machine Learning (2012)
8. Bourguignon, F., Ferreira, F.H.G., Leite, P.G.: Beyond oaxaca-blinder: accounting for differences in household income distributions. J. Econ. Inequal. **6**(2), 117–148 (2008)
9. Cho, K., van Merrienboer, B., Gulcehre, C., Bahdanau, D., Bougares, F., Schwenk, H., Bengio, Y.: Learning phrase representations using rnn encoder-decoder for statistical machine translation (2014). arXiv preprint arXiv:1406.1078
10. Eckmann, J.P., Kamphorst, S.O., Ruelle, D.: Recurrence plots of dynamical systems. Europhys. Lett. **5**(9), 973–977 (1987)
11. Graves, A.: Generating sequences with recurrent neural networks (2014). arXiv preprint arXiv:1308.0850v5
12. Hochreiter, S., Schmidhuber, J.: Long short-term memory. Neural Comput. **9**(8), 1735–1780 (1997)

13. Martinez Jr., A., Perales, F.: The dynamics of multidimensional poverty in contemporary australia. Soc. Indic. Res. **130**(2), 479–496 (2017)
14. Kostenko, W., Scutella R., Wilkins, R.: Estimates of poverty and social exclusion in Australia: a multidimensional approach. In: 6th Joint Economic and Social Outlook Conference, Melbourne (2009)
15. Organisation of Economic Co-operation and Development.: Is work the best antidote to poverty? Chapter 3 in OECD employment outlook 2009: trackling the Jobs crisis (2009)
16. Rosanna, S., Roger, W.: Measuring poverty and social exclusion in Australia: a proposed multidimensional framework for identifying socio-economic disadvantage. Melbourne Institute of Applied Economic and Social Research, Australia (2009)
17. Rosanna, S., Roger, W., Weiping, K.: Intensity and persistence of individual's social exclusion in australia. Aust. J. Soc. Issues **48**(3), 273–298 (2013)
18. Rumelhart, D.E., Hinton, G.E., Williams, R.J.: Learning representations by back-propagating errors. Nature **323**, 533–536 (1986)
19. Shorrocks, A.F.: Decomposition procedures for distributed analysis: a unified framework based on the shapley value. J. Econ. Inequal. **11**(1), 179–191 (2013)
20. Credit Suisse: Global wealth report 2014 zurich: Credit suisse group (2015). https://publications.credit-suisse.com/tasks/render/file/?fileID=60931FDE-A2D2-F568-B041B58C5EA591A
21. Summerfield, M., Freidin, S., Hahn, M., La, N., Li, N., Macalalad, N., O'Shea, M., Watson, N., Wilkins, R., Wooden, M.: HILDA user manual release 15. Melbourne Institute of Applied Economic and Social Research, University of Melbourne (2016)
22. Sutskever, I., Vinyals, O., Le, Q.V.: Sequence to sequence learning with neural networks. In: Advances in Neural Information Processing Systems (2014)
23. Tieleman, T., Hinton, G.: Lecture 6.5-RMSPROP: Divide the gradient by a running average of its recent magnitude. Technical report Neural networks ofr machine learning (2012)
24. Wang, Y., Huang, X., Lin, W.: Clustering via geometric median shift over Riemannian manifolds. Inf. Sci. **220**, 292–305 (2013)
25. Wang, Y., Lin, X., Lin, W., Zhang, Q., Zhang, W.: Shifting multi-hypergraphs via collaborative probabilistic voting. Knowl. Inf. Syst. **46**(3), 515–536 (2016)
26. Wang, Y., Lin, X., Lin, W., Zhang, W.: Robust landmark retrieval. In: ACM Multimedia, Effective Multi-query Expansions (2015)
27. Wang, Y., Lin, X., Lin, W., Zhang, W.: Effective multi-query expansions: collaborative deep networks for robust landmark retrieval. IEEE Trans. Image Proc. **26**(3), 1393–1404 (2017)
28. Wang, Y., Lin, X., Lin, W., Zhang, W., Zhang, Q.: Towards subspace clustering for multi-modal data. In: ACM Multimedia, Exploiting Correlation Consensus (2014)
29. Wang, Y., Lin, X., Lin, W., Zhang, W., Zhang, Q.: Learning Bridging Mapping for Cross-modal Hashing. In: ACM SIGIR, LBMCH (2015)
30. Wang, Y., Lin, X., Lin, W., Zhang, W., Zhang, Q., Huang, X.: Robust subspace clustering for multi-view data by exploiting correlation consensus. IEEE Trans. Image Proc. **24**(11), 3939–3949 (2015)
31. Wang, Y., Lin, X., Zhang, Q.: Towards metric fusion on multi-view data: a cross-view based graph random walk approach. In: ACM CIKM(2013)
32. Wang, Y., Zhang, W., Wu, L., Lin, X., Fang, M., Pan, S.: Iterative views agreement: an iterative low-rank based structured optimization method to multi-view spectral clustering. In: IJCAI (2016)

33. Wang, Y., Zhang, W., Lin, W., Lin, X., Zhao, X.: Unsupervised metric fusion over multiview data by graph random walk-based cross-view diffusion. IEEE Trans. Neural Netw. Learn. Syst. **28**(1), 57–70 (2017)
34. Watson, N., Wooden, M. Identifying factors affecting longitudinal survey response chapter 10. Methodol. Longitud. Surv. **1**, 157–182 (2009)
35. Whiteford, P.: Australia: Inequality and Prosperity and their Impacts in a Radical Welfare State. Crawford School of Public Polic, The Australian National University, Social Policy Action Research Centre, Mimeo (2013)
36. Williams, R., Zipse, D.: Gradient-based learning algorithms for recurrent networks and their computational complexity. Back Propag. Theory Archit. Appl. **1**, 433–486 (1995)
37. Lin, W., Shen, C., van den Hengel, A.: Deep linear discriminant analysis on fisher networks: a hybrid architecture for person re-identification. Pattern Recogn. **65**, 238–250 (2017)
38. Lin, W., Wang, Y.: Robust hashing for multi-view data: jointly learning low-rank kernelized similarity consensus and hash functions. Image Vis. Comput. **57**, 58–66 (2017)
39. Wu, L., Wang, Y., Gao, J., Li, X.: Deep adaptive feature embedding with local sample distributions for person re-identification (2017). arXiv preprint arXiv:1706.03160
40. Wu, L., Wang, Y., Li, X., Gao, J.: What-and-where to match: Deep spatially multiplicative integration networks for person re-identification (2017). arXiv preprint arXiv:1707.07074
41. Wu, L., Wang, Y., Pan, S.: Exploiting attribute correlations: a novel trace lasso-based weakly supervised dictionary learning method. IEEE Trans. Cybern. **99**, 1–12 (2016)
42. Wu, L., Wang, Y., Shepherd, J.: Efficient image and tag co-ranking: a bregman divergence optimization method. In: Proceedings of the 21st ACM International Conference on Multimedia. ACM (2013)

FRISK: A Multilingual Approach to Find twitteR InterestS via wiKipedia

Coriane Nana Jipmo, Gianluca Quercini(✉), and Nacéra Bennacer

LRI, CentraleSupélec, Université Paris-Saclay, 91190 Gif-sur-Yvette, France
{coriane.nanajipmo,gianluca.quercini,nacera.bennacer}@lri.fr

Abstract. Several studies have shown that the users of Twitter reveal their *interests* (i.e., what they like) while they share their opinions, preferences and personal stories.

In this paper we describe FRISK a multilingual unsupervised approach for the categorization of the interests of Twitter users. FRISK models the tweets of a user and the interests (e.g., *politics*, *sports*) as bags of articles and categories of Wikipedia respectively, and ranks the interests by relevance, measured as the graph distance between the articles and the categories. To the best of our knowledge, existing unsupervised approaches do not address multilingualism and describe the users' interests through bags of words (e.g., *phone*, *apps*), without a precise categorization (e.g., *technology*).

We evaluated FRISK on a dataset including 1,347 users and more than three million tweets written in four different languages (English, French, Italian and Spanish). The results indicate that FRISK shows quantitative promise, also compared to approaches based on text classification (SVM, Naive Bayes and Random Forest) and LDA.

Keywords: Interests · Multilingual text processing · Wikipedia · Twitter

1 Introduction

Popular online social networking sites, such as Facebook and Twitter, are a major vehicle of social interactions. In particular, the users of Twitter share their thoughts, opinions, preferences and personal stories by *posting* (i.e., writing) *tweets*, short messages that anyone can read. Twitter is a gigantic corpus of textual data contributed by millions of individuals from different countries and, as such, is likely to reveal important insights about the individuals themselves.

Several studies have shown that the tweets posted by Twitter users are a good indicator of their *interests*, in fact they are likely to talk about what they like often [5,10,13–16,18–21]. For example, those who are primarily interested in politics will mostly tweet about elections, legislation and major political events. Understanding the interests of individuals, which is the focus of this paper, is key to many applications that need to characterize the individuals to recommend

G. Cong et al. (Eds.): ADMA 2017, LNAI 10604, pp. 243–256, 2017.
https://doi.org/10.1007/978-3-319-69179-4_17

them some services [12], find other individuals with similar interests [17], and even predict their future interests [2].

Not surprisingly, a lot of studies focused on the problem of determining the interests of individuals based on what they write in Twitter and, for that matter, other online social platforms. The existing approaches can be categorized along different axes, based on the data that they exploit (content written by the individuals themselves vs. their friends) and the methods that they use (supervised vs. unsupervised). In particular, supervised methods use text classifiers that assign individuals to one class or a probability distribution over a set of classes that represent their interests [13,14]. Supervised methods have the merit of providing a clear categorization of the interests, because a class, that has a specific label (e.g., *politics*, *economics*), corresponds to an interest. However, they have two major shortcomings. First, they need a training set, where individuals are manually categorized by their interests based on a visual inspection of what they write, which is a time-consuming task. Second, they are language-dependent because a classifier trained on posts written in English cannot be used to predict the interests of a person who writes in French.

In this paper, we present FRISK (Find twitteR InterestS via wiKipedia), a multilingual and unsupervised approach for the categorization of the interests of Twitter users. More specifically, FRISK models the tweets of a user and the interests (e.g., *politics*, *sports*) as bags of articles and categories of Wikipedia respectively, and ranks the interests by relevance, measured in terms of the graph distance between the articles and the categories. The ability of ranking the interests is particularly important because a Twitter user might have several. Unlike the existing unsupervised approaches [10,15,16,18–21], that describe the interests through bags of words (e.g., *phone*, *developers*, *apps*), FRISK gives a precise categorization of the interests (e.g., *technology*), in the same way as supervised approaches do, but with the advantage of being independent of the language and without training data. The categorization of the interests is particularly important to applications that need to precisely identify groups of individuals that share the same interests.

We claim the following contributions:

- FRISK is *multilingual*. It can determine the interests based on the tweets without making any assumption as to their language.
- FRISK is *unsupervised*. It does not need any training set, which is generally difficult (i.e., time-consuming and expensive) to obtain. Unlike existing unsupervised approaches, FRISK gives a precise categorization of the interests.
- FRISK is *effective* and *robust*. Despite the noise and the ambiguous terms in the tweets, FRISK shows quantitative promise, also compared to supervised approaches (SVM, Naive Bayes and Random Forest) based on text classification. We used a dataset including 1,347 users with a total of more than three million tweets written in four different languages (English, French, Italian and Spanish).

The remainder of this paper is organized as follows. After an overview of the existing approaches presented in Sect. 2, we introduce some basic notation and concepts in Sect. 3; we describe FRISK in detail in Sect. 4 and we discuss the evaluation results in Sect. 5. Finally, Sect. 6 concludes the presentation.

2 Related Work

The scientific literature describes many approaches to infer the interests of social media users based on what they, or their friends, write [5, 10, 13–16, 18–21], the tags that they use to organize their favorite resources (e.g., bookmarks of Web pages) [9, 17] and the celebrities that they like or follow [3, 7]. We focus here on the approaches that are based on the textual content posted in Twitter. Since few Twitter users mention their interests in their biographies [5], researchers usually turn their attention to the tweets.

Supervised machine learning techniques trained on textual and profile features, such as gender and location, proved to be effective [13, 14], but they are language-dependent and need a training set that is difficult to obtain. As opposed to that, FRISK, the approach that we propose in this paper, is unsupervised.

As for the unsupervised approaches, Vu and Perez use regular expressions to extract key-phrases from the tweets and rank them by their frequency based on popular measures such as tf-idf or TextRank [15]. Many researchers resort to a technique known as *Latent Dirichlet Allocation* (LDA) [16, 19, 20], a probabilistic topic model for uncovering the topics of a collection of textual documents [4]. While Weng et al. apply LDA as is to the tweets [19], Xu et al. describe a variation of LDA that filters out noisy tweets that do not necessarily reflect the interests of the user (e.g., tweets about everyday activities) [20]. The main shortcoming of all these approaches is that they describe an interest as a bag of words, or a probability distribution over words, without giving the exact categorization of the interest (e.g., *politics*). Moreover, our experiments show that LDA does not perform well in a multilingual context.

Among the approaches that use Wikipedia, Zarrinkalam et al. model the relationships among the concepts, represented as Wikipedia articles, mentioned in a user's tweets in a certain time interval and identify the interests as clusters of concepts [21]. These clusters are unnamed and often hard to interpret. Michelson and Macskassy describe the interests of a Twitter user as a bag of Wikipedia categories (e.g., *Football in England*) determined from the named entities (e.g., *Arsenal*, *Walcott*) mentioned in the tweets [10]. As opposed to FRISK, their approach ignores the tweets that do not contain any named entity, resulting in a loss of information.

3 Background

FRISK uses Wikipedia, the largest online multilingual encyclopedia with 284 active language editions, to represent both the tweets of a user and the interests. Any Wikipedia edition in a language α consists of a set of interlinked pages. A *page* has one of four types: article, disambiguation, redirect or category. An *article* discusses a specific topic and consists of a *title* (e.g., *Paris*), a textual content, *links* to related articles (e.g., *Eiffel Tower* and *Louvre*) and *cross-language links* to articles that cover the same topic (e.g., *Parigi*) in other language editions (e.g., the Italian Wikipedia). A *disambiguation page* with title t (e.g., *Campaign*) contains links to Wikipedia articles that are possible interpretations of t (e.g., *Advertising campaign, Political campaign*). A *redirect page*, or simply *redirect*, with title t (e.g., *Paris, France*) has no content itself and provides a link to another article whose title is an alias of t (e.g., *Paris*). Henceforth, we will use the title to refer to a page. Each page (e.g., the article *Political campaign*), except redirects, is included in one or more *categories* (e.g., *Category:Political campaigns*). The motivation for categories is to help readers browse the pages, and to this extent they are organized in a hierarchy, as each may branch into *subcategories*, as well as possibly being included in one or more categories.

In this paper we model Wikipedia as a directed graph $\mathcal{W} = (PA, LI)$, where the nodes in PA correspond to the pages and the edges in LI are pairs of nodes connected by a link. Unless otherwise specified, we will treat the terms node and Wikipedia page as synonyms. A node p_α belongs to a Wikipedia edition in a specific language α and has one of the four types specified above. A cross-language link (p_α, p_β) (or simply *crosslink*) connects two pages p_α and p_β that cover the same topic in two different language editions α and β. The meaning of an *intra-language* link (or simply, link), connecting a page p_α to a page q_α within the same language edition, depends on the types of p_α and q_α. If p_α is a disambiguation page, q_α corresponds to one of the possible interpretations of p_α; if p_α is a redirect page, q_α is the page to which p_α redirects; if p_α is an article and q_α is a category, p_α is contained in the category q_α; finally, if both p_α and q_α are categories, p_α is contained in q_α (q_α is *parent* of p_α, or, alternatively, p_α is a *subcategory* of q_α).

4 Our Approach

FRISK ranks the interests of a Twitter user by relevance based on the tweets authored by that user. The rationale is that the words occurring in the tweets (e.g., *campaign, elections, player, game*) are important clues as to what the user likes (e.g., *politics, sports*); the more the words related to an interest, the higher the relevance of that interest.

The key to the approach is the computation of a relevance score of an interest from the words of the tweets by using a Wikipedia-based representation. We observe that a Wikipedia article (e.g., *Political campaign*) identifies a specific meaning of a word (e.g., *campaign*) and thus a set of tweets can be represented as the bag (i.e., collection) of the Wikipedia articles associated to its words. At the same time, a Wikipedia article is organized into a hierarchy of categories (e.g., *Category: Political activism, Category: Politics*) that identify the broad domain (e.g., *politics*) of that article and, as such, the interest of a person who reads the article. An interest can therefore be described as a bag of Wikipedia categories. FRISK computes the relevance score of an interest to a Twitter user in terms of the graph distance between the articles associated to the tweets of that user and one of the categories representing the interest.

Formally, the input of FRISK is a set $\mathcal{I}$ of interests, each described by a bag of Wikipedia categories, and a set $\mathcal{T}_u$ of tweets authored by a user u; the number of tweets $|\mathcal{T}_u|$ will be discussed in Sect. 5. The main steps of FRISK are:

1. *BOW representation.* The tweets $\mathcal{T}_u$ are turned into a bag of words $\mathcal{BOW}_u$.
2. *BOA representation.* $\mathcal{BOW}_u$ is turned into a bag of Wikipedia articles $\mathcal{BOA}_u$.
3. *Interests Ranking.* Interests are ranked by relevance.

The remainder of the section describes each step in greater detail.

BOW Representation. The tweets in $\mathcal{T}_u$ are pre-processed to remove stop words (i.e. frequent words, such as *the, will, be, at, of*), numbers, special characters (e.g., /, \, #) and URLs. Mentions (i.e., references to Twitter users intended to be the recipient of the tweet) are removed from the tweets because they will almost never map to any Wikipedia article, with very few exceptions (e.g., *@neo4j*). We keep *hashtags* (i.e., keywords preceded by the character "#" used to specify the topic of a tweet) while removing the character "#", as they might map to Wikipedia articles, although we found that it does not occur frequently, due to the fact that an hashtag might be composed of multiple words without spaces (e.g., "#androidgames"). The output of this step is a bag of words representation $\mathcal{BOW}_u$ of the tweets $\mathcal{T}_u$. For instance, the bag of words of the tweet "Going to the store without a budget #creditchat" is {store; budget; creditchat}.

BOA Representation. When it comes to transforming the bag of words $\mathcal{BOW}_u$ into a bag of articles $\mathcal{BOA}_u$, the challenge is that natural language is inherently ambiguous; thus, a word w (e.g., *gender*) might have several *meanings* (e.g., distinction between male and female, or grammatical gender), that are described by different Wikipedia articles, also referred to as the *interpretations* of w. Since FRISK does not make any assumption as to the language of the tweets, it looks for the interpretations of w across all Wikipedia language editions. In order to address the problem of ambiguity, in a previous work of ours we observed that the Wikipedia article that has the word w as its title is usually the *default* (i.e., most common) interpretation of w and, as such, the correct interpretation in many cases [8]. This stems from the fact that for an ambiguous word (e.g., *election*) the article that corresponds to the default interpretation (e.g., the one describing the political decision-making process) is chosen by millions of Wikipedia users that agree that the word is normally used with that meaning. For this reason, FRISK always selects the default interpretation of w, if it exists, as the correct one.

However, if the word w (e.g., *campaign*) is ambiguous and the Wikipedia users cannot find any agreement as to its default interpretation, a disambiguation page exists having w as its title and listing all the possible interpretations of w (e.g., *Political campaign, Advertising campaign*). In this case, FRISK selects the interpretation (Wikipedia article) with the highest indegree, based on the observation that the number of Wikipedia articles that link to an interpretation is an indication of the importance, or *popularity*, of that interpretation.

Algorithm 1. Calculate $\mathcal{BOA}_u$

```
1: function COMPUTEBOA(𝓑𝓞𝓦_u, 𝓦): 𝓑𝓞𝓐_u
2:     𝓑𝓞𝓐_u ← ∅
3:     for each w ∈ 𝓑𝓞𝓦_u do
4:         AW = ∅
5:         A = getArticlesByTitle(w, 𝓦)
6:         for each a ∈ A do
7:             if isRedirect(a) then a ← resolveRedirect(a, 𝓦)
8:             if isDisambiguationPage(a) then
9:                 I ← getInterpretations(a, 𝓦)
10:                a ← getMostPopular(I, 𝓦)
11:            if language(a) ≠ "English" then a ← geEnglishArticle(a, 𝓦)
12:            if |categories(a)| ≥ 5 then AW ← AW ∪ {a}
13:        𝓑𝓞𝓐_u ← 𝓑𝓞𝓐_u ∪ {getMostPopular(AW, 𝓦)}
```

The function that computes $\mathcal{BOA}_u$ (Algorithm 1) iterates over each word w in $\mathcal{BOW}_u$ and obtains the set A of articles that have w as their title across all language editions of Wikipedia $\mathcal{W}$ (Line 5). For each article $a \in A$, if a is a redirect page, the article that is the target of the redirection is obtained (Line 7). If a is a disambiguation page (i.e., there is no default interpretation of the word w), the function gets all the interpretations (i.e., all the articles to which the disambiguation page links) and selects the most popular (Line 10); otherwise, a is the default interpretation and is selected. The English version of the selected article is obtained by using the crosslinks (Line 11), so as all articles in $\mathcal{BOA}_u$ belong to the same language edition. Finally, the article is added to the set AW of articles that are associated to the current word w, provided that it is in at least five categories (Line 12). Indeed, we experimentally observed that articles that are in less than five categories have often a negative impact on the determination of the relevance of an interest to the user u.

At this point, the set AW may contain more than one article for a given word. For instance, given the word *store*, the page titled *Store* in the English Wikipedia is a disambiguation page whose most popular interpretation is the article titled *Retail.* However, the article titled *Store* in the Italian Wikipedia redirects to the article titled *Štore* (a small town in Eastern Slovenia). Since only one article is the correct interpretation of the word, only the most popular is retained (Line 13). The bag of articles of the tweet "Going to the store without a budget #creditchat" is {Retail, Budget}; the words *store* and *budget* are associated to the articles titled *Retail* and *Budget* respectively, while no article is found for the word *creditchat.*

Interest Ranking. In order to rank the interests by relevance to the user u, a relevance score S_i^u is computed for each interest $i \in \mathcal{I}$. To this extent, FRISK represents i (e.g., *sports*) as the bag of Wikipedia categories $\mathcal{BOC}_i$ whose titles contain the name of the interest (e.g., *Category: Sports by year*, *Category: Sport in France*).

The relevance score S_i^u is obtained as the sum of the relevance scores of all articles $a \in \mathcal{BOA}_u$ to the interest i. This is shown in Eq. 1

$$S_i^u = \sum_{a \in \mathcal{BOA}_u} \frac{1}{\min_{c \in \mathcal{BOC}_i} dist(a, c)} \quad (1)$$

where the relevance score of an article a to the interest i is computed as the inverse of the minimum distance between a and any of the categories $c \in \mathcal{BOC}_i$ that represent the interest. Since a and c are both nodes in the Wikipedia graph, the distance $dist(a, c)$ is defined as the length of the shortest directed path from a to c. The rationale of this choice is that if an article a is relevant to the interest, then it is either contained in a category describing the interest or in one of its direct ascendants, resulting in a short distance.

5 Evaluation

For the evaluation of FRISK we adopted the following methodology. First, we collected a multilingual dataset, which we called MULTIDS, that includes 1,347 Twitter users who tweet in one of four selected languages—English, French, Italian and Spanish; second, we manually determined the interest—one among *Politics*, *Economy*, *Games*, *Gastronomy* and *Sports*—of each user by reading their tweets; finally, we verified whether the interests output by FRISK are consistent with the interests determined manually for all users, to evaluate the predictive capability of FRISK. We compared FRISK against three text classifiers and LDA in a multilingual and monolingual context and evaluated FRISK used in combination with TagMe, a tool to annotate short texts with Wikipedia [6]. All the steps of the evaluation are detailed in the remainder of the section.

5.1 Data Collection

The data collection consisted of two steps: first, we obtained a set of Twitter users and categorized them by interest; then we retrieved their most recent tweets (up to 5000) by using the Twitter search API. In order to collect the set of users, we submitted queries to the Twitter search engine, using keywords that are representative of five selected interests —*Politics*, *Economy*, *Games*, *Gastronomy* and *Sports*. For the five interests (between parentheses in the following list) we obtained the following keywords from the category hierarchy provided by Google AdWords[1]: politics, government, campaigns, elections (*Politics*); economy, finance (*Economy*); game, board games, video games (*Games*); sports, basketball, baseball, bowling, football (*Sports*); drink, food, restaurant (*Gastronomy*). To retrieve users communicating in languages other than English, we translated these keywords. Finally, we filtered out the users who did not have any of the five selected interests by reading the tweets of all users, a long manual process needed to make sure that the ground truth was reliable. At the

[1] developers.google.com/adwords/api/docs/appendix/productsservices.

end of the collection, the dataset, that we name MULTIDS, consists of more than 3 million tweets and 1,347 users distributed uniformly over the four languages and the five interests.

5.2 Results

We define precision (P_i), recall (R_i) and f-measure (F_i), the standard metrics to evaluate the prediction ability of an algorithm, for any given interest $i \in \mathcal{I}$:

$$P_i = \frac{|TP_i|}{|TP_i| + |FP_i|} \quad R_i = \frac{|TP_i|}{|TP_i| + |FN_i|} \quad F_i = \frac{2 \times P_i \times R_i}{P_i + R_i}$$

where TP_i (true positives) is the set of users whose actual and predicted interest is i; FP_i (false positives) is the set of users whose predicted and actual interest are i and j respectively, $i \neq j$; FN_i (false negatives) is the set of users whose predicted and actual interest are j and i respectively, $j \neq i$.

The values of precision (P), recall (R) and f-measure (F) averaged over the five interests depend on the number of tweets $\mathcal{T}_u$ that FRISK uses to predict the interests of a user u (Fig. 1a). As we expected, the higher the number of the tweets, the higher the overall accuracy of FRISK, although using more than 200 tweets is useless, since both precision and recall stabilize beyond that point. The fact that FRISK does not need too high a number of tweets to obtain a good accuracy is particularly important because its computation time also increases with the number of tweets. We also observe that both precision and recall are high (83% and 80%, respectively) when only using 50 tweets, which indicates that FRISK can determine the interest of users who are not very active.

The overall accuracy of FRISK is stable across the interests, with the exception for the precision and recall for *Politics* and *Economy* respectively (Fig. 1b).

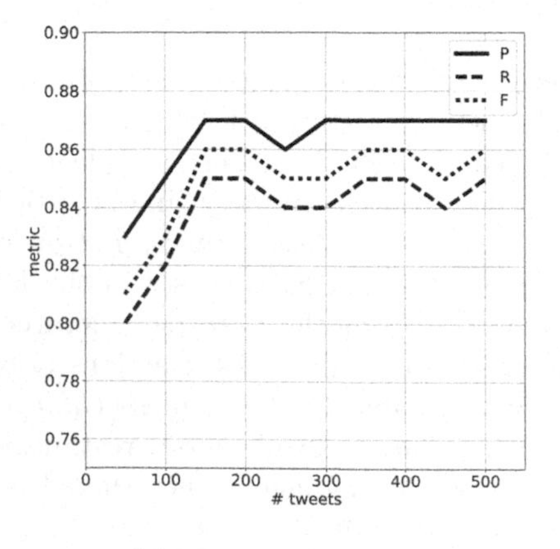

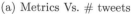

(a) Metrics Vs. # tweets

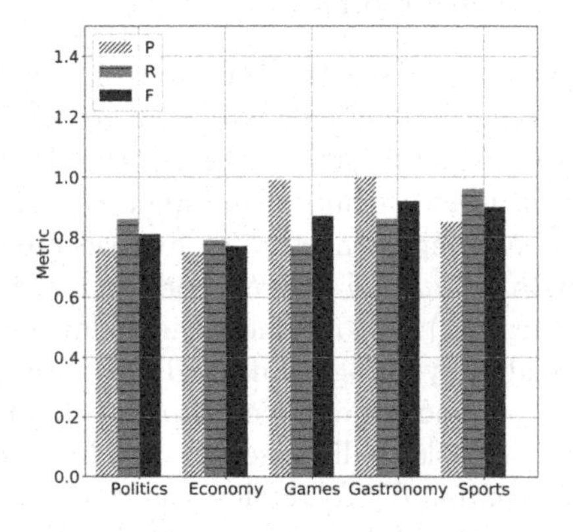

(b) Metrics per interest

Fig. 1. Results of FRISK on MULTIDS.

This might occur because the two interests, unlike the others, are somehow related; after all, the politics of a country influences its economy, and the other way round.

FRISK Vs. Text Classification. In a recent work, Raghuram and colleagues proposed a supervised approach to categorize the interests of Twitter users by using traditional classifiers [13]. Here we want to verify whether the promising results that they reported in a monolingual context (which are coherent with our findings described below) can be generalized to a multilingual context. In order to train the text classifiers, we randomly split MULTIDS to obtain a training set MULTIDS_TRAIN with 753 users and a test set MULTIDS_TEST with 594 users. In either set, an instance is a Twitter user represented as a tf-idf vector obtained from that user tweets, after removing stop words and special characters. Each user is assigned to one class, representing the interest of the user. In both sets, users are uniformly distributed over the five classes (to avoid class imbalance) and across the four languages.

We used scikit-learn, a popular machine learning library in Python, to train several text classifiers, of which we selected the best three: a Support Vector Machine (SVM) with linear kernel and hyper-parameter $C = 1.0$, a Multinomial Naive Bayes classifier with Laplacian smoothing parameter $\alpha = 1.0$ and a Random Forest using the Gini impurity as the function to measure the quality of a split. We found that the number of tweets has little or no impact on the f-measure, while the higher the number of users, the higher the f-measure; our experiments indicate that the f-measure does not improve significantly with more than 400 users. Based on these observations, for the training of the three classifiers we set the number of users to 400 (100 per language) and the number of tweets per user to 150.

The comparison on MULTIDS_TEST (Table 1) shows that FRISK clearly outperforms the three text classifiers in all metrics, considering that precision, recall and f-measure (0.86, 0.84 and 0.85 respectively) averaged over all interests are much higher than the values obtained by the SVM (0.60, 0.58 and 0.59 respectively), the best of the text classifiers. Despite the large number of training instances, the ability of the three text classifiers of predicting the interests in a

Table 1. FRISK vs. text classifiers on MULTIDS_TEST.

Interest	FRISK			SVM			Naive Bayes			R. Forest		
	P	R	F	P	R	F	P	R	F	P	R	F
Politics	0.75	0.87	**0.81**	0.65	0.37	0.47	0.64	0.40	0.49	0.43	0.22	0.29
Economy	0.72	0.77	**0.74**	0.54	0.46	0.50	0.54	0.49	0.51	0.33	0.42	0.37
Games	0.99	0.76	**0.86**	0.87	0.79	0.83	0.56	0.80	0.65	0.62	0.71	0.66
Gastronomy	1.0	0.84	**0.91**	0.53	0.90	0.66	0.50	0.61	0.55	0.37	0.52	0.42
Sports	0.86	0.94	**0.90**	0.40	0.40	0.40	0.41	0.34	0.37	0.30	0.21	0.24
Average	0.86	0.84	**0.85**	0.60	0.58	0.59	0.53	0.53	0.53	0.41	0.42	0.41

Table 2. The topic model learned on MULTIDS_TRAIN.

Interest 1	Interest 2	Interest 3	Interest 4	Interest 5
jeu, bien	day, finance	politica, calcio	juego, nuevo	videogames, food
faire, j'ai	win, watch	solo, sapevatelo	economia, gracias	xbox, trailer
merci, nouveau	support, minister	ecco, dopo	millones, partido	gameplay, nintendo
monde, faut	team, week	prima, renzi	ver, ser	playstation, foodie
après, contre	release, world	cosa, italia	día, españa	foodporn, wars
entreprises, français	work, donald	ora, anni	juegos, gran	super, play
soir, bonjour	check, president	roma, grazie	mundo, mejor	day, sale
jour, jeux	big, campaign	sempre, lavoro	ahora, gobierno	lego, week
ans, demain	clinton, top	ancora, tramite	nueva, semana	world, gamedev

multilingual context is limited. Since the text classifiers perform well in a monolingual context, as we will show below, a possible alternative would be to train four monolingual classifiers and predict the interests of a user by using the classifier trained on the user language. However, this solution is not multilingual, because the language of the user must be known, and cannot deal with users that use multiple languages at the same time. Also, we note that FRISK does not need any training data, which is time-consuming to obtain.

FRISK Vs. LDA. We compare FRISK against the approach proposed by Weng and colleagues that apply LDA to discover the interests of Twitter users [19]. To this extent, we used the collapsed variational Bayes approximation to the LDA objective [1] implemented in the Stanford Topic Modeling Toolbox[2] to learn a topic model with five topics (one for each interest) over MULTIDS_TRAIN. The learning phase is necessary to determine the best values of the LDA parameters, namely the Dirichlet prior on the per-document topic distributions, and the Dirichlet prior on the per-topic word distribution (for both, we found that the best value was 0.01). For all tweets, we lowercased the words and we removed the stopwords in the four languages so as to avoid to include words that are used too frequently in the topic model. The learned topic model consists of five groups of words (shown in Table 2), one for each interest; the groups are unlabeled, meaning that one has to guess which group corresponds to which interest based on the words that occur in it.

From the table one can see that some interests are easily recognizable based on the words that describe them; this is the case of "Interest 2" and "Interest 5" that correspond to *Politics* (cf. words such as "minister", "donald", "president" and "clinton") and *Games* (cf. words such as "videogrames", "xbox", and "nintendo") respectively,

However, the other groups of words do not seem to identify unambiguously the other interests. For instance, "Interest 3" includes words in Italian, some of which (e.g., "calcio" that means "soccer") indicate the interest *Sports*, others (e.g., "politica", that means "politics", and "renzi", the family name of the former

[2] https://nlp.stanford.edu/software/tmt/tmt-0.4/.

Italian prime minister) indicate the interest *Politics*. "Interest 1" is a collection of words in French, some of them (e.g., "jeu" and "jeux" that translate to "game" and "games" respectively) indicate either the interest *Games* or *Sports*, others (e.g., "entreprises" that translates to "companies") indicate the interest *Economy*. Finally, "Interest 4" is a group of words in Spanish that again do not point unambiguously to any of the five interests that we selected.

We played with the parameters of LDA, especially with the number of topics, to try to obtain groups of words that would identify our five interests. In particular, based on the observation that each group of words in Table 2 is only in one language, we set the number of topics to 20, in the hope to obtain four groups of words (one in each language) for each interest; however, we did not obtain that result.

In the end, we applied the learned topic model to the Twitter users in MULTIDS_TEST and we computed the precision/recall/f-measure for the two interests *Games* and *Politics* that are identified unambiguously in the training phase. For the interest *Politics*, we obtain a precision/recall/f-measure of 0.29, 0.37 and 0.33 respectively; for the interest *Games*, we obtain 0.55, 0.34 and 0.42. In both cases, the values are well below those obtained with FRISK.

Monolingual Dataset. We finally compare FRISK, the three text classifiers and LDA in a monolingual context, where the language of the users is known. For this purpose, we split MULTIDS into four datasets (MONOEN, MONOFR, MONOIT, MONOES), one per language, and each dataset is split into a training (used to train the three classifiers and a topic model) and a test set. We also included in the evaluation a variation of FRISK (that we term FRISKTM), one that creates $\mathcal{BOA}_u$, for each user u, with TagMe, a tool to annotate short texts with Wikipedia [6]. TagMe associates each word of the tweet to at most one Wikipedia article; in case of ambiguity, it uses the context to select one of the possible interpretations of a word.

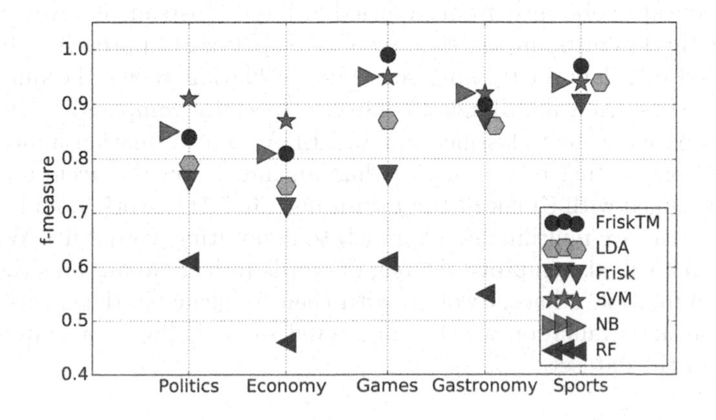

Fig. 2. Evaluation on MONOEN.

Figure 2 shows the f-measure obtained with the different approaches on the test set of MonoEN, that only includes users who tweet in English. The results on the other languages are similar and are omitted because of space constraints. The f-measure of Frisk (represented as a black circle) is comparable to the values obtained in a multilingual context (with the only exception of *Games*), which indicates that Frisk does not depend on the language. Among the text classifiers, Random Forest (RF) performs poorly while SVM and Naive Bayes outperform Frisk across the five interests. The results seem to confirm the findings of Raghuram and colleagues [13] who reported a good accuracy of traditional classifiers in a monolingual context.

Interestingly, the accuracy of FriskTM is comparable to that of SVM and Naive Bayes, which is probably the effect of TagMe considering the context of a tweet to assign an interpretation to its words. The only problem is that TagMe is not truly multilingual in the sense that it needs to know the language of the tweets in order to create $\mathcal{BOA}_u$. An alternative multilingual annotation tool that we considered is Babelfy [11] that, however, does not use only Wikipedia to annotate the words and the result is that many words (annotated with other sources, e.g., WordNet) are not represented in the corresponding bag of articles.

Finally, LDA leads to a good accuracy across the five interests, comparable to or slightly better than, that of Frisk but in general worse than SVM, Naive Bayes and FriskTM. We observe that, unlike the multilingual context, the topics discovered by LDA in a monolingual context are groups of words that unambiguously identify the five interests that we selected for the evaluation.

6 Concluding Remarks

In this paper we presented Frisk a multilingual unsupervised approach to categorize the interests of Twitter users. Unlike existing unsupervised approaches, Frisk determines the interests of Twitter users in a multilingual context and does not merely represent the interests of individuals as unlabeled bag-of-words or bag-of-concepts obtained from knowledge bases. Instead, it gives a categorization of the interests, in the same way as supervised approaches, but without the need of a labeled training set. The evaluation shows the quantitative promise of Frisk in a multilingual context, especially compared to supervised approaches based on text classification and LDA. Our evaluation indicates that the method of creating bag of articles has an impact on the accuracy (cf. the accuracy obtained with FriskTM). Our immediate future work intends to investigate an alternative multilingual approach to annotating words with Wikipedia. This approach will also improve the bag of words to include n-grams (i.e., terms composed of multiple adjacent words) with their frequency in the tweets. Finally, a more thorough evaluation will be conducted by including more interests and languages in the dataset.

References

1. Asuncion, A., Welling, M., Smyth, P., Teh, Y.W.: On smoothing and inference for topic models. In: Proceedings of the Twenty-Fifth Conference on Uncertainty in Artificial Intelligence, UAI 2009, pp. 27–34. AUAI Press (2009)
2. Bao, H., Li, Q., Liao, S.S., Song, S., Gao, H.: A new temporal and social PMF-based method to predict users' interests in micro-blogging. Decis. Support Syst. **55**(3), 698–709 (2013)
3. Bhattacharya, P., Zafar, M.B., Ganguly, N., Ghosh, S., Gummadi, K.P.: Inferring user interests in the twitter social network. In: RecSys, pp. 357–360 (2014)
4. Blei, D.M., Ng, A.Y., Jordan, M.I.: Latent dirichlet allocation. J. Mach. Learn. Res. **3**, 993–1022 (2003)
5. Ding, Y., Jiang, J.: Extracting interest tags from twitter user biographies. In: Jaafar, A., Mohamad Ali, N., Mohd Noah, S.A., Smeaton, A.F., Bruza, P., Bakar, Z.A., Jamil, N., Sembok, T.M.T. (eds.) AIRS 2014. LNCS, vol. 8870, pp. 268–279. Springer, Cham (2014). doi:10.1007/978-3-319-12844-3_23
6. Ferragina, P., Scaiella, U.: TAGME: on-the-fly annotation of short text fragments (by wikipedia entities). In: CIKM, pp. 1625–1628 (2010)
7. He, W., Liu, H., He, J., Tang, S., Du, X.: Extracting interest tags for non-famous users in social network. In: CIKM, pp. 861–870. ACM (2015)
8. Jipmo, C.N., Quercini, G., Bennacer, N.: Catégorisation et Désambiguïsation des Intérêts des Individus dans le Web Social. In: EGC, pp. 523–524 (2016)
9. Li, X., Guo, L., Zhao, Y.E.: Tag-based social interest discovery. In: WWW, pp. 675–684 (2008)
10. Michelson, M., Macskassy, S.A.: Discovering users' topics of interest on twitter: a first look. In: 4th Workshop on Analytics for Noisy Unstructured Text Data, pp. 73–80. ACM (2010)
11. Moro, A., Raganato, A., Navigli, R.: Entity linking meets word sense disambiguation: a unified approach. TACL **2**, 231–244 (2014)
12. Pennacchiotti, M., Silvestri, F., Vahabi, H., Venturini, R.: Making your interests follow you on twitter. In: CIKM, pp. 165–174 (2012)
13. Raghuram, M.A., Akshay, K., Chandrasekaran, K.: Efficient user profiling in twitter social network using traditional classifiers. In: Berretti, S., Thampi, S.M., Dasgupta, S. (eds.) Intelligent Systems Technologies and Applications. AISC, vol. 385, pp. 399–411. Springer, Cham (2016). doi:10.1007/978-3-319-23258-4_35
14. Spasojevic, N., Yan, J., Rao, A., Bhattacharyya, P.: LASTA: large scale topic assignment on multiple social networks. In: KDD, pp. 1809–1818 (2014)
15. Vu, T., Perez, V.: Interest mining from user tweets. In: CIKM, pp. 1869–1872 (2013)
16. Wang, T., Liu, H., He, J., Du, X.: Mining user interests from information sharing behaviors in social media. In: Pei, J., Tseng, V.S., Cao, L., Motoda, H., Xu, G. (eds.) PAKDD 2013. LNCS, vol. 7819, pp. 85–98. Springer, Heidelberg (2013). doi:10.1007/978-3-642-37456-2_8
17. Wang, X., Liu, H., Fan, W.: Connecting users with similar interests via tag network inference. In: CIKM, pp. 1019–1024. ACM (2011)
18. Wen, Z., Lin, C.Y.: Improving user interest inference from social neighbors. In: CIKM, pp. 1001–1006 (2011)
19. Weng, J., Lim, E.P., Jiang, J., He, Q.: TwitterRank: finding topic-sensitive influential twitterers. In: WSDM, pp. 261–270 (2010)

20. Xu, Z., Lu, R., Xiang, L., Yang, Q.: Discovering user interest on twitter with a modified author-topic model. In: WI-IAT, vol. 1, pp. 422–429 (2011)
21. Zarrinkalam, F., Fani, H., Bagheri, E., Kahani, M., Du, W.: Semantics-enabled user interest detection from twitter. In: WI-IAT, vol. 1, pp. 469–476 (2015)

A Solution to Tweet-Based User Identification Across Online Social Networks

Yongjun Li(✉), Zhen Zhang, and You Peng

School of Computer, Northwestern Polytechnical University,
Xiàn, Shaanxi 710072, China
lyj@nwpu.edu.cn

Abstract. User identification can help us build better users' profiles and benefit many applications. It has attracted many scholars' attention. The existing works with good performance are mainly based on the rich online data. However, due to the privacy settings, it is costless or even difficult to obtain the rich data. Besides some profile attributes do not require exclusivity and are easily faked by users for different purposes. This makes the existing schemes are quite fragile. Users often publicly publish their activities on different social networks. This provides a way to overcome the above problem. We aim to address the user identification only based on users' tweets. We first formulate the user identification based on tweets and propose a tweet-based user identification model. Then a supervised machine learning based solution is presented. It consists of three key steps: first, we propose several algorithms to measure the spatial similarity, temporal similarity and content similarity of two tweets; second, we extract the spatial, temporal and content features to exploit information redundancies; Afterwards, we employ the machine learning method for user identification. The experiment shows that the proposed solution can provide excellent performance with F1 values reaching 89.79%, 86.78% and 86.24% on three ground truth datasets, respectively. This work shows the possibility of user identification with easily accessible and not easily impersonated online data.

Keywords: User identification · Tweet · Social network · Machine learning · Online behavior analysis

1 Introduction

In the last decade, many types of social networking sites have emerged and grown rapidly in Monthly Active Users(MAU). As of April 2017, Twitter has more than 319 million MAUs, and Facebook has 1,968 million MAUs. Sina Microblog has also more than 313 million MAUs [1]. These social sites have changed the way we interact with each other, and make it simple to stay connected in our lives.

Due to the differences in the services provided by online social networks (OSNs), people tend to use different OSNs for different purposes. As we may expect, a user's activities and connections are scattered into several different sites. If we integrate these sites, his better and more complete profile can be

G. Cong et al. (Eds.): ADMA 2017, LNAI 10604, pp. 257–269, 2017.
https://doi.org/10.1007/978-3-319-69179-4_18

built to improve online services, such as community discovery, recommendation, and information diffusion.

To integrate these OSNs, it is necessary to identify users across sites. There are some existing works discussing possible solutions to this problem. Many existing works addressed this problem based on the rich user profile attributes, including screen name, birthday, hometown, etc. [3–10]. Owing to privacy settings, it is high costless or even difficult to obtain the above attributes. On the other hand, these attributes are easily faked by users for different purposes. These limitation make the existing schemes quite fragile [2]. Some researchers leveraged the friend network to identify users [2,11–21]. Taking into account personal privacy, most of users do not make their friend network public. Even if we can obtain the user's friend network, these connections are also sparse. The existing methods based on friend network are also plagued by the above limitations [2]. Some researchers also employed user tweets to identify users based on posting time, location and writing style [22–25]. However, in existing works, the tweets are always used with profiles or friend network together, so these solutions face similar problems as described above.

The tweets posted on different sites by the same user usually contain rich information redundancies. Meanwhile, users often make some of their tweets public and easily accessible. Intuitively, we can identify users solely based on the users' tweets, and break through these limitations. However, the tweets-based method is surely very challenging. The first challenge is that writing style, usually used in the existing works, is difficult to extract from short tweets. The number of tweets the user posting publicly on different sites are serious imbalance. In this study, we calculate semantic similarity of tweets rather than writing style. On the other side, we consider the similarity of any two tweets from different sites to overcome the problem of imbalance. We present a novel framework to tackle the user identification. This method could be applied jointly with other feature-based algorithms for more accurate results.

The rest of the paper is organized as follows. We first introduce the related works in Sect. 2. Then in Sect. 3, we describe the preliminary concepts, and give the problem formulation. In Sect. 4, we present the solution framework and tweet-based user identification across OSNs. Then Sect. 5 shows the experiment results on social networks. In Sect. 6, we conclude the paper.

2 Related Works

In OSN, a user usually creates an identity and constitutes its three major dimensions namely Profile, Content and Network. Each dimension is composed of a set of attributes which describes her and differentiates her from others [26]. The existing works are mainly based on these three dimensions or the hybrid dimensions.

In some existing works, the researchers presented methods which solely use profile attributes to identify users across sites. Liu et al. [3] matched user accounts in an unsupervised approach using usernames. Zafarani et al. [4] presented a MOBIUS method to identify users based on the naming patterns of usernames. Perito et al. [27] introduced the idea of using username to match the accounts of a user across sites. Liu et al. [29] analyzed usernames' characteristics including length, special character, numeric character etc., and proposed a weighting function of user identification. However, username are not always available, and even in some situation, the username is a numeric string automatically assigned by sites. This makes these existing schemes fragile. Motoyama et al. [6] extended the profile attribute set, and used name, city, school, location, age, email etc. to match user accounts. Iofciu et al. [5] used the similarity between users' profiles to identify users. Abel et al. [7] aggregated user profiles and matched users across systems. Raad et al. [8] addressed the user identification by providing a matching framework based on all the prole's attributes. The proposed framework allowed users to give more importance to some attributes and assign each attribute a different similarity measure. The hybrid methods concluded that user accounts could be accurately matched based on a set of attributes. However, the profile attributes are not exclusive and easily faked by users for different purposes.

Some existing works studied the user identification problem solely based on user network. Zhou et al. [2] proposed a friend relationship-based user identification algorithm. It calculates a match degree for all candidate user matched pairs, and only pairs with top ranks are considered as identical users. Narayanan et al. [19] solely used network structure to analyze privacy and anonymity, which is closely related to user identification issue. Korula et al. [21] presented a mapping algorithm based on the degrees of unmapped users and the number of common neighbors, using two control parameters to finetune performance. Owing to the privacy setting, in many cases, the users' friend networks are not public and accessible across sites. Researchers attempted hybrid approaches to solve this issue. Bartunov et al. [20] considered both the profile and friend network, and proposed an approach based on conditional random fields to identify users. Bennacer et al. [30] also used the friend network and the publicly available profile to iteratively match profiles across OSNs. Malhotra et al. [31] used user profile and friend network to generate the user's digital footprints, and applied automated classifiers for user identification. The above studies show that the friend network has forceful and robust features for user identification. However, this information is often sparse, because only a small portion of users are willing to make their friend network public.

A set of researchers used the content dimension for user identification. Goga et al. [23] used three attributes extracted from the content, timestamp, location and description, to identify users. Kong et al. [22] considered the content and social relationship to solve this issue, and proposed Multi-Network Anchoring to match user accounts. They calculated the combined similarities of user's social, spatial, temporal and text information, and employed SVM classifier to identify users. Almishari et al. [32] studied likability of community-based reviews and show that a high percentage of ostensibly anonymous reviews can be accurately linked to their authors. This study focuses on one single popular site(Yelp). Besides, Jiang et al. [28] assume multiple accounts belonging to the same person contain the same or similar camera fingerprint information, and identify the user by matching his cameras. In these existing content-based works, only Goga et al. [23] solely used the content to identify users across OSNs. At this point, this works is the same as our work, and we also find that the location of tweets is the most powerful feature to match accounts. Our work also focuses on spatial, temporal and text information extracted from tweets, but it is different from Goga et al.'s work in the information processing.

3 Problem Formulation

In this paper, we focus on studying the tweet-based user identification problem across OSNs. The task of tweet-based user identification is to predict whether a pair of user accounts from two OSNs belongs to the same individual. This problem can easily be generalized to the cases with more than two OSNs.

Suppose we are given an OSN $G^1 = \{V^1, E^1\}$, where V^1 is a set of nodes and E^1 is a set of links. For node $v_i^1 \in V^1$, it represents an offline individual. This individual has a unique account u_i^1 on G^1, and also posts some short public tweets on his page. These tweets are denoted as TW_i^1. The kth tweet of v_i^1 is denoted by $tw_{ik}^1 \in TW_i^1$. The tweet tw_{ik}^1 is triple $tuple(t_{ik}^1, l_{ik}^1, w_{ik}^1)$, where t_{ik}^1 is posting time of tweet tw_{ik}^1, l_{ik}^1 is the posting location or place, and w_{ik}^1 is the set of words that user has used in tweet tw_{ik}^1. Similarly, we define another network as $G^2 = (V^2, E^2)$. u_i^2 denotes the account of $v_i^2 \in V^2$ on G^2. TW_i^2 denotes his tweets on G^2 and tw_{ik}^2 denotes the kth tweet.

The tweets posted by a user on different OSNs provide rich information redundancies and can help identify users across sites. When considering tweet-based user identification, we first need to analyze and measure these information redundancies and solve the following general problem based on analysis results.

Given two tweet sets TW_i^1 and TW_k from two different OSNs, do they belong to the same offline individual?

Tweet-Based User Identification. Suppose we have two OSNs G^1 and G^2, with a small set of identified users across two OSNs, $A = (v_i^1, v_j^2), v_i^1 \in V^1, v_j^2 \in V^2$. $\forall(v_i^1, v_j^2) \in A$, we also know the tweet sets TW_i^1 and TW_j^2. Given two tweet sets TW_m^1 and TW_n^2, where $(v_m^1, v_n^2) \notin A$, the task of tweet-based user identification is to determine whether node v_m^1 and v_n^2 belong to the same individual.

The key issue of tweet-based user identification is to learn a identification function of two user accounts. The main difference from the existing works is that we identify users solely based on users' public tweets. This suggests that we should analyze information redundancies of tweets accurately.

4 Model and Solution Framework

For tweet-based user identification, we have the following basic intuition. If two users post several similar tweets, including similar content, similar posting time or similar location, their two accounts belong to the same individual with high probability.

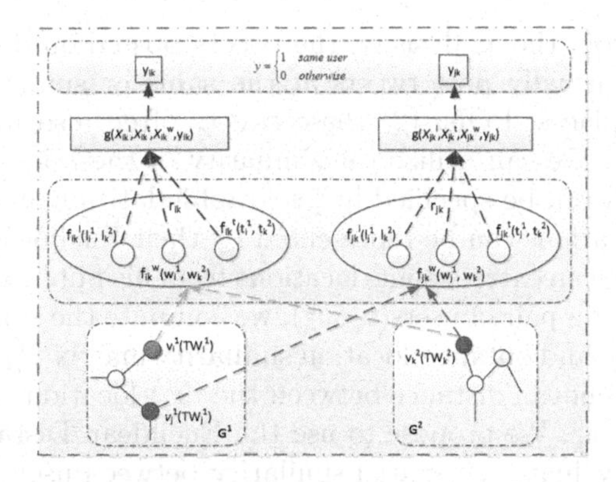

Fig. 1. Graphical representation of T-UIM

4.1 Tweet-Based User Identification Model

Based on the above intuitions, we propose a tweet-based user identification model (T-UIM). Figure 1 shows the graphical representation of the T-UIM. A pair of $users(v_i^1, v_k^2)$ from two OSNs G^1 and G^2 is mapped into a node r_{ik} in T-UIM. Based on the information source, the node r_{ik} is further subdivided into three distinct sub-nodes r_{ik}^l, r_{ik}^t and r_{ik}^w. The sub-nodes represent the similarity of two tweet sets (TW_i^1, TW_k^2) in content, posting time and location dimension, respectively. The similarity in content dimension is denoted by vector X_{ik}^w. Accordingly, we have vectors X_{ik}^l and X_{ik}^t. A pair of tweet sets is represented as three feature vectors extracted based on three distinct dimensions. The tweet-based user identification problem is converted into the binary classification problem. In other words, the identification of (v_i^1, v_k^2) is changed to the classification of node r_{ik}. We denote the classification result of node r_{ik} by y_{ik}. If $y_{ik} = 1$, the two accounts (u_i^1, u_k^2) belong to the same offline individual; otherwise, these two accounts belong to two distinct person. We can employ the supervised machine learning method to solve the user identification.

4.2 The Framework of T-UIM

The framework of T-UIM is shown in Fig. 2. A pair of user tweet sets (TW_i^1, TW_k^2) is represented as a bag of feature vectors $X_{ik} = \{X_{ik}^l, X_{ik}^t, X_{ik}^w\}$. Assume we have s set of identified users $\{X_{ik}, y_{ik}\}$ for training. Based on the labeled data and the identification model T-UIM, we design a cascaded three-level classifier to identify the user across OSNs.

Feature Extraction Across Networks. In social media, a user often posts hundreds of tweets publicly, containing rich information about: where, when, and what. In the following, we propose to exploit the spatial, temporal and text content information redundancies of two different tweet sets for user identification.

Spatial Features. From the analysis on the tweets posted on different OSNs, we find that (1) users usually post tweets at the same or similar locations, such as home, working places, POIs; (2) these tweets often also mention the same or similar locations. We can utilize the similarity of these locations to identify users. Each location can be specified by geographic latitude and longitude. The similarity of two locations can be represented by their Euclidean distance. For a user on one OSN, we can extract some locations from his public tweets and obtain a set of locations. For a pair of users(v_i^1, v_k^2), we compute the similarities between two sets of locations, and obtain a location similarity matrix $P_{ik}^l = \{p_{mn}\}$, where p_{mn} denotes the Euclidean distance between the mth location of user v_i^1 and the nth location of user v_k^2. We propose to use the Euclidean Distance Distribution of $P_{ik}^l(Euc2D)$ to evaluate the spatial similarity between user v_i^1 and user v_k^2.

Temporal Features. As said in [22], an individual usually post public tweets on different OSNs at similar time slots. Such temporal distribution indicates the user's online activity patterns. For example, some users like to post tweets at night, while other users publish tweets on the way to work. Such users' online patterns are very helpful for user identification. For each user, we can extract the posting time from his public tweets and obtain a sequence of posting time. The similarity of posting time can be represented as the difference in time. Similar to spatial feature, for a pair of users (v_i^1, v_k^2), we can compute the difference between two sequences of time, and get a time similarity matrix $P_{ik}^t = \{p_{mn}\}$, where p_{mn} denotes the difference in the mth posting time of user v_i^1 and the nth time of user v_k^2.Considering the difference in users' online behavior patterns, we compute the time similarity in two different granularities: date and time, and get two corresponding matrices P_{ik}^{t1} and P_{ik}^{t2}. We extract the time difference distribution from P_{ik}^{t1} and P_{ik}^{t2} (DateD and TimeD) to represent the temporal features.

Content Features. We notice that an individual often posts the tweets of similar or same content in different OSNs. This indicates that users usually publish his offline behaviors on multiple different OSNs. These tweets contain many of the same words or synonyms. The similarity of tweet content can be represented by the semantic similarity of content or the number of common words. The tweet content can also help to identify users. Similarly, for a pair of users (v_i^1, v_k^2), we can compute the similarity of two tweets, and get a content similarity matrix $P_{ik}^w = \{p_{mn}\}$. We remove the stop words from tweet, and convert it into a bag-of-words vector. We compute five kinds of similarities: (1) Jaccard coefficient(JacD); (2) the longest common subse-quence(LcsD); (3) the cosine similarity of the two average weight vectors (AwvD); (4) the cosine similarity of the two TFIDF-based weight vectors(TfidfD); (5) the cosine similarity of the two part-of-speech-based weight vectors (PoSD).

Base Classifier Construction. On information dimension $r \in \{l, t, w\}$, we train n base classifier $f_s^r(\cdot)(1 \le s \le n)$ with a set of training data $\{X_{ik}^r, y_{ik}\}$. Based on these base classifiers, for a pair of users (v_i^1, v_k^2) and the feature vector X_{ik}^r, we can obtain n confidence score $p_{sr} = f_s^r(X_{ik}^r)(1 \le s \le n)$ for user v_i^1 and user v_k^2

belonging to the same user. In practice, the number of unidentified user pairs is much larger than the number of identified users. In these unidentified users, there are also plenty of information redundancies for improving the performance of base classifiers. Following the idea of co-training, we re-train the base classifiers with identified users and unidentified users. After training the base classifiers with identified users, we employ them to identify user pairs on unidentified users. Based on the voting method, we select the unidentified user pairs that more than half of base classifiers agree on the identification result, and put them into training set. We conduct the training process iteratively until convergence. The re-training process is marking out by the (color) dotted line as shown in Fig. 2. The purpose for building n base classifiers is expected to improve identification performance with respect to both accuracy and generalization.

Fusion Classifier Construction. In framework of T-UIM, we design two level fusion classifiers. On information dimension $r \in \{l, t, w\}$, we design the fusion classifier $g_r(\cdot)$ to fusion the classification results of n base classifiers. If a base classifier $f_s^r(\cdot)$ outperforms other base classifiers on dimension r, we take $f_s^r(\cdot)$ as the fusion classifier $g_r(\cdot)$. Otherwise, suppose the classification results of n base classifiers are $\{f_s^r(X_{ik}^r), 1 \leq s \leq n\}$. We train the classifier $g_r(\cdot)$ with a set of data $\{\{f_s^r(X_{ik}^r), 1 \leq s \leq n\}, y_{ik}\}$. Then we use the 2nd level fusion classifier $g'(\cdot)$ to fusion the classification results of $g_l(\cdot)$, $g_t(\cdot)$, $g_w(\cdot)$. The purpose for designing the fusion classifiers is expected to overcome the defect in single base classifier or single information dimension, and generalize the tweet-based user identification.

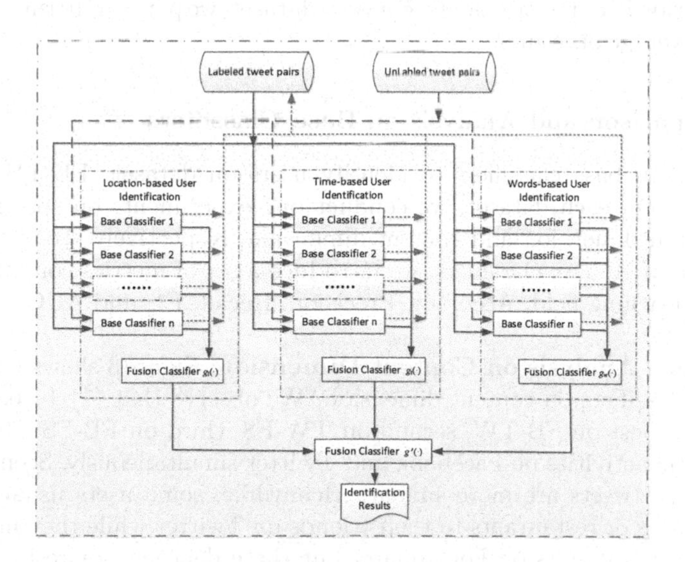

Fig. 2. Framework of T-UIM

5 Experiments and Analysis

Some OSN sites provide the cross-site linking function, such as Foursquare, Google+. Take Foursquare for instance. A user is allowed to make his Facebook and/or Twitter accounts public on his profile page. When a Foursquare user links his profile to his accounts of Facebook and/or Twitter, he should authorize Foursquare to access his Facebook and/or Twitter account. Only after Foursquare verifies the ownership, the user could formally link his public profile to Facebook and/or Twitter account. It is credible to use this method to obtain the ground truth data of a user on different OSN sites. Based on the cross-site function, we could obtain the ground truth data from Facebook, Twitter and Foursquare sites.

Based on the obtain data, we can construct three datasets that only contain positive instances. Three datasets are named as FB-FS, FS-TW and FB-TW, respectively. FS, FB and TW are abbreviations of Foursquare, Facebook and Twitter, respectively. In order to improve the performance of classifiers, we add as many negative instances as positive instances to these three datasets.

We select ten classifiers including Bagging(Bag), Multinomial Nave Bayes(MNB), Gaussian Nave Bayes(GNB), Logistic Regression(LR), Logistic Regression with builtin Cross-Validation(LRCV), Support Vector Machine (SVM), Decision Tree(DT), Random Forest(RF), GraBoosting(GraB), AdaBoost (AdaB) as base classifiers. The ten base classifiers could be implemented by scikit-learn[1]. All parameters of these classifiers are default values. We perform the 10-fold cross-validation in our experiments. For each dataset, we perform 10 runs, and then report the average of results.

5.1 Comparison and Analysis on Base Classifiers

We first use 10 base classifiers to identify users on datasets FB-TW, FB-FS, and TW-FS. On each dataset, we conduct our experiments on spatial dimension, temporal dimension and content dimension, respectively. To evaluate the performance of 10 base classifiers, we introduce a set of metrics commonly used in machine learning field: Accuracy, Precision, Recall, F1, and AUC.

Performance Analysis on Content Dimension. Figure 3 shows the metrics of 10 base classifiers on content dimension. We observe that (1) 10 base classifiers perform best on FB-TW, second on TW-FS, third on FB-FS. Users often post the same activities on Facebook and Twitter simultaneously. Seen from the content, these tweets are more similar. Meanwhile, some users usually recommend delicacies or restaurants to their friends on Twitter while they mark these delicacies or restaurants on Foursquare, but these delicacies or restaurants are often popular and also marked by other users. This causes a little confusion on identifying users. However, due to the different function between Facebook and Foursquare, users rarely simultaneously share the same activities on two sites.

[1] http://scikit-learn.org/stable/.

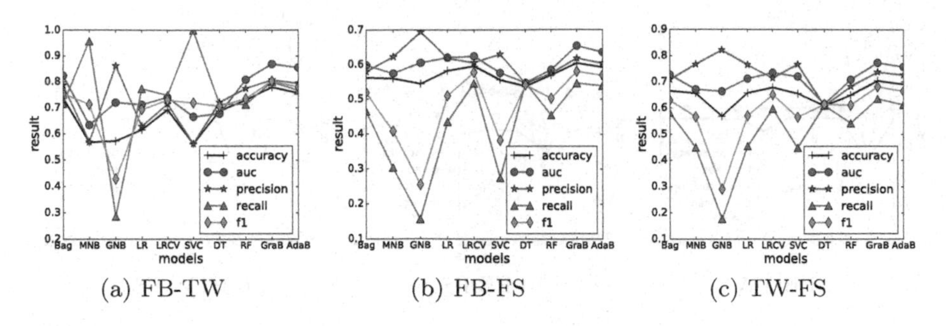

(a) FB-TW (b) FB-FS (c) TW-FS

Fig. 3. Metric comparison of 10 base classifiers on content dimension.

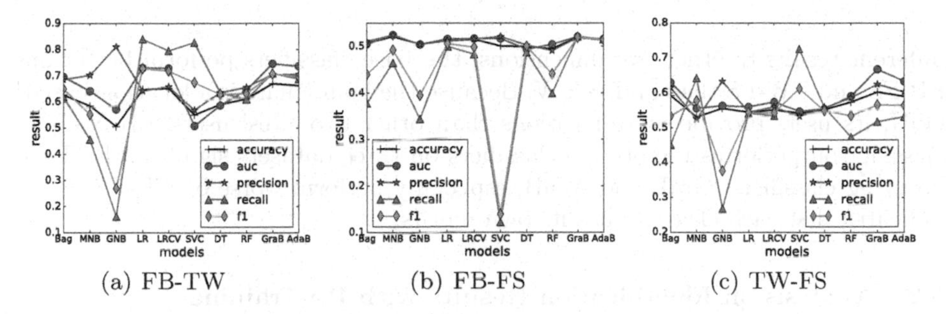

(a) FB-TW (b) FB-FS (c) TW-FS

Fig. 4. Metric comparison of 10 base classifiers on time dimension.

(2) No one base classifier significantly outperforms the other 9 classifiers on three datasets, but GNB significantly do worst on three datasets. For the other 9 classifiers, excluding GNB, each in his own way makes a contribution to identify user. Compared with other classifiers, GraB performs better on three datasets, mainly because GraB is a boosting classifier. (3) All F1 values of 10 classifiers are less than 0.8.

Performance Analysis on Temporal Dimension. Figure 4 shows the metrics of 10 base classifiers on posting time dimension. It illustrates that (1) all base classifiers also perform best on FB-TW, second on FS-TW, and third on FB-FS. The reason for results is same as the reason on content dimension. (2) Compared with results on content dimension, the classifiers perform badly on posting time dimension. At the same date or time, there are many users posting their activities on OSNs. This will lower the identification ability of posting time. (3) The performance of each base classifier on posting time is also not good enough. GraB is with comparatively better results.

Performance Analysis on Location Dimension. Figure 5 shows the metrics of 10 base classifiers on location dimension. We find that (1) 10 base classifiers perform better on location dimension than on other two dimensions. The AUC values are significantly better on location than on other two dimensions. This indicates the location attribute has better identification ability. (2) With the

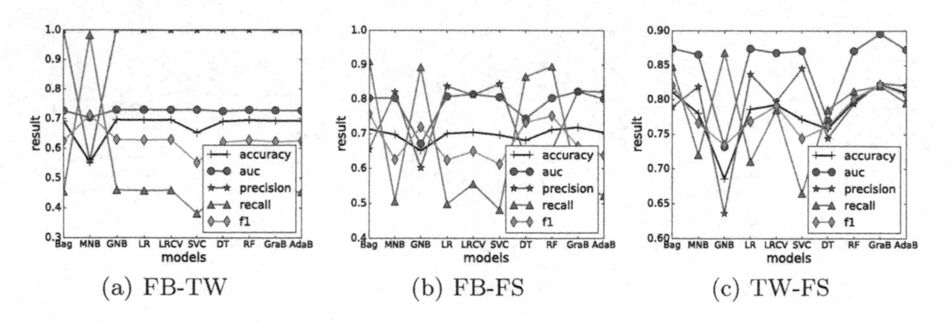

(a) FB-TW (b) FB-FS (c) TW-FS

Fig. 5. Metric comparison of 10 base classifiers on location dimension.

different results of other two dimensions, the base classifiers perform better on FB-FS and TW-FS than on FB-TW. Because the Foursquare is a location-based OSN, its users provide more locations than other two sites' users. (3) No one classifier outperforms the other 9 classifiers on three datasets significantly. Two boosting classifiers, GraB and AdaB, especially perform worse on FB-FS. This indicates that each classifier has its own merits.

5.2 Analysis on Identification Results with Re-Training

We illustrate the evaluation results of $g'(\cdot)$ after re-training in Table 1. $g'(\cdot) + RT$ represents the evaluation results of $g'(\cdot)$ after re-training. We find that the evaluation results of $g'(\cdot)$ after re-training are slightly better. This indicates that the re-training process is helpful for improving identification results, but its effect is not significant. One reason may be that the features come from the same view of training data. We will conduct our research on re-training the base classifiers across information dimensions in the future work.

Table 1. Evaluation results of $g'(\cdot)$ with re-training process

Dataset	Method	Acc.	Pre.	Rec.	F1
FB-TW	$g'(\cdot)$+RT	**0.8538**	**0.8767**	**0.8591**	**0.8678**
	$g'(\cdot)$	0.8463	0.8661	0.8574	0.8617
FB-FS	$g'(\cdot)$+RT	**0.8597**	**0.8466**	0.8808	**0.8624**
	$g'(\cdot)$	0.8010	0.7455	**0.9292**	0.8256
FS-TW	$g'(\cdot)$+RT	**0.8946**	0.8719	**0.9258**	**0.8979**
	$g'(\cdot)$	0.8663	**0.8787**	0.8485	0.8634

5.3 Comparison with Existing Works

To study the effectiveness of our method, we compare T-UIM with two existing works and their combination: MNA [22], CRMP [24] and MNA+CRMP. For each

Table 2. Evaluation results comparison on T-UIM and the existing works

Dataset	Method	Acc.	Pre.	Rec.	F1
FB-TW	MNA	0.7980	0.8277	0.8062	0.8168
	CRMP	0.6228	0.6820	0.6082	0.6430
	MNA+CRMP	0.8055	0.8323	0.8163	0.8242
	T-UIM	**0.8538**	**0.8767**	**0.8591**	**0.8678**
FB-FS	MNA	0.7418	0.7421	0.7415	0.7415
	CRMP	0.6997	0.7002	0.7665	0.7046
	MNA+CRMP	0.7530	0.7507	0.7583	0.7544
	T-UIM	**0.8597**	**0.8466**	**0.8808**	**0.8624**
FS-TW	MNA	0.8210	0.8202	0.8228	0.8213
	CRMP	0.7453	0.7677	0.7048	0.7345
	MNA+CRMP	0.8484	0.8449	0.8540	0.8493
	T-UIM	**0.8946**	**0.8719**	**0.9258**	**0.8979**

classifier and dataset, we also perform the 10-fold cross-validation. The results are illustrated in Table 2. We find that our method is capable to achieve the best accuracy, recall, precision and F1 on three datasets. This indicates that these suitable features we selected are capable to identify user across OSNs effectively. Besides, it is also shown that MNA and CRMP achieve good performance on three datasets. The combination of MNA and CRMP outperforms better than MNA and CRMP. Three baseline methods perform worse on FB-FS than on other two datasets.

6 Conclusion

In this study we have formalized and studied the problem of user identification across OSNs. As a key and inseparable part of OSN, the tweets posted across OSNs by the same individual usually contain rich information redundancies. This makes the tweet-based user identification possible. Therefore, we proposed a cascaded three-level machine learning-based user identification solution. We developed several algorithms to measure the similarity of tweets on spatial dimension, temporal dimensions and content dimensions. Finally, we verified our solution on three ground truth networks. The results show that our solution can provide excellent performance. Our algorithm could be applied jointly with other profile-based or friendship-based algorithms. The integration of these algorithms is helpful for more accurate identification results.

References

1. Global Social Media Ranking (2017). https://www.statista.com/statistics/272014/global-social-networks-ranked-by-number-of-users/

2. Zhou, X.P., Liang, X., Zhang, H.Y., et al.: Cross-platform identification of anonymous identical users in multiple social media networks. IEEE Trans. Knowl. Data Eng. **28**(2), 411–424 (2016)
3. Liu, J., Zhang, F., Song, X.Y., et al.: What's in a name?: an unsupervised approach to link users across communities. In: Proceedings of the Sixth ACM International Conference on Web Search and Data Mining, pp. 495–504 (2013)
4. Zafarani, R., Liu, H.: Connecting users across social media sites: a behavioral-modeling approach. In: Proceedings of the 19th ACM SIGKDD International Conference on Knowledge Discovery and Data Mining, pp. 41–49 (2013)
5. Iofciu, T., Fankhauser, P., Abel, F., et al.: Identifying users across social tagging systems. In: Proceedings of 5th International AAAI Conference on Weblogs and Social Media, pp. 522–525 (2011)
6. Motoyama, M., Varghese, G.: I seek you: searching and matching individuals in social networks. In: Proceedings of 7th International Workshop on Web Information and Data Management, pp. 67–75 (2009)
7. Abel, F., Herder, E., Houben, G.-J., et al.: Cross-system user modeling and personalization on the social web. User Model. User Adapt. Interact. **23**(2), 169–209 (2013)
8. Raad, E., Dipanda, A., Chbeir, R.: User profile matching in social networks. In: Proceedings of 16th International Conference on Network-Based Information Systems, pp. 297–304 (2010)
9. Vosecky, J., Hong, D., Shen, V.Y.: User identification across multiple social networks. In: Proceedings of 1st International Conferences on Networked Digital Technologies, pp. 360–365 (2009)
10. Jain, P., Kumaraguru, P., Joshi, A.: @ i seek 'fb. me': identifying users across multiple online social networks. In: Proceedings of the 22nd International Conference on World Wide Web Companion, pp. 1259–1268 (2013)
11. Vosecky, J., Hong, D., Shen, V.Y.: User identification across social networks using the web profile and friend network. Int. J. Web Appl. **2**(1), 23–34 (2010)
12. Buccafurri, F., Lax, G., Nocera, A., Ursino, D.: Discovering links among social networks. In: Flach, P.A., Bie, T., Cristianini, N. (eds.) ECML PKDD 2012. LNCS (LNAI), vol. 7524, pp. 467–482. Springer, Heidelberg (2012). doi:10.1007/978-3-642-33486-3_30
13. Tan, S., Guan, Z.Y., Cai, D., et al.: Mapping users across networks by manifold alignment on hypergraph. In: Proceedings of 28th AAAI Conference on Artificial Intelligence, pp. 159–165 (2014)
14. You, G.-W., Hwang, S.-W., Nie, Z.Q., et al.: SocialSearch: enhancing entity search with social network matching. In: Proceedings of the 14th International Conference on Extending Database Technology, pp. 515–519 (2011)
15. Goga, O.: Matching user accounts across online social networks: methods and applications. Ph.D. Dissertation, Universite Pierre etmarie curie – Pairs 6, Franch (2014)
16. Vesdapunt, N., Hector, G.-M.: Identifying users in social networks with limited information. In: Proceedings of the IEEE 31st International Conference on Data Engineering, pp. 627–638 (2015)
17. Huang, S.R., Zhang, J., Lu, S.Y., et al.: Social friend recommendation based on network correlation and feature co-clustering. In: Proceedings of the 5th ACM on International Conference on Multimedia Retrieval, pp. 315–322 (2015)
18. Zafarani, R., Tang, L., Liu, H.: User identification across social media. ACM Trans. Knowl. Discov. Data **10**(2), 1–30 (2015)
19. Shmatikov, V., Narayanan, A.: De-anonymizing social networks. In: Proceedings of IEEE Symposium on Security and Privacy, pp. 173–187 (2009)

20. Bartunov, S., Korshunov, A., Park, S.-T., et al.: Joint link-attribute user identity resolution in online social networks. In: Proceedings of 6th SNA-KDD Workshop (2012)
21. Korula, N., Lattanzi, S.: An efficient reconciliation algorithm for social networks. Proc. VLDB Endow. **7**(5), 377–388 (2013)
22. Kong, X.N., Zhang, J.W., Yu, P.-S.: Inferring anchor links across multiple heterogeneous social networks. In: Proceedings of the 22nd ACM International Conference on Information & Knowledge Management, pp. 179–188 (2013)
23. Goga, O., Lei, H., Hari, S., et al.: Exploiting innocuous activity for correlating users across sites. In Proceedings of the 22nd International Conference on World Wide Web, pp. 447–458 (2013)
24. Sajadmanesh, S., Rabiee, H.R., Khodadadi, A.: Predicting anchor links between heterogeneous social networks. In: Proceedings of 2016 IEEE/ACM International Conference on Advances in Social Networks Analysis and Mining, pp. 158–163 (2016)
25. Zhang, J.W., Kong, X.N., Yu, P.-S.: Predicting social links for new users across aligned heterogeneous social networks. In: Proceedings of IEEE 13th International Conference on Data Mining, pp. 1289–1294 (2013)
26. Jain, P., Kumaraguru, P.: Finding nemo: searching and resolving identities of users across online social networks. arXiv preprint 2012. arxiv:1212.6147
27. Perito, D., Castelluccia, C., Kaafar, M., et al.: How unique and traceable are usernames? In: Proceedings of 11th International Conference on Privacy Enhancing Technologies, pp. 1–17 (2011)
28. Jiang, X., Wei, S.K., Zhao, R.Z., et al.: Camera fingerprint: a new perspective for identifying user's identity. arXiv preprint arxiv: 1610.07728 (2016)
29. Liu, D., Wu, Q.Y., Han, W.H.: User identification across multiple websites based on usern-ame features. Chin. J. Comput. **38**(10), 2028–2040 (2015)
30. Bennacer, N., Nana Jipmo, C., Penta, A., Quercini, G.: Matching user profiles across social networks. In: Jarke, M., Mylopoulos, J., Quix, C., Rolland, C., Manolopoulos, Y., Mouratidis, H., Horkoff, J. (eds.) CAiSE 2014. LNCS, vol. 8484, pp. 424–438. Springer, Cham (2014). doi:10.1007/978-3-319-07881-6_29
31. Malhotra, A., Totti, L., Meira, W., et al.: Studying user footprints in different online social networks. In: Proceedings of the 2012 International Conference on Advances in Social Networks Analysis and Mining, pp. 1065–1070 (2012)
32. Almishari, M., Tsudik, G.: Exploring linkability of user reviews. In: Foresti, S., Yung, M., Martinelli, F. (eds.) ESORICS 2012. LNCS, vol. 7459, pp. 307–324. Springer, Heidelberg (2012). doi:10.1007/978-3-642-33167-1_18

Machine Learning

Supervised Feature Selection Algorithm Based on Low-Rank and Manifold Learning

Yue Fang[1,2], Jilian Zhang[3], Shichao Zhang[1,2(✉)], Cong Lei[1,2], and Xiaoyi Hu[1,2]

[1] Guangxi Key Lab of Multi-source Information Mining and Security, Guilin 541004, China
zhangsc@gxnu.edu.cn

[2] College of CS and IT,Guangxi Normal University, Guilin 541004, China

[3] College of Cyber Security, Jinan University, Guangzhou 510632, China

Abstract. In this paper we show that manifold learning could effectively find the essential dimension of nonlinear high-dimensional data, but it could not use class label information of the data because it is an unsupervised learning method. This paper explores a novel supervised feature selection algorithm based on low-rank and manifold learning. Specifically, we obtain the coefficient matrix according to the relationship between data and class label. Then we combine sparse learning and manifold learning to conduct feature selection. Finally, we use the low-rank representation to further adjust the result of feature selection. Experimental results show that our new method obtains the best results on the four public datasets when compared with six existing methods.

Keywords: Manifold learning · Low-rank representation · Sparse learning · Supervised feature selection

1 Introduction

With the advancement of Internet technology, high-dimensional data are increasing rapidly, such as biological gene sequence data, text data, face images, medical image data and climate data [15,23,25]. Analysis and processing of these large-scale and high-dimensional data is a great challenge. Therefore, dimensionality reduction is necessary to cut down the storage and computational overhead for high-dimensional image data [8,22,24].

Dimensionality reduction methods fall into two categories [24,27] (i.e., one is feature selection, the other is subspace learning). The essence of the two methods is to find key information from the high-dimensional data, so as to enhance the performance of machine learning algorithm for high-dimensional data. Feature selection is to remove irrelevant or redundant features from the original feature set, and select a subset of features so that the feature space is optimally reduced according to some determined criteria. Existing feature selection methods are mainly divided into three categories: wrappers methods [16], filters methods [11] and embedded methods [14]. Feature selection methods select a few and representative features,without considering the manifold structure of the data [9].

G. Cong et al. (Eds.): ADMA 2017, LNAI 10604, pp. 273–286, 2017.
https://doi.org/10.1007/978-3-319-69179-4_19

In contrast, subspace learning takes the local or global structure of the data into account [21]. Common subspace learning techniques include Linear Discriminant Analysis (LDA) [10], Local Discriminant Embedding (LDE) [2] and Locality Preserving Projection (LPP) [6]. Recently, Zhu et al. utilized two subspace learning methods, namely, LDA and LPP, to consider both the local and global information of the data. However, using subspace learning alone will lose the additional information of the data, such as class labels. Inspired by the above research, this paper combines manifold learning method and low rank to conduct supervised feature selection to achieve better performance.

This paper proposes a new Supervised Feature Selection Algorithm Based on Low-Rank and Manifold Learning (HEL_FS for short) algorithm, to overcome the above limitations. We first perform a sparse learning ($\ell_{2,1}-$norm regularizer and an $\ell_{2,p}-$norm regularizer) on the coefficient matrix, to capture more important features. Then, we embed LPP and hypergraph Laplacian regularization term into the unified feature selection model, so as to utilize the manifold (local and global) structure of the data. The hypergraph regularization term can keep the stability of local structure data in the low-dimensional space. Then we use low-rank on weight matrix to explore the global structure among different features.

The main contributions of the paper include:

- HEL_FS algorithm considers data sparsity for feature selection via utilizing the double sparse expressing norm, that is, using $\ell_{2,1}-$norm and $\ell_{2,p}-$norm to select significant samples for loss function and punish the coefficient matrix, respectively. The more spare the coefficient matrix, the more important the selected features.
- We use subspace learning methods, that is, use hypergraph regularization term and low-rank constraint to explore the local and global structures of the data, respectively. Then, we embed the classical subspace learning method (*e.g.*, LDA) into feature selection framework to generate a stable feature selection model.
- HEL_FS algorithm embeds manifold learning into the supervised learning framework, improving the classification accuracy for high dimensional data, and achieving better performance.

The paper is organized as follows. In Sect. 2, we give detailed description of our proposed feature selection method via using low rank and its corresponding optimization method. After that, we present our experiment results in Sect. 3. Finally, we conclude the paper and give our future work in Sect. 4.

2 Our Approach

In this section, we give some notations in Table 1 and explain the details of the proposed method HEL_FS in Sect. 2.1, and then we give the optimization algorithm in Sect. 2.2.

Table 1. Notation

Symbols	Description
$\mathbf{X}$	The feature matrix of a data set
$\mathbf{x}$	A vector of $\mathbf{X}$
$\mathbf{x}^i$	The i-th row of $\mathbf{X}$
$\mathbf{x}_j$	The j-th column of $\mathbf{X}$
x_{ij}	The element in the i-th row and the j-th column of $\mathbf{X}$
$\lVert\mathbf{X}\rVert_{2,1}$	The $\ell_{2,1}$-norm of $\lVert\mathbf{X}\rVert_{2,1} = \sum_{i=1}^{n}\sqrt{\sum_{j=1}^{d} x_{ij}^2}$
$\lVert\mathbf{X}\rVert_{2,p}$	The $\ell_{2,p}$-norm of $\lVert\mathbf{X}\rVert_{2,p} = (\sum_{i=1}^{n}(\sum_{j=1}^{d} x_{ij}^2)^{p/2})^{1/p}$
$rank(\mathbf{X})$	The rank of $\mathbf{X}$
$\mathbf{X}^T$	The transpose of $\mathbf{X}$
$\mathrm{tr}(\mathbf{X})$	The trace of $\mathbf{X}$
$\mathbf{X}^{-1}$	The inverse of $\mathbf{X}$

2.1 The HEL_FS Algorithm

Given a sample matrix $\mathbf{X} \in \mathbb{R}^{n\times d}$ and a label matrix $\mathbf{Y} \in \mathbb{R}^{n\times c}$, where n, d and c are the number of training samples, features, and classes, respectively. Let $\mathbf{x}^1, \mathbf{x}^2, ..., \mathbf{x}^n$ be n samples, where $\mathbf{x}^i \in \mathbb{R}^{1\times d}$ and $\mathbf{X} = [\mathbf{x}^1; \mathbf{x}^2; ...; \mathbf{x}^n]$.

Some methods [18] always construct the sample similarity matrix at first, then utilize a response matrix $\mathbf{Y} = [\mathbf{y}_1, \mathbf{y}_2, ..., \mathbf{y}_c]$ obtained through class label information. Thus, the classic supervised feature selection problem is written as follows:

$$\min_{\mathbf{Z}} l(\mathbf{Y} - \mathbf{XZ}) + \alpha R(\mathbf{Z}) \tag{1}$$

Where $\mathbf{Z} \in \mathbb{R}^{d\times c}$ is the coefficient matrix for the d features and c classes, $l(\mathbf{Y} - \mathbf{XZ})$ is the loss function, $R(\mathbf{Z})$ is a regularization term on $\mathbf{Z}$ and α is regularization parameter. According to the previous literature [26], $l(\mathbf{Y} - \mathbf{XZ})$ is used to obtain the relevant minimum fitting error that reflects the deviation between the response label $\mathbf{Y}$ and the predicted term $\mathbf{XZ}$. Therefore, we can use the Frobenius norm on coefficient matrix and response matrix to build the initial model as follows:

$$\min_{\mathbf{Z}} \lVert\mathbf{Y} - \mathbf{XZ}\rVert_F^2 + \alpha\lVert\mathbf{Z}\rVert_F^2 \tag{2}$$

Equation (2) is a convex function and its function graph is smooth, so it can be easily optimized, and the ideal coefficient matrix $\mathbf{Z}$ can be solved by $\mathbf{Z}^* = \left(\mathbf{X}^T\mathbf{X} + \alpha\mathbf{I}\right)^{-1}\mathbf{X}^T\mathbf{Y}$, where the $\mathbf{I} \in \mathbb{R}^{d\times d}$ is a unitary matrix. Since data matrix $\mathbf{X}$ always contains outlier samples that influence the performance of classification, the Frobenius norm is unable to remove outliers for loss function and to punish coefficient matrix for regularization term. Thus, we use an $\ell_{2,1}-$norm and an $\ell_{2,p}-$norm regularizers to select significant samples (i.e., removing the useless samples from the model) for loss function and punish the coefficient matrix (i.e., using a sparsity constraint) on the regularization term, respectively. Meanwhile, in our model we employ the representative LPP based on hypergraph to increase the generalized ability of our model as shown in Eq. (2). And then we define the objective function as follows:

$$\min_{\mathbf{Z}} ||\mathbf{Y} - \mathbf{XZ}||_{2,1} + \alpha||\mathbf{Z}||_{2,p} + \beta tr(\mathbf{Z}^T\mathbf{X}\mathbf{L}_H\mathbf{X}^T\mathbf{Z}) \tag{3}$$

The parameters of α and β can be tuned in a specific range. The $\ell_{2,p}-$norm regularizer $||\mathbf{Z}||_{2,p}$ penalizes coefficient matrix $\mathbf{Z}$, the coefficient matrix can be more sparse (i.e., selecting or un-selecting in predicting the feature matrix $\mathbf{X}$) by tuning the parameter p, where p is in the range of 0 to 2, and decides related structure among features. And $\mathbf{L}_H$ is a normalized hypergraph Laplacian matrix which can be constructed via the method in [5].

However, the coefficient matrix $\mathbf{Z}$ in Eq. (3) does not take advantage of correlated structure among the label matrix. To address this issue, we explore the correlated structure by introducing one low-rank constraint on $\mathbf{Z}$ [17], that is,

$$rank(\mathbf{Z}) = r \leq \min(n, c) \tag{4}$$

In real applications, samples or features have some latent correlations, and outliers of samples or redundancy of features usually make the rank increased. Thus, the low rank constraint on Eq. (4) can easily explore low-dimensional and latent structures in original and complex data [13]. We use the two r-rank matrices to explore the low rank on $\mathbf{Z}$. Hence Eq. (4) can be rewritten as:

$$\mathbf{Z} = \mathbf{AB} \tag{5}$$

Where $\mathbf{A} \in \mathbb{R}^{d\times r}$ and $\mathbf{B} \in \mathbb{R}^{r\times c}$. Then, the final objective function is written as:

$$\begin{aligned} \min_{\mathbf{A},\mathbf{B}} ||\mathbf{Y} - \mathbf{XAB}||_{2,1} + \alpha||\mathbf{AB}||_{2,p} + \beta tr(\mathbf{B}^T\mathbf{A}^T\mathbf{X}\mathbf{L}_H\mathbf{X}^T\mathbf{AB}) \\ s.t., rank(\mathbf{AB}) \leq \min(n, c) \end{aligned} \tag{6}$$

Where $\mathbf{X} \in \mathbb{R}^{n\times d}$ and $\mathbf{Y} \in \mathbb{R}^{n\times c}$, respectively, represent the feature matrix and the label matrix, $\mathbf{A} \in \mathbb{R}^{d\times r}$ and $\mathbf{B} \in \mathbb{R}^{r\times c}$ are coefficient matrices, α, β and p are parameters. We describe our algorithm as follows.

First, Eq. (6) applies an $\ell_{2,1}-$norm and an $\ell_{2,p}-$norm regularizers to yield sparse results, moreover, the $\ell_{2,1}-$norm regularization term is used to choose significant samples for penalty function and the $\ell_{2,p}-$norm regularization is utilized to punish the coefficient matrix, respectively. On the one hand, we use the $\ell_{2,1}-$norm penalty function to improve our model robust. Thus, each row of $(\mathbf{Y} - \mathbf{XAB})$ can be used for prediction. Using $\ell_{2,1}-$norm on the loss function, predicted values are less affected by the outliers. On the other hand, the $\ell_{2,p}-$norm regularization on $\mathbf{AB}$ is used to penalize $\mathbf{AB}$, thus most of the row elements in the coefficient matrix $\mathbf{AB}$ are changed to 0, the features corresponding to nonzero elements in $\mathbf{AB}$ are preserved. This is the feature selection process.

Second, we use the hypergraph Laplacian regularizer (i.e., $tr(\mathbf{B}^T\mathbf{A}^T\mathbf{X}\mathbf{L}_H\mathbf{X}^T\mathbf{A}\mathbf{B})$) to keep the local relationship between samples in the low-dimensional space, which actually conducts subspace learning, and low rank constraint on $\mathbf{Z}$ (i.e., $\mathbf{Z} = \mathbf{AB}$) is used to take advantage of global structures of the data for subspace learning as well. Thus, Eq. (6) utilizes low-rank constraint and sparse regularization simultaneously for subspace learning (i.e., LDA introduced in Eq. (11)) and feature selection, respectively.

Finally, we use the method for feature selection and subspace learning in a unified framework. Recently, feature selection can produce explainable result and subspace learning can output stable result [21]. In this way, our proposed method can output the optimal results.

2.2 Optimization

We give the details of solving our suggested function in Eq. (6). The $\ell_{2,1}$–norm and $\ell_{2,p}$–norm are used to remove the outlier samples and punish the coefficient matrix, respectively, the objective function is convex but not smooth, and it is hardly to solve directly in a closed form. Meanwhile, our suggested function is not convex since it has two variables (i.e., $\mathbf{A}$, $\mathbf{B}$) to be optimized. Thus, we use the optimizing framework proposed by Iteratively Reweighted Least Square (IRLS) [3] to iteratively optimize each parameter while fixing the other parameter until the algorithm converges. Specifically, when the predefined stopping criterion is satisfied, our procedure is terminated. The details of optimization consist of two steps: (1) Update $\mathbf{B}$ while fixing $\mathbf{A}$. (2) Update $\mathbf{A}$ while fixing $\mathbf{B}$.

According to the IRLS method, we use two diagonal matrices $\mathbf{D}$ and $\mathbf{Q}$ for brevity, their diagonal elements are written as follows:

$$d_{ii} = \frac{1}{2||u^i||_2^{\frac{1}{2}}} \quad s.t.,\ i = 1, 2, ..., n \tag{7}$$

$$q_{ii} = \frac{1}{(2/p)(||g^i||)_2^{2-p}} \quad s.t.,\ i = 1, 2, ..., d, 0 < p < 2 \tag{8}$$

where u^i and g^i, represent the i-th row of the matrix $\mathbf{U}^* = (\mathbf{Y} - \mathbf{X}\mathbf{A}^*\mathbf{B}^*)$ and $\mathbf{G}^* = \mathbf{A}^*\mathbf{B}^*$, respectively. $\mathbf{A}^*$and $\mathbf{B}^*$ are the optimal solution of $\mathbf{A}$ and $\mathbf{B}$, respectively. Therefore, the objective function in Eq. (6) is written as:

$$\begin{aligned}&\min_{\mathbf{A},\mathbf{B}} tr((\mathbf{Y} - \mathbf{XAB})^T\mathbf{D}(\mathbf{Y} - \mathbf{XAB})) + \\ &\alpha tr(\mathbf{B}^T\mathbf{A}^T\mathbf{QAB}) + \beta tr(\mathbf{B}^T\mathbf{A}^T\mathbf{X}\mathbf{L}_H\mathbf{X}^T\mathbf{AB})\end{aligned} \tag{9}$$

We utilize IRLS method to solve our objective function, and iteratively optimize each of the parameters while fixing the rest.

Let $J(\mathbf{AB})$ represent Eq. (9), and let its derivative about $\mathbf{B}$ to zero, we have:

$$\begin{aligned}&\tfrac{\partial J(\mathbf{A},\mathbf{B})}{\partial \mathbf{B}} = -2\mathbf{A}^T\mathbf{X}^T\mathbf{DY} + 2\mathbf{A}^T\mathbf{X}^T\mathbf{DXAB} \\ &+2\alpha\mathbf{A}^T\mathbf{QAB} + 2\beta\mathbf{A}^T\mathbf{X}^T\mathbf{L}_H\mathbf{XAB} = \mathbf{0}\end{aligned} \tag{10}$$

Then, we use **A** to represent **B**, Eq. (10) becomes:

$$\mathbf{B} = (\mathbf{A}^T(\mathbf{X}^T\mathbf{D}\mathbf{X} + \alpha\mathbf{Q} + \beta\mathbf{X}^T\mathbf{L}_H\mathbf{X})\mathbf{A})^{-1}\mathbf{A}^T\mathbf{X}^T\mathbf{D}\mathbf{Y} \tag{11}$$

The optimization of **B** can conduct LDA learning result. However, in Eq. (11), the matrices **D**, **Q** and **A** are both unknown, thus the variable of **B** cannot be directly optimized. We iteratively update above steps until our procedure terminated when the stopping condition is reached. Thus, we optimize **A** by substituting Eq. (11) into Eq. (9), we get the following:

$$\max_{\mathbf{A}} tr((\mathbf{A}^T(\mathbf{X}^T\mathbf{D}\mathbf{X} + \alpha\mathbf{Q} + \beta\mathbf{X}^T\mathbf{L}_H\mathbf{X})\mathbf{A})^{-1}\mathbf{A}^T\mathbf{X}^T\mathbf{D}\mathbf{Y}\mathbf{Y}^T\mathbf{D}^T\mathbf{X}\mathbf{A}) \tag{12}$$

It is worth noting that:

$$\mathbf{S}_t = \mathbf{X}^T + \alpha\mathbf{Q} + \beta\mathbf{X}^T\mathbf{L}_H\mathbf{X},\ \ \mathbf{S}_b = \mathbf{X}^T\mathbf{D}\mathbf{Y}\mathbf{Y}^T\mathbf{D}^T\mathbf{X} \tag{13}$$

Where $\mathbf{S}_t$ and $\mathbf{S}_b$ are the between-class and total-class scatter matrices of data in the LDA subspace, respectively. Equation (12) only obtains one unknown variable **A**, therefore, the solution of Eq. (12) is

$$\mathbf{A} = \arg\max_{\mathbf{A}}\{tr((\mathbf{A}^T\mathbf{S}_t\mathbf{A})^{-1}\mathbf{A}^T\mathbf{S}_b\mathbf{A})\} \tag{14}$$

Therefore, the problem of LDA can be solved exactly by Eq. (14), and the top $\underline{r}$ eigenvectors corresponding to $\underline{r}$ nonzero eigenvalues of ${\mathbf{S}_t}^{-1}\mathbf{S}_b$ is the global optimal solution. We can use this strategy to yield **A** by solving Eq. (14) and then yield **B** by Eq. (11). We list the details of optimizing **A** and **B** in Algorithm 1.

Algorithm 1: The approach to solve **A** and **B**.

Input: Data matrix $\mathbf{X} \in \mathbb{R}^{n\times d}$, Label matrix $\mathbf{Y} \in \mathbb{R}^{n\times c}$, α, β and p;
Output: $\mathbf{A} \in \mathbb{R}^{d\times r}$ and $\mathbf{B} \in \mathbb{R}^{r\times c}$;

1 Initial $\underline{t}$=0;
2 Initial randomly the matrix $\mathbf{A}(0)$ and $\mathbf{B}(0)$;
3 Initial $\mathbf{D}(t) = \mathbf{I} \in \mathbb{R}^{n\times n}$;
4 Initial $\mathbf{Q}(t) = \mathbf{I} \in \mathbb{R}^{d\times d}$;
5 **repeat**
6 | Update $\mathbf{A}(t+1)$ by solving Eqn (14);
7 | Update $\mathbf{B}(t+1)$ by solving Eqn (11);
8 | Update $\mathbf{Q}(t+1)$ by calculating Eqn (8);
9 | Update $\mathbf{D}(t+1)$ by calculating Eqn (7);
10 **until** The difference between two iterative target values cannot exceed 10^{-5}.;

---

3 Experiments

We compare our HEL_FS method with six existing methods. It is worth noting that we first transform large and high-dimensional data into low-dimensional data by using dimensionality reduction methods, and then use LIBSVM toolbox[1] to classify the transformed data.

3.1 Experimental Setting

We compare our algorithm with six existing methods on four publicly available datasets. Specifically, dataset Chess, ALLAML, Yale and ORL can be downloaded from the UCI Machine Learning Repository[2] and the Feature Selection Datasets can be found on the Web[3]. We give statistics of the datasets in Table 2.

We use FSSI, FSASL, CSFS, FRFS0, RSR and JELSR algorithms as our competitors in our experiments, and we summarize these algorithms below.

FSSI: (Feature Selection Sharing Information) [12] assumes that different feature selection tasks were similar, and uses $F-$norm regularization and $\ell_{2,1}-$norm regularization for the loss function and coefficient matrix, respectively.

FSASL: (Feature Selection Adaptive Structure Learning) [4] uses structure learning and feature selection simultaneously. The structures are adaptively obtained from the results of selecting features. And moreover, the important features are obtained to keep the meaningful data structures.

CSFS: (Convex Semi-supervised Feature Selection) [1] combines feature selection with sparsity and semi-supervised learning into a single framework, and adopts the least square loss function to minimize the classification error.

FRFS0: (Non-convex Regularized Self-representation) [19] is a novel-convex regularized self-representation model that uses $\ell_{2,p}-$norm regularization and $\ell_{2,1}-$norm regularization to choose features and regularize the loss term, respectively, to guarantee the algorithm converged.

RSR: (Regularized self-representation) [20] chooses one of the most representative of the response matrix by self-expression method, and meanwhile, embeds a sparse learning into the model for selecting features. The value of element of

Table 2. The details of datasets for feature selection.

Datasets	Samples	Features	Classes	Types
ALLAML	72	7129	2	Biological
Chess	3196	36	2	Text
Yale	165	1024	15	Face image
ORL	400	1024	20	Face image

[1] http://www.csie.ntu.edu.tw/cjlin/libsvm/.
[2] http://archive.ics.uci.edu/ml/.
[3] http://featureselection.asu.edu/datasets.php.

coefficient matrix represents the strength of the corresponding attribute significance.

JESLR: (Joint Embedding Learning and Sparse Regression) [7] integrates the advantages of embedding learning and sparse regression, and uses the $\ell_{2,1}-$norm regularization and the local linear proximate weights to obtain a transfer matrix for feature selection.

In our experiments, we employ 10-fold cross-validation 10 times to select different types of samples. In other words, we split data into ten subsets randomly and select one of those sets as test data and the rest as training data. The final classification accuracy is averaged over the results of the 10 trials. Then, the 5-fold inner cross-validation is used to choose the best parameters c and g for the model selection by setting $\alpha, \beta \in \{10^{-3}, ..., 10^{3}\}$ and $c, g \in \{2^{-5}, ..., 2^{5}\}$ in SVM.

Three kinds of evaluation metrics are employed to assess the classification result of the competitors and our HEL_FS method. The evaluation metrics include classification accuracy, standard deviation, and coefficient of variation.

The classification ACCuracy (ACC) is defined as:

$$ACC = \frac{N_{correct}}{N} \tag{15}$$

Where N and $N_{correct}$ are the number of data samples and correct classified samples, respectively.

The Standard Deviation (STD) is defined as:

$$STD = \sqrt{\frac{1}{n_{run}} \sum_{i=1}^{N} (ACC_i - \mu)^2} \tag{16}$$

Where n_{run} is the number of the runs of experiments, i.e., $n_{run} = 10$ in our experiments, and μ is the value of average of ACC. A large ACC means good classification performance and a small STD suggests good running stability.

The Coefficient of Variation (CV) is also regarded as evaluation metric and it is defined as:

$$CV = \frac{STD}{ACC} \tag{17}$$

Where STD is the square root of an unbiased estimate of each sample, i.e., standard deviation. A small CV symbolizes good the precision and repeatability.

3.2 Experimental Results and Analysis

We show the average classification accuracy of our HEL_FS method and six competing methods in Table 3. The results of coefficient of variation of all methods are listed in Table 4. Also, we report the results of classification accuracy of each

Table 3. Classification accuracy (ACC ± STD (%)) for all datasets.

Datasets	FSSI	FSASL	CSFS	FRFS0	RSR	JELSR	HEL_FS
ALLAML	83.03 ± 3.93	82.14 ± 4.08	90.89 ± 3.61	87.50 ± 3.82	88.75 ± 2.92	79.28 ± 3.40	**91.42 ± 2.82**
Chess	87.70 ± 1.64	94.24 ± 1.10	89.70 ± 2.09	90.20 ± 1.24	90.50 ± 1.50	90.90 ± 1.95	**95.00 ± 1.10**
Yale	77.54 ± 2.95	70.51 ± 3.48	69.70 ± 3.02	69.89 ± 2.46	74.82 ± 3.25	70.29 ± 3.34	**81.14 ± 2.45**
ORL	94.50 ± 1.64	91.00 ± 2.15	90.50 ± 2.04	95.50 ± 2.00	87.75 ± 2.33	95.75 ± 1.66	**97.50 ± 1.64**
Average value	85.69 ± 2.54	84.47 ± 2.68	85.20 ± 2.69	85.77 ± 2.38	85.46 ± 2.50	84.06 ± 2.59	**91.27 ± 2.00**

Table 4. Coefficient of variation (%) for all datasets.

Datasets	FSSI	FSASL	CSFS	FRFS0	RSR	JELSR	HEL_FS
ALLAML	4.73	4.97	3.98	4.36	3.29	4.29	**3.08**
Chess	1.87	1.17	2.33	1.37	1.66	2.15	**1.15**
Yale	3.80	4.93	4.34	3.52	4.34	4.74	**3.02**
ORL	1.74	2.37	2.25	2.09	2.65	1.73	**1.68**
average value	3.03	3.36	3.22	2.84	2.99	3.23	**2.23**

fold in 10-fold cross-validation for all data sets in Fig. 1 to show the stability of each method. Figure 2 shows the convergence of our HEL_FS method on four data sets. Figure 3 represents the ACC results of the HEL_FS method at different number of ranks.

From Table 3, we see that the HEL_FS method obtains the best classification accuracy among all methods on most of the datasets. For example, the HEL_FS method increases by 5.50% on average, compared with the FRFS0 method, which obtains the best result among the comparison feature selection methods but does not use class label and not consider the local correlation between data. And, our method increases on average by 7.21%, compared with the JELSR algorithm which achieved the worse performance among the comparison feature selection methods. As well as, our proposed method achieves the minimum average standard deviation, compared with all the comparison methods for most of all datasets. This means that the HEL_FS method exhibits the best stability over all competing methods. In terms of the coefficient of variation in Table 4, the proposed method achieved the large coefficient variation on the datasets (such as ALLAML and Yale) and the small coefficient variation on the datasets (such as Chess and ORL), but it obtained smaller variation than all comparison methods. This verifies the fact that our method achieves the best stability.

Figure 2 shows the behavior of the proposed objective values of Algorithm 1 on four data sets to the increase of the iterations, where we set the stop criteria of Algorithm 1 as $\frac{\|obj(t+1)-obj(t)\|_2^2}{obj(t)} \leq 10^{-3}$, where $obj(t)$ represents the t-th iteration objective function value of Eq. (6). From Fig. 2, we can get the conclusion:

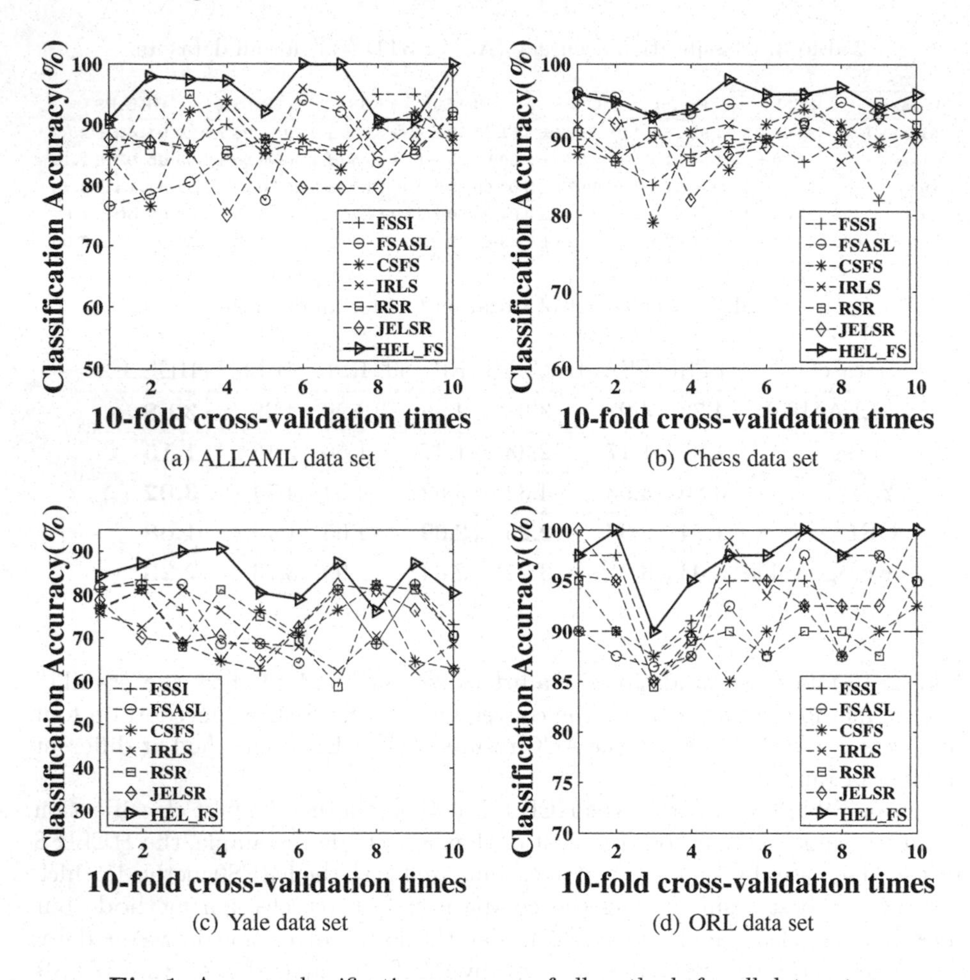

(a) ALLAML data set

(b) Chess data set

(c) Yale data set

(d) ORL data set

Fig. 1. Average classification accuracy of all methods for all data sets.

(1) the proposed Algorithm 1 to optimize the objective function listed in Eq. (6) monotonically decreases the objective function values until Algorithm 1 converges; (2) the proposed Algorithm 1 efficiently reaches to its convergence within 20 iterations.

We investigate the influence of the effect of different numbers of ranks (*i.e.*, $r \in \{1, 2, 3, 4, 5, 6, 7, 8, 9\}$) in Eq. (6) at different datasets, and reported the ACC results in Fig. 3, where the horizontal axis indicates the number of kept ranks, while the full rank of these datasets is 36, 18, 24 and 40, from (a) to (d), respectively. From Table 2, we know that the number of real classes in the binary datasets (such as ALLAML, Chess) is less than 9. Since real datasets always

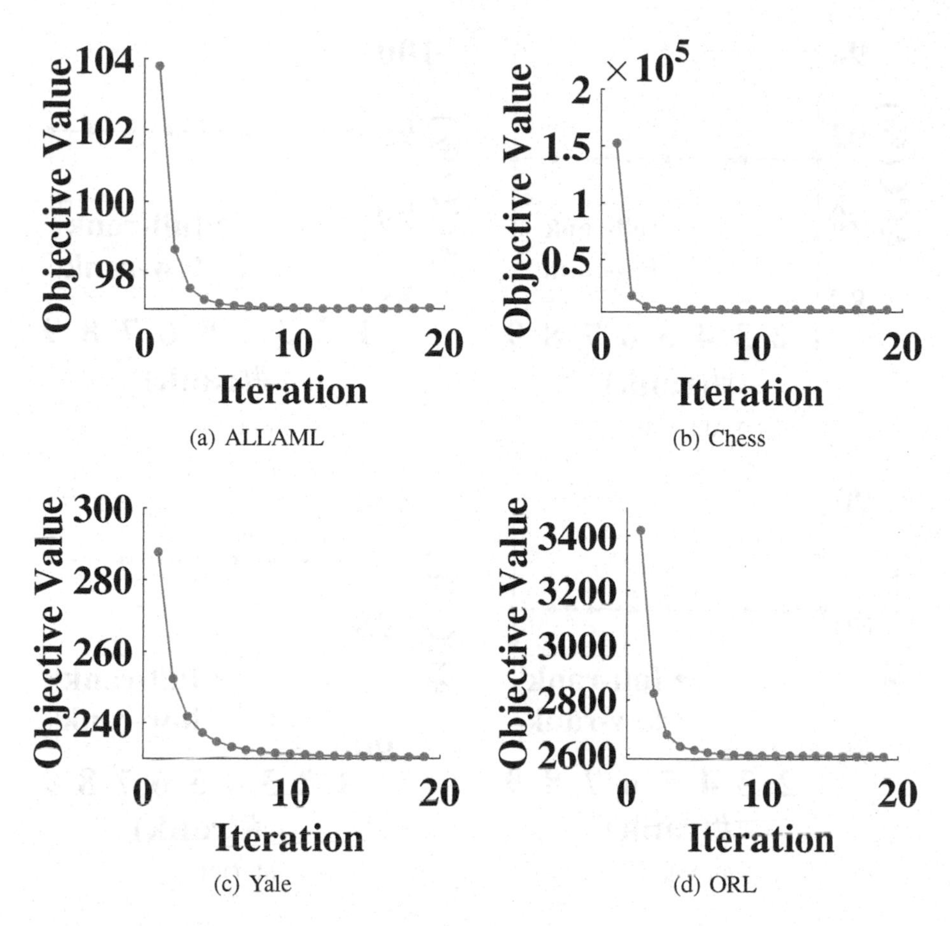

(a) ALLAML

(b) Chess

(c) Yale

(d) ORL

Fig. 2. The four data sets and their corresponding objective values of the proposed objective function with different iterations.

contain noise and redundancy, thus, we let the rank of their feature matrices to be 9 since the real rank of these corresponding datasets is large than 9.

From Fig. 3, we know that the classification accuracy with a low-rank constraint for the most part exceeded the classification accuracy of the full-rank. For instance, the average classification accuracy of the proposed method with low rank constraints increased by 0.96, 0.56, 0.97 and 0.67%, respectively, compared to the results of full-rank constraint on the datasets ALLAML, Chess, Yale and ORL. It is obvious that analyzing high-dimensional data with a low-rank constraint in feature selection is meaningful. Due to the fact that the low-rank constraint conducting subspace learning helps search the low-dimensional space of high-dimensional data by considering the global feature correlation.

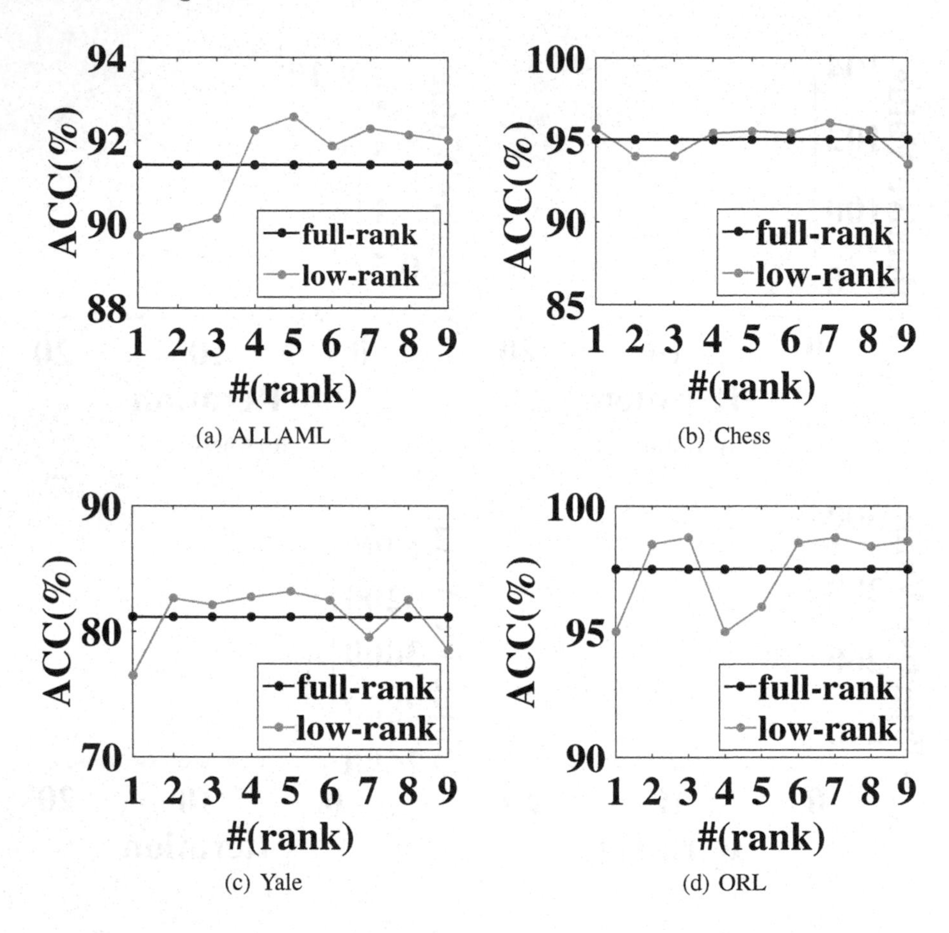

(a) ALLAML (b) Chess

(c) Yale (d) ORL

Fig. 3. ACC results of our proposed method at different number of ranks.

4 Conclusion

This paper proposed a comprehensive supervised spectral features selection method by combining feature selection with subspace learning simultaneously. Moreover, we use sparse learning to choose significant samples, then, utilize the low rank constraint, hypergraph expressing and LDA method to select more representative features. The HEL_FS method extends the use of subspace learning in classification applications, but also makes up for the deficiency of the low rank feature selection in maintaining the geometry structure of data. The results on the twelve datasets verified that the HEL_FS method achieved the best classification result, compared to the state-of-the-art feature selection methods in terms of three basic types of evaluation metric for both binary classification and multi-classification problems.

In the future, our will use semi-supervised feature selection method to extend our proposed framework on high-dimensional data with incomplete data since the labels are often hard to get in real applications.

Acknowledgments. This work was supported in part by the China Key Research Program (Grant No: 2016YFB1000905), the China 973 Program (Grant No: 2013CB329404), the China 1000-Plan National Distinguished Professorship, the Nation Natural Science Foundation of China (Grants No: 61573270, 61672177, and 61363009), the Guangxi Natural Science Foundation (Grant No: 2015GXNSFCB139011), the Guangxi High Institutions Program of Introducing 100 High-Level Overseas Talents, the Guangxi Collaborative Innovation Center of Multi-Source Information Integration and Intelligent Processing, the Research Fund of Guangxi Key Lab of MIMS (16-A-01-01 and 16-A-01-02), and the Guangxi Bagui Teams for Innovation and Research, and Innovation Project of Guangxi Graduate Education under grant YCSW2017065, XYCSZ2017064 and XYCSZ2017067.

References

1. Chang, X., Nie, F., Yang, Y., Huang, H.: A convex formulation for semi-supervised multi-label feature selection. In AAAI, pp. 1171–1177 (2014)
2. Chen, H.T., Chang, H.W., Liu, T.L.: Local discriminant embedding and its variants. In: CVPR, pp. 846–853 (2005)
3. Daubechies, I., Devore, R., Fornasier, M., Gntrk,C.S.: Iteratively reweighted least squares minimization for sparse recovery. Commun. Pure Appl. Math. **63**(1), 1–38 (2008)
4. Du, L., Shen, Y.D.: Unsupervised feature selection with adaptive structure learning. Comput. Sci. **37**(7), 209–218 (2015)
5. Gao, S., Tsang, I.W., Chia, L.T.: Laplacian sparse coding, hypergraph laplacian sparse coding, and applications. IEEE Trans. Pattern Anal. Mach. Intell. **35**(1), 92–104 (2013)
6. He, X., Niyogi, P.: Locality preserving projections. NIPS **16**(1), 186–197 (2003)
7. Hou, C., Nie, F., Li, X., Yi, D.: Joint embedding learning and sparse regression: a framework for unsupervised feature selection. IEEE Trans. Cybern. **44**(6), 793 (2014)
8. Hu, R., Zhu, X., Cheng, D., He, W., Yan, Y., Song, J., Zhang, S.: Graph self-representation method for unsupervised feature selection. Neurocomputing **220**, 130–137 (2017)
9. Li, X., Ng, M.K., Gao, C., Ye, Y., Wu, Q.: MR-NTD: manifold regularization nonnegative tucker decomposition for tensor data dimension reduction and representation. IEEE Trans. Neural Netw. Learn. Syst. **28**(8), 1787–1800 (2017)
10. Luo, D., Ding, C.H.Q., Huang, H.: Linear discriminant analysis: New formulations and overfit analysis. In: AAAI, (2011)
11. Qin, Y., Zhang, S., Zhu, X., Zhang, J., Zhang, C.: Pop algorithm: Kernel-based imputation to treat missing values in knowledge discovery from databases. Expert Syst. Appl. **36**(2), 2794–2804 (2009)
12. Yang, Y., Ma, Z., Hauptmann, A.G., Sebe, N.: Feature selection for multimedia analysis by sharing information among multiple tasks. IEEE Trans. Multim. **15**(3), 661–669 (2013)
13. Zhang, J., Chen, D., Liang, J., Xue, H., Lei, J., Wang, Q., Chen, D., Meng, M., Jin, Z., Tian, J.: Incorporating MRI structural information into bioluminescence tomography: system, heterogeneous reconstruction and in vivo quantification. Biomed. Opt. Express **5**(6), 1861 (2014)
14. Zhang, S.: Shell-neighbor method and its application in missing data imputation. Appl. Intell. **35**(1), 123–133 (2011)

15. Zhang, S., Jin, Z., Zhu, X.: Missing data imputation by utilizing information within incomplete instances. J. Syst. Softw. **84**(3), 452–459 (2011)
16. Zhang, S., Qin, Z., Ling, C.X., Sheng, S.: "missing is useful": missing values in cost-sensitive decision trees. IEEE Trans. Knowl. Data Eng. **17**(12), 1689–1693 (2005)
17. Zhang, S., Wu, X., Zhang, C.: Multi-database mining. IEEE Comput. Intell. Bull. **2**, 5–13 (2003)
18. Zhao, Z., Wang, L., Liu, H.: Efficient spectral feature selection with minimum redundancy. In: AAAI (2011)
19. Zhu, P., Zhu, W., Wang, W., Zuo, W., HuQ.: Non-convex regularized self-representation for unsupervised feature selection. Image Vis. Comput. **60**, 22–29 (2016)
20. Zhu, P., Zuo, W., Zhang, L., Hu, Q., Shiu, S.C.K.: Unsupervised feature selection by regularized self-representation. Pattern Recognit. **48**(2), 438–446 (2015)
21. Zhu, X., Huang, Z., Shen, H.T., Cheng, J., Xu, C.: Dimensionality reduction by mixed kernel canonical correlation analysis. Pattern Recognit. **45**(8), 3003–3016 (2012)
22. Zhu, X., Li, X., Zhang, S.: Block-row sparse multiview multilabel learning for image classification. IEEE Trans. Cybern. **46**(2), 450–461 (2016)
23. Zhu, X., Li, X., Zhang, S., Ju, C., Wu, X.: Robust joint graph sparse coding for unsupervised spectral feature selection. IEEE Trans. Neural Netw. Learn. Syst. **28**(6), 1263–1275 (2017)
24. Zhu, X., Li, X., Zhang, S., Xu, Z., Yu, L., Wang, C.: Graph PCA hashing for similarity search. IEEE Trans. Multim. (2017)
25. Zhu, X., Suk, H., Wang, L., Lee, S., Shen, D.: A novel relational regularization feature selection method for joint regression and classification in AD diagnosis. Med. Image Anal. **38**, 205–214 (2017)
26. Zhu, X., Suk, H.I., Shen, D.: A novel multi-relation regularization method for regression and classification in AD diagnosis. Med. Image Comput. Comput. Assist. Interv. **17**(Pt 3), 401–408 (2014)
27. Zhu, X., Zhang, L., Huang, Z.: A sparse embedding and least variance encoding approach to hashing. IEEE Trans. Image Process. **23**(9), 3737–3750 (2014)

Mixed Membership Sparse Gaussian Conditional Random Fields

Jie Yang[1(✉)], Henry C.M. Leung[1], S.M. Yiu[1(✉)], and Francis Y.L. Chin[2]

[1] Department of Computer Science, The University of Hong Kong, Hong Kong, Hong Kong
{jyang2,cmleung2,smyiu}@cs.hku.hk

[2] Department of Computing, Hang Sang Management College, Hong Kong, Hong Kong
francischin@hsmc.edu.hk

Abstract. Building statistical models to explain the association between responses (output) and predictors (input) is critical in many real applications. In reality, responses may not be independent. A promising direction is to predict related responses together (e.g. Multi-task LASSO). However, not all responses have the same degree of relatedness. Sparse Gaussian conditional random field (SGCRF) was developed to learn the degree of relatedness automatically from the samples without any prior knowledge. In real cases, features (both predictors and responses) are not arbitrary, but are dominated by a (smaller) set of related latent factors, e.g. clusters. SGCRF does not capture these latent relations in the model. Being able to model these relations could result in more accurate association between responses and predictors. In this paper, we propose a novel (mixed membership) hierarchical Bayesian model, namely M^{2}GCRF, to capture this phenomenon (in terms of clusters). We develop a variational Expectation-Maximization algorithm to infer the latent relations and association matrices. We show that M^{2}GCRF clearly outperforms existing methods for both synthetic and real datasets, and the association matrices identified by M^{2}GCRF are more accurate.

1 Introduction

Building statistical models to explain the association between responses (output) and predictors (input) is crucial in many real applications such as bioinformatics, finance and computer vision. For example, gene pathway analysis [12] in bioinformatics aims at studying the relationship of gene expressions in various pathways. The expressions of genes for pathway P_1 can be considered as predictors, and the genes in pathway P_2 are treated as responses. Understanding the association between the expression levels of P_1 and P_2 provides us insights on the mechanism behind the pathways. For each response (gene in P_2), we can infer a statistical model from the predictors (genes in P_1). However, genes in P_2 are not totally independent, a more promising approach is to group *related* genes together and study multiple statistical models at the same time. It was

G. Cong et al. (Eds.): ADMA 2017, LNAI 10604, pp. 287–302, 2017.
https://doi.org/10.1007/978-3-319-69179-4_20

shown that learning multiple statistical models [5] for related responses (genes in P_2 for example) simultaneously can be superior to learning them individually. There are also examples in finance and computer vision that motivate us to study related responses together (e.g. [2]).

Multi-task learning [5] was proposed to exploit the *relatedness* among responses. Figure 1(a) shows the multi-task learning framework, Q models are built by predicting Q responses $\{y_1, ..., y_Q\}$ from P predictors $\{x_1, ..., x_P\}$ simultaneously. In this paper, we only consider linear models with unique empirical predictors for all tasks[1], i.e. multi-output regression with weight $B_{P\times Q}$. Most existing works in this framework assume that tasks are *all related*, but without much difference for each task. Multi-task LASSO [14,21] simply learns all tasks together by assuming B are mainly zeros. Multi-task group LASSO [6] assumes that most rows of B are zeros. Dirty Model [10] and rMTFL [8] assume that all responses are related with similar predictors but with some outliers. All methods above assume that tasks are related in a *similar* degree which is not valid in practice. Some other works make use of prior knowledge about the relatedness of tasks. For example, [4,13] model this knowledge as a *prior* tree in which tasks represented by adjacent vertices share similar regression weights. Prior knowledge may not always be available. Sparse Gaussian conditional random field (SGCRF) [16,19,23] was developed to learn the degree of relatedness among tasks automatically without prior knowledge. To achieve this, the association matrices (of predictor-response Θ_{xy} and response-response Θ_{yy}) are estimated together in SGCRF (compared to methods mentioned in the above which only estimate B). SGCRF has considered the relationship between responses and predictors as well as the relationship among responses. Figure 1(b) shows examples of relationship among responses (e.g. (y_1, y_2), (y_1, y_3), (y_2, y_4) etc.) in which the degrees of relatedness are captured by Θ_{yy} in SGCRF.

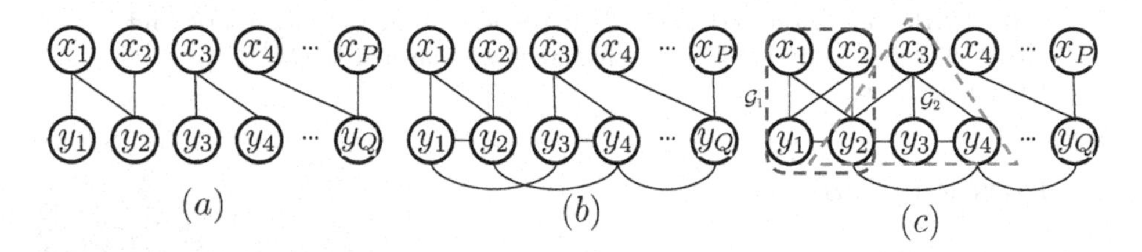

Fig. 1. Different kinds of multi-task learning frameworks. (a) considers the the associations of predictors and responses B_{xy}, e.g. Dirty Model and rMTFL; (b) considers both Θ_{xy} and Θ_{yy}, e.g. SGCRF; (c) shows the framework of M^{2}GCRF. M^{2}GCRF explicitly considers the relatedness of both Θ_{xy} and Θ_{yy}, in which x and y are related in terms of low-level cluster structures.

In reality, features (both responses and predictors) are usually not drawn from arbitrary domains, they are usually dominated by related latent factors.

[1] A task refers to the prediction task for a response based on the set of given predictors.

In gene regulatory networks, genes regulate in a group manner [3]. For stock market, weather and government policy affect energy-related stocks while weather and other factors (e.g. pollution) affect agriculture related stocks. Thus, the following hypothesis could be more relevant for real applications: (1) Both the predictors and responses features are dominated by latent clusters. Co-clustering of predictors and responses can boost the estimation of Θ_{xy} and Θ_{yy}. Performing clustering on the two association matrices Θ_{xy} and Θ_{yy} simultaneously can improve prediction as estimating Θ_{xy} can gain insights from clustering Θ_{yy} and vice versa. (2) Non-unique cluster strength. Features form clusters with stronger association for features inside (*intra-cluster association*) and weaker association for features in inter-clusters (*inter-cluster association*). (3) Clusters can overlap. Figure 1(c) shows an example: predictors $\{x_1, x_2\}$ and responses $\{y_1, y_2\}$ belong to cluster $\mathcal{G}_1$ while predictor $\{x_3\}$ and responses $\{y_2, y_3, y_4\}$ are from cluster $\mathcal{G}_2$. The links in the same cluster are dense while the links between features from different clusters are sparse. A feature may belong to multiple clusters (e.g. y_2 belongs to $\mathcal{G}_1$ and $\mathcal{G}_2$). No existing work captures this realistic scenario. We extend SGCRF and propose a novel (mixed membership [1]) hierarchical Bayesian framework, namely M^{2}GCRF, to model this observation. To realize our framework, we develop a variational Expectation-Maximization (EM) algorithm to estimate cluster structures and association matrices. We demonstrated that M^{2}GCRF outperforms other existing methods for both synthetic and real datasets (one from bioinformatics, three from stock markets and one from supply chain management). We also show that the association matrices identified by M^{2}GCRF are more accurate in the simulation.

To evaluate the performance of M^{2}GCRF, we selected two interesting case studies with different characteristics. The first set of experiments are datasets from bioinformatics and daily stock data. These datasets (e.g. datasets from bioinformatics) are well-known to have small sample size but with more parameters to learn. For instance, for a typical gene expression dataset, we only have several *hundred* samples, however, we need to estimate $50 * 50(\Theta_{xy}) + (\frac{50*49}{2} + 50)(\Theta_{yy}) = 3775$ parameters even for a GCRF with only 50 predictors and 50 responses. In this case, complex models tend to overfit. Technically speaking, to tackle this problem, SGCRF tries to learn a sparse GCRF, but the parameter space may still be large for real world applications as the number of samples may be relatively small. M^{2}GCRF, on the other hand, tries to further reduce the parameter space of SGCRF by the assumption that predictors and responses in the same cluster would behave similarly, thus the parameters among them will be very similar; while for those not in the same cluster, they are less likely to interact. Therefore, we make use of the concept of latent structures to define a much simpler GCRF which is sparse and of lower dimensions to overcome the overfitting problem. For the second set of experiments, we tend to pick a relatively larger dataset (e.g. a supply chain management dataset). The aim of this set of experiments is to show that M^{2}GCRF is able to benefit from the more accurate association matrix as the sample size increases and tends to capture more complicated latent structures from the data, thus also improve the result of SGCRF. The followings summarize our contributions: (1) M^{2}GCRF is the first model to

Table 1. Summary of notations

Class	Notation	Description
Data	X, Y	Predictor and response matrices
Notations	$\oint f(s)ds$	Integrals or sums of $f(s)$ $\forall s_i \in s$
	$\|\|A\|\|_1$	Norm one of matrix A
	$\|A\|$	Determinant of matrix A
	A^T, $\boldsymbol{a}^T$	Transpose of matrix A, vector $\boldsymbol{a}$
Model	$\mathbf{Dir}(\cdot)$, $\mathbf{Mul}(\cdot)$	Dirichlet and Multinomial distribution
	$\mathbf{Exp}(\cdot)$, $\mathbf{Lap}(\cdot)$	Exponential and Laplacian distribution
	$\alpha_x, \alpha_y, \eta_x, \eta_y$	Hyper-parameters
	$\boldsymbol{\pi}_x, \boldsymbol{\pi}_y, \boldsymbol{\beta}_x, \boldsymbol{\beta}_y$	Global variables
	N, K	Number of samples and clusters
	$\boldsymbol{z}_x, \boldsymbol{z}_y$	Local variables
	Θ_{xy}, Θ_{yy}	Association matrix
	P, Q	Number of predictors and responses
	$\mathcal{K}, \mathcal{P}, \mathcal{Q}$	All clusters, predictors and responses
	$\boldsymbol{x}$, $\boldsymbol{y}$	A sample of predictor and response
	$\boldsymbol{\tau}_x, \boldsymbol{\tau}_y, \boldsymbol{\gamma}_x, \boldsymbol{\gamma}_y$	Variational parameters
	$\boldsymbol{\Phi}_x, \boldsymbol{\Phi}_y$	Variational parameters
	λ_0	Parameter of L_1 regularization

co-cluster Θ_{xy} and Θ_{yy}; (2) M^{2}GCRF considers non-uniform cluster strengths (i.e. intra- and inter- cluster associations), which is more realistic; (3) M^{2}GCRF considers overlapping clusters; (4) A hierarchical Bayesian model is proposed to capture (1) to (3); (5) A novel variational EM algorithm is proposed for parameter estimation. The idea of clustering features is not completely new (e.g. [9,18,24,25]). However, they did not capture the association among responses, i.e., they only consider B and without considering co-clustering Θ_{xy} and Θ_{yy}. There are other models extending SGCRF, for example [7] learns a SGCRF with sparse and low-rank regularization, which is different from M^{2}GCRF.

Sparse Gaussian Conditional Random Fields

The notations are given in Table 1. We first provide a brief summary for Gaussian conditional random fields. Let $\boldsymbol{x} \in \mathbb{R}^P$ and $\boldsymbol{y} \in \mathbb{R}^Q$ denote the predictor and response features for a prediction task. A GCRF is a log-linear model of multivariate Gaussian distribution which is defined as:

$$\boldsymbol{y}|\boldsymbol{x}; \Theta_{xy}, \Theta_{yy} \sim \mathcal{N}(-\Theta_{yy}^{-1}\Theta_{xy}^T\boldsymbol{x}, \Theta_{yy}^{-1}) \tag{1}$$

i.e.,

$$p(\boldsymbol{y}|\boldsymbol{x}; \Theta_{xy}, \Theta_{yy}) = \frac{1}{Z(x)} e^{-\boldsymbol{y}^T\Theta_{yy}\boldsymbol{y} - 2\boldsymbol{x}^T\Theta_{xy}\boldsymbol{y}} \tag{2}$$

The quadratic term Θ_{yy} in Eq. (2) represents the conditional dependencies of response $\boldsymbol{y}$ and the linear term Θ_{xy} represents the dependence of response $\boldsymbol{y}$ over predictor $\boldsymbol{x}$. GCRF is parameterized by $\Theta_{xy} \in \mathbb{R}^{P\times Q}$, which connects the predictors and responses, and $\Theta_{yy} \in \mathbb{R}^{Q\times Q}$, which corresponds to the inverse covariance matrix. An illustration for representing the associations Θ_{xy} and Θ_{yy} is shown in Fig. 1(b). In other words, the predictor $\boldsymbol{y}$ of GCRF follows a multivariate Gaussian distribution with mean $-\Theta_{yy}^{-1}\Theta_{xy}^{T}\boldsymbol{x}$ and covariance Θ_{yy}^{-1}, and the partition function is given by

$$\frac{1}{Z(\boldsymbol{x})} = c|\Theta_{yy}|e^{-\boldsymbol{x}^T\Theta_{xy}\Theta_{yy}^{-1}\Theta_{xy}^{T}\boldsymbol{x}} \tag{3}$$

where c is a constant. For a prediction task with N data samples, we can arrange the samples as the rows of predictors $X \in \mathbb{R}^{N\times P}$ and responses $Y \in \mathbb{R}^{N\times Q}$. Thus the log-likelihood $f(\Theta_{xy}, \Theta_{yy}) = \log P(Y|X;\Theta_{xy}, \Theta_{yy})$ without the constant term c is given by

$$f(\Theta_{xy}, \Theta_{yy}) = \log|\Theta_{yy}| - \mathrm{Tr}(S_{yy}\Theta_{yy} + 2S_{yx}\Theta_{xy} + \Theta_{yy}^{-1}\Theta_{xy}^{T}S_{xx}\Theta_{xy}) \tag{4}$$

where Θ_{yy} is positive definite, $\mathrm{Tr}(\cdot)$ represents the trace of a matrix and S terms are the empirical covariances

$$S_{yy} = \frac{1}{N}Y^TY, S_{yx} = \frac{1}{N}Y^TX, S_{xx} = \frac{1}{N}X^TX \tag{5}$$

Without regularization, it is straightforward to verify that the optimization problem of maximizing log-likelihood $f(\Theta_{xy}, \Theta_{yy})$ is simply a re-parameterization of solving the least squares problem. We can additionally learn a SGCRF by regularizing Θ_{xy} and Θ_{yy} with L_1 penalty [21], i.e. to maximize $f(\Theta_{xy}, \Theta_{yy}) - \lambda_0(||\Theta_{xy}||_1 + ||\Theta_{yy}||_1)$ where $\Theta_{yy} \succ 0$ and $\lambda_0 > 0$ for controlling the sparsity level of Θ_{xy} and Θ_{yy}.

2 Model

M^{2}GCRF estimates the association matrices Θ_{xy} and Θ_{yy} and captures the cluster structures for both predictors and responses, simultaneously. We assume that each element of Θ_{xy} and Θ_{yy} is generated from independent Laplacian distributions, which is equivalent to applying L_1 regularization [21], i.e. maximize $f(\Theta_{xy}, \Theta_{yy}) - \sum_{p,q}\lambda_{xy}^{pq}|\Theta_{xy}^{pq}| - \sum_{q\hat{q}}\lambda_{yy}^{q\hat{q}}|\Theta_{yy}^{q\hat{q}}|$. Intuitively, λ_{xy}^{pq} and $\lambda_{yy}^{q\hat{q}}$ are determined by the clustering memberships of the corresponding features, e.g. λ_{xy}^{pq} is related to the clusters of predictor p and response q. We explicitly model the cluster relationships with *cluster assignment*, *intra-cluster association* and *inter-cluster association* assumptions: (1) *Cluster assignment*: we generate the clustering probability profile of predictors and responses from two global Dirichlet distributions, respectively. (2) *Intra-cluster association*: features in a same cluster may have strong intra-cluster association, which may be different from features in one other cluster. Consequently two global exponential prior distributions are used to model the cluster strengths of Θ_{xy} and Θ_{yy} respectively.

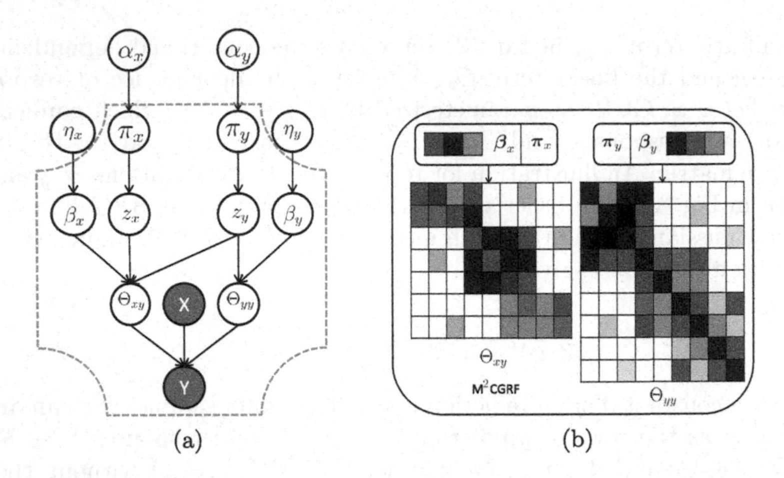

Fig. 2. (a) The generative process for M²GCRF; (b) An example of M²GCRF for $K = 3$, note that the clusters for both Θ_{xy} and Θ_{yy} overlap.

(3) *Inter-cluster association*: features in one cluster may interact with those in another in similar manner with weaker associations.

An M²GCRF for K clusters is generated as follows: (1) At *global level*, Dirichlet distributions $\mathbf{Dir}(\frac{\alpha_x}{K}\boldsymbol{1}^K)$ and $\mathbf{Dir}(\frac{\alpha_y}{K}\boldsymbol{1}^K)$ are used to generate the cluster proportions $\boldsymbol{\pi}_x$ and $\boldsymbol{\pi}_y$ for predictors and responses, respectively. Exponential distributions $\mathbf{Exp}(\eta_x)$ and $\mathbf{Exp}(\eta_y)$ are used to generate the intra-cluster associations for $\boldsymbol{\beta}_x$ and $\boldsymbol{\beta}_y$. Additionally, $\zeta > 0$ is for the intra-cluster associations. (2) At *feature level*, cluster proportion matrices $\boldsymbol{\pi}_x$ $(P \times K)$ and $\boldsymbol{\pi}_y$ $(Q \times K)$ describe the probability that predictors and responses belong to each cluster, e.g. $\boldsymbol{\pi}_{x,pk}$ represents the probability of pth predictor belongs to the kth cluster. (3) At *association level*, the cluster indicators $\boldsymbol{z}_x$ $(P \times Q \times K)$ and $\boldsymbol{z}_y$ $(Q \times Q \times K)$ are sampled from multinomial distributions $\mathbf{Mul}(\boldsymbol{\pi}_{xp})$ and $\mathbf{Mul}(\boldsymbol{\pi}_{yq})$, namely $\boldsymbol{z}_{x,p\to q}$ $(K \times 1)$ and $\boldsymbol{z}_{y,q\to\hat{q}}$ $(K \times 1)$ for Θ_{xy}^{pq} and $\Theta_{yy}^{q\hat{q}}$. For example, $\boldsymbol{z}_{x,1\to 2} = (1, ..., 0)$ indicates Θ_{xy}^{12} belongs to the 1st cluster since $\boldsymbol{z}_{x,1\to 2}^1 = 1$; similarly, $\boldsymbol{z}_{y,1\to 2} = (0, 1, ..., 0)$ represents Θ_{yy}^{12} belongs to 2nd cluster since $\boldsymbol{z}_{y,1\to 2}^2 = 1$. We sample Θ_{xy}^{pq} and $\Theta_{yy}^{q\hat{q}}$ from Laplacian distributions $\mathbf{Lap}(\lambda_{xy}^{pq})$ and $\mathbf{Lap}(\lambda_{yy}^{q\hat{q}})$. Note that λ_{xy}^{pq} and $\lambda_{yy}^{q\hat{q}}$ are generated from the mixture effects of clusters. In this paper, we assume the associations of features in a same cluster tend to be large, i.e. M²GCRF generates small λ_{xy}^{pq} and $\lambda_{yy}^{q\hat{q}}$ for features in a same cluster and the associations of features in different clusters tend to be small, i.e. M²GCRF generates large λ_{xy}^{pq} and $\lambda_{yy}^{q\hat{q}}$ for features in diverse clusters. We set $\lambda_{xy}^{pq} = \lambda_0 \times f_x(\boldsymbol{z}_{x,p\to q}, \boldsymbol{\beta}_x, \boldsymbol{z}_{y,q\to p})$ and $\lambda_{yy}^{q\hat{q}} = \lambda_0 \times f_y(\boldsymbol{z}_{y,q\to\hat{q}}, \boldsymbol{\beta}_y, \boldsymbol{z}_{y,\hat{q}\to q})$ where the regularization parameter $\lambda_0 > 0$ and

$$
\begin{aligned}
f_x(\boldsymbol{z}_{x,p\to q}, \boldsymbol{\beta}_x, \boldsymbol{z}_{y,q\to p}) &= \sum_k \boldsymbol{z}_{x,p\to q}^k \boldsymbol{\beta}_{x,k} \boldsymbol{z}_{y,q\to p}^k + (1 - \sum_k \boldsymbol{z}_{x,p\to q}^k \boldsymbol{z}_{y,q\to p}^k)\zeta \\
f_y(\boldsymbol{z}_{y,q\to\hat{q}}, \boldsymbol{\beta}_y, \boldsymbol{z}_{y,\hat{q}\to q}) &= \sum_k \boldsymbol{z}_{y,q\to\hat{q}}^k \boldsymbol{\beta}_{y,k} \boldsymbol{z}_{y,\hat{q}\to q}^k + (1 - \sum_k \boldsymbol{z}_{y,q\to\hat{q}}^k \boldsymbol{z}_{y,\hat{q}\to q}^k)\zeta.
\end{aligned}
\tag{6}
$$

Algorithm 1. Generative process for M²GCRF

Input:
$\alpha_x, \alpha_y, \eta_x, \eta_y$ /*Hyper-parameters*/
Output:
A mixed membership GCRF;
1 Global level
2 for $k \in \mathcal{K}$ do
3 Draw cluster strength $\boldsymbol{\beta}_{x,k} \sim \mathbf{Exp}(\eta_x)$ and $\boldsymbol{\beta}_{y,k} \sim \mathbf{Exp}(\eta_y)$;
4 Feature level
5 for $p \in \mathcal{P}$ do
6 Draw cluster probabilities $\boldsymbol{\pi}_{x,p} \sim \mathbf{Dir}(\frac{\alpha_x}{K}\boldsymbol{1}^K)$;
7 for $q \in \mathcal{Q}$ do
8 Draw cluster probabilities $\boldsymbol{\pi}_{y,q} \sim \mathbf{Dir}(\frac{\alpha_y}{K}\boldsymbol{1}^K)$;
9 Association level
10 for $(p,q) \in \mathcal{P} \times \mathcal{Q}$ do
11 Draw mem. indicator $\boldsymbol{z}_{x,p\to q} \sim \mathbf{Mul}\ (\boldsymbol{\pi}_{x,p})$;
12 for $(q,\hat{q}) \in \mathcal{Q} \times \mathcal{Q}$ do
13 Draw mem. indicator $\boldsymbol{z}_{y,q\to\hat{q}} \sim \mathbf{Mul}\ (\boldsymbol{\pi}_{y,q})$;
14 for $(p,q) \in \mathcal{P} \times \mathcal{Q}$ do
15 $\Theta_{xy}^{pq} \sim \mathbf{Lap}(\lambda_0 \times f_x(\boldsymbol{z}_{x,p\to q}, \boldsymbol{\beta}_x, \boldsymbol{z}_{y,q\to p}))$;
16 for $(q,\hat{q}) \in \mathcal{Q} \times \mathcal{Q}$ do
17 $\Theta_{yy}^{q\hat{q}} \sim \mathbf{Lap}(\lambda_0 \times f_y(\boldsymbol{z}_{y,q\to\hat{q}}, \boldsymbol{\beta}_y, \boldsymbol{z}_{y,\hat{q}\to q}))$;
18 Generate sample
19 $\boldsymbol{y}|\boldsymbol{x} \sim \mathcal{N}(-\Theta_{yy}^{-1}\Theta_{xy}^T\boldsymbol{x}, \Theta_{yy}^{-1})$.

Lastly we draw samples of response $\boldsymbol{y}$ given a predictor $\boldsymbol{x}$, from a Gaussian distribution $\mathcal{N}(-\Theta_{yy}^{-1}\Theta_{xy}^T\boldsymbol{x}, \Theta_{yy}^{-1})$. Gathering all above steps together gives us the full generative process of M²GCRF as demonstrated in Algorithm 1 and Fig. 2(a). An example of M²GCRF is shown in Fig. 2(b). The darkness of cells indicate the strength of association. Θ_{xy} and Θ_{yy} are generated from $K = 3$ clusters, with cluster proportions $\boldsymbol{\pi}_x$, $\boldsymbol{\pi}_y$ and strengths $\boldsymbol{\beta}_x$, $\boldsymbol{\beta}_y$. The cluster strengths $\boldsymbol{\beta}_x$ for predictors are medium, strong and weak. Consequently, Θ_{xy} consists of three clusters with strengths of medium, strong and weak from left to right.

3 Parameter Estimation

The classical maximum a posterior (MAP) approach is applied to estimate the association matrices $\hat{\Theta}_{xy}$ and $\hat{\Theta}_{yy}$ as

$$\hat{\Theta}_{xy}, \hat{\Theta}_{yy} = \underset{\Theta_{yy}\succ 0}{\operatorname{argmax}}\ P(\Theta_{xy}, \Theta_{yy}|X, Y, \alpha_x, \alpha_y, \eta_x, \eta_y) \quad (7)$$

To simply the notations, we denote the association matrices $\Theta = \{\Theta_{xy}, \Theta_{yy}\}$, the latent variables $\Xi = \{\boldsymbol{\beta}_x, \boldsymbol{\beta}_y, \boldsymbol{\pi}_x, \boldsymbol{\pi}_y, \boldsymbol{z}_x, \boldsymbol{z}_y\}$ and hyper-parameters as

$H=\{\alpha_x, \alpha_y, \eta_x, \eta_y\}$. By Bayes' law it follows immediately as

$$\begin{aligned}\hat{\Theta} &= \underset{\Theta_{yy}\succ 0}{\text{argmax}} \log P(\Theta|X,Y;H) = \underset{\Theta_{yy}\succ 0}{\text{argmax}} \log \frac{P(\Theta,Y|X;H)}{P(Y|X;H)} \\ &= \underset{\Theta_{yy}\succ 0}{\text{argmax}} \log P(\Theta,Y|X;H) = \underset{\Theta_{yy}\succ 0}{\text{argmax}} \log \sum\!\!\!\!\!\!\int P(\Theta,Y,\Xi|X;H)\, d\Xi\end{aligned} \tag{8}$$

Note that as defined in Table 1, we have

$$\sum\!\!\!\!\!\!\int P(\Theta,Y,\Xi|X;H)\, d\Xi = \int\!\!\int\!\!\int\!\!\int \sum_{\boldsymbol{z}_x,\boldsymbol{z}_y} P(\Theta,Y,\Xi|X;H)\, d\boldsymbol{\pi}_x d\pi_y d\boldsymbol{\beta}_x d\beta_y.$$

Since the integrations and summation over all possible values of the hidden variables Ξ in Eq. (8) are intractable, i.e. unsolvable in closed form, we propose to use approximate inference algorithm to tackle the problem. We introduce an Expectation-Maximization (EM) algorithm [15] for MAP estimation as shown in Eq. (8). In particular, we can use Jensen's inequality to approximate $\log P(\Theta,Y|X;H)$ by *any distribution* over latent variables $P(\Xi)$ as follows:

$$\begin{aligned}\log P(\Theta,Y|X;H) &= \log \sum\!\!\!\!\!\!\int P(\Theta,Y,\Xi|X;H)\, d\Xi = \log \sum\!\!\!\!\!\!\int P(\Xi) \frac{P(\Theta,Y,\Xi|X;H)}{P(\Xi)}\, d\Xi \\ &\geq \sum\!\!\!\!\!\!\int P(\Xi) \log \frac{P(\Theta,Y,\Xi|X;H)}{P(\Xi)}\, d\Xi = \mathbb{E}_{P(\Xi)}\left[\log P(\Theta,Y,\Xi|X;H) - \log P(\Xi)\right] \\ &\triangleq \mathcal{L}(\Theta, P(\Xi)).\end{aligned} \tag{9}$$

In EM, the objective function $\mathcal{L}(\Theta, P(\Xi))$ is maximized iteratively w.r.t. Θ by fixing $P(\Xi)$ in the M step, and $P(\Xi)$ by fixing Θ in the E step. In the tth E step we can set $P^{(t)}(\Xi) = P(\Xi|X,Y;H,\hat{\Theta}^{(t)})$, which is the posterior distribution of Ξ given the data points $\{X,Y\}$ and latest estimation of association matrices $\hat{\Theta}^{(t)}$). However, it is intractable for an analytic representation of the posterior distribution $P(\Xi|X,Y;H,\hat{\Theta}^{(t)})$. The objective function $\mathcal{L}(\Theta, P(\Xi))$ for EM is still intractable. Thus an approximation extensional algorithm termed variational EM is proposed for the estimation of $P(\Xi|X,Y;H,\hat{\Theta}^{(t)})$ and Θ alternatively from the data. To achieve this, we approximate the posterior of latent variables $P(\Xi|X,Y;H,\hat{\Theta}^{(t)})$ with a simplified distribution $\tilde{P}(\Xi)$ by the mean field assumption [11].

3.1 Variational EM

We derive a variational EM algorithm to estimate the optimal association matrices $\hat{\Theta}$ in Eq. (8) by alternatively maximizing the lower bound of the posterior distribution of Θ, i.e. $\mathcal{L}(\Theta, P(\Xi))$, with respect to Θ and an approximated posterior distribution of latent variables Ξ, i.e. $\tilde{P}(\Xi)$.

Variational Expectation Step (Mean Field). In the E step, we maximize the objective function $\tilde{\mathcal{L}}(\hat{\Theta}^t, \tilde{P}(\Xi))$ with respect to Ξ given the latest estimation of association matrices $\hat{\Theta}^{(t)}$. By the mean field assumption, we define the approximated distribution $\tilde{P}(\Xi)$ in a factorized way:

$$\tilde{P}(\Xi) = \tilde{P}(\boldsymbol{\beta}_x|\boldsymbol{\tau}_x)\tilde{P}(\boldsymbol{\beta}_y|\boldsymbol{\tau}_y)\tilde{P}(\boldsymbol{\pi}_x|\gamma_x)\tilde{P}(\boldsymbol{\pi}_y|\boldsymbol{\gamma}_y)\tilde{P}(\boldsymbol{z}_x|\Phi_x)\tilde{P}(\boldsymbol{z}_y|\Phi_y). \tag{10}$$

Algorithm 2. Variational inference for M^{2}GCRF

Input:
α_x, α_y, η_x, η_y, K, Θ_{xy}, Θ_{yy} ; /* Hyper-params */
/* Cluster # and Associations */

Output:
$\boldsymbol{\tau}_x$, $\boldsymbol{\tau}_y$, $\boldsymbol{\gamma}_x$, $\boldsymbol{\gamma}_y$, $\boldsymbol{\Phi}_x$, $\boldsymbol{\Phi}_y$; /* Varia. params */

1 Initialize each element of $\boldsymbol{\tau}_x$ and $\boldsymbol{\tau}_y$ to be η_x and η_y;
2 Initialize each element of $\boldsymbol{\gamma}_x$ and $\boldsymbol{\gamma}_y$ to be α_x and α_y;
3 Initialize each element of $\boldsymbol{\Phi}_x$ and $\boldsymbol{\Phi}_y$ to be $\frac{1}{K}$;
4 $t \leftarrow 0$; /* Iteration # */
/* Update $\boldsymbol{\Phi}_x$, $\boldsymbol{\Phi}_y$, $\boldsymbol{\gamma}_x$, $\boldsymbol{\gamma}_y$, $\boldsymbol{\tau}_x$, $\boldsymbol{\tau}_y$ */
5 **repeat**
6 Estimate $\boldsymbol{\Phi}_x^{(t+1)}$ and $\boldsymbol{\Phi}_y^{(t+1)}$ with other parameters fixed;
7 Estimate $\boldsymbol{\gamma}_x^{(t+1)}$ and $\boldsymbol{\gamma}_y^{(t+1)}$ with other parameters fixed;
8 Estimate $\boldsymbol{\tau}_x^{(t+1)}$ and $\boldsymbol{\tau}_y^{(t+1)}$ with other parameters fixed;
9 $t \leftarrow t+1$;
10 **until** *convergence*;
11 $\boldsymbol{\tau}_x = \boldsymbol{\tau}_x^{(t)}, \boldsymbol{\tau}_y = \boldsymbol{\tau}_y^{(t)}, \boldsymbol{\gamma}_x = \boldsymbol{\gamma}_x^{(t)}, \boldsymbol{\gamma}_y = \boldsymbol{\gamma}_y^{(t)}, \boldsymbol{\Phi}_x = \boldsymbol{\Phi}_x^{(t)}, \boldsymbol{\Phi}_y = \boldsymbol{\Phi}_y^{(t)}$;

By selecting all $\tilde{P}$ distributions to be in the same family as the prior distribution defined in Algorithm 1, the variational objective function of variational EM algorithm is

$$\begin{aligned}\tilde{\mathcal{L}}(\Theta, \tilde{P}(\Xi)) &= \mathbb{E}_{\tilde{P}(\Xi)}\big[\log P(\Theta, Y, \Xi | X; H) - \log \tilde{P}(\Xi)\big] \\ &= \mathbb{E}_{\tilde{P}(\Xi)}\big[\log P(\Theta, Y, \Xi | X; H)\big] - \mathbb{E}_{\tilde{P}(\Xi)}\big[\log \tilde{P}(\Xi)\big].\end{aligned} \tag{11}$$

The objective function $\tilde{\mathcal{L}}(\Theta, \tilde{P}(\Xi))$ can be easily derived by calculating the expectations in Eq. (11). In the following, we derive a coordinate ascent algorithm (Algorithm 2) to optimize the variational objective with respect to the variational parameters $\boldsymbol{\tau}_x$, $\boldsymbol{\tau}_y$, $\boldsymbol{\gamma}_x$, $\boldsymbol{\gamma}_y$, $\boldsymbol{\Phi}_x$, $\boldsymbol{\Phi}_y$, given the latest estimation of Θ_{xy} and Θ_{yy}. We first estimate the variational parameters $\boldsymbol{\Phi}_x$ and $\boldsymbol{\Phi}_y$ of multinomial distributions for generating the cluster indicators $\boldsymbol{z}_x$ and $\boldsymbol{z}_y$. Then, we estimate the variational parameters $\boldsymbol{\gamma}_x$ and $\boldsymbol{\gamma}_y$ of Dirichlet distributions. Finally, we estimate the variational parameters $\boldsymbol{\tau}_x$ and $\boldsymbol{\tau}_y$ of the exponential distributions for generating cluster strengths. By repeatedly applying the above three steps until convergence (from our experiments, the algorithm usually converges in less than 100 iterations), we obtain the latest estimation of variational parameters.

Variational Maximization Step. In the M step, we maximize the variational objective function $\tilde{\mathcal{L}}(\Theta, \tilde{P}^{(t)}(\Xi))$ with respect to Θ_{xy} and Θ_{yy} using a second order active set method proposed in [23], given latest estimation of variational parameters. $\tilde{\mathcal{L}}(\Theta, \tilde{P}^{(t)}(\Xi))$ can be calculated as

$$\tilde{\mathcal{L}}(\Theta, \tilde{P}^{(t)}(\Xi)) = f(\Theta_{xy}, \Theta_{yy}) - \sum_{p,q} \tilde{\lambda}_{xy}^{pq(t)} |\Theta_{xy}^{pq}| - \sum_{q,\hat{q}} \tilde{\lambda}_{yy}^{q\hat{q}(t)} |\Theta_{yy}^{q\hat{q}}| + c \tag{12}$$

where

$$\tilde{\lambda}_{xy}^{pq(t)} = \lambda_0 \times \Big(\sum_k \Phi_{x,p\to q}^{k(t)} \tau_{x,k}^{(t)} \Phi_{y,q\to p}^{k(t)} + (1 - \sum_k \Phi_{x,p\to q}^{k(t)} \Phi_{y,q\to p}^{k(t)}) \zeta \Big)$$

and

$$\tilde{\lambda}_{yy}^{q\hat{q}(t)} = \lambda_0 \times \Big(\sum_k \Phi_{y,q\to \hat{q}}^{k(t)} \tau_{y,k}^{(t)} \Phi_{y,\hat{q}\to q}^{k(t)} + (1 - \sum_k \Phi_{y,q\to \hat{q}}^{k(t)} \Phi_{y,\hat{q}\to q}^{k(t)}) \zeta \Big),$$

c is a constant independent from Θ_{xy} and Θ_{yy}. We follow the specialized second-order active set method in [23] for estimating the SGCRF's parameters. The basic idea is to iteratively form a second-order approximation to the objective function as given in Eq. (12) (without the L_1 regularization term), and then solve an L_1 regularized quadratic program to find a regularized analog of the Newton step. More details can be found in [23].

3.2 Hyper-parameter Optimization

We use Type-II Maximum Likelihood to optimize the hyper-parameters α_x, α_y, η_x and η_y, i.e. by taking steps towards the direction of $\frac{\partial \tilde{\mathcal{L}}(\Theta, \tilde{P}(\Xi))}{\partial \alpha_x}$, $\frac{\partial \tilde{\mathcal{L}}(\Theta, \tilde{P}(\Xi))}{\partial \alpha_y}$, $\frac{\partial \tilde{\mathcal{L}}(\Theta, \tilde{P}(\Xi))}{\partial \eta_x}$ and $\frac{\partial \tilde{\mathcal{L}}(\Theta, \tilde{P}(\Xi))}{\partial \eta_y}$ until converged.

4 Experiments

We compare the performances of M^2GCRF with independent LASSO, Dirty Model/rMTFL and SGCRF on both synthetic and real world data sets. Independent LASSO builds separate models for each response. Dirty Model/rMTFL assume that all tasks are similar, but with some outliers. SGCRF considers associations of predictor-response along with these of response-response. We initialize our hyper-parameters as $\alpha_x = 1.0$, $\alpha_y = 1.0$, $\eta_x = 0.1$, $\eta_y = 0.1$ for all experiments.

4.1 Synthetic Datasets

Data Generation. We generate 20×4 datasets (20 each for $N = 100$, 150, 200, or 300 samples) for $P = 50$ predictors, $Q = 50$ responses and $K = 7$ clusters. We begin by generating the association matrices Θ_{xy} and Θ_{yy}. There are $K = 7$ clusters in total (five 10×10 diagonal and two 8×8 corner clusters) in both Θ_{xy} and Θ_{xy}). To specify various strengths for different clusters in Θ_{xy},

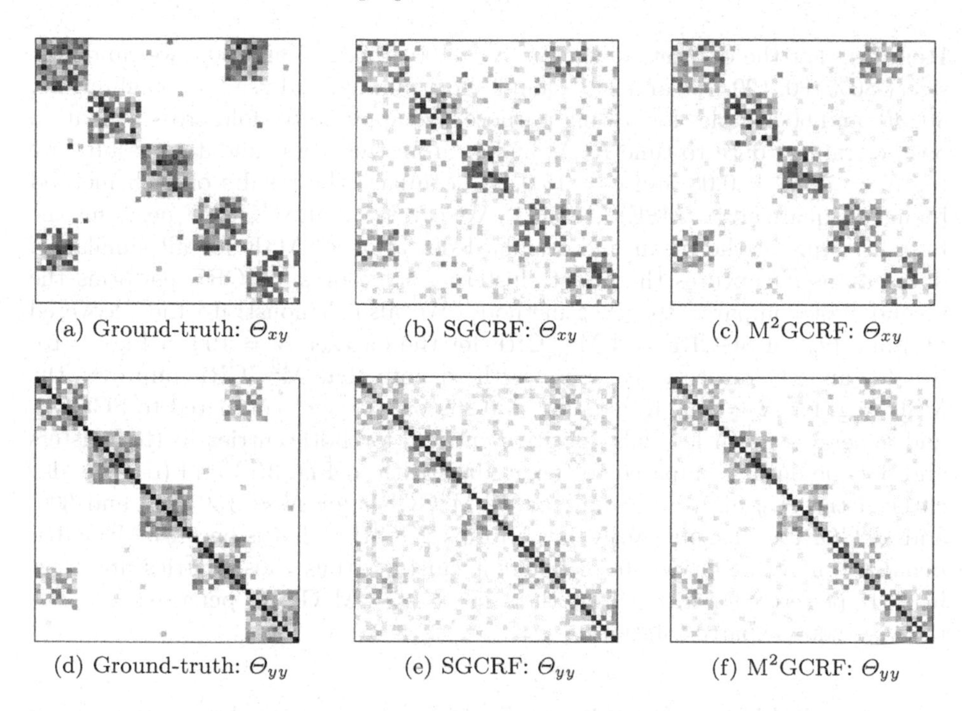

(a) Ground-truth: Θ_{xy} (b) SGCRF: Θ_{xy} (c) M^{2}GCRF: Θ_{xy}

(d) Ground-truth: Θ_{yy} (e) SGCRF: Θ_{yy} (f) M^{2}GCRF: Θ_{yy}

Fig. 3. (a), (b) and (c) illustrate the ground-truth, SGCRF and M^{2}GCRF estimated Θ_{xy}, respectively. The strength of association is proportional to the darkness of the cells. M^{2}GCRF estimated Θ_{xy} is more accurate than SGCRF. (d), (e) and (f) illustrate the ground-truth, SGCRF and M^{2}GCRF estimated Θ_{yy}, respectively. M^{2}GCRF predicts significantly better Θ_{yy} than SGCRF.

we restrict the proportion of non-zeros in each cluster. For each cluster in Θ_{xy}: (1) We sample a value p randomly from $\{\frac{3}{5}, \frac{4}{5}, \frac{5}{5}\}$ for the proportion of non-zeros in Θ_{xy}; (2) For each entry in the cluster, we set it to be 0 with probability $(1-p)$, and draw it from a Gaussian distribution $\mathcal{N}(0,1)$ with probability p. An illustration of the ground-truth of Θ_{xy} and Θ_{yy} for $N = 100$ is shown in Fig. 3(a) and (d). To add some noise, we set the entries not in clusters to be zero with probability 0.99, and sample them from $\mathcal{N}(0,1)$ with probability 0.01. We sample Θ_{xy} in a similar way, by additionally adding a large enough positive value to the diagonal elements of Θ_{xy} to enforce $\Theta_{xy} \succ 0$. In our simulation, we set this value to be 8.0. Later we sample each element of X independently from $\mathcal{N}(0,1)$. Each sample of Y is generated from the multivariate Gaussian distribution $\mathcal{N}(-\Theta_{yy}^{-1}\Theta_{xy}\boldsymbol{x}, \Theta_{yy}^{-1})$, where $\boldsymbol{x}$ is the predictor of each sample, i.e. each row of X. Note that Θ_{xy}, Θ_{yy}, X and Y for the datasets are different since we use different randomized seeds for generation. Note that we have considered overlapping clusters in simulation, e.g. from Fig. 3(a), the top 8 rows predictors can belong to two clusters, the left top cluster and the right top one; similarly, the predictors in the bottom left one also belong to two clusters.

Results. For the datasets of sample $N = 100$, 150, 200 and 300, we randomly select 80% (80, 120, 160 and 240) samples for training, and use the remaining 20, 30, 40, and 60 samples for testing purpose. We apply a five-fold cross validation on the training data to tune K, λ_0 and ζ. From the cross validation results, we set $K = 7$, $\lambda_0 = 0.08$ and $\zeta = 15.0$. We compare the results of each method by mean-square error (MSE) (Table 2). We can see that M^{2}GCRF performs the best in terms of the mean and standard deviation of MSE for all simulation datasets, as it captures the latent clustering structures. SGCRF performs the second best compared to other methods. We also demonstrate the recovered Θ_{xy} and Θ_{yy} of SGCRF and M^{2}GCRF for the dataset $N = 100$ in Fig. 3 (b), (c), (e) and (f) respectively. It is worth to note that M^{2}GCRF improves the MSE (e.g. for $N = 100$, from 0.284 to 0.269 on average) compared to SGCRF, and generates much less false positive entries (for both entries in the clusters and outside ones), compared to the ground-truth in Fig. 3(a) and (d). We also checked the Θ_{xy} and Θ_{yy} estimated by M^{2}GCRF for $N = 150$, 200 and 300, and M^{2}GCRF still significantly outperforms SGCRF. That is because M^{2}GCRF penalizes more for entries from different clusters, thus those entries are more likely to be zeros; for entries from the same cluster, M^{2}GCRF penalizes less thus recovers not-so-sparse solutions.

Table 2. MSE results (smaller better) for synthetic dataset

Method	$N = 100$	150	200	300
Ind. LASSO	0.851 ± 0.416	0.528 ± 0.127	0.497 ± 0.153	0.380 ± 0.117
Dirty Model	0.480 ± 0.092	0.294 ± 0.037	0.292 ± 0.159	0.223 ± 0.050
rMTFL	0.360 ± 0.081	0.268 ± 0.037	0.281 ± 0.161	0.219 ± 0.050
SGCRF	0.284 ± 0.063	0.231 ± 0.037	0.227 ± 0.036	0.207 ± 0.026
M^{2}GCRF	$\mathbf{0.269 \pm 0.059}$	$\mathbf{0.218 \pm 0.030}$	$\mathbf{0.215 \pm 0.035}$	$\mathbf{0.193 \pm 0.025}$

Effect of K: In our simulation, we also tried to specify different number of clusters to check the sensitivity of K. The result shows that as long as K is near the ground-truth, the output of M^{2}GCRF is robust (i.e., if we set K a little bit larger than the ground-truth, interestingly, M^{2}GCRF will keep some clusters empty and still recover the ground-truth; if we set K to be a little bit smaller than the ground-truth, it will merge multiple clusters to a single cluster).

4.2 Real Datasets

We apply M^{2}GCRF to a gene expression dataset, three stock datasets from US stock market and a supply chain management dataset to demonstrate the performance of M^{2}GCRF for real scenarios.

Table 3. MSE results for gene, stock and SCM datasets

Method	Gene	STK13	STK14	STK15	SCM20D
Ind. LASSO	0.759 ± 0.112	1.254	1.101	1.150	0.495 ± 0.067
Dirty Model	0.685 ± 0.093	0.164	0.229	0.237	0.421 ± 0.033
rMTFL	0.662 ± 0.083	0.234	0.241	0.268	0.420 ± 0.031
SGCRF	0.632 ± 0.073	0.205	0.224	0.253	0.424 ± 0.037
M^2GCRF	$\mathbf{0.616 \pm 0.067}$	**0.130**	**0.167**	**0.190**	$\mathbf{0.411 \pm 0.023}$

Gene Expression. We apply M^2GCRF to a gene expression data with a microarray dataset pertaining to isoprenoid biosynthesis in Arabidopsis thaliana (A. thaliana) [22]. Of particular relevance is to develop an understanding of the crosswalks among the different isoprenoid pathways: the non-mevalonate pathways and the mevalonate pathway. In the dataset considered, the predictors are the expression levels of $P = 19$ genes in the non-mevalonate pathways, the responses are the expression levels of $Q = 21$ genes in the mevalonate pathway. There are $N = 118$ samples in total. We standardize the features by log operator, and scale them with zero mean and unit standard deviation. We randomly generate 20 datasets with 100 samples for training and the remained 18 for testing. Five-fold cross validation is used to tune the parameters K, λ_0 and ζ. MSE results in Table 3 show that M^2GCRF performs the best (M^2GCRF obtains the best MSE 0.616 on average, better than SGCRF with 0.632, and third best method rMTFL with 0.662) as its ability of capturing more detailed interactions.

Stock Datasets. We obtain three datasets of the daily closing prices for 50 stocks from US stock market in year 2013, 2014 and 2015, each with N = 252, 252 and 253 samples from Yahoo Finance. We train a first-order autoregressive model to predict next day's stock price by using the current day's price. The predictors are the stock prices from day_1 to day_{N-1}, the responses are the stock prices from day_2 to day_N. All features are log transformed, centered and normalized with standard deviation of one. For all datasets, we choose the first 126 days for training, and the remaining days are for testing. Also, we use five-fold cross validation to tune the parameters, e.g. the optimal parameters are $K = 7$, $\lambda_0 = 0.04$ and $\zeta = 10$ for year 2015. MSE results in Table 3 show that M^2GCRF performs the best (e.g. obtain an MSE of 0.19, compared to SGCRF with 0.253, which is the second best for STK15). Benefiting from considering the latent stock clusters, M^2GCRF also improves the prediction over other models, e.g. Ind. LASSO, Dirty Model and rMTFL.

Supply Chain Management Dataset. The Supply Chain Management (SCM) datasets are derived from the Trading Agent Competition in Supply Chain Management (TAC SCM) tournament from 2010 [17,20]. We apply

M^2GCRF on SCM20D dataset which in total has $N = 8966$ observations. There are $P = 61$ predictors which represent for the observed prices for a specific tournament day. In addition, the datasets contain $Q = 16$ responses with each response corresponds to the mean price for 20-days in the future (SCM20D) for each product in the simulation. Similarly, we standardize each predictor and responses to have zero mean and unit standard deviation. We randomly select 5966 observations for training, and the remained 3000 samples for testing, for 20 rounds with different random seeds. Five-fold cross validation is used to tune the parameters K, λ_0 and ζ of M^2GCRF, e.g. from cross validation M^2GCRF performs best by setting $K = 3$, $\lambda_0 = 0.01$ and $\zeta = 10$ for the dataset with splitting random seed = 10099. As we can see from the MSE results in Table 3, M^2GCRF performs best (with the best mean MSE of 0.411 and the best standard deviation of 0.023), and SGCRF only obtain an MSE of 0.424 with much larger standard deviation of 0.037. This is because for the response variables, the mean prices of different products may be associated, e.g. the prices of different products may go up or go down in a similar way. M^2GCRF is able to capture this kind of relationship, thus improves the prediction. Dirty model and rMTFL perform similarly with mean around 0.042, and a little bit higher standard deviation than M^2GCRF. The Ind. LASSO performs worst with mean of 0.495 and standard deviation of 0.067 which is reasonable as it fits sparse regression for each response separately which does not capture the associations among different response variables.

5 Conclusions

In this paper, we proposed a hierarchical Bayesian model that explores clustering over the association matrices of SGCRF. M^2GCRF integrates mixed membership modeling with SGCRF to estimate clusters and association matrices. In the future work, we are interested in a non-parametric way for automatically estimating K from data, e.g. Dirichlet process. Also more sophisticated variational inference algorithm should be investigated to further improve the approximation accuracy of the posterior distribution.

Acknowledgement. This work was supported by Hong Kong RGC Ref No. UGC/IDS14/16 and RGC Project No. CityU C1008-16G, AoE/M-403/16.

References

1. Airoldi, E.M., Blei, D.M., Fienberg, S.E., Xing, E.P.: Mixed membership stochastic blockmodels. J. Mach. Learn. Res. **9**, 1981–2014 (2008)
2. Allenby, G.M., Rossi, P.E.: Marketing models of consumer heterogeneity. J. Econometr. **89**(1), 57–78 (1998)
3. Boutanaev, A.M., Kalmykova, A.I., Shevelyov, Y.Y., Nurminsky, D.I.: Large clusters of co-expressed genes in the drosophila genome. Nature **420**(6916), 666–669 (2002)

4. Chen, X., Shi, X., Xu, X., Wang, Z., Mills, R., Lee, C., Xu, J.: A two-graph guided multi-task lasso approach for eqtl mapping. In: International Conference on Artificial Intelligence and Statistics, pp. 208–217 (2012)
5. Evgeniou, T., Pontil, M.: Regularized multi-task learning. In: Proceedings of the 10th ACM SIGKDD International Conference on Knowledge Discovery and Data mining, pp. 109–117. ACM (2004)
6. Friedman, J., Hastie, T., Tibshirani, R.: A note on the group lasso and a sparse group lasso (2010). arXiv:1001.0736
7. Frot, B., Jostins, L., McVean, G.: Latent variable model selection for gaussian conditional random fields (2015). arXiv:1512.06412
8. Gong, P., Ye, J., Zhang, C.: Robust multi-task feature learning. In: Proceedings of the 18th ACM SIGKDD International Conference on Knowledge Discovery and Data Mining, pp. 895–903. ACM (2012)
9. Gupta, S., Phung, D., Venkatesh, S.: Factorial multi-task learning: a bayesian nonparametric approach. In: Proceedings of the 30th International Conference on Machine Learning, pp. 657–665 (2013)
10. Jalali, A., Sanghavi, S., Ruan, C., Ravikumar, P.K.: A dirty model for multi-task learning. In: NIPS, pp. 964–972 (2010)
11. Jordan, M.I., Ghahramani, Z., Jaakkola, T.S., Saul, L.K.: An introduction to variational methods for graphical models. Mach. Learn. **37**(2), 183–233 (1999)
12. Karlebach, G., Shamir, R.: Modelling and analysis of gene regulatory networks. Nat. Rev. Mol. Cell Biol. **9**(10), 770–780 (2008)
13. Kim, S., Xing, E.P.: Tree-guided group lasso for multi-task regression with structured sparsity. In: Proceedings of the 27th International Conference on Machine Learning, pp. 543–550 (2010)
14. Lee, S., Zhu, J., Xing, E.P.: Adaptive multi-task lasso: with application to eQTL detection. In: NIPS, pp. 1306–1314 (2010)
15. Logothetis, A., Krishnamurthy, V.: Expectation maximization algorithms for map estimation of jump Markov linear systems. IEEE Trans. Signal Process. **47**(8), 2139–2156 (1999)
16. McCarter, C., Kim, S.: Large-scale optimization algorithms for sparse conditional gaussian graphical models. In: Proceedings of the 19th International Conference on Artificial Intelligence and Statistics, pp. 528–537 (2016)
17. Pardoe, D., Stone, P.: The 2007 tac scm prediction challenge. In: Ketter, W., La Poutré, H., Sadeh, N., Shehory, O., Walsh, W. (eds.) AMEC/TADA -2008. LNBIP, vol. 44. Springer, Heidelberg (2010). doi:10.1007/978-3-642-15237-5
18. Passos, A., Rai, P., Wainer, J., Daume, H.: Flexible modeling of latent task structures in multitask learning. In: Proceedings of the 29th ICML Conference, pp. 1103–1110 (2012)
19. Sohn, K.A., Kim, S.: Joint estimation of structured sparsity and output structure in multiple-output regression via inverse-covariance regularization. In: International Conference on Artificial Intelligence and Statistics, pp. 1081–1089 (2012)
20. Spyromitros-Xioufis, E., Tsoumakas, G., Groves, W., Vlahavas, I.: Multi-target regression via input space expansion: treating targets as inputs. Mach. Learn. **104**(1), 55–98 (2016)
21. Tibshirani, R.: Regression shrinkage and selection via the lasso. J. R. Stat. Soc. Ser. B (Methodological), 267–288 (1996)
22. Wille, A., Zimmermann, P., Vranová, E., Fürholz, A., Laule, O., Bleuler, S., Hennig, L., Prelic, A., von Rohr, P., Thiele, L., et al.: Sparse graphical gaussian modeling of the isoprenoid gene network in arabidopsis thaliana. Genome Biol. **5**(11), R92 (2004)

23. Wytock, M., Kolter, Z.: Sparse gaussian conditional random fields: algorithms, theory, and application to energy forecasting. In: Proceedings of the 30th International Conference on Machine Learning, pp. 1265–1273 (2013)
24. Zhong, L.W., Kwok, J.T.Y.: Convex multitask learning with flexible task clusters. In: Proceedings of the 29th International Conference on Machine Learning, p. 49 (2012)
25. Zhou, Q., Zhao, Q.: Flexible clustered multi-task learning by learning representative tasks. IEEE Trans. PAMI **38**(2), 266 (2016)

Effects of Dynamic Subspacing in Random Forest

Md Nasim Adnan(✉) and Md Zahidul Islam

School of Computing and Mathematics, Charles Sturt University,
Bathurst, NSW 2795, Australia
{madnan,zislam}@csu.edu.au

Abstract. Due to its simplicity and good performance, Random Forest attains much interest from the research community. The splitting attribute at each node of a decision tree for Random Forest is determined from a predefined number of randomly selected attributes (a subset of the entire attribute set). The size of an attribute subset (subspace) is one of the most important factors that stems multitude of influences over Random Forest. In this paper, we propose a new technique that dynamically determines the size of subspaces based on the relative size of the current data segment to the entire data set. In order to assess the effects of the proposed technique, we conduct experiments involving five widely used data set from the UCI Machine Learning Repository. The experimental results indicate the capability of the proposed technique on improving the ensemble accuracy of Random Forest.

Keywords: Decision tree · Decision forest · Random forest

1 Introduction

Data mining has entered into our day to day life; we now predict the diagnoses of patients, credit approvals/denials and even elections. These predictions are carried out by classifier(s) based on previously known information. Likewise, classifiers are used in business, science, education, security and many other arena. As classifiers enter such influential and sensitive ambit, the importance of improving their efficiency is paramount.

A classifier is a function that maps a set of non-class attributes $\boldsymbol{m} = \{A_1, A_2, ..., A_m\}$ to a predefined class attribute C from an existing data set $\boldsymbol{D}$. A data set generally contains two types of attributes such as numerical (e.g. Age) and categorical (e.g. Gender). Among categorical attributes, one is chosen to be the "class" attribute. All other attributes are termed as "non-class" attributes. A classifier is built from an existing data set (i.e. training data set) where the values of the class attribute are present and then the classifier is applied on unseen/test records to predict their class values.

There are different types of classifiers in literature such as Artificial Neural Networks [25,51,52], Bayesian Classifiers [14,37], Nearest-Neighbor classifiers [26,46], Support Vector Machines [18] and Decision Trees [17,40,41]. Some

G. Cong et al. (Eds.): ADMA 2017, LNAI 10604, pp. 303–312, 2017.
https://doi.org/10.1007/978-3-319-69179-4_21

classifiers such as Artificial Neural Network and Support Vector Machines work similar to a "black box" where they only give predictive results without providing any reasoning for the results [27,32]. On the other hand, a decision tree expresses the patterns that exist in a data set into a flow-chart like representation that closely resembles human reasoning. Each path of the flow-chart represents a logic rule which can be used for knowledge discovery as well as predicting unlabeled records. In this way, decision trees avoid the knowledge discovery bottleneck and thus very popular to the real-world users [38,39].

It is worth to mention that decision trees require no domain knowledge for any parameter setting and therefore more appropriate for exploratory knowledge discovery [21]; and unlike some classifiers (such as Artificial Neural Networks, Nearest-Neighbor Classifiers and Support Vector Machines) decision trees are readily applicable on both categorical and numerical data that further increases their application domain. In addition, decision trees are able to deal with high dimensional, redundant as well as correlated attributes [11,21,33].

Hunt's Concept Learning System (CLS) [23] can be credited as the pioneering work for inducing top-down decision trees. According to CLS, the induction of a decision tree starts by selecting a non-class attribute A_i to split a training data set $\boldsymbol{D}$ into a disjoint set of horizontal partitions [24,40,46]. The purpose of this splitting is to create a purer distribution of class values in the succeeding partitions than the distribution in $\boldsymbol{D}$. The purity of class distribution in succeeding partitions is checked for all contending non-class attributes and the attribute that gives purer class distribution than others is selected as the splitting attribute. The process of selecting the splitting attribute continues recursively in each subsequent partition $\boldsymbol{D}_i$ until either every partition gets the "purest class distribution" or a stopping criterion is satisfied. By "purest class distribution" we mean the presence of a single class value for all records. A stopping criterion can be the minimum number of records that a partition must contain; meaning that if an splitting event creates one or more succeeding partitions with less than the minimum number of records, the splitting is not considered.

A decision tree consists of nodes (denoted by rectangles) and leaves (denoted by ovals) as shown in Fig. 1. The node of a decision tree symbolizes a splitting event where the splitting attribute (label of the node) partitions a data set according to its domain values. As a result, a disjoint set of horizontal segments of the data set are generated and each segment contains one set of domain values of the splitting attribute. For example, in Fig. 1 "Trouble Remembering" is selected as the splitting attribute in the root node. "Trouble Remembering" has two domain values: "Y" and "N" and thus it splits the data set into two disjoint horizontal segments in such as way that the records of one segment contain "Y" value for "Trouble Remembering" attribute and the records of another segment contain "N" value. The domain values of the splitting attribute designated for the respective horizontal segments are represented by the labels of edges leaving the node.

The use of an ensemble of classifiers is a comparatively newer area of research [3–7,20,42]. Interestingly, an ensemble of classifiers is found to be more effective

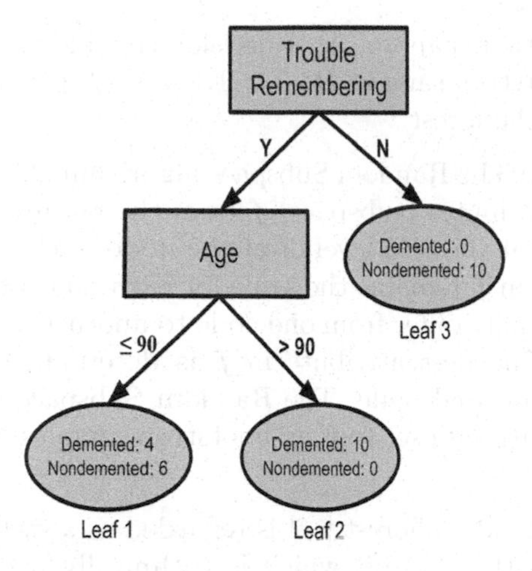

Fig. 1. Decision Tree

for unstable classifiers such as decision trees [46,49]. Decision trees are considered to be an unstable classifier as slight change(s) in a training data set can cause significant differences between the resulting decision trees obtained from the original and modified data sets. A decision forest is an ensemble of decision trees where an individual decision tree acts as a base classifier. The ensemble classification is performed by taking a vote based on the predictions made by each decision tree of the forest [46].

In order to achieve better ensemble accuracy, decision trees to be voted should be as different/diverse as possible; otherwise if they were identical, there could be little or no improvement from the ensemble [44]. Hence, diversity is considered as the cornerstone of ensemble systems and this is the reason why unstable classifiers are good for ensembles. However, to establish the scope of generating too diverse decision trees may be the cause of generating less accurate decision trees as optimization on the two conflicting objectives can be difficult to attain simultaneously [22]. In literature, we find a considerable study on the accuracy-diversity trade-off and find that individual accuracy should not be ignored for diversity [8,28,47].

Several decision forest algorithms exist aiming to generate more diverse as well as accurate decision trees by manipulating the training data set. We explain some of the renowned algorithms as follows.

Bagging: Bagging [15] generates a new training data set $\boldsymbol{D}_i$ where the records of $\boldsymbol{D}_i$ are selected randomly from the original training data set $\boldsymbol{D}$. A new training data set $\boldsymbol{D}_i$ contains the same number of records as in $\boldsymbol{D}$. Thus, some records of $\boldsymbol{D}$ can be selected multiple times and some records may not be selected at all. This approach of generating a new training data set is known as bootstrap sampling. Approximately, 63.2% of the original records are selected in a bootstrap sample and the remaining 36.8% records are repeated [21]. In Bagging, a predefined number ($|T|$) of bootstrap samples $\boldsymbol{D}_1, \boldsymbol{D}_2, ..., \boldsymbol{D}_{|T|}$ are generated using the above mentioned approach. A decision tree induction algorithm is then applied on each bootstrap sample $\boldsymbol{D}_i$ ($i = 1, 2, \ldots, |T|$) in order to generate $|T|$ number of trees for the forest.

Random Subspace: The Random Subspace algorithm [22] algorithm randomly draws a subset of attributes (subspace) $\boldsymbol{f}$ from the entire attribute space $\boldsymbol{m}$. $\boldsymbol{f}$ can be drawn either at the tree level or at the node level. When selected at the tree level, attributes in $\boldsymbol{f}$ remains the same for each node of a tree; on the other hand attributes in $\boldsymbol{f}$ may differ from one node to another in a tree when selected at the node level. The best attribute in $\boldsymbol{f}$ is determined to be the splitting attribute for the associated node. The Random Subspace algorithm is applied on the original training data set (not on bootstrap samples) for building decision trees.

Random Forest: Random Forest [16] is regarded as a state-of-the-art decision forest building algorithm [12,13] which is technically a combination of Bagging and Random Subspace algorithms. In the simplest form of Random Forest, attributes in $\boldsymbol{f}$ is randomly selected at the node level and the size of $\boldsymbol{f}$ is chosen to be $int(log_2|\boldsymbol{m}|) + 1$ [16] (popularly known as the hyperparameter [13]).

Since its inception in 2001, Random Forest attains much interest from the research community and thereby numerous enhancements have been proposed in recent years [2–5,9,12,45,53]. In particular, the selection of more suitable subspace ($\boldsymbol{f}$) invites much attention [13,19,20,36,43,48,50]. In Forest-RK [13], the authors proposed for random selection of $|\boldsymbol{f}|$ between 1 to $|\boldsymbol{m}|$ while in Extremely Randomized Trees [20], $|\boldsymbol{f}|$ is chosen to be $\sqrt{|\boldsymbol{m}|}$ for the classification problem. The Extremely Randomized Trees algorithm improvises more randomness for numerical attributes by selecting the cut-points fully at random while ensuring a minimum number of records in either sides of a cut-point. Another algorithm [19] suggested setting the cut point midway between two training records that had been picked randomly.

In [50], the authors applied the stratified sampling of attributes for Random Forest to deal with high dimensional data set. The key idea behind the stratified sampling is to divide the attributes $\boldsymbol{m}$ into two groups. One group will contain the good attributes $\boldsymbol{m}_G$ and the other group will contain the bad attributes $\boldsymbol{m}_B$. The attributes having the informativeness capacity higher than the average informativeness capacity are placed in the group of good attributes $\boldsymbol{m}_G$ and all other attributes are placed in the group of bad attributes $\boldsymbol{m}_B$. Then $int(log_2|\boldsymbol{m}|) + 1$ number of attributes are selected randomly from each group in proportion to the size of the groups.

We understand that with the traversal from the root node down the tree, the number of records in data segments become smaller and smaller as a result of the recursive partitioning [1,24,46]. A data segment is partitioned according to its splitting attributes domain values and thus the resultant partitions tend to have very weak relationship with the same attribute (specially when the attribute is a categorical attribute). As shown earlier, in Fig. 1 "Trouble Remembering" is selected as the splitting attribute in the root node. "Trouble Remembering" has two domain values: "Y" and "N" and thus it splits the data set into two disjoint horizontal segments in such as way that the records of one segment contain "Y" value for "Trouble Remembering" attribute and the records of another segment contain "N" value. Hence, any of the two disjoint horizontal segments can not be split further by the "Trouble Remembering" attribute. As a consequence, fewer attributes become relevant for a data segment that has been generated through a number of partitioning involving different splitting attributes and hence the probability of drawing relevant attributes in $\boldsymbol{f}$ becomes progressively lower down the tree.

We now understand that if this problem of Random Forest is not addressed accordingly, poor-quality splitting attributes may be selected down the tree from which poor-quality partitions may generated. This may decrease individual accuracies of trees in a forest which in turn may affect the ensemble accuracy negatively. Yet, none of the above mentioned variants on subspacing of Random Forest addresses this issue. In this paper, we propose a new technique that dynamically increases the size of $\boldsymbol{f}$ down the tree based on the relative size of the current data segment to the entire training data set so that the probability of drawing relevant attributes in $\boldsymbol{f}$ does not get decreased.

The remainder of this paper is organized as follows: In Sect. 2 we explain the proposed technique. Section 3 discusses the experimental results in detail. Finally, we offer some concluding remarks in Sect. 4.

2 Our Technique

In the proposed technique, the number of attributes in $\boldsymbol{f}$ is dynamically increased with the decrease of records in the current data segment according to Eq. 1:

$$int(log_2(|\boldsymbol{m}| \times \frac{|\boldsymbol{D}|}{|\boldsymbol{D}_i|})) + 1 \tag{1}$$

Here, $|\boldsymbol{D}_i|$ denotes the number of records present in the current data segment and $|\boldsymbol{D}|$ denotes the number of records present in the entire training data set. The term $(\frac{|\boldsymbol{D}|}{|\boldsymbol{D}_i|})$ dynamically increases the number of attributes in $\boldsymbol{f}$ with the relative decrease of records in $\boldsymbol{D}_i$ to $\boldsymbol{D}$. For example, let $\boldsymbol{D} = 1000$ with $\boldsymbol{m} = 16$ and let $\boldsymbol{D}_i = 50$. Conventionally, $|\boldsymbol{f}|$ will remain as 5 for the $\boldsymbol{D}_i$ with 50 records in Random Forest even if the $\boldsymbol{D}_i$ is a result of a number of partitioning involving several splitting attributes. However, according to the proposed technique $|\boldsymbol{f}|$ is increased to 9 in this case.

Random Forest is modified through the proposed technique and its new form is presented in the following.

for ($i = 1$ **to** $|T|$) **do** /* $|T|$ is the number of trees in Random Forest */

Step 1: Generate a bootstrap sample from the training data set.

Step 2: Generate a decision tree from the bootstrap sample with subspaces generated from the proposed technique.

end for.

3 Experimental Results

We conduct the experimentation on five well known data sets that are publicly available from the UCI Machine Learning Repository [31]. We already know, when a data segment is partitioned by the splitting attribute, the resultant partitions tend to have very weak relationship with the splitting attribute specially when the attribute is categorical. Hence, in order to exhibit the effectiveness of the proposed technique we select all five data sets with all-categorical attributes. The data sets are listed in Table 1.

Table 1. Description of the data sets

Data Set name (DS)	Non-Class attributes	Records	Distinct class Values
Car Evaluation (CE)	06	1728	4
Chess (CHS)	36	3196	2
Hayes-Roth (HR)	04	132	3
Nursery (NUR)	08	12960	5
Tic-Tac-Toe Endgame (TTT)	09	958	2

We implement Random Forest (RF) and the Modified Random Forest (MRF) maintaining the following settings. We use Gini Index as a measure of classification capacity in accordance with RF. The minimum Gini Index value is set to 0.01 for any attribute to qualify for splitting a node. Each leaf node of a tree requires at least two records and no further post-pruning is applied. We apply majority voting in order to aggregate results for the forests. The entire experimentation is conducted by a single machine with Intel(R) 3.4 GHz processor and 4 GB Main Memory (RAM) running under 64-bit Windows 8.1 Operating System. All the results reported in this paper are obtained using 10-fold-cross-validation (10-CV) [10,29,30] for every data set.

In 10-CV, at first a data set is randomly divided into 10 horizontal segments/partitions. The segments are mutually exclusive meaning that they do not have any overlapping records. Each segment in turn is considered to be the testing data set (out of bag samples) while for the same turn the remaining nine segments are considered to be the training data set. Thus, we get 10 training data sets and 10 corresponding testing data sets. A classifier is then built from each training data set and its performance indicator (such as prediction accuracy) is tested on each corresponding testing data set. The average result obtained from all 10 testing data sets is termed to be 10-CV. The best results reported in this chapter are stressed through **bold-face**.

Ensemble Accuracy (EA) is one of the most important performance indicators for any decision forest algorithm [2,3,6]. In Table 2, we present the EA (in percent) of RF and MRF for all data sets considered.

Table 2. EA

DS	RF	MRF
CE	92.8	**93.9**
CHS	94.9	**97.0**
HR	71.1	**74.2**
NUR	95.0	**97.4**
TTT	84.5	**90.6**
Avg.	87.7	**90.6**

From Table 2, we see that MRF provides the best EA for all data sets considered. We know, EA of a decision forest mainly depends on two factors: individual tree accuracy and diversity among the trees. Hence, in order to explain reasons behind the improvement, we first compute individual accuracy (in percent) of each tree in a forest to compute the Average Individual Accuracy (AIA) for the forest as was done in literature [3–5, 9].

Margineantu and Dietterich [34] proposed a visualization method for classifier ensembles called Kappa that has been used extensively as a measure of diversity in literature [9, 29, 35, 42, 53]. Kappa typically estimates the diversity between *two trees* T_i and T_j. Diversity among *more than two trees* is computed by first computing the Kappa (K) value of a single tree T_i with the ensemble of trees except the tree in consideration (i.e. with $T - T_i$ where T is the set of all trees in the forest) [9]. The combined prediction of the forest (computed through the majority voting) can be regarded as a single tree T_j. Then Kappa is computed between T_i and T_j as shown in Eq. 2, where $Pr(a)$ is the probability of the observed agreement between two classifiers T_i and T_j, and $Pr(e)$ is the probability of the random agreement between T_i and T_j. Once the Kappa for every single tree T_i of a decision forest is computed we then compute the Average Individual Kappa (AIK) for the forest.

$$K = \frac{Pr(a) - Pr(e)}{1 - Pr(e)} \tag{2}$$

According to Eq. 2, when $K = 1$ two trees agree on every example. When $K = 0$ they disagree on every examples except agreements by chance. Rarely, K can be negative when two trees disagree in most examples suppressing agreements by chance. Thus, the lower the Kappa (K)/AIK value, the higher the diversity. The results related to AIA and AIK are reported in Table 3.

From Table 3, we observe that MRF achieves higher AIA for all data sets considered. This indicates that trees generated by MRF are individually more accurate; and we understand that this is due to the fact that MRF can effort better-quality splitting down the tree.

Table 3. AIA and AIK

	AIA		AIK	
DS	RF	MRF	RF	MRF
CE	83.5	**88.9**	**0.68**	0.82
CHS	68.0	**71.9**	**0.49**	0.56
HR	55.3	**56.2**	**0.33**	0.34
NUR	71.6	**80.8**	**0.65**	0.79
TTT	54.9	**59.4**	**0.32**	0.38
Avg.	66.6	**71.4**	**0.49**	0.58

4 Conclusion

In this paper, we propose a novel technique that dynamically increases the size of subspaces down the tree based on the relative size of the current data segment to the entire training data set so that the probability of drawing relevant attributes in subspaces does not get decreased. Aided by the proposed technique, Random Forest is able to generate better-quality trees (individually more accurate). This in turn helps Random Forest to attain higher ensemble accuracy. In future, we plan to apply the proposed technique on other decision forest algorithms.

References

1. Adnan, M.N., Islam, M.Z.: ComboSplit: Combining various splitting criteria for building a single decision tree. In: Proceedings of the International Conference on Artificial Intelligence and Pattern Recognition, pp. 1–8 (2014)
2. Adnan, M.N., Islam, M.Z.: A comprehensive method for attribute space extension for random forest. In: Proceedings of 17th International Conference on Computer and Information Technology, Dec (2014)
3. Adnan, M.N., Islam, M.Z.: Complement random forest. In: Proceedings of the 13th Australasian Data Mining Conference (AusDM), pp. 89–97 (2015)
4. Adnan, M.N., Islam, M.Z.: Improving the random forest algorithm by randomly varying the size of the bootstrap samples for low dimensional data sets. In: Proceedings of the European Symposium on Artificial Neural Networks, Computational Intelligence and Machine Learning, pp. 391–396 (2015)
5. Adnan, M.N., Islam, M.Z.: One-vs-all binarization technique in the context of random forest. In: Proceedings of the European Symposium on Artificial Neural Networks, Computational Intelligence and Machine Learning, pp. 385–390 (2015)
6. Adnan, M.N., Islam, M.Z.: Forest CERN: A New Decision Forest Building Technique. In: Bailey, J., Khan, L., Washio, T., Dobbie, G., Huang, J.Z., Wang, R. (eds.) PAKDD 2016. LNCS (LNAI), vol. 9651, pp. 304–315. Springer, Cham (2016). doi:10.1007/978-3-319-31753-3_25
7. Adnan, M.N., Islam, M.Z.: Knowledge discovery from a data set on dementia through decision forest. In: Proceedings of the 14th Australasian Data Mining Conference (AusDM) (2016). Accepted

8. Adnan, M.N., Islam, M.Z.: Optimizing the number of trees in a decision forest to discover a subforest with high ensemble accuracy using a genetic algorithm. Knowl. Based Syst. **110**, 86–97 (2016)
9. Amasyali, M.F., Ersoy, O.K.: Classifier ensembles with the extended space forest. IEEE Trans. Knowl. Data Eng. **16**, 145–153 (2014)
10. Arlot, S.: A survey of cross-validation procedures for model selection. Stat. Surv. **4**, 40–79 (2010)
11. Barros, R.C., Basgalupp, M.P., de Carvalho, A.C.P.L.F., Freitas, A.A.: A survey of evolutionary algorithm for decision tree induction. IEEE Trans. Syst. Man Cybern. Part C Appl. Rev. **42**(3), 291–312 (2012)
12. Bernard, S., Adam, S., Heutte, L.: Dynamic random forests. Pattern Recognit. Lett. **33**, 1580–1586 (2012)
13. Bernard, S., Heutte, L., Adam, S.: Forest-RK: A New Random Forest Induction Method. In: Huang, D.-S., Wunsch, D.C., Levine, D.S., Jo, K.-H. (eds.) ICIC 2008. LNCS, vol. 5227, pp. 430–437. Springer, Heidelberg (2008). doi:10.1007/978-3-540-85984-0_52
14. Bishop, C.M.: Pattern Recognition and Machine Learning. Springer, New York (2008)
15. Breiman, L.: Bagging predictors. Mach. Learn. **24**, 123–140 (1996)
16. Breiman, L.: Random forests. Mach. Learn. **45**, 5–32 (2001)
17. Breiman, L., Friedman, J., Olshen, R., Stone, C.: Classification and Regression Trees. Wadsworth International Group. San Diego (1985)
18. Burges, C.J.C.: A tutorial on support vector machines for pattern recognition. Data Min. Knowl. Discov. **2**, 121–167 (1998)
19. Cutler, A., Zhao, G.: Pert: perfect random tree ensembles. Comput. Sci. Stat. **33**, 204–497 (2001)
20. Geurts, P., Ernst, D., Wehenkel, L.: Extremely randomized trees. Mach. Learn. **63**, 3–42 (2006)
21. Han, J., Kamber, M.: Data Mining Concepts and Techniques. Morgan Kaufmann Publishers (2006)
22. Ho, T.K.: The random subspace method for constructing decision forests. IEEE Trans. Pattern Anal. Mach. Intell. **20**, 832–844 (1998)
23. Hunt, E., Marin, J., Stone, P.: Experiments in Induction. Academic Press, New York (1966)
24. Islam, M.Z., Giggins, H.: Knowledge discovery through sysfor - a systematically developed forest of multiple decision trees. In: Proceedings of the 9th Australlasian Data Mining Conference (2011)
25. Jain, A.K., Mao, J.: Artificial neural network: a tutorial. Computer **29**(3), 31–44 (1996)
26. Kataria, A., Singh, M.D.: A review of data classification using k-nearest neighbour algorithm. Int. J. Emerg. Technol. Adv. Eng. **3**(6), 354–360 (2013)
27. Kotsiantis, S.B.: Decision trees: a recent overview. Artif. Intell. Rev. **39**, 261–283 (2013)
28. Kuncheva, L.I., Whitaker, C.J.: Measures of diversity in classifier ensembles and their relationship with ensemble accuracy. Mach. Learn. **51**, 181–207 (2003)
29. Kurgan, L.A., Cios, K.J.: Caim discretization algorithm. IEEE Trans. Knowl. Data Eng. **16**, 145–153 (2004)
30. Li, J., Liu, H.: Ensembles of cascading trees. In: Proceedings of the third IEEE International Conference on Data Mining, pp. 585–588. (2003)
31. Lichman, M.: UCI machine learning repository. http://archive.ics.uci.edu/ml/datasets.html. Accessed 15 Mar 2016

32. Liu, S., Patel, R.Y., Daga, P.R., Liu, H., Fu, G., Doerksen, R.J., Chen, Y., Wilkins, D.E.: Combined rule extraction and feature elimination in supervised classification. IEEE Trans. NanoBioscience **11**(3), 228–236 (2012)
33. Maimon, O., Rokach, L. (eds.): The Data Mining and Knowledge Discovery Handbook. Springer, New York (2005)
34. Margineantu, D.D., Dietterich, T.G.: Pruning adaptive boosting. In: Proceedings of the 14th International Conference on Machine Learning, pp. 211–218 (1997)
35. Maudes, J., Rodriguez, J.J., Osorio, C.G., Pedrajas, N.G.: Random feature weights for decision tree ensemble construction. Inf. Fusion **13**, 20–30 (2012)
36. Menze, B., Petrich, W., Hamprecht, F.: Multivariate feature selection and hierarchical classification for infrared spectroscopy: serum-based detection of bovine spongiform encephalopathy. Anal. Bioanal. Chem. **387**, 1801–1807 (2007)
37. Mitchell, T.M.: Machine Learning. McGraw-Hill, New York (1997)
38. Murthy, S.K.: On growing better decision trees from data. Ph.D. thesis, The Johns Hopkins University, Baltimore, Maryland (1997)
39. Murthy, S.K.: Automatic construction of decision trees from data: a multi-disciplinary survey. Data Min. Knowl. Discov. **2**, 345–389 (1998)
40. Quinlan, J.R.: C4.5: Programs for Machine Learning. Morgan Kaufmann Publishers, San Mateo (1993)
41. Quinlan, J.R.: Improved use of continuous attributes in c4.5. J. Artif. Intell. Res. **4**, 77–90 (1996)
42. Rodriguez, J.J., Kuncheva, L.I., Alonso, C.J.: Rotation forest: a new classifier ensemble method. IEEE Trans. Pattern Anal. Mach. Intell. **28**, 1619–1630 (2006)
43. Saeys, Y., Abeel, T., Van de Peer, Y.: Robust feature selection using ensemble feature selection techniques. In: Daelemans, W., Goethals, B., Morik, K. (eds.) ECML PKDD 2008. LNCS, vol. 5212, pp. 313–325. Springer, Heidelberg (2008). doi:10.1007/978-3-540-87481-2_21
44. Shipp, C.A., Kuncheva, L.I.: Relationships between combination methods and measures of diversity in combining classifiers. Inf. Fusion **3**, 135–148 (2002)
45. Robnik-Šikonja, M.: Improving Random Forests. In: Boulicaut, J.-F., Esposito, F., Giannotti, F., Pedreschi, D. (eds.) ECML 2004. LNCS (LNAI), vol. 3201, pp. 359–370. Springer, Heidelberg (2004). doi:10.1007/978-3-540-30115-8_34
46. Tan, P.N., Steinbach, M., Kumar, V.: Introduction to Data Mining. Pearson Education, Boston(2006)
47. Tang, E.K., Suganthan, P.N., Yao, X.: An analysis of diversity measures. Mach. Learn. **65**, 247–271 (2006)
48. Tuv, E., Borisov, A., Runger, G., Torkkola, K.: Feature selection with ensembles, artificial variables, and redundancy elimination. J. Mach. Learn. Res. **10**, 1341–1366 (2009)
49. Williams, G.J.: Combining decision trees: Initial results from the MIL algorithm. In: Proceedings of the First Australian Joint Artificial Intelligence Conference, pp. 273–289, Sydney, Australia, 2–4 Nov 1988, 1987
50. Ye, Y., Wu, Q., Huang, J.Z., Ng, M.K., Li, X.: Stratified sampling of feature subspace selection in random forests for high dimensional data. Pattern Recognit. **46**, 769–787 (2014)
51. Zhang, G., Patuwo, B.E., Hu, M.Y.: Forecasting with artificial neural networks: the state of the art. Int. J. Forecast. **14**, 35–62 (1998)
52. Zhang, G.P.: Neural networks for classification: a survey. IEEE Trans. Syst. Man Cybern. **30**, 451–462 (2000)
53. Zhang, L., Suganthan, P.N.: Random forests with ensemble of feature spaces. Pattern Recognit. **47**, 3429–3437 (2014)

Diversity and Locality in Multi-Component, Multi-Layer Predictive Systems: A Mutual Information Based Approach

Bassma Al-Jubouri(✉) and Bogdan Gabrys

Data Science Institute, Bournemouth University, Dorset BH12 5BB, UK
{baljubouri,bgabrys}@bournemouth.ac.uk
http://staffprofiles.bournemouth.ac.uk/display/i7217997
http://bogdan-gabrys.com

Abstract. This paper discusses the effect of locality and diversity among the base models of a Multi-Components Multi-Layer Predictive System (MCMLPS). A new ensemble method is introduced, where in the proposed architecture, the data instances are assigned to local regions using a conditional mutual information based on the similarity of their features. Furthermore, the outputs of the base models are weighted by this similarity metric. The proposed architecture has been tested on a number of data sets and its performance was compared to four benchmark algorithms. Moreover, the effect of changing three parameters of the proposed architecture has been tested and compared.

Keywords: Ensemble diversity · Ensemble methods · Local learning · Conditional mutual information · Feature selection

1 Introduction

Ensemble learning have shown many theoretical and practical benefits compared to the use of a single best model [13,18]. As opposed to using a single predictor, ensemble methods have statistical benefits acquired from combining the output of several predictors. It provides a divide and conquer strategy that a single predictor is incapable of achieving when the problem is too difficult and provides a more accurate representation of the data when the data is generated from different sources (data fusion).

An early example of the use of ensemble methods in literature is presented in [7], where the feature space is partitioned using two or more classifiers. In the nineties, two of the most widely used ensemble methods where proposed, these are: Boosting [19] and Bagging [3]. Schapire introduced Boosting algorithm in [19] where the author showed that a strong learner can be built by combining a number of weak learners. The introduction of Boosting has led to the development of AdaBoost and its many variations to solve multi-class and regression problems. Meanwhile, Breiman introduced Bagging in [3], where the base predictors are trained on bootstrap replicas of the training data. In addition to these

G. Cong et al. (Eds.): ADMA 2017, LNAI 10604, pp. 313–325, 2017.
https://doi.org/10.1007/978-3-319-69179-4_22

two algorithms, many well performing ensemble methods were developed and used in a wide area of applications, such as stacked generalization [20], mixture of experts [10] and negative correlation learning [8] among others.

In literature, it has been shown that there are two conditions for an ensembles to perform better than a single predictor. These are that the base predictors should be diverse (their error correlation is reduced) and that they have a reasonable level of performance [18]. In ensemble learning diversity has been acknowledged as an important characteristic [6]. An ensemble with diverse models can have better performance due to the complementary behaviour of its components [21], however, as shown in [17] the diversity measure used has to be chosen carefully so it works with the used combiner.

The work presented in this paper builds on our broader investigations of multilevel structures of classifiers and predictors [11,14,16,18] and directly follows from our previous work presented in [1]. It discusses diversity as a characteristic of an MCMLPS, and investigates its effect on the accuracy of prediction.

The organization of this paper is: in Sect. 2 a new type of ensemble system is introduced. Section 3 explores the methodology and the design cycle of the proposed locally trained MCMLPS. Section 4 discusses the experimental work in the paper and the obtained results. It compares the testing accuracy of the system with four benchmark algorithms and studies the relation between the overall accuracy of the ensemble and the amount of disagreements among the base predictors. Section 5 explores a number of variations in the parameters of the proposed systems. Finally Sect. 6 draws the main conclusions in the paper.

2 Multi-Component, Multi-Layer Predictive Systems

The MCMLPS used in this study was introduced in [1] and it is shown in Fig. 1; where $w_{11},\ldots,w_{nk}$, are the weights of the first layer, n represent the number of the base ensembles and k represent the number of the models inside the base ensembles. Furthermore, $w_1,\ldots,w_n$ are the weights of the second layer for the n base ensembles. $M_1,\ldots,M_k$ are the base predictors of the first layer ensembles, $g_1,\ldots,g_n$ are the ensembles created from combining the base predictors, $h(x)$ is the second layer combiner and $\hat{Y}$ is the final prediction of the system. Let X be the data set containing the training objects, C represent the number of classes, θ_c represent the actual class and M_k^n represent the output prediction of the model (shown in the first layer of the ensemble in Fig. 1), where $M_k^n = 1$ for class θ_c and 0 otherwise and $c = 1,..,C$. The outputs of the base predictors M_k^n and the ensemble g_n are given as c-dimensional binary vectors where $[M_1^j,..,M_k^j]^T \in \{0,1\}^c$ and $[g_1,..,g_j]^T \in [0,1]^c$, j=1,...,n respectively. Equations 1 and 2 show the mathematical representation for the ensembles generated from the first layer:

$$g_j(x) = \Sigma_{i=1}^k w_{1j} M_i^{(j)}(x) \tag{1}$$

and let

$$d_{j,c}(x) = \begin{cases} 1 & if\ g_j(x) \ = \theta_c, \\ 0 & otherwise. \end{cases} \tag{2}$$

Then the second layer ensemble is as:

$$h(x) = \Sigma_{j=1}^{m} w_{2j} d_{j,c} \tag{3}$$

and the final prediction of the system is:

$$\hat{Y} = \arg\max_{c} h(x). \tag{4}$$

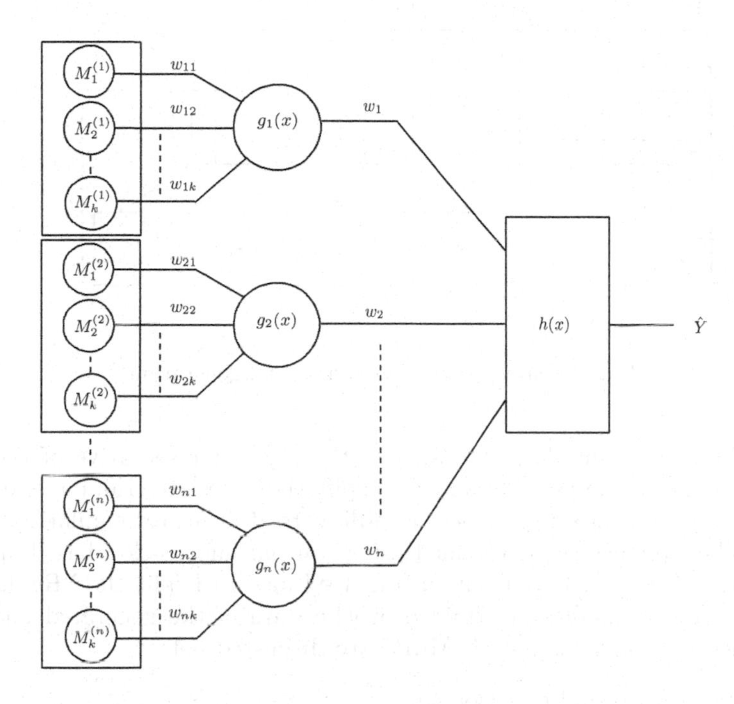

Fig. 1. The multi-component multi-layer predictive system.

3 Designing MCMLPS: Methodology

Despite the similarities between the MCMLPS presented in this paper with that presented in [1], there is a key difference between these systems. The approach introduced in [1] is an unsupervised learning approach, where the base predictors are trained on disjoint sets of the data for which only subsets of the features are selected. Meanwhile, the MCMLPS presented in this paper is a supervised learning approach in which the base predictors are trained on subsets of the features for all of the training data. Moreover, it uses a different similarity metric. The methodology used to built the MCMLPS encompasses the following phases: (a) data preparation and partitioning, (b) model generation and combination.

In order to validate and examine the generalization ability of the proposed architecture, the Density Preserving Sampling (DPS) [5] is used to partition the

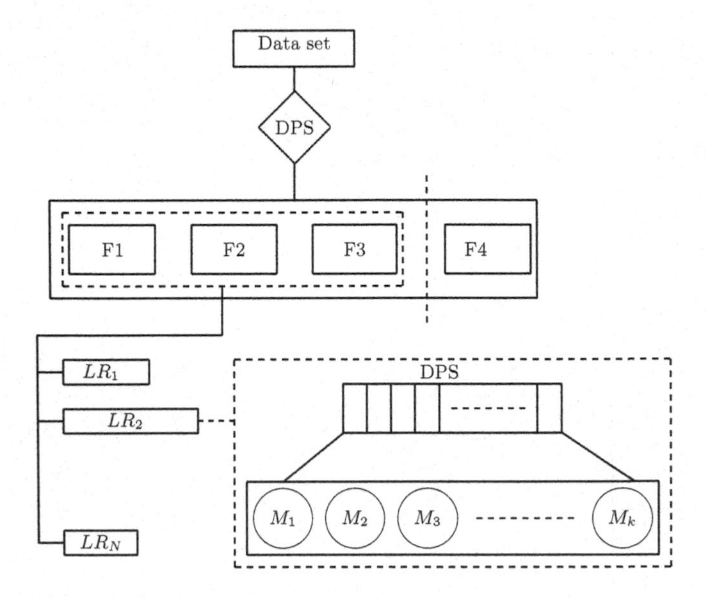

Fig. 2. Data preparation and model generation.

data. DPS divides the data into subsets that are representative of the whole data set [5]. In this work DPS is used to split the data into training and testing sets. The training data is assigned according to its features similarity to a set of LRs. The similarity is determined using mutual information based approach (discussed in Subsect. 3.1). Then DPS is used again to split the LRs data into K folds, where K models are trained on the data of the generated folds. The general design phases for the MCMLPS are discussed below:

- Data preparation and partitioning:
  The data goes through three partitioning stages, first the whole data is split into training and testing sets, then the training set is allocated to the LRs and finally within the LRs the data is split into K subsets which are used to train the local models. Figure 2 shows the preparation and partitioning of the data, where, $F_1, ...F_4$ are the folds generated from the first DPS split, $LR_1, ...LR_N$ are the LRs and $M_1, ...M_k$ are the local models within the regions trained using data from the second DPS split.

  The points given below summarise the procedure used in this phase:

  - Apply DPS to split the data into 4 representative folds.
  - Use 3 out of 4 folds for training and the last fold for testing.
  - Find the similarity matrix for the training data using the mutual information of the features.
  - Choose N rows from the similarity matrix to be the seeds for the LRs.
  - Add the training data to the LRs according to the similarity of data features to the LRs seeds.

- Apply k fold DPS to the LRs data.

– Model generation, testing and combining:
Once the data is assigned to the relevant LRs, the second DPS is applied to generate the K folds within the LRs and K models are trained on the LR folds. Furthermore, for all new instances N weights values are computed with respect to the N LRs. This phase can be summarized as follow:

- Train a predictive model on each of the K LRs folds.
- Compute the weights of the LRs votes using the similarity between the LRs seeds and the testing data.

In the first layer, N ensembles are generated from combining the models of the N LRs. While, in the second layer a single ensemble that combines the first layer N ensembles is generated. The combining method used is a weighted majority vote with the similarity of the LRs features used as the weights in both layers. The procedure is repeated for all four folds $F1, ...F4$, so that each time a different fold is used for testing.

3.1 Conditional Mutual Information Based LRs

This approach aims to split the feature space into a number of subsets based on their Conditional Mutual Information (CMI). The features with the highest CMI values are chosen to be the seeds for the LRs. The CMI is measured using the following equation [4]:

$$J_{cmi}(X_k) = I(X_k; Y) - I(X_k; S) + I(X_k, S|Y) \tag{5}$$

where X_k is a single feature, Y is the output and S are the remaining features (all the features apart from X_k). $I(X_k; Y)$ is the mutual information between the feature X_k and the class Y, $I(X_k; S)$ is the redundancy of feature X_k with respect to the remaining features and $I(X_k, S|Y)$ is the conditional redundancy (the class dependency of X_k with the existing feature set S). According to [4] the equation given above shows that including correlated features can be useful, if the correlation of the features with the class is higher than their inner correlation. The benefits of including correlated features have been explored before by [9], where it has been observed that "correlation does not imply redundancy" .

Once the CMI values of the features are computed using Eq. 5, the highest N features are selected to be the seeds for the LRs. In order to add new features to the LRs, the similarity of the features to the LRs seeds need to be calculated. Equation 6 is used to determine the similarity between the features and the LRs seeds.

$$J_{cmi+}(X_k) = I(X_k; Y) + I(X_k; J_{cmi}(X_k)) + I(X_k, J_{cmi}(X_k)|Y) \tag{6}$$

In this equation the pairwise mutual information of the features with the LR seeds is calculated and the features that have the highest CMI with respect to the seeds are added to the LRs. By adding rather than subtracting the redundancy term $I(X_k; J_{cmi}(X_k))$ this approach aims to group together similar features in the LRs. Each LR is assigned with a subset of the features, where all the features are ranked according to their mutual information with the seed of the LR and only the highest ranking features are assigned to the LR. The ratio of the features assigned to the LRs is α, where $1 > \alpha > 0$.

In order to use this approach to build an MCMLPS, initially the data is split using the method presented in Fig. 2. DPS is also used to split the data into training and testing. Then the following steps are taken to split the training data into the N LRs:

1. Calculate the CMI among the training data features using Eq. 5.
2. Choose the highest scoring N features to be the seeds of the LRs.
3. For the remaining features, use Eq. 6 to rank the features according to their similarity to the LRs seeds.
4. Based on the features mutual information with the seeds, assign α of the total number of features to the LRs.

In both layers weighted majority vote is used to combine the respective predictions, where the mutual information of the LRs features is used as the weighing vector. The weights of the predictions of the LRs models are calculated using the summation of the mutual information values of the LR features.

4 Results

The MI based MCMLPS introduced in this paper is applied to the data sets shown in Table 1. The data sets used are taken from the UCI machine learning archive [12]. The performance of this system is compared to correlation based MCMLPS [1], Rotation Forest (RF) [15], Bagging [3] and AdaBoost [19]. The settings for these benchmark algorithms is as follows:

- MI based MCMLPS: 6 LR's are used with each having 8 models (48 Decision Trees (DT's) in total) trained on α subset of the features.
- Correlation based MCMLPS: 6 LR's are used with each having 8 models trained on disjoint subsets of the data. The number of features used in the LRs is determined through a separate optimization routine [1].
- RF: the number of classifier are 6 and the number of disjoint features subspaces are 6.
- AdaBoost and Bagging: 48 DT were used as the weak learners for both algorithms.

In order to be able to compare the results obtained from this system with the correlation based MCMLPS, both the number of the LRs and the number of models inside the LRs are set to the same numbers (6 LRs with 8 models inside each one of the LRs). Furthermore the α value (the ratio of the features assigned to the LRs) is set to 30% of the features. The base predictors used are CART DTs and feedforward Neural Networks (NNs). The following subsections discuss

Table 1. Data sets used in the experiments.

Data sets	Features	Examples	Classes
Ionosphere	34	351	2
Pima	8	768	2
Wisconsin Breast Cancer (WBC)	30	569	2
Heart	13	270	2
Sonar	60	208	2
Chess	36	3196	2
German credit card	24	1000	2
Spam base	57	4601	2
Gaussian 8D	8	5000	2
Vehicle	18	846	4
Waveform	40	5000	3

the internal accuracies of the LRs base predictors and compare the overall system performance with the benchmark algorithms. This is followed by a subsection that investigates the level of disagreement among the LRs prediction of the proposed MI based MCMLPS and compare its overall performance with benchmark algorithms.

4.1 Internal Accuracy and Benchmark Comparison

In this section the internal accuracies of the LRs base predictors (CART DTs) are measured and compared across the four DPS folds. An example of the LRs base predictors internal accuracies for the Gaussian 8 dimensional data set is shown in Fig. 3. Figure 3 shows that, there are no single LRs that outperform the other LRs on all of the four folds. In the MI approach even small data sets like the Ionosphere data set, has a lower variation in its internal accuracies compared to the results of the correlation based MCMLPS [1]. A possible explanation for this is that the LRs in this case are trained on a subset of the features for the whole data set rather than being trained on disjoint subsets of the data. The overall testing accuracy of the MI based MCMLPS averaged over the four DPS iterations are shown in Table 2. In addition, the Table shows the test accuracies of the four benchmark algorithms (correlation based MCMLPS, RF, Bagging and AdaBoost algorithms). The results show that, this approach for generating the LRs has generally improved the testing accuracy obtained from the correlation based MCMLPS.

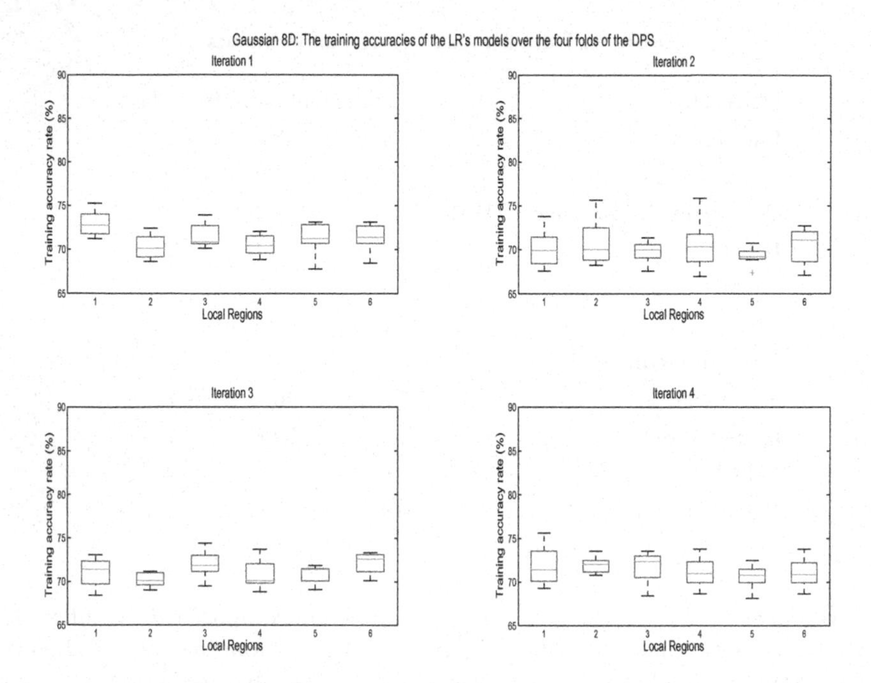

Fig. 3. Training accuracies of the local regions models for the Gaussian 8D data set when CART DTs are used as the base predictors.

Furthermore, it can be seen in Table 2 that Bagging has the highest test accuracy on all the data sets except for the waveform data set, where the RF has the highest accuracy. Nevertheless, our proposed MCMLPS has a comparable accuracy to the Bagging algorithm, with accuracy difference ranges from having the same accuracy for WBC data set to 6.2 for the heart data set. Furthermore, Table 3 shows the test accuracy of the MI based MCMLPS compared to the correlation base MCMLPS and the RF, when the type of the base predictors is changed from CART DTs to feedforward NNs. In the RF algorithm, the testing accuracy increases on every single data set when the feedforward NNs are used as the base predictors. On the other hand, the MI based MCMLPS showed mixed responses, where the accuracy increased for only 4 out of 11 data sets.

4.2 Disagreement Among the Base Predictors

The disagreements among the LRs votes and the final prediction, when CART DTs as well as feedforward NNs are used as the base predictors for the MI based MCMLPs, are shown in Fig. 4. The total disagreement values are found by measuring the disagreement between the final prediction of the system and the prediction of the individual LRs ensembles. In Fig. 4 it can be noticed that, in the proposed architecture, when CART DTs are used as the base predictors there are varied levels of disagreements within the LRs models and even a higher

Table 2. Benchmark comparison: Testing accuracy using CART DTs as the base predictors for both correlation based and MI based MCMLPS.

Data sets	MI based MCMLPS	Correlation based MCMLPS	RF	Bagging	AdaBoost
Gaussian 8D	86.94	88.16	80.70	88.78	87.08
German	74.60	70.00	65.30	77.30	75.90
Ionosphere	92.30	77.19	92.61	93.44	93.16
Spam base	93.81	85.20	85.50	95.37	93.20
Pima	75.78	76.62	73.30	77.60	77.08
WBC	95.61	86.29	91.56	95.61	95.25
Heart	78.89	76.65	77.06	85.18	83.34
Sonar	84.62	63.46	74.04	87.02	83.17
Chess	98.78	93.74	70.46	98.99	94.84
Vehicle	74.35	67.61	61.37	77.07	51.07
Waveform	81.80	65.68	91.46	85.74	80.78

Table 3. Benchmark comparison: Testing accuracy using feedforward NNs as the base predictors for the MI based MCMLPS.

Data sets	MI based MCMLPS	Energy based MCMLPS	RF
Gaussian 8D	84.22	88.45	88.4
German credit cards	77.50	70.00	70.00
Ionosphere	90.03	74.25	93.15
Spambase	90.44	90.55	85.75
Pima indians diabetes	76.04	76.30	76.80
WBC	94.90	91.55	95.61
Heart	82.61	77.02	81.12
Sonar	82.21	62.50	79.81
Chess	94.65	96.75	73.06
Vehicle	79.67	78.50	81.75
Waveform	85.36	85.05	92.65

level of disagreement across the LRs. On the other hand, when feedforward NNs are used as the base predictors, similar models are generated in the individual LRs, yet there is still a high level of disagreement across the LRs. The high level of disagreement of the proposed architecture can be beneficial when applied on noisy data sets.

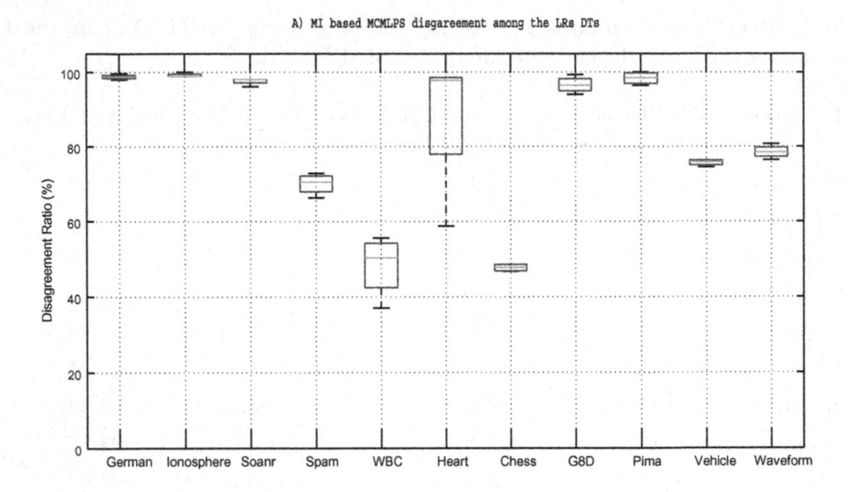

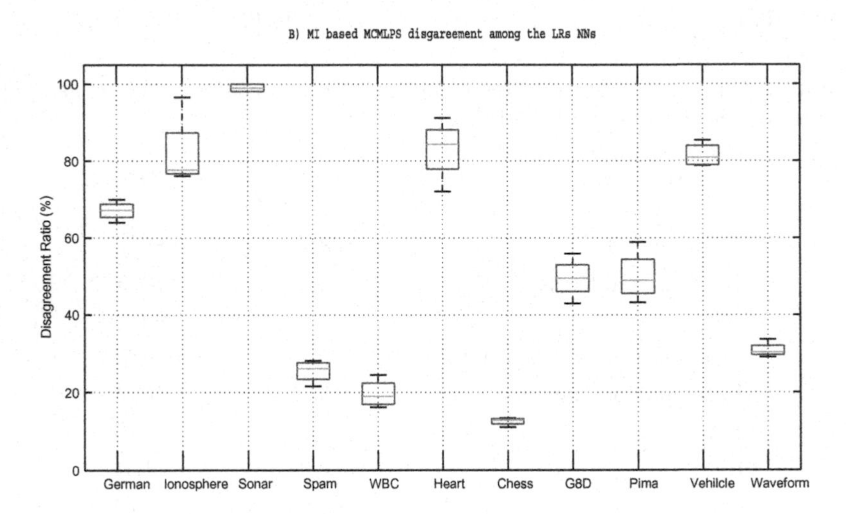

Fig. 4. Disagreements among the LRs of MI based MCMLPS when CART DTs and feedforward NNs are used as the base predictors.

5 Variation of the Conditional Mutual Information

This section investigates the effect of changing three aspects of the proposed MI based architecture. These are: modifying the equation used to find the LR seeds, partitioning the data using Cross Validation (CV) instead of DPS and changing the ratio of features allocated to the LRs. Table 4 compares the testing accuracy for the proposed architecture when the data is sampled using DPS as well as CV and when the conditional redundancy is included or excluded from the CMI equation.

Table 4. Benchmark comparison: Testing accuracy using feedforward NNs as the base predictors for the MI based MCMLPS.

Data sets	DPS with conditional redundancy	DPS ignore conditional redundancy	CV with conditional redundancy
Gaussian 8D	86.94	83.48	84.74
German credit cards	74.60	77.40	76.20
Ionosphere	92.30	91.16	88.28
Spambase	93.81	92.85	92.63
Pima indians diabetes	75.78	72.14	75.52
WBC	95.61	91.20	91.56
Heart	78.89	71.84	77.44
Sonar	84.62	76.92	78.85
Chess	98.78	80.88	95.08
Vehicle	74.35	74.35	63.01
Waveform	81.80	81.70	81.22

5.1 Ignoring the Conditional Redundancy with Respect to the Class

In this case the conditional mutual information term $I(X_k, S|Y)$ is removed from Eq. 5. This transforms the feature selection process to mutual information feature selection proposed by Battiti [2] given in Eq. 7:

$$J_{cmi}(X_k) = I(X_k; Y) - \beta I(X_k; X_j) \tag{7}$$

where β is a configurable parameter for which, according to Battiti [2], the optimal value is often 1. The aim of this section is to compare the case where correlated features are considered as redundant and are removed from the feature selection process with the case where the conditional redundancy between the features is assessed with respect to the class. The results showed that, apart from the German credit card data set, the cases where the conditional redundancy is considered in selecting the features, have higher accuracies than the cases where the conditional redundancy are removed during features selection.

5.2 Using CV Instead of DPS

In this subsection stratified CV is used to partition the data set into training and testing sets and then to partition the LRs data into K folds. Table 4 shows the testing accuracies averaged over the four iterations, and it can be seen that using DPS to split the data produce higher accuracies than that obtained from using stratified CV.

5.3 Changing the Ratio of Features Used in the LRs

In the previous experiments, the ratio of features used in the LRs of the MI based MCMLPS was set to 30%. Using a higher or lower feature ratio have been tested on the data sets used in these experiments. It has been found that lowering this ratio from 30% to 10% decreases the accuracy of the LRs prediction as well as the overall accuracy of the system. Meanwhile, increasing it to 80% result in a slight improving in the prediction accuracy for some of the data sets used in this experiment and it remained unchanged for the rest.

6 Conclusions and Future Work

This paper introduces a local learning based algorithm for MCMLPS. The architecture consists of multiple LRs. Each LR has multiple models trained on subsets of the features. These subsets of features are assigned to the LRs according to the similarity calculated using their conditional mutual information.

Investigating the internal performance of the proposed architecture showed that the overall testing accuracies of the architecture exceeded the average internal accuracies of its LRs models. The amount of variation in the internal accuracy depends mainly on the size and dimensionality of the data. The results showed that both the number of LRs and the number of models developed within the LRs need to be optimised with respect to the data set size and dimensionality.

This paper also explored changing three aspects of the proposed architecture. The first aspect is modifying the equation used to find the LR seeds, where removing the correlation redundancy term from the CMI equation resulted in deterioration of the performance of the proposed architecture. This result support the claim in [4], that including correlated features can be useful if their correlation with the class is higher than their inner correlation. The second aspect is partitioning the data using CV instead of DPS. Changing the sampling technique did have a negative effect on the performance of the proposed architecture, where mainly the accuracy obtained from DPS is higher than that obtained from CV. Finally, increasing the ratio of the features used in the LRs may improve the accuracy of the MCMLPS for certain data sets.

The locality of the proposed architecture and the high level of disagreement among its base predictors can be beneficial in noisy environments. For example, when the noise is applied to only a part of the data, it will not have the same effect on all of the MCMLPS base predictors. The robustness of the proposed architecture to external noise will be investigated in future work.

References

1. Al-Jubouri, B., Gabrys, B.: Local learning for multi-layer, multi-component predictive system. Procedia Comput. Sci. **96**, 723–732 (2016)
2. Battiti, R.: Using mutual information for selecting features in supervised neural net learning. IEEE Trans. Neural Netw. **5**(4), 537–550 (1994)

3. Breiman, L.: Bagging predictors. Mach. Learn. **24**(2), 123–140 (1996)
4. Brown, G., Pocock, A., Zhao, M.J., Luján, M.: Conditional likelihood maximisation: a unifying framework for information theoretic feature selection. J. Mach. Learn. Res. **13**, 27–66 (2012)
5. Budka, M., Gabrys, B.: Density-preserving sampling: robust and efficient alternative to cross-validation for error estimation. IEEE Trans. Neural Netw. Learn. Syst. **24**(1), 22–34 (2013)
6. Cunningham, P., Carney, J.: Diversity versus quality in classification ensembles based on feature selection. In: López de Mántaras, R., Plaza, E. (eds.) ECML 2000. LNCS, vol. 1810, pp. 109–116. Springer, Heidelberg (2000). doi:10.1007/3-540-45164-1_12
7. Dasarathy, B.V., Sheela, B.V.: A composite classifier system design: concepts and methodology. Proc. IEEE **67**(5), 708–713 (1979)
8. Eastwood, M., Gabrys, B.: The dynamics of negative correlation learning. J. VLSI Signal Proc. **49**, 251–263 (2007)
9. Guyon, I., Gunn, S., Nikravesh, M., Zadeh, L.A.: Feature Extraction: Foundations and Applications, vol. 207. Springer, Heidelberg (2008)
10. Jacobs, R.A., Jordan, M.I., Nowlan, S.J., Hinton, G.E.: Adaptive mixtures of local experts. Neural Comput. **3**(1), 79–87 (1991)
11. Kadlec, P., Gabrys, B.: Architecture for development of adaptive on-line prediction models. Memet. Comput. **1**(4), 241–269 (2009)
12. Lichman, M.: UCI machine learning repository (2013). http://archive.ics.uci.edu/ml
13. Polikar, R.: Ensemble based systems in decision making. IEEE Circuits Syst. Mag. **6**(3), 21–45 (2006)
14. Riedel, S., Gabrys, B.: Pooling for combination of multi level forecasts. IEEE Trans. Knowl. Data Eng. **12**(21), 1753–1766 (2009)
15. Rodriguez, J.J., Kuncheva, L.I., Alonso, C.J.: Rotation forest: a new classifier ensemble method. IEEE Trans. Pattern Anal. Mach. Intell. **28**(10), 1619–1630 (2006)
16. Ruta, D., Gabrys, B., Lemke, C.: A generic multilevel architecture for time series prediction. IEEE Trans. Knowl. Data Eng. **23**(3), 350–359 (2011)
17. Ruta, D., Gabrys, B.: New Measure of Classifier Dependency in Multiple Classifier Systems. In: Roli, F., Kittler, J. (eds.) MCS 2002. LNCS, vol. 2364, pp. 127–136. Springer, Heidelberg (2002). doi:10.1007/3-540-45428-4_13
18. Ruta, D., Gabrys, B.: Classifier selection for majority voting. Inf. Fusion **6**(1), 63–81 (2005)
19. Schapire, R.E.: The strength of weak learnability. Mach. Learn. **5**(2), 197–227 (1990)
20. Wolpert, D.H.: Stacked generalization. Neural Netw. **5**(2), 241–259 (1992)
21. Xue, F., Subbu, R., Bonissone, P.: Locally weighted fusion of multiple predictive models. In: International Joint Conference on Neural Networks, 2006. IJCNN'06, pp. 2137–2143. IEEE (2006)

Hybrid Subspace Mixture Models for Prediction and Anomaly Detection in High Dimensions

Jenn-Bing Ong(✉) and Wee-Keong Ng

School of Computer Science and Engineering, Nanyang Technological University, Singapore, Singapore
{ongj0063,awkng}@ntu.edu.sg

Abstract. Robust learning of mixture models in high dimensions remains an open challenge and especially so in current big data era. This paper investigates twelve variants of hybrid mixture models that combine the G-means clustering, Gaussian, and Student t-distribution mixture models for high-dimensional predictive modeling and anomaly detection. High-dimensional data is first reduced to lower-dimensional subspace using whitened principal component analysis. For real-time data processing in batch mode, a technique based on Gram-Schmidt orthogonalization process is proposed and demonstrated to update the reduced dimensions to remain relevant in fulfilling the task objectives. In addition, a model-adaptation technique is proposed and demonstrated for big data incremental learning by statistically matching the mixture components' mean and variance vectors; the adapted parameters are computed based on weighted average that takes into account the sample size of new and older statistics with a parameter to scale down the influence of older statistics in each iterative computation. The hybrid models' performance are evaluated using simulation and empirical studies. Results show that simple hybrid models without the Expectation-Maximization training step can achieve equally high performance in high dimensions that is comparable to the more sophisticated models. For unsupervised anomaly detection, the hybrid models achieve detection rate $\gtrsim 90\%$ with injected anomalies from 1% to 60% using the KDD Cup 1999 network intrusion dataset.

Keywords: Mixture models · Coarse filtering · Model adaptation · Parameter rating · Dimensionality reduction · Incremental learning · Diffusion map

1 Introduction

Mixture models have been widely used in many applications such as speaker verification, background subtraction for real-time tracking, and biological applications. Efficient algorithm to learn mixture of Gaussians in high dimensions with small error bound has recently been demonstrated [6]. However, practical algorithms for robust and adaptive learning of high-dimensional mixture models

G. Cong et al. (Eds.): ADMA 2017, LNAI 10604, pp. 326–339, 2017.
https://doi.org/10.1007/978-3-319-69179-4_23

is still an open challenge [13]. This paper extends the work of a robust subspace mixture model initially developed by [2] for anomaly detection to predictive modeling in high dimensions. High-dimensional data is reduced to lower dimensional subspace using whitened principal component analysis. Diffusion Map (DM)-based coarse-filtering technique is robust to noise perturbation [5] and Student-t distribution Mixture Model (SMM) is robust to outliers [10], both provide a robust statistics of the model developed by [2]. The estimated SMM parameters are then used to form a Gaussian Mixture Model (GMM) statistics for predictive density estimation to ensure robustness and sensitivity to outliers. This paper aims to further investigate and improve the model performance and computing efficiency for high-dimensional predictive modeling and anomaly detection. The contributions of this paper are as follow[1].

- Twelve variants of hybrid mixture models that combine G-means clustering or K-Means clustering using Gaussian algorithm (KM) developed by [7], GMM, and SMM have been compared for predictive modeling and anomaly detection. Results show that simple hybrid models without the Expectation-Maximization (EM) step can achieve equally high prediction accuracy and anomaly detection rates comparable to the sophisticated models.
- For unsupervised anomaly detection, the noise can be removed by a DM-based coarse-filtering technique developed by [2]. However, without the coarse filtering, the hybrid models achieve detection rate $\gtrsim 90\%$ with injected anomalies from 1% to 60% in the KDD Cup 1999 network intrusion dataset. The top-down approach produces results that do not fluctuate with data sampling in contrast to the models using the DM-based coarse-filtering technique that process data in smaller chunks.
- For real-time batch data processing, a technique based on Gram-Schmidt orthogonalization process is proposed and demonstrated to update the reduced dimensions to remain relevant in fulfilling the task objectives. Existing work usually assumes same reduced dimensions for each batch of data or assumes spherical-Gaussian covariance so that the covariance remains conserved after re-projection from one set of dimension vectors to another.
- A model-adaptation technique is proposed and tested for incremental learning of GMM and SMM model parameters. This technique is different from previous [2,11,12] in that the adapted model parameters are computed by taking account the data size of new and older statistics, and a parameter is introduced in the technique to scale down the influence of older statistics in each iterative computation.
- Application of the parameter rating technique developed by [2] is demonstrated using KDD Cup 1999 network intrusion dataset (10% subset); the parameter ratings may be used to suggest mitigating actions for the different intrusion types or to label the data.

The organization of this paper is as follows. Data pre-processing for dimensionality reduction and coarse filtering are provided in Sect. 2. The data processing

[1] For reproducibility, the Matlab scripts to run the simulation and experimental studies in this paper are obtainable from https://github.com/jennbing/hybrid-models.

to form the hybrid mixture models, model adaptation, and the parameter rating techniques are covered in Sect. 3. Section 4 evaluates the model performance by simulation/experimental studies and Sect. 5 concludes the work.

2 Data Pre-processing

2.1 Dimensionality Reduction Using Whitened PCA

Principal component analysis (PCA) is a linear mapping from a high-dimensional space to a subspace that captures the most variability in the data specified by a set of orthogonal/principal components (PCs). To extract the relevant components from different datasets, different number of PCs with the highest eigenvalues are tested to find the minimum required for better model performance. For batch processing, it is important to ensure that these minimum number of PCs are sufficient for each batch of data to fulfill particular objective; e.g., predictive modeling or anomaly detection. Suppose there exists additional PCs in new batch of data which are not spanned by the older set of PCs, the new dimensions can be appended by using the Gram-Schmidt orthogonalization process to remove the projections on older set of PCs. On the other hand, older PC may be discarded if the absolute value of the Pearson correlation with the set of new PCs is low (<0.5). The threshold can be determined from empirical experiments to ensure good model performance. The reason this updating technique is proposed because the projection of non-spherical Gaussian covariance from a set of orthonormal vectors to another is not conserved, therefore the PCs can only be appended or discarded, but not re-projected, during the updating process.

2.2 Coarse Filtering Using Technique Based on Diffusion Map

Diffusion Map (DM) is a non-linear technique that helps to discover the underlying manifold of high-dimensional data [5]. Given a set of d-dimensional data X, the similarity measure between two data points is defined as

$$\chi(x_i, x_j) = \exp\left(-\frac{||x_i - x_j||^2}{\epsilon}\right) \tag{1}$$

where $|| \bullet ||$ is the Euclidean distance of the vectors in the ambient space $\mathbb{R}^d$. The scaling parameter is computed by the average smallest neighbouring distance [9]. The transition probability between two data points can be computed by normalizing Eq. 1. The diffusion distance is small if there are many short paths connecting two data points, which implies large transition probability between the two points. DM provides a representation in which the data points are clustered according to their connectivity, which is robust to noise perturbations [5]. In the diffusion space, inliers are expected to be clustered together, whereas outliers might be spread between several small clusters or scattered randomly. The inliers can then be identified by discovering the biggest connected component in the diffusion space using technique proposed in [2].

3 Hybrid Mixture Models

This section explains the methods to estimate the hybrid models' parameters, some of the algorithms can be found in [2]. Table 1 tabulates the sequence of data processing of the hybrid mixture models. The acronym for each hybrid model follows the sequence of data processing. For example, the sequence of KEG model is (1) K̲M (2) E̲M (3) G̲MM. For anomaly detection, the data is first coarse-filtered with a technique based on diffusion map described in Sect. 2.2 to remove anomalies before model training. GMM and SMM parameters are estimated using the EM algorithms described in [3] and [10] respectively. The EM initialization is provided by the K-means clustering using Gaussian algorithm (KM) developed by [7] that repeatedly splits every clusters until each approximates the Gaussian distribution statistically. The statistical test, which is based on the one-dimensional Anderson-Darling statistics, is valid for multi-dimensional Gaussian distribution. In addition, the mixture model parameters can also be learnt using KM directly and is theoretically shown to require near-optimal sample requirement with well-separated mixture components [4]. The reason this simple model is explored because EM algorithm often converges to local minimum in high dimensions. For computing efficiency, variance vectors are used in the mixture modeling instead of full covariance matrices. For KESG, the estimated SMM parameters are used to form GMM statistics; while for KEGS, the estimated GMM parameters form the SMM statistics assuming the degree of freedom is 1, this is justifiable because real data usually spreads out. Similar applies to other models. In addition, a model-adaptation technique is introduced for incremental learning of big data and the computation of a parameter rating

Table 1. Sequence of data processing of the proposed hybrid mixture models. The acronym for each hybrid model follows the sequence of data processing. For example, the sequence for DKEGS model is (1) D̲M (2) K̲M (3) E̲M (4) G̲MM (5) S̲MM.

Models	DM	KM	EM	GMM	SMM	Remark
KG		1		2		Prediction
KS		1			2	
KEG		1	2	3		
KES		1	2		3	
KESG		1	2	4	3	
KEGS		1	2	3	4	
DKG	1	2		3		Anomaly detection
DKS	1	2			3	
DKEG	1	2	3	4		
DKES	1	2	3		4	
DKESG	1	2	3	5	4	
DKEGS	1	2	3	4	5	

technique developed by [2] is presented here in order to examine the source of anomalies occurrences in the original feature space.

3.1 Model Adaptation

Box's M test is used to statistically compare the sample variance from new and older statistics. After finding a match of a pair of mixture components' variance, Hotelling's T^2 test is used to compare and match the corresponding sample mean. The adapted parameters are estimated using Maximum A-Posteriori (MAP) estimation. Similar model adaptation technique has been developed for GMM by [12]. Our proposed technique differs from previous [2,11,12] in that the adapted parameters are computed by taking account the sample size of new and older statistics, and a parameter $f^{\rho}(\mathbf{c})$ is introduced in the technique to scale down the influence of older statistics in the iterative computation. Equation 2 summarizes the model adaptation for both GMM and SMM. Although Box's M test and Hotelling's T^2 test assume the pair of mixture components are multidimensional Gaussian-distributed, short of other alternatives, these statistical tests provide a more stringent criteria for matching SMM mixture components. Additionally, the EM algorithm to estimate the mixture model parameters does not guarantee to find a global optimum since the problem is non-convex and the final solutions depend on the initial parameter values. Therefore, a technique to combine the statistics of a mixture of parametric models for predictive density estimation is proposed in [2]. The technique can be easily parallelized in the expense of computational resources due to model independence [2]. Our model-adaptation technique can also be used to merge the model parameters estimated from multiple trial estimation on a given dataset, this saves the memory space from storing duplicate parameters from different trials.

$$
\begin{aligned}
Mixing\ coefficient : \tilde{\omega}_i &= \left(\alpha_i^{\omega}\omega_i^{new} + (1-\alpha_i^{\omega})\omega_i\right)\gamma \\
Sample\ mean : \tilde{\mu}_i &= \alpha_i^{\mu}\mu_i^{new} + (1-\alpha_i^{\mu})\mu_i \\
Sample\ variance : \tilde{\sigma}_i^2 &= \alpha_i^{\sigma}\left((\sigma_i^{new})^2 + (\mu_i^{new})^2\right) + (1-\alpha_i^{\sigma})(\sigma_i^2+\mu_i^2) - \tilde{\mu}^2 \\
Degree\ of\ freedom : \tilde{v}_i &= \alpha_i^{v}v_i^{new} + (1-\alpha_i^{v})v_i
\end{aligned} \tag{2}
$$

where γ is a normalization factor which ensures the adapted weights sum to unity, α_i^{ρ} is the data-dependent adaptation coefficient that are computed by $\alpha_i^{\rho} = \frac{n_i^{new}}{n_i^{new}+f^{\rho}(\mathbf{c})n_i}$, where $\rho \in \{\omega, \mu, \sigma, v\}$, $n_i^{new} = N^{new}\omega_i^{new}$ and $n_i = N\omega_i$ is the sample size estimates of the i-th mixture component, $f^{\rho}(\mathbf{c})$ is a function of the context ranges from 0 to 1 that characterizes the decay of the influence of older statistics in the iterative computation. The sample mean and variance vectors have been matched statistically between a pair of mixture components before adaptation, therefore $f^{\rho}(\mathbf{c})$ has a larger impact on the mixing coefficients and degree of freedom than the sample mean and variance. Additionally, the weights of unmatched components may be scaled down appropriately, one way to do this is by applying the normalization factor on the unmatched components but keeping the weights of the matched components unchanged.

3.2 Parameter Rating

To understand the source of anomaly occurrences in the original feature space, a technique was developed by [2] for parameter rating from the learnt subspace. An anomaly is detected when its logarithmic probability is extremely low. Let z_a be the observed anomaly in the projected subspace span by the PCs, the associated mixture component of the anomaly is given by

$$i^* \triangleq \underset{i}{\operatorname{argmax}} \{q_i^{\tilde{K}}(z_a) | 1 \leqslant i \leqslant M\} \tag{3}$$

$$q_i^{\tilde{K}}(z_j) = \frac{\omega_i N(z_j; \mu_i, \Sigma_i)}{\sum_{\tilde{k}=1}^{\tilde{K}} \omega_i N(z_{\tilde{k}}; \mu_i, \Sigma_i)} \tag{4}$$

where $N(z_{\tilde{k}}; \mu_i, \Sigma_i)$ is the probability density of a Gaussian mixture component, M is the number of mixture components, and $\tilde{K}$ is the number of samples. The explanatory vector, which represents the parameters that account for the anomaly, is computed by

$$\bar{x}_a = \phi_{i^*}(x_a) \triangleq \sigma_{q_{i^*}^{\tilde{K}}}^{-\frac{1}{2}}[S] \left| x_a - E_{q_{i^*}^{\tilde{K}}}[S] \right| \tag{5}$$

$$\begin{aligned} E_{q_{i^*}^{\tilde{K}}}[S] &= \sum_{\tilde{k}=1}^{\tilde{K}} q_{i^*}^{\tilde{K}}(z_{\tilde{k}}) x_{\tilde{k}} \\ \sigma_{q_{i^*}^{\tilde{K}}}[S] &= \sum_{\tilde{k}=1}^{\tilde{K}} q_{i^*}^{\tilde{K}}(z_{\tilde{k}})(x_{\tilde{k}} - E_{q_{i^*}^{\tilde{K}}})^2 \end{aligned} \tag{6}$$

$\bar{x}_a$ represents the scaled geometric difference vector between the anomaly and the sample mean associated with the mixture component i^*. The parameters are rated by their responsibility for the anomaly occurrence by sorting the entries in $\bar{x}_a$ in a descending order. In cases that a low confidence in the responsibility of a specific mixture component for an observed anomaly, Eq. 7 presents a soft parameter rating technique proposed by [2] that takes into account the deviation from all the mixture components.

$$\begin{aligned} q_i^M(z_j) &= \frac{\omega_i N(z_j; \mu_i, \Sigma_i)}{\sum_{m=1}^{M} \omega_m N(z_j; \mu_m, \Sigma_m)} \\ \bar{x}_a &= \mathbf{E}_q[\phi(x_a)] = \sum_{i=1}^{M} q_i^M(z_a)(\phi_i(x_a)) \end{aligned} \tag{7}$$

Both soft and hard parameter rating techniques can be applied when the SMM statistics is used, in this case, $N(z_{\tilde{k}}; \mu_i, \Sigma_i)$ should be replaced by SMM distribution. The soft parameter rating technique (Eq. 7) is more computing-efficient than the hard one (Eq. 6) because there is no need to search for the associated mixture component for each anomaly. Notice that Eq. 4 is modified from Eq. 3 in [2]; the summation in the denominator is over the sample points instead of the mixture components as in [2], this makes more sense in computing the mean and variance in Eq. 6.

4 Experimental Evaluation

4.1 Simulation Studies

Figure 1(a) shows two simulated multidimensional Gaussian-distributed centers with white noise added. The noise constitutes one-third of the sample size. Two hybrid models for anomaly detection (see Table 1) are used to remove the white noise, the models differ in sophistication and therefore computing efficiency. Although KG is less sophisticated and hence more computing-efficient compared to DKESG, both models perform equally well in removing the white noise with appropriate logarithmic-probability threshold to identify the outliers. It will be

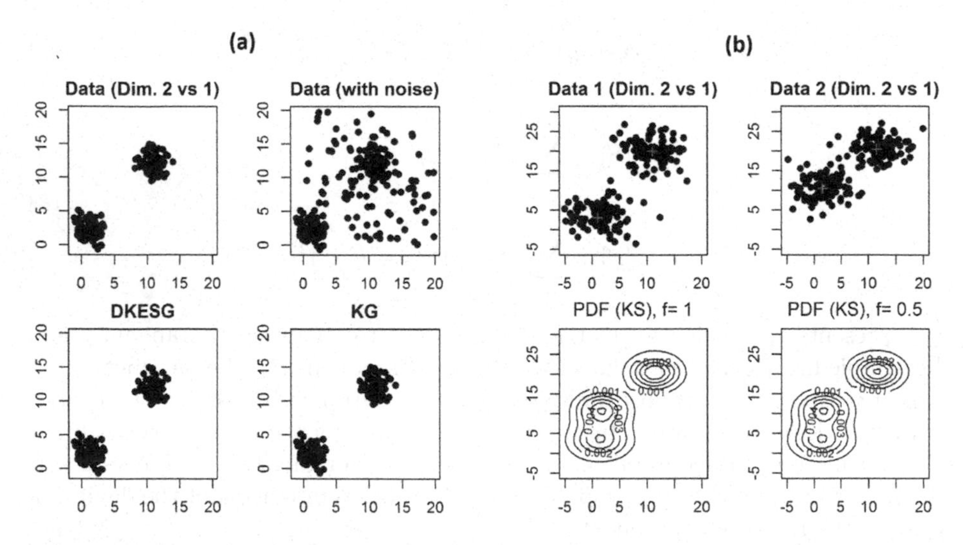

Fig. 1. **(a)** Top: Simulated multidimensional Gaussian-distributed data with two mixture components (left) and injected white noise (right). The first and second dimensions are plotted here and the distribution centers are $\mu_1 = (1, 2, ..., 10)$ and $\mu_2 = (11, 12, ..., 20)$ respectively with variance $\sigma^2 = (1, 1.5, ..., 5.5)$. The white noise comes from a uniform distribution within the range 0 to 20 in all dimensions. Bottom: Two hybrid models are used to remove the noise, DKESG is more sophisticated and hence less computing-efficient compared to KG but both models perform equally well in removing the noise. **(b)** Top: Two datasets with a common but slightly shifted multidimensional Gaussian-distributed center. The distribution centers are marked as red cross. Bottom: The predictive density of KS model after adaptation of the two datasets with the decay of influence of the older statistics, $f^{\rho}(\mathbf{c})$ set as 1 and 0.5 respectively.

shown later using empirical data that even without the EM step, simple hybrid model like KS shows high performance in anomaly detection. The model adaptation is demonstrated in Fig. 1(b) with two datasets sharing a common but slightly deviated multidimensional Gaussian-distributed center between the two datasets; the common distribution centers are $(11, 20)$ and $(11.5, 20.5)$ respectively. Each dataset also includes another non-colocated centers, which are $(1, 3)$ and $(1.5, 10.5)$ respectively. The standard deviation of all the distributions are set to 3. With high confidence level ($p \leqslant 0.0001$) during the matching of model mean and variance vectors using statistical methods, the results show that the proposed model-adaptation technique in Sect. 3.1 provides reasonable predictive density estimation with slight variation near the center of the common distribution between using parameter $f^{\rho}(\mathbf{c}) = 1$ and 0.5 to scale down the older statistics in model adaptation (see Sect. 3.1).

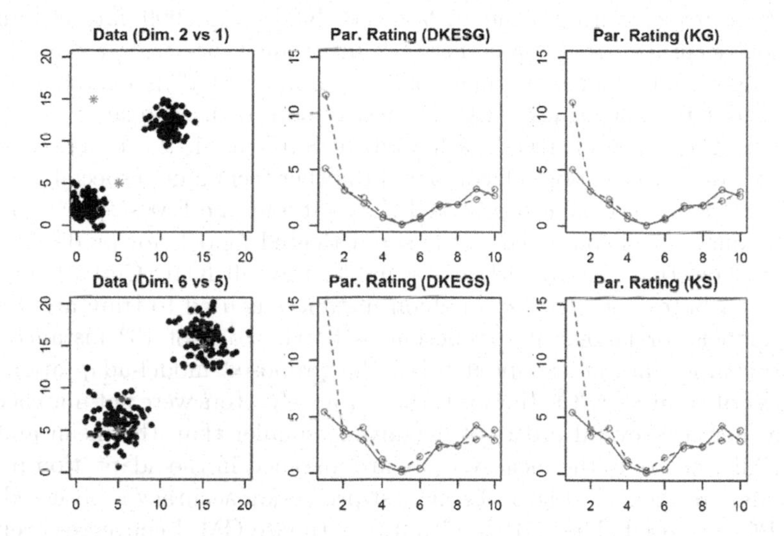

Fig. 2. First column from left: The first and second dimensions (top) and fifth and sixth dimensions (bottom) of simulated 10 dimensional data with two multidimensional Gaussian-distributed centers and two anomalies marked as red star. The two anomalies are $x_1 = (5, 5, ..., 5)$ and $x_2 = (2, 15, 15, ..., 15)$ respectively, which overlap with the distributions at about the 5th dimension but deviate at other dimensions. Remaining plots are the parameter rating using selected hybrid models. The blue lines correspond to the soft parameter rating using Eq. 7 and red circles are hard parameter rating using Eq. 6. (Color figure online)

Figure 2 simulates the data with the same multidimensional Gaussian distributions as in Fig. 1(a) top left plot, but with two anomalies inserted into the dataset to evaluate the parameter rating technique. All the selected hybrid models perform equally well by showing high parameter rating at the dimensions where deviation from the Gaussian distributions occur. However, large sample size is required to form a reliable judgement of the parameter ratings because the EM algorithm is sensitive to initial parameter values and better statistics with higher confidence level can be obtained with larger sample size.

4.2 Empirical Studies

Table 2 tabulates the prediction accuracy of the hybrid mixture models on five popular datasets obtained from UCI Machine Learning Repository [1]. Training and testing on Adult dataset are conducted on two different given datasets (train: 32561, test: 16281), prediction accuracy on other datasets are computed using 10-fold cross validation on a single dataset. The highest prediction accuracy recorded in the repository are Adult (Forward Sequential Selection Naive-Bayes: 85.95%), Wine (Regularized Discriminant Analysis: 100%), and Breast Cancer (separating plane: 97.5%). For KDD Cup 1999 dataset, different prediction accuracy for different network intrusion types were reported using genetic algorithm [8]; i.e., normal (69.5%), probe (71.1%), denial of service (99.4%), user to root attacks (18.9%), and remote to user attacks (5.4%). On average, 88.2% detection rate is achieved in [8]. Overall, the proposed hybrid models perform reasonably well compared to other techniques especially in high-dimensional regime. It is also observed that without the EM step, KG and KS perform equally well compared to the sophisticated models for predictive modeling. To show that the algorithm is scalable, the full KDD Cup 1999 dataset with 41 attributes and close to 5 million instances is used to train and test the hybrid models for large-scale prediction in batch mode of 10^5 instances. The mixture components are adapted using the proposed model-adaptation technique described in Sect. 3.1. However, the variance vectors were not matched here because they are several orders of magnitude smaller than the mean and fluctuate wildly, i.e., only the mean vectors are matched in the adaptation process. The results are shown in Fig. 3, the highest prediction accuracy is observed when all the PCs are used. The EM algorithm to estimate GMM converges even with reduced dimensions $\gtrsim$ 40 and produce higher prediction accuracy compared to the ones without the EM step (compare KEG and KEGS to KG and KS).

Table 2. Prediction accuracy of the hybrid mixture models using different datasets obtained from UCI Machine Learning Repository [1].

Dataset	KG	KS	KEG	KES	KEGS	KESG
Iris (Instances: 150, Attributes: 4)	0.97	0.97	0.97	0.97	0.97	0.97
Wine (178, 13)	0.94	0.94	0.94	0.93	0.94	0.93
Adult (48842, 14)	0.81	0.81	0.81	0.80	0.81	0.80
Wisconsin Diagnostic Breast Cancer (569, 32)	0.96	0.96	0.96	0.94	0.96	0.94
KDD Cup 1999 (10% subset: 494020, 41)	0.90	0.90	0.86	N/A	0.86	N/A

The prediction accuracy fluctuates with the data sampling, this is likely a characteristic of the dataset which contains both predictable and less-predictable events. New PCs not spanned by the older set of PCs are appended using the Gram-Schmidt orthogonalization process described in Sect. 2.1, the unused PCs are not discarded in the updating process. It is observed that the SMM-based hybrid models (KS, KES, and KESG) do not perform well in reduced dimensions $\gtrsim 30$.

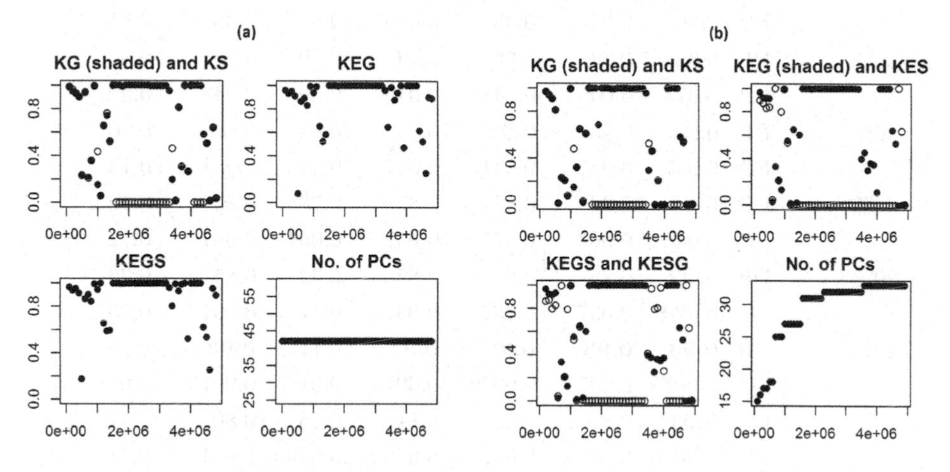

Fig. 3. Prediction accuracy of the hybrid models for batches of 10^5 instances using KDD Cup 1999 network intrusion dataset **(a)** with same number of PCs and **(b)** changing number of PCs for each batch of data.

Table 3 tabulates the detection rate and false positive rate of the hybrid mixture models using the KDD Cup 1999 dataset (10% subset). Normal-type network data of 95000 instances are extracted from the dataset and injected with different percentages of injected anomalies. The number of PCs required for anomaly detection is lesser compared to predictive modeling, in particular, only seven PCs were used here. The data is coarse-filtered with the technique based on diffusion map described in Sect. 2.2 to remove the anomalies before model training. The logarithmic-probability threshold for anomaly detection is set as the percentile of injected anomalies. It is observed that $\gtrsim$80% detection rate is possible with 1% to 60% injected anomalies with coarse-filtering technique based on DM. Higher percentage of injected anomalies biases the training model and lower percentage increases the false positive rate, hence present different challenges to unsupervised anomaly detection. However, the detection rates fluctuate with the data-sampling process because the DM-based coarse-filtering technique processes limited amount of data points at one time due to the need to compute the similarity distance between each pair of data points (see Sect. 2.2).

Table 3. Model performance in anomaly detection using KDD Cup 1999 computer network intrusion dataset (10% subset) with different percentages of injected anomalies. The dataset contains "normal" and "attack" data. The "normal" data is first extracted from the dataset and "attack" data is then artificially injected. The percentages of injected anomalies are calculated based on the ratio of artificially injected "intrusion" data into the extracted "normal" data.

Anomalies		KS	DKG	DKS	DKEG	DKES	DKEGS	DKESG
60%	DR	0.93	**0.94**	0.77	**0.94**	0.47	0.77	0.46
	FP	0.10	0.086	0.35	0.086	0.80	0.35	0.81
50%	DR	0.93	**0.96**	0.95	**0.96**	0.50	0.95	0.51
	FP	0.073	0.045	0.048	0.045	0.50	0.048	0.49
40%	DR	0.93	0.93	**0.94**	0.93	0.84	**0.94**	0.80
	FP	0.047	0.047	0.041	0.047	0.11	0.041	0.13
30%	DR	**0.90**	0.84	0.82	0.85	0.78	0.84	0.72
	FP	0.043	0.067	0.075	0.062	0.094	0.067	0.12
20%	DR	**0.92**	0.85	0.85	0.85	0.32	0.85	0.36
	FP	0.020	0.037	0.037	0.037	0.17	0.037	0.16
10%	DR	**0.93**	**0.93**	**0.93**	**0.93**	0.11	**0.93**	0.90
	FP	0.0079	0.0073	0.0079	0.0073	0.017	0.0079	0.011
5%	DR	**0.91**	0.81	0.80	0.81	0.16	0.80	0.17
	FP	0.0050	0.0099	0.011	0.0099	0.044	0.011	0.014
1%	DR	0.89	**0.92**	**0.92**	**0.92**	0.00	**0.92**	0.00
	FP	0.0012	0.00085	0.00075	0.00085	0.010	0.00075	0.010

Without coarse filtering, KS detection rate achieves $\gtrsim$90% and because of the top-down approach, the measured detection rates are robust to data sampling process.

Figure 4 shows the soft parameter rating for different network intrusion types using KDD Cup 1999 dataset (10% subset). The model is trained with normal-type network data and the KS statistics is used to compute the parameter rating. This is because KG statistics is too sparse due to the rapidly-decaying GMM tail distribution. For large number of anomalies, the soft parameter rating technique (Eq. 7) is more computing-efficient than the hard one (Eq. 6) because there is no need to search for the associated mixture component for each anomaly. Results show that there is overlap between the sources of anomaly occurrences from different network intrusion types; the parameter rating may be used to suggest mitigating actions for each intrusion type.

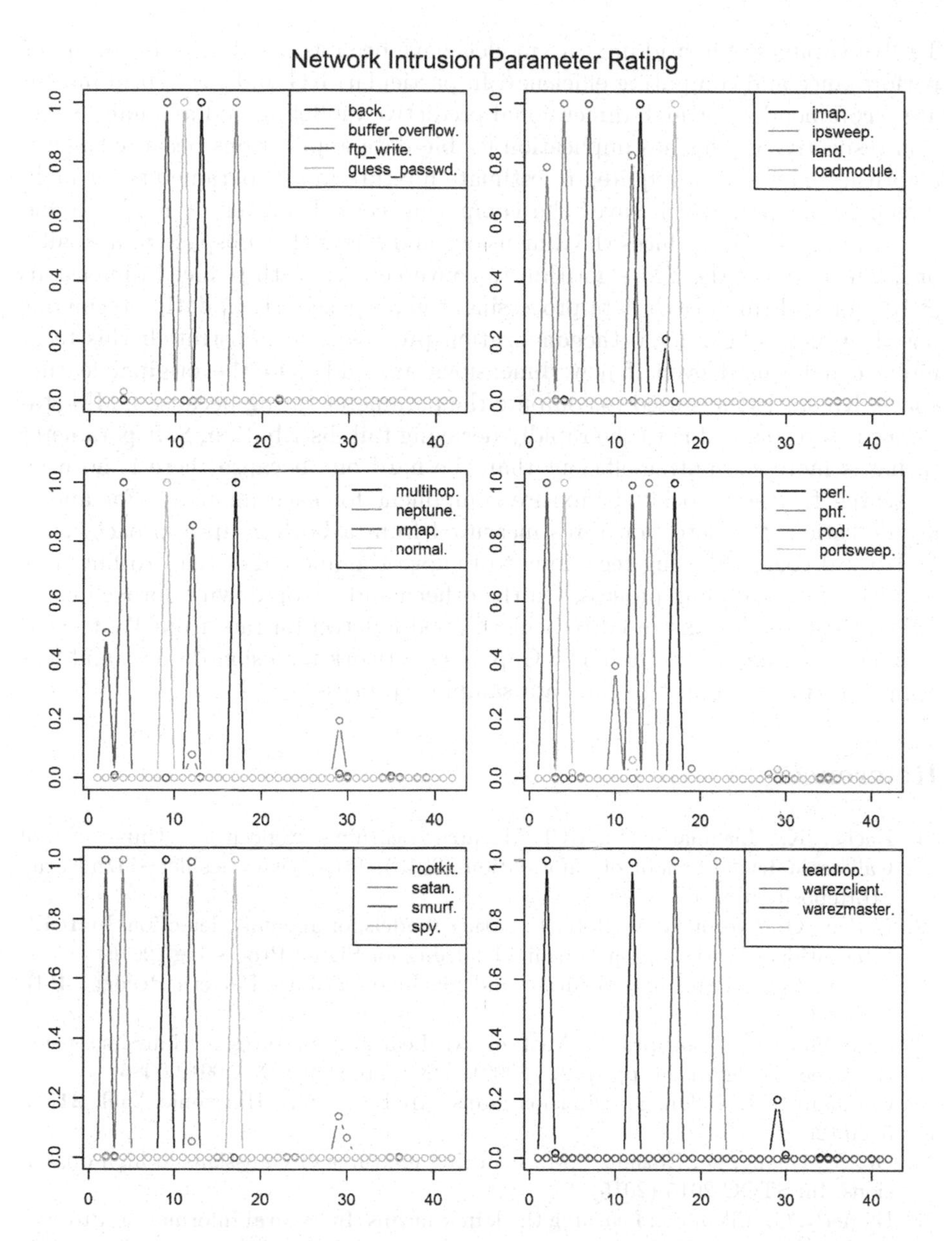

Fig. 4. Parameter rating of each network intrusion type of KDD Cup 1999 dataset (10% subset). The ratings are normalized to the range $[0, 1]$. Results show that majority of the sources of anomaly occurrences come from dimensions $\lesssim 20$ and may be used to suggest mitigating actions.

5 Conclusion

Twelve variants of hybrid mixture models have been assessed in terms of model performance and computing efficiency. In particular, KG and KS hybrid models are recommended for high-dimensional predictive modeling and anomaly detection respectively. This has implication for big-data applications because the EM algorithm may not be required to estimate mixture model parameters for high-dimensional data, which saves the computing cost. However, it is also found that whitened PCA reduces the dimensions and scales the subspace to a smaller one, which allows the EM algorithm to converge even with reduced dimensions $\gtrsim 10$. For real-time batch data processing, the proposed PC-updating technique based on Gram-Schmidt orthogonalization process is demonstrated; this technique can be used even if new dimensions are added in the original feature space. KS statistics is used to compute the parameter rating because GMM statistics is too sparse due to the rapidly-decaying tail distribution. Soft parameter rating is more computing-efficient than the hard one because there is no need to search for the associated mixture component for each anomaly. For anomaly detection, the detection rates measured from a bottom-up approach using DM-based coarse-filtering technique to remove the anomalies tend to fluctuate with the data sampling process. On the other hand, a top-down approach using KS statistics is demonstrated to achieve $\gtrsim 90\%$ detection rate from 1% to 60% of injected anomalies in the KDD Cup 1999 network intrusion dataset and this approach is more robust to the data sampling process.

References

1. Bache, K., Lichman, M.: UCI Machine Learning Repository. University of California Irvine School of Information (2013). http://www.ics.uci.edu/mlearn/MLRepository.html
2. Barkan, O., Averbuch, A.: Robust mixture models for anomaly detection. In: IEEE International Workshop on Machine Learning for Signal Processing (2016)
3. Bishop, C.M.: Pattern recognition and machine learning. Pattern Recogn. **4**(4), 738 (2006)
4. Chaudhuri, K., Dasgupta, S., Vattani, A.: Learning mixtures of Gaussians using the k-means algorithm, pp. 1–22 (2009). arXiv preprint arXiv:0912.0086
5. Coifman, R.R., Lafon, S.: Diffusion maps. Appl. Comput. Harmonic Anal. **21**(1), 5–30 (2006)
6. Ge, R., Huang, Q., Kakade, S.M.: Learning mixtures of Gaussians in high dimensions. In: STOC 2015 (2015)
7. Hamerly, G., Elkan, C.: Learning the k in k-means. In: Neural Information Processing Systems, pp. 281–288 (2003)
8. Hoque, M.S., Mukit, M.A., Bikas, M.A.N., Sazzadul Hoque, M.: An implementation of intrusion detection system using genetic algorithm. Int. J. Netw. Secur. Appl. **4**(2), 109–120 (2012)
9. Lafon, S.: Diffusion maps and geometric harmonics. Ph.D. thesis, Yale University, U.S.A, p. 97 (2004)

10. Peel, D., McLachlan, G.J.: Robust mixture modelling using the t distribution. Stat. Comput. **10**(4), 339–348 (2000)
11. Reynolds, D.A., Quatieri, T.F., Dunn, R.B.: Speaker verification using adapted Gaussian mixture models. Digit. Signal Proc. **10**(1–3), 19–41 (2000)
12. Song, M., Wang, H.: Highly efficient incremental estimation of Gaussian mixture models for online data stream clustering. Intell. Comput. Theory Appl. **5803**, 174–183 (2005)
13. Vempala, S.S.: Technical perspective modeling high-dimensional data. Commun. ACM **55**(2), 112 (2012)

Classification and Clustering Methods

StruClus: Scalable Structural Graph Set Clustering with Representative Sampling

Till Schäfer(✉) and Petra Mutzel

Department of Computer Science, TU Dortmund University, Dortmund, Germany
{till.schaefer,petra.mutzel}@cs.tu-dortmund.de

Abstract. We present a structural clustering algorithm for large-scale datasets of small labeled graphs, utilizing a frequent subgraph sampling strategy. A set of representatives provides an intuitive description of each cluster, supports the clustering process, and helps to interpret the clustering results. The projection-based nature of the clustering approach allows us to bypass dimensionality and feature extraction problems that arise in the context of graph datasets reduced to pairwise distances or feature vectors. While achieving high quality and (human) interpretable clusterings, the runtime of the algorithm only grows linearly with the number of graphs. Furthermore, the approach is easy to parallelize and therefore suitable for very large datasets. Our extensive experimental evaluation on synthetic and real world datasets demonstrates the superiority of our approach over existing structural and subspace clustering algorithms, both, from a runtime and quality point of view.

1 Introduction

The ability to represent topological and semantic information causes graphs to be among the most versatile data structures in computer science. In the age of Big Data, huge amounts of graph data are collected and the demand to analyze them increases with its collection. We focus on the special case of clustering large sets of small labeled graphs. Our primary motivation stems from the need to cluster large-scale molecular databases for drug discovery, such as PubChem, ChEMBL, ChemDB[1] or synthetically constructed de-novo databases [19], which contain up to several billions of molecules. However, the presented approach is not limited to this use case. Clustering techniques aim to find homogeneous subsets in a set of objects. Classical approaches do not interpret the objects directly, but abstract them by utilizing some intermediate representation, such as feature vectors or pairwise distances. While the abstraction over pairwise distances is beneficial in terms of generality, it can be disadvantageous in the case of *intrinsic high dimensional* datasets [8,14]. In this case the *concentration effect* may cause the

This work was supported by the German Research Foundation (DFG), priority programme *Algorithms for Big Data (SPP 1736)*.

[1] https://pubchem.ncbi.nlm.nih.gov/, https://www.ebi.ac.uk/chembl/, http://cdb.ics.uci.edu/.

G. Cong et al. (Eds.): ADMA 2017, LNAI 10604, pp. 343–359, 2017.
https://doi.org/10.1007/978-3-319-69179-4_24

pairwise distances to loose their relative contrast; i.e., the distances converge towards a common value [5]. The concentration effect is closely related to a bad *clusterability* [1]. Furthermore, metric pruning is ineffective in such a setting.

In order to apply these classical clustering approaches on sets of graphs, the graphs are usually transformed into feature vectors or graph theoretic similarity measures are used. Typical feature extraction methods for graphs are: counting *graphlets*, that is, small subgraphs [28,33], counting *walks* [32], and using *eigenvectors* of adjacency matrices (spectral graph theory) [11]. The enumeration of all subgraphs is considered intractable even for graphs of moderate size, because there exist up to exponentially many subgraphs w.r.t. the graph size. Many efficient clustering algorithms have been proposed for vector space. Therefore, the transformation to feature vectors might look beneficial in the first place. However, the above mentioned feature extraction methods tend to produce a large number of independent features, which results in datasets with a high intrinsic dimensionality [20,30]. Additionally, the extracted features only approximate the graph structure, which implies that feature vectors cannot be transformed back into a graph. Hence, the interpretability of clustering algorithms which perform vector modifications (e.g., calculating centroids) is limited. Besides the utilization of vectors, graphs can be compared directly using graph theoretic distances such as *(maximum) common subgraph* derived distances [7,9,34] or the *graph edit distance* [6]. The computation of the previously mentioned graph theoretic distances is NP-hard and as shown in [20] their application results in datasets with a high intrinsic dimensionality as well. High quality clustering methods for non-vectorial and high dimensional datasets furthermore require a superlinear number of distance computations. These factors render graph theoretic distance measures in combination with generic clustering algorithms infeasible for large-scale datasets. Subspace and projected clustering methods tackle high dimensional datasets by identifying subspaces in which well separated clusters exist. However, generic subspace algorithms still suffer from the above mentioned problems, i.e., (a) a complete subgraph feature space is infeasible, (b) lossy feature representations have a limited interpretability/accuracy, and (c) non-vectorial representations require a superlinear number of distance computations.

Structural clustering avoids an intermediate representation by vectors or distances but uses graph theoretic concepts such as subgraph isomorphism or (maximum) common subgraph isomorphism directly in the clustering process. Our *structural projection* clustering algorithm approaches the dimensionality problems of the subgraph space by explicitly selecting cluster representatives in the form of common subgraphs. This selection could also be interpreted as a subspace projection in the binary vector space that contains one feature for each subgraph in the dataset. We would like to point out that the structural perspective on the data allows the integration of domain specific requirements, e.g., an approximate (common) subgraph isomorphism with label costs [4]

Our **main contributions** in this paper are: We present a novel structural projection clustering algorithm for datasets of small labeled graphs which scales linearly with the dataset size. A set of subgraph representatives provides an intuitive description of each cluster, supports the clustering process, and helps to interpret the clustering results. Up to our knowledge, this is the first approach actively selecting representative sets based on a ranking function which involves homogeneity and separation constraints. Additionally, it is the first approach which balances cluster homogeneities with the help of dynamically sized representatives and an adaptive minimum support threshold. To speed up the computation, we suggest a new error bounded sampling strategy for support counting in the context of frequent subgraph sampling. To the best of our knowledge this is the first fully structural clustering algorithm for general graphs that scales to very large datasets. Our experimental evaluation shows that our new approach outperforms competitors in terms of runtime and quality.

The paper is structured as follows: Sect. 2 provides an overview of related clustering algorithms. Basic definitions are given in Sect. 3. Section 4 presents the main algorithm and a runtime analysis. Our experimental evaluation in which we compare our new algorithm to SCAP [26], PROCLUS [2] and Kernel K-Means [13] is presented in Sect. 5.

2 Related Work

Several clustering algorithms for graph and molecule data have been proposed in the last years. Tsuda and Kudo [30] presented an EM algorithm using a binomial mixture model over very high dimensional binary vectors, indicating the presence of all frequent substructures. Two years later, Tsuda and Kurihara [31] presented a similar graph clustering algorithm using a Dirichlet Process mixture model which prunes the set of frequent substructures to achieve smaller feature vectors. Ferrer et al. [10] presented a K-Median like graph clustering algorithm, that maps each graph into the euclidean space utilizing the edit distance to pivot elements. Median graphs are approximated by their distance to the euclidean median. Seeland et al. [25] presented a parallel greedy overlapping clustering algorithm. It adds a graph to a cluster whenever a common substructure of a user-defined minimum size exists. Jouili et al. [18] adopted the idea of median-shift clustering to the domain of graphs. However, none of the previously mentioned algorithms are suitable for large datasets as a result of their high computational complexity. XProj [3] is a structural clustering algorithm for XML documents, i.e., labeled trees. It uses a projection-based approach and uses heuristic frequent subtrees of a fixed size as cluster representatives. In contrast to the previously mentioned approaches it scales well to very large datasets. However, it still requires the enumeration of all frequent substructures, their approximate subtree isomorphism test has no error bound and the generalization to graphs would result in a huge performance degradation. Furthermore, there exist some hybrid approaches, that pre-cluster the dataset by using a vector-based representation and refine the results using structural clustering algorithms. The most relevant with respect to large-scale datasets is the SCAP algorithm proposed by Seeland et al. [26]. Huang et al. [16] presented another type of hybridization, where a feature selection phase eliminates redundant patterns and the clustering is then done with the help of kernel k-means.

Giving a comprehensive overview on vectorial subspace algorithms is out of the scope of this article. However, there are two algorithms that are of special interest: In [36] it is shown that frequent pattern mining is suitable for feature selection in vector space. This relates to XProj and our approach in the way, that the selection of a frequent subgraph as a representative is another way of selecting a subspace in the feature space of substructures. In the later evaluation we will compare ourself to the PROCLUS [2] algorithm. It is a fast projected clustering algorithm with noise detection, that selects features by minimizing variance. Although the algorithm was proposed about two decades ago, it has been studied intensively and still performed very well in recent subspace clustering algorithm surveys [22,23]. Therefore, it suits well as a baseline for our algorithm evaluation.

Since *StruClus* introduces a novel sampled representative mining approach it is important to mention that there exist several other representative (e.g., [15,24]) and discriminative (e.g., [29,35]) subgraph miners. However, with the exception of ORIGAMI [15], all of them enumerate the (pruned) search space and our multiple hypothesis testing correction for support sampling is not applicable.

3 Preliminaries

An *undirected labeled graph* $G = (V, E, l)$ consists of a finite set of *vertices* $V(G) = V$, a finite set of *edges* $E(G) = E \subseteq \{\{u, v\} \subseteq V \mid u \neq v\}$ and a labeling function $l : V \uplus E \to L$, where L is a finite set of *labels*. $|G|$ is used as a short term for $|V(G)|+|E(G)|$. A *path* of length n is a sequence of vertices $(v_0, \ldots, v_n)$ such that $\{v_i, v_{i+1}\} \in E$ and $v_i \neq v_j$ for $i \neq j$. Let G and H be two undirected labeled graphs. A *(label preserving) subgraph isomorphism* from G to H is an injection $\psi : V(G) \to V(H)$, were $\forall v \in V(G) : l(v) = l(\psi(v))$ and $\forall u, v \in V(G) :$ $\{u, v\} \in E(G) \Rightarrow \{\psi(u), \psi(v)\} \in E(H) \wedge l(\{u, v\}) = l(\{\psi(u), \psi(v)\})$. If there exists a subgraph isomorphism from G to H we say G is *supported* by H, G is a *subgraph* of H, H is a *supergraph* of G or write $G \subseteq H$. The coverage of a graph G by a graph $H \subseteq G$ is defined as $\text{cov}(H, G) := \frac{|H|}{|G|}$. If there exists a subgraph isomorphism from G to H and from H to G, the two graphs are isomorphic. A *common subgraph* of G and H is a graph S, that is subgraph isomorphic to G and H. Furthermore, the *support* $\sup(G, \mathcal{G})$ of a graph G over a set of graphs $\mathcal{G}$ is the fraction of graphs in $\mathcal{G}$, that support G. G is said to be *frequent*, if its support is larger or equal than a *minimum support threshold* $sup_{\min}$. A frequent subgraph G is *maximal*, if there exists no frequent supergraph of G. For a set of graphs $\mathcal{G}$, we write $\mathcal{F}(\mathcal{G})$ for the set of all frequent subgraphs and $\mathcal{M}(\mathcal{G})$ for the set of all maximal frequent subgraphs. A *clustering* of a graph dataset —i.e., multiset— $\mathcal{X}$ is a partition $\mathcal{C} = \{C_1, \ldots, C_n\}$ of $\mathcal{X}$. Each *cluster* $C \in \mathcal{C}$ consists of a set of graphs and is linked to a *set of cluster representatives* $\mathcal{R}(C) = \{R_1, \ldots, R_k\}$ which are itself undirected labeled graphs.

4 The StruClus Algorithm

The *StruClus* algorithm emerges around sets of representatives $\mathcal{R}(C)$ for each cluster $C \in \mathcal{C}$. Representatives serve as an intuitive description of a cluster

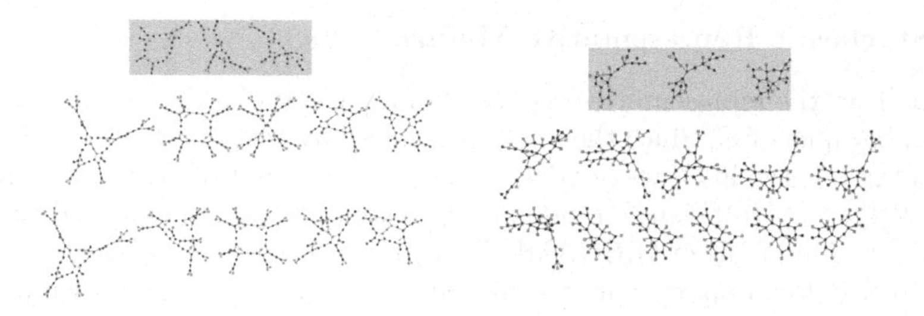

Fig. 1. Real world clusters with representatives (grey boxes) generated by *StruClus*.

and define the substructures, i.e., subspace over which intra cluster similarity is measured. With the exception of a single *noise* cluster the following invariant holds after each iteration:

$$\forall C \in \mathcal{C} : \forall G \in C : \exists R \in \mathcal{R}(C) : R \subseteq G \tag{1}$$

Figure 1 shows a real world example of two clusters with representatives. The **objective of *StruClus*** is to maximize cluster homogeneity, i.e., the coverage of graphs $G \in C \in \mathcal{C}$ by their representatives $R \in \mathcal{R}(C)$, while minimizing the number of clusters and keeping a minimum separation between them. A formal definition is given below by Eqs. 7 and 8. The representative sets $\mathcal{R}(C)$ are constructed using maximal frequent subgraphs of C (see Sect. 4.1). Having a representative set has the advantage, that graphs composed of multiple common substructures or slight variations of a single graph can be represented by a cluster. To be meaningful and human interpretable, the cardinality of $\mathcal{R}(C)$ is bounded by a user defined value $\mathcal{R}_{\max}$. A high level description of the *StruClus* algorithm is given in Algorithm 1. Initially, it partitions the dataset using a lightweight pre-clustering algorithm. Afterwards, the clustering is refined using an optimization loop similar to the K-Means algorithm. In order to achieve a good homogeneity and cluster separation, we use a cluster splitting and merging strategy in each iteration.

Algorithm 1. *StruClus* Algorithm

```
1: apply pre-clustering {Section 4.5}
2: while not convergent {Section 4.6} do
3:    split clusters {Section 4.4}
4:    merge clusters {Section 4.4}
5:    update representatives {Section 4.2}
6:    assign graphs to closest cluster {Section 4.3}
7: end while
```

Please note that we will present the algorithm not in order (see order in Algorithm 1) to make it easier to follow some algorithm design decisions.

4.1 Stochastic Representative Mining

We construct the representative set $\mathcal{R}(C)$ of a cluster $C \in \mathcal{C}$ using maximal frequent subgraphs of C. Since the set $\mathcal{M}(C)$ may have exponential size w.r.t. the maximal graph size in C, we restrict ourselves to a subset of candidate representatives $\mathcal{S}(C) \subseteq \mathcal{M}(C)$ using a randomized maximal frequent connected subgraph sampling technique from ORIGAMI [15] combined with a new stochastic sampling strategy for support counting. In a second step, the final representative set $\mathcal{R}(C) \subseteq \mathcal{S}(C)$ is selected using a ranking function (see Sect. 4.2.1).

ORIGAMI constructs a maximal frequent connected subgraph $S \in \mathcal{S}(\mathcal{G})$ over a set of graphs $\mathcal{G}$ by extending a graph with frequent paths of length one leading to a graph S'. In the first step, all frequent paths of length one $\mathrm{P}(\mathcal{G})$ are enumerated with a single scan of $\mathcal{G}$. Then, for each extension, a random vertex of S' is chosen and a random, label preserving path $p \in \mathrm{P}(\mathcal{G})$ is connected to it in a forward (creating a new vertex) or backward (connecting two existing vertices) fashion. After each extension, the support $\sup(S', \mathcal{G})$ is evaluated by solving a subgraph isomorphism test for all graphs in $\mathcal{G}$. If $\sup(S', \mathcal{G}) \geq sup_{\min}$, the extension is permanently added to S' or otherwise removed. If no further extension is possible without violating the minimum support threshold, a maximal frequent subgraph S has been found. This process is justified by the *monotonicity property* of subgraphs $\mathcal{G}_{\subseteq}$ of graphs in $\mathcal{G}$:

$$\forall G, H \in \mathcal{G}_{\subseteq} : G \subseteq H \Rightarrow \sup(G, \mathcal{G}) \geq \sup(H, \mathcal{G}) \tag{2}$$

While ORIGAMI greatly improves performance in comparison with enumeration algorithms, the $|\mathcal{G}|$ subgraph isomorphism tests for each extension remain a major performance bottleneck for *StruClus*. For this reason, we have added a stochastic sampling strategy for support counting. Initially, we draw a random sample $\mathcal{H} \subseteq \mathcal{G}$. Then $\hat{\theta} = \sup(S', \mathcal{H})$ is an estimator for the parameter θ of a binomial distribution $\mathrm{B}(\cdot, \theta)$, where $\theta = \sup(S', \mathcal{G})$ is the true probability of the underlying Bernoulli distribution. We are interested if the true value of $\sup(S', \mathcal{G})$ is smaller than the minimum support threshold. Without loss of generality, let us focus on the case $\hat{\theta} < sup_{\min}$ in the following. We can take advantage of a binomial test under the null hypothesis, that $\theta \geq sup_{\min}$ and thereby determine the probability of an error, if we assume $\sup(S', \mathcal{G}) < sup_{\min}$. With a predefined significance level α we can decide if the sample gives us enough confidence to justify our assumption. If the null hypothesis cannot be discarded, we double the sample size $|\mathcal{H}|$ and repeat the process. In the extreme case we will therefore calculate the exact value of $\sup(S', \mathcal{G})$. The statistical test is repeated for each extension and each sample size doubling. As a consequence, a multiple hypothesis testing correction is necessary to bound the real error for S to be a maximal frequent substructure of $\mathcal{G}$. With the value of Proposition 1 we are able to apply a Bonferroni correction to our significance level.

Proposition 1. *Let $\mathcal{G}$ be a set of undirected labeled graphs, $|\mathcal{H}_{\min}|$ the minimal sample size, $P(\mathcal{G})$ the set of all frequent paths of length one, $sup_{\min}$ a minimum support threshold, and $V_{\max}$ the $(1 - sup_{\min})$-quantile of the sorted (increasing* *order) graph sizes in $\mathcal{G}$. Then the maximal number of binomial tests to construct a maximal frequent substructure over $\mathcal{G}$ is bounded by:*

$$\left\lceil \log \frac{|\mathcal{G}|}{|\mathcal{H}_{\min}|} \right\rceil \left(\binom{V_{\max}}{2} + V_{\max} \right) |P(\mathcal{G})|$$

Proof. The sample size is doubled $\left\lceil \log \frac{|\mathcal{G}|}{|\mathcal{H}_{\min}|} \right\rceil$ times if the test never reaches the desired significance level. The size of some $S \in \mathcal{M}(\mathcal{G})$ is bounded by the size of each supporting graph. In the worst case S is supported by the ($|\mathcal{G}|\ sup_{\min}$)-largest graphs of $\mathcal{G}$. The size of the smallest supporting graph is then equal to the ($1 - sup_{\min}$)-quantile of the sorted graph sizes in increasing order. The number of backward extensions is bounded by the number of edges in the complete graph times the number of applicable extensions $p \in \mathrm{P}(\mathcal{G})$. To conclude that S is maximal, $|\mathrm{P}(\mathcal{G})|$ additional (infrequent) forward extensions for each vertex need to be performed.

4.2 Update Representatives

4.2.1 Representative Selection

In its role as a cluster description, a good representative $R \in \mathcal{R}(C)$ should (a) be supported by a large fraction of C and (b) maximize coverage $\mathrm{cov}(R, G)$ for each graph $G \in C$ supporting R. The two criteria are related to cluster homogeneity in the following way: A uniform cluster, that is, a cluster that contains only isomorphic graphs, can achieve optimal values for both criteria. Vice versa, the monotonicity property (2) implies non-optimal values for inhomogeneous clusters for at least one criteria. As homogeneous clusters are desired and we want to avoid the extreme cases in which one criteria has a high value while the other criteria has a very low value, we use a product of the two criteria for our ranking function. In order to discriminate clusters from each other, a cluster representative should have a low support in the rest of the dataset. For this reasons, we use the following ranking function for a dataset $\mathcal{X}$, cluster C and representative $R \in \mathcal{R}(C)$:

$$C_R := \{G \in C \mid R \subseteq G\}$$

$$\mathrm{rank}(R) := \frac{|C_R|\ |R|}{\sum_{G \in C_R} |G|} \left(\sup(R, C) - \sup(R, \mathcal{X})\right) \qquad (3)$$

Finally, we select the $\mathcal{R}_{\max}$ highest ranked subgraphs from $\mathcal{S}(C) \cup \mathcal{R}(C_{-1})$ as cluster representatives $\mathcal{R}(C)$, where $\mathcal{R}(C_{-1})$ are the cluster representatives from the previous iteration.

4.2.2 Balancing Cluster Homogeneity

Besides the representative selection, the minimum support threshold $sup_{\min}$ for representative mining has an influence on the cluster homogeneity, as it is a bound for criteria (a) (see Sect. 4.2.1). However, unsupported graphs will be assigned to a different cluster and the effect of a low minimum support value on (a) is only temporary. On the contrary, a minimum support below 1 increases the representatives size, i.e., the coverage value (b) (see monotonicity property (2)). In other words: the lower the minimum support, the higher the increase in homogeneity per iteration. Clearly, this process of sorting out graphs needs to be stopped at some point to have clusters of meaningful size. Thus, we will choose the minimum support cluster specific and aim for a balanced homogeneity over all clusters. Since an appropriate homogeneity level depends on the dataset, we use an average coverage score as baseline adjustment. For the ease of computation, we assume all representatives to be subgraph isomorphic to the cluster graphs:

$$\mathrm{aCov}(C) = \frac{\frac{1}{|\mathcal{R}(C)|}\sum_{R\in\mathcal{R}(C)}|R|}{\frac{1}{|C|}\sum_{G\in C}|G|} \tag{4}$$

$$\mathrm{relCov}(C,\mathcal{C}) = \frac{\mathrm{aCov}(C)}{\frac{1}{|\mathcal{C}|}\sum_{C'\in\mathcal{C}}\mathrm{aCov}(C')} \tag{5}$$

Finally, we map the relative coverage $\mathrm{relCov}(C,\mathcal{C})$ with a linear function to the cluster specific minimum support threshold $\mathrm{minSup}(C,\mathcal{C})$. To lower the asymptotic complexity of the algorithm, we bound $\mathrm{minSup}(C,\mathcal{C})$ by a constant ls from below (see Sect. 4.7).

4.3 Cluster Assignment

Each graph G in the dataset is assigned to its *most similar cluster* in the assignment phase. As a measure for similarity, we are summing up the squared sizes of the representatives of a cluster, which are subgraph isomorphic to G. We square the representative sizes, to prefer a high coverage, i.e., our objective, over a high number of representatives to be subgraph isomorphic to the assigned graph. After the representative update, a graph may be not supported by any representative. For this reason, we create a noise cluster in each iteration, where all unsupported graphs are collected.

4.4 Cluster Splitting and Merging

Without cluster splitting, noise clusters are the only way to create new clusters. For very inhomogeneous clusters it is furthermore possible that no representatives can be found to increase the relative coverage to an average level (see Sect. 4.2.2). Thus, convergence to a balanced and homogeneous clustering may be slow or impossible. For this reason, we use a cluster splitting step. It collects all graphs from clusters with a relative coverage value below an a priori specified threshold, i.e., $\{G \in C \in \mathcal{C} \mid \mathrm{relCov}(C,\mathcal{C}) < \mathrm{relCov}_{\min}\}$, and applies the pre-clustering algorithm on them. The resulting clusters are added back to the clustering.

On the contrary to cluster splitting, which focuses on cluster homogeneity, cluster merging ensures a minimum separation between clusters. Although the pre-clustering ensures well separated initial clusters (see Sect. 4.5) it may happen that two clusters converge towards each other or that newly formed clusters are similar to existing ones. Many classical measures define separation over the distance between cluster elements. Since this definition does not take the cluster specific subspace into account, it is not suitable for projected clustering. The representatives $\mathcal{R}(C)$ describe the subspace as well as the elements of C. Thus, we will define *separation* between two clusters C and C' solely over the representatives sets $\mathcal{R}(C)$ and $\mathcal{R}(C')$. This definition is also beneficial from a runtime perspective. To compare two representatives R, R' we calculate the size of their maximum common subgraph (MCS) and use its relative size as similarity:

$$\mathrm{sim}(R, R') := \frac{|\mathrm{mcs}(R, R')|}{\max\{|R|, |R'|\}} \tag{6}$$

The maximum of the representatives sizes is chosen as denominator to discriminate distinct clusters with subgraph isomorphic representatives, which differ largely in size. Finally, we merge two clusters C and C' if the following condition holds:

$$|\{(R, R') \in \mathcal{R}(C) \times \mathcal{R}(C') \mid \mathrm{sim}(R, R') \geq sim_{\max}\}| \geq \frac{|\mathcal{R}(C)| + |\mathcal{R}(C')|}{2} \tag{7}$$

The calculated MCS between two representatives $R \in \mathcal{R}(C), R' \in \mathcal{R}(C')$ is supported by all the graphs $G \in C \cup C'$, that support either R or R'. We choose the merge threshold close to the number of representatives per cluster to support a large fraction of graphs in the merged cluster. The coverage for the graphs in the merged cluster is furthermore bounded by $\max\{\mathrm{cov}(G, R), \mathrm{cov}(G, R')\}\ \mathrm{sim}(R, R')$ if we reuse the MCSs as representatives. After merging two clusters, we run a regular representative update, since better representatives than the MCSs may exist.

4.5 Pre-clustering

The pre-clustering serves as an initial partitioning of the dataset. A random partitioning of all graphs would be problematic as representatives will most likely have a low coverage and are not cluster specific. This will result in a high number of clusters to be merged to a few inhomogeneous clusters and in a slow convergence of the *StruClus* algorithm. To pre-cluster the dataset $\mathcal{X}$, we compute maximal frequent subgraphs $\mathcal{S}(\mathcal{X}) \subseteq \mathcal{M}(\mathcal{X})$, as described in Sect. 4.1. These frequent subgraphs serve as representative candidates for the initial clusters. To avoid very similar representatives we will first greedily construct maximal sets of dissimilar graphs. As a measure of similarity we re-use the similarity (6) and the threshold $sim_{\max}$ to respect the separation constraint. In other words, we are picking all graphs G from $\mathcal{S}(\mathcal{X})$ in a random order and add G to our dissimilar set $\mathcal{D}$, if $\nexists H \in \mathcal{D}$ with $\mathrm{sim}(G, H) < sim_{\max}$. This process is repeated several times and the largest set $\mathcal{D}_{\max}$ is used to create one cluster for each $H \in \mathcal{D}$ with H as single representative. Afterwards we run a regular assignment phase.

4.6 Convergence

StruClus will terminate as soon as its objective (see Sect. 4) converges. Since separation is a binary constraint and is maintained by the merging step, the convergence criteria $\mathrm{z}(\mathcal{C})$ only contains the coverage and the number of clusters.

$$\mathrm{z}(\mathcal{C}) := \frac{\sum_{C \in \mathcal{C}} |C| \ \mathrm{aCov}(C)}{|\mathcal{C}|} \tag{8}$$

As a consequence of the cluster splitting and merging, the convergence criteria will fluctuate and contain local optima. We will therefore smooth the criteria. Let $\mathcal{C}_i$ be the clustering after the i-th iteration and w an averaging width. Algorithm 1 will terminate after the first iteration c for which the following condition holds:

$$c \geq 2w \wedge \frac{\sum_{c-w<i\leq c} \mathrm{z}(\mathcal{C}_i)}{\sum_{c-2w<i\leq c-w} \mathrm{z}(\mathcal{C}_i)} \leq 1 + \epsilon \tag{9}$$

4.7 Runtime Analysis

The subgraph isomorphism problem and the maximum common subgraph problem are both NP-complete. Thus, *StruClus* scales exponentially w.r.t. the size of the graphs in the dataset $\mathcal{X}$. Nevertheless, these problems can be solved sufficiently fast for small graphs, e.g., molecular structures. We will therefore consider the graph size a constant in the following analysis and focus on the scalability w.r.t. the dataset size. Let $\mathcal{V}_{\max}$ be the maximal number of vertices for a graph in $\mathcal{X}$ and $\mathcal{C}_{\max}$ the maximal number of clusters during the clustering process.

Representative Mining. As described in Proposition 1 the number of extensions to mine a single maximal frequent subgraph from a set of graphs $\mathcal{G} \subseteq \mathcal{X}$ is bounded by $\left(\binom{V_{\max}}{2} + V_{\max}\right) |\mathrm{P}(\mathcal{G})| < \left(V_{\max}^2 + V_{\max}\right) |\mathrm{P}(\mathcal{G})|$. The value $V_{\max}$ is obviously a constant as it is bounded by $\mathcal{V}_{\max}$. Also $|\mathrm{P}(\mathcal{G})|$ is only bounded by $\mathcal{V}_{\max}$ and the lowest minimum support threshold ls, as a fraction of $\frac{\lceil ls \ |\mathcal{G}| \rceil}{\mathcal{V}_{\max}^2}$ of all edges in $\mathcal{G}$ must be isomorphic to be frequent. Thus, there exist at most $\frac{\mathcal{V}_{\max}^2}{ls}$ frequent paths of length one. For each mined maximal frequent subgraph we calculate the support over $\mathcal{G}$ and this involves $\mathcal{O}(|\mathcal{G}|)$ subgraph isomorphism tests. Thus, the runtime to mine a single maximal frequent subgraph is in $\mathcal{O}(|\mathcal{G}|)$.

Other Parts. The runtimes of the representative update, cluster assignment and pre-clustering are in $\mathcal{O}(\mathcal{C}_{\max} \ |\mathcal{X}|)$, cluster splitting in $\mathcal{O}(\mathcal{C}_{\max} + |\mathcal{X}|)$, cluster merging in $\mathcal{O}(\mathcal{C}_{\max}^2 + |\mathcal{X}|)$, and converge in $\mathcal{O}(\mathcal{C}_{\max})$.

Overall Runtime. A single iteration of Algorithm 1 has a runtime of $\mathcal{O}(\mathcal{C}_{\max} \ |\mathcal{X}|)$, and hence is linear. This is justified by the observation that $\mathcal{O}(\mathcal{C}_{\max}^2) \leq \mathcal{O}(\mathcal{C}_{\max} \ |\mathcal{X}|)$.

5 Evaluation

In the following evaluation we compare *StruClus* to SCAP [26] (the only other scalable structural clustering algorithm for labeled graphs), PROCLUS [2] (representative for the vectorial projected clustering algorithms) and Kernel K-Means [13] (representative for non-subspace vectorial clustering algorithms) w.r.t. their runtime and the clustering quality. Furthermore, we investigate the influence of our support sampling strategy and the parallel scaling of our implementation.

Hardware and Software. Tests are run on a Xeon E5-2640 v3 (Turbo Boost disabled) with 64 GiB RAM. The Java implementations of *StruClus*, PROCLUS and Kernel K-Means were running in an Hotspot VM 1.8.0_66. SCAP was compiled with GCC 4.9.3 (O3 optimization). *StruClus* and SCAP are parallelized.

Test Setup and Evaluation Measures. Tests were repeated 30 times if the runtime was below 2 h, 15 times otherwise. Quality is measured by ground truth comparisons using the Normalized Variation of Information (NVI) [21] and Fowlkes-Mallows (FW) [12] measures. We use Purity [17] for comparison with SCAP, as NVI and FW are not suited for overlapping clusterings.

Table 1. Real world dataset statistics. Cumulated values are given as min/max/average.

Dataset	Size	Classes	# vertices	# edges	# vertex labels	# edge labels
AnchorQuery	65 700	12	11 / 90 / 79.19	11 / 99 / 86.02	6	5
Heterocyclic	10 000	39	9 / 69 / 42.99	10 / 79 / 47.35	25	5
ChemDB	5 000 000	–	1 / 684 / 50.74	0 / 745 / 53.20	86	5

Datasets. We use synthetic datasets of different sizes and three real world datasets. The synthetic datasets have ≈35 vertices and ≈51 edges on average with 10 vertex and 3 edge labels (weights drawn from an exponential distribution). They contain 100 clusters and 5% random noise graphs. Each graph was generated by connecting 3 cluster specific and up to 2 common/noise seed patterns. The graphs have an edge probability of 10% and the seeds contain 10 vertices on average (poison distributed). AnchorQuery is a real-world molecular de-novo database. Each molecule is the result of a chemical reaction of purchasable building blocks. We have used 12 reaction types, i.e., class labels, from AnchorQuery[2]. Heterocyclic is a similar dataset, but contains heterocyclic compounds and 39 distinct reaction types. ChemDB is a collection of purchasable molecules from 150 chemical vendors. The dataset has no ground truth and will serve as proof that *StruClus* scales to large real world datasets. Table 1 shows additional statistics about the real world datasets. For PROCLUS the graphs data was transformed to vectors by counting connected subgraphs of size 3, resulting in 7 000–10 000 features on the synthetic datasets. The application to

[2] http://anchorquery.csb.pitt.edu/reactions/.

the AnchorQuery and Heterocyclic datasets result in feature counts of 274 and 133. The same vectors were used as features space representation for Kernel K-Means. Additionally, we have evaluated various other graph kernels with explicit feature mapping, such as Weisfeiler-Lehman and random walk kernels [27]. We observed clusterings with lower quality and omitted the results for this reason.

Algorithm Parameterization. SCAP has the following parameters: (a) the minimum size for s common substructure, that must be present in a single cluster and (b) a parameter for the granularity of the fingerprint-based pre-partitioning. (a) was set to 8. (b) was set to the highest value that results in a reasonable clustering quality, as it trades quality for speed. For the synthetic datasets this was 0.2. PROCLUS has two parameters: (c) the number of clusters and (d) the mean dimensionality of the cluster subspaces. (c) was set to the number of clusters in the ground truth. (d) was set to 20, for which we got best quality results. The number of clusters is the only parameter of Kernel K-Means and was set in exact the same manner as for PROCLUS. Note, that the a priory selection of this optimal value gives PROCLUS and Kernel K-Means an advantage over their competitors during the evaluation.

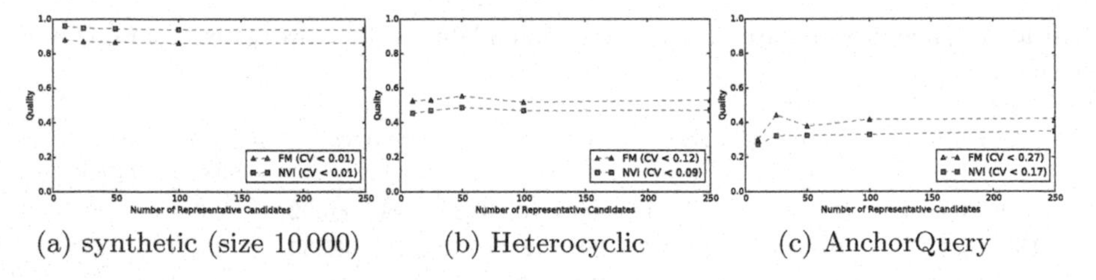

(a) synthetic (size 10 000) (b) Heterocyclic (c) AnchorQuery

Fig. 2. Influence of the number of candidate representatives on the clustering quality. CV is the max. coef. of variation (per measurement category).

The parameters of *StruClus* can be set dataset independent and are largely insensitive to the concrete values. We demonstrate this ability by using the same parameter set for all experiments. This contrasts the dataset dependent parameters (a) and (c) of SCAP, PROCLUS and Kernel K-Means. The parameters of *StruClus* were set as follows: (e) The maximal error for support counting is set to 50%. We can afford errors, because the selection of the final representatives will filter out bad candidates. Nevertheless, the used significance level has a theoretical influence on the runtime: A high error causes many bad candidates and an increased number of candidates to mine, but it also leads to small sample sizes to reject the null hypothesis. We have never observed a significant empirical runtime difference for different error rates in the range $[1, 90]$. Thus, the algorithm performance is insensitive to this parameter. (f) The number of representative candidates $|\mathcal{S}(\cdot)|$ has been set to 25. This parameter has a linear influence on the runtime. Figure 2 displays the influence of this parameter on the clustering quality for the different datasets. It shows, that the clustering quality is insensitive to the parameter in the range $[10, 250]$. (g) The maximal number of representatives per cluster was set to $\mathcal{R}_{\max} = 3$ to be human interpretable. (h) The splitting threshold for homogeneity balancing was set to $\text{relCov}_{\min} = 0.6$. This value should always be set well below 1, since *StruClus* would destroy clusters with a high or average homogeneity otherwise. Contrariwise, very low values would lead to unbalanced clusterings with a low quality. During our experimental evaluation values in the interval $[0.4, 0.8]$ have led to high quality clusterings independently of the clustered dataset. (i) The parameter $sim_{\max}$ is a constraint for the desired separation. Thus, there is no *optimal* value. We have chosen a value of 0.7 (j) Convergence was determined with an averaging width of $w = 3$. We show the convergence behavior of *StruClus* in Fig. 3, by plotting the relevant factors for convergence alongside with quality scores for each iteration. The plot shows that the quality of the clusterings does not increase significantly after the convergence and that the fluctuation in the number of clusters (caused by cluster splitting and merging) make it necessary to smooth the convergence criteria.

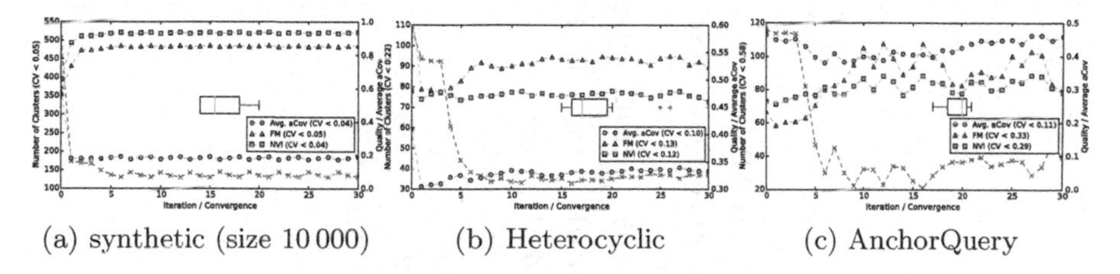

(a) synthetic (size 10 000) (b) Heterocyclic (c) AnchorQuery

Fig. 3. Convergence: The box plots show the number of iterations. CV is the max. coef. of variation (per category). *Avg.* aCov is the avg. value of Eq. (4) for all clusters.

Quality and Runtime Comparisons. As shown in Table 2, *StruClus* outperforms all competitors in terms of quality on the synthetic datasets. For small synthetic datasets, SCAP was the fastest algorithm. This changes for larger dataset sizes. *StruClus* outperforms SCAP by a factor of ≈13 at size 500 000. Furthermore, we were unable to cluster the largest dataset with SCAP in less than 2 days. PROCLUS and Kernel K-Means were the slowest algorithms with a huge gap to their next competitor. The sublinear growth of *StruClus*'s runtime for the smaller datasets is caused by our sampling strategy for support counting. Running *StruClus* with exact support counting yields a linear growth in runtime. It is important to mention that the clustering quality is not significantly influenced by the support counting strategy. The implementation of *StruClus* scales well with the number of cores: With 8 cores we get a speedup of 7.15. Including Hyper-Threading, we get a speedup of 9.11.

The evaluation results w.r.t. the real world datasets are summarized in Table 3. We were unable to cluster the AnchorQuery and the ChemDB datasets with PROCLUS, Kernel K-Means and SCAP (even for high values of parameter (b)) in less than 2 days. For the chemical reaction datasets, *StruClus* also needs more time compared to a synthetic dataset of similar size. This runtime increase can be partially explained by the larger graph sizes. However, other parameters of the datasets, such as the sizes of maximal common substructures have an influence on the runtime as well. Figure 3c reveals a large average aCov value

Table 2. Results: synthetic datasets. CV is the max. coef. of variation (per column).

Size	*StruClus*				*StruClus* (Exact Support)			SCAP		PROCLUS			Kernel K-Means		
	Runtime (hours)	NVI	FM	Purity	Runtime (hours)	NVI	FM	Runtime (hours)	Purity	Runtime	NVI	FM	Runtime (hours)	NVI	FM
	CV< 0.08	<0.03	<0.07	<0.03	<0.07	<0.02	<0.04	<0.06	<0.02	<0.32	<0.11	<0.22	<0.01	<0.01	<0.01
1 000	0.05	**0.90**	0.75	**0.90**	0.05	**0.90**	**0.77**	**<0.01**	0.83	0.13	0.58	0.26	0.02	0.77	0.54
5 000	0.15	0.94	0.85	**0.98**	0.27	**0.95**	**0.86**	**<0.01**	0.84	4.99	0.50	0.24	2.87	0.84	0.67
10 000	0.19	**0.95**	**0.87**	**0.99**	0.59	0.93	0.85	**0.03**	0.83	11.91	0.49	0.24	10.32	0.86	0.78
50 000	**0.33**	**0.94**	**0.87**	**0.99**	2.69	0.92	0.85	0.38	0.83	–	–	–	–	–	–
100 000	**0.47**	0.93	0.86	**0.99**	–	–	–	1.21	0.86	–	–	–	–	–	–
500 000	**1.35**	0.93	0.86	**0.99**	–	–	–	18.15	0.83	–	–	–	–	–	–
1 000 000	**2.73**	0.91	0.84	0.98	–	–	–	–	–	–	–	–	–	–	–

Table 3. Results: real world datasets. CV is the max. coef. of variation (per column).

Dataset	*StruClus*				SCAP		PROCLUS			Kernel K-Means		
	Runtime (hours)	NVI	FM	Purity	Runtime (hours)	Purity	Runtime (hours)	NVI	FM	Runtime (hours)	NVI	FM
	CV<2.91	<0.09	<0.12	<0.08	<0.02	<0.01	<0.03	<0.05	<0.08	<0.01	<0.01	<0.01
AnchorQuery	**2.47**	0.36	0.43	0.85	–	–	–	–	–	–	–	–
Heterocyclic	1.07	**0.46**	**0.53**	**0.66**	**0.01**	0.58	**0.01**	0.29	0.29	*3.03* (Subset)	*0.27*	*0.29*
ChemDB	**≈19**	–	–	–	–	–	–	–	–	–	–	–

for the AnchorQuery dataset. Thus, in addition to the large graph sizes, the common substructures (and representatives) are much larger than in the other datasets. The high runtime of the SCAP algorithm on the AnchorQuery dataset is a bit surprising, as the common substructures processed by SCAP are limited in their size (maximum 8 vertices). We consider a larger frequent pattern search space to be the reason for this runtime increase. *StruClus* had some runtime outliers on the Heterocyclic dataset. They were caused by small temporary clusters with large (>60 vertices) representatives. Kernel K-Means was surprisingly slow on the Heterocyclic dataset and took more than 24 h for a single run. We have therefore created a random subset with a size of 5000 graphs for it. *StruClus* always outperforms the competitors w.r.t. the quality scores. For the AnchorQuery dataset *StruClus* created 30.67 clusters on average. The high score for the Purity measure shows that *StruClus* splitted some of the real clusters, but keeps a well intra cluster homogeneity. ChemDB was clustered by *StruClus* in ≈19 h with ≈117 clusters. As a consequence of the high runtime of the ChemDB measurement, we repeated the test only 3 times. The aCov value for the final clustering was 0.49 on average. This highlights the ability of *StruClus* to cluster large-scale real-world datasets with highly descriptive representatives.

Reproducible Results Statement. The GPLv3 licensed implementation[3] of *StruClus*, including the test setups and the datasets[4], is made publicly available.

6 Conclusion

We have presented a new structural clustering algorithm for large-scale datasets of small labeled graphs. With explicitly selected cluster representatives, we were able to achieve a linear worst case runtime w.r.t. the dataset size. A novel support counting sampling with multiple hypothesis testing correction accelerates the algorithm significantly without influencing the clustering quality. We have shown, that cluster homogeneity can be balanced with a dynamic minimum support for representatives of variable size. A cluster merging and splitting step was introduced to achieve well separated clusters even in the high dimensional pattern space. In combination with the homogeneity and separation aware representative selection this leads to high quality clustering results. Our experimental

[3] https://ls11-www.cs.tu-dortmund.de/people/schaefer/publication_data/struclus_adma2017.tar.gz.

[4] https://ls11-www.cs.tu-dortmund.de/people/schaefer/publication_data/struclus_adma2017_datasets.tar.gz.

evaluation has shown that *StruClus* outperforms the competitors w.r.t. clustering quality, while attaining significantly lower runtimes for large scale datasets. We would like to thank Nils Kriege for his subgraph isomorphism implementation, Madeleine Seeland, Andreas Karwath, and Stefan Kramer for their SCAP implementation and Oliver Koch and Lina Humbeck for the chemical reaction datasets.

References

1. Ackerman, M., Ben-David, S.: Clusterability: a theoretical study. In: Proceedings of AISTATS, pp. 1–8 (2009)
2. Aggarwal, C.C., Procopiuc, C.M., Wolf, J.L., Yu, P.S., Park, J.S.: Fast algorithms for projected clustering. In: Proceedings of SIGMOD, pp. 61–72 (1999)
3. Aggarwal, C.C., Ta, N., Wang, J., Feng, J., Zaki, M.J.: XProj: a framework for projected structural clustering of XML documents. In: Proceedings of KDD, pp. 46–55 (2007)
4. Anchuri, P., Zaki, M.J., Barkol, O., Golan, S., Shamy, M.: Approximate graph mining with label costs. In: Proceedings of KDD, pp. 518–526, Chicago, Illinois, USA (2013)
5. Beyer, K.S., Goldstein, J., Ramakrishnan, R., Shaft, U.: When is "Nearest Neighbor" meaningful? In: Proceedings of ICDT, pp. 217–235 (1999)
6. Bunke, H.: On a relation between graph edit distance and maximum common subgraph. Pattern Recognit. Lett. **18**(8), 689–694 (1997)
7. Bunke, H., Shearer, K.: A graph distance metric based on the maximal common subgraph. Pattern Recognit. Lett. **19**(3–4), 255–259 (1998)
8. Chávez, E., Navarro, G.: A probabilistic spell for the curse of dimensionality. In: Buchsbaum, A.L., Snoeyink, J. (eds.) ALENEX 2001. LNCS, vol. 2153, pp. 147–160. Springer, Heidelberg (2001). doi:10.1007/3-540-44808-X_12
9. Fernández, M.-L., Valiente, G.: A graph distance metric combining maximum common subgraph and minimum common supergraph. Pattern Recognit. Lett. **22**(6–7), 753–758 (2001)
10. Ferrer, M., Valveny, E., Serratosa, F., Bardají, I., Bunke, H.: Graph-based k-means clustering: a comparison of the set median versus the generalized median graph. In: Jiang, X., Petkov, N. (eds.) CAIP 2009. LNCS, vol. 5702, pp. 342–350. Springer, Heidelberg (2009). doi:10.1007/978-3-642-03767-2_42
11. Foggia, P., Percannella, G., Vento, M.: Graph matching and learning in pattern recognition in the last 10 years. IJPRAI 28(1) (2014)
12. Fowlkes, E.B., Mallows, C.L.: A method for comparing two hierarchical clusterings. J. Am. Stat. Assoc. **78**(383), 553–569 (1983)
13. Girolami, M.A.: Mercer kernel-based clustering in feature space. IEEE Trans. Neural Netw. **13**(3), 780–784 (2002)
14. Gupta, A., Krauthgamer, R., Lee, J.R.: Bounded geometries, fractals, and low-distortion embeddings. In: Proceedings of FOCS, pp. 534–543 (2003)
15. Hasan, M.A., Chaoji, V., Salem, S., Besson, J., Zaki, M.J.: ORIGAMI: mining representative orthogonal graph patterns. In: Proceedings of ICDM, pp. 153–162 (2007)
16. Huang, X., Cheng, H., Yang, J., Yu, J.X., Fei, H., Huan, J.: Semi-supervised clustering of graph objects: a subgraph mining approach. In: Lee, S., Peng, Z., Zhou, X., Moon, Y.-S., Unland, R., Yoo, J. (eds.) DASFAA 2012. LNCS, vol. 7238, pp. 197–212. Springer, Heidelberg (2012). doi:10.1007/978-3-642-29038-1_16

17. Hui, X., Zhongmon, L.: Clustering validation measures. In: Data Clustering: Algorithms and Applications, pp. 571–605 (2013)
18. Jouili, S., Tabbone, S., Lacroix, V.: Median graph shift: a new clustering algorithm for graph domain. In: Proceedings of ICPR, pp. 950–953 (2010)
19. Kalinski, C., Umkehrer, M., Weber, L., Kolb, J., Burdack, C., Ross, G.: On the industrial applications of MCRs: molecular diversity in drug discovery and generic drug synthesis. Mol. Divers. **14**(3), 513–522 (2010)
20. Kriege, N., Mutzel, P., Schäfer, T.: Practical SAHN clustering for very large data sets and expensive distance metrics. JGAA **18**(4), 577–602 (2014)
21. Meilă, M.: Comparing clusterings–an information based distance. J. Multivar. Anal. **98**(5), 873–895 (2007)
22. Müller, E., Günnemann, S., Assent, I., Seidl, T.: Evaluating clustering in subspace projections of high dimensional data. In: Proceedings of VLDB, pp. 1270–1281 (2009)
23. Patrikainen, A., Meila, M.: Comparing subspace clusterings. IEEE Trans. Knowl. Data Eng. **18**(7), 902–916 (2006)
24. Ranu, S., Hoang, M., Singh, A.: Answering top-k representative queries on graph databases. In: Proceedings of SIGMOD, pp. 1163–1174, Snowbird, Utah, USA (2014)
25. Seeland, M., Berger, S.A., Stamatakis, A., Kramer, S.: Parallel structural graph clustering. In: Gunopulos, D., Hofmann, T., Malerba, D., Vazirgiannis, M. (eds.) ECML PKDD 2011. LNCS (LNAI), vol. 6913, pp. 256–272. Springer, Heidelberg (2011). doi:10.1007/978-3-642-23808-6_17
26. Seeland, M., Karwath, A., Kramer, S.: Structural clustering of millions of molecular graphs. In: Symposium on Applied Computing, pp. 121–128 (2014)
27. Shervashidze, N., Schweitzer, P., van Leeuwen, E.J., Mehlhorn, K., Borgwardt, K.M.: Weisfeiler-Lehman graph kernels. J. Mach. Learn. Res. **12**, 2539–2561 (2011)
28. Shervashidze, N., Vishwanathan, S.V.N., Petri, T., Mehlhorn, K., Borgwardt, K.M.: Efficient graphlet kernels for large graph comparison. In: Proceedings of AISTATS, pp. 488–495 (2009)
29. Thoma, M., Cheng, H., Gretton, A., Han, J., Kriegel, H., Smola, A.J., Song, L., Yu, P.S., Yan, X., Borgwardt, K.M.: Discriminative frequent subgraph mining with optimality guarantees. Stat. Anal. Data Min. **3**(5), 302–318 (2010)
30. Tsuda, K., Kudo, T.: Clustering graphs by weighted substructure mining. In: Proceedings of ICML, pp. 953–960 (2006)
31. Tsuda, K., Kurihara, K.: Graph mining with variational dirichlet process mixture models. In: Proceedings of the International Conference on Data Mining, pp. 432–442 (2008)
32. Vishwanathan, S.V.N., Schraudolph, N.N., Kondor, R.I., Borgwardt, K.M.: Graph kernels. J. Mach. Learn. Res. **11**, 1201–1242 (2010)
33. Wale, N., Watson, I.A., Karypis, G.: Comparison of descriptor spaces for chemical compound retrieval and classification. Knowl. Inf. Syst. **14**(3), 347–375 (2008)
34. Wallis, W.D., Shoubridge, P., Kraetzl, M., Ray, D.: Graph distances using graph union. Pattern Recognit. Lett. **22**(6/7), 701–704 (2001)
35. Yan, X., Cheng, H., Han, J., Yu, P.S.: Mining significant graph patterns by leap search. In: Proceedings of SIGMOD, pp. 433–444 (2008)
36. Yiu, M.L., Mamoulis, N.: Frequent-pattern based iterative projected clustering. In: Proceedings of ICDM, pp. 689–692 (2003)

Employing Hierarchical Clustering and Reinforcement Learning for Attribute-Based Zero-Shot Classification

Bin Liu, Li Yao(✉), Junfeng Wu, and Xiaosheng Feng

Science and Technology on Information System and Engineering Laboratory, National University of Defense Technology, Changsha 410073, China
913381959@qq.com

Abstract. Zero-shot classification (ZSC) is a hot topic of computer vision. Because the training labels are totally different from the testing labels, ZSC cannot be dealt with by classical classifiers. Attribute-based classifier is a dominant solution for ZSC. It employs attribute annotations to bridge training labels and testing labels, making it able to realize ZSC. Classical attribute-based classifiers treat different attributes equally. However, the attributes contribute to classification unequally. In this paper, a novel attribute-based classifier for ZSC named HCRL is proposed. HCRL utilizes hierarchical clustering to obtain a hierarchy from the attribute annotations. Then the attribute annotations are decomposed into hierarchical rules which contain only a few attributes. The discriminative abilities of the rules reflect the significances of attributes to classification, but there are no training samples for evaluating the rules. The discriminative abilities are determined by reinforcement learning during the testing and the most discriminative rules are picked out for classification. Experiments conducted on 2 popular datasets for ZSC show the competitiveness of HCRL.

Keywords: Reinforcement learning · Image classification · Attribute · Zero-Shot classification · Hierarchical clustering

1 Introduction

Zero-shot classification (ZSC) is a hot topic in the area of computer vision recently [1–6]. Different from traditional image classifications, ZSC are the cases where labels of training samples are totally different from labels of testing samples. In reality, it is difficult to obtain labeled training samples for all classes, because there are so many object classes. There are even classes without one training sample, because new classes are defined on the fly [3]. So, developing classifiers for ZSC can significantly extend the ability of machine learning for handling practical problems.

ZSC cannot be handled by traditional classifiers, because the classes in the testing phase (seen classes) are totally different from the classes in the training phase (unseen classes). The concept of zero-shot learning is proposed [7] for solving ZSC problems. As understandable features, attributes can be shared by multiple object classes. Knowledge about the attributes for describing the unseen classes can be obtained by

G. Cong et al. (Eds.): ADMA 2017, LNAI 10604, pp. 360–372, 2017.
https://doi.org/10.1007/978-3-319-69179-4_25

learning from examples of the seen classes. Therefore, knowledge of the unseen classes for ZSC can be obtained by transferring the knowledge about the attributes [8]. Based on this assumption, the attribute-based method for ZSC is proposed [3]. The attribute-based method became a popular method for ZSC since it was proposed [4, 9]. It realizes ZSC by employing attribute annotations of the object classes which are from human prior knowledge or data mining, and by training attributes' classifiers upon the low-level features extracted from the images. In the attribute-based method in [3], all object classes are annotated by the same set of attributes, i.e., all attributes are treated equally. Therefore, different contributions of the attributes to the classification are not considered.

In fact, not every attribute plays a part in ZSC [3]. Choosing the best attributes combination benefits ZSC [10]. In the attribute annotations, the attributes which distinguish a set of classes from another set of classes in the scope are called discriminative attributes [11]. The non-discriminative attributes are useless in ZSC; hence the best combination has to exclude them. In addition, not all discriminative attributes show the same ability in distinguishing different couples of classes [12]. CAAP predicts class-attribute associations for ZSC and discriminates negative and positive associations between the discriminative attributes and the unseen classes [6]. The enriched descriptions for unseen classes make CAAP more competitive. HAT trains attributes' predictors at different levels of abstraction based on a hierarchy [12] and plans to distinguish contributions of attributes using adaptive weights.

A method named HCRL (Hierarchical Clustering and Reinforcement Learning) is proposed for ZSC. The concept of hierarchical rule is introduced to enable reinforcement learning to be used in ZSC. Hierarchical rules are obtained from attribute annotations with the guidance of a hierarchy obtained by hierarchical clustering from attribute annotations. One predictor is trained for each attribute appeared in the rules, enabling it to predict the object's attributes using the low-level features extracted from images. Reinforcement learning is used by HCRL to determine the discriminative abilities of the hierarchical rules and to obtain a policy which selects the most discriminative hierarchical rules for ZSC.

There are 3 main contributions of the paper. Firstly, rules only containing attributes necessary for classification are obtained from attribute annotations, through the introduction of hierarchical rule. Secondly, by decomposing the attribute annotations into hierarchical rules, there are many choices for classification by using the rules, making reinforcement learning applicable. Thirdly, the most discriminative rules are picked out for classification by reinforcement learning and the most discriminative attributes can be obtained.

HCRL achieves competitive performances on 2 popular ZSC datasets compared with baseline zero-shot classifiers, indicating that the most discriminative rules are used for classification. The most discriminative attributes of one dataset are analyzed, further validating the statement that the different significances of attributes at levels in the hierarchy are reflected by the value function of reinforcement learning.

2 Related Work

As an important approach to deal with ZSC, attribute-based methods categorize samples of unseen classes through sharing attributes between seen classes and unseen classes. The attribute-based method for ZSC is first proposed in [3] and DAP is one of the realizations of attribute-based method. The attribute-based method realizes ZSC via describing object classes by attributes and building predictors upon low-level features for these attributes by support vector machine [13]. Utilizing attributes which are human-understandable features as the bridge, the low-level features extracted from images can be associated to human prior knowledge, making it able to realize ZSC based on attributes.

One recent work on ZSC which considers the class-attribute associations and the associations between the discriminative attributes and the unseen classes is CAAP [6]. However, the associations are not quantized; therefore, the most discriminative attribute cannot be obtained. HAT [12] trains discriminative attributes' predictors at different levels of abstraction based on a biological hierarchy and refines the attributes' predictors. However, it does not distinguish contributions of attributes, too.

Hierarchical clustering organizes samples into hierarchy based on similarities. Hierarchical clustering algorithms are divided into two categories: agglomerative and divisive. Agglomerative clustering obtains hierarchy from bottom to top. It treats each sample as a single cluster and merges clusters step by step until all samples are merged into a single cluster. Divisive clustering obtains hierarchy in a top-down way. It puts all samples in one cluster at first and then split them into clusters until the expected number of clusters is obtained. To split the cluster, divisive clustering usually employs heuristics, which may lead to inaccurate results. For this reason, there are more options for using agglomerative clustering than divisive clustering [14]. There are many agglomerative clustering algorithms, such as BIRCH, single-link, complete-link and average-link [14]. Single-link, complete-link and average-link are grouped into the linkage algorithms [15]. These hierarchical methods merge clusters based on distances between clusters. Average-link is a medium between single-link and complete-link. It overcomes the problem of being sensitive to outliers [14]. Therefore, it will be used to obtain the hierarchy for HCRL.

Reinforcement learning is an important machine learning techniques [16]. It perceives state of the environment and chooses the best actions to change the state of environment. Its most important properties are trials and rewards [17]. Monte Carlo methods for reinforcement learning are the ones which exploit online experience statistically [18]. It provides a general way to determine the values of actions by statistics and obtains the policy for selecting the best actions. By determining the discriminative abilities of hierarchical rules using reinforcement learning, the most discriminative hierarchical rules can be picked out for ZSC.

3 The Proposed Method

The proposed HCRL, which combines hierarchical clustering and reinforcement learning for ZSC, first learns hierarchical rules from the attribute annotations based on the clustered hierarchy. Then, a predictor for each attribute appeared in the rules is learned, making it able to predict the attribute value from the low-level features extracted from the images for testing. Finally, a policy is obtained by reinforcement learning, aiming at selecting the most discriminative rules for classification. An overview of HCRL is shown in Fig. 1.

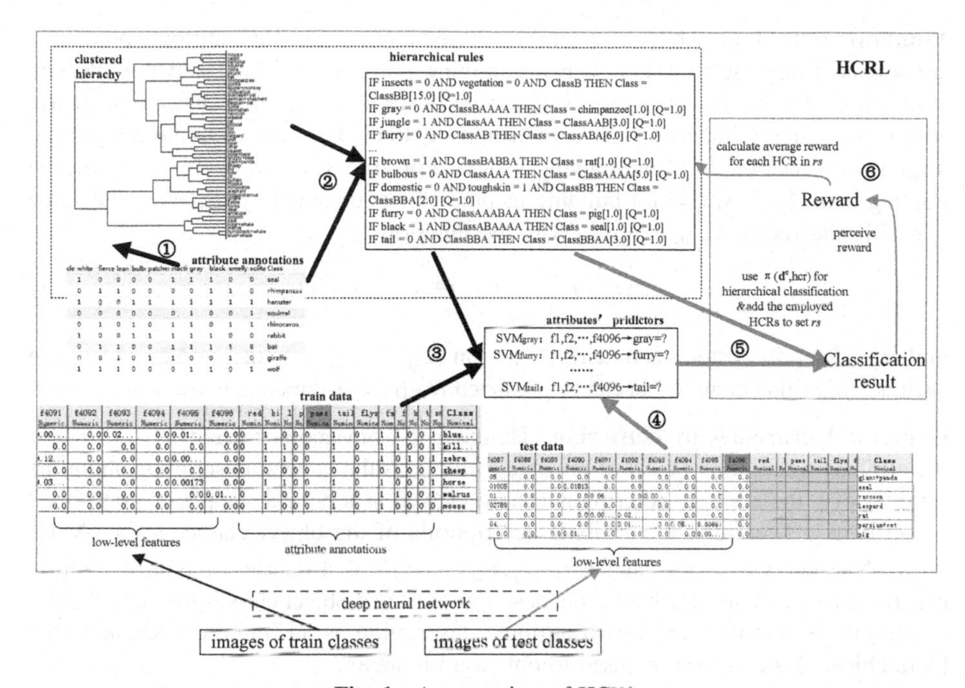

Fig. 1. An overview of HCRL

As shown in Fig. 1, HCRL first obtains a hierarchy by a linkage algorithm of hierarchical clustering (step ①), and use the hierarchy to obtain hierarchical rules (step ②). Then, one predictor for each attribute appeared in the hierarchical rules is trained by SVM (step ③), making it able to predict the attributes of an object from the low-level features (step ④). Therefore, the category to which the object belongs can be determined by classification using the hierarchical rules (step ⑤). After the classification, a reward is perceived and the reward is used to update the indices which evaluate the discriminative abilities of the hierarchical rules used in the classification (step ⑥).

3.1 Preliminaries

To illustrate the proposed approach, necessary definitions are given first. In the following, the meanings of the symbols refer to the meanings of their first appearance if not pointed out specifically.

Describing Object Classes by Attributes in ZSC. Given a set of object classes $C = \{c_1, c_2, \ldots, c_n\}$ in ZSC, the set of training classes is $Y = \{y_1, y_2, \ldots, y_k\}$, and the set of testing classes is $Z = \{z_1, z_2, \ldots, z_l\}$, where $Y \cap Z = \emptyset$ and $Y \cup Z = C$ hold.

Therefore, the train set contains samples labeled as element of Y but no samples labeled as element of Z. An m-dimension vector $\mathbf{v}_j = (v_{j1}, v_{j2}, \ldots, v_{jm})(v_{ji} \in [0,1], 1 \leq i \leq m)$ describes the object class $c_j \in C$. The value v_{ji} in the vector $\mathbf{v}_j$ represents the "*relative strength of association*" [19] between the object class c_j and the attribute a_i in the set of attributes $A = \{a_1, a_2, \ldots, a_m\}$.

Notation. In DAP [3] which is an attribute-based method for ZSC, attribute predictors are trained using the (α + 1)-dimension training data $(\mathbf{F}_{\text{train}}, \mathbf{Y}_{\text{train}})$ and the attribute annotations for the object classes $\mathbf{v}$ (attribute descriptions), where $\mathbf{F}_{\text{train}}$ is a matrix composed of the α-dimension low-level features extracted from the training images and $\mathbf{Y}_{\text{train}}$ is the label vector of the training images. For an attribute $a_i \in A(1 \leq i \leq m)$, the training data $(\mathbf{F}_{\text{train}}, \mathbf{v}_{\text{i,train}})$ for building its predictor is obtained by replacing the value $y_j \in Y$ in the vector $\mathbf{Y}_{\text{train}}$ with v_{ji}. With the function

$$SVM_{a_i} : \mathbf{f} \rightarrow v\,(\mathbf{f} \in R^{\alpha}, v \in [0,1]) \tag{1}$$

built by a support vector machine (SVM) upon $(\mathbf{F}_{\text{train}}, \mathbf{v}_{\text{i,train}})$ as the predictor of a_i, the attribute a_i's value of an object can be predicted from the α-dimension low-level feature.

Generate hierarchies by clustering. Thinking it from another perspective, because the attribute description $(\mathbf{v}_z, z)$ of the object class z is the general description about the samples of z, the attribute description can be viewed as a typical sample of z described by attributes. Therefore, the attribute descriptions of the object classes $DS = (\mathbf{V}, \mathbf{C})$ where $\mathbf{V} = (\mathbf{v}_1, \mathbf{v}_2, \ldots, \mathbf{v}_l)^{\mathrm{T}}$ and $\mathbf{C} = (c_1, c_2, \ldots, c_l)^{\mathrm{T}}$, is a dataset of typical samples described by attributes. Each attribute description of one object class is the central point of the class's samples. Treat each attribute description as an initial cluster, and then hierarchical clustering can be used to obtain a hierarchy.

In the following, the concept of hierarchical rule will be introduced. Then, how to generate hierarchical rules and obtain a policy for picking out the most discriminative rules by reinforcement learning in the proposed HCRL will be described.

3.2 Learning Hierarchical Rules

The classical attribute-based method DAP classifies objects by attribute annotations which employ all attributes in A to describe object classes. Different from DAP, HCRL classifies objects using hierarchical rules. These rules only use attributes which are necessary to discriminate the object classes. First, the concept of hierarchical rule is defined.

Hierarchical Rule. A tree $H = \, <N, E>$ defines a hierarchy over the classes in C and their super classes. The leaf nodes of the tree are the classes in C and the root is denoted as *root*. A rule of the form

$$\textbf{IF}\; a_i\, rel_i\, v_{i\lambda}, \ldots, a_j\, rel_j\, v_{j\lambda}, class = super\_t\; \textbf{THEN}\; class = t \tag{2}$$

where *super_t* is t's father in the hierarchy H, is called hierarchical rule. t is called the rule's descendant.

Objects are classified by hierarchical rules from general types to specific types hierarchically. The hierarchical rules only discriminate classes who own the same super-class. Therefore, fewer attributes are necessary for discriminating the classes. The hierarchical rules can be obtained through learning hierarchically according to the hierarchy H from training data. Algorithm 1 is proposed to generate hierarchical rules.

Algorithm 1: HR_Learning(hier,ds,cls)
/*learn hierarchical rules of cls from dataset ds guided by the clustered hierarchy*/

Input: Hierarchy hier, DataSet ds, Root cls←"root"
Output: RulesSet rs←∅

1 tmpds←copy(ds), subs←getSubCls(hier,cls); //create a copy of ds & get children of cls
/*steps 2-7: replace instances' labels which cls is the father of to cls's child and remove instances whose label is not a child of cls */
2 **for all** inst∈tmpds **do**
3 lbl_set←subs ∩ super(hier,labelOf(inst); //obtain super-classes of inst's label in subs
4 **if** lbl_set≠∅ **then** inst.label←element(lbl_set); //replace label guided by the hierarchy
5 **else** tmpds←tmpds\{inst};
// remove instances guided by the hierarchy
6 **end if**
7 **end for**
8 attrs_set←∅, ml_rules←∅; //create an empty set of attributes and an empty set of rules
9 **do** /*step 9-12: learning rules with different attributes*/
10 attrs_set←attrs_set ∪ attrsInHRs(ml_rules); //exclude attributes already in rules
11 ml_rules←CR_learning(tmpds, attrs_set); //learning rules without using attributes in attrs_set
12 **while** ml_rules≠∅ //some rules are learned using new attributes
/*steps 13-16: form hierarchical rules which derive cls's child (r's head) from cls*/
13 **for all** r∈ml_rules **do**
14 hr←formHR(r, cls); //add $class = cls$ to the antecendent of r to form the new hierarchical rule
15 rs←rs ∪ { hr}; //add hr to the rules set rs
16 **end for**
/*steps 17-20: hierarchical learning: learning rules for cls's subclasses */
17 tmpds1←copy(ds); //create a new copy of ds for learning
18 **for all** sub∈subs **do**
19 rs←rs ∪HR_Learning (hier, tmpds1,sub);
20 **end for**

The attribute descriptions for the object classes will be decomposed by Algorithm 1 into hierarchical rules. A single hierarchical rule uses fewer attributes than a single attribute description. As pointed out in Sect. 3.1, the attribute annotations of the object classes $DS = (\mathbf{V}, \mathbf{C})$ constitute a dataset of typical samples. Therefore, they can be used to obtain classification rules. All the generated hierarchical rules whose descendant is an unseen class or ancestor of an unseen class in the hierarchy H can take role in the zero-shot classification. These rules constitute a set, denoted as Rs. The attributes appeared in the rules in *Rs* constitute the set $\{a'_1, a'_2, ..., a'_\lambda\}$, denoted as A'. It is easy to see that $A' \subseteq A$ holds.

Algorithm 1 generates rules which derive children of *cls* from *cls*, through replacing labels in the training data *ds* with their super classes who are children of *cls* on the hierarchy *hier*. Steps 2–7 modify the labels in the training data and reside samples whose labels are children of *cls* for rule learning. Therefore, only rules that derive children of *cls* from *cls* are obtained in steps 9–12. Correspondingly in steps 13-16 which convert the generated rules to hierarchical rules, the antecedent should contain the condition *class* = *cls*. Steps 17–20 generate rules that derive from children of *cls* by calling the algorithm recursively.

3.3 Applying Reinforcement Learning for Rule Selection

The learning for hierarchical rules decomposes attribute annotations for object classes into rules. These rules provide many choices for classifying an object. Hence, reinforcement learning can be applied for choosing the most discriminative rules to classify the object. In this section, reinforcement learning will be applied to obtain the best policy which picks out the most discriminative rules for classification.

Treat the dataset of unclassified objects *E* as the environment. For an unclassified object $e \in E$, its attributes' values can be estimated by the attribute predictors from the low-level features, using the trained function in (1). Denoting its attributes' values as $(a'_1, a'_2, ..., a'_\lambda) = (v^e_1, v^e_2, ..., v^e_\lambda)$ and giving its known type which is *root*, then its description $\mathbf{d}_e = (v^e_1, v^e_2, ..., v^e_\lambda, root)$ is seen as the initial state of the environment. Given a set of hierarchical rules $rs \subseteq Rs$ which derives *e*'s type from the general type to the more specific types based on the description $\mathbf{d}_e$, then a hierarchical rule $hcr \in rs$ is seen as an action. $\forall hcr \in Rs$, a *q-value* is setup for *hcr*, denoted as q_{hcr}. The classification which derives *e*'s type from *root* to z_e ($z_e \in Z$) is then an episode in the context of reinforcement learning.

The value function $Q(\mathbf{d}, hcr)$ for the state **d** and action *hcr* means the value of the hierarchical rule *hcr* in the state **d**. Therefore, if we let **d** represent a category of descriptions which are satisfied by *hcr*, i.e., $Q(\mathbf{d}, hcr)$ means the value of *hcr* in any state **d** which satisfies *hcr*. Therefore, it is appropriate to approximate $Q(\mathbf{d}, hcr)$ using q_{hcr}, i.e., $Q(\mathbf{d}, hcr) \approx q_{hcr}$.

When HCRL classifies the object *e* hierarchically, the rules are selected for classifying the object *e* by the **ε-greedy** policy. Hence the following steps are executed. First, one rule hcr_1 whose antecedents are satisfied by $\mathbf{d}^0_e = \mathbf{d}_e$ is picked out. There may be several candidate rules, so the rule with the biggest *q-value* is chosen with the probability of $(1 - \varepsilon)$ and other rules are chosen with the whole probability of ε. Then, the rule hcr_2 whose antecedents are satisfied by $\mathbf{d}^1_e = (v^e_1, v^e_2, ..., v^e_\lambda, desc(hcr_1))$ is picked out similarly. Similar steps shall be executed until the rule hcr_β is selected, where $desc(hcr_\beta) = z_e$ and $z_e \in Z$.

The reward function is defined as

$$r(\mathbf{d}_e, rs) = \begin{cases} \phi, \phi > 0 \\ \varphi, \varphi \leq 0 \end{cases} \quad (3)$$

If the object is classified correctly, $\hat{r} = r(\mathbf{d}_e, rs)$ is assigned to the value ϕ; otherwise, $\hat{r}$ is assigned to the value φ. $\hat{r}$ is used to update the *q-values* of the rules in *rs* using Monte Carlo method of reinforcement learning, following the formula

$$q_{hcr}^{k+1} \leftarrow q_{hcr}^{k} + (\hat{r} - q_{hcr}^{k})/(k+1) \quad (4)$$

where k is the number of episodes where *hcr* already participated in and (k + l) is the order of the classification where *hcr* is participating in. According to the law of large numbers, $q_{hcr} = \lim_{k \to +\infty} q_{hcr}^{k}$, therefore, the discriminative ability of *hcr* is determined.

4 Experiments

HCRL's performances are validated by experiments in this section. Experiments on 2 benchmark datasets for ZSC are conducted using HCRL, to compare HCRL with baseline zero-shot classifiers. The hierarchical rules whose *q-values* have been determined by reinforcement learning are also analyzed to obtain the most discriminative attributes. By comparing these attributes and the associative attributes in CAAP [6], our statement that HCRL can obtain the most discriminative attributes are further checked.

4.1 Datasets and Experiment Setup

The two benchmark datasets for ZSC, Animals with Attributes (AwA) [3] and aPascal-aYahoo (aPaY) [11], are used for the experiments. There are 30475 images of 50 animals classes in AwA. Each class of AwA is annotated with 85 attributes. Samples of 40 classes in AwA are used for training, and samples of the other 10 classes are the test samples. The aPaY dataset provides 15339 images of 32 classes. Every sample in aPaY is annotated with 64 attributes. Samples of 20 classes in aPaY are used for training, and samples of the other 12 classes are the test samples.

To obtain attribute descriptions for the classes in aPaY and CUB, the same method as that proposed in [3] is used. Each class is annotated with the attributes using the average values of its samples. The resulting class-attribute matrices are then binarized by thresholding at its global mean value, to obtain the binary attribute descriptions of the classes. Only the binary attribute descriptions are used for experiments. The training data contains 3 parts: the low-level features extracted from images, the labels of the images and the attribute descriptions for the labels. The test data only contains the low-level features extracted from images for testing. The 4096-dimension VGG19-fc7 features provided by Lampert et al. are used for the experiments on

AwA[1]. For aPaY, the 1024-dimension GoogLeNet features provided by [12] are used for the experiments.

We use the statistical toolbox in MATLAB[2] to obtain hierarchies. The function *Y = pdist(X, 'euclidean')* is used to calculate the Euclidean distances between any two attribute descriptions and *linkage(Y, 'ward')* is employed to obtain a hierarchy based on the calculated distances. Hierarchical rules are learned by employing Algorithm 1. In the step 11 of Algorithm 1, decision trees are obtained by calling C4.5 [20] to extract rules with precision equaling to 1. The hierarchical rules for AwA and aPaY are all learned from the binary attribute descriptions for the classes. The initial *q-value* of each rule is set to be 1.

The attributes' predictors are learned in the same way in **Notation** in Sect. 3.1. One 2-order polynomial SVM is learned for each attribute used in the rules by the SMO [21] implemented in WEKA[3]. For memory limitation, 3% (728 samples) and 5% (634 samples) of the training data obtained by sampling with replacement are used to train attributes' predictors for AwA and aPaY respectively.

Half of the testing samples in both datasets are used for reinforcement learning and exploration probability is set to be (0.4/*square root of the number of objects which have been classified*). The proposed HCRL are implemented in WEKA, making it easy to obtain important indices of evaluation, such as accuracy and confusion matrices.

4.2 Results and Analysis

Comparing HCRL with other zero-shot classifiers. Conducting experiments on 2 benchmark datasets, AwA and aPaY, the highest accuracies achieved by HCRL and baseline zero-shot classifiers are shown in Table 1.

Table 1. The highest accuracies achieved by various methods

	HCRL	CAAP [6]	JACP [22]	HAT [12]	SSE-INT [1]	DAP [3]
AwA	69.9	67.5	44.1	74.9	71.5	57.2
aPaY	37.9	37.0	24.4	45.4	44.2	35.5

HCRL achieves the competitive accuracies of ZSC on AwA and aPaY, compared to baseline zero-shot classifiers. It achieves higher accuracies than the classical attribute-based method DAP on the 2 datasets. The comparisons between HCRL and DAP further indicate that the more discriminative rules are picked out by the reinforcement learning to classify objects. Among the above zero-shot classifiers, HAT performs best. It incorporates a semantic hierarchy and refines attributes' classifiers for ZSC. HCRL obtains the hierarchy by clustering. Therefore, more prior information

[1] http://attributes.kyb.tuebingen.mpg.de/.

[2] http://www.mathworks.com/.

[3] http://www.cs.waikato.ac.nz/ml/weka/.

(semantic hierarchy) is used by HAT than HCRL. The hierarchy for AwA used by HCRL is shown in Fig. 2.

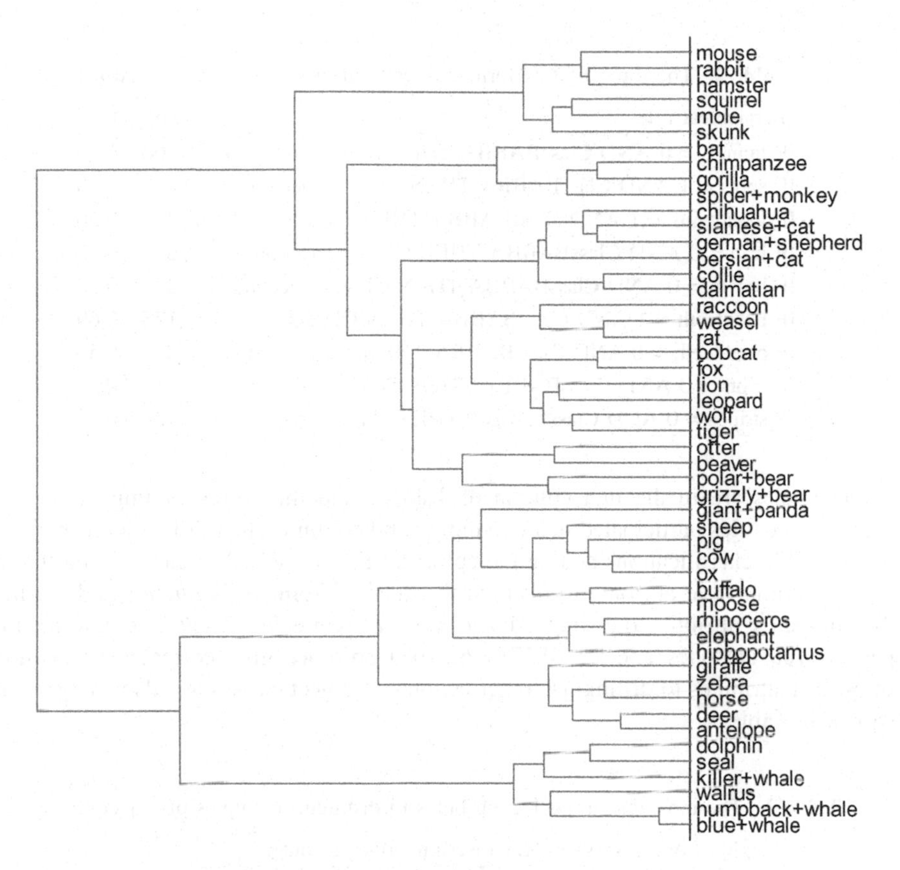

Fig. 2. Hierarchy for AwA used by HCRL.

From Fig. 2, it can be seen that the clustered hierarchy is not as accurate as the semantic hierarchy used by HAT. For example, *giant+panda* is clustered into the group which contains *pig*, *sheep* and *cow* and does not contain *bear* or *raccoon*, while *giant+panda* are closer to *bear* or *raccoon* than *pig*, *sheep* and *cow*. This is also a factor that affects the performance of HCRL.

Analyzing the most discriminative attributes in AwA. The experiment results on AwA and aPaY indicate that rules composed of the most discriminative attributes are used for classifying objects by HCRL. Through analyzing the hierarchical rules whose discriminative abilities have been determined by reinforcement learning, the most discriminative attributes can be discovered. Some of AwA's attributes with the most discriminative ability are shown in the following.

By hierarchical clustering, *raccoon* and *rat* are grouped into one cluster in Fig. 2. Several attributes distinguish the two object classes. Hence, multiple hierarchical rules are formed to discriminate *raccoon* and *rat*. The top 5 hierarchical rules sorted by descending order using discriminative abilities determined by reinforcement learning are shown in Table 2.

Table 2. The top 5 best-performed rules to discriminate *raccoon* and *rat*

Hierarchical rule	#eps	Q
IF tunnels = 0 AND ClassBABBA THEN Class = raccoon	108	0.57
IF spots = 1 AND ClassBABBA THEN Class = raccoon	2	0.50
IF mountains = 1 AND ClassBABBA THEN Class = raccoon	2	0.50
IF lean = 0 AND ClassBABBA THEN Class = raccoon	6	0.33
IF brown = 0 AND ClassBABBA THEN Class = raccoon	3	0.33
IF buckteeth = 1 AND ClassBABBA THEN Class = rat	178	0.69
IF chewteeth = 0 AND ClassBABBA THEN Class = rat	2	0.50
IF spots = 0 AND ClassBABBA THEN Class = rat	11	0.36
IF stripes = 0 AND ClassBABBA THEN Class = rat	12	0.33

The rules are in the first column of Table 2 and the corresponding numbers of episodes the rules participated in are in the second column. The third column shows the ratio of right classifications among the episodes. From Table 2, it can be seen that the most discriminative attribute to distinguish *raccoon* from *rat* is *tunnels* and the most discriminative attribute to distinguish *rat* from *raccoon* is *buckteeth*. The first rule took part in 108 episodes and 62 ($0.57 \approx 62/108$) episodes give correct classifications. Important attributes to distinguish other couples of object classes are also analyzed and shown in Table 3.

Table 3. The most discriminative attributes to distinguish couples of object classes

Couple of object classes	Key discriminative attributes
persian+cat/giant+panda	meat; scavenger; oldworld; domestic; fast
pig/hippopotamus	newworld; gray; active; smelly; bush
seal/humpback+whale	plankton; gray; skimmer; white; blue; inactive
leopard/rat&raccoon	oldworld; red; active; bush; hunter; tail; forest

From Table 3, it can be known that the most important attributes for distinguishing *persian+cat* from *giant+panda* include *meat*, *scavenger*, *oldworld* and etc. The most important attributes for distinguishing other couples such as *pig/hippopotamus*, *seal/humpback+whale* and *leopard/rat&raccoon* are also listed. The positive attributes associated with *leopard* found by CAAP are *fast*, *lean*, *oldworld*, *active* and *tail*. The most discriminative attributes found by HCRL include *oldworld*, *active* and *tail*, and the most discriminative attribute is *oldworld*. Therefore, the results of HCRL and CAAP are consistent. This comparison further validates the statement HCRL can obtain the most discriminative attributes for classification.

5 Conclusions

A method named HCRL which employs hierarchical clustering and reinforcement learning is proposed for zero-shot classification. The concept of hierarchical rule is introduced. HCRL utilizes hierarchical clustering to obtain a hierarchy for learning hierarchical rules. The hierarchical rules only contain attributes necessary for classification, i.e., discriminative attributes. By decomposing the attribute descriptions of the object classes into hierarchical rules, multiple choices exist when classifying object using the rules, making it possible to applying reinforcement learning. Experiments conducted on two benchmark datasets for ZSC show that that HCRL achieves competitive accuracies, preliminarily showing HCRL's power for solving ZSC problems. By analyzing the hierarchical rules whose discriminative abilities have been determined, HCRL is able to show the most discriminative attributes for distinguishing a set of classes from another set of classes.

The proposed approach not only is suitable for ZSC, but also owns the potential for solving general classification problems. The main drawback of HCRL is that it can handle only hundreds of training samples, and we will try to make HCRL more scalable to handle more training data. In addition, all the attributes' classifiers used by HCRL in each experiment are built upon the same sampled training set. Therefore, the attributes' classifiers can be refined further at each level in the hierarchy like that in HAT in [12]. In the future work, we will explore to train the attributes' classifiers at each level in the hierarchy for refinement.

Acknowledgments. The presented work is framed within the National Natural Science Foundation of China (No. 71371184).

References

1. Zhang, Z., Saligrama, V.: Zero-shot learning via semantic similarity embedding. In: IEEE International Conference on Computer Vision, pp. 4166–4174 (2015)
2. Socher, R., Ganjoo, M., Sridhar, H., Bastani, O., Manning, C.D., Ng, A.Y.: Zero-shot learning through cross-modal transfer. In: Advances in Neural Information Processing Systems, pp. 935–943 (2013)
3. Lampert, C.H., Nickisch, H., Harmeling, S.: Attribute-based classification for zero-shot visual object categorization. IEEE Trans. Pattern Anal. Mach. Intell. **36**, 453–465 (2014)
4. Ji, Z., Yu, Y., Pang, Y., Guo, J., Zhang, Z.: Manifold regularized cross-modal embedding for zero-shot learning. Inf. Sci. **378**, 48–58 (2017)
5. Changpinyo, S., Chao, W.L., Gong, B., Sha, F.: Synthesized classifiers for zero-shot learning. In: IEEE Conference on Computer Vision and Pattern Recognition, pp. 5327–5336 (2016)
6. Alhalah, Z., Tapaswi, M., Stiefelhagen, R.: Recovering the missing link: predicting class-attribute associations for unsupervised zero-shot learning. In: IEEE Conference on Computer Vision and Pattern Recognition, pp. 5975–5984 (2016)
7. Larochelle, H., Erhan, D., Bengio, Y.: Zero-data learning of new tasks. In: AAAI Conference on Artificial Intelligence, AAAI 2008, Chicago, Illinois, USA, July, pp. 646–651 (2008)

8. Rohrbach, M., Stark, M., Schiele, B.: Evaluating knowledge transfer and zero-shot learning in a large-scale setting. In: Computer Vision and Pattern Recognition, pp. 1641–1648 (2011)
9. Wang, X., Chen, C., Cheng, Y., Wang, Z.J.: Zero-shot image classification based on deep feature extraction. IEEE Trans. Cogn. Dev. Syst. **99**, 1–14 (2017)
10. Hoo, W.L., Chan, C.S.: Recognizing unknown objects with attributes relationship model. Expert Syst. Appl. **42**, 9279–9283 (2015)
11. Farhadi, A., Endres, I., Hoiem, D., Forsyth, D.: Describing objects by their attributes. In: IEEE Conference on Computer Vision and Pattern Recognition, CVPR 2009, pp. 1778–1785 (2009)
12. Alhalah, Z., Stiefelhagen, R.: How to transfer? Zero-Shot object recognition via hierarchical transfer of semantic attributes. In: IEEE Winter Conference on Applications of Computer Vision, pp. 837–843 (2015)
13. Kivinen, J., Smola, A.J., Williamson, R.C.: Learning with Kernels. MIT Press, Cambridge (2002)
14. Han, J., Kamber, M., Pei, J.: Data Mining: Concepts and Techniques. Morgan Kaufmann Publishers Inc., Waltham (2011)
15. Rafsanjani, M.K., Varzaneh, Z.A., Chukanlo, N.E.: A survey of hierarchical clustering algorithms. Int. J. Appl. Math. Comput. Sci. **5**, 229–240 (2012)
16. Jordan, M.I., Mitchell, T.M.: Machine learning: trends, perspectives, and prospects. Science **349**, 255–260 (2015)
17. Mozer, S.: C, M., Hasselmo, M.: Reinforcement Learning: An Introduction. IEEE Trans. Neural Networks **16**, 285–286 (1998)
18. Sutton, R., Barto, A.: Reinforcement Learning: An Introduction. MIT Press, Cambridge (1998)
19. Kemp, C., Tenenbaum, J.B., Griffiths, T.L., Yamada, T., Ueda, N.: Learning systems of concepts with an infinite relational model. In: National Conference on Artificial Intelligence, pp. 381–388 (2006)
20. Quinlan, J.R.: C4.5: Programs for Machine Learning. Morgan Kaufmann Publishers Inc., San Francisco (2014)
21. Keerthi, S., Shevade, S., Bhattacharyya, C., Murthy, K.: Improvements to Platt's SMO algorithm for SVM classifier design. Neural Comput. **13**, 637–649 (2006)
22. Qiao, L., Tuo, H., Fang, Z., Feng, P., Jing, Z.: Joint probability estimation of attribute chain for zero-shot learning. In: IEEE International Conference on Image Processing, pp. 1863–1867 (2016)

Environmental Sound Recognition Using Masked Conditional Neural Networks

Fady Medhat(✉), David Chesmore, and John Robinson

Department of Electronic Engineering, University of York, York, UK
{fady.medhat,david.chesmore,john.robinson}@york.ac.uk

Abstract. Neural network based architectures used for sound recognition are usually adapted from other application domains, which may not harness sound related properties. The ConditionaL Neural Network (CLNN) is designed to consider the relational properties across frames in a temporal signal, and its extension the Masked ConditionaL Neural Network (MCLNN) embeds a filterbank behavior within the network, which enforces the network to learn in frequency bands rather than bins. Additionally, it automates the exploration of different feature combinations analogous to handcrafting the optimum combination of features for a recognition task. We applied the MCLNN to the environmental sounds of the ESC-10 dataset. The MCLNN achieved competitive accuracies compared to state-of-the-art convolutional neural networks and hand-crafted attempts.

Keywords: Boltzmann Machine · RBM · Conditional RBM · CRBM · Deep Neural Network · DNN · Conditional Neural Network · CLNN · Masked Conditional Neural Network · MCLNN · Environmental Sound Recognition · ESR

1 Introduction

Handcrafting the features required for the sound recognition problem has been investigated for decades. It is still an open area of research that consumes a lot of effort in an attempt to design the best features to be fed to a recognition system. Deep architectures of neural networks are currently being considered to be a replacement to the feature handcrafting stage. There is an endeavor to use these deep architectures that achieved wide success for images [1], on signals like sound to extract features automatically that can be further classified using a conventional classifier such as a Support Vector Machine (SVM) [2]. Handcrafted features still hold their position, but the performance gap between them and the use of the deep neural architectures as automatic feature extractors is getting narrower.

The work by Soltau et al. [3] marks an early attempt in using neural networks based architectures for feature extraction in sound recognition. In their work, they used a

This work is funded by the European Union's Seventh Framework Programme for research, technological development and demonstration under grant agreement no. 608014 (CAPACITIE).

G. Cong et al. (Eds.): ADMA 2017, LNAI 10604, pp. 373–385, 2017.
https://doi.org/10.1007/978-3-319-69179-4_26

three-stage recognition system. The first stage is an event detection phase to extract musical events, where they dropped the output nodes of a neural network and used the hidden nodes as features for the succeeding stages. A more recent attempt by Lee et al. [4] used Convolutional Deep Belief Networks [5] for several audio recognition tasks. Hamel et al. [6] introduced another attempt to extract features using a Deep Belief Network (DBN) architecture, where the features extracted with the DBN were further classified using an SVM, a similar attempt was in [7]. Hinton et al. [8] proposed the use of deep neural network architectures to replace the Gaussian Mixture Model (GMM) in a GMM-HMM combination for speech recognition. Graves et al. [9] used a deep recurrent neural network for speech recognition. An overlapping usage to music genre classification was in the work of Oord et al. [10], where they used Convolutional Neural Network (CNN) [11] for automatic music recommendation. Dieleman et al. [12] aimed to bypass the need for an intermediate signal representation like spectrograms by using a CNN over the raw signal, where their findings showed that spectrograms provided better performance.

Several neural based architectures were proposed for the sound recognition problem in music, speech and environmental sound, but they are usually adapted to the sound problem after they gain wide acceptance by the research community in other applications especially image recognition. Despite these successful attempts, they may not harness the full properties of the sound signal represented in a spectrogram. For example, recent efforts [13, 14] proposed the need to restructure the widely used Convolutional Neural Network (CNN) to fit the sound recognition problem. This need is attributed to the inability of the vanilla CNN to preserve the spatial locality of the learned features across the frequency domain in a time-frequency representation. Similarly, DBNs have a shortcoming in ignoring the inter-frames relation, where it treats each frame as an isolated entity.

The ConditionaL Neural Network (CLNN) [15] is designed to exploit the time-frequency representation of the sound signals. The model structure also extends its application to other multi-dimensional temporal representations. The CLNN takes into consideration the influence the successive frames, in a temporal signal, have on each other. The Masked Conditional Neural Network (MCLNN) [15] extends the functionality of the CLNN to include a binary masking operation using a systematic sparseness to automate the exploration of different feature combinations concurrently, which is usually a manual mix-and-match process of various features combinations. Additionally, the MCLNN embeds a filterbank behavior, which lends filterbank's properties such as the frequency shift-invariance to the neural network structure. In this work, we extend the work in [16] with an analysis of the masking effect in the MCLNN compared to the CLNN.

2 Related Work

The Conditional Restricted Boltzmann Machine (CRBM) [17] is an extension to the RBM [18] that takes into consideration the temporal nature of the successive feature vectors. The CRBM has been introduced initially to model the human motion by training it on a temporal signal captured from the movement of the human joints.

Figure 1 shows the structure of a CRBM. The main difference compared to the RBM involves the inclusion of the directed links from previous visible frames $(\hat{v}_{-n}, \ldots, \hat{v}_{-2}, \hat{v}_{-1})$ to both the visible feature vector $\hat{v}_0$ and the hidden nodes $\hat{h}$. The figure depicts the $\hat{W}$ links present in a normal RBM to hold the bidirectional relation between the hidden and the visible nodes. Additionally, the $\hat{B}$ links to hold the conditional relation between the previous n states of the visible vectors and the current hidden one, and the $\hat{A}$ links to hold the autoregressive relations between the previous visible states and the current visible vector $\hat{v}_0$. The Interpolating CRBM (ICRBM) [19] extended the work of the CRBM by considering both the future frames in addition to the past ones used in the CRBM. The ICRBM was applied for the phone recognition task in [19], and it surpassed the accuracy of the CRBM. The CLNN discussed in the next section extends from both the CRBM and the ICRBM by considering both the future and past frames without the autoregressive links.

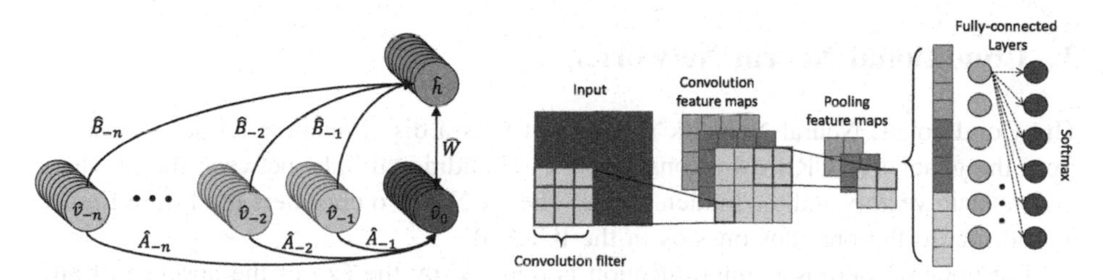

Fig. 1. The Conditional RBM structure

Fig. 2. Convolutional Neural Network.

The Convolutional Neural Network (CNN) [11] achieved breakthrough results [1, 20] for the image recognition problem. The model is based on two primary operations namely; Convolution and Pooling. The convolution operation involves a set of filters (weight matrices) of small sizes, e.g. 5×5, to convolve the 2-dimensional input image as shown in Fig. 2. The pooling (e.g. mean or max pooling) operation is a subsampling procedure to decrease the resolution of the feature maps generated from the convolution stage. The feature maps generated from these interleaved convolution and pooling operations are flattened to a single feature vector to be fed to a fully-connected network of neurons or a conventional classifier, e.g. Random Forest, SVM for the final classification decision.

Long Short-Term Memory [21] is a Recurrent Neural Network (RNN) model that makes use of internal memory to capture the previous states influence on the current input. Choi et al. [22] tried a hybrid model of both the CNN to extract localized features and the LSTM to capture long-term dependencies in the Convolutional RNN (CRNN) for several music tasks.

Convolutional DBN (ConvDBN) [5] by Lee et al. extended the CNN terminologies like weight sharing and pooling to the unsupervised learning of the DBN. In their work, they adopted a convolution layer like the one in the CNN to the ConvDBN in addition to a probabilistic max-pooling layer. The ConvDBN was used in [4] for speech and music recognition.

The deep neural network architectures proposed earlier are examples of the most successful attempts, but they are adapted to the sound recognition problem after they gain wide acceptance in other domains primarily image recognition. This may not optimally harness properties of multidimensional temporal signals. For example, convolutional models dependent on weight sharing, which does not preserve the spatial locality of the learned features and models such as DBN treats each temporal frame as an isolated entity, ignoring the inter-frames relation.

The ConditionaL Neural Networks (CLNN) considers the inter-frame relation, and the Masked ConditionaL Neural Networks extends the CLNN architecture by embedding a filterbank-like behavior within the network. This enforces the network to learn about frequency bands allowing it to sustain frequency shifts as in a normal filterbank. Additionally, the masking used in the MCLNN automates the exploration of different feature combination similar to the manual process of finding the optimum combination of features.

3 Conditional Neural Networks

The ConditionaL Neural Network (CLNN) [15] is a discriminative model that stems from the generative CRBM by considering the conditional links between the previous visible state vectors and the hidden nodes. The CLNN also considers the future frames in addition to the previous ones as in the ICRBM.

For notation purposes, multiplication is denoted by the ($\times$) or the absence of any sign between terms, e.g. ($x\ W$) or ($l \times e$). Element-wise multiplication between vectors or matrices of the same sizes is denoted by ($\circ$). The hat operator is used to denote vectors when used in combination with lowercase literals ($\hat{x}$) and to denote matrices with uppercase ones ($\hat{W}$). Subscripts in the absence of the hat operator are used to indicate individual elements in a vector or a matrix e.g. x_i is the ith element in vector ($\hat{x}$) and $W_{i,j}$ is the element at position [i, j] within a matrix. ($\hat{W}_u$) denotes a matrix at index u within a tensor.

The CLNN is formed of a vector-shaped hidden layer of e dimensions and accepts an input of a dimension [l, d], where l is the feature vector length and d is the number of frames in a window of width following (1)

$$d = 2n + 1, \quad n \geq 1 \tag{1}$$

where d is the window's width and n is the order. The order n refers to the number of frames to consider in a single temporal direction. The 2 is for both the past and future frames, and the central frame is considered by the 1. Each feature vector within the window of frames is fully-connected to the same hidden layer of length e neurons. The activation of a single hidden node can be given in (2)

$$y_{j,t} = f\left(b_j + \sum_{u=-n}^{n} \sum_{i=1}^{l} x_{i,u+t} W_{i,j,u}\right) \tag{2}$$

where $y_{j,t}$ is the activation at the jth hidden neuron (index t discussed later) and f is the transfer function applied at the neuron level. b_j is the bias at the jth neuron. $x_{i,u+t}$ is i^{th} element of the vector of length l at index $u + t$, where u is the index of the feature vector in a window of width d, i.e. u takes the values within the interval $[-n, n]$. $W_{i,j,u}$ is the weight between the ith feature in the input vector at index u and the jth hidden neuron. The window of frames is extracted from a larger chunk of the spectrogram, which we will refer to as the segment. The index t in the above equation refers to the position of the frame within the segment, which is also the window's central frame (at $u = 0$). The window's additional $2n$ frames are also extracted from the segment together with the window's central frame at index t. The vector form of (2) is formulated in (3)

$$\hat{y}_t = f\left(\hat{b} + \sum_{u=-n}^{n} \hat{x}_{u+t} \cdot \hat{W}_u\right) \tag{3}$$

where the activation vector $\hat{y}_t$ for the vector $\hat{x}_t$ condition on the $2n$ vectors in the window of frames is given by the output of the transfer function f. The bias vector of the hidden layer is $\hat{b}$. $\hat{x}_{u+t}$ is the input feature vector at index $u+t$ within the window, where t is the window's middle frame and also the index of the frame in the segment. The index u is used to specify the position of the input frame in the window, where the middle frame is positioned at $u = 0$. $\hat{W}_u$ is the weight matrix at position u within the weight tensor of size [feature vector length l, hidden layer width e, window's depth d]. The vector-matrix multiplication between the vector of length l at index u in a window and its corresponding weight matrix at index u within the weight tensor, generates d frames summed together per dimension to produce a single resultant vector of e dimensions. A logistic transfer function provides the conditional distribution of the prediction of the window's middle frame conditioned on the $2n$ neighboring frames formulated in $p(\hat{y}_t|\hat{x}_{-n+t}, \ldots \hat{x}_{-1+t}, \hat{x}_t, \hat{x}_{1+t}, \ldots \hat{x}_{n+t}) = \sigma(\ldots)$, where σ is a Sigmoid or the final layer output Softmax function.

The output of a CLNN layer is $2n$ fewer frames than its input. Therefore, in a deep CLNN architecture, the input segment should account for the consumed frames at each layer. Accordingly, the width of a segment of frames is given in (4)

$$q = (2n)m + k \quad , n, m \text{ and } k \geq 1 \tag{4}$$

where the segment of width q (the length follows the feature vector length l) is given by the order n, the number of layers m and the extra frames k. The extra frames k account for the frames that should remain beyond the CLNN layers to be flattened to a single vector or globally pooled as in [23] but for time-frequency representations, it is a single dimensional pooling.

Figure 3 shows a two-layer CLNN model. Each CLNN layer has an order $n = 1$, accordingly, a window considers one past and one future frame in addition to the central one. Each CLNN layer possesses a weight tensor $\hat{W}^b$, where b (the layer index) = 1, 2,..., m. The number of matrices in the tensor matches the number of frames in the window. Accordingly, at $n = 1$, $\hat{W}^b_0$ will processes the central frame, $\hat{W}^b_{-1}$

processes the previous frame and $\hat{W}_1^b$ processes one future frame. The second CLNN operates on the frames from the first CLNN layer. The figure also depicts a number of frames remaining beyond the two CLNN layers used in the flattening or pooling operation, which behaves as a form of aggregation over a texture window studied in [24] for music.

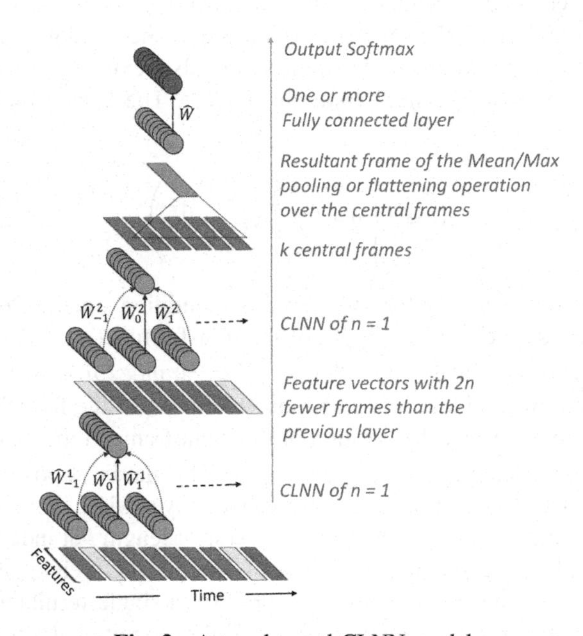

Fig. 3. A two-layered CLNN model.

4 Masked Conditional Neural Networks

Time-frequency representations such as spectrograms are widely adapted for signal analysis. These intermediate representations provide an insight of the change of energy across different frequency components as the signal progresses through time. Though these representations are efficient, they are sensitive to frequency shifts, especially for sound, since the same sound signal can be affected by different propagation factors that can alter its spectrogram representation. This is encountered through the use of a filterbank, which is one of the central operating blocks in a Mel-Scaled transformation such as an MFCC. A filterbank is a group of filters with their central frequency spaced from each other following a specific distance, e.g. Mel-spaced in MFCC. The filters allow each group of frequency bins to be treated as a band of frequencies, which permits the spectrogram transformation to be frequency shift-invariant.

The Masked ConditionaL Neural Network (MCLNN) [15] extends the CLNN by adopting a filterbank-like behavior within the network by enforcing a systematic sparseness through a binary mask. The binary mask is designed using two parameters:

the Bandwidth *bw* and the Overlap *ov*. The bandwidth specifies the number of consecutive ones, column-wise, as shown in Fig. 4a and the overlap specifies the superposition of the ones between one column and another. This binary mask, when enforced over the network connections, allows each hidden node to be an expert in a localized region of the feature vector. Thus, preserving the spatial locality of the features especially for time-frequency representations. Figure 4b shows the sparseness pattern enforced on the links matching the mask in Fig. 4a (ignoring the temporal aspect for simplicity). The linear indices of the 1's locations to generate a masking pattern follows (5)

$$lx = a + (g - 1)(l + (bw - ov)) \tag{5}$$

where the linear index lx of a 1's positions is dependent on the feature vector length, the bandwidth bw and the overlap ov. The values of a range within the interval $[0, bw - 1]$ and g within interval $[1, \lceil (l \times e)/(l + (bw - ov)) \rceil]$.

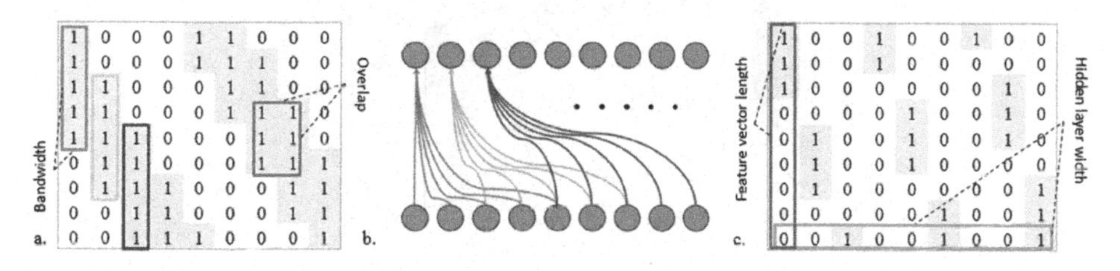

Fig. 4. Examples of the Mask patterns. (a) A bandwidth of 5 with an overlap of 3, (b) The allowed connections matching the mask in a. across the neurons of two layers, (c) A bandwidth of 3 and an overlap of −1

The overlap can be assigned negative values as depicted in Fig. 4c, which refers to the non-overlapping distance between groupings of ones across columns. The figure also shows the exploration of different feature combinations concurrently within the network. This is depicted in the presence of the shifted version of the filterbank-like pattern across the 1st set of three columns compared to the 2nd and the 3rd sets. In this setting, the input to the 1st neuron (mapping to the first column) is the first three features, the 4th neuron is observing the first two features, and the 7th neuron has an interest in the first feature only. This behavior enforces different hidden nodes to consider a different combination of features through disabling the effect of various regions of the input and enabling others.

The mask is applied through an element-wise multiplication between the mask pattern and each matrix within the weight tensor following (6)

$$\hat{Z}_u = \hat{W}_u \circ \hat{M} \tag{6}$$

where $\hat{W}_u$ is the original weight matrix at index u masked by the mask $\hat{M}$. The original weight matrix in (3) is substituted with the masked version $\hat{Z}_u$.

Figure 5 shows an MCLNN step. The figure depicts the number of matrices matching the number of frames. The highlighted regions in each matrix represent the active connection following the binary mask pattern. The output generated from each of the vector-matrix multiplication is d vectors of e dimensions each. The vectors are summed together feature-wise to generate one representative vector for the window then the nonlinearity is applied through the transfer function over this single vector.

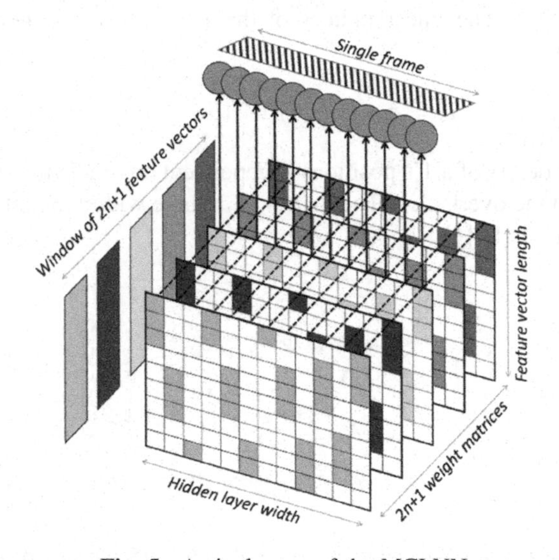

Fig. 5. A single step of the MCLNN

5 Experiments

We extend the evaluation of the MCLNN in [16] to different experimental settings affecting the model performance. We evaluated the MCLNN using the ESC-10 dataset of environmental sounds.

The ESC-10 [25] is a dataset of 10 environmental sounds categories evenly pre-distributed into 5-folds with 40 samples per category: Dog Bark, Rain, Sea Waves, Baby Cry, Clock Tick, Person Sneeze, Helicopter, Chainsaw, Rooster and Fire Cracking. The dataset is released with all files unified to 5 s in length, with clips having shorter events padded with silence. As an initial pre-processing step, we trimmed the silence and cloned the files several times to extract 5 s.

All files were transformed to a 60 bins logarithmic Mel-scaled spectrogram with the Delta (1st derivative between the frames) concatenated column-wise to generate 120 frequency bins vector. The transformation used an FFT window of 1024 and 50% overlap.

We adopted a two-layer MCLNN architecture followed by a single dimension global mean pooling [23] layer to pool across the extra frames k and two fully connected layers of 100 nodes before the final Softmax. Parametric Rectifier Linear Units (PRELU) [26] were used as the transfer function for all the model's nodes. Dropout

[27] was used for regularization. A summary of the hyper-parameters used is given in Table 1. The whole model was trained using ADAM [28] to minimize the categorical cross-entropy, and the final decision of a clip's class is decided by a probability voting across the frames of the clip following (7).

$$Category = argmax_{j=1 \ldots c}\left(\sum_{i=1}^{r} o_{ji}\right) \tag{7}$$

where each clip has a number of prediction vectors r matching the number of segments. The vector has c elements corresponding to the number of classes. All activation vectors are summed, and the class with the maximum value is the clip's category.

Table 1. MCLNN model parameters for ESC-10

Layer	Type	Nodes	Mask bandwidth	Mask overlap	Order n
1	MCLNN	300	20	−5	15
2	MCLNN	200	5	3	15

The mask overlap and bandwidth are different across the two MCLNN layers as listed in Table 1. We found through several experiments that using wide bandwidth with negative overlap in the first layer in combination with narrow bandwidth and positive overlap in the second layer increases the accuracy. This is accounted to the ability of the wide bandwidth to collectively consider more frequency bins, which suppress the effect of the smearing of the energy. Also, the negative overlap increases the sparseness, which decreases the effect of noisy bins in the input. On the other hand, the second layer's narrow bandwidth and positive overlap allow considering a smaller number of bins collectively as a band, which focuses on the distinct features that can enhance the accuracy.

Experiments were applied using cross-validation over the dataset's original 5-fold, where 3 training folds are standardized, and the mean and standard deviation of the training data were used to standardize the testing and validation folds.

Table 2 lists several accuracies achieved using both the CLNN and the MCLNN. MCLNN achieved an accuracy of 85.5% at k = 40 and an accuracy of 83% at k = 1. The deep CNN architecture used in Piczak-CNN [29] is a model of two convolutions and two pooling layers followed by two densely connected layers of neurons of 5000 neurons each. Piczak-CNN experimented with different segment sizes, where he used short segments of 41 frames and long segments formed of 101 frames. Piczak reported higher accuracy using the long segments compared to the short segments. Piczak-CNN achieved 80% using 25 million parameters with the long segment of 101 frames. Additionally, the work of Piczak [29] applied 10 augmentation variants for each sound file, which involves applying 10 deformations to the sound file with different time delays and shifted pitches. This increases the size of the dataset and consequently the accuracy as studied by Salamon et al. in [30]. On the other hand, MCLNN achieved the listed accuracies using 3 million parameters (12% of the parameters used in the

Piczak-CNN) without any augmentation. MCLNN achieved 85.5% for long segments containing 101 frames ($m = 2$, $n = 15$, $k = 40$ and middle frame. $q = (2n)m + k = (2 \times 15) \times 2 + 41 = 101$), which is the same size of Piczak-CNN, 83% for segments of size 61 frames and 82% for segments of size 86 frames. The segment size is controlled by the extra frames k with the rest of the model parameters unchanged. Moreover, to avoid the influence of the intermediate data representation on the MCLNN reported accuracies, we adopted the same spectrogram representation (60 Mel + Delta) used by the Piczak-CNN.

Table 2. Accuracies reported on the ESC-10

Classifiers and features	Acc.%
MCLNN (k = 40) + Mel-Spectrogram (this work)[a]	**85.50**
MCLNN (k = 1) + Mel-Spectrogram [16][a]	83.00
MCLNN (k = 25) + Mel-Spectrogram (this work)[a]	**82.00**
Piczak-CNN + Mel-Spectrogram (*101 frames*) [29][b]	80.00
Piczak-CNN + Mel-Spectrogram (*41 frames*) [29][b]	78.20
CLNN (k = 25) + Mel-Spectrogram (this work)[a]	**77.50**
CLNN (k = 40) + Mel-Spectrogram (this work)[a]	**75.75**
CLNN (k = 1) + Mel-Spectrogram (this work)[a]	**73.25**
Random Forest + MFCC [25][a]	72.70

[a] *Without augmentation*
[b] *With augmentation*

In a different evaluation to the MCLNN against the CLNN, we used the same architecture of the MCLNN, but without the mask to benchmark the CLNN. The highest CLNN accuracy is 77.5% at k = 25, and the lowest one at k = 1 is 73.25%, both are higher than the work reported in [25]. The MCLNN demonstrate accuracies that surpass the ones of the CLNN with the same architectures and segment sizes, which emphasizes the important role of the mask due to the properties discussed earlier.

Figure 6 shows the confusion across the ESC-10 classes. The Clock tick sound is confused with fire cracking and dog barks due to the nature of the short duration of this category. There is also high confusion among the Chainsaw sound and both the Rain and Sea Waves due to the common low tones across these classes. The Baby Cry sound was detected with an accuracy of 97.5% and the lowest accuracy of 65% was for the Clock Ticks due to its short event duration.

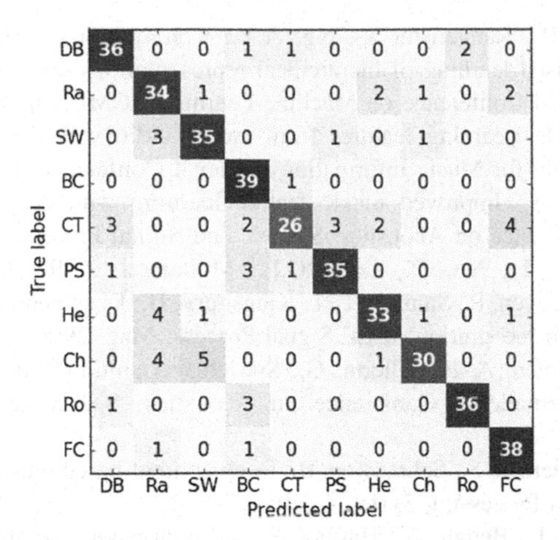

Fig. 6. Confusion matrix for the ESC-10 dataset. Classes: Dog Bark (DB), Rain (Ra), Sea Waves (SW), Baby Cry (BC), Clock Tick (CT), Person Sneeze (PS), Helicopter (He), Chainsaw (Ch), Rooster (Ro) and Fire Cracking (FC)

6 Conclusions and Future Work

In this work, we have explored different experimental settings for the ConditionaL Neural Network (CLNN) designed for multidimensional temporal signal recognition and the Masked Conditional Neural Network (MCLNN) that extends upon the CLNN by enforcing a systematic binary mask. The mask plays the role of a filterbank embedded within the network, and it automates the handcrafting of the features through considering a different combination of features concurrently. We have used the MCLNN for environmental sound recognition using ESC-10 dataset, and it achieved accuracies that surpassed state-of-the-art convolutional neural networks using fewer parameters. Future work will consider different order n across the layers and deeper MCLNN architectures. We will also consider applying the MCLNN to temporal signals other than sound.

References

1. Krizhevsky, A., Sutskever, I., Hinton, G.E.: ImageNet classification with deep convolutional neural networks. In: Neural Information Processing Systems, NIPS (2012)
2. Vapnik, V., Lerner, A.: Pattern recognition using generalized portrait method. Autom. Remote Control **24**, 774–780 (1963)
3. Soltau, H., Schultz, T., Martin, W., Waibel, A.: Recognition of music types. In: International Conference on Acoustics, Speech, and Signal Processing, ICASSP (1998)
4. Lee, H., Largman, Y., Pham, P., Ng, A.Y.: Unsupervised feature learning for audio classification using convolutional deep belief networks. In: Neural Information Processing Systems (NIPS) (2009)

5. Lee, H., Grosse, R., Ranganath, R., Ng, A.Y.: Convolutional deep belief networks for scalable unsupervised learning of hierarchical representations. In: Proceedings of the 26th Annual International Conference on Machine Learning, ICML, pp. 1–8 (2009)
6. Hamel, P., Eck, D.: Learning features from music audio with deep belief networks. In: International Society for Music Information Retrieval Conference, ISMIR (2010)
7. Sigtia, S., Dixon, S.: Improved music feature learning with deep neural networks. In: International Conference on Acoustics, Speech, and Signal Processing, ICASSP (2014)
8. Hinton, G., Deng, L., Yu, D., Dahl, G.E., Mohamed, A.-R., Jaitly, N., Senior, A., Vanhoucke, V., Nguyen, P., Sainath, T.N., Kingsbury, B.: Deep neural networks for acoustic modeling in speech recognition. IEEE Signal Process. Mag. **29**(6), 82–97 (2012)
9. Graves, A., Mohamed, A.-R., Hinton, G.: Speech recognition with deep recurrent neural networks. In: International Conference on Acoustics, Speech and Signal Processing, ICASSP. (2013)
10. Oord, A.V.D., Dieleman, S., Schrauwen, B.: Deep content-based music recommendation. In: Neural Information Processing Systems, NIPS (2013)
11. LeCun, Y., Bottou, L., Bengio, Y., Haffner, P.: Gradient-based learning applied to document recognition. Proc. IEEE **86**, 2278–2324 (1998)
12. Dieleman, S., Schrauwen, B.: End-to-end learning for music audio. In: International Conference on Acoustic, Speech and Signal Processing, ICASSP (2014)
13. Abdel-Hamid, O., Mohamed, A.-R., Jiang, H., Deng, L., Penn, G., Yu, D.: Convolutional neural networks for speech recognition. IEEE/ACM Trans. Audio Speech Lang. Process. **22**, 1533–1545 (2014)
14. Pons, J., Lidy, T., Serra, X.: Experimenting with musically motivated convolutional neural networks. In: International Workshop on Content-based Multimedia Indexing, CBMI. (2016)
15. Medhat, F., Chesmore, D., Robinson, J.: Masked conditional neural networks for audio classification. In: International Conference on Artificial Neural Networks (ICANN) (2017)
16. Medhat, F., Chesmore, D., Robinson, J.: Masked conditional neural networks for automatic sound events recognition. In: IEEE International Conference on Data Science and Advanced Analytics (DSAA) (2017)
17. Taylor, G.W., Hinton, G.E., Roweis, S.: Modeling human motion using binary latent variables. In: Advances in Neural Information Processing Systems, NIPS, pp. 1345–1352 (2006)
18. Fahlman, S.E., Hinton, G.E., Sejnowski, T.J.: Massively parallel architectures for AI: NETL, Thistle, and Boltzmann Machines. In: National Conference on Artificial Intelligence, AAAI (1983)
19. Mohamed, A.-R., Hinton, G.: Phone recognition using restricted Boltzmann Machines In: IEEE International Conference on Acoustics Speech and Signal Processing, ICASSP (2010)
20. Szegedy, C., Wei, L., Yangqing, J., Sermanet, P., Reed, S., Anguelov, D., Erhan, D., Vanhoucke, V., Rabinovich, A.: Going deeper with convolutions. In: IEEE Conference on Computer Vision and Pattern Recognition, CVPR, pp. 1–9 (2015)
21. Hochreiter, S., Schmidhuber, J.: Long short-term memory. Neural Comput. **9**, 1735–1780 (1997)
22. Choi, K., Fazekas, G., Sandler, M., Cho, K.: Convolutional recurrent neural networks for music classification. In: arXiv preprint arXiv:1609.04243 (2016)
23. Lin, M., Chen, Q., Yan, S.: Network in network. In: International Conference on Learning Representations, ICLR (2014)
24. Bergstra, J., Casagrande, N., Erhan, D., Eck, D., Kégl, B.: Aggregate features and AdaBoost for music classification. Mach. Learn. **65**, 473–484 (2006)

25. Piczak, K.J.: ESC: dataset for environmental sound classification. In: ACM International Conference on Multimedia, pp. 1015–1018 (2015)
26. He, K., Zhang, X., Ren, S., Sun, J.: Delving deep into rectifiers: surpassing human-level performance on ImageNet classification. In: IEEE International Conference on Computer Vision, ICCV (2015)
27. Srivastava, N., Hinton, G., Krizhevsky, A., Sutskever, I., Salakhutdinov, R.: Dropout: a simple way to prevent neural networks from overfitting. J. Mach. Learn. Res. JMLR **15**, 1929–1958 (2014)
28. Kingma, D., Ba, J.: ADAM: a method for stochastic optimization. In: International Conference for Learning Representations, ICLR (2015)
29. Piczak, K.J.: Environmental sound classification with convolutional neural networks. In: IEEE international workshop on Machine Learning for Signal Processing (MLSP) (2015)
30. Salamon, J., Bello, J.P.: Deep convolutional neural networks and data augmentation for environmental sound classification. IEEE Signal Process. Lett. **24**(3), 279–283 (2016)

Analyzing Performance of Classification Techniques in Detecting Epileptic Seizure

Mohammad Khubeb Siddiqui(✉), Md Zahidul Islam, and Muhammad Ashad Kabir

School of Computing and Mathematics, Charles Sturt University, Bathurst, NSW, Australia
{msiddiqui,zislam,akabir}@csu.edu.au

Abstract. Epileptic seizure detection is a challenging research topic. The objective of this research is to analyze the performance of various classification techniques while detecting the epileptic seizure in a shorter time. In this paper, we apply four different types of classifiers-two are black-box (SVM & KNN) and other two are non-black-box (Decision tree & Ensemble) on two epileptic patient seizure data sets. Our finding shows that non-black box classifiers, specifically ensemble classifiers, do better than other classifiers. The experimental results indicate that the ensemble classifier can assist for seizure detection in a shorter epoch length of time (i.e., 0.5 s) with high accuracy rate. Significantly in comparison to other classifiers the ensemble classifier provides high accuracy and less chance of false detection rate.

Keywords: Classification techniques · Black-box classifier · Non-black box classifier · Data mining · Seizure detection · Epilepsy

1 Introduction

A human body typically acts as per the instructions of the brain. Brain is one of the most complex and important organs of the body. It is made up of millions of small nerve cells called neurones, each of which can send and receive messages in a very likewise manner to one of the units in an electronic device such as computer [13]. In the brain, messages are passed from cell to cell by various chemicals (neurotransmitters). If a brain signal is transmitted and the cells fail to respond then it may cause the epileptic seizure. A seizure occurs when a sudden and uncontrolled electrical activity happens, either in a particular or whole region of the brain. Epilepsy is a common neurological disorder which can take the form of recurring seizures [6]. Epilepsy can affect anyone at any age but most people with epilepsy will experience their first seizure before the age of twenty. It is estimated that approximately 65 million people worldwide currently struggling with epilepsy [10].

An electroencephalogram called EEG is used for monitoring the brain signals. On the surface of the brain, small discs called electrodes or channels are placed

G. Cong et al. (Eds.): ADMA 2017, LNAI 10604, pp. 386–398, 2017.
https://doi.org/10.1007/978-3-319-69179-4_27

in a non-invasive manner to collect the electrical signals from the brain [25]. It displays the important information about the brain function on the screen. Doctors may get help to diagnose the epilepsy from EEG, as it may expose some sort of abnormal activities which are commonly found in epilepsy [21].

Data mining is widely used for discovering sensible patterns from large data sets which are helpful for solving real world problems [11,15,27]. In the present work, classification techniques are applied to analyze the EEG seizure data set for performance analysis and fast seizure detection. We used four prominent classifiers of classification technique in which two are black-box (Support Vector Machine-SVM and K-Nearest Neighbors-KNN) and two are non-black box (Decision Tree and Decision Forest).

The main contributions of this paper are listed as follows:

1. We apply different classifiers such as black-box and non-black box classifiers of a supervised learning method on EEG data sets for seizure detection.
2. We identify through our results that non-black box (ensemble) classifier performs better than black-box classifiers.
3. We assign the class values -*Seizure and non-seizure* to the class attribute of our processed data sets.
4. We also identify that an ensemble (a decision forest) classifier outperforms other classifiers (a Decision Tree, KNN and SVM) for all data sets with various epoch lengths.
5. Our work also shows the importance of epoch reduction [24] for seizure detection.

Structure of the paper is as follows. Section 2 presents a literature review. Section 3 describes the methodology for analyzing the performance of classifiers and seizure detection. Section 4 reports our experimental results and a discussion on achieved results. In Sect. 5 we conclude the paper.

2 Related Work

Data mining has been widely used for seizure detection because of its high accuracy rate and capability to extract hidden patterns in terms of knowledge [9,23,24].

A KNN classifier was applied on EEG data set to classify the 342 seizure and non-seizure recordings for seizure detection on different patients without any early information. Features such as sample entropy, RMS, and median frequency are suitable for classifying the seizure and non-seizure cases [12]. Hybrid approach of LDA, KNN, CVE, and SVM classifiers is used and it is found that the onset seizures can be predicted earlier than 65 s [10]. The KNN classifier had been applied on EEG brain data sets to discriminate the seizure and non-seizure class values, and it also shows the suitable channels for seizure detection [5]. Suitable feature importance from EEG data set for seizure detection is presented [18]. Approximate entropy(AE) and sample entropy(SE) features were extracted for classifiers SVM and extreme learning machine (ELM). Result shows that the SE and ELM give better performance [26].

Four different types of entropy features were applied on seven different types of classifiers-fuzzy surgeon classifier, SVM, K-NN, Probabilistic neural network, Gaussian mixture model, Decision tree and Naïve Bayes for seizure detection [2]. However, they did not applied the ensemble classifier. As a result the seizure detection accuracy is not good. Other than black-box classifiers, some studies are also done by applying non-black box classifiers. A decision tree classifier was used for seizure detection but the logic rules are limited because of its limitation in extracting limited number of logic rules from the EEG data sets [8]. A decision forest classifier could perhaps overcome with these limitations because it is the ensemble of decision trees and it produces more sensible logic rules with a good accuracy rate. In the present work, we apply nine features with an ensemble classifiers for better accuracy and F-measure.

Random forest classifier was applied on EEG data sets for identifying which channels are contributing most in detecting the seizure and non-seizure events with dimension reduction [5]. In another study, random forest was applied on time and frequency domain features of IEEG (Intra-cranial EEG). It is found that seizure can be detected with 93.8% of sensitivity rate [9]. Spectro-temporal transformation had been used for feature extraction and these features were used as an input data set to random forest classifier for seizure detection with 98.30% accuracy [19].

Previous researches applied different data mining/machine learning classifiers such as black-box and non-black box for detecting the seizure. More or less they give competent results. Although, some of the research also carried out using decision tree and decision forest. Here, the point of argument is that none of the previous researches had done the work on training the EEG data set for quick seizure detection using prominent classifiers altogether.

3 Methodology

In this section, we present our approach for detecting the seizure using various classification techniques. It comprises of four steps: Data set exploration, Feature extraction, Data preprocessing and Classification.

3.1 Data Set Exploration

In this paper, we have used a publicly available EEG data set from CHB-MIT [1]. The data set contains number of recordings for patients having epileptic seizures [22].

Primary data sets contain EEG Signals obtained through 23 channels that were used to collect the brain signals. All signals of the data set were sampled at the frequency of 256 Hz. The International 10–20 system was used for these recordings [12]. Below Table 1 describes about primary data set: patient ID - a numerical number to identify a patient, Seizure Recording - number of seizure recordings for each patient, and Seizure duration - total time duration of seizures in all the recordings of patient.

Table 1. Primary data set description

Patient ID	Number of Seizure Recordings	Seizure duration (s)
P1	7	430
P2	4	170

3.2 Feature Extraction

Feature extraction is a crucial step in seizure detection as it helps to find the different statistical properties from a seizure data set. Features have been extracted from various types of transformation techniques such as frequency and time [18]. In this work, we apply *nine* time-domain features shown in Table 2. We used the same set of features in our previous papers [23,24].

Table 2. Time domain features used in Data processing

Features	Equations
Min	$min(x(n))$; minimum value of the data
Max	$max(x(n))$; maximum value of the data
Mean	$1/N \cdot \sum_{n=1}^{N} x(n)$; n is a record and N is total number of records
Entropy	$p(x) \cdot \sum_{n=1}^{N} log_2(p(x))$; $p(x)$ is probability for $x(n)$
Line Length	$\sum_{n=2}^{N} \lvert x(n-1) - x(n) \rvert$; sum of distance between two consecutive points
Std Dev	$1/N \cdot \sum_{n=1}^{N} (x(n) - \mu_x)^2$; mean is represented by μ_x
Kurtosis	$1/N \cdot \sum_{n=1}^{N} (x(n) - \mu_x)^4 / [1/N \sum_{n=1}^{N} - \mu_x)^2]^2$
Skewness	$1/N \cdot \sum_{n=1}^{N} (x(n) - \mu_x)^3 / [1/N \sum_{n=1}^{N} (x(n) - \mu_x)^2]^{3/2}$
Energy	$1/N \cdot \sum_{n=1}^{N} x(n)^2$

3.3 Preparing Data Sets

In this paper, we have used the set of EEG recordings of two different patients. All of these recordings contain both seizure and non-seizure events. Patient 1 contains 7 recordings and seizure duration is 430 s. Similarly, patient 2 contains 4 recordings and seizure duration is 170 s.

Primary data sets are the raw data sets. Each data set contains 23 columns where each column represents the channel that gives information about the EEG signal. The total number of records in each data set is approximately, $256\,\text{Hz} \times 60 \times 60 = 921600$ cycles/hour. We processed the data sets by using *nine* time-domain features where each column produces nine-features. Hence, we get altogether $23 \times 9 = 207$ non-class attributes for all epoch data sets.

We process all of the recordings of each patient into two epochs 10 s and 0.5 s. As a result, we get total four data sets- two data sets for each patient.

Assigning Class-Value to Class Attribute. Motive of this section, is to declare the class values (specifically seizure records) to the class attribute. In supervised learning methods [7,16] class attribute is the key attribute of a data set. The class attribute is typically discrete in nature. Lets say, there are 1000 records in a data set and the class attribute consists of two distinct class values such as seizure and non-seizure, all of these 1000 records are classified either by seizure or non-seizure.

Table 3. Data set dimension

Patient ID	Epochs' data set	Attribute size	Number of records
P1	D_1	208	2520
	D_2	208	50400
P2	D_3	208	1440
	D_4	208	28800

The data set which we used in our initial experiments is without class-attribute. Here, the challenge is that how to classify the records of taken data set based on two class values- seizure and non-seizure. In order to achieve this, we need to align the seizure timings of EEG signals to the records of primary data sets. This is very crucial for applying the classification techniques on the data sets. As a result, to solve this issue we are explaining from below equations:

We have prepared data sets based on epoch lengths same we did in our previous work [24]. The data set of two patients are in a descending order of time frames called epochs. In the present work, the data sets have epoch length 10 s and 0.5 s. The record size of these data sets can be measured from Eq. 1. Where TR is total number of records in the primary EEG data set and E_l is the required epoch length (e.g., 10 s).

$$E_l = \frac{TR}{E_l} \tag{1}$$

It is very important to find the record number at which the actual seizure starts in our created epoch data set. In order to do this, Eq. 2 is used which refers to the exact position of the record number in the data set aligned to the EEG signals where-from the actual seizure starts for epoch data set. It is calculated as (R_{st}), the ratio of (SZ_{st}) to (E_l). Where R_{st} is the record number where from seizure is started in the epoch data set, SZ_{st} tells the seizure start time of EEG signal in primary data set and E_l is the epoch length from Eq. 1 .

$$R_{st} = \frac{SZ_{st}}{E_l} \tag{2}$$

Similarly, Eq. 3 has been applied to find the record number at which the seizure terminates in our created epoch data set, aligned to the EEG signals where-from the actual seizure ends for epoch data set. It is calculated as (R_{et}) which is the ratio of (SZ_{et}) to (E_l). Where R_{et} represents the record number at which the seizure terminates, SZ_{et} represents the seizure end time of EEG signal in primary data set and E_l is the epoch length.

$$R_{et} = \frac{SZ_{et}}{E_l} \tag{3}$$

From Eqs. 2 and 3, Eq. 4 calculates the total number of seizure records (R_{sz}) in epoch data sets. It is the difference of R_{et} to R_{st} of epoch data sets. Where (R_{sz}) is used as one of the class value in the class attribute for all epoch data sets.

$$R_{sz} = R_{et} - R_{st} \tag{4}$$

Finally, including the class attribute with class values, total number of columns are 208 for all the processed data sets (refer to Table 3).

3.4 Classification

Classification is a supervised learning method of data mining and it plays a crucial role in knowledge discovery and finding meaningful patterns from a data set of different domains [14]. In this work, we employ four popular classifiers: decision tree, decision forest (ensemble), KNN, and SVM [11]. Classification process is carried out on four main components of data set:

1. Class attribute: Is a target attribute which is discrete in nature- it represents the class-values.
2. Non-Class attribute: It is independent attributes of the data set also called as predictors e.g., in this work the data sets contain 207 non-class attributes and each attribute represents the statistical information of EEG signals.
3. Training data set: The data mining classifier is applied on the data set which contains both non-class attribute and class attributes. The values of class attribute are not hidden.
4. Testing data set: Testing data set is used to detect the performance of a classifier. This is done by using n-fold cross validation(CV) (mostly 10 fold). In 10-fold CV data is trained and validated for 10 times [17].

4 Experimental Results

The objective of this experiment is to analyze the performance of both the black-box and non-black box classifiers in detecting seizure in a shorter time. The experiment is conducted using MATLAB. We applied four major classifiers: Decision trees, Ensemble, SVM, and KNN. Each classifier has sub-classifiers viz **Decision trees**- Simple DT, Medium DT, and Complex DT; **SVM**- Linear, Quadratic, Cubic, Medium Gaussian, and Coarse Gaussian; **KNN**- Fine, Medium Cosine, Cubic and Weighted; **Ensemble**- Bagged trees, Subspace Discriminant, Subspace KNN and RUSBoosted trees.

Performance of these classifiers have been computed by using the evaluation matrices parameters such as precision, recall and F-measure [20]. It is based on four possible classification outcomes. True Positive (TP) = The seizure cases that are actually positive and predicted positive. True Negative (TN) = The seizure cases that are actually negative and predicted negative. False Negative (FN) = The seizure cases that are actually positive but predicted to be negative. False Positive (FP) = The seizure cases that are actually negative but predicted to be positive.

Precision is the ratio of true positives to the cases that are predicted as positive. It is the percentage of selected cases that are correct.

$$Precision = \frac{TP}{TP + FP} \times 100\% \tag{5}$$

Recall is the ratio of true positives to the cases that actually positive. It is the percentage of corrected cases that are selected.

$$Recall = \frac{TP}{TP + FN} \times 100\% \tag{6}$$

F-measure is the mean of Precision and Recall. It takes both false positives and false negatives into an account. F-measure is calculated as:

$$F\text{-}measure = \frac{2 \cdot Precision \cdot Recall}{Precision + Recall} \tag{7}$$

The experiment is carried out by using 10-fold cross-validation on all epoch testing data set. For every classifier, we show the value of its sub-classifier which persists to high F-measure (refer to Table 4). In Table 5 we choose the sub-classifier of the main classifier that has maximum F-measure values. For example, in data set D_1 decision tree selects the **simple decision tree** because it gives maximum F-measure value compared to medium and complex tree sub-classifiers. Similarly, we have chosen the F-measure for other classifiers too.

Result are discussed in Sects. 4.1, 4.2, 4.3 and 4.4 respectively. Table 5 has been graphically represented in Fig. 1, X-axis represents the epoch data sets($D_1 \cdots D_4$) with their applied classifiers and Y-axis represents the value of F-measure.

4.1 Non-black Box - Decision Tree vs. Ensemble (Decision Forest)

We compare the performance of two non-black box classifiers-Decision tree and Ensemble on epochs' data sets. Here, the decision tree means a single decision tree and ensemble means a group of decision trees also called as decision forest. Our experimental result shows that F-measure of ensemble classifier is far better than a single decision tree (refer to Tables 4, 5 and Fig. 1).

From the result of both patients' data sets shown in Table 5, the F-measure value of ensemble classifier outperforms the decision tree as shown in Fig. 1. In 10 s epoch length data set of patient (P1) the F-measure value of ensemble classifier is 84.06 followed by decision tree (i.e., 72.46), which is less in comparison to ensemble because decision tree generates limited number of logic rules with less accuracy rate. Decision forest generates a set of logic rules, each tree of a decision forest behaves as a classifier due to this reason it provides more logic rules. As a result, we get high performance in terms of classification accuracy with high F-measure.

4.2 Black-Box - SVM vs. KNN

From Tables 4, 5 and Fig. 1 we analyze the results for all four data sets of both the patients and find that SVM is dominant to KNN. In three data sets the accuracy and F-measure values of SVM is higher compared to KNN. Here, KNN is not performing well in terms of both accuracy and f-measure, because the data set has too many data points. We have used high dimension data set of 208 attributes and 50,400 records [3]. However, just in a single data set D_1 the value of both accuracy and F-measure are equal i.e., 99.1 and 81.69 respectively.

4.3 Black-Box vs. Non-black Box

The concept of a 'black-box' is used to describe a scenario in which a user can learn as much as possible about an internal system of a classifier. Black-box classifiers are unable to explain their classification steps for several class values. They have limited meaningful patterns because it is hard to interpret them and unable to expose their knowledge. Non-black box means the acquired knowledge by the classifier can be expressed in a readable human-understandable form. Since, one of its classifier is ensemble thus it generates a set of logic rules. As a result, it is widely used in knowledge discovery purposes [4,16].

In the present work, from Tables 4 and 5, we observe for both the patients' data sets the accuracy and F-measure values for non-black box classifier (ensemble) is outperforming compared to black-box classifiers (SVM and KNN) shown in Fig. 1. The F-measure value of ensemble for data set D_1 is 84.06 which is higher than other classifiers. Similarly, for remaining data sets the ensemble classifier outperforms compared to other classifiers (refer to Table 5).

It is true that not every time a particular classifier behaves well for all types of data set. The performance of a classifier also depends on the data set dimension. Overall, it is estimated that ensemble classifier works better than the black-box classifiers in terms of both accuracy and knowledge discovery [17]. To the best of our knowledge, generally non-black box classifier(ensemble) outperforms compared to other classifiers of black-box. Even, ensemble also performs better than a single decision tree which is non-black box classifier.

4.4 Epoch Length Reduction

In our submitted work [24] we applied two different classifiers (SysFor and Forest CERN) of decision forest with epoch reduction method on an ECoG data set.

Table 4. Individual classifier and it's sub-classifiers performance on Epochs' data sets

Patient ID	Data set-Epoch length	Classifier	Sub-classifier	Accuracy	Precision	Recall	F-measure
P1	D_1-10 s	Tree	Complex	99	75.76	64.1	69.44
			Medium	99	75.76	64.1	69.44
			Simple	99.1	83.33	64.1	**72.46**
		SVM	Linear	99.4	90.63	74.36	**81.69**
			Quadratic	99.4	90.32	71.79	80
			Cubic	99.3	87.1	69.23	77.14
			Medium Gaussian	98.5	100	17.95	30.43
			Coarse Gaussian	99.2	92.31	61.54	73.85
		KNN	Fine	99.4	90.63	74.36	**81.69**
			Medium	99.2	92.31	61.54	73.85
			Cosine	99.3	78.57	84.62	81.48
			Cubic	99.1	91.67	56.41	69.84
			Weighted	99.3	92.59	64.1	75.76
		Ensemble	Bagged trees	99.5	96.67	74.36	**84.06**
			Subspace Discriminant	99.2	86.67	66.67	75.36
			Subspace KNN	99.3	81.58	79.49	80.52
			RUSBoosted trees	98.2	50	94.87	65.49
	D_2-0.5 s	Tree	Complex	99	75.36	69.69	72.41
			Medium	99.1	81.26	67.15	**73.53**
			Simple	99	1	59.62	69.73
		SVM	Linear	99.3	93.16	69.36	79.52
			Quadratic	99.4	94.51	72.35	81.95
			Cubic	99.4	93.18	74.12	**82.56**
			Medium Gaussian	99.1	95.21	52.77	67.9
			Coarse Gaussian	99.4	96.26	68.36	79.95
		KNN	Fine	99.2	85.44	70.13	77.04
			Medium	99.3	97.32	64.27	77.42
			Cosine	99.1	72.25	82.08	76.85
			Cubic	99.2	96.71	62.96	76.26
			Weighted	99.3	95.45	67.37	**78.99**
		Ensemble	Bagged trees	99.4	93.66	71.9	**81.35**
			Subspace Discriminant	98.7	69.01	60.84	64.67
			Subspace KNN	99.2	92.68	63.05	75.05
			RUSBoosted trees	97.6	43.62	92.26	59.23
P2	D_3-10 s	Tree	Complex	98.7	61.54	63.16	62.34
			Medium	98.7	61.54	63.16	62.34
			Simple	98.9	71.88	60.53	**65.71**
		SVM	Linear	98.7	66.67	47.37	55.38
			Quadratic	98.8	67.65	60.53	63.89
			Cubic	98.8	65.79	65.79	**65.79**
			Medium Gaussian	98.8	100	34.21	50.98
		KNN	Fine	98.7	64.71	57.89	**61.11**
			Medium	98.7	90.91	26.32	40.82
			Cosine	98.8	92.86	34.21	50
			Cubic	98.2	50	2.63	5
			Weighted	98.8	88.24	39.47	54.55
		Ensemble	Bagged trees	99.2	88.89	63.16	**73.85**
			Subspace Discriminant	98.9	66.67	73.68	70
			Subspace KNN	99.1	80.65	65.79	72.46
			RUSBoosted trees	98.2	49.33	97.37	65.49
	D_4-0.5 Sec	Tree	Complex	99.1	77.82	70.24	**73.84**
			Medium	99.1	80.65	65.93	72.55
			Simple	99	84.52	59.18	69.62
		SVM	Linear	99.3	93.72	69.36	79.72
			Quadratic	99.4	94.51	72.35	81.95
			Cubic	99.4	93.21	74.45	**82.78**
			Medium Gaussian	99.1	95.56	52.32	67.62
			Coarse Gaussian	99.3	95.77	67.59	79.25
		KNN	Fine	99.2	86.31	70.46	77.59
			Medium	99.3	96.65	63.83	76.88
			Cosine	99.1	72.49	82.19	77.03
			Cubic	99.2	95.38	61.73	74.95
			Weighted	99.3	96.18	66.92	**78.93**
		Ensemble	Bagged trees	99.4	93.73	71.13	**80.88**
			Subspace Discriminant	98.7	68.92	60.84	64.63
			Subspace KNN	99.2	94.36	62.94	75.51
			RUSBoosted trees	97.6	43.83	92.26	59.42

Table 5. Classifier performance on Epochs' data sets

Patient ID	Data set-Epoch length	Classifier	Accuracy	Precision	Recall	F-measure
P1	10 s	Decision Tree	99.1	83.33	64.1	72.46
		SVM	99.4	90.63	74.36	81.69
		KNN	99.4	90.63	74.36	81.69
		Ensemble	99.5	96.67	74.36	**84.06**
	0.5 s	Decision Tree	99.1	81.26	67.15	73.53
		SVM	99.4	93.18	74.12	82.56
		KNN	99.3	95.45	67.37	78.99
		Ensemble	99.4	91.13	78.43	**84.3**
P2	10 s	Decision Tree	98.9	71.88	60.53	65.71
		SVM	98.8	65.79	65.79	65.79
		KNN	98.7	64.71	57.89	61.11
		Ensemble	99.2	88.89	63.16	**73.85**
	0.5 s	Decision Tree	99.1	77.82	70.24	73.84
		SVM	99.4	93.21	74.45	82.78
		KNN	99.3	96.18	66.92	78.93
		Ensemble	99.4	90.93	77.65	**83.77**

We explored that a seizure can be detected in a short epoch length by training the data set. However, in this work we are using two epochs (10 and 0.5 s) but with two patients of EEG data sets.

If we conclude that a seizure can be detected in a small epoch length with good accuracy then we can use the same epoch length which results in fast seizure detection. On the other hand, if we can reduce the epoch length let say up to 0.5 s then the future record will be produced in approximately 0.5 s. From the experimental results shown in Table 5 and Fig. 1 both patients' data sets(D_2 and D_4) are epoch length of 0.5 s. The accuracy and F-measure values are higher than D_1 and D_3 epoch length of 10 s. This implies that a seizure can also be detected in a shorter time of 0.5 s. Thus, we can make a prediction within a time of 0.5 s which is about 20 times faster than 10 s.

Hence, it reconfirms the results of our paper under-review [24] that the ensemble classifiers model can be used for fast seizure detection by reducing the epoch length of EEG data set to 0.5 s.

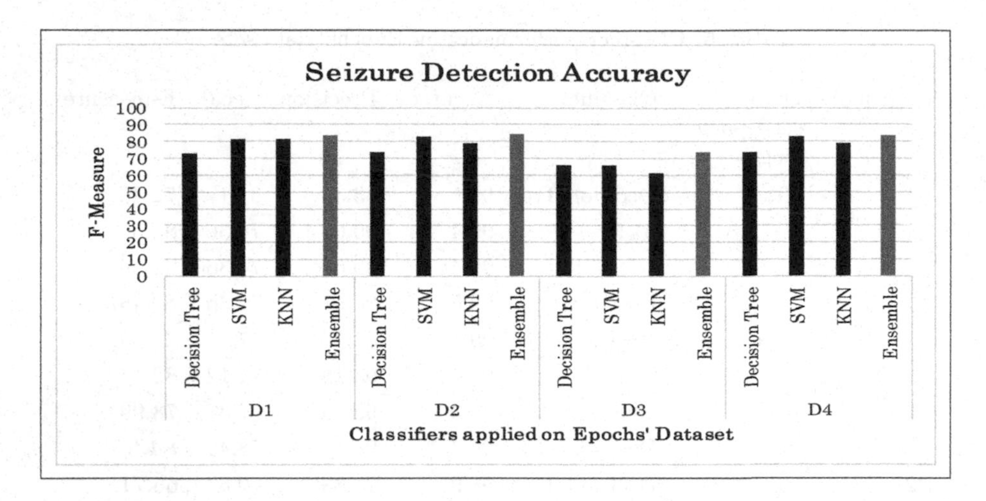

Fig. 1. Seizure Detection Accuracy on Epochs' data set by Black-box and Non-black box classifiers

5 Conclusion and Future Work

Classifier performance is typically a serious concern for data miners. Generally, EEG data set is of high dimension. Hence, some classifiers may not perform well in terms of accuracy and their true prediction rate. As demonstrated in Table 5 and Fig. 1 we make a comparative analysis among these classifiers. It is observed that for all the data sets ensemble classifiers outperform other classifiers. However, the results described in Tables 4 and 5 indicate that from the data sets of both the patients we get good accuracy and F-measure with shorter epoch length of 0.5 s by using an ensemble classifier instead of using other classifiers. It implies that an ensemble classifier can be potentially applied for detecting the seizure quickly in a clinical practice.

Acknowledgments. We acknowledge the contribution of Mr. Sajid Saeed Khan, Faculty member of the English Department of Amiruddaula Islamia College, Lucknow University, Lucknow in carefully proof reading the paper.

References

1. CHB-MIT scalp EEG database. https://physionet.org/pn6/chbmit/. Accessed 20 June 2015
2. Acharya, U.R., Molinari, F., Sree, S.V., Chattopadhyay, S., Ng, K.H., Suri, J.S.: Automated diagnosis of epileptic EEG using entropies. Biomed. Signal Process. Control **7**(4), 401–408 (2012)
3. Aditya, S., Tibarewala, D.: Comparing ANN, LDA, QDA, KNN and SVM algorithms in classifying relaxed and stressful mental state from two-channel prefrontal EEG data. Int. J. Artif. Intell. Soft Comput. **3**(2), 143–164 (2012)

4. Adnan, M.N., Islam, M.Z.: Forest CERN: a new decision forest building technique. In: Bailey, J., Khan, L., Washio, T., Dobbie, G., Huang, J.Z., Wang, R. (eds.) PAKDD 2016. LNCS, vol. 9651, pp. 304–315. Springer, Cham (2016). doi:10.1007/978-3-319-31753-3_25
5. Birjandtalab, J., Pouyan, M.B., Cogan, D., Nourani, M., Harvey, J.: Automated seizure detection using limited-channel EEG and non-linear dimension reduction. Comput. Biol. Med. **82**, 49–58 (2017)
6. de Boer, H.M., Mula, M., Sander, J.W.: The global burden and stigma of epilepsy. Epilepsy Behav. **12**(4), 540–546 (2008)
7. Breiman, L.: Random forests. Mach. Learn. **45**(1), 5–32 (2001). http://dx.doi.org/10.1023/A:1010933404324
8. Chen, C.L., Liu, J.L., Syu, J.Y.: Application of chaos theory and data mining to seizure detection of epilepsy
9. Donos, C., Dümpelmann, M., Schulze-Bonhage, A.: Early seizure detection algorithm based on intracranial EEG and random forest classification. Int. J. Neural Syst. **25**(05), 1550023 (2015)
10. Dorai, A., Ponnambalam, K.: Automated epileptic seizure onset detection. In: 2010 International Conference on Autonomous and Intelligent Systems (AIS), pp. 1–4. IEEE (2010)
11. Fayyad, U.M., Piatetsky-Shapiro, G., Smyth, P., Uthurusamy, R. (eds.): Advances in Knowledge Discovery and Data Mining. American Association for Artificial Intelligence, Menlo Park (1996)
12. Fergus, P., Hussain, A., Hignett, D., Al-Jumeily, D., Abdel-Aziz, K., Hamdan, H.: A machine learning system for automated whole-brain seizure detection. Appl. Comput. Inf. **12**(1), 70–89 (2016)
13. Furness, J.B., Costa, M.: The enteric nervous system. Churchill Livingstone Edinburgh etc. (1987)
14. Gorunescu, F.: Data Mining: Concepts, Models and Techniques, vol. 12. Springer Science & Business Media, Heidelberg (2011). doi:10.1007/978-3-642-19721-5
15. Islam, M.Z., D'Alessandro, S., Furner, M., Johnson, L., Gray, D., Carter, L.: Brand switching pattern discovery by data mining techniques for the telecommunication industry in Australia. Australas. J. Inf. Syst. **20** (2016)
16. Islam, M.Z., Giggins, H.: Knowledge discovery through SysFor: a systematically developed forest of multiple decision trees. In: Proceedings of the Ninth Australasian Data Mining Conference, vol. 121, pp. 195–204. Australian Computer Society, Inc. (2011)
17. Li, J., Liu, H.: Ensembles of cascading trees. In: Third IEEE International Conference on Data Mining, ICDM 2003, pp. 585–588. IEEE (2003)
18. Logesparan, L., Casson, A.J., Rodriguez-Villegas, E.: Optimal features for online seizure detection. Med. Biol. Eng. Comput. **50**(7), 659–669 (2012)
19. Orellana, M.P., Cerqueira, F.: Personalized epilepsy seizure detection using random forest classification over one-dimension transformed EEG data. bioRxiv p. 070300 (2016)
20. Powers, D.M.: Evaluation: from Precision, Recall and F-measure to ROC, Informedness, Markedness and Correlation (2011)
21. Rosenow, F., Klein, K.M., Hamer, H.M.: Non-invasive EEG evaluation in epilepsy diagnosis. Expert Rev. Neurother. **15**(4), 425–444 (2015)
22. Shoeb, A., Edwards, H., Connolly, J., Bourgeois, B., Treves, S.T., Guttag, J.: Patient-specific seizure onset detection. Epilepsy Behav. **5**(4), 483–498 (2004)

23. Siddiqui, M.K., Islam, M.Z.: Data mining approach in seizure detection. In: 2016 IEEE Region 10 Conference (TENCON), Singapore, pp. 3579–3583. Institute of Electrical and Electronics Engineers (IEEE), November 2016
24. Siddiqui, M.K., Islam, M.Z., Kabir, M.A.: Brain data mining on an ECoG dataset for Quick Seizure detection and Localization, March 2017. Submitted to Neural Computing and Applications
25. Teplan, M., et al.: Fundamentals of EEG measurement. Meas. Sci. Rev. **2**(2), 1–11 (2002)
26. Zhang, Y., Zhang, Y., Wang, J., Zheng, X.: Comparison of classification methods on EEG signals based on wavelet packet decomposition. Neural Comput. Appl. **26**(5), 1217–1225 (2014)
27. Almazyad, A.S., Ahamad, M.G.: Siddiqui. M.K., Almazyad, A.S.: Effective hypertensive treatment using data mining in Saudi Arabia. J. Clin. Monit. Comput. **24**(6), 391–401 (2010). Springer

A Framework for Clustering and Dynamic Maintenance of XML Documents

Ahmed Al-Shammari(✉), Chengfei Liu, Mehdi Naseriparsa, Bao Quoc Vo, Tarique Anwar, and Rui Zhou

Swinburne University of Technology, Melbourne, VIC 3122, Australia
{aalshammari,cliu,mnaseriparsa,bvo,tanwar,rzhou}@swin.edu.au

Abstract. Web data clustering has been widely studied in the data mining communities. However, dynamic maintenance of the web data clusters is still a challenging task. In this paper, we propose a novel framework called XClusterMaint which serves for both clustering and maintenance of the XML documents. For clustering, we take both structure and content into account and propose an efficient solution for grouping the documents based on the combination of structure and content similarity. For maintenance, we propose an incremental approach for maintaining the existing clusters dynamically when we receive new incoming XML documents. Since the dynamic maintenance of the clusters is computationally expensive, we also propose an improved approach which uses a lazy maintenance scheme to improve the performance of the clusters maintenance. The experimental results on real datasets verify the efficiency of the proposed clustering and maintenance model.

Keywords: Clustering · XML documents · Structure and content similarity · Dynamic maintenance

1 Introduction

XML has become a standard data exchange format these days, which provides interoperability and simplicity among Web-based services such as financial transactions, transportation, and healthcare services [10]. In general, these services are required to meet the minimum response time for transferring large amounts of XML data between users and the application providers. Therefore, identifying groups of users with similar requests can potentially reduce the required response time. Clustering is one of the most crucial techniques for organising the disseminated documents into groups based on their similarities [7,14]. Several studies have proposed different XML clustering models to support the compression and aggregation techniques in reducing the latency and bandwidth over the Web services [1,2]. For clustering XML documents, the similarities between them are computed and the measures are used to group them into clusters. When the new documents arrive, the existing clusters are to be updated and maintained dynamically in an efficient manner. For the dynamic maintenance, some clustering techniques such as the partitioning-based are inapplicable in the dynamic

G. Cong et al. (Eds.): ADMA 2017, LNAI 10604, pp. 399–412, 2017.
https://doi.org/10.1007/978-3-319-69179-4_28

environment [11]. There are two reasons behind this. Firstly, these approaches assume a fixed number of clusters. However, in the dynamic environment the number of clusters may change frequently over a period of time. Secondly, the partitioning-based approach completely recalculates the cluster properties to update the clusters each time with the new XML documents. This complete re-calculation approach is inefficient. Conversely, the agglomerative (bottom-up) clustering method does not require a predefined number of clusters [4,5]. There has not been much works on developing methods for efficient maintenance of XML document clusters in a dynamic environment. Some studies have proposed clustering models for XML documents based on the structure and content similarity [12]. These models are inefficient for clustering XML documents because they require a long execution time to calculate the pairwise distance between the documents. For instance, fractal clustering models [2] use a fractal similarity method that needs to calculate the scale and offset factors to find the similarity between the XML documents. To address the above limitations, we introduce a novel framework for clustering and maintenance of the XML documents called XClusterMaint. The XClusterMaint framework includes the followings: (1) clustering, and (2) the clusters maintenance. The main contributions of this paper are summarised as follows:

- We propose a fast clustering model for the XML documents based on a combination of the structure and content similarity. The proposed model requires a low computational cost in comparison with the existing clustering models.
- We introduce an incremental approach for the dynamic maintenance of existing clusters when new documents arrive. The maintenance includes adding the new documents to their closest cluster, and updating the cluster properties.
- We further improve the performance of the dynamic maintenance of clusters by proposing a lazy maintenance scheme. It keeps track only of the unstable cluster spaces to minimize the computations.
- We validate the proposed framework with extensive experiments on real-world datasets and demonstrate the efficiency of our clustering and maintenance approaches.

The rest of the paper is organised as follows. Section 2 presents the related work, which is followed by the problem definition in Sect. 3, and a high-level solution sketch in Sect. 4. Thereafter, we present the initial clustering of XML documents in Sect. 5, and the dynamic cluster maintenance in Sect. 6. The experimental results are presented in Sect. 7, and the paper is finally concluded in Sect. 8.

2 Related Work

This section highlights the basic findings and gaps in the studies related to clustering methods. Many studies have addressed the problem of XML document clustering. XML document includes two main features: structure and content. However, most current XML clustering algorithms do not concentrate on both of these features due to their demand of more processing time and computational storage. Clustering of static XML documents based on the similarity/distance measure has attracted a great deal of attention. Static clustering approaches can be generally separated into the following categories: content-based approaches, structure-based approaches, and hybrid approaches. Clustering XML by structure and content features is more efficient and useful whenever XML documents share overlapping [6]. In addition, in a heterogeneous environment clustering by both features achieves a high performance in comparison with other approaches using content/structure only [12,15]. We focus on the clustering XML documents algorithms by considering both structure and content similarity since there is no work done on the dynamic maintenance of the XML documents clustering in the literature.

Yongming et al. (2008) [15] introduced a clustering technique for XML documents based on similarity measures which exploits both the structure and content features of XML data. The leaf path and nested elements of XML data are the major features forming the vector-based dataset before the clustering process is performed. Experiments showed that the performance of the extended vector space model is greater than the basic VSM, showing higher purity and lower entropy. Al-Shammary and Khalil (2011) [2] proposed Fractal clustering algorithms by structure and content similarity. These models do not require a pre-defined number of clusters. In the pre-processing, XML is transformed as a vector by using the tf.idf weighting scheme. Then, Fractal coefficient is used to find the similarity among vectors and finally group them based on minimum fractal mean square error. The experimental results have shown better performance of the proposed self-similarity model than other clustering techniques such as k-means and PCA combined with k-means.

However, partitioning-based clustering algorithms are inapplicable in the dynamic environment. The main reason is that the proposed algorithms assume a fixed number of clusters [11]. On the other hand, clustering algorithms [2,6] have also shown some drawbacks such as the lack of incremental maintenance for the existing clusters and disregard the content similarity of XML documents. Therefore, our work focuses on proposing a framework for both clustering and maintenance of the clusters over XML documents.

3 Problem Statement

Suppose we have a given set of XML documents $\mathcal{D} = \{\mathrm{d}_1, \mathrm{d}_2, \mathrm{d}_3, ..., \mathrm{d}_{|\mathcal{D}|}\}$. We use two aspects to reflect an XML document: (a) data structure, and (b) data content. Therefore for a document $d_i \in \mathcal{D}$, we generate two vectors called $\vec{v}_i^s$ and $\vec{v}_i^c$ to represent the document structure and content properties respectively. Then, we combine these vectors to generate the XML vector that represents the corresponding XML document. The first problem that we address in this paper is defined as grouping these documents $\mathcal{D}$ based on their structure and content similarity to generate the initial set of clusters $\mathcal{C} = \{c_1, ..., c_{|\mathcal{C}|}\}$. These clusters contain the summarised information of the documents. To assign the

XML vectors into their proper clusters, we have to measure the distance between these vectors.

Definition 1 ***(Vector distance).*** *For two XML vectors $\vec{v}_1$ and $\vec{v}_2$, the vector distance (dist) is defined as their Euclidean distance presented in Eq. 1*

$$dist(\vec{v}_1, \vec{v}_2) = \sqrt{\sum_{i=1}^{n} \left(\vec{v}_1.w_i - \vec{v}_2.w_i\right)^2} \quad (1)$$

Here w_i is the weight of the ith entry in the XML vector. After measuring the distance between the XML vectors, we group these vectors into a set of clusters based on their distance measure.

Definition 2 ***(Cluster).*** *A cluster $c \in \mathcal{C}$ contains a set of XML vectors, and has the following properties: (a) the centroid m_c which is defined as the central mean vector of the c which is presented in Eq. 2, (b) the radius r_c^1 which is required a pre-defined to the set of clusters $\mathcal{C}$.*

$$\vec{m}_c = \frac{\sum_{i=1}^{|c|} \vec{v}_i}{|c|} \quad (2)$$

The second problem is incrementally maintaining the generated clusters when the new incoming documents arrive. Given a set of clusters $\mathcal{C}$ and an incoming document d_{new}, maintenance of the existing clusters defined as a set of updates for the cluster properties with tracking the affected XML vectors. In the tracking process, we may assign the affected XML vectors to the nearest clusters or we may initialise new clusters for these vectors. However, dynamic maintenance of the clusters incurs high computational costs. Therefore, there is a need for an efficient maintenance approach to improve the performance of the clusters maintenance.

4 The Solution Sketch

Figure 1 shows our proposed framework called XClusterMaint. Technically, XClusterMaint that takes care of both the clustering and the clusters maintenance. In the clustering, we start with traversing the order labelled XML tree, and then we generate the XML vector which is a combination of the structure and content vectors respectively. Technically, the term frequency-inverse document frequency (tf.idf) weighting scheme [8] is used to assign the weights to the terms of XML document, and the weights are stored in a vector matrix. Afterwards, Euclidean distance [3] is used for the similarity measurement by computing the minimum distance between the XML vectors. Then, the similar XML vectors are distributed into the clusters based on the agglomerative clustering model. The steps of clustering are presented in Sect. 5. In the clusters maintenance, an incremental approach is proposed for maintaining the properties of the existing clusters when the new incoming document arrives. Finally, we improve the efficiency of the clusters maintenance based on lazy maintenance scheme. The steps of clusters maintenance are presented in Sect. 6.

5 Clustering of XML Documents

In this section we focus on the main steps of the clustering of XML documents. The steps are as follows: (a) generating the vectors for the XML documents, (b) computing the similarity of the documents using their vectors, and (c) allocating the documents to their proper clusters.

5.1 Generating the XML Vectors

Any XML document in the dataset is modelled as a rooted tree. The XML tree has two kinds of nodes: (a) structure node and (b) content node. The structure refers to the nested tags (elements) that organise the content information while the content refers to the data values of the elements. We use depth-first search algorithm for traversing and indexing XML nodes level by level since all the nodes obtain a unique number as their index. To generate the XML vectors, we firstly generate the structure vector $\vec{v}^s$ and content vector $\vec{v}^c$.

Definition 3 ***(XML vector).*** *An XML document $d_i \in \mathcal{D}$ represented as a vector $\vec{v}_i = (\vec{v}_i^s.w_1, \vec{v}_i^s.w_2, ..., \vec{v}_i^s.w_m, \vec{v}_i^c.w_{m+1}, ..., \vec{v}_i^c.w_n)$ where $\vec{v}_i^s.w_j$ reflects the weight (total frequency) of the XML term j in the structure vector $(1 \leq j \leq m)$ and $\vec{v}_i^c.w_{m+k}$ reflects the weight of the XML term k in the content vector $(1 \leq k \leq n-m)$*[1].

We select m terms for the structure vector and $n - m$ for the content vector, where m and n are usually application dependent and constrained by storage. For each term t in the structure or content vector, we use the tf.idf scheme to calculate the weight. The tf measures the frequency of the term t in the document denoted by $tf(t, d)$ while the idf measures the importance of the term

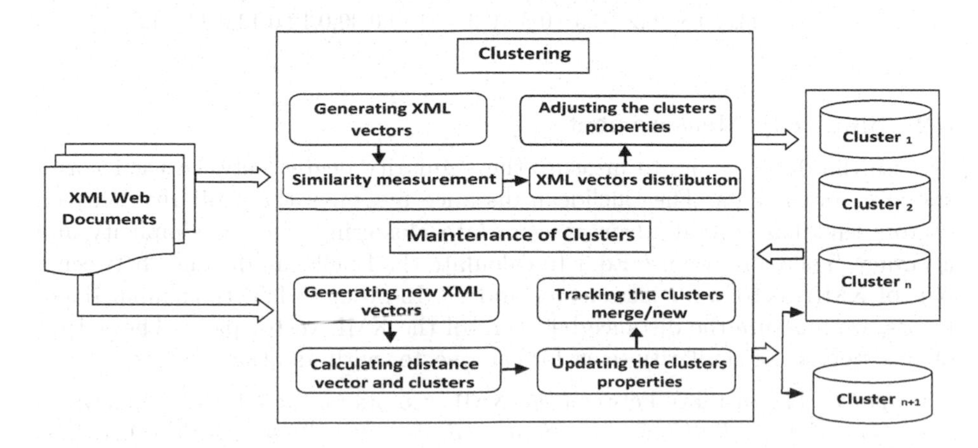

Fig. 1. The main components of XClusterMaint framework

[1] For simplicity, in this paper, we set $m = \frac{n}{2}$.

in the entire set of documents denoted by $idf(t) = log\frac{N}{df(t)}$ where $df(t)$ presents the number of documents that contain t in the dataset and N is the total number of XML documents in the dataset. Formula 3 presents the tf.idf formula for a term t in the document d.

$$w_{t,d} = tf(t,d) \times idf(t) \tag{3}$$

After generating $\vec{v}^s$ and $\vec{v}^c$, we combine these vectors to generate the XML vector of a document. This vector is used to measure the similarity score between the documents. The Eq. 4 presents the combination formula where α is the tuning parameter which trades off between the importance of the structure and content terms of the document.

$$\vec{v} = (\alpha \times \vec{v}^s, (1-\alpha) \times \vec{v}^c) \tag{4}$$

For example purpose, assume we have 6 documents in the dataset. The XML vector for each document is generated by applying the combination formula presented in Eq. 4 using the tuning parameter $\alpha = 0.6$. For each vector, there are 3 weights for the structural terms and 3 weights for the content terms. Figure 1 presents the vectors for these documents.

Table 1. Vectors generation

Vectors	Structure			Content			Generating the vectors
	w_{t_1}	w_{t_2}	w_{t_3}	w_{t_1}	w_{t_2}	w_{t_3}	
v_1	0.3	0.6	0.2	0.4	0.9	0.3	(0.18,0.36,0.12,0.16,0.36,0.12)
v_2	0.2	0.3	0.3	0.6	0.3	0.2	(0.12,0.18,0.18,0.24,0.12,0.08)
v_3	0.3	0.6	0.2	0.6	0.9	0.3	(0.18,0.36,0.12,0.24,0.36,0.12)
v_4	0.3	0.6	0.4	0.4	0.9	0.3	(0.18,0.36,0.24,0.16,0.36,0.12)
v_5	0.2	0.2	0.3	0.6	0.3	0.2	(0.12,0.12,0.18,0.24,0.12,0.08)
v_6	0.2	0.5	0.2	0.3	0.8	0.3	(0.12,0.30,0.12,0.12,0.32,0.12)

5.2 Similarity Measurement

We use the data vectors to measure the similarity degree between their corresponding documents. The Euclidean distance measures the similarity between vectors that has several advantages in data clustering, such as simplicity and accuracy. Therefore, we use Eq. 1 to calculate the Euclidean distance between a pair of XML vectors, for instance $\vec{v}_1$ and $\vec{v}_2$. In order to find the similar documents, we measure the distance between all the XML vector pairs. The output of this step is the similarity score for each vector with all other vectors.

Example 1. The distance between the XML vectors in Table 1 are as follows: $dist(\vec{v}_2,\vec{v}_5) = 0.06$, $dist(\vec{v}_1,\vec{v}_3) = 0.08$, $dist(\vec{v}_1,\vec{v}_6) = 0.1019$, $dist(\vec{v}_1,\vec{v}_4) = 0.12$, $dist(\vec{v}_3,\vec{v}_4) = 0.1442$, $dist(\vec{v}_3,\vec{v}_6) = 0.1523$, $dist(\vec{v}_4,\vec{v}_6) = 0.1574$, $dist(\vec{v}_5,\vec{v}_6) = 0.2049$, $dist(\vec{v}_2,\vec{v}_6) = 0.2720$, $dist(\vec{v}_2,\vec{v}_3) = 0.3143$, $dist(\vec{v}_1,\vec{v}_2) = 0.3243$, $dist(\vec{v}_3,\vec{v}_5) = 0.3521$, $dist(\vec{v}_1,\vec{v}_5) = 0.3611$.

5.3 XML Vectors Distribution

After measuring the pairwise similarity between the XML vectors, we initialize the clusters for these vectors. To initialize the clusters, we start with sorting the pairwise distance between every two vectors, as shown in Example 1. The pair with the minimum distance is first checked whether it is less than a given threshold δ. The two vectors of this pair are merged into a cluster if it is true. This process is carried out to all the other vector pairs $(\vec{v}_i,\vec{v}_j)$ for which $\text{dist}(\vec{v}_i,\vec{v}_j) < \delta$, in the order of increasing pairwise distance. After this first round, the pairwise distance between the centroids of every two clusters are computed and sorted in increasing order. Following the same process as the first round, the clusters are merged if their distance is less than δ. These rounds are continued until all the pairs satisfying the pairwise distance condition have been processed. Considering Example 1 and $\delta = 0.21055$, the distance between $\vec{v}_1$ and $\vec{v}_3$, $\vec{v}_6$, and $\vec{v}_4$ is less than δ. While, the distance between $\vec{v}_1$ and $\vec{v}_2$, $\vec{v}_1$ and $\vec{v}_5$ is greater than δ. As a result, $\vec{v}_2$ and $\vec{v}_5$ have a high similarity and they will assign to the first clusterc_1. While, $\vec{v}_1$ $\vec{v}_3$, $\vec{v}_6$, and $\vec{v}_4$ will assign to the second cluster c_2.

6 Maintenance of the Clusters

As we mentioned earlier, the existing clustering algorithms are inapplicable for the dynamic maintenance of the clusters. Therefore, we propose two approaches for the incremental maintenance: (1) Baseline approach, and (2) Improved approach. When new XML documents arrive, these approaches maintain the properties of the existing clusters incrementally. The first approach uses an Eager Maintenance scheme of the Clusters (EMC) that tracks the entire XML vectors in the cluster. The second approach uses a Lazy Maintenance scheme of the Clusters (LMC) which tracks only a part of the XML vectors. The technical details for the proposed approaches are presented in Sects. 6.1 and 6.2 respectively. Maintenance of the clusters starts with the generating new XML vectors. Then, a decision is made to either assign the new XML vector $\vec{v}$ to the nearest cluster $c \in \mathcal{C}$ by calculating the minimum distance between the new vector and the existing clusters or initialise new cluster. Once the new XML vector is assigned to its nearest cluster, the new cluster centroid will be adjusted. The process of adjusting the new cluster centroid is performed incrementally by using the following formula:

$$\vec{m}_{c_{new}} = \frac{|c| \times \vec{m}_c + \vec{v}}{|c| + 1} \tag{5}$$

Where $|c|$ is the cluster size before adding the new XML vectors.

6.1 Baseline Maintenance Approach

We first present the baseline maintenance approach which is implemented based on EMC. We introduce a second yet smaller radius r_c^2, such that $(r_c^2 < r_c^1)^2$ to divide a cluster $c \in \mathcal{C}$ into two spaces as followings:

- Stable space (S): This space contains the XML vectors that reside in the second radius of a cluster r_c^2. The distance between these vectors and their centroid is less than or equal the second radius, where $dist(\vec{v}, \vec{m}_c) \leq r_c^2$.
- Boundary space (B): This space contains the XML vectors that reside out of the second radius r_c^2 but in the first radius r_c^1, i.e., $r_c^2 < dist(\vec{v}, \vec{m}_c) \leq r_c^1$. These vectors may be unstable and should be considered in the cluster maintenance. For instance, when the new centroid moves to a specific side, some of these vectors may be outside of the cluster boundary since the distance between these vectors and the new centroid is bigger than r_c^1 as shown in Fig. 2.

Basically, EMC uses two sets of maintenance operations as follows:

- $moveOut(\vec{v}, S, c)$ this operation moves the XML vector $\vec{v}$ from the stable space to the boundary space of the cluster c.
- $moveIn(\vec{v}, S, c)$ this operation moves the XML vector $\vec{v}$ from the boundary space to the stable space of the cluster c.
- $moveOut(\vec{v}, B, c)$ this operation moves the XML vector $\vec{v}$ from the boundary space to the outside of the cluster c.
- $moveIn(\vec{v}', B, c)$ this operation receives the XML vector $\vec{v}'$ from the outside of the cluster to the boundary space of the cluster c.

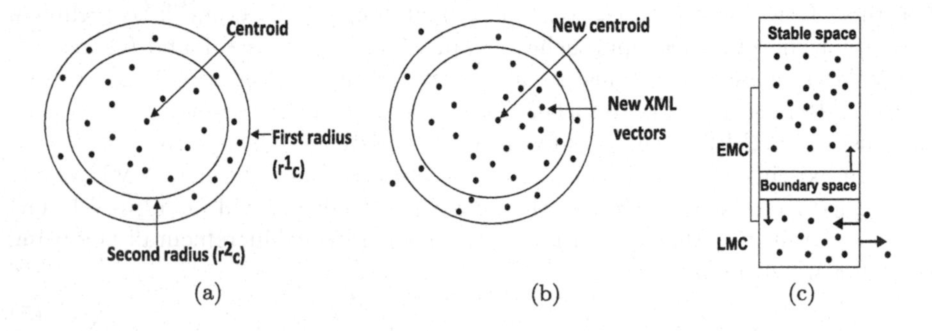

Fig. 2. Maintenance of the cluster

The EMC maintains the existing clusters by tracking the XML vectors in the stable and unstable spaces in the maintenance process. It includes two checking conditions: (1) cluster merge and (2) cluster initialisation. Firstly, a decision is

[2] r_c^2 is usually a fraction of r_c^1, i.e. $r_c^2 = \lambda r_c^1, \lambda \in (0, 1)$. In the paper, we find $\lambda = 0.8$ is fairly good.

made to merge the vectors that are located outside of the first cluster boundary to the nearest cluster. Secondly, a decision is made to initialise a new cluster if the minimum distance between the vector and the existing centroids is bigger than a distance threshold θ such that $min(dist(\vec{v}, \vec{m}_{c_i}, 1 \leq i \leq |\mathcal{C}|)) > \theta$.

6.2 Improved Maintenance Approach

The improved maintenance approach uses the Lazy Maintenance of the Clusters scheme (LMC) for maintaining the existing set of the clusters efficiently. LMC scheme only tracks the XML vectors in the unstable space. Therefore, this approach does not require to check the XML vectors in the stable space of a cluster, which cause it to accelerate the process of the cluster maintenance (see Fig. 2). The EMC and LMC tracking spaces are presented in Fig. 2. Clearly, the EMC works on both spaces while the LMC only works on the boundary space. According to this approach, we guarantee that the entire XML vectors do not require an adjustment in the stable space of the cluster. LMC uses a set of maintenance operations are as follows:

- $moveOut(\vec{v}, B, c_{new})$ this operation moves the XML vectors from the boundary space to the outside of the cluster.
- $moveIn(\vec{v}', B, c_{new})$ this operation receives the XML vectors from the outside of the cluster to the boundary space.

Theorem 1. *Let* c *and* c_{new} *denote the cluster before and after adding the new incoming documents respectively. Then* r_c^1-r_c^2 *denote the boundary threshold* δ, *and* $\vec{m}_c$ *is the old cluster centroid. There is no adjustment required for the stable space of the cluster* c_{new} *if the distance between the centroids* $dist(\vec{m}_c, \vec{m}_{c_{new}}) \leq \delta$.

Proof. Assume $\vec{v}$ is a vector that resides in the stable space of the cluster c such that $dist(\vec{v}, \vec{m}_c) = r_c^2$. Then if the distance of $\vec{v}$ with the new cluster c_{new} is $dist(\vec{v}, \vec{m}_{c_{new}}) > r_c^1$, thus $\vec{v}$ is out of cluster c_{new}. We prove that this can never happen. Since the new centroid $m_{c_{new}}$ is moved within the distance of (r_c^1-r_c^2), the maximum distance for the new vector $\vec{v}$ will be $dist(\vec{v}, \vec{m}_{c_{new}}) = r_c^2 + (r_c^1 - r_c^2) = r_c^1$ which means in the worst case it resides in the boundary of c_{new}. As a result, the distance of $\vec{v}$ in the new cluster c_{new} is $dist(\vec{v}, \vec{m}_{c_{new}}) \leq r_c^1$. Therefore, the primary assumption is not true and the vectors of the stable space will never move out of the c_{new}; thus, no adjustment required.

Basically, there are two possibilities might be happened after adjusting a new cluster centroid. Firstly, the new centroid of the cluster might be changed slightly. Secondly, The new centroid of the first cluster might be changed dramatically (it takes a sudden jump). For the first possibility, we proposed incremental maintenance of clusters is capable of maintaining the accumulated clusters incrementally. Secondly, recalculation for centroid is required if the distance between old and new centroids is bigger than the boundary threshold δ. Therefore, we propose a local re-calculation approach to recalculate the cluster properties. In particular, this approach is performed locally for a part of clusters. The distance between a pair of cluster centroids is calculated based on the vector distance formula 1.

Algorithm 1. Improved Maintenance

Input : $\mathcal{C} = \{c_1, c_2, c_3, ..., c_{|\mathcal{C}|}\}$, new document d_{new}, minimum distance threshold θ, tuning Parameter α

Output: Updated set of clusters $\mathcal{C}_{new}$

1 $\vec{v}_{new} \leftarrow createVector(d_{new}, \alpha)$
2 $c_{near} \leftarrow$findNearestCluster($\vec{v}_{new}$,$\mathcal{C}$)
3 **if** $dist(\vec{v}_{new}, \vec{m}_{c_{near}}) \geq \theta$ **then**
4 | Initialize a new cluster and assign $\vec{v}_{new}$ to the new cluster c_{new}
5 | $\mathcal{C}_{new} \leftarrow \mathcal{C} \cup c_{new}$
6 **else**
7 | $c_{new} \leftarrow c_{near}$
8 | Assign vector $\vec{v}_{new}$ to c_{new}
9 | Update($\vec{m}_{c_{new}}$)
10 | **for** *each* $\vec{v}_i$ *in* c_{new} **do**
11 | | **if** $dist(\vec{v}_i, \vec{m}_{c_{new}}) > r_c^1$ **then**
12 | | | $moveOut(\vec{v}_i, B, c_{new})$
13 | **for** *each vector* $\vec{v}'$ *near to cluster* c **do**
14 | | **if** $dist(\vec{v}', \vec{m}_{c_{new}}) <= r_c^1$ **then**
15 | | | $moveIn(\vec{v}', B, c_{new})$
16 | $\delta \leftarrow$Determine the boundary threshold r_c^1-r_c^2
17 | **if** $dist(\vec{m}_{c_{near}}, \vec{m}_{c_{new}}) > \delta$ **then**
18 | | Recalculate the properties of the cluster c_{new}
19 $\mathcal{C}_{new} \leftarrow c_{new} \cup (\mathcal{C} \setminus c_{near})$
20 **return** $\mathcal{C}_{new}$

Algorithm 1 presents the maintenance steps for the proposed framework using the improved maintenance approach. In lines 1–2, we do the preparation for the maintenance. Lines 3–5 check the distance between the XML vectors and the centroid. If the distance is bigger than the distance threshold θ, we initialize a new cluster. In lines 7–9, we assign the XML vectors to the nearest cluster c_{near}. In lines 10–15, we track the XML vectors in the boundary space by using a set of maintenance operations. Lines 16–18 verify the distance between the old and new cluster centroids. If the distance is bigger than the boundary threshold δ, we do the local recalculation for the cluster.

7 Experimental Results

This section highlights the experimental results for the XClusterMaint framework. The comparison analysis between the clustering models is discussed in

Sect. 7.1. For the effectiveness test, we prove the correctness of the incremental maintenance approaches based on the cluster radius. Therefore, this paper addresses the efficiency of the clusters maintenance which is presented in Sect. 7.2. The experiments are implemented with Visual Basic 2012 and executed by a processor Intel, Core (i5)-3570 CPU 3.40 GHz. We conducted experiments on the real datasets. Specifically, we use four datasets that include 16,000 documents. These documents contain the information of the scheduled flights [9]. The datasets have the following sizes: 400 MB, 980 MB, 920 MB, and 640 MB.

7.1 Comparison with Fractal Clustering Model

We quantify the effects of the proposed clustering model according to the execution time in comparison with the fractal clustering model which is discussed in the literature 2. The execution time is the actual processing time that covers the entire processes for the clustering. It is an essential indicator to verify the efficiency of the proposed framework. The results show that our clustering model requires less execution time for clustering 4000 XML documents in comparison with fractal clustering model as shown in Fig. 3. Technically, both clustering models use tf.idf formula to represent the structure and content of XML documents as vectors. However, the main reason behind this difference is that the fractal clustering model needs further execution time to capture the similar vectors by computing the offset and scale factors of fractal similarity to determine the similar vectors.

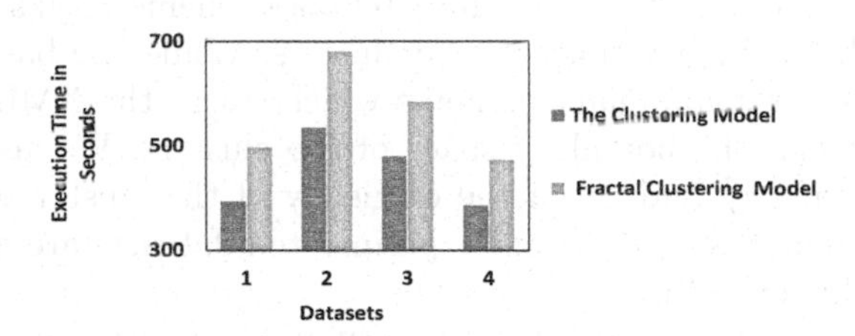

Fig. 3. Comparison of the execution time for the XML clustering models

7.2 Efficiency of the Clusters Maintenance

Figure 4 shows the execution time of our proposed approaches by varying the number of inserted XML documents in the experimented datasets. We note that both datasets 2 and 3 require a long execution time in comparison with datasets 1 and 4. When the number of XML documents is set from 1000 to 4000 with an increase of 500 documents at each iteration. We set the radius $r_c^1 = 0.682$ and $r_c^2 = 0.547$ respectively. The value of the first cluster radius r_c^1 is predefined depending on the maximum distance between the centroid $\vec{m}_c$ and the contained XML vectors in each cluster. While the value of the second cluster radius

r_c^2 is determined depending on the average of the minimum and maximum distances. Based on the Euclidean distance, the maximum distance is 0.682 and the minimum distance is 0.413. We note that the improved maintenance approach requires a less execution time for maintaining the clusters in comparison with the baseline maintenance approach.

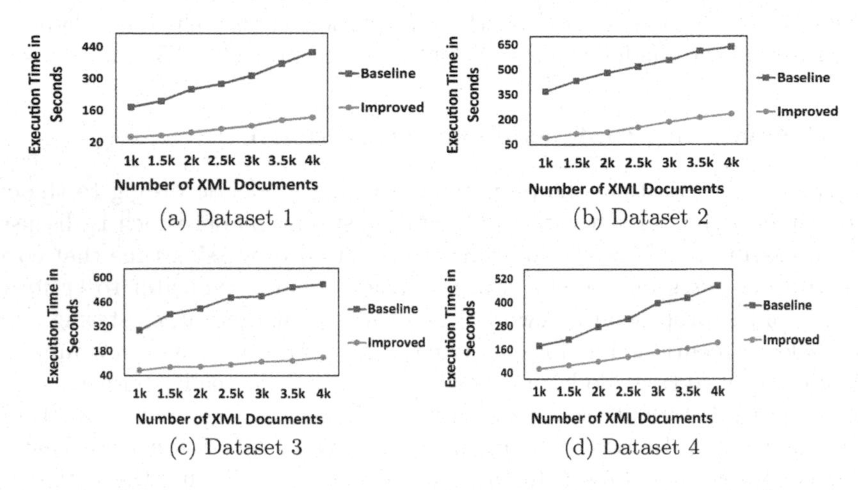

Fig. 4. Execution time for the baseline and improved maintenance approaches

The main reason is that the lazy maintenance scheme tracks only the XML vectors inside the boundary space of the clusters. While the baseline approach depends on the eager maintenance scheme which tracks the XML vectors inside the stable space and the boundary space of the clusters. We also examine the effect of the varying r_c^1 and r_c^2 on the efficiency of the cluster maintenance as shown in Fig. 5. The first and second experimented datasets are used in the test of varying the cluster radius.

Figures 5a and c present the effect of varying r_c^1 on the maintenance performance in two datasets. We set the value of the first radius and the second radius as $r_c^1 = 0.506$, 0.612, 0.718 and 0.824; and $r_c^2 = 0.412$, 0.515, 0.618 and 0.721 respectively. We note that when the value of r_c^1 increases, the execution time decreases for both maintenance approaches on both datasets. That's because when the value of the r_c^1 gets bigger, the number of generated clusters is smaller. Therefore, most XML vectors are assigned to the small set of the existing clusters without having to initialize the new clusters. Figures 5b and d present the effect of varying of the second radius r_c^2 on the maintenance performance. We fix $r_c^1 = 0.824$, and vary $r_c^2 = 0.412$, 0.515, 0.618 and 0.721. Clearly, varying r_c^2 has almost no effect on the performance of the baseline maintenance approach. That's because the baseline approach works on all the vectors in the stable and boundary spaces for maintenance. In the improved approach; however, by varying r_c^2 to a smaller value, the number of vectors in the stable space decreases which leads to bigger execution time. Conversely, by setting r_c^2 to a bigger value,

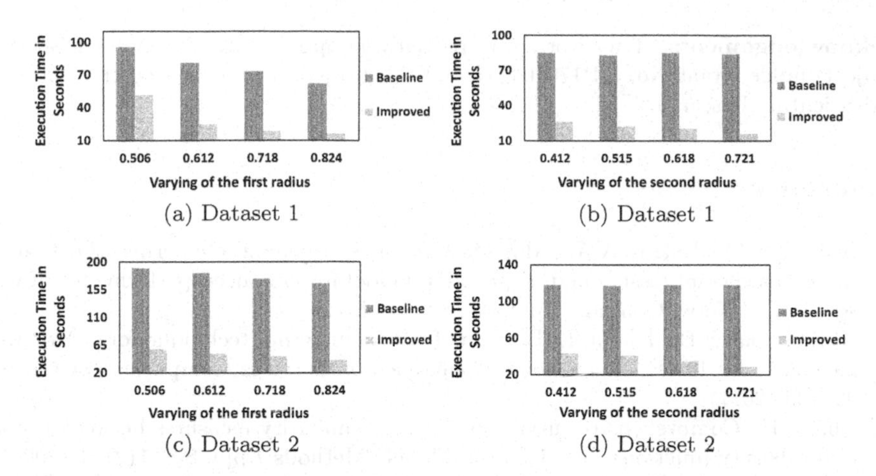

Fig. 5. Execution time for the baseline and improved maintenance approaches with varying the values of r_c^1 and r_c^2

the number of vectors inside the stable space increases. As a result, only small number of vectors in the boundary space are checked for the maintenance which leads to improving the performance on both datasets.

8 Conclusion

In this paper, we introduce a novel framework called XClusterMaint that serves both the clustering and the clusters maintenance of XML documents. For clustering, we generate a set of initial clusters for the XML documents based on the combination of structure and content similarity. For maintenance, we maintain the properties of the existing clusters dynamically by using two incremental approaches for the clusters maintenance: (1) Baseline approach, and (2) Improved approach. In the first approach, we use the Eager Maintenance scheme of the Cluster (EMC) which tracks the XML vectors that reside in the stable and boundary spaces by using two sets of maintenance operations. In the second approach, we use the Lazy Maintenance scheme of the Cluster (LMC) to improve the performance of the cluster maintenance. The LMC scheme tracks only the XML vectors that reside in the boundary space by using a set of maintenance operations. Our experiments verify that the proposed LMC scheme is more efficient than EMC scheme. The resultant development for the clustering and maintenance of XML documents would be capable of improving the performance of real world applications by reducing the required response time. For future work, we will consider further extensions for the XML documents clustering as well as the clusters maintenance to be more effective in the dynamic environment.

Acknowledgements. This work was partially supported by the ARC Discovery Project under Grant No. DP170104747 and the Iraqi Ministry of Higher Education and Scientific Research.

References

1. Abbas, A.M., Bakar, A.A., Ahmad, M.Z.: Fast dynamic clustering SOAP messages based compression and aggregation model for enhanced performance of web services. J. Netw. Comput. Appl. **41**, 80–88 (2014)
2. Al-Shammary, D., Khalil, I.: Dynamic fractal clustering technique for SOAP web messages. In: IEEE International Conference on Services Computing (SCC), pp. 96–103 (2011)
3. Cha, S.H.: Comprehensive survey on distance/similarity measures between probability density functions. Int. J. Math. Models Methods Appl. Sci. **1**(2), 1 (2007)
4. Cheng, W., Zhang, X., Pan, F., Wang, W.: HICC: an entropy splitting-based framework for hierarchical co-clustering. Knowl. Inf. Syst. **46**(2), 343–367 (2016)
5. Cochez, M., Mou, H.: Twister tries: approximate hierarchical agglomerative clustering for average distance in linear time. In: Proceedings of the 2015 ACM SIGMOD International Conference on Management of Data, pp. 505–517 (2015)
6. Costa, G., Manco, G., Ortale, R., Ritacco, E.: Hierarchical clustering of XML documents focused on structural components. Data Knowl. Eng. **84**, 26–46 (2013)
7. Ding, R., Wang, Q., Dang, Y., Fu, Q., Zhang, H., Zhang, D.: Yading: fast clustering of large-scale time series data. Proc. VLDB Endow. **8**(5), 473–484 (2015)
8. Salton, G., McGill, M.J.: Introduction to Modern Information Retrieval. McGraw-Hill, New York (1983)
9. OpenFlights, 15 December 2016. https://datahub.io/dataset/open-flights
10. Phan, K.A., Tari, Z., Bertok, P.: Similarity-based soap multicast protocol to reduce bandwidth and latency in web services. IEEE Trans. Serv. Comput. **1**(2), 88–103 (2008)
11. Silva, J.A., Faria, E.R., Barros, R.C., Hruschka, E.R., de Carvalho, A.C., Gama, J.: Data stream clustering: a survey. ACM Comput. Surv. (CSUR) **46**(1), 13 (2013)
12. Tran, T., Nayak, R., Bruza, P.: Combining structure and content similarities for XML document clustering. In: Proceedings of the 7th Australasian Data Mining Conference, vol. 87, pp. 219–225 (2008)
13. Wang, D., Li, T.: Document update summarization using incremental hierarchical clustering. In Proceedings of the 19th ACM International Conference on Information and Knowledge Management, pp. 279–288 (2010)
14. Yan, J., Cheng, D., Zong, M., Deng, Z.: Improved spectral clustering algorithm based on similarity measure. In: International Conference on Advanced Data Mining and Applications, pp. 641–654 (2014)
15. Yongming, G., Dehua, C., Jiajin, L.: Clustering XML documents by combining content and structure. In: International Symposium on Information Science and Engineering, ISISE 2008, vol. 1, pp. 583–587 (2008)

Language-Independent Twitter Classification Using Character-Based Convolutional Networks

Shiwei Zhang(✉), Xiuzhen Zhang, and Jeffrey Chan

School of Computer Science and Information Technology,
RMIT University, Melbourne 3001, Australia
{shiwei.zhang,xiuzhen.zhang,jeffrey.chan}@rmit.edu.au

Abstract. Most research on Twitter classification is focused on tweets in English. But Twitter supports over 40 languages and about 50% of tweets are non-English tweets. To fully use the Twitter contents, it is important to develop classifiers that can classify multilingual tweets or tweets of mixed languages (for example tweets mainly in Chinese but containing English words). The translation-based model is a classical approach to achieving multilingual or cross-lingual text classification. Recently character-based neural models are shown to be effective for text classification. But they are designed for limited European languages and require identification of languages to build an alphabet to encode and quantize characters. In this paper, we propose UniCNN (Unicode character Convolutional Networks), a fully language-independent character-based CNN model for the classification of tweets in multiple languages and mixed languages, not requiring language identification. Specifically, we propose to encode the sequence of characters in a tweet into a sequence of numerical UTF-8 codes, and then train a character-based CNN classifier. In addition, a character-based embedding layer is included before the convolutional layer for learning distributed character representation. We conducted experiments on Twitter datasets for multilingual sentiment classification in six languages and for mixed-language informativeness classification in over 40 languages. Our experiments showed that UniCNN mostly performed better than state-of-the-art neural models and traditional feature-based models, while not requiring the extra burden of any translation or tokenization.

Keywords: Twitter · Language independent · Convolutional neural networks

1 Introduction

With about 313 million monthly active users and about one billion tweets posted every month, Twitter is one of the most popular social media platforms, and is also a great resource for extracting useful information and knowledge. Twitter classification is a form of document categorization where tweets (Twitter posts) are analyzed and classified into different categories. Twitter classification tasks such as sentiment classification [18], information type classification

G. Cong et al. (Eds.): ADMA 2017, LNAI 10604, pp. 413–425, 2017.
https://doi.org/10.1007/978-3-319-69179-4_29

and account type classification [5] all require advanced techniques for natural language processing (NLP) of the textual contents of tweets. Most research on Twitter classification is for the English language and is focused on addressing the linguistics challenges presented by Twitter, such as limited short text length (140 characters), incorrect spelling, the widespread use of abbreviations and slangs and multilingual content [9].

As an internationally popular microblogging services, Twitter supports more than 40 languages and about 50% of tweets are non-English tweets.[1] There are also tweets of mixed languages. To fully analyze the Twitter contents, it is therefore important to develop language-independent classification model for tweets of multiple languages and for tweets of mixed languages.

A traditional multilingual text (document) classification approach requires a parallel corpus for each language in the classification task by translation into English [6]. Classification models are then trained on the translated English corpus for each language. The effectiveness of this translation-based approach may be limited due to that the classification model misses the language-specific linguistic features and also depends on the accuracy of translation.

Neural network models have shown very promising results for document categorization. It is believed that the non-linearity of neural networks can outperform traditional machine learning models [11]. Popular neural networks for NLP tasks include convolutional network (CNN), recurrent neural network (RNN) and CNN-long short term memory (CNN-LSTM). CNN can utilize the internal structure of data and has been applied for various NLP tasks, including sentence classification [13], text categorization [12], sentiment classification [7] and machine translation [16].

Recently character-level convolutional neural networks [14,25] were proposed for multilingual text classification and it was shown that using characters as input, the performance of convolutional neural networks is improved when the network is deeper [4]. However, to the best of our knowledge, all existing neural models are designed for European languages of overlapping alphabets and require language identification to build the alphabet to encode and quantize characters. None of them is fully language independent and can not deal with the over 40 languages of Twitter posts.

In this paper, we propose UniCNN (Unicode UTF-8 encoded character CNN), a fully language-independent character-based convolutional neural network model for classifying tweets of multiple languages and tweets of mixed languages. To achieve complete language independence, we propose to encode characters in any language using the UTF-8 code. The advantages of using UTF-8 encoding instead of characters are:

- Language identification is not required any more. The UTF-8 code for characters is a universal alphabet for *any* languages.
- It allows neural networks to read tweets (documents) of mixed languages. Since we are using the whole character set of UTF-8 as the alphabet, UniCNN can encode tweets containing characters for different languages, for example tweets in Chinese but containing some English phrases.

[1] http://latimesblogs.latimes.com/technology/2010/02/twitter-tweets-english.html.

We experimented UniCNN for two Twitter classification tasks, sentiment classification and informativeness classification. The sentiment classification task includes six Twitter datasets of six different European languages. The informativeness classification task included a Twitter dataset of over 40 languages where many tweets are in mixed languages. We benchmarked UniCNN against several baseline models. Wilcoxon signed-rank test showed that UniCNN significantly outperformed character-based neural models and classical translation-based models using word-level feature unigram and bigram. UniCNN performed on par with the translation-based word-level neural model, a state-of-the-art word-level neural model that uses external data sources for training word embeddings.

2 Related Work

The recently proposed character-based convolutional neural models are the most related to our research [16,21]. Character-based CNN models need an alphabet to encode and quantize characters to build the neural networks. All existing character-based CNN models are designed for the alphabet of European languages like English, German, Polish and Spanish. To apply these models to multilingual text classification requires first identifying language, whether or not automatically, to build the alphabet to encode and quantize characters. Any foreign characters in mixed-language documents outside the alphabet are ignored. But the foreign language characters may contain important signals for classification. Although not designed for text classification, a character-level CNN with highway network and Bidirectional GRU for machine translation was proposed by Lee et al. [16], that accepts a sequence of characters in the source language and outputs a sequence of characters in the target language. It is shown that their character-based translation model can be better than subword-level translation model in the multilingual many-to-one translation task (which are German, Czech, Finnish and Russian to English). It is notable that their model still needs to first perform language identification on the fly.

Another character-based convolutional neural network [21] was proposed to focus on cross-language Twitter sentiment classification. However, their character-based model is limited by the semantic and syntactic structural differences among languages and requires the prior knowledge of the language to build the alphabet for developing the one-hot vector representation.

In the wider context of NLP research, since multilingual is commonly seen for natural language applications, building cross-language models is highly desirable for several NLP tasks, including multilingual Part-of-Speech (POS) Tagging [10], language-independent sentiment classification [18] and named entity recognition (NER) [10,24]. Word-based neural models are popularly applied for these tasks. To achieve multilingual and cross-lingual analysis, tokenization and translation are generally needed. The model presented by Yang et al. [24] is based on gated recurrent units and conditional random fields, which generates representation of words based on characters and is designed for leveraging morphological similarities between languages, such as English and Spanish. An attention-based LSTM

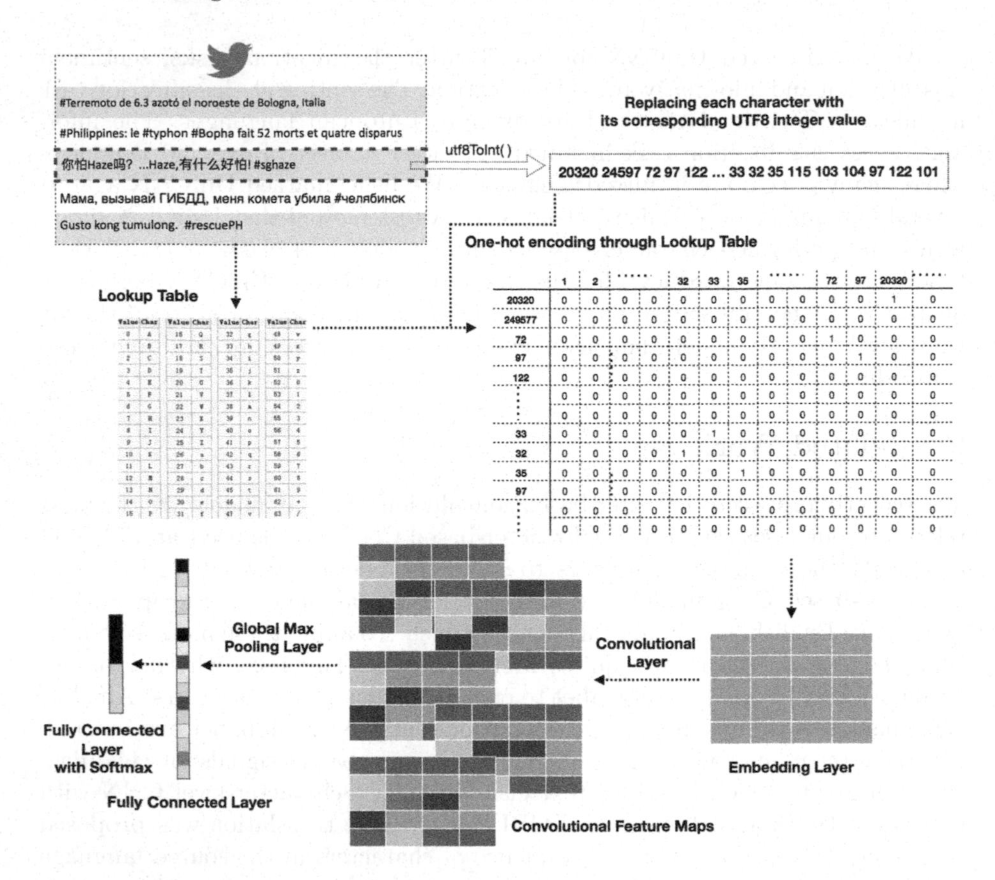

Fig. 1. The Complete Structure of UniCNN (A lookup table is built firstly on whole dataset, and each character will be transformed into a sequence of UTF-8 integers and then mapped into a one-hot vector, and followed by a matrix multiplication with the embedding matrix. Embeddings of each character will be concatenated as a matrix passed into a convolutional neural network.)

neural model has been proposed by [26], which is able to learn distributed document representations in Chinese and English. Gillick et al. [10] described a LSTM-based model that can read text as bytes rather than characters or words. Their model is much more compact than word-based models, which can be used in Part-of-Speech tagging and Named Entity Recognition in multilingual environment without using a string tokenizer.

With traditional classification models based on feature engineering, to build multilingual or cross lingual models, a typical method requires translation of texts from low-resourced languages into a rich-resourced language, usually English [2,6], or building a parallel corpus that builds a bridge between languages. Other methods focus on creating language independent features or language independent models. The method proposed by work [18] uses Naïve Bayes as the classifier and n-gram as features, which is mainly designed for languages that use spaces as word separators.

Table 1. Examples of characters and their numerical UTF-8 codes

!	*	+	2	9	<	?	@	A	H	Q	a	h
33	42	43	50	57	60	63	64	65	72	81	97	104

3 UniCNN: Unicode UTF-8 Encoded Character-Based CNN

We aim for a fully language-independent Twitter classification mode. Towards this objective, we need to address two research questions:

1. Is there a fully language independent approach that does not require identification of languages to encode characters for text classification neural models?
2. Is there an efficient character-based CNN structure that suits the language-independent alphabet that potentially contain a wide range of characters?

Figure 1 depicts our proposed UniCNN model. The model comprises two parts: first the scheme for encoding characters with UTF-8 codes to address the first research question and then the CNN structure to address the second research question.

3.1 Character Embedding with UTF-8 Codes

The Unicode standard is a character coding system designed to encode texts in different languages. It currently has an alphabet of 136,755 characters catering for 139 written languages on the earth. Unicode currently has three major different forms, namely UTF-8, UTF-16 and UTF-32 (UTF-8 stands for Unicode Transformation Format - 8-bit). In our work, we use UTF-8, since Twitter only accepts UTF-8 encoded text and all other encodings must be converted to UTF-8.[2] Additionally, since 2010, UTF-8 has become the dominant unicode format on the web.[3] UTF-8 uses one to four bytes for encoding characters. English uses one byte and actually the first 128 characters of UTF-8 has a one-to-one correspondence with ASCII, which contains not only English characters but also punctuations and numbers. Other languages use two or three bytes, such as Arabic, Chinese and Japanese. In our model, we use the corresponded decimal value of each character as the unit of input representation instead of characters themselves. Table 1 shows some examples of characters with their corresponding numerical values in UTF-8.

In our work, each character is represented by its numerical value in UTF-8, which transforms a sentence or tweet to a vector of n numerical values (n is the number of characters in a sentence or tweet). In Fig. 2, this character cloud is generated on dataset CrisisLexT26 [19], more details about dataset will be discussed in experiment part. As you see, the character diversity in this tweets corpus is beyond the imagination. The traditional character-based convolutional

[2] https://dev.twitter.com/basics/counting-characters.
[3] http://www.utf-8.com.

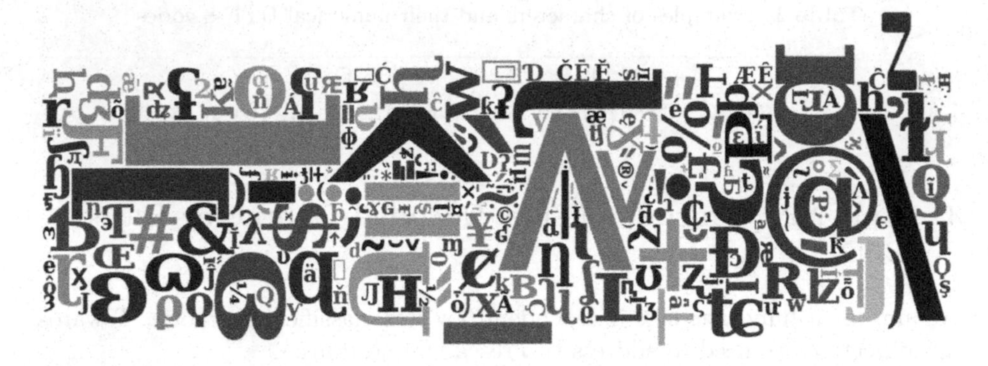

Fig. 2. Character Cloud generated on experiment dataset CrisisLexT26 (The number of characters and character diversity are beyond imagination. However, each character in this figure can be mapped into an integer value by UTF-8 encoding.)

neural network will filter out most of them when we have a pre-defined alphabet. However, with the assistance of UTF-8 encoding, unexpected character will be easily handled. Another advantage of this input transformation is that it does not require a step of building an alphabet, since it uses the whole set of UTF-8 characters as the alphabet. By applying UTF-8 encoding, each character is replaced by its UTF-8 integer value, and then a sentence can be simply transformed to a sequence of numerical values regardless of how they separate words and what written languages are.

Before approaching to the embedding layer, a lookup table is built firstly based on the whole dataset. After a tweet has been transformed into a sequence of numbers by using UTF-8 encoding, this sequence is mapped into one-hot vector through the lookup table and then passed to the embedding layer. The embedding layer learns the distributed character representation. In this layer, each one-hot encoding does matrix multiplication with an embedding matrix $W \in \mathbb{R}^{v \times d}$ (v is the number of unique characters in the dataset, and d is the embedding dimensionality), and the result are concatenated as a matrix, see

Table 2. The dataset statistics

Classification	Dataset	# Tweets	Positive	Negative
Sentiment	English	31,151	16,582	14,569
	German	29,570	17,269	12,301
	Polish	89,389	53,324	36,065
	Slovak	35,987	24,367	11,620
	Slovenian	42,264	20,325	21,939
	Swedish	21,739	9,313	12,426
Informativeness	CrisisLexT26 (40+ languages)	27,968	16,841	11,127

Fig. 1. The embedding weights will be randomly initialized at the beginning and trained in the neural network with the respect to the loss function. Additionally, a *dropout* is applied after the embedding layer to reduce the over-fitting of character embeddings [8].

3.2 Convoluitonal Neural Network

In our work, we use the traditional architecture of convolutional neural network which is convolution-and-pooling, with slight modifications, see Fig. 1. It is commonly believed that the convolution-and-pooling architecture can capture local aspects that can be used for prediction tasks [11]. In terms of pooling layer, we choose global max pooling which returns the largest value in a convolutional feature map. For a given input $x \in \mathbb{R}^{d_{in}}$, the output of convolutional layer is given by $p_i = g(x_i W + b)$. $b \in \mathbb{R}^{d_{out}}$ is the bias, and $W \in \mathbb{R}^{d_{in} \times d_{out}}$ is a matrix of weights. After convolution-and-pooling layers, there are two fully connected layers. The non-linearity function g we use a rectified linear unit (ReLU), and the regularization method in our model uses the most popular one *dropout*. The results of many experiments show that the combination of *ReLU* and *dropout* performs very well [11]. The final fully connected layer produces output transformed by the *softmax* function. Finally, the loss function of our model uses cross-entropy loss $\sum_i y_i log(\hat{y}_i)$ (y_i is the true distribution, while $\hat{y}_i$ is the predicted distribution) and the training optimizer we use Adam [15].

Character-based neural network is believed to capture the similarities of subwords, such as "cats" and "cat", compared with word-based models [23]. The idea of character-based model is to obtain word representations or character representations from the character composition [14]. So, we take the advantages of character-based convolutional neural networks, and add Unicode encoding part so as to bypass the burden of language translation and achieve the real language-independence.

4 Experiments

We evaluated our model on two Twitter classification tasks: Twitter sentiment classification and informativeness classification. The following section will introduce the dataset used for each task, data preprocessing and then evaluation.

4.1 Dataset and Preprocessing

For Twitter sentiment classification, we use human annotated Twitter corpora from [17]. This dataset has 1.6 million annotated tweets in 13 European languages, which might be the largest Twitter sentiment collection at the moment. In our work, we pick tweets in 6 languages from these corpora, namely English, Polish, German, Slovak, Slovenian and Swedish, since these subsets have acceptable self-agreement and inter-agreement rate [17] (the self-agreement is the agreement for multiple annotations by the same annotator, the inter-agreement is the

	Informative	Non-informative
	Forte terremoto de magnitude 7,9 atinge a Costa Rica: ~http	Мама, вызывай ГИБДД, меня комета убила #челябинск
T	Strong earthquake of magnitude 7.9 hits Costa Rica: ~http	Mom, call traffic police, I killed a comet #Chelyabinsk
	#Terremoto de 6.3 azotó el noroeste de Bologna, Italia	你怕Haze吗? ...Haze,有什么好怕! #sghaze
T	#Terremoto 6.3 earthquake struck northwest of Bologna, Italy	Are you afraid of Haze? ... Haze, what is so afraid #sghaze
	#Philippines: le #typhon #Bopha fait 52 morts et quatre disparus	Gusto kong tumulong. #rescuePH
T	#Philippines: #typhon #Bopha has 52 dead and four missing	I want to help. #rescuePH

Fig. 3. Examples of informative and non-informative tweets with their translation. (Row highlighted with T is the translation.)

agreement for multiple annotations by different annotators). The high value of both self-agreement and inter-agreement rate means high quality of the annotated work. The basic statistics of the used sentiment dataset are given in Table 2. At the step of data pre-processing, we removed hashtags, URLs and user mentions, since these elements are noisy characters when applying character-based convolutional neural networks.

For Twitter informativeness classification, we used CrisisLexT26 [19]. This dataset contains 27,933 tweets related to 26 crisis events that happened between 2012 and 2013. The number of languages in this dataset is more than 40 languages, such as Russian, Chinese, Japanese, English, Spanish and so on. In terms of informativeness classification, tweets are labelled as "Related and Informative", "Related and not informative", "Not Related" and "Not applicable". For clarity, we mapped the problem into a binary classification problem, where the "Related and Informative" class is the "Informative" class and the rest is the "Uninformative" class, see Fig. 3 for examples. At step of data pre-processing, instead of discarding noise, such as hashtags, URLs and user mentions, we decided to replace all hashtags with the string "#hashtag", all user mentions with the string "@user" and all URLs with "url".

4.2 Experiment Setup

Each dataset is randomly divided into two parts, and 80% is used for training and 20% for testing. We evaluate the accuracy of classification models.

The parameter settings for CNN are as follows: For hyper-parameters settings of convolutional neural network and embedding layer, we performed a grid search by investigating the flowing values: number of filters $\in \{256, 512, 1024, 2048\}$, dropout rate $\in \{0.2, 0.3, 0.4, 0.5\}$, character embedding dimensions $\in \{50, 100, 150\}$. Based on experiment results on English sentiment dataset, we decided to use 1024 filters for first convolutional layer, 2048 filters for second convolutional layer, 0.4 and 0.2 as the dropout rate for the dropout layer after the embedding layer and the dropout layer after two convolutional layers respectively. The dimensions of character embedding has been set to 100. All neural models are programmed using a

Python deep learning library Keras [3] with Tensorflow [1] as the backend, and each model is trained on a single GTX 1080TI with 11 GB RAM.

We compare UniCNN against the following baselines:

- SVM_Unigram and SVM_Bigram. In our work, we apply word-based n-grams. Specifically, we choose unigrams (1-word) and bigrams (2-words). The classifier we use Support Vector Machine (SVM) with a linear kernel. The data representation is Frequency-Inverse Document Frequency (TF-IDF), which is a well-known weighting scheme in NLP. We name the approaches as *SVM_Unigram* and *SVM_Bigram* separately.
- Translation-based Neural Models. Apparently, we need to translate all tweets from source languages into a target language, which is English in this case. The translation work is completed by using Google cloud translation API. In our work, there are two translation-based models, namely TransCNN(word) and TransCNN(char) for both experiments. *TransCNN(word):* uses our standard convolutional neural network as the classifier, but with Glove2Vec [20] as the input representation, which are pre-trained word vectors. Pre-trained Glove2Vec has several different versions, such as vectors trained on Wikipedia data or vectors trained on tweets. In our experiment, we use the word vectors that were trained on 2 billion tweets, which has 27 billion tokens (or words). Additionally, when training the neural model, word vectors are left to be trainable. *TransCNN(char):* also uses our standard convolutional neural network, but the input representation uses one-hot vector of each character, which is different from former model. The alphabet for one-hot encoding contains 94 characters, the list is given below.

  ```
  0123456789abcdefghijklmnopqrstuvwxyzABCDEFGHIJK
  LMNOPQRSTUVWXYZ<=>?@:;!\"#$%&'()*+,-./ []^_`\\{|}~
  ```

  Additionally, it also uses our standard embedding layer, which uses the randomly initialized weights that will be trained with the respect to loss function.

4.3 Results

In this section we report and analyze the results of all models listed in Table 3. Not only the experiment results of our UniCNN are compared with the other four models, but also comparison between translation-based models and comparison between n-gram based models and neural models. We also applied the Wilcoxon signed-rank test [22]. The Wilcoxon signed-rank test p-value of our UniCNN with the other four approaches are also shown in Table 3.

UniCNN vs. Other Models. In terms of classification accuracy, Table 3 shows that UniCNN is better than TransCNN(char), the translation-based character CNN, and SVM_Unigram and SVM_Bigram, the traditional SVM models using unigram and bigram features. UniCNN has comparable accuracy with Trans_CNN(word), the translation-based word-embedding CNN model. The superior performance of UniCNN over TransCNN(char) can be attributed to

Table 3. The Accuracy of UniCNN versus the other approaches

	UniCNN	TransCNN(char)	TransCNN(word)	SVM_Unigram	SVM_Bigram
Translation	No	Yes	Yes	No	No
Tokenization	No	No	Yes	Yes	Yes
Sentiment Classification					
English	0.7794	0.7825	**0.7957**	0.7623	0.6049
German	**0.7577**	0.7274	0.7367	0.7291	0.6031
Polish	**0.7908**	0.7682	0.7324	0.7220	0.6251
Slovak	0.7545	0.7309	0.7260	**0.7628**	0.7035
Slovenian	**0.7659**	0.7379	0.7623	0.7438	0.5752
Swedish	**0.7752**	0.7432	0.7218	0.7403	0.6178
Informativeness Classification					
CrisisLexT26	0.8418	0.8345	**0.8503**	0.8412	0.7937
p-value	-	0.0313	0.1563	0.0469	0.0156

the limitation enforced by translation, and that over the SVM models shows the power of deep features extracted from CNN. The reason why UniCNN has comparable performance with TransCNN(word) can be explained by the semantic structure representation brought by the word vectors.

On the other hand, it should be noted that UniCNN is a fully language-independent model that does not require translation or tokenization. In contrast, all other models require some form of translation or tokenization, which incurs extra computation.

N-Grams vs. Neural Models. In general, all translation-based neural models and our UniCNN performs better than N-gram based models in most experiments, but SVM_Unigram can still achieve accepted results. Especially in informativeness task, SVM_Unigram is pretty comparable with the state-of-art model, convolutional neural network with pre-trained word vectors, and our UniCNN. However, it must be noted that the CrisisLexT26 has been translated into English before applying n-gram models. Unlike sentiment dataset which are using space as the word separator, instead, CrisisLexT26 is a language mixed dataset whose languages are different in structure, such as English and Chinese. In sentiment tasks, the result of SVM_Unigram is not much worse than neural models, even achieved the highest accuracy in Slovak sentiment task. However, the results of SVM_Bigram are much lower than those of other models in almost all tasks. In addition, using GPU and Tensorflow really facilitates the training procedure of neural network. The whole training process takes about a few minutes for each neural model, while N-gram based models takes more than an hour even several hours depend on the data size.

TransCNN(word) vs. UniCNN. Using pre-trained word vectors as the input and re-train them in neural models has been widely adopted in many NLP tasks, and is currently the state-of-art technique for NLP classification tasks. In our experiment, the result is consistent with current trend. In English sentiment task, TransCNN(word) has achieved the highest accuracy 0.7957, while our UniCNN achieved 0.7794. However, when other languages are translated into English, the results of TransCNN(word) are much lower than results of our UniCNN. For example, in Polish sentiment task, the accuracy of our UniCNN is 0.7908 which is 0.05 more than the accuracy of TransCNN(word) (0.7324). Actually, our UniCNN outperformed all baselines in sentiment tasks apart from English sentiment task, which indicates that when there is not a pre-trained word vectors available in the source language, using UniCNN is more likely to achieve better results than using translated texts with the state-of-art model. On the other hand, since pre-trained word vectors are trained on a large dataset in an unsupervised manner for learning semantic meaning of words, using pre-trained word vectors can be an effective way to improve accuracy of various NLP classification tasks.

TransCNN(char) vs. UniCNN. Both are character-based neural models, but with differences in input and alphabet. The first difference is that the input text is the translated tweets for TransCNN(char), while for UniCNN the input are the tweets in source language. The second difference is that TransCNN(char) has a pre-defined alphabet of characters, while UniCNN does not. Generally, our UniCNN outperforms TransCNN(char) across all tasks except the English sentiment task. It is mainly because the English sentiment dataset is not a translated dataset. Therefore, using UniCNN is more likely to achieve better results than TransCNN(char), when translation is needed.

TransCNN(word) vs. TransCNN(char). Both are translation-based models, but TransCNN(word) is a word-based neural model, while TransCNN(char) is a character-based neural model. The results of these two translation-based neural models are not constant. In English, German and Slovenian sentiment tasks, TransCNN(word) slightly outperformed TransCNN(char), while TransCNN(char) performed better in the rest three sentiment tasks. It is uncertain why the result of word-based model and character-based model is not constant. But we can conclude that with translated text as the training and testing dataset, there are not much differences between word-based convolutional neural model and character-based convolutional neural model.

For the informativeness task, the experiment result of all these models except SVM_bigram are pretty close. In terms of resource consumption, our UniCNN is clearly the winner, since it is translation free. Translation-based models require much higher consumption in time and money. The cost of Google Translation API is $20 per million characters and translation speed is roughly two tweets per second. In contrast, our UniCNN is much faster and requires zero cost.

5 Conclusion

In this paper, we proposed a character-based convolutional neural network with Unicode UTF-8 encoding for language independent classification. Our proposal of UTF-8 character encoding does not require language identification and therefore is a fully language independent approach. Furthermore the character-based convolutional neural network on learning distributed character representations leads to promising classification accuracy. In this work, we focused on short text classification (tweets), and have tested our method on two Twitter classification tasks. Experiments showed that our method is fully language independent. Most importantly, our UniCNN model is the first neural model that can work with tweets written in mixed languages. Lastly, our model does not need language knowledge to pre-define an alphabet. In our future work, we are planning to work on designing neural network structure and objective function so that a neural model can learn both semantic and sentiment meaning in multilingual environments.

References

1. TensorFlow: large-scale machine learning on heterogeneous systems (2015). http://tensorow.org/
2. Bel, N., Koster, C.H.A., Villegas, M.: Cross-lingual text categorization. In: Koch, T., Sølvberg, I.T. (eds.) ECDL 2003. LNCS, vol. 2769, pp. 126–139. Springer, Heidelberg (2003). doi:10.1007/978-3-540-45175-4_13
3. Chollet, F., et al.: Keras. (2015). https://github.com/fchollet/keras
4. Conneau, A., Schwenk, H., Barrault, L., Lecun, Y.: Very deep convolutional networks for text classification. In: EACL (2017)
5. Cui, L., Zhang, X., Qin, A., Sellis, T., Wu, L.: CDS: collaborative distant supervision for Twitter account classification. Exp. Syst. Appl. **83**, 94–103 (2017)
6. Denecke, K.: Using SentiWordNet for multilingual sentiment analysis. In: ICDEW. IEEE (2008)
7. Dos Santos, C.N., Gatti, M.: Deep convolutional neural networks for sentiment analysis of short texts. In: COLING (2014)
8. Gal, Y., Ghahramani, Z.: A theoretically grounded application of dropout in recurrent neural networks. In: NIPS (2016)
9. Giachanou, A., Crestani, F.: Like it or not: a survey of Twitter sentiment analysis methods. ACM Comput. Surv. (CSUR) **49**, 1–41 (2016)
10. Gillick, D., Brunk, C., Vinyals, O., Subramanya, A.: Multilingual language processing from bytes. arXiv preprint arXiv:1512.00103 (2015)
11. Goldberg, Y.: A primer on neural network models for natural language processing. J. Artif. Intell. Res. **57**, 345–420 (2016)
12. Johnson, R., Zhang, T.: Effective use of word order for text categorization with convolutional neural networks. arXiv preprint arXiv:1412.1058 (2014)
13. Kim, Y.: Convolutional neural networks for sentence classification. In: EMNLP (2014)
14. Kim, Y., Jernite, Y., Sontag, D., Rush, A.M.: Character-aware neural language models. In: AAAI (2016)
15. Kingma, D., Ba, J.: Adam: A method for stochastic optimization. In: ICLR (2015)

16. Lee, J., Cho, K., Hofmann, T.: Fully character-level neural machine translation without explicit segmentation. In: TACL (2017)
17. Mozetič, I., Grčar, M., Smailović, J.: Multilingual Twitter sentiment classification: the role of human annotators. PloS ONE **11**, e0155036 (2016)
18. Narr, S., Hulfenhaus, M., Albayrak, S.: Language-independent Twitter sentiment analysis. In: KDML (2012)
19. Olteanu, A., Vieweg, S., Castillo, C.: What to expect when the unexpected happens: social media communications across crises. In: CSCW. ACM (2015)
20. Pennington, J., Socher, R., Manning, C.D.: Glove: global vectors for word representation. In: EMNLP (2014)
21. Wehrmann, J., Becker, W., Cagnini, H.E., Barros, R.C.: A character-based convolutional neural network for language-agnostic Twitter sentiment analysis. In: IJCNN. IEEE (2017)
22. Wilcoxon, F.: Individual comparisons by ranking methods. Biometrics Bull. **1**, 80–83 (1945)
23. Yang, Z., Dhingra, B., Yuan, Y., Hu, J., Cohen, W.W., Salakhutdinov, R.: Words or characters? Fine-grained gating for reading comprehension. In: ICLR (2017)
24. Yang, Z., Salakhutdinov, R., Cohen, W.: Multi-task cross-lingual sequence tagging from scratch. arXiv preprint arXiv:1603.06270 (2016)
25. Zhang, X., Zhao, J., LeCun, Y.: Character-level convolutional networks for text classification. In: NIPS (2015)
26. Zhou, X., Wan, X., Xiao, J.: Attention-based LSTM network for cross-lingual sentiment classification. In: EMNLP (2016)

Behavior Modeling and User Profiling

Modeling Check-In Behavior with Geographical Neighborhood Influence of Venues

Thanh-Nam Doan(✉) and Ee-Peng Lim

School of Information Systems, Singapore Management University, Singapore, Singapore
{tndoan.2012,eplim}@smu.edu.sg

Abstract. With many users adopting location-based social networks (LBSNs) to share their daily activities, LBSNs become a gold mine for researchers to study human check-in behavior. Modeling such behavior can benefit many useful applications such as urban planning and location-aware recommender systems. Unlike previous studies [4,6,12,17] that focus on the effect of distance on users checking in venues, we consider two venue-specific effects of geographical neighborhood influence, namely, *spatial homophily* and *neighborhood competition*. The former refers to the fact that venues share more common features with their spatial neighbors, while the latter captures the rivalry of a venue and its nearby neighbors in order to gain visitation from users. In this paper, through an extensive empirical study, we show that these two geographical effects, together with *social homophily*, play significant roles in understanding users' check-in behaviors. From the observation, we then propose to model users' check-in behavior by incorporating these effects into a matrix factorization-based framework. To evaluate our proposed models, we conduct check-in prediction task and show that our models outperform the baselines. Furthermore, we discover that *neighborhood competition* effect has more impact to the users' check-in behavior than *spatial homophily*. To the best of our knowledge, this is the first study that quantitatively examine the two effects of geographical neighborhood influence on users' check-in behavior.

1 Introduction

Motivation. The popularity of smartphones and wearable devices in recent years has helped to create new location based social networking applications for users to publish their visits (or check-ins) to different venues. For example, Foursquare is used by 50 millions users each month and it covers more than 65 million venues around the world with 8 billion check-ins worldwide[1]. By analyzing these check-in data, we can reveal the behavior of user visitation. Then,

This research is supported by the National Research Foundation, Prime Minister's Office, Singapore under its International Research Centres in Singapore Funding Initiative.

[1] https://foursquare.com/about.

G. Cong et al. (Eds.): ADMA 2017, LNAI 10604, pp. 429–444, 2017.
https://doi.org/10.1007/978-3-319-69179-4_30

one may derive useful insights for urban planning, business recommendation and other applications [27].

The behavior of user visitation in LBSN is a complex outcome of multiple effects. For example, *distance effect* [6,23] says that users want to visit venues near their home locations while *social homophily* [3,9] states that a user's choice of venues is partially under the influence of her friends.

Research Objectives. In this paper, we study the geographical neighborhood influence of venues. Specifically, we focus on *spatial homophily* and *neighborhood competition* effects. We analyze and model them in check-in behavior data. *Spatial homophily* says that venues and other nearby ones share more common user visitation patterns than venues far away. *Neighborhood competition* suggests that a venue competes with its neighbors so as to earn check-ins from users. Since the visitation behavior of users are the mixture of multiple effects, understanding the geographical neighborhood influence provides an additional dimension to reveal the properties of users' movement. Despite of their crucial roles, these two effects have not been well studied in previous works. Quantifying the effects' contribution to geographical neighborhood influence is therefore potentially useful for disclosing the visitation behavior of users.

Learning *spatial homophily* and *neighborhood competition* effects from check-in data gives rise to several useful applications. These two effects are essential for businesses to decide their new store locations as models incorporating them can more accurately predict venues to be visited by users. Latent variables associated with these effects also provide useful insights about users and venues which in turn help marketing teams to enhance advertising strategies to attract more customers to stores or shopping locations. We further improve the models by including *social homophily*.

There are however several research challenges in studying *spatial homophily* and *neighborhood competition*. Firstly, it is not easy to illustrate the impacts of these two effects using real datasets so special empirical data analyses are required. Secondly, the check-in's from users to venues are the results of multiple user and venue factors interacting with one another. Exactly how the interaction takes place is still an open research question. The challenge is therefore to create some generative stories to describe this interaction. Finally, there is no obvious ground truth in real datasets for evaluation of proposed models. We will need to adopt an indirect approach to conduct model evaluation.

To overcome the above challenges, we carry out the research as follows:

- We carefully gather Foursquare check-in data of users and venues from two cities, Singapore and Jakarta. To study the effects of *spatial homophily* and *neighborhood competition*, we determine the exact home locations of a subset of users through some stringent criteria. This gives us reliable datasets to embark on this research.
- We conduct an empirical analysis of the check-in data and demonstrate the existence of *spatial homophily* and *neighborhood competition* effects. The presence of *social homophily* is also demonstrated in our analysis.

- We extend matrix factorization to model the check-in behavior of users incorporating *spatial homophily* and *neighborhood competition* effects. Moreover, we also provide multiple options to model these two effects. Our proposed models are further enhanced by incorporating *social homophily* effects.
- The performance of our methods is evaluated on real datasets so as to demonstrate its superior accuracy. In our experiments, we show that our proposed models outperform the baselines with reasonable results in check-in prediction task. We also found that the number of neighbors of a venue does not affect the performance of our models much in a dense dataset but in a sparse one, it is the factor that we need to consider. Moreover, we discover that in geographical neighborhood influence, *neighborhood competition* contributes more than *spatial homophily* to users' check-in prediction. To the best of our knowledge, this is the first work which weighs these two effects in LBSNs.

Paper Outline. The remainder of the paper is organized as follows. Section 2 covers the literature review of previous works related to our research. Section 3 shows the data science aspect of our works to study check-in related factors. Section 4 describes the preliminary of matrix factorization and our proposed models. Sections 5 shows their performance on real datasets. Lastly, Sect. 6 concludes the paper and suggests some future works.

2 Related Works

Influence of Multiple Effects. The visitation of users to venues occurs under the influence of multiple effects [4,7,12,17]. In this section, we only focus on surveying previous research works on *Spatial Homophily*, *Neighborhood Competition* and *Social Homophily* effects.

Spatial Homophily: It is the effect that a venue is more similar to its nearby venues rather than further away ones. Liu et al. [21] studied Gowalla dataset and underscored the crucial impact of regional information in check-in prediction in LBSNs. Hu et al. [11] analyzed spatial homophily using Yelp data and then applied matrix factorization framework to predict the ratings of users to venues. Doan et al. [6] used spatial homophily of venues as features to predict the visitation between users and venues in LBSNs.

Neighborhood Competition: Venues compete with their neighbors to attract users' visitation. Liu et al. [19] used the competition effect in their model through the popularity score of each venue which represents the competitiveness of a venue in its neighborhood. Then, the authors embed this feature into the combination of *Latent Dirichlet Allocation* model [1] and *Bayesian Non-negative Matrix Factorization* [26] to study latent factors of users and venues. In [5], PageRank model has been adapted to measure the competitiveness of venues by deriving transition probabilities among venues. Doan et al. [7] provided the first neighborhood competition evidence via real datasets. Moreover, they showed that using the effect could improve the performance of check-in prediction task and home prediction task.

Table 1. Dataset statistics

	SG	H_SG	JK	H_JK
# users	55,891	856	14,974	455
# venues	75,346	12,020	38,183	4,380
# check-in's	1.11M	63,777	119,618	9,557
# user-venue pairs with > 0 check-ins	541,588	28,298	81,188	5,422

Social Homophily: Social homophily is widely used in LBSN to understand users' check-in behavior [9,17,25]. The work in [6] derived features based on this effect to predict number of check-ins between users and venues. Cheng et al. [3] captured this effect using a regularizer to penalize the difference between users and their friends. Cho et al. [4] extended their periodic mobility model by considering the influence of users' friends. Their results concluded that using *social homophily* could more accurately predict users' movement behavior.

Matrix Factorization for Check-In Prediction. Matrix factorization methods [14,22] is one of the most widely adopted techniques to predict the number check-ins between users and venues in LBSNs [11,16,18,21]. Cheng et al. [3] first extended classical matrix factorization for check-in prediction by adding regularization to model friendship network. Li et al. [15] illustrated the importance of *social friends*, *neighboring friends* and *location friends* and used them to study users' movement in LBSNs under matrix factorization framework. Gao et al. [8] introduced tensor factorization to model check-in behavior involving timestamps. Liu et al. [20] learned the topic preferences of users using LDA [1] and used the learnt topics in matrix factorization to predict check-ins between users and venues.

Unlike the above works, this paper considers the spatial homophily of venues and neighborhood competition in the design of our proposed matrix factorization models. Moreover, our models are also extended to include social homophily.

3 Data Exploration

3.1 Datasets

To study user check-in behavior and how it is affected by user and venue characteristics, we need to gather Foursquare datasets that capture complete check-in data of both users and venues. We thus crawled check-in data of users and venues from two populated Asian cities, Singapore and Jakarta.

SG Dataset. This dataset consists of 1.11 millions check-ins by 55,891 Singapore Foursquare users on 75,346 venues between August 2012 and June 2013 (see Table 1). The users and venues are determined to be located in Singapore based on their profile declared locations and venues' geo-locations respectively.

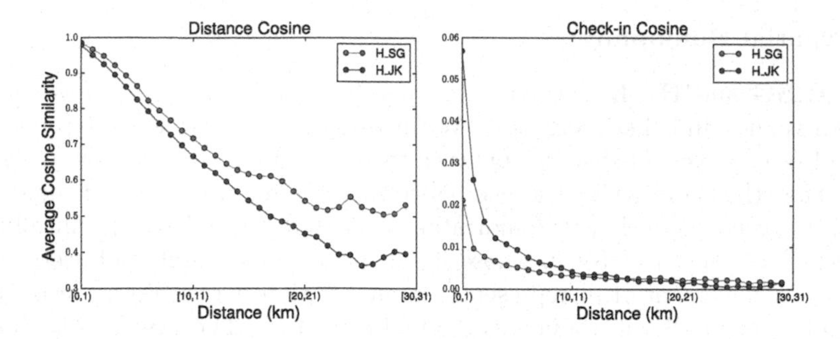

Fig. 1. Spatial homophily through cosine similarity of all venue pairs over their distance in **H_SG** and **H_JK**.

JK Dataset. Similarly, we crawled another Foursquare dataset for the users and venues in Jakarta the largest city in Indonesia from July 2014 to May 2015. There are 119,618 check-ins performed by 14,974 users on 38,183 venues. The numbers are generally smaller than those of **SG** dataset.

Users with Home Locations. Among the users in the **SG** (and **JK**) dataset, we identify a subset of users whose home locations can be determined using the method described in Sect. 3.2. We then construct another dataset to include users with home locations and the venues that they perform check-ins on. This leads us to the **H_SG** and **H_JK** datasets.

3.2 Home Location Identification

To understand the effect of users' decision on check-in venues, we selected a subset of users whose home locations can be clearly identified using both their check-ins and check-in messages as follows:

- We selected a subset of venues under the "home (private)" category which is a sub-category of the "residence" category. We found 8447 and 1985 venues satisfying this criteria in the **SG** and **JK** datasets respectively.
- We further identified 3276 and 891 users performing check-ins at only one "home (private)" venue each in the **SG** and **JK** datasets respectively. This rules out users who performed check-ins at multiple "home (private)" venues.
- We finally selected an even smaller set of users who also shouted some home relevant messages during their check-ins to their "home (private)" venues.

We finally had 856 users with exact home locations in the **SG** dataset. We denote the Foursquare dataset of these users and their check-in venues by **H_SG**. These users have 63,777 check-ins on 12,020 venues as shown in Table 1. In a similar way, we obtained the **H_JK** dataset.

3.3 Spatial Homophily

Using **H_SG** and **H_JK** datasets, we want to examine the *spatial homophily* between venues and their neighbors. We investigate the visitor overlap between a pair of venues over the distance between them to explore *spatial homophily*. We expect that the shorter the distance between two venues, the higher the visitor overlap between them. It is the indicator for *spatial homophily*. Specifically, for each venue j, it has a vector v_j whose size is equal to the number of users in the dataset. Each element of v_j represents the interaction between a corresponding user and venue j. We introduce two definitions of v_j. The first one is that v_j contains the number of check-ins of every user to venue j. The second one is that each element of v_j is the distance from the corresponding user to venue j.

Before calculating the *cosine similarity* between every pair of venues, we divide the distance of venue pairs into bins of width of one kilometer each. For example, the i-th bin covers distance range between $i-1$ and i km. We exclude all venue pairs whose distance between them is greater than 31 Km in both datasets due to the sparsity of such venue pairs. The average cosine similarity of all venue pairs whose distance within the bin is calculated and reported. The *cosine similarity* of a venue pair (j, k) is calculated by formula $\frac{(v_j \circ I^{jk}) \bullet (v_k \circ I^{jk})}{\|v_j \circ I^{jk}\| \|v_k \circ I^{jk}\|}$ where $\circ$ and $\bullet$ are Hadamard and inner products of vectors respectively. I^{jk} is the binary vector to indicate if a user makes check-ins to both venues j and k. Since we have two version of v_j, there are two corresponding *cosine similarities*: *distance cosine* and *check-in cosine*.

Figure 1 depicts the *cosine similarity* of all venue pairs for different distance bins of **H_SG** and **H_JK**, then we observe that: (i) the similarity between a pair of venues decreases if the distance between them increases, (ii) the trends are consistent regarding datasets or types of *cosine similarity* and (iii) despite of having the same trend, *distance cosine* and *check-in cosine* have different shapes. While the former is nearly linear, the latter one follows a log-series distribution. In our model, we will formalize *spatial homophily* by the two types of similarities.

3.4 Neighborhood Competition

To demonstrate the effect, we adopt the method originally proposed by Weng et al. [28] to study competition among memes. We divide the check-in history into weeks. We then measure the following entropies for each week.

- **System entropy (E_S):** $E_S(t) = -\sum_v f_v(t) \log f_v(t)$ where $f_v(t)$ is the fraction of check-ins in week t performed on venue v, i.e., $f_v(t) = \frac{\#cks(v,t)}{\sum_v \#cks(v,t)}$. The system entropy essentially measures the degree to which the distribution of check-ins concentrates on a small fraction of venues.
- **Average neighbor entropy (E_N):** We first define the entropy of the neighborhood N_j of venue j to be $E_j(t) = -\sum_{v \in N_j \cup \{j\}} f_{v,N_j}(t) \log f_{v,N_j}(t)$ and $f_{v,N_j}(t)$ is the ratio of the number of check-ins of v over the total check-ins of $N_j \cup \{j\}$ in week t. We then take the average of all neighborhood entropies,

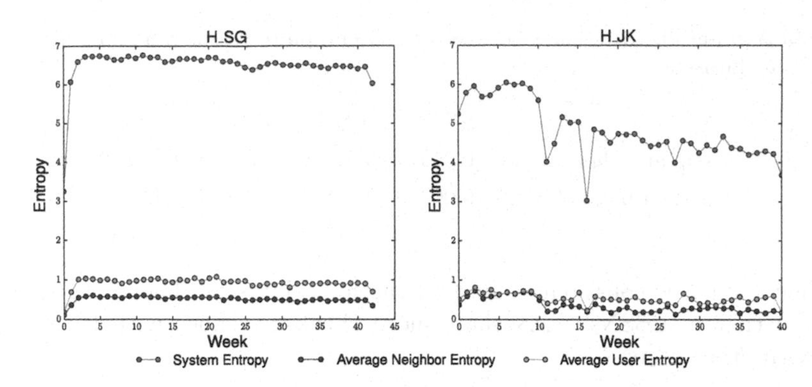

Fig. 2. Weekly entropies in **H_SG** and **H_JK** datasets.

i.e., $E_N(t) = Avg_j E_j(t)$. We choose N_j is the top-10 nearest neighbors of venue j. Similar to system entropy E_S, E_N captures the degree to which the distribution of check-ins of a neighborhood concentrates on one of its venues.

- **Average user entropy (E_U):** We next define the average user entropy as $E_U(t) = Avg_{u \in U} E_u(t)$ where entropy of user u is $E_u(t) = -\sum_v f_{u,v}(t) \log f_{u,v}(t)$ and $f_{u,v}(t) = \frac{\#cks(u,v,t)}{\#cks(u,t)}$. This entropy quantifies the concentration of users' attention on the venues they perform check-ins on.

Figure 2 shows the three entropies over weeks in both **H_SG** and **H_JK** datasets. The first important observation is that the value of E_U is much smaller than the value of E_S. It clearly suggests that each user's attention is limited to very small fraction of venues in the entire city. Venues therefore have to compete to gain attraction from users. Secondly, we observed from Fig. 2 that E_S is much larger than E_N in both datasets. This implies that the check-in distribution in the neighborhood of one venue and its neighbors is not as uniform as the one of the whole system. In other words, the neighbors of a venue create stronger competition than the further away ones. Therefore, modeling the competition between a venue and its neighbors is more reasonable than that between this venue and the whole system.

3.5 Social Homophily

Social homophily is the tendency that users and their friends share more common check-in venues than that between users and other ones. We illustrate the effect by calculating the average Jaccard similarity score of all pairs of users and their friends. Then, we compute the same score for equal number of random pairs of users. Specifically, each user u is represented by a set s_u containing all venues that u has visited and the Jaccard similarity of u and u' is $J(u, u') = \frac{|s_u \cap s_{u'}|}{|s_u \cup s_{u'}|}$.

Table 2 shows that the average Jaccard scores between users and their friends are significantly higher than that between random pairs of users. Moreover,

Table 2. Average Jaccard scores between user-friend pairs versus random pairs of users across four datasets.

	SG	H_SG	JK	H_JK
Users and their friends	0.01411	0.01818	0.00697	0.01812
Random pairs of users	0.00448	0.00867	0.00097	0.00085

the phenomenon is consistent across all the four datasets. Therefore, we could conclude that in LBSNs, users share more check-in venues with their friends than with other users.

4 Modeling Check-In Behavior

4.1 Preliminaries

Our proposed model is built upon matrix factorization technique [14]. In matrix factorization, the check-in count matrix is factorized into user-specific matrix and venue-specific matrix. Formally, we assume that $R \in \mathbb{R}^{m \times n}$ is the check-in count matrix where R_{ij} is the number of check-ins user i performs on venue j. R_{ij} is undefined when user i does not perform any check-ins on venue j. m and n are the number of users and number of venues respectively. We then factorize R into two matrices $U \in \mathbb{R}^{f \times m}$ and $V \in \mathbb{R}^{f \times n}$ which satisfy $R \approx U^T V$. Therefore, the predicted number of check-ins between any pair of user i and venue j is $\hat{R}_{ij} = U_i^T V_j$. According to Table 3, V_j represents the latent features or intrinsic characteristics of venue j such as quality, location of venue j while U_i is the vector of user i's preferences over these latent features.

Nevertheless, users have some biases when performing check-ins to venues. Some users are eager to perform check-ins generating many check-ins at each visited venue while others are selective generating zero or very few check-ins. Similarly, venues also have some degree of biases because of their locations or amounts of advertisement. Hence, we represent these biases as b_i and b_j which are incorporated into the model together with a global bias μ as shown below [13]:

$$\hat{R}_{ij} = \mu + b_i + b_j + U_i^T V_j \tag{1}$$

Learning the latent parameters is an optimization problem as follow:

$$\min_{U_*, V_*, b_*} \sum_{(i,j) \in \mathcal{K}} (R_{ij} - \hat{R}_{ij})^2 + \lambda_1(\|U_i\|^2 + \|V_j\|^2) + \lambda_2(b_i^2 + b_j^2)$$

where λ_1 and λ_2 are regularization parameters to avoid overfitting. To learn the parameters, stochastic gradient descent (SGD) [2] is usually adopted.

Geographical Neighborhood Matrix Factorization (N-MF). Hu et al. [11] incorporated geographical neighborhood influence defined by the average of extrinsic characteristics of neighbors. Formally, Eq. 1 becomes

$$\hat{R}_{ij} = \mu + b_i + b_j + U_i^T (V_j + \frac{\beta}{|N_j|} \sum_{k \in N_j} Q_k) \tag{2}$$

where N_j denotes the neighbors of venue j, and Q_k is the extrinsic characteristics of neighbor k. In this model, also known as Geographical Neighborhood Matrix Factorization (N-MF), the extrinsic characteristics Q_k of a venue k share the same dimension as its intrinsic characteristics V_k but the former is meant for characteristics noticeable by visitors. In this paper, we extend N-MF further to incorporate neighborhood competition.

4.2 Extended Neighborhood Matrix Factorization

In Sect. 3, we show that the check-ins of each venue are affected by *spatial homophily* and *neighborhood competition* effects. Hence, we propose *Extended Neighborhood Matrix Factorization (EN_MF)* model to include the two effects to check-in behavior. We extend Eq. 2 as follow:

$$\hat{R}_{ij} = \mu + b_i + b_j + U_i^T V_j + \frac{\beta}{|N_j|} \sum_{k \in N_j} G_{ijk} U_i^T Q_k \tag{3}$$

In *EN_MF*, we assume that the size of N_j is identical for any venue j. In Eq. 3, Q_k denotes the extrinsic characteristics of venue k which is a neighbor of venue j and its product with U_i contributes to the number of check-ins between user i and venue j. First of all, we need to explain that Q_j has the same number of latent dimensions as V_j. Each Q_{jt} element captures the ability of a venue j to bring check-ins from users interested in t-th latent factor to its neighbors. G_{ijk} denotes the neighborhood influence weight which is defined to be a combination of venue j winning over the neighboring venue k (*neighborhood competition*), and similarity with the neighboring venue k (*spatial homophily*) as user i chooses venue j over its neighbor k for check-ins. Formally, G_{ijk} is:

$$G_{ijk} = \alpha\sigma(U_i^T Q_j > U_i^T Q_k) + (1 - \alpha) sim(j, k) \tag{4}$$

The two parameters β ($\beta > 0$) and α ($\alpha \in [0, 1]$) in Eqs. 3 and 4 are:

- β controls the geographical neighborhood influence of neighboring venues.
- α is the tradeoff between spatial homophily and neighborhood competition.

$sim(j, k)$ in Eq. 4 measures the effect of *spatial homophily* of the neighbor k of venue j to the selection of venue j by users. By including $sim(j, k)$, our model covers the spatial homophily effect among venues. We explore $sim(j, k)$ function further by considering these following options to capture our observations in Sect. 3.3:

- *Check-in cosine similarity:* Cosine similarity between check-in counts of users of two venues j and k.
- *Distance cosine similarity:* Cosine similarity of distance of common users between venue j and venue k.

$\sigma(U_i^T Q_j > U_i^T Q_k)$ in Eq. 4 captures the competition between venue j and its neighbor k. The intuition behind is that from the perspective of user i, the

Table 3. Table of notations.

Notation	Meaning
N_j	Set of neighbors of venue j
$\mathcal{K}$	Set of user-venue pairs with known check-ins
F	Set of user-friend pairs
R_{ij}, $\hat{R}_{ij}$	Observed and predicted numbers of check-ins of user i to venue j, respectively
μ	Mean of all known R_{ij} check-ins
b_i, b_j	Biases of user i and venue j respectively
U_i	Latent vector of user i
V_j/Q_j	Intrinsic/Extrinsic characteristic vector of venue j
β	Parameter to control the effect of neighborhood venues
α	Relative weight between spatial homophily and neighborhood competition

extrinsic characteristics of venue j are ranked higher than those of its neighbor k. User i therefore selects venue j to visit instead of its neighbor k. In other words, user i prefers venue j over k by comparing the extrinsic characteristics of j and k. Function σ returns the probability that user i is more attracted to venue j than k. In this work, we consider two options for function σ:

- Sigmoid function: We adopt this option from the study of personal ranking using matrix factorization [24]. Formally, $\sigma(U_i^T Q_j > U_i^T Q_k) = \frac{1}{1+\exp(-(U_i^T Q_j - U_i^T Q_k))}$
- Cumulative density function of standard normal distribution (CDF): Similar to Sigmoid function, we use CDF to map the value of $U_i^T Q_j - U_i^T Q_k$ into the range $[0, 1]$.

Finally, our task is to learn the parameters U_*, V_*, Q_* and b_* through solving the following optimization problem by using gradient descent method [2]:

$$\min_{U_*,V_*,Q_*,b*} \sum_{(i,j)\in\mathcal{K}} (R_{ij} - \hat{R}_{ij})^2 + \lambda_1(\|U_i\|^2 + \|V_j\|^2) + \lambda_2(b_i^2 + b_j^2) + \lambda_3\|Q_j\|^2 \quad (5)$$

Note: The special thing is that our model is the generalization of *N-MF* model proposed by Hu et al. [11]. Specifically, if we set $\alpha = 0$ and the $sim(j, k) = 1$ for all venues j, k, then our model reduces to *N-MF* model (see Eq. 2).

Extension Incorporating Social Homophily (FEN_MF): Similar to [3], we model social homophily by adding a social regularizer $\lambda_f \sum_{(i,i')\in F} \|U_i - U_{i'}\|^2$ to Eq. 5. It says that if two users i and i' have social connection, their latent features U_i and $U_{i'}$ tend to have similar values and λ_f is the parameter to control the impact of social homophily.

5 Experiments

5.1 Experimental Setting

In this experiment, we evaluate the performance of our model using check-in prediction task.

Setup: We sort the check-ins of the **H_SG** and **H_JK** datasets in chronological order and divide each dataset into ten folds. For each run of experiment, we hide one fold as test set and use the remaining nine folds as training set.

We order check-ins of the **SG** and **JK** chronologically then divide the data into two parts: the first 80% is for training and the remaining 20% is for testing. There are no home location for all users in these datasets so to apply the *distance cosine similarity*, we approximate the home locations of users by deriving the centers of the mass from all check-in venues of the users.

Evaluation Metric: We adopt two popular error metrics, *Mean Absolute Error* (MAE) and *Root Mean Square Error* (RMSE). The smaller the value of MAE and RMSE, the more accurate the model is. In general, RMSE penalizes more on the large errors and less on smaller ones than MAE. Suppose T is the test set containing user-venue check-in pairs (i, j)'s, the two metrics are:

$$MAE = \frac{1}{|T|} \sum_{(i,j) \in T} |R_{ij} - \hat{R}_{ij}|; \; RMSE = \sqrt{\frac{1}{|T|} \sum_{(i,j) \in T} (R_{ij} - \hat{R}_{ij})^2} \quad (6)$$

We report the average MAE and $RMSE$ of all ten folds. For the case of reading, we use MAE and $RMSE$ to refer to average MAE and average $RMSE$ respectively henceforth.

Proposed Models: Our proposed models to be evaluated are:

- $EN\_MF^{DS}_{Sigmoid}$: In this model, *distance cosine similarity* is used for *spatial homophily* and the *Sigmoid function* is adopted for *neighborhood competition*.
- $EN\_MF^{CS}_{Sigmoid}$: This model uses *check-in cosine similarity* for *spatial homophily* and *Sigmoid function* for *neighborhood competition*.
- $EN\_MF^{DS}_{CDF}$: In this model, *distance cosine similarity* is adopted for *spatial homophily* and *CDF* is to model *neighborhood competition* effect.
- $EN\_MF^{CS}_{CDF}$: This model uses *check-in cosine similarity* and *CDF* to model *spatial homophily* and *neighborhood competition* respectively.

$FEN\_MF^{DS}_{Sigmoid}$, $FEN\_MF^{CS}_{Sigmoid}$, $FEN\_MF^{DS}_{CDF}$ and $FEN\_MF^{CS}_{CDF}$ are the extension of $EN\_MF^{DS}_{Sigmoid}$, $EN\_MF^{CS}_{Sigmoid}$, $EN\_MF^{DS}_{CDF}$ and $EN\_MF^{CS}_{CDF}$ respectively by adding social homophily.

Baselines: The baseline models are described below:

- *User Mean:* To predict the number of check-ins between a user and a venue, it outputs the average number of check-ins of this user performs to a venue.

- *Bias Matrix Factorization (B-MF)*: This matrix factorization model was proposed by Koren [13]. In this model, the biases of users and venues are considered and it is briefly mentioned in Sect. 4.1.
- *Neighborhood influence Matrix Factorization (N-MF)*: Hu et al. [11] proposed a model to incorporate only the effect of *spatial homophily*. It is the special case of our model (see Sect. 4.2).

Parameter Setting: We adopt a parameter setting similar to that of [11] for *EN_MF*, *FEN_MF* models and *N-MF* since it provides overall good performance for the baselines. That is, the number of latent factors is $f = 20$, and neighborhood importance is $\beta = 0.8$. The regularization parameters: $\lambda_1 = 0.8$, $\lambda_2 = 0.4$, $\lambda_3 = 0.6$ and $\lambda_f = 0.01$. The learning rate of SGD γ is assigned to 0.00001. Besides the above parameters, we also set $\alpha = 0.5$ to give equal weights to both: *spatial homophily* and *neighborhood competition* effects. For *EN_MF*, *FEN_MF* and *N-MF*, we consider the top 10 nearest venues as neighbors of a venue since it generates a good result across multiple variants (more details in later sections).

5.2 Experiment Results

We conduct the experiment to compare the performance of our proposed *EN_MF* and FEN_MF with several baselines. We then evaluate the impact of neighborhood size to the prediction accuracy of *EN_MF*. Next, we also tune parameter α to measure the contribution of *neighborhood competition* and *spatial homophily* to the prediction accuracy of *EN_MF*. We do not report the performance of FEN_MF on the last two experiments since its behavior is similar to EN_MF.

Check-In Prediction Task. The performance of all the four variants of EN_MF and FEN_MF as well as the baselines on the four datasets **SG**, **H_SG**, **JK** and **H_JK** are listed in Table 4.

Firstly, all four variants of EN_MF and FEN_MF perform better than the baselines. Specifically, FEN_MF could improve up to 13.49% in MAE and 16.8% in RMSE compared to the baselines. It suggests that incorporating *spatial homophily* and *neighborhood competition* as well as *social homophily* effectively reduce prediction errors. The performance is superior than baseline models that do not consider any effects (i.e. *User Mean*, *B-MF*) or the one (i.e. *N-MF*) that incorporates only the *spatial homophily* effect. We further apply hypothesis testing to examine if our improvements are significantly better than the baselines. Specifically, the *null hypothesis* is the performance of our methods and the baselines are not different while the *alternative hypothesis* is our methods are significantly better than the baselines. To achieve the goal, we apply the paired t-tests [10] to compare each variant of EN_MF and FEN_MF to *N-MF*. The population size in our tests is 10 (the number of folds in our experiment). Since the *p-values* of all tests are less than 0.05, we conclude that EN_MF and FEN_MF are significantly better than the baselines. Next, we also perform significant test to compare between each variant of EN_MF and the corresponding variant of FEN_MF. From the result of the test, we found that FEN_MF model variants significantly improve those of EN_MF.

Table 4. Performance of check-in prediction task. The best results are highlighted.

Method	H_SG		H_JK		SG		JK	
	MAE	RMSE	MAE	RMSE	MAE	RMSE	MAE	RMSE
User Mean	1.9621	17.2189	1.7530	12.7721	1.642	12.1344	1.0923	13.2112
B-MF	1.8122	15.2199	1.6892	11.2758	1.4812	11.4354	0.9873	12.8085
N-MF	1.7522	14.7212	1.4016	9.4293	1.4033	11.4266	0.9784	12.7491
$EN\_MF^{DS}_{Sigmoid}$	1.6974	14.3460	1.2475	9.2948	1.39	11.4156	0.9638	12.7005
$EN\_MF^{CS}_{Sigmoid}$	1.6975	14.3424	1.2471	9.2942	1.3872	11.4150	0.9624	12.7057
$EN\_MF^{DS}_{CDF}$	1.6965	14.3463	1.2475	9.2936	1.3899	11.4148	0.9635	12.7058
$EN\_MF^{CS}_{CDF}$	1.6964	14.3421	1.2469	9.2946	1.3873	11.4177	0.9628	12.7095
$FEN\_MF^{DS}_{Sigmoid}$	1.6957	14.3451	1.21795	**8.2367**	1.3890	11.4135	0.9633	12.6996
$FEN\_MF^{CS}_{Sigmoid}$	1.6942	14.342	1.2172	8.3744	1.3872	11.4147	**0.9624**	**12.6953**
$FEN\_MF^{DS}_{CDF}$	1.6959	14.346	1.2175	8.2832	1.3890	**11.4133**	0.9632	12.6970
$FEN\_MF^{CS}_{CDF}$	**1.6941**	**14.3417**	**1.2164**	8.2789	**1.3871**	11.4150	0.9625	12.6992

Secondly, Table 4 shows that $FEN\_MF^{CS}_{CDF}$ has the best overall performance on the **H_SG** and **H_JK** datasets. Recall that it uses *check-in cosine similarity* and *CDF* to model the effects of *spatial homophily* and *neighborhood competition* respectively. This model produces the lowest prediction errors in both datasets except the case of RMSE in **H_JK**. Hence, using *CDF* is more appropriate for modeling *neighborhood competition* than *Sigmoid function*. Similarly, characterizing *spatial homophily* by *check-in cosine similarity* is more accurate than using *distance cosine similarity*. For the large datasets **SG** and **JK**, it is hard to find the best model.

Thirdly, the MAE and RMSE errors in Table 4 are higher than those reported by Hu et al. [11] since they used Yelp dataset to evaluate prediction performance of *N-MF*. Specifically, *N-MF* predicts the ratings of users to venues and the ratings can obtain a discrete value from 1 to 5. In contrast, we apply *N-MF* and our models to predict the number of check-ins between users and venues and such number can be much larger than 5. Hence, the figures reported in Table 4 are significantly higher than the ones showed in [11].

Next, Table 4 shows that EN_MF performs better than *N-MF* by incorporating additional neighborhood effects. *User Mean* method does not cover any information of venues so its results are not better than that of *B-MF* which includes the interaction between users and venues. However, *N-MF* outperforms *B-MF* because it considers spatial homophily.

Lastly, social homophily can improve the prediction performance and this phenomenon happens across all variants. However, the improvement of using social homophily is small, consistent with the result reported in previous works [3].

Choice of Neighborhood Size. In our models, the neighbors of a venue are the top-n nearest neighbors of this venue. To measure the impact of n, we vary n to quantify the importance of neighborhood size to the prediction errors of all

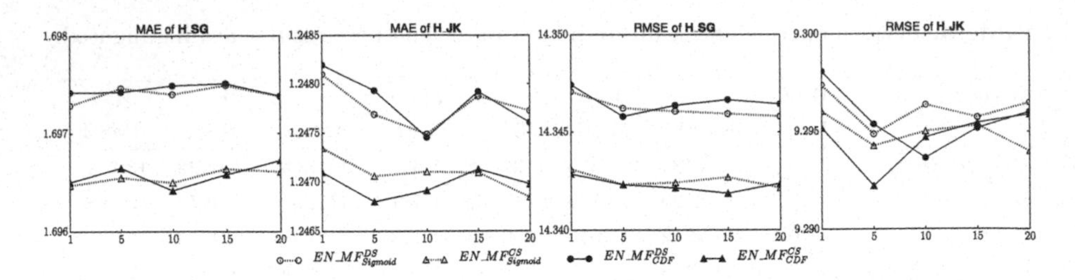

Fig. 3. Performance of variants of EN_MF with different numbers of neighbors.

variants of EN_MF. Figure 3 depicts the finding in both **H_SG** and **H_JK** datasets. For other parameters of *EN_MF*, we use their default values (see Sect. 5.1). There are three useful observations from Fig. 3.

First of all, in **H_SG**, the prediction errors of all variants of EN_MF are more stable than the ones of **H_JK** dataset and it is hard to observe the trending of our error metrics when n is varied for the dataset **H_SG**. Secondly, we can group the variants into two groups: *check-in* and *distance cosine similarity* groups since the first one usually has lower prediction errors than the other. This result is consistent on both the two datasets and both error metrics except in the case of RMSE in **H_JK**. It suggests that we should use *check-in cosine similarity* to model the *spatial homophily* of two venues to achieve smaller prediction errors. Thirdly, from **H_JK** dataset, we observe that three out of four variants of EN_MF achieve the lowest RMSE value at when number of neighbors of a venue is 5 while only $EN\_MF^{CS}_{CDF}$ obtains the lowest MAE at $n = 5$.

The reason behind the differences between **H_SG** and **H_JK** is the sparsity of **H_JK**. From Table 1, the number of venues of **H_JK** is one third of that of **H_SG**. Therefore, increasing the number of neighbors of a venue j is equal to the fact of considering more further away venues as neighbors of j. Consequently, it reduces the accuracy of EN_MF.

Hence, we could conclude that in datasets whose venues are dense (e.g. **H_SG**), the number of neighbors in our model does not affect the prediction performance as much as datasets whose venues are sparse (e.g. **H_JK**).

Spatial Homophily vs. Neighborhood Competition. The role of α in Eq. 3 is to control the impact of two effects: *spatial homophily* and *neighborhood competition*. Specifically, if $\alpha \rightarrow 0$, the effect of *neighborhood competition* is eliminated in EN_MF model. Otherwise (i.e. $\alpha \rightarrow 1$), the effect of *spatial homophily* is left out in EN_MF.

In this section, we want to quantify the influence of both effects. For that reason, we vary the value of α from 0.1 to 0.9 with step 0.1 and measure the prediction errors of EN_MF and its variants. We use the default values for other parameters during the experiment (see Sect. 5.1). As shown in Fig. 4, the prediction errors of all versions of EN_MF reduce when we increase α. The exceptions are the cases of $EN\_MF^{DS}_{Sigmoid}$ and $EN\_MF^{DS}_{CDF}$ on **H_SG** dataset. For example, the MAE and RMSE of these two models increase when α changes

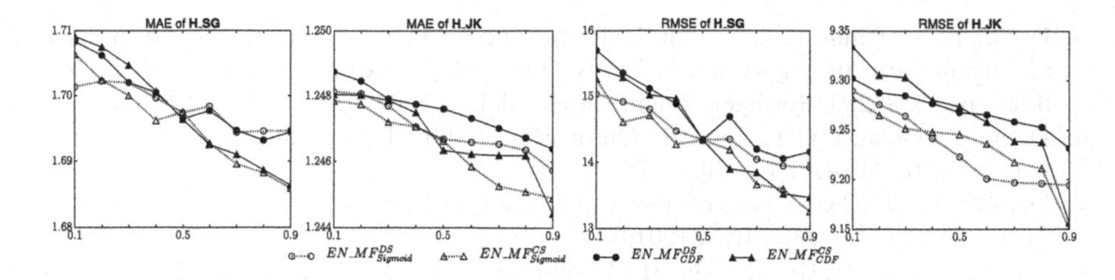

Fig. 4. Prediction errors of variants of EN_MF with different values of α.

from 0.5 to 0.6 but these errors drop when α increases to 0.7. However, the errors of $EN\_MF^{DS}_{Sigmoid}$ and $EN\_MF^{DS}_{CDF}$ decrease when we increase the value of α. Hence, in general, we could conclude that *spatial homophily* effect contributes less to the accuracy of check-in prediction than *neighborhood competition*. Despite this findings, the contribution of *spatial homophily* is not negligible because the worst performing in both datasets still perform better than the baselines. The other observation from Fig. 4 is that we cannot conclude which model has the best performance since there are no clear winner among them.

6 Conclusion and Future Works

In this paper, we have examined and modeled the geographical neighborhood influence of venues to users' check-in behavior by inspecting *spatial homophily* and *neighborhood competition* effects. Considering different options to characterize these effects give us the best setting to model such behavior. Moreover, we find out that *spatial homophily* is not as important as *neighborhood competition* on predicting the check-in behavior. Last but not least, *social homophily* helps our model to improve the accuracy of check-in prediction task.

There are several directions to extend this research further. In our model, we have not considered factors such as venue type, distance between venues and others that may affect the choices of venues to visit. Furthermore, we have not yet integrated temporal information as one may influence users' decision to visit venues. Thus, these interesting factors should be studied in the future especially to address data sparsity issues.

References

1. Blei, D.M., Ng, A.Y., Jordan, M.I.: Latent dirichlet allocation. J. Mach. Learn. Res. **3**, 993–1022 (2003)
2. Boyd, S., Vandenberghe, L.: Convex Optimization. Cambridge University Press, New York (2004)
3. Cheng, C., Yang, H., King, I., Lyu, M.R.: Fused matrix factorization with geographical and social influence in location-based social networks. In: AAAI (2012)
4. Cho, E., Myers, S.A., Leskovec, J.: Friendship and mobility: user movement in location-based social networks. In: KDD (2011)

5. Doan, T.-N., Chua, F.C.T., Lim, E.-P.: Mining business competitiveness from user visitation data. In: Agarwal, N., Xu, K., Osgood, N. (eds.) SBP 2015. LNCS, vol. 9021, pp. 283–289. Springer, Cham (2015). doi:10.1007/978-3-319-16268-3_31
6. Doan, T., Chua, F.C.T., Lim, E.: On neighborhood effects in location-based social networks. In: WI-IAT (2015)
7. Doan, T., Lim, E.: Attractiveness versus competition: towards an unified model for user visitation. In: CIKM (2016)
8. Gao, H., Tang, J., Hu, X., Liu, H.: Exploring temporal effects for location recommendation on location-based social networks. In: RecSys (2013)
9. Gao, H., Tang, J., Liu, H.: gSCorr: modeling geo-social correlations for new check-ins on location-based social networks. In: CIKM (2012)
10. Hsu, H., Lachenbruch, P.A.: Paired t test. In: Wiley Encyclopedia of Clinical Trials (2008)
11. Hu, L., Sun, A., Liu, Y.: Your neighbors affect your ratings: On geographical neighborhood influence to rating prediction. In: SIGIR (2014)
12. Huff, D.L.: A probabilistic analysis of shopping center trade areas. Land Econ. **39**, 81–90 (1963)
13. Koren, Y.: Factorization meets the neighborhood: a multifaceted collaborative filtering model. In: KDD (2008)
14. Koren, Y., Bell, R., Volinsky, C., et al.: Matrix factorization techniques for recommender systems. Computer **42**, 30–37 (2009)
15. Li, H., Ge, Y., Zhu, H.: Point-of-interest recommendations: learning potential check-ins from friends. In: KDD (2016)
16. Li, H., Richang, H., Zhiang, W., Ge, Y.: A spatial-temporal probabilistic matrix factorization model for point-of-interest recommendation. In: SDM (2016)
17. Li, R., Wang, S., Deng, H., Wang, R., Chang, K.C.C.: Towards social user profiling: unified and discriminative influence model for inferring home locations. In: KDD (2012)
18. Liang, D., Charlin, L., McInerney, J., Blei, D.M.: Modeling user exposure in recommendation. In: WWW (2016)
19. Liu, B., Fu, Y., Yao, Z., Xiong, H.: Learning geographical preferences for point-of-interest recommendation. In: KDD (2013)
20. Liu, B., Xiong, H.: Point-of-interest recommendation in location based social networks with topic and location awareness. In: SDM (2013)
21. Liu, Y., Wei, W., Sun, A., Miao, C.: Exploiting geographical neighborhood characteristics for location recommendation. In: CIKM (2014)
22. Mnih, A., Salakhutdinov, R.: Probabilistic matrix factorization. In: NIPS (2007)
23. Qu, Y., Zhang, J.: Trade area analysis using user generated mobile location data. In: WWW (2013)
24. Rendle, S., Freudenthaler, C., Gantner, Z., Schmidt-Thieme, L.: BPR: Bayesian personalized ranking from implicit feedback. In: UAI (2009)
25. Scellato, S., Noulas, A., Mascolo, C.: Exploiting place features in link prediction on location-based social networks. In: KDD (2011)
26. Schmidt, M.N., Winther, O., Hansen, L.K.: Bayesian non-negative matrix factorization. In: Independent Component Analysis and Signal Separation (2009)
27. Smarzaro, R., de Melo Lima, T.F., Davis Jr., C.A.: Could data from location-based social networks be used to support urban planning? In: WWW (2017)
28. Weng, L., Flammini, A., Vespignani, A., Menczer, F.: Competition among memes in a world with limited attention. Scientific reports (2012)

An Empirical Study on Collective Online Behaviors of Extremist Supporters

Jung-jae Kim(✉), Yong Liu, Wee Yong Lim, and Vrizlynn L.L. Thing

Institute for Infocomm Research, Singapore, Singapore
{jjkim,liuyo,weylim,vriz}@i2r.a-star.edu.sg

Abstract. Online social media platforms such as Twitter have been found to be misused by extremist groups, including Islamic State of Iraq and Syria (ISIS), who attract and recruit social media users. To prevent their influence from expanding in the online social media platforms, it is required to understand the online behaviors of these extremist group users and their followers, for predicting and identifying potential security threats. We present an empirical study about ISIS followers' online behaviors on Twitter, proposing to classify their tweets in terms of political and subjectivity polarities. We first develop a supervised classification model for the polarity classification, based on natural language processing and clustering methods. We then develop a statistical analysis of term-polarity correlations, which leads us to successfully observe ISIS followers' online behaviors, which are in line with the reports of experts.

Keywords: Extremist online behavior · Social media analysis · Polarity-based classification

1 Introduction

Online social media platforms, such as Facebook, Twitter, YouTube, and Flicker, have emerged and been widely used in our daily lives during the last decade. The users of these platforms are encouraged to make connections and share information (e.g., personal statuses, news, videos, pictures) with each other. Due to the high popularity and reachability of the online social media platforms, terrorist organizations have been found to utilize the platforms to spread their ideas, recruit members, and plan terrorist activities [11]. As their influence grows in the social media, more users may be attracted to, follow, and even join these terrorist organizations. For public safety, there is thus the need of understanding how they work in the social media and timely analyzing what are their propaganda.

Recently, several studies focus on analysing terrorist users' online behaviors for identifying potential security threats. For examples, Scanlon and Gerber [26, 27] applied supervised learning methods, e.g., support vector machine (SVM) [9], and natural language processing techniques, e.g., topic modeling with latent Dirichlet allocation (LDA) [3], to detect the recruitment activities of violent groups within extremist social media websites. Rudas et al. [25] investigated the role of extremists in the value production environment such as Wikipedia.

G. Cong et al. (Eds.): ADMA 2017, LNAI 10604, pp. 445–459, 2017.
https://doi.org/10.1007/978-3-319-69179-4_31

The recent rise and actions of an extremist group, called Islamic State of Iraq and the Levant (ISIL/ISIS), have received widespread news coverage over the world. Simultaneously, researchers have also studied the identification and behavioral analysis of ISIS supporters in the social media, who can be security threats. For instance, Magdy et al. [19] collected the Arabic tweets referring to ISIS and classified them into two categories, i.e., pro-ISIS and anti-ISIS, to study the antecedents of ISIS supports. Furthermore, they exploited the social media users' online content and social network dynamics to predict their future attitudes towards Islam and Muslims [18]. Also, Rowe and Saif [24] characterized the online radicalisation signals generated by social media users before, during, and after they adopt pro-ISIS behaviors.

In this paper, we also analyze ISIS supporters' online posts on social media platforms. Differing from the previous studies that predict who are or will become ISIS supporters, we aim at studying how known ISIS supporters collectively behaved on the social media platform Twitter for promoting terrorism[1]. The collective analysis is proposed based on the report that the social media users of Jihadists are largely controlled by feed accounts [15], subsequentially influencing their followers. This study may help spontaneously employ relevant counter-measures that can protect citizens from falling into the trap of their propaganda.

Previous approaches to understanding users' behaviors in social media platforms focus on classifying social media texts into pre-defined labels, including sentiment [29,31], commercial (e.g. Movie, Sport, Music) [2,30] and application-specific categories (e.g. election [21], natural disaster [23]), which can form into a taxonomy [1,12]. Several works employ unsupervised text mining methods to identify insights from social media texts. For instance, Chen et al. [8] incrementally clustered tweets to detect emerging topics, and Hamroon et al. [13] extracted triples of (subject, intention verb (e.g. 'intend'), object). Such unsupervised approaches, however, cannot straightforwardly identify certain characteristics of the ISIS supporter tweets we observe as below.

We examined samples among 14,546 tweets that were written in English by known ISIS followers between 2015 January and 2016 May.[2] We observed that there is subtle difference when the known ISIS followers wrote about 'us' and 'them', such that they *promote*, *support*, or *defend* the activities of 'us' (ISIS) but *blame* or *criticize* the activities of 'them' (e.g. US, Syria, Russia, Saudi). Also, we observed that when the ISIS followers express their opinion, they often use religious terms considering their audience [22].

Based on those observations, we propose first to classify the tweets according to the following two polarity dimensions: (1) 'us' vs. 'them', whether the tweet describes about ISIS ('us') or about its opponents ('them'), and (2) 'subjective' vs. 'objective', whether the tweet expresses subjective opinion or reports events without emotional words. We then employ statistical measures for term-polarity correlations, estimating how well a term differentiates between two opposite categories in each polarity dimension. We finally identify the behaviors of the

[1] https://blog.twitter.com/2016/combating-violent-extremism.

[2] https://www.kaggle.com/kzaman/how-isis-uses-twitter.

supporters by comparing keywords of the opposite categories, citing relevant reports of experts. This approach of comparing opposite categories differentiates our work from other visual text analytic works that explore emerging topics [17,28] and events [5] from text data.

To our best knowledge, our work is the first attempt to understand the online behaviors of extremist user group like ISIS supporters by polarizing their social media posts and capturing their different attitudes towards the opposite ends of the polarity dimensions. The major contributions of the work are as follows:

- We propose to classify extremist user online posts in terms of political and subjectivity polarities.
- We present a temporal method for analyzing term-polarity correlations to support spontaneous counter-measures against the extremist user activities.
- We identify online behaviors of extremist user group by comparing terms associated with opposite ends of a given polarity dimension.

2 Methods

2.1 Tweet Classification Scheme for Analyzing ISIS Follower Online Behaviors

To understand the online behaviors of the ISIS followers, we define the following two polarity dimensions for classifying the ISIS follower tweets: (1) poltical polarity - 'us' (tweets about ISIS), 'them' (tweets about ISIS opponents), and 'other' (the other tweets), and (2) subjectivity polarity - 'subjective' (tweets with emotional or religious words), 'objective' (tweets reporting events or information), and 'other' (the other tweets). Table 1 shows example tweets of the classes.

The proposed classification scheme is different from previous works on political and sentimental classification tasks. Previous works on political classification task focus on answering which of the two parties the author of a given article belongs to [32] or which of the two opposite ideologies (i.e. Democrat, Republican) a given article supports [14]. In contrast, the ISIS followers like other extremists side with ISIS and share similar ideology. The political polarity of our work rather classifies if a given tweet is about whom ('us' or 'them'), in order to understand how differently the followers describe about 'us' and 'them', thus revealing their propaganda. Also, as the ISIS followers have stance biased toward ISIS, we do not identify if a given tweet has positive or negative emotion, which might be inferred from the political polarity. Instead, we address the task of identifying if a tweet is subjective or not, in order to detect the explicit or concealed emotional appeal to their audience.

Three annotators including two of the authors worked together for the manual labeling of 280 tweets. They followed and maintained annotation guidelines throughout the labeling process. Example guidelines are as follows:

- If a tweet does not have specific information, label it as 'other', not as 'objective'.

Table 1. Example tweets of the polarity-driven classes

Political	Subjectivity	Example tweet
us	objective	#ISIS continues its rampage in #Palmyra and two #Iranian Colonels reportedly killed in there... #Syria
us	subjective	@saladinisback1 If you wants but IS have different view and other project just like Taliban in Afghanistan, mostly religious
them	objective	RT @_SalmanHashimi: American machine gun left behind by the #Peshmerga after the fled despite having US air cover: https://t.co/IISLdHO8pV
them	subjective	They should call Saudi & UAE pilots to stop bombing them first. #Saudi Council of Senior Scholars calls to aid civilians in #Fallujah #Iraq
other	objective	RT @HeartHasStereo: Situation in north Syria now https://t.co/6Dz9st9qEt
other	subjective	RT @IslamicEyes: Nabi SAW said, "No one who has the weight of a seed of arrogance in his heart will enter Paradise. (Muslim)
other	other	@Ibn__Al_Farooq_ yes...

- Only if the follower adds his/her opinion to report of activity, label the tweet as 'subjective'; otherwise, label it as 'objective'.

Table 2 shows the number of manually annotated tweets for the classes defined by the two polarities. Note that there is no tweet that is manually labeled with the 'other' class of the subjectivity polarity and with either 'us' or 'them' class of the political polarity, which may indicate that the ISIS followers wrote tweets about 'us' and 'them' *purposefully*, either delivering certain information or expressing opinion explicitly.

Table 2. Counts of manually labeled tweets

	us	them	other
objective	54	40	62
subjective	7	17	47
other	0	0	52

2.2 Tweet Classification

To classify the ISIS follower tweets with regards to the two polarities, we represent tweets as feature vectors and employ a machine learning method (e.g. SVM) for learning a classification model from the tweet vector representations. We consider the following three representations of tweets without requiring any gazetteer.

TF-IDF (term frequency-inverse document frequency): TF-IDF is a well-known way of vector representation of texts, based on term frequencies within and across documents. We consider both unigrams and bigrams as terms.

This method has such a limitation that it does not capture lexical semantics of short texts like tweets well. Note that the proposed tweet classification should consider term (dis-)similarity (e.g. 'ISIS', 'islamic state' vs. 'US', 'Saudi').

Topic modeling: Topic modeling based on LDA (Latent Dirichlet allocation) [3] builds a low dimensional vector space model for documents based on *topics*. A *topic* is a distribution over the vocabulary of a given corpus, and each document is represented as the distribution of topics. The words in a topic are closely related to each other, but do not necessarily reflect lexical relationship involved in the tweet classification task.

Clustering: Clustering is the task of grouping similar instances and can be applied to identifying lexical similarity. We first utilize clustering methods to group similar *information units* (IUs) like words into clusters and then represent each tweet as the set of clusters to which the IUs of the tweet belong. We employ and compare clustering methods of K-Means, DBSCAN [10], and Greedy Variance Minimization (GVM)[3].

We consider two IU types: word and dependency. A dependency consists of two elements: a word and a dependency type [16]. For the example of triple relationship "nsubj(destroy, ISIS)" produced by the Stanford dependency parser [6], which means that ISIS destroys (something), we can identify two dependencies: (ISIS, nsubj) and (destroy, nsubjI), where 'I' in 'nsubjI' indicates that 'nsubjI' is an inverse relation of 'nsubj'. We identify the words and dependencies in a given tweet by using the Stanford dependency parser.

We estimate the similarity between IUs based on the embeddings (or vector representations) of the IUs. We employ Word2Vec [20] and word2vecf [16] to learn embeddings of words and dependencies, respectively, from a corpus of tweets. We then use the embeddings of each IU type as input for clustering methods, which produce clusters of words and dependencies.

We compare two tweet corpora as input of Word2Vec and word2vecf for learning the embeddings of IUs: (1) the tweets of the known ISIS followers, which is closely relevant but small, and (2) a big corpus of tweets that are crawled with relevant keyword searches, which is thus loosely relevant but big. We describe the details of the second corpus in Sect. 3.1 and show that the word/dependency embeddings learnt from the big corpus of tweets generate better clusters as features of the classification task than those learnt from the ISIS follower tweets.

We compare combinations of the three representations (i.e. TF-IDF, topic modeling, clustering) for the classification task in the Results section. We also compare the clusters of words and dependencies and their union.

With the best representation of tweets, we train machine learning models (see Sect. 3.1 for details) and apply them to automatically identify the polarity-based classes of unannotated tweets. We utilize both manually and automatically labeled tweets for the analysis discussed in the next section.

[3] http://www.tomgibara.com/clustering/fast-spatial/.

2.3 Analyzing Online Behavior of ISIS Followers

In the following sub-sections, we discuss how we can utilize the classification of ISIS follower tweets to understand the online behaviors of the followers when they wrote the tweets. The notations used in the sub-sections are listed below.

T: The set of all the tweets written by known ISIS followers
D: The set of all the relevant dates when the followers wrote their tweets

- The function *labels*(*tweet*) returns two classes of the two polarities as the labels of the given tweet
- The function *date*(*tweet*) returns the date of posting the given *tweet*

Which polarity categories did ISIS followers adhere to when writing tweets? The polarity-driven tweet classification helps answer this question by separating opposite categories in each polarity dimension (see Observations (1) and (2) in the Results section).

What did ISIS followers highlight in their tweets, differentiating two opposite categories? This question is not to locate the top-frequent keywords in the tweets (e.g. ISIS, Syria, US), but to identify the keywords that are highlighted more for one side than for the other side and vice versa. Such keywords may help us understand how the followers tried to differentiate ISIS from 'them'.

To answer this question, we devise a statistical function that considers the proposed classification and gives higher weights to potential 'answers' than the other terms as illustrated in Eq. (1).

$$\begin{aligned} f(word, cat_1, cat_2) &= \log\left(1 + count(word, cat_1) + count(word, cat_2)\right) \\ &\quad \times \left(\frac{count(word, cat_1)}{count(cat_1)} - \frac{count(word, cat_2)}{count(cat_2)}\right) \\ count(word, cat) &= |\{\forall t \in T | word \in t \wedge cat \in labels(t)\}| \\ count(cat) &= |\{\forall t \in T | cat \in labels(t)\}| \end{aligned} \tag{1}$$

The main function f in Eq. (1) takes three arguments: a word and two orthogonal categories in each dimension (e.g. 'us'/'them'), and returns an estimate of how well the word differentiates the first category from the second category. Basic ideas of the estimation are (1) to prefer terms that appear relatively more often in the tweets of the first category than the second category, and (2) to prefer more frequent terms to less frequent terms in the two categories.

We apply this function to all the unique words in the tweets and rank the words for the two dimensions, f(*word*, 'us', 'them') and f(*word*, 'objective', 'subjective'). The ranking results are summarized in Observations (4)–(6).

At a given time, what did ISIS followers highlight in their tweets, differentiating two opposite categories? Equation (1) can be used to identify key differentiating words in the whole set of the known ISIS follower tweets, but cannot identify keywords at a given time. Such temporal analysis is important due to the need of spontaneously employing relevant counter-measures against the ISIS follower propaganda at the given time.

To address the need, we revise the functions as illustrated in Eq. (2). The difference is that the new function f_t in Eq. (2) requires one more argument, a specific time (i.e. date), and takes into account only the tweets posted on and/or before the given date, giving older tweets lower weights by using an exponential decay function.

$$\begin{aligned} f_t(w, c_1, c_2, t_0) &= \log\left(1 + count_t(w, c_1, t_0) + count_t(w, c_2, t_0)\right) \\ &\quad \times \left(\frac{freq_t(w, c_1, t_0)}{freq_t(c_1, t_0)} - \frac{freq_t(w, c_2, t_0)}{freq_t(c_2, t_0)}\right) \\ freq_t(w, c, t_0) &= \sum_{\forall t \in T, w \in t \wedge c \in labels(t) \wedge date(t) \leq t_0} e^{-\lambda(t_0 - date(t))} \\ freq_t(c, t_0) &= \sum_{\forall t \in T, c \in labels(t) \wedge date(t) \leq t_0} e^{-\lambda(t_0 - date(t))} \\ count_t(w, c, t_0) &= |\{\forall t \in T | w \in t \wedge c \in labels(t) \wedge date(t) \leq t_0\}| \end{aligned} \tag{2}$$

We also apply this function to rank all the unique words at selected times and summarize the results in Observations (7) and (8).

3 Results

3.1 Classification Performance

The manually labeled tweets (Sect. 2.1) are used for training machine learning models of the automatic classification, which are then applied to automatically label the tweets that are not manually labeled. All the tweets are pre-processed (i.e. removing punctuations, non-alphanumeric tokens, converting to lowercase).

We compare the three vector representations of tweets described in Sect. 2.2 (i.e. TF-IDF, Topic modeling, clustering) and their combinations. As for the clustering-based representation, we also compare the results of different clustering methods (i.e. K-Means, DBSCAN, GVM) and also the clustering results of different IU types (i.e. word only, word + dependency) whose embeddings are learnt from different tweet corpora (i.e. ISIS follower tweets only, a big tweet corpus crawled with relevant keywords).

We apply two classification methods of support vector machine (SVM) and XGBoost [7] to the three vector representations of tweets. We also apply feature selection by using Chi-square test (threshold: 50%, which showed the best result).

Table 3 summarizes the performance results in terms of micro-averaged F-score with the following settings: Tweets are represented with TF-IDF and the results of different clustering methods, and feature selection is employed. We used k-fold cross-validation for the evaluation (k = 10). The first column shows the type of IUs used for the clustering-based tweet representation. The second column indicates the clustering method for experiment. The columns 3–4 and 5–6 are the evaluation results on the political and subjectivity polarities, respectively.

The best F-scores of the political and subjectivity polarities are 71.4% and 78.9%, respectively (p-value = 0.01). In general, the combination of word and

Table 3. Evaluation results of tweet classification ('dep' indicates 'dependency')

IU type	Clustering	Political polarity		Subjectivity polarity	
	Method	SVM	XGBoost	SVM	XGBoost
word	KMeans	69.6%	69.4%	73.6%	77.4%
word	GVM	68.9%	70.6%	73.2%	76.6%
word	DBSCAN	59.6%	69.8%	56.4%	63.5%
dep	KMeans	70.0%	71.0%	75.0%	72.6%
dep	DBSCAN	59.3%	69.0%	56.4%	64.3%
word+dep	KMeans	71.1%	71.4%	**80.4%**	76.6%
word+dep	GVM	**72.5%**	68.7%	79.3%	76.2%
word+dep	DBSCAN	59.3%	64.3%	56.4%	58.3%

dependency IUs shows better results than individual IU types. Note that all the reported results are obtained when using both unigrams and bigrams, which show higher results in our experiments than using either unigrams or bigrams. Both K-Means and GVM clustering methods are helpful for the classification task. The evaluation results discussed below are thus based on the tweet representation with combination of word and dependency IUs that are clustered by using K-Means and GVM, called as 'default' setting.

Table 4. Evaluation results of tweet classification in terms of F-score

Configuration	Political		Subjectivity	
	SVM	XGBoost	SVM	XGBoost
Only TF-IDF	59.3%	65.1%	56.4%	59.5%
Only topic modeling	62.9%	68.3%	65.7%	69.0%
Only clustering	71.0%	69.8%	79.3%	76.2%
Default with topic modeling	71.4%	69.4%	78.2%	74.6%
Default without feature selection	68.2%	70.2%	78.2%	75.4%
Clustering with ISIS follower tweets	71.8%	67.5%	78.6%	77.8%

Table 4 shows the evaluation results with settings different from the 'default' setting, based on which we discuss about the impact of the parameters proposed in this paper. The first three rows (i.e. 'Only TF-IDF', 'Only topic modeling', 'Only clustering') show the performance of our system when using only one of the three tweet representations. The clustering-based tweet representation shows the highest performance, and the topic modeling-based representation the second best. However, the combination of all the three representations (the fourth row) does not outperform the combination of TF-IDF and clustering-based representation except the topic modeling-based representation. This may

Table 5. Evaluation results for each of the polarity-driven classes

Class	Political polarity			Class	Subjectivity polarity		
	Precision	Recall	F-score		Precision	Recall	F-score
us	72.3%	48.1%	55.2%	Objective	81.5%	98.8%	89.2%
them	73.3%	40.4%	46.9%	Subjective	75.1%	70.6%	72.0%
other	73.3%	94.9%	82.4%	Other	70.0%	35.1%	46.5%

indicate that the clustering results cover the topic modeling results significantly. We also tested our system without feature selection (the fifth row), and found feature selection enhances the system performance significantly.

Table 5 shows the performance of the best model for each polarity-driven class. As for the political polarity, the precision for the three classes is similar, but their recall is different such that the recall of the 'other' class is the highest, which may mean some tweets are misclassified into the 'other' class. The political polarity generally shows lower performance than the subjectivity polarity. This may be due to the fact that a tweet may include entity names of both sides. Note that we label such a tweet with the category of the side that plays more active role (e.g. attack) than the other side (e.g. killed).

Table 6. Counts of automatically labeled tweets

	us	them	other
objective	2,786	1,680	5,425
subjective	30	137	3,112
other	1	3	1,088

As explained in the Methods section, we perform clustering by measuring similarity between information units based on embeddings learnt from a corpus. We tested two corpora for this purpose: (1) ISIS follower tweets and (2) *big tweet corpus* including the ISIS follower tweets. The *big tweet corpus* was constructed in 2016 October by crawling 3,846,457 tweets that contain any of relevant keywords[4]. We collected the keywords as follows: We first crawled tweets that contain terrorism-related keywords (e.g. 'terrorism'), but found that they are quite different from the ISIS follower tweets, thus not useful for the behavioral analysis. We then applied Naive Bayes to classify between the ISIS follower tweets and the terrorism-related tweets and identified the words that differentiate the former from the latter the most, which were used as the search keywords. The clustering with embeddings learnt from the big tweet corpus shows better performance than those learnt only with the ISIS follower tweets (the last row of Table 4), even though the two corpora were constructed at different times.

[4] islamicstate, syria, syrian, isis, iraqi, iraq, aleppo, assad, mosul, palmyra, ramiallolah, fallujah, ramadi, homs, kuffar, kafir, kufr, amaq, sheikh, shia, damascus, deir ezzor, abu bakr al-baghdadi, #albaghdadi, raqqah, nusayri, azaz, awlaki, anwar al-awlaki, islamic, islam, yarmouk, khanaser, khanase, tadmur, daraa.

3.2 Online Behavior Analysis Results

We apply the best classification model to all unlabeled tweets, whose automatic classification results are summarized in Table 6. We analyze all the tweets, both manually and automatically labeled, and describe our observations below.

Which polarity categories did ISIS followers adhere to when writing tweets? We plot the counts of tweets that were posted on each date and belong to the pre-defined categories as in Figs. 1 and 2, where the X-axis indicates the series of relevant dates, and Y-axis tweet counts. Note that the plots include dates from 2016 January to 2016 May, omitting the year 2015, because the year 2015 have much fewer tweets than the year 2016.

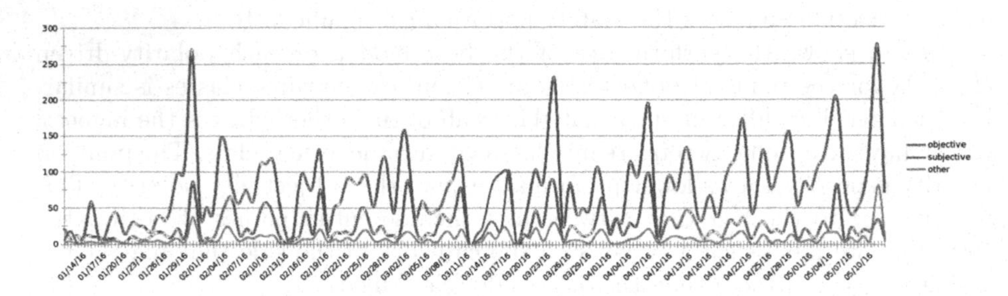

Fig. 1. Counts of tweets belonging to 'objective' and 'subjective' categories over time

Observation 1. *The ISIS followers almost always wrote more 'objective' tweets than 'subjective' ones (Fig. 1).*

This may suggest that the followers want to paint them as 'neural' (i.e. non-obvious ISIS supporters), which may have better appeal to the audience. These 'objective' tweets of ISIS followers, however, were not always based on facts. For instance, they "twisted small, one-sided skirmishes into significant battlefield victories", thus "spreading panic" in Mosul, before ISIS conquered the city in 2014 June [4].

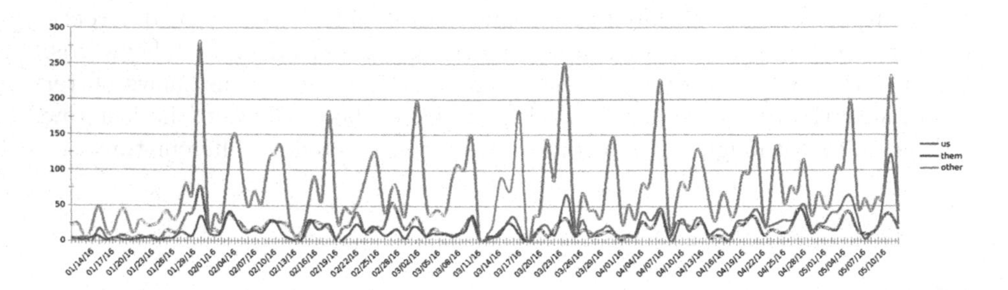

Fig. 2. Counts of tweets belonging to 'us' and 'them' categories over time

Observation 2. *The ISIS followers wrote about the activities of 'us' more frequently than those of 'them' (Fig. 2).*

This obvious tendency as followers may show that the followers think that the media do not publish enough of the ISIS activities, and thus want to advertise them to the public to keep a balance between the two sides. Note also that when they reported about the activities of 'them', they wrote more subjective tweets about 'them' (8%), mostly with negative emotion, than about 'us' (1%).

What did ISIS followers highlight in their tweets, differentiating opposite categories? We apply the functions of Eq. (1) to all the tweets with the following two pairs of arguments: (1) $f(word$, 'us', 'them') vs. $f(word$, 'them', 'us') and (2) $f(word$, 'objective', 'subjective') vs. $f(word$, 'subjective', 'objective'). The resultant top-ranked words are listed in Table 7. We group the top-ranked keywords as follows: (1) Entity-referring words ('islamic' and 'state' indicate 'Islamic State'; 'rebels' include SAF, FSA, and YPG), (2) military words, (3) location-indicating words, (4) religious words, and (5) other words (e.g. near, today), which are not listed in the tables.

Table 7. Top-20 differentiating keywords: 'us' vs. 'them', 'objective' vs. 'subjective'

	us	them
Entity	isis, state, islamic, iraq, iraqi, amaqagency, islamicstate	us, ypg, rebels, syria, saudi, russia, assad, usa, fsa, turkish, nusra
Military	army, fighters, soldiers, killed, attack	airstrikes, fight, bomb, kill
Location	area, near, west, fallujah, ramadi, east	aleppo
Religious	-	-
	objective	subjective
Entity	isis, syria, iraq, islamicstate, islamic, iraqi, state	is
Military	killed, army, forces, soldiers, attack	-
Location	aleppo, near, city	-
Religious	-	allah, muslims, islam, muslim

Observation 3. *The ISIS followers used more location-related words, which refer to the locations of military operations, when writing about 'us' than about 'them' (6 keywords compared to 1 keyword) (Table 7).*

The frequent military location keywords along with the military action keywords (e.g. 'army', 'attack') may indicate that the ISIS followers highlighted military activities of ISIS, though often exaggerated. In comparison, the two military keywords of 'them', 'airstrikes' and 'bomb', were used to criticize the civilian casaulities caused by the airstrikes of 'them'.

Observation 4. *When the ISIS followers wrote about 'them', they specified who are 'them', individually criticizing 'them' (11 out of 20 top-ranked keywords) (Table 7).*

The entity-referring keywords show who belong to which side from the perspective of ISIS, who consider most except them as 'them'. They criticized 'them' individually and specifically in their tweets. Note that all the entity-referring keywords of 'us' (e.g. Amaq News Agency[5]) are closely related to ISIS, with the exception of 'Iraq' where most of ISIS activities at the time happened.

Observation 5. *The top-ranked keywords of 'objective' tweets mainly indicate the people and locations of military activities (Table 7).*

This observation, together with the fact that most of the tweets about 'us' are 'objective', is in line with the fact that ISIS' online propaganda is intertwined with their real-life military operations [4].

Observation 6. *The top-ranked keywords of 'subjective' tweets are mostly religious words (Table 7).*

As shown in Table 6, most of the subjective tweets are about 'them', which together with Observation 6 may indicate that the ISIS followers criticize 'them' with religious terms, even non-Muslim 'them' (e.g. USA, Russia).

At a specific time, what did ISIS followers highlight in their tweets, differentiating opposite categories? We chose two specific dates for the temporal analysis, which are commonly cited in the Web pages[6] that list important events related to ISIS, as follows: Iraqi troops retook the city of Ramadi from ISIS around December 28, 2015, and ISIS claimed responsibility for the terrorist attacks in Brussels on March 22, 2016. We chose the six dates before/after the two dates as shown in Table 8.

We utilized the functions of Eq. (2) ($\lambda = 0.5$) as follows: (1) f(word, 'us', 'them', date) with each of the three dates around December 28, 2015, and (2) f(word, 'us', 'other', date) with each of the three dates around March 22, 2016. We compare 'us' with the 'other' class of the poltical polarity because the tweets about the Brussels attack are not about 'them' and thus classified to 'other'. The resultant top-ranked words are listed in Table 8.

Observation 7. *The temporal analysis captures the significance of the location keyword 'ramadi' for the class 'us' around December 28, 2015 (Table 8).*

The keyword 'ramadi' was ranked high not only on December 29, 2015, but also on an earlier date of December 26, because the city was retaken on December 28 as the result of attacks for several months[7]. Note that the rank of the keyword 'ramadi' for the 'us' class went down after the retake.

[5] https://www.nytimes.com/2016/01/15/world/middleeast/a-news-agency-with-scoops-directly-from-isis-and-a-veneer-of-objectivity.html.
[6] https://www.wilsoncenter.org/article/timeline-rise-and-spread-the-islamic-state, http://edition.cnn.com/2014/08/08/world/isis-fast-facts/.
[7] http://edition.cnn.com/2015/12/28/middleeast/iraq-military-retakes-ramadi/.

Observation 8. *The temporal analysis captures the significance of the location keyword 'brussels' for the class 'other' after March 22, 2016 (Table 8).*

Unlike the attacks on Ramadi for several months, the terrorist attack on Brussels happened exactly on March 22, 2016, which explains the sudden appearance of the keyword 'brussels' after the attack. Even though ISIS claimed that they are responsible for the Brussels attack, the keyword 'brussels' is not strongly associated with the 'us' class. Instead, another location keyword of 'palmyra' had been ranked high before and even after the Brussels attack, which may reflect the fact that ISIS military activities were focused on Palmyra at the time. These results may imply that the ISIS followers highlighted 'important' events, which can be different from the highlights of the other media.

Table 8. Top differentiating keywords of temporal analysis

	12–26		12–29		12–31	
	us	them	us	them	us	them
1	is	breaking	is	russia	is	syria
2	iraqi	russia	iraqi	syria	isis	russia
3	isis	saudi	forces	breaking	iraq	russian
4	fighters	islamic	killed	airstrikes	ramiallola	saudi
5	regime	us	army	alive	forces	civilians
6	battles	ramiallolah	baghdad	tel	targeting	trained
7	damascus	fallujah	**ramadi**	airport	civilian	sakirkhader
8	fierce	isf	alshabaab	bomb	led	hit
9	**ramadi**	executed	hands	casualties	iraqi	yemen
10	west	military	amisom	defence	neighborhoods	warplane
12					**ramadi**	
	03–19		03–23		03–25	
	us	other	us	other	us	other
1	is	is	isis	muslims	isis	allah
2	killed	takfir	killed	people	killed	**brussels**
3	syria	us	syria	**brussels**	army	is
4	army	make	attack	news	*palmyra*	kronykal
5	iraq	allah	attacks	muslim	state	time
6	soldiers	milksheikh2	*palmyra*	police	islamic	muslim
7	near	islam	iraq	world	syria	people
8	*palmyra*	muslim	soldiers	say	attack	think
9	west	like	today	twitter	forces	muslims
10	russian	muslims	abu	like	south	years

4 Conclusion

We present a classification scheme and statistical measures to analyze the online behaviors of the ISIS followers when they wrote their tweets. By comparing the opposite categories in the two polarity dimensions, we could identify the behavioral patterns in form of top-weighted keywords. In particular, the temporal analysis helps us understand what might be the highlights of the ISIS follower tweets at a given time in comparison to the other media.

Acknowledgement. This material is based on research work supported by the Singapore National Research Foundation under NCR Award No. NRF2014NCR-NCR001-034.

References

1. Alhadi, A.C., Gottron, T., Staab, S.: Exploring user purpose writing single tweets. In: WebSci. ACM (2011)
2. Banerjee, N., Chakraborty, D., Joshi, A., Mittal, S., Rai, A., Ravindran, B.: Towards analyzing micro-blogs for detection and classification of real-time intentions. In: ICWSM (2012)
3. Blei, D.M., Ng, A.Y., Jordan, M.I.: Latent Dirichlet allocation. J. Mach. Learn. Res. **3**, 993–1022 (2003)
4. Brooking, E.T., Singer, P.W.: War goes viral: how social media is being weaponized across the world. The Atlantic (2016). https://www.theatlantic.com/magazine/archive/2016/11/war-goes-viral/501125/
5. Chae, J., Thom, D., Jang, Y., Kim, S., Ertl, T., Ebert, D.S.: Public behavior response analysis in disaster events utilizing visual analytics of microblog data. Comput. Graph. (Pergamon) **38**(1), 51–60 (2014)
6. Chen, D., Manning, C.D.: A fast and accurate dependency parser using neural networks. In: EMNLP, pp. 740–750 (2014)
7. Chen, T., Guestrin, C.: XGBoost : Reliable large-scale tree boosting system. In: SIGKDD Conference on Knowledge Discovery and Data Mining, pp. 785–794 (2016)
8. Chen, Z., Liu, B., Hsu, M., Castellanos, M., Ghosh, R.: Identifying intention posts in discussion forums. In: HLT-NAACL, pp. 1041–1050 (2013)
9. Cristianini, N., Shawe-Taylor, J.: An Introduction to Support Vector Machines and Other Kernel-Based Learning Methods. Cambridge University Press, Cambridge (2000)
10. Daszykowski, M., Walczak, B.: Density-based clustering methods. Compr. Chemometr. **2**, 635–654 (2010)
11. Fisher, A.: Swarmcast: how Jihadist networks maintain a persistent online presence. Perspect. Terror. **9**(3), 3–20 (2015)
12. Gómez-Adorno, H., Pinto, D., Montes, M., Sidorov, G., Alfaro, R.: Content and style features for automatic detection of users' intentions in tweets. In: Ibero-American Conference on Artificial Intelligence, pp. 120–128 (2014)
13. Hamroun, M., Gouider, M.S., Said, L.B.: Customer intentions analysis of twitter based on semantic patterns. In: WISDOM (2015)
14. Iyyer, M., Enns, P., Boyd-Graber, J., Resnik, P.: Political ideology detection using recursive neural networks. In: ACL, pp. 1113–1122 (2014)

15. Klausen, J.: Tweeting the Jihad: social media networks of western foreign fighters in Syria and Iraq. Stud. Conflict Terror. **38**(1), 1–22 (2015)
16. Levy, O., Goldberg, Y.: Dependency-based word embeddings. In: ACL, pp. 302–308 (2014)
17. Liu, S., Wang, X., Chen, J., Zhu, J., Guo, B.: TopicPanorama: a full picture of relevant topics. In: IEEE Conference on Visual Analytics Science and Technology, pp. 183–192 (2014)
18. Magdy, W., Darwish, K., Abokhodair, N., Rahimi, A., Baldwin, T.: ISISisNotislam or DeportAllMuslims?: Predicting unspoken views. In: ACM Conference on Web Science, pp. 95–106 (2016)
19. Magdy, W., Darwish, K., Weber, I.: FailedRevolutions: using twitter to study the antecedents of ISIS support. First Monday **21**(2), 1481–1492 (2016)
20. Mikolov, T., Sutskever, I., Chen, K., Corrado, G., Dean, J.: Distributed representations of words and phrases and their compositionality. In: Advances in Neural Information Processing Systems, pp. 3111–3119 (2013)
21. Mohammad, S.M., Kiritchenko, S., Martin, J.: Identifying purpose behind electoral tweets. In: Proceedings of the Second International Workshop on Issues of Sentiment Discovery and Opinion Mining (2013)
22. Prentice, S., Taylor, P.J., Rayson, P., Hoskins, A., O'Loughlin, B.: Analyzing the semantic content and persuasive composition of extremist media: a case study of texts produced during the Gaza conflict. Inf. Syst. Front. **13**(1), 61–73 (2011)
23. Purohit, H., Dong, G., Shalin, V., Thirunarayan, K., Sheth, A.: Intent classification of short-text on social media. In: IEEE International Conference on Smart City/SocialCom/SustainCom (SmartCity), pp. 222–228 (2015)
24. Rowe, M., Saif, H.: Mining Pro-ISIS radicalisation signals from social media users. In: International Conference on Weblogs and Social Media, pp. 329–338 (2016)
25. Rudas, C., Surányi, O., Yasseri, T., Török, J.: Understanding and coping with extremism in an online collaborative environment: a data-driven modeling. PLoS ONE **12**(3), e0173561 (2017)
26. Scanlon, J.R., Gerber, M.S.: Automatic detection of cyber-recruitment by violent extremists. Secur. Inf. **3**(1), 1–10 (2014)
27. Scanlon, J.R., Gerber, M.S.: Forecasting violent extremist cyber recruitment. IEEE Trans. Inf. Forensics Secur. **10**(11), 2461–2470 (2015)
28. Sun, G., Wu, Y., Liu, S., Peng, T.Q., Zhu, J.J., Liang, R.: EvoRiver: visual analysis of topic coopetition on social media. IEEE Trans. Visual. Comput. Graph. **20**(12), 1753–1762 (2014)
29. Tang, J., Liu, H.: An unsupervised feature selection framework for social media data. IEEE Trans. Knowl. Data Eng. **26**(12), 2914–2927 (2014)
30. Wang, J., Cong, G., Zhao, W.X., Li, X.: Mining user intents in Twitter: a semi-supervised approach to inferring intent categories for tweets. In: AAAI, pp. 318–324 (2015)
31. Wang, X., Liu, Y., SUN, C., Wang, B., Wang, X.: Predicting polarities of tweets by composing word embeddings with long short-term memory. In: ACL/IJCNLP, pp. 1343–1353 (2015)
32. Yu, B., Kaufmann, S., Diermeier, D.: Classifying party affiliation from political speech. J. Inf. Technol. Pol. **5**(1), 33–48 (2008)

Your Moves, Your Device: Establishing Behavior Profiles Using Tensors

Eric Falk(✉), Jérémy Charlier, and Radu State

University of Luxembourg, SnT, 6 Rue Richard Coudenhove-Kalergi,
1359 Luxembourg City, Luxembourg
{eric.falk,jeremy.charlier,radu.state}@uni.lu

Abstract. Smartphones became a person's constant companion. As the strictly personal devices they are, they gradually enable the replacement of well established activities as for instance payments, two factor authentication or personal assistants. In addition, Internet of Things (IoT) gadgets extend the capabilities of the latter even further. Devices such as body worn fitness trackers allow users to keep track of daily activities by periodically synchronizing data with the smartphone and ultimately with the vendor's computational centers in the cloud. These fitness trackers are equipped with an array of sensors to measure the movements of the device, to derive information as step counts or make assessments about sleep quality. We capture the raw sensor data from wrist-worn activity trackers to model a biometric behavior profile of the carrier. We establish and present techniques to determine rather the original person, who trained the model, is currently wearing the bracelet or another individual. Our contribution is based on CANDECOMP/PARAFAC (CP) tensor decomposition so that computational complexity facilitates: the execution on light computational devices on low precision settings, or the migration to stronger CPUs or to the cloud, for high to very high granularity. This precision parameter allows the security layer to be adaptable, in order to be compliant with the requirements set by the use cases. We show that our approach identifies users with high confidence.

1 Introduction

Over the last years everyday tasks have been facilitated by the use of smartphones. Indeed, numerous functions have been ported to the mobile format: vendors launch smartphone based payment methods, major applications as social media apps employ advanced smartphones based multi-factor authentication [3], and mobile banking has become a must have for financial institutions [23]. In the meantime traditional password authentication schemes are becoming undesirable because of their cumbersomeness [7]. Smartphones are the ideal medium for novel authentication schemes as they are already esteemed as a highly personal equipment. Recent devices are equipped with biometric authenticators as fingerprint scanners. Still, secure authentication on smartphones is challenging.

Problem Statement: It has recently been shown that a smartphone's fingerprint reader can be compromised [25]. The authors showed that it is possible to

G. Cong et al. (Eds.): ADMA 2017, LNAI 10604, pp. 460–474, 2017.
https://doi.org/10.1007/978-3-319-69179-4_32

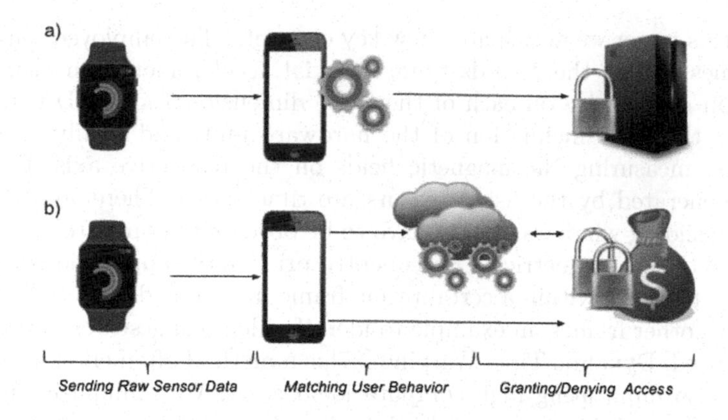

Fig. 1. Depiction of the target applications

generate a “MasterPrint” for the impersonation of multiple users at once. It has furthermore been established that over 90% of the PINs and passwords can be guessed by so called “Smudge Attacks”, where attackers use finger smear traces on the touchscreen [5], neither are those methods prone to “Shoulder Surfers”. Are the current smartphone authentication methods really synonymous with the sensibility of the information and services they unlock? This question occupies the research community and industry, both investigating alternatives as biometric shaking movements [32] or gait recognition [20]. To increase the trust in the user authentication on smartphones, an identification method with strong biometric verifications must be implemented. Although, it should be transparent for the end-user to make the authentication processes as seamless as possible. With the methodology presented in this work, we are convinced to fulfill these requirements. In Fig. 1 the envisioned application is illustrated. In the use case show by panel Fig. 1a the user signs-in to a device with the smartphone sending a user authenticity confidence score to the target device. An authentication score is computed by the smartphone itself, using the raw sensor data from a wrist-worn activity tracker. Due to the limited computational capabilities of the smartphone the confidence score is computed on less precise data. Should the confidence score be situated below a fixed threshold, the target device or service can request further authentication challenges. Alternatively, in Fig. 1b the user is authenticating with a online banking service requiring a more precise authenticity score. The smartphone is initiating the sign-in, but the score is computed by a cloud application on the more precise sensor data continuously forwarded by the user device. The cloud application is synchronizing with the online banking application for a more confident user authenticity score. In this work we describe the first step on the way to the described target application, namely the methodology to confidently identify users and detect impersonators.

Contributions: A substantial amount of research work has been done on identifying specific activities based on data from built-in movement sensor data. A survey of the related work is provided in Sect. 2. Nevertheless, to properly motivate this paper we anticipate a few key concepts. The employed sensor data is oftentimes among the records from: tri-axial accelerometers, measuring the acceleration of a device on each of the three dimensional axis, 3D gyroscopes, calculating the axial inclination of the hardware unit, and finally, from magnetometers, measuring the magnetic fields on the respective axis. By nature the data generated by the listed sensors are time series. Therefore, to extract knowledge, sliding windows of data have to be observed in order to examine the evolution of the sensor metrics. Consequently, prior to the application of learning algorithms, the data within a certain time frame has to be discretized and overlapped with other frames, in example to identify identical gestures performed at different speed. Dynamic Time Warping [27] is a method often employed for this purposes, also implicating high computational costs. We relinquish this initial step by immediately investigating the data distribution of the momentary device orientations rather than the evolution of it's acceleration or inclination. With this work we contribute in the following aspects: **(a)** From the sensor data we extract *9DOF Quaternions* a 4 dimensional vector describing the device orientation in the earth referential. Our assumption is that for each carrier the distribution of device positions is unique. **(b)** We describe how we transform continuous 4 dimensional quaternion data for the use with four-way tensors dedicated to the representation of the data distribution. **(c)** We outline how the knowledge gained from *Candecomp/Parafac* (CP) tensor decomposition on novel incoming data is used, in combination with subsequent similarity measures, to identify the wristband carrier. **(d)** Finally, we provide an evaluation of our model on "real world" test data recorded during a small scale user study.

The remainder of the paper is organized as follows, in the related work chapter (Sect. 2), our contribution is placed in the context of academic advances. In Sect. 3, methodology, we blueprint the proposed approach. In the evaluation section (Sect. 4), we describe the data collection and pre-processing steps, and we analyze the performance of our method using data samples recorded in a small scale user study. Finally, this work is concluded and future directions are discussed in Sect. 5.

2 Related Work

Regarding behavioral biometric authentication, scientific contributions are extensively surveyed and analyzed in the work of Rybnicek et al. [26]. Publications related to the underlying paper evolve along three thematic axis. Firstly, works considering sensor data to infer human activities are of interest. Secondly, contributions proposing biometric or sensor based security mechanisms are of relevance. Finally, use cases employing tensor decomposition for machine learning purposes, as classification or anomaly detection, are related. To place the underlying work in the correct context, among the scientific advances from the three previously mentioned areas, the latter are reviewed in that respective order.

One of the most recent contributions analyzed sensor data, captured from smart glasses, to recognize a specific person based on a set performed head gestures [31]. The authors employ a mixture of *K-Nearest-Neighbors* (kNN) [15], *Support Vector Machines* (SVM) [8], and *k-Dimensional Trees* (k-D Trees) [6] algorithms. They are applied on raw accelerometer and gyroscope data for recorded and labeled head gestures. The experiments are conducted in a controlled environment in order to obtain labeled datasets. Similarly the authors of [22] propose the *RisQ* system to detect smoking sessions and determine their durations. Decision Trees [9] are therefore applied on sequences of 9DOF quaternions logged by sensor wristbands.

Considering security mechanism diverging from classical password schemes, a multitude of techniques have been proposed by academics over the last years. *EyeVeri* [28] for instance presents algorithms to identify users by eye tracking through the front camera of cell phones. As a proposal closer to the underlying work, the *ShakeIn* [32] system trains a SVM model of a shaking movement using smartphone sensor data. The hand-held is only unlocked if the shaking pattern is repeated and matches the trained model of the authorized user. In [12] Feng et al. introduce *Fast* a challenge response system for unlocking the smartphone. A user is asked to perform a certain gesture on the touchscreen (i.e. pinch), micro movements of the fingers are recorded by a sensor glove specifically build for that purpose.

Tensor decompositions are very popular in data compression and classification domains. In [19], Mahfoodh and Radha proposed to use a tensor decomposition approach for the compression and the classification of a collection of images. It allowed to save more data storage than per image compression as correlations are likely to exist between images. Another popular tensor decomposition for data compression is the Tucker decomposition [29]. In [24], the authors introduced a tensor-product based representation of images and highlighted their processing. In [21], Papalexakis et al. used the CP tensor decomposition for the analysis of the local based social networks. This allowed the identification of hidden communities of users according to locations as tensors allow interaction analysis across several dimensions. In [2], Acar et al. proceeded to a data mining oriented analysis of internet chatroom communications for n-way analysis in multidimensional streaming data.

The related publications in the respective fields is indeed much more resourceful. We provided a brief overview which allows us to position our contribution in the context of related academic research. We presented several common denominators exist: firstly, all contributions employ a meticulously labeled dataset, with timed activities, and secondly for the authentication mostly supervised classifiers are used, recognizing a specific sequence or combination of movements. In this regards our aim is to propose a seamless system where the model training and evaluation is performed online without a prior calibration on special gestures. We will not label our dataset except for an identifier for the user. We cannot rely on classifiers for the evaluation of novel data, we require an unsupervised approach. The method of choice is built around tensor decomposition, since it is clear from the related work that the former is oftentimes performing well for the statistical modeling of data distributions. Furthermore is tensor decomposition computationally inexpensive for small tensor sizes. The novelty of this approach is the application of CP tensor decomposition on a set of totally unlabeled wristband sensor data, and the evaluation of the methodology for continuous authentication.

3 Methodology

The concepts of importance for this work are 9DOF quaternions and tensors, more specifically CP tensor decomposition. In a follow-up step the results from the CP decomposition are assessed using *Kullback Leibner Divergence* (KL), the Simpson's rule and the Cosine Similarity. The workflow underlying our methodology is described in the following.

3.1 9DOF-Quaternions

The sensors determining the orientation of an object are commonly called *Inertial Measurement Units* (IMU). Oftentimes employed in robotics or aerospace technology, identical sensors are now to be found in user devices as smartphones or body worn devices called wearables. IMUs typically include tri-axial accelerometers, tri-axis gyroscopes and tri-axis magnetometers. The above array of sensors is commonly called *MARG* sensors. Although physically only 6 *Degrees Of Freedom* (DOF) exist: 3 for rotations and 3 for translation. The term 9DOF in the context of inertial sensor hardware designates the degrees of freedom obtained when combining data from all sensors. Combining the 3DOFs from accelerometers, the 3DOFs from gyroscopes and 3DOFs from the magnetometers. The device orientation is expressed as a so called quaternion [4]. With 9DOF quaternions the device's orientation can be encoded with the consideration of the earth's cardinal points: north, south, east and west. Algorithms to derive 9DOF quaternions from MARG sensors are described in [14]. A quaternion q is expressed by:

$$q = a + bi + cj + dk \tag{1}$$

with $a \in \mathbb{R}$ being the scalar part describing the rotation to perform, and $\{b, c, d\}$ being factors of the imaginary parts characterizing the 3D vector around which the rotation is to be performed (also called the vector part). With $\{i, j, k\} \in \mathbb{C}$. To illustrate how quaternions encode orientation: given q from Eq. 1, and the Euler rotation around the X, Y, Z axis of respective angles Φ, Θ, Ψ q is:

$$\mathbf{q} = \begin{pmatrix} a \\ b \\ c \\ d \end{pmatrix} = \begin{pmatrix} \sin\Theta \cdot \sin\Psi \cdot \cos\Phi + \cos\Theta \cdot \cos\Psi \cdot \sin\Phi \\ \sin\Theta \cdot \cos\Psi \cdot \cos\Phi + \cos\Theta \cdot \sin\Psi \cdot \sin\Phi \\ \cos\Theta \cdot \sin\Psi \cdot \cos\Phi - \sin\Theta \cdot \cos\Psi \cdot \sin\Phi \\ \cos\Theta \cdot \cos\Psi \cdot \cos\Phi - \sin\Theta \cdot \sin\Psi \cdot \sin\Phi \end{pmatrix} \tag{2}$$

It can furthermore be shown that the values returned by the cos, sin products and additions are in the interval $[-1, 1]$ [4]. One of the assumptions of this work is that by considering the data distribution of the orientation of a sensor wristband it will be possible to uniquely identify the carrier. Assuming that most of the daily activities of a person are redundant, in example sitting at a desk or walking, the data distribution will describe a limited amount of large clusters with a multitude of small clusters. We estimate that this data distribution is unique for each person, due to different behavior, but also because of minimalistic differences in the posture and movements. In the next subsection we describe how we capture the data density using CP tensor decomposition.

3.2 CP Decomposition

Multidimensional arrays have been well known to computer scientists since the early age of computers. However, from linear algebra perspective, operations on multidimensional arrays had to be theoretically formalized. The idea was to formally extend the *Singular Value Decomposition* (SVD) of a matrix to n dimensions with $n \in \mathbb{N}$. SVD is the eigendecomposition of positive semi definite normal matrix factorization applied to real or complex matrices. The SVD n-dimension extension with CP decomposition has been introduced by Harshman and Caroll and Chang, respectively in [13] and [11]. Before we provide the in-depth explanation about how we apply CP decomposition for behavior profiling we introduce the operations involved in CP decomposition in general.

Common CP Decomposition Operations. Notations and formulations use Kolda and Bader's terminology from [16]. The chosen notation obeys the following rules: **(a)** Scalars are denoted by lower case letters: a. **(b)** Vectors are symbolized by boldface lowercase letters: **a**. **(c)** Matrices are denoted by boldface capital letters: **A**. **(d)** Euler script notations such as $\mathcal{X}$ are used for tensors.

Let $\mathcal{X} \in \mathbb{R}^{I_1 \times I_2 \times I_3 \times \ldots \times I_n}$ be defined as a n-th multidimensional array such as $\mathcal{X}$ is a tensor of order n. $\mathcal{X}$ can also be called a n-way tensor. The rank of a tensor $\mathcal{X} \in \mathbb{R}^{I_1 \times I_2 \times I_3 \times \ldots \times I_n}$, denoted by R, is the number of linear components that could fit $\mathcal{X}$ exactly such that

$$\mathcal{X} = \sum_{r=1}^{R} \mathbf{a}_r^{(1)} \circ \mathbf{a}_r^{(2)} \circ \ldots \circ \mathbf{a}_r^{(N)} \tag{3}$$

with the outer product between vectors denoted by $\circ$. The Frobenius norm of a tensor $\mathcal{X}$, denoted by $\parallel \mathcal{X} \parallel$, is defined as the square root of the sum of all tensor entries squared. Unfolding, or matricization, is the transformation of a n-way tensor into a matrix. The mode-n unfolding of the tensor $\mathcal{X} \in \mathbb{R}^{I_1 \times I_2 \times \ldots \times I_N}$, denoted $\mathbf{X}_{(n)}$, maps the $(i_1, ..., i_d)$ tensor element to a (i_n, j) matrix element.

The Khatri-Rao product between $\mathbf{A} \in \mathbb{R}^{I \times K}$ and $\mathbf{B} \in \mathbb{R}^{J \times K}$ is the column-wise Kronecker product, denoted by $\mathbf{A} \odot \mathbf{B}$, resulting in a matrix $\mathbf{C}$ of size $\mathbb{R}^{IJ \times K}$.

Description of CP Decomposition. The CP decomposition has been introduced by Harsman and Caroll and Chang in [13] and in [11]. A N-way tensor can be decomposed as a sum of rank-one tensors. In terms of equations, the tensor $\mathcal{X} \in \mathbb{R}^{I_1 \times I_2 \times \ldots \times I_N}$ of rank R can be decomposed using Eq. 4.

$$\mathcal{X} = \sum_{r=1}^{R} \mathbf{a}_r^{(1)} \circ \mathbf{a}_r^{(2)} \circ \cdots \circ \mathbf{a}_r^{(N)} \tag{4}$$

A three-way tensor $\mathcal{X} \in \mathbb{R}^{I_1 \times I_2 \times I_3}$ is represented in Fig. 2 with the notation $a^{(1)} = a$, $a^{(2)} = b$ and $a^{(3)} = c$. The sum of the rank-one tensors is determined by the resolution of the minimization equation

$$\min_{\hat{\mathcal{X}}} ||\mathcal{X} - \hat{\mathcal{X}}|| \tag{5}$$

with the approximate tensor denoted by $\hat{\mathcal{X}}$ and the original tensor denoted by $\mathcal{X}$. The *Alternating Least Squares* (ALS) method described by Harshman in [13] and Carroll and Chang in [11] allows the resolution of the Eq. 5 with an iterative multiplicative update rule. The update rule iterates each of the tensor order until a stopping criteria is satisfied. In the methodology, the stopping criteria ϵ is equal to the evolution of the norm of the approximate tensor with a 0.001 threshold.

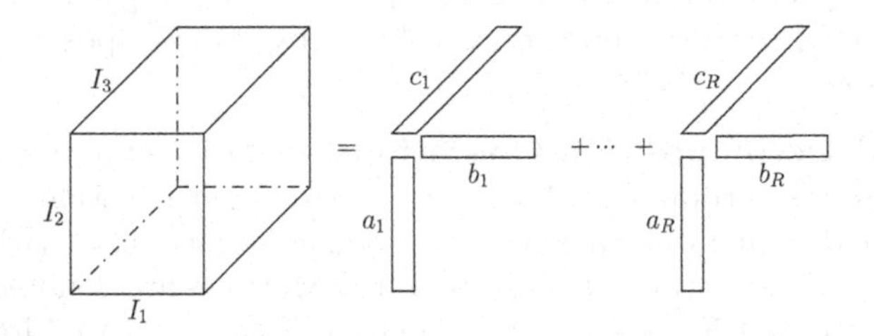

Fig. 2. Sum of rank-one tensors of a three-way tensor resulting from CP decomposition

However, the standard ALS procedure often leads to positive and negative entries in the rank-one tensors. It means that, although the convergence is well achieved, the post- treatment of the calculation is more complex. Therefore the CP decomposition is applied using the Lee and Seung's non-negative algorithm from [18]. For a three-way tensor $\mathcal{X} \in \mathbb{R}^{I_1 \times I_2 \times I_3}$ of rank R, the matrices $\mathbf{A} \in \mathbb{R}^{I_1 \times R}$, $\mathbf{B} \in \mathbb{R}^{I_2 \times R}$ and $\mathbf{C} \in \mathbb{R}^{I_3 \times R}$ are updated according to Eqs. 6.

$$\begin{cases} a_{ir} \leftarrow a_{ir} \dfrac{[\mathbf{X}_{(1)}\mathbf{Z}]_{ir}}{[\mathbf{A}\mathbf{Z}^T\mathbf{Z}]_{ir}} \quad , \quad \mathbf{Z} = (\mathbf{C} \odot \mathbf{B}) \\ b_{ir} \leftarrow b_{ir} \dfrac{[\mathbf{X}_{(2)}\mathbf{Z}]_{ir}}{[\mathbf{B}\mathbf{Z}^T\mathbf{Z}]_{ir}} \quad , \quad \mathbf{Z} = (\mathbf{C} \odot \mathbf{A}) \\ c_{ir} \leftarrow c_{ir} \dfrac{[\mathbf{X}_{(3)}\mathbf{Z}]_{ir}}{[\mathbf{C}\mathbf{Z}^T\mathbf{Z}]_{ir}} \quad , \quad \mathbf{Z} = (\mathbf{B} \odot \mathbf{A}) \end{cases} \tag{6}$$

The system of equations 6 has also been introduced by Welling and Weber in [30] and was first applied to image decompositions.

3.3 Identification of the Behavior Profiles

After the quaternion data has been used to build tensors for the CP decomposition, the similarity of the decompositions has to be assessed. Different data characteristics should be investigated for the comparison of the behavior profiles. First, a user could have performed the same activity recorded in different data sets which lead to similar data measures. Then, the same user could have an activity slightly different from one dataset to another one, for instance, different meetings scheduled at different time in different rooms. And, finally, the measures could come from two different users. Each of the measures described in the following is applied to the vectors of the rank one tensors obtained from CP decomposition. These vectors contain the information of a user's behavior profile.

Kullback-Leibler Divergence. The Kullback-Leibler (KL) divergence has been introduced in [17] by Kullback and Leibler as a directed divergence. The KL divergence is a measure of the difference between two probability distributions, P and Q, and it is denoted by $D_{KL}(P||Q)$. For discrete distributions, the KL divergence from Q to P is expressed as in Eq. 7.

$$D_{KL}(P||Q) = \sum_{k} P(k) log(\frac{P(k)}{Q(k)}) \tag{7}$$

Simpson's Rule and the Euclidean Distance. The Simpson's rule is a method of numerical integration. The integration interval $[a, b]$ is subdivided in n smaller intervals. On each of the n intervals the function is approximated with parabolas. In addition, for two vectors P and Q, the Euclidean distance is defined as the difference of the square root of the vectors. These two measures help to describe a unique behavior profile.

Cosine Similarity. The cosine similarity is a measure to evaluate the similarity of two vectors. For two vectors, P and Q, the cosine similarity is expressed by Eq. 8.

$$\text{cosine sim} = \frac{P \cdot Q}{\parallel P \parallel \ \parallel Q \parallel} \tag{8}$$

A cosine similarity of one means the vector P and Q are identical. By opposition, a cosine similarity of zero underlines no similarity between the two vectors.

To summarize our methodology: we arrange the quaternion data extracted from the movement sensors to build tensors. We apply the CP decomposition on the said quaternion data before using the extracted rank 1 vectors as input for an ensemble of distance and similarity measures namely: KL divergence, the Simpson's rule and the cosine similarity. The following section describes the user study we conducted to evaluate the methodology, together with the required data pre-processing steps and the impact certain parameters have on predictions.

4 Evaluation

In this section we apply the methodologies described in the previous section to a "real-world" dataset collected on our premises. As hardware, we employed the Shimmer 3 IMU sensor [10]. The data was collected with a pool of ten candidates each wearing the sensor mounted to the wrist of the dominant hand. We only collected data from right handed persons since we expected that by comparison data from left handed individuals would have innate disparity. For each user, the data was collected over 5 sessions of 4 h and 20 min, with the first and last 10 min being removed from the logged data. For each of the 10 subjects we posses 20 h of exploitable sensor data. The participants could move freely and were not asked to return an activity log. The time frames in which the data was recorded were the same on the 5 weekdays namely from 9:50am to 2:10pm, so that a large variation of activities was recorded between office work, meetings, or lunch time. The recordings are all collected from subjects active in the same line of work, implying similar activities for all participants. Records were sampled with a frequency of 60 Hz, which is also the sampling frequency of smartphone sensors on the highest setting. Hence, one hour of recordings contains $60 \cdot 60 \cdot 60 = 216.000$ rows. Finally, we were in possession of 6 different sensor bracelets, each day the respective subjects got a different device handed out, to ensure no hardware related bias impacts the behavior profiles. In other words, we want to make sure not to identify an unique device rather than the carrier. The average height of the participants is 182.4 cm (min: 170, max: 197, median: 179, sd: 8.5). The average age of the participants is 30 years (min: 26, max: 34, median: 29, sd: 2.7). For the extraction of 9DOF quaternions a detailed description of the algorithm is given in [1]. For the following we divided the data into one hour intervals. With 20 h of recordings from 10 users we possess 200 data samples. With *training set* we designate the dataset used: **(a)** to build a reference tensor for a user (2/3 of the training set), with which all other tensors are compared for identification, **(b)** for threshold calibration (1/3 of the training set).

4.1 From Quaternions to Tensors

Values for each quaternion unit are within the interval $I = [-1; 1]$. The set of quaternions is discretized according to a step length, denoted by h, with $h = 0.1$. This means the interval I is described as a union of subintervals of length h such as $I = I_1 \cup I_2 \cup \cdots \cup I_{20} = [-1; -0.9[\cup[-0.9; -0.8[\cup \cdots \cup [0.9; 1]$. Then, for each of the subintervals and for each unit, the number of quaternions is enumerated. Finally, for each unit, the list of the subintervals counts is aggregated within the tensor $\mathcal{X} \in \mathbb{R}^{M_1 \times M_2 \times M_3 \times M_4}$, with M_1 the dimension representing the discretization of the quaternions real numbers, M_2 the dimension of the i-unit discretization, M_3 the dimension of the j-unit discretization, and M_4 the dimension of the k-unit discretization.

In order to perform the CP decomposition on light devices, the tensor size should be limited but not too limited as it influences result quality. If the subintervals are decomposed with a 0.1 step length the resulting tensor has a size of $20 \times 20 \times 20 \times 20$. A step length of 0.04 would result in a $50 \times 50 \times 50 \times 50$, not to decompose by light devices anymore, but therefore containing a fine grained level of details.

In addition, in the initial simulations, different tensor ranks have been used for the CP decomposition. The accuracy of the tensor rank was measured as the difference between the original tensor and the approximated tensor. Observations showed that a tensor rank of five offers a good compromise between the accuracy of the results and the speed of calculation.

4.2 From Tensors to Behavior Profiles

After the quaternions discretization, the CP decomposition is applied to the four-way tensors containing the data. The identification of the behavior profiles is based on the results of the CP decomposition for each dimension, with the vectors a_i representing quaternions real numbers, b_i quaternions on i unit, c_i quaternions on j unit and d_i quaternions on k unit with subscript $i = \{1, ..., R\}$. For each dimension a_i, b_i, c_i and d_i, the set of measures described in the previous section is applied for the behavior profile identification. Between two data sets that have been factorized using CP decomposition, the sum over the rank R for each of the dimensions of the rank-one tensors is performed as the addition between the rank-one tensors is commutative as illustrated in Fig. 3. Then, for two decomposed tensors from two data sets, the Euclidean distance of the Simpson's rule is computed as well as the Kullback-Leibler divergence and the cosine similarity. Formal identification of the user behavior profile is assessed when at least two out of the three criteria are verified.

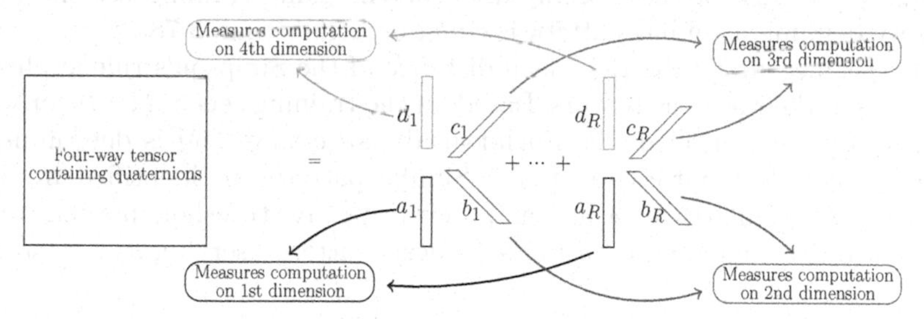

Fig. 3. The four-way tensor containing the discretized quaternions is decomposed using the CP model. Each dimension of the rank-one tensors highlights quaternion characteristics. The set of measures is applied to the sum of the vectors of each dimension of the rank-one tensors before comparison

4.3 Measures Computations for Pattern Comparison

In this section we investigate the adequacy of the employed measures on the vectors extracted from the tensors. A dataset of 30 samples is randomly chosen out of the 200 one hour sets after the quaternion discretization, evenly distributed over the subjects.

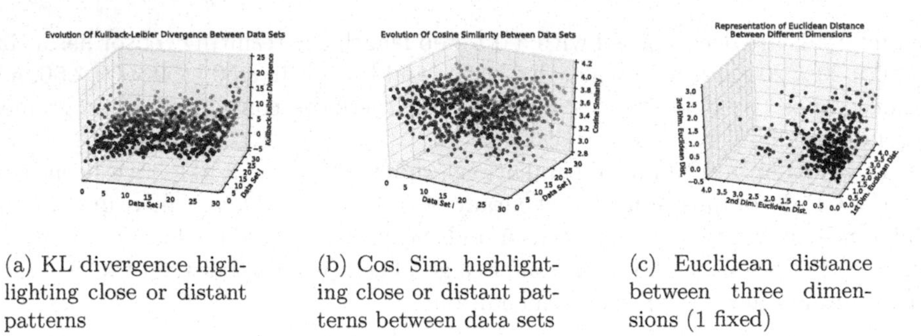

(a) KL divergence highlighting close or distant patterns

(b) Cos. Sim. highlighting close or distant patterns between data sets

(c) Euclidean distance between three dimensions (1 fixed)

Fig. 4. Shapes of the similarity measures graphs

The first of the three measures to highlight similar patterns is the KL divergence (7). A pairwise comparison of the KL divergences is performed resulting in a matrix of 900 entries. On Fig. 4a identical datasets are recognized at the zero level. In later experiments, with varying sizes of the training set as well as changing numbers of records in the dataset, a threshold of similarity is defined at 4 as the tensor is a 4-way tensor.

The cosine similarity, a symmetric distance, is the second measure used for the analysis of similar patterns between two datasets. For the same 30 data sets 450 cosine similarity are computed evolving between 0 and 4 due to the 4-way tensor and the non-negative algorithm. On Fig. 4b similar patterns between the tensor decompositions can be observed around the value 4. Again, the determination of the threshold for binary decisions: are two records similar or not depends of the size of the training set. For the same training set the cosine similarity defining a similar pattern is equal or higher than 3.78.

The last measure is the Euclidean distance of the Simpson's rule applied on the vectors of the rank-one tensors. Based on the training sets, and sets for which the same user is confirmed, the Euclidean distance threshold is determined as the 90% percentile and it is equal to 3.5. Similar patterns are identified around 0. Using the three similarity measures and their respective threshold novel incoming data records are compared to a user's "genesis pattern" serving as a reference.

4.4 Identification of Similar Behavior Profiles

The objective of this work is to assess rather a person different from the rightful owner is wearing a sensor wristband. A threshold per similarity measure has been set as described in the above. A training set of a fixed amount of one hour samples is transformed into a reference tensor to evaluate novel data. In the following we describe the results for a training set of 9 h, we later emphasize on the impact the training set size has on the predictions. The adequacy of the threshold is then evaluated with data from the same and also different users. To align our contribution with related publications we express the results with the terminology prevalent in the field: **(a)** True Acceptance Rate (TAR): The

Table 1. Results 0.1 discretization.

TAR	FAR	TRR	FRR
97%	12%	88%	3%

Table 2. Results 0.4 discretization.

TAR	FAR	TRR	FRR
100%	3%	97%	0%

ratio of users legitimately authenticated with the system. **(b)** False Acceptance Rate (FAR): The ratio of attempts erroneously granted access. **(c)** True Rejection Rate (TRR): The percentage of correctly rejected authentication attempts. **(d)** False Rejection Rate (FRR): The percentage of falsely rejected requests. The rendered decisions are binary, to assess if two dataset are coming from the same user, at least two similarity measures must be below their respective thresholds. With a training set of 9 hours per user, 11 untouched samples remained per user. To assess TAR/FAR for a total of 50 samples, in addition to the 11 h we selected 39 further 1 h sets starting from random timestamps in respective user datasets. For TRR/FRR we randomly sampled 50 one hour sets from other users. In total we ran $10 \times (50 + 50) = 1000$ comparisons.

The results of the computations are shown in Table 1. Our methodology achieves a TAR of 97% and a FAR of 12%. For TRR and FRR respective rates of 88% and 3% are achieved, indicating that in the majority of cases adversaries are successfully rejected, but denials remain less accurate. The quality of TAR and FAR rates depend on the size of the initial training sets. For less than five hours as training set the values for TAR and FRR can go down to 68% and 32% respectively. However, reliable results are obtained for training sets having more than 6 h worth of recordings. This is probably due to the fact that with a to small training set size not sufficiently enough independent records are available for the threshold calibration.

The most important metrics from a security aspect are a low FAR and FRR, to disable the use of the device by unauthorized individuals. If a users login is falsely rejected the device can still present additional challenges, such as passwords, for the login. The FAR of 12% is to increased for a security use case. We therefore repeat the experiment with a finer quaternion step discretization of 0.04. Because the data previously assigned to one of the 0.1 intervals, is now distributed over at least two 0.04 intervals. It is esteemed that the tensors will carry a finer grained precision. The objective is to observe if a smaller discretization step could lead to lower FAR rates and better overall accuracy. With 0.04 discretization steps the tensor size becomes $50 \times 50 \times 50 \times 50$. In Table 2, the results of this simulation are displayed. For the same datasets and methodology as for the previous experiment, with a 0.04 discretization a TAR of 100% is observed and consequently a FRR of 0%. For the task of recognizing a same user a perfect score has been achieved. Likewise FAR and TRR have strongly improved, scores of 3% and 97% have been obtained, which gives a higher confidence for a security use case. With a smaller discretization steps it is possible to implement safer access control mechanisms. However, the computational complexity is not supported by light devices. More powerful multi-core CPUs are required for that level of precision.

5 Conclusion and Future Work

In this paper, 9DOF Quaternions have been used for the determination of a device orientation in a Galilean referential. Quaternions have then been transposed to four dimensional tensors. The CP tensor decomposition has been applied for further data analysis with a set of three similarity measures, the KL divergence, the cosine similarity, and the Euclidean distance on the Simpson's rule for the identification of similar CP decompositions. For each similarity measure the calibration of their respective thresholds has been defined on data sets for which the user identity is confirmed. For the matching of the behavior profiles majority voting consensus requires that at least two measures are below their respective calibrated threshold, in order to acknowledge that two CP decompositions are from the same user. When changing the quaternion discretization step the accuracy of predictions is impacted. With a setting where computations are still feasible on a light device a good confidence in predictions is obtained. With a fine grained discretization for more powerful CPU workloads, almost perfect scores have been achieved with regards to TAR, FAR, TRR and FRR.

We showed that our introduced approach for behavioral authentication is performing well on data free of any activity labels. Although with this work we barely scratched on the surface of what can be achieved with the proposed methodology. We believe that the shown results are encouraging, especially since the impact of a large number of parameters has not been investigated yet. We are for instance interested in examining how the prediction performance evolves when recordings are divided into smaller sliding windows of 30, 15 or even 5 min. We are also planning on further investigating the impact of quaternion discretization to totally assess the relation between prediction accuracy, computational complexity, and training set size. Finally, we are outlining to extend our field study with a larger amount of subjects, but also in a context of streaming analytics, with varying tensor sizes for large scale CPU and even GPU calculations.

References

1. Shimmer 9DoF documentation (2016). https://goo.gl/9msLu6
2. Acar, E., Çamtepe, S.A., Krishnamoorthy, M.S., Yener, B.: Modeling and multiway analysis of chatroom tensors. In: Kantor, P., Muresan, G., Roberts, F., Zeng, D.D., Wang, F.-Y., Chen, H., Merkle, R.C. (eds.) ISI 2005. LNCS, vol. 3495, pp. 256–268. Springer, Heidelberg (2005). doi:10.1007/11427995_21
3. Al-Bajjari, A.L., Yuan, L.: Optimized authentication scheme for web application. In: 2016 IEEE 9th International Conference on Service-Oriented Computing and Applications (SOCA), pp. 52–58, November 2016
4. Altmann, S.: Rotations, Quaternions, and Double Groups. Dover Books on Mathematics. Dover Publications, New York (2005)
5. Aviv, A.J., Gibson, K., Mossop, E., Blaze, M., Smith, J.M.: Smudge attacks on smartphone touch screens. In: Proceedings of the 4th USENIX Conference on Offensive Technologies, WOOT 2010, pp. 1–7. USENIX Association, Berkeley (2010)

6. Bentley, J.L.: Multidimensional binary search trees used for associative searching. Commun. ACM **18**(9), 509–517 (1975)
7. Bonneau, J., Herley, C., van Oorschot, P.C., Stajano, F.: The quest to replace passwords: a framework for comparative evaluation of web authentication schemes. In: 2012 IEEE Symposium on Security and Privacy, pp. 553–567, May 2012
8. Boser, B.E., Guyon, I.M., Vapnik, V.N.: A training algorithm for optimal margin classifiers. In: Proceedings of the Fifth Annual Workshop on Computational Learning Theory, pp. 144–152. ACM, New York (1992)
9. Breiman, L.: Random forests. Mach. Learn. **45**(1), 5–32 (2001)
10. Burns, A., Greene, B.R., McGrath, M.J., O'Shea, T.J., Kuris, B., Ayer, S.M., Stroiescu, F., Cionca, V.: Shimmer; a wireless sensor platform for noninvasive biomedical research. IEEE Sens. J. **10**(9), 1527–1534 (2010)
11. Carroll, J.D., Chang, J.J.: Analysis of individual differences in multidimensional scaling via an n-way generalization of Eckart-Young decomposition. Psychometrika **35**(3), 283–319 (1970)
12. Feng, T., Liu, Z., Kwon, K.A., Shi, W., Carbunar, B., Jiang, Y., Nguyen, N.: Continuous mobile authentication using touchscreen gestures. In: 2012 IEEE Conference on Technologies for Homeland Security, pp. 451–456, November 2012
13. Harshman, R.A.: Foundations of the PARAFAC procedure: models and conditions for an "explanatory" multi-modal factor analysis (1970)
14. Hu, J.S., Sun, K.C.: A robust orientation estimation algorithm using MARG sensors. IEEE Trans. Instrum. Meas. **64**(3), 815–822 (2015)
15. Keller, J.M., Gray, M.R., Givens, J.A.: A fuzzy k-nearest neighbor algorithm. IEEE Trans. Syst. Man Cybernet. SMC **15**(4), 580–585 (1985)
16. Kolda, T.G., Bader, B.W.: Tensor decompositions and applications. SIAM Rev. **51**(3), 455–500 (2009)
17. Kullback, S., Leibler, R.A.: On information and sufficiency. Ann. Math. Stat. **22**(1), 79–86 (1951)
18. Lee, D.D., Seung, H.S.: Learning the parts of objects by non-negative matrix factorization. Nature **401**(6755), 788–791 (1999)
19. Mahfoodh, A.T., Radha, H.: Compression of image ensembles using tensor decomposition. In: Picture Coding Symposium, pp. 21–24. IEEE (2013)
20. Nickel, C., Wirtl, T., Busch, C.: Authentication of smartphone users based on the way they walk using k-nn algorithm. In: 2012 Eighth International Conference on Intelligent Information Hiding and Multimedia Signal Processing, pp. 16–20, July 2012
21. Papalexakis, E.E., Pelechrinis, K., Faloutsos, C.: Location based social network analysis using tensors and signal processing tools. In: 2015 IEEE 6th International Workshop on Computational Advances in Multi-Sensor Adaptive Processing (CAMSAP), pp. 93–96. IEEE (2015)
22. Parate, A., Chiu, M.C., Chadowitz, C., Ganesan, D., Kalogerakis, E.: RISQ: recognizing smoking gestures with inertial sensors on a wristband. In: Proceedings of the 12th Annual International Conference on Mobile Systems, Applications, and Services, MobiSys 2014, pp. 149–161. ACM, New York (2014)
23. Pietro, R.D., Me, G., Strangio, M.A.: A two-factor mobile authentication scheme for secure financial transactions. In: International Conference on Mobile Business (ICMB 2005), pp. 28–34, July 2005
24. Rövid, A., Szeid, L., Rudas, I., Várlaki, P.: Image processing on tensor-product basis. Obuda Univ. e-Bull. **2**(1), 247–258 (2011)

25. Roy, A., Memon, N., Ross, A.: MasterPrint: exploring the vulnerability of partial fingerprint-based authentication systems. IEEE Trans. Inf. Forensics Secur. **PP**(99), 1 (2017)
26. Rybnicek, M., Lang-Muhr, C., Haslinger, D.: A roadmap to continuous biometric authentication on mobile devices. In: 2014 International Wireless Communications and Mobile Computing Conference (IWCMC), pp. 122–127, August 2014
27. Silva, D.F., Batista, G.: Speeding up all-pairwise dynamic time warping matrix calculation, pp. 837–845
28. Song, C., Wang, A., Ren, K., Xu, W.: EyeVeri: a secure and usable approach for smartphone user authentication. In: IEEE INFOCOM 2016 - The 35th Annual IEEE International Conference on Computer Communications, pp. 1–9, April 2016
29. Tucker, L.R.: Some mathematical notes on three-mode factor analysis. Psychometrika **31**(3), 279–311 (1966)
30. Welling, M., Weber, M.: Positive tensor factorization. Pattern Recogn. Lett. **22**(12), 1255–1261 (2001)
31. Yi, S., Qin, Z., Novak, E., Yin, Y., Li, Q.: GlassGesture: exploring head gesture interface of smart glasses. In: IEEE INFOCOM 2016 - The 35th Annual IEEE International Conference on Computer Communications, pp. 1–9, April 2016
32. Zhu, H., Hu, J., Chang, S., Lu, L.: ShakeIn: secure user authentication of smartphones with habitual single-handed shakes. IEEE Trans. Mob. Comput. **PP**(99), 1 (2017)

An Approach for Identifying Author Profiles of Blogs

Chunxia Zhang[1(✉)], Yu Guo[1], Jiayu Wu[1], Shuliang Wang[1], Zhendong Niu[2], and Wen Cheng[3]

[1] School of Software, Beijing Institute of Technology, Beijing, China
{cxzhang,2220160601,2220160656,slwang2011}@bit.edu.cn
[2] School of Computer Science, Beijing Institute of Technology, Beijing, China
zniu@bit.edu.cn
[3] School of Aerospace Engineering, Beijing Institute of Technology, Beijing, China
572705622@qq.com

Abstract. Author profile identification has been an important research problem in the areas of web mining, network public opinion monitoring and social network analysis. The aim of this problem is to identify characteristics or traits of authors of textual information such as blogs, microblogs or reviews in social network platforms or commercial platforms. The technology of author profile identification can be employed into many applications including cyberspace forensics, electronic commerce and information security. In this paper, we propose a hybrid framework or technique to solve the author profile identification problem. In this framework, we design a distributed integrated representation approach of blogs based on Doc2vec and term frequency-inverse document frequency, and apply the convolutional neural network to predict age, gender and education status of authors of blogs. The benefit of our technique is that it predicts three different traits of authors in a uniform way, is an unsupervised method which can learn representation vectors of blog posts based on unlabeled data, and does not need any syntactic and semantic parsing of sentences. Experimental results on blogs show that our approach achieves a promising performance.

Keywords: Author profile identification · Doc2vec · Convolutional neural network · Age prediction · Gender prediction · Education status prediction

1 Introduction

The task of author profile identification or author profiling is to identify characteristics or traits of authors of textual information such as blogs, microblogs, or reviews in social network platforms or commercial platforms. The traits of authors consist of age, gender, location, education status and native language and so on. Author profile identification is an important research problem in the areas of web mining, network public opinion monitoring, social network analysis and opinion mining.

G. Cong et al. (Eds.): ADMA 2017, LNAI 10604, pp. 475–487, 2017.
https://doi.org/10.1007/978-3-319-69179-4_33

The author profile identification technology can be used into many application areas including cyberspace forensics, electronic commerce and information security [1–5]. For example, the author profiling technique can be great helpful to distinguish identity of Internet crimers who may commit network theft and fraud, terrorism, or child predation through social media [1,6]. In addition, the author profiling can be highly beneficial for targeted marketing and advertising, product and service development, product and service review mining [7]. However, it is difficult to fulfill the author profile identification task through manual recognition and detection [6]. Therefore, this paper aims to identify age, gender and educational status of authors of blogs.

As a text genre in social media, blogs have two main characteristics: (1) sentences within blogs maybe contain a lot of non-standard, informal or spoken words, phrases and language usages. For instance, there are abbreviations, internet slangs, or emoticons in texts of blogs. (2) Unlike novels, books or other traditional documents, there are various topics within blog posts, and blog entries are relatively short with personal or subjective thoughts and views.

The key difficulties of solving the author profile identification problem are given as follows: (1) which features are extracted to identify different traits of authors of blogs such as age, gender and education status, and those features are independent of specific topics of blog posts; (2) how to design a uniform generation method of blog representation and a uniform identification method to predict different traits of authors of Internet documents.

In this paper, we propose a hybrid framework or technique to fulfill the author profile identification task. In this framework, we design a distributed integrated representation approach of blogs based on Doc2vec and term frequency-inverse document frequency (TF-IDF), and apply the convolutional neural network to recognize age, gender and education status of authors of blogs. First, we utilize a document representation method based on Doc2vec to generate the distributed representation of blog posts. Second, we construct the representation of blog posts based on TF-IDF. Third, we build the distributed integrated representation of blog posts in terms of the former two kinds of generated representation. Finally, we use the convolutional neural network (CNN) to predict traits of authors of blogs. Experimental results on blogs show that our technique obtains a high performance and outperforms the baseline method.

The main contributions of this paper are given as follows. (1) We propose a distributed integrated representation method for blogs. That method does not rely on any syntactic and semantic parsing of blog posts, and can capture semantic associations between words in sentences and topics of blog posts. Moreover, that representation approach is an unsupervised one which can learn blog post vectors based on unlabeled data. (2) This paper offers a promising technique to identify the age, gender and education status of authors of blogs in a uniform way, that is, it provides a unified pipeline to accomplish the author profile identification task. Experimental results demonstrate that our hybrid technique including Doc2vec, TF-IDF and convolutional neural network outperforms the baseline method, and achieves the higher performance than those of the blog representation method based on TF-IDF or Doc2vec by using decision tree, random forest, and sequential minimal optimization.

The rest of the paper is organized as follows. Section 2 discusses related works about author profile identification. Section 3 presents our approach to solving the author profile identification task. Experimental results are given in Sect. 4. Section 5 concludes the paper and discusses future works.

2 Related Works

The problem of author profile identification or author trait prediction in most works is treated as a two-class or multi-class text classification problem. There have been lots of works on gender identification of authors of blogs, microblogs, news texts, e-mails or PhD theses [1,2,8–16].

Argamon et al. [2] first built style-related features about function words and part-of-speech, and content-based features about the most frequent words to express documents. Further, they used the Bayesian Multinomial Regression to identify age, gender, personality and native language of writers of blogs. Mukherjee and Liu [12] proposed a kind of features about part-of-speech sequence patterns to represent documents, and used support vector machine classification, support vector machine regression and Naive Bayes to identify the gender of blog authors. In addition, the work of Mikros [11] was to predict the gender of authors of Greek blogs. They built features about the most frequent words, character n-grams and stylometric variables, and adopted support vector machine to classify the gender of writers. Furthermore, Ansari et al. [9] constructed three mutual independent features about frequency counter, TF-IDF of tokens and part-of-speech, and then used ZeroR and Naive Bayes to classify gender of blog authors.

Ramnial et al. [8] extracted features about combined-words, words endings, function words, part-of-speech tags and statistics of characters, words, sentences and punctuations as stylometric features of PhD theses, and applied two classifiers of k-nearest neighbour and support vector machine to predict the gender of writers of those PhD theses. Wang et al. [10] first developed two classifiers based on features about user names and microblog texts, respectively. Further, they employed the Bayes rule to integrate two classifiers to recognize the gender of microblog authors. Moreover, Cheng et al. [1] proposed 545 character-based features, word-based features including psycho-linguistic words, syntactic features, structural features and function words including gender-preferential words to represent documents. Three machine learning approaches of support vector machine, Bayesian logistic regression and AdaBoost decision tree were utilized to distinguish the gender of authors of news texts and e-mails.

Relatively, there is a small amount of works on age and education status predication of writers of Internet texts [2,16,17]. Nguyen et al. [17] used a logical and linear regression algorithm to classify Twitter users into three age categories (20−, 20–40, 40+). In addition, Alvarez-Carmona et al. [16] extracted features based on second order attributes and latent semantic analysis to express texts in Twitter, and applied the support vector machine to predict the gender, age and personality of authors.

3 An Approach of Identifying Author Profiles of Blogs

3.1 Problem Formulation

The definition of author profile identification task in this paper is given as follows.

Definition 1 (Author Profile Identification Task). Given a set of authors with known age, gender and education status and their blogs, the author profile identification or author profiling task is to identify the age, gender and education status of authors of anonymous blog posts. In other words, an anonymous blog post is assigned to one of four classes in the set C_{age}, one of two classes in the set C_{gender}, and one of three class in the set $C_{education}$, as shown in (1), respectively.

$$\begin{aligned} C_{age} &= \{25-,\ 26-40,\ 41-60,\ 60+\} \\ C_{gender} &= \{male,\ female\} \\ C_{education} &= \{postgraduate,\ undergraduate,\ others\} \end{aligned} \quad (1)$$

3.2 Overview of Our Framework

In general, our author profile identification framework or technique of age, gender and education status consists of four steps, as shown in Fig. 1. (1) Crawling and

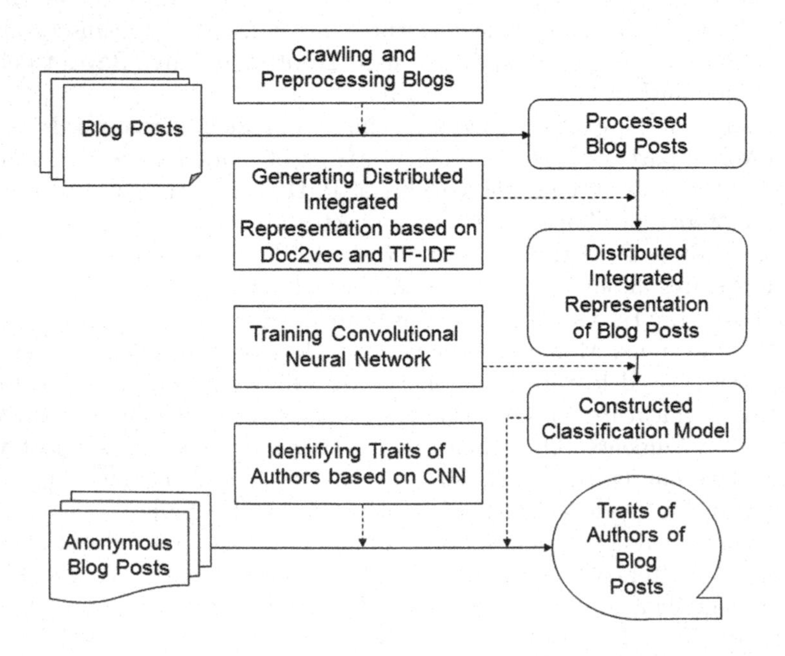

Fig. 1. The framework of our author profile identification of blogs

processing blogs to obtain a set of blogs of authors with known age, gender and education status. (2) Building text representation based on Doc2vec and TF-IDF to generate the distributed integrated representation of blog posts. (3) Training the convolutional neural network (CNN) to construct the classification model. (4) Identifying traits of authors of anonymous blog posts based on the trained CNN classification model.

3.3 Generating Distributed Integrated Representation of Blog Posts Based on Doc2vec and TF-IDF

The process of generating vectors of blog posts in this paper is illustrated on the upper part of Fig. 2 [18]. For a blog post, we first learn its distributed representation vector u based on Doc2vec [18]. Second, we build the vector w of each blog post based on TF-IDF values of feature words. Third, we fuse those two vectors to generate the distributed integrated representation of blog posts.

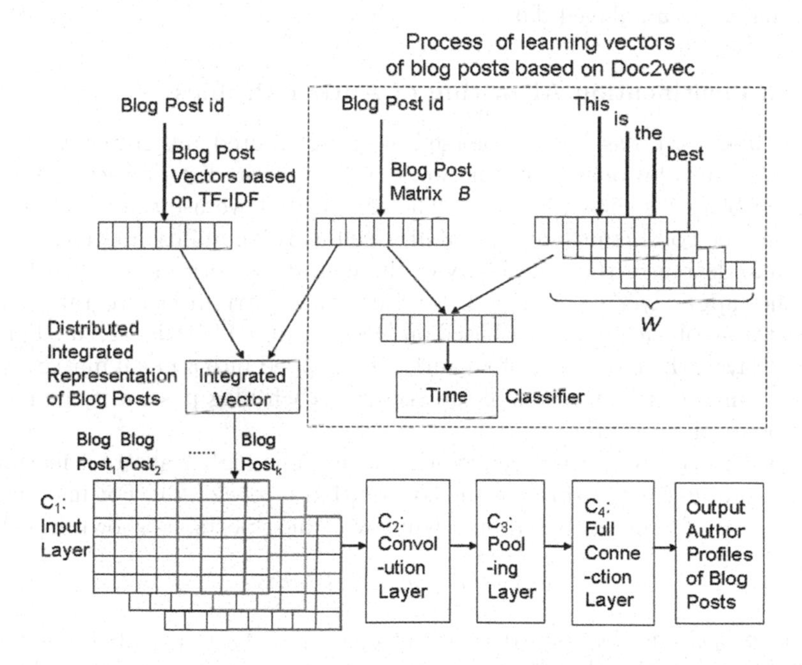

Fig. 2. The process of our approach to identify author profiles of blogs.

In Fig. 2, each blog post within blogs of an author is viewed as a document. Every blog post and every word in blog posts corresponds to a unique vector. The matrix B in Fig. 2 is composed of vectors of different blog posts, where a column in B denotes a blog post. In addition, the matrix W in Fig. 2 is made up of vectors of different words, where a column in W expresses a word.

The core idea of Doc2vec is to extend word embedding to document embedding, that is, it is an extension of Word2vec [18–21]. Actually, document embedding can generate vectors of sentences, paragraphs, or documents. Word2vec aims to build the word embedding based on contexts of words in sentences. In other words, the goal of word2vec is to construct a vector for each word according to its contextual words within sentences. The difference between Doc2vec and Word2vec is that a document vector is introduced into word2vec to capture the topic of the document or the missing information of the current context [18].

The reasons that we employed Doc2vec and TF-IDF to generate distributed vectors of blog posts are given as follows [18–21]. (1) Doc2vec is an unsupervised approach which can generate vector representations of different length of blog posts. (2) The distributed vector representations of blog posts are intended to capture semantic associations between words in sentences. (3) The blog representation based on TF-IDF highlights the differences between stylistic word features of blogs with different traits of authors. (4) We do not need any syntactic and semantic parsing on sentences in blogs, since Doc2vec learns document vectors based on unlabeled data.

3.4 An Identification Algorithm of Author Profiles

When a blog post has been expressed as a distributed integrated vector, we employ the convolutional neural network (CNN) to predict profiles or traits of authors of blogs, as shown in Fig. 2. The reason that we use the CNN model is that it has the good fault tolerance ability, self learning ability and local sensing ability, and decreases the complexity of the neural network models [22,23].

In the input layer C_1 in Fig. 2, we build the distributed integrated vector representation of each blog post based on Doc2vec and TF-IDF [22,23]. Through the input layer, the blog posts of an author is mapped into a $m \times n$ matrix, where m is the number of dimensions of the vector of each blog post, n is the number of blog posts of this author.

The layer C_2 in Fig. 2 is a convolution layer. The higher abstract features of blog posts are extracted through the convolution layer [22,23]. For instance, we can generate a feature d_i based on a window of blog posts, as shown in (2).

$$d_i = f(W * v_{i:i+h-1} + b) \tag{2}$$

Here, $v_{i:i+h-1}$ is the concatenation of $v_i, v_{i+1}, ..., v_{i+h-1}$, v_i is the vector of the i-th blog post, the filter W and b are parameters of the convolutional kernel, and f is a non-linear function. Further, we build a feature map shown in (3) by executing convolution on all possible windows of blog posts.

$$d = (d_1,\ d_2,\ ...,\ d_{n-h+1}) \tag{3}$$

In the pooling layer C_3 in Fig. 2, we obtain distinct features v_{max} of blog posts, shown in (4), by performing the max-pooling operation over the feature map [22,23].

$$v_{max} = max\{v_1,\ v_2,\ ...,\ v_n\} \tag{4}$$

Further, those distinct features are input into the full connection layer C_4 in Fig. 2 with dropout and softmax. And we can get the probability distribution over different trait classes for blog posts [22,23]. Now, we give our author profile identification algorithm in Algorithm 1.

Algorithm 1. *Identifying Author Profiles of Blogs*

Input: The blog posts B of anonymous authors.
Output: The age, gender and education status of authors of blog posts in B.

1: **for** $b_i \in B$, i=1, 2,..., n **do**
2: Use a word segmentation tool to separate words in sentences in the blog post b_i.
3: Generate the distributed vector representation u_i of b_i based on Doc2vec.
4: Build the vector w_i of b_i based on TF-IDF.
5: Construct the distributed integrated representation (u_i,w_i) of b_i.
6: **end for**
7: Classify the author of each blog post into one class in C_{age}, C_{gender} and $C_{education}$ based on the convolutional neural network(CNN) in a uniform pipeline.

4 Experiments

4.1 Experimental Results

In our experiments, we downloaded Chinese blogs of fifty-two famous persons with about 8700 blog posts from the website "http://www.sina.com.cn/" for evaluation of our technique. That website is one of the biggest portal sites in China, and Sina blog is one of the most popular blog channels in China. The number of blog posts of each author is ranging from 15 to 675. In order to build datasets as balanced as possible, we selected three different sets of downloaded blog posts as the datasets for gender, education status and age identification. The dataset used in the experiment of gender identification of authors of blog posts include more than 5100 blog posts of twenty-four persons, the dataset for education status identification consists of more than 4900 blog posts of thirty-four persons, and the dataset for age identification contains more than 5200 blog posts of thirty-two persons. The ten-fold cross validation is used to evaluate the performance of our author profiles identification technique. The baseline method is one which builds vectors of blog posts based on TF-IDF and employs the decision tree J48 to deal with the author profile identification task.

Table 1 gives the identification accuracy of gender, education status and age of authors of blogs by using our proposed technique in this paper and nine approaches which are combinations of three kinds of representation methods of blog posts and three types of prediction methods of authors' traits. Those three kinds of representation methods of blog posts include representations based on TF-IDF, Doc2vec, and the integration of TF-IDF and Doc2vec. Those three types of prediction methods of authors' traits consist of the decision tree J48 (DT), random forest (RF), and sequential minimal optimization (SMO). For example, the fifth method "Doc2vec ⊕ SMO" in Table 1 means one which constructs vectors of blog posts according to Doc2vec and utilizes SMO to recognize author profiles of authors of blog posts. Here, SMO is an optimization method for training support vector machines [24]. In Table 1, the dimensions of representation vectors of blog posts based on TF-IDF for gender, education status and age identification is 501, 503, 503, respectively. And the dimensions of representation vectors of blog posts based on Doc2vec in Table 1 is 1000.

Table 1. The identification accuracy of gender, education status and age of authors of blogs

NO.	Accuracy (%)	Gender	Education status	Age
1	Baseline (TF-IDF ⊕ DT)	90.6371	87.0040	90.0661
2	TF-IDF ⊕ SMO	86.1583	82.4899	89.0652
3	TF-IDF ⊕ RF	85.3861	83.5830	87.6865
4	Doc2vec ⊕ DT	83.9575	61.8421	66.0812
5	Doc2vec ⊕ SMO	98.2046	90.0607	96.3362
6	Doc2vec ⊕ RF	94.4981	83.1781	94.0321
7	Doc2vec ⊕ TF-IDF ⊕ DT	89.4208	82.2672	91.1237
8	Doc2vec ⊕ TF-IDF ⊕ SMO	98.0309	97.6721	98.3947
9	Doc2vec ⊕ TF-IDF ⊕ RF	95.2317	94.1498	95.5052
10	Our Approach (Doc2vec ⊕ TF-IDF ⊕ CNN)	99.9676	97.7473	96.3197

The experimental results in Table 1 indicate that the following facts. (1) our hybrid technique achieves the highest identification accuracy of gender and education status than those of other nine kinds of approaches, and obtains the higher identification accuracy of age than those of other seven types of methods (i.e., the 1st, 2nd, 3rd, 4th, 6th, 7th and 9th methods). (2) Our distributed integrated representation of TF-IDF and Doc2vec gets the higher accuracy than those of blog post representation based on TF-IDF or Doc2vec by using SMO and RF for age and education status identification.

4.2 Parameters Analysis

We analyse the performance influence of different dimensions of representation vectors of blog posts. The vector of blog posts based on Doc2vec are set as 50, 100, 200, 300, 500, 800 and 1000 dimensions. The vector of blog posts based on TF-IDF are set up from 301 to 5003 dimensions. Figures 3, 4 and 5 give the accuracy curves of our hybrid technique and the accuracy curves of DT, RF and

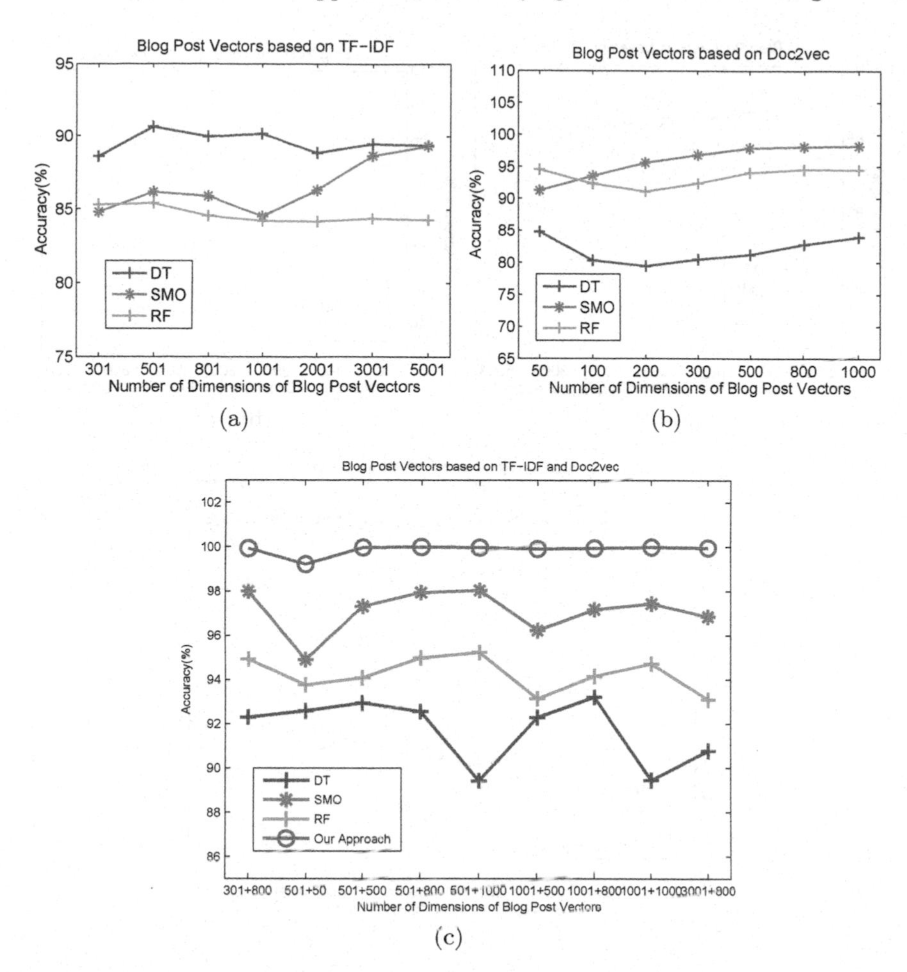

Fig. 3. The gender identification accuracy of different methods. (a) The accuracies with different dimensions of the blog post vectors obtained by TF-IDF; (b) The accuracies with different dimensions of the blog post vectors obtained by Doc2vec; (c) The accuracies achieved by combing together the features obtained respectively by TF-IDF and Doc2vec with different dimensions of the blog post vectors. For example, "301 + 800" means that the features of 301 dimensions obtained by TF-IDF and the features of 800 dimensions obtained by Doc2vec are combined together.

SMO by representing blog posts based on TF-IDF, Dov2vec and the distributed integrated representation of TF-IDF and Doc2vec, respectively.

We can see the following facts from Figs. 3, 4 and 5. (1) The gender prediction accuracy of SMO is higher than those of DT and RF based on two kinds of blog representation methods in most cases of Fig. 3(b) and (c). Those two kinds of blog representation methods include representations based on Doc2vec and the integration of TF-IDF and Doc2vec. This fact holds for the education status identification in most cases of Fig. 4(b) and (c) and for the age identification

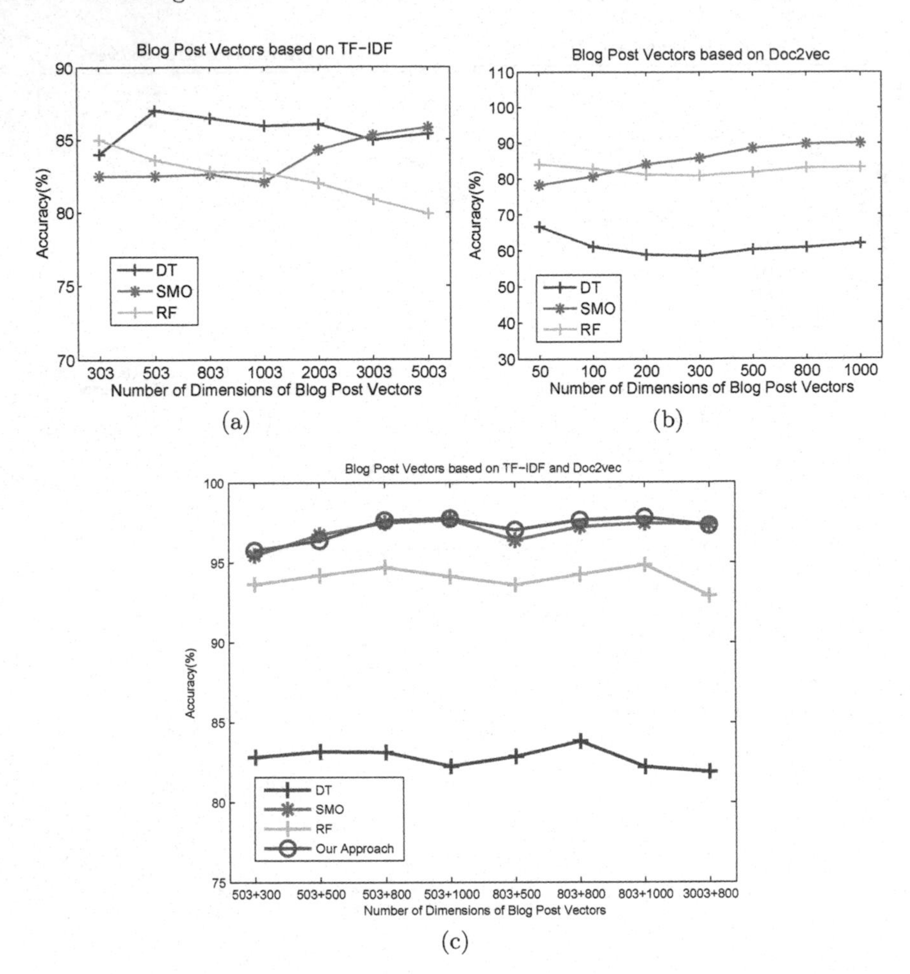

Fig. 4. The education status identification accuracy of different methods. (a) The accuracies with different dimensions of the blog post vectors obtained by TF-IDF; (b) The accuracies with different dimensions of the blog post vectors obtained by Doc2vec; (c) The accuracies achieved by combing together the features obtained respectively by TF-IDF and Doc2vec with different dimensions of the blog post vectors. For instance, "503 + 300" means that the features of 503 dimensions obtained by TF-IDF and the features of 300 dimensions obtained by Doc2vec are combined together.

in most cases of Fig. 5(b) and (c). (2) In general, our hybrid technique obtains the highest accuracy of the gender and education status identification in Figs. 3 and 4. Specifically, the identification accuracy of gender of blog authors by using our approach gets about 99.987%, while the identification accuracy of education status with our algorithm achieves about 97.826%.

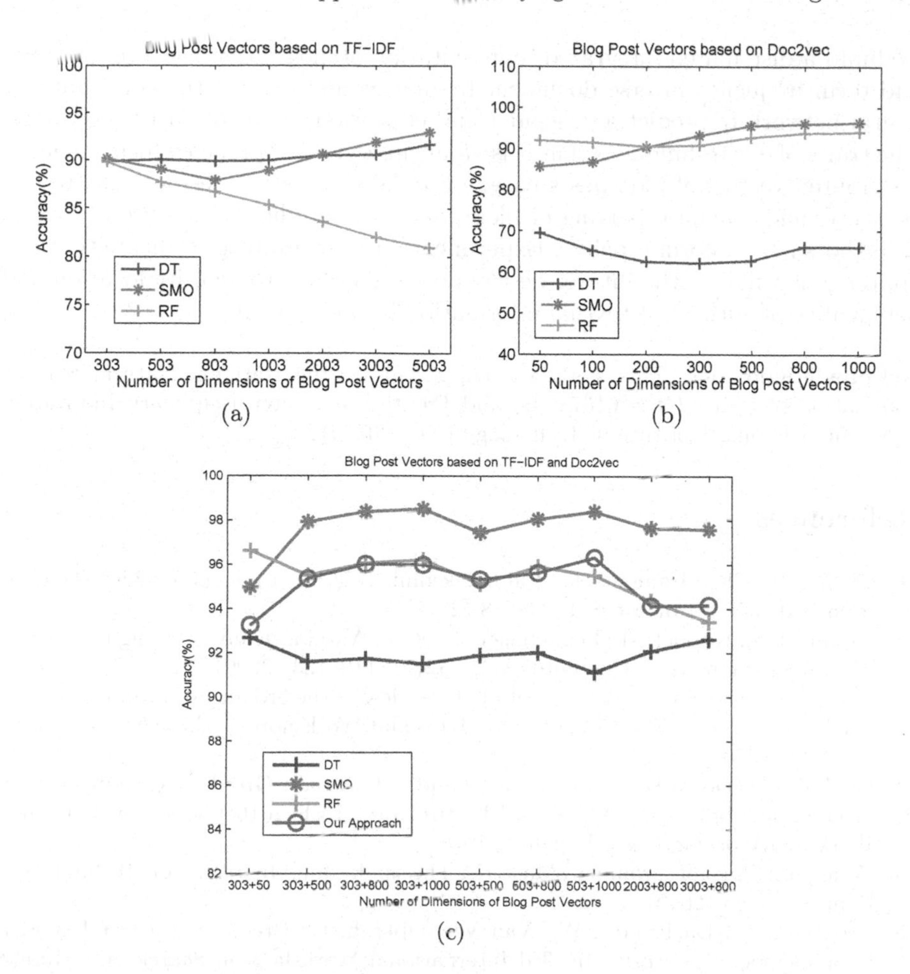

Fig. 5. The age identification accuracy of different methods. (a) The accuracies obtained by TF-IDF with different dimensions of the blog post vectors; (b) The accuracies obtained by Doc2vec approach with different dimensions of the blog post vectors; (c) The accuracies achieved by combing together the features obtained respectively by TF-IDF and Doc2vec approach with different dimensions of the blog post vectors. For example, "303 + 50" means that the features of 303 dimensions obtained by TF-IDF and the features of 50 dimensions obtained by Doc2vec are combined together.

5 Conclusion

More and more efforts have been paid on author profile identification or author profiling from Internet documents such as microblogs, blogs and product reviews. The author profile identification technology has wide applications containing cyberspace forensics, electronic commerce, information recommendation and information security. In this paper, a hybrid framework or technique is proposed to solve the author profile identification task. Specifically, in this framework, we build a distributed integrated representation of blog posts based on Doc2vec and term frequency-inverse document frequency, and employ the convolutional neural network to predict age, gender and education status of authors of blogs. The traits of our technique is that it is an unsupervised approach which can learn distributed vectors of blog posts based on unlabeled data, does not require any syntactic and semantic parsing of blog posts, and predict three different traits of authors in a uniform pipeline. Experimental results on blogs indicate that our approach is valid. In the future, we will design methods to identify location and personality of authors of textual information in social media.

Acknowledgements. This work was supported by the National Natural Science Foundation of China (NO. 61672098) and Frontier and Interdisciplinary Innovation Program of Beijing Institute of Technology (NO. 3080012291701).

References

1. Cheng, N., Chandramouli, R., Subbalakshmi, K.P.: Author gender identification from text. Digital Invest. **8**(1), 78–88 (2011)
2. Argamon, S., Koppel, M., Pennebaker, J., et al.: Automatically profiling the author of an anonymous text. Commun. ACM **52**(2), 119–123 (2009)
3. Rangel, F., Rosso, C., Fabio, M., et al.: Overview of the 3rd author profiling task at PAN 2015. In: CLEF 2015 Evaluation Labs and Workshop Working Notes Papers, pp. 1–8 (2015)
4. Op Vollenbroek, M.B., Carlotto, T., Kreutz, T., et al.: GronUP: Groningen user profiling notebook for PAN at CLEF 2016. In: CLEF 2016 Evaluation Labs and Workshop Working Notes Papers (2016)
5. Wang, L.: Author profiling. Master's Thesis. Beijing Institute of Technology, Beijing, China (2013)
6. Peersman, C., Daelemans, W., Van Vaerenbergh, L.: Predicting age and gender in online social networks. In: 3rd International Workshop on Search and Mining User-Generated Contents, pp. 37–44 (2011)
7. Zhang, C., Zhang, P.: Predicting gender from blog posts (2010). http://web.stanford.edu/~pyzhang/papers/gender_prediction.pdf
8. Ramnial, H., Panchoo, S., Pudaruth, S.: Gender profiling from PhD theses using k-nearest neighbour and sequential minimal optimisation. In: Berretti, S., Thampi, S.M., Dasgupta, S. (eds.) Intelligent Systems Technologies and Applications. AISC, vol. 385, pp. 369–377. Springer, Cham (2016). doi:10.1007/978-3-319-23258-4_32
9. Ansari, Y.Z., Azad, S.A., AKhtar, H., et al.: Gender classification of blog authors. Int. J. Sustain. Dev. Green Econ. (2013). Special Issue
10. Wang, J., Li, S., Huang, L.: User gender classification in Chinese microblog. J. Chin. Inf. Process. **28**(6), 150–155 (2014)
11. Mikros, G.K.: Authorship attribution and gender identification in Greek blogs. Meth. Appl. Quant. Linguist. **21**, 21–32 (2012)
12. Mukherjee, A., Liu, B.: Improving gender classification of blog authors. In: The Conference on Empirical Methods in Natural Language Processing, pp. 207–217 (2010)
13. Miller, Z., Dickinson, B., Hu, W.: Gender prediction on twitter using stream algorithms with N-gram character features. Int. J. Intell. Sci. **2**(4), 143–148 (2012)

14. Wang, F.: A study on gender classification of blog authors. Master's Thesis. Beijing Jiaotong University. Beijing, China (2012)
15. Yang, J.: Research on gender recognition technology of Chinese e-mail authors based on SVM. Master's Thesis. Hebei Agricultural University, Hebei, China (2007)
16. Alvarez-Carmona, M., Lopez-Monroy, P., et al.: INAOE's participation at PAN'15: author profiling task-notebook for PAN at CLEF 2015. In: CLEF 2015 Evaluation Labs and Workshop Working Notes Papers (2015)
17. Nguyen, D., Gravel, R., Trieschnigg, D., et al.: How old do you think I am? A study of language and age in Twitter. In: 7th International AAAI Conference on Weblogs and Social Media, pp. 1–10 (2013)
18. Le, Q., Mikolov, T.: Distributed representations of sentences and documents. In: 31st International Conference on Machine Learning, pp. 1188–1196 (2014)
19. Lau, J.H., Baldwin, T.: An empirical evaluation of Doc2vec with practical insights into document embedding generation (2016). https://arxiv.org/pdf/1607.05368.pdf
20. Word embedding. https://en.wikipedia.org/wiki/Word_embedding
21. Word2vec. https://en.wikipedia.org/wiki/Word2vec
22. Kim, Y.: Convolutional Neural Networks for Sentence Classification (2014). http://www.aclweb.org/anthology/D14-1181
23. Hu, B., Lu, Z., Li, H., et al.: Convolutional neural network architectures for matching natural language sentences(2014). http://www.hangli-hl.com/uploads/3/1/6/8/3168008/hu-etal-nips2014.pdf
24. Sequential minimal optimization. https://en.wikipedia.org/wiki/Sequential_minimal_optimization

Generating Topics of Interests for Research Communities

Nagendra Kumar[(✉)], Rahul Utkoor, Bharath K.R. Appareddy, and Manish Singh

Indian Institute of Technology Hyderabad, Sangareddy 502285, India
{cs14resch11005,cs14btech11037,cs15mtech11001,msingh}@iith.ac.in

Abstract. With ever increasing number of publication venues and research topics, it is becoming difficult for users to find out topics of interest for conferences or research areas. Although we have many popular topic modeling techniques, we still find that conferences are listing their topics of interest using a manual approach. Topics that are generated by existing topic modeling algorithms are good for text categorization, but they are not ideal for displaying to users because they generate topics that are not so readable and are often redundant. In this paper, we propose a novel technique to generate topics of interest using association mining and natural language processing. We show that the topics of interest that are generated by our technique is much more similar to manually written topics of interest compared to existing topic modeling algorithms. Our results show that the proposed method generates meaningful, interpretable topics, and leads to 13.9% higher precision than existing techniques.

1 Introduction

Computer Science is a vast and ever-expanding engineering stream. It includes many research areas, such as Databases, Data Mining, Computer Networks, Machine Learning, and so on. Each of these research areas consists of various sub-areas (topics). For example, VLDB 2017 conference[1], which is one of the top conferences in Databases, lists Provenance, Workflows, Distributed Database Systems, Social Networks, etc., as topics of interest. Although there are many popular topic finding algorithms, such as LDA [4], Topical N-Gram (TNG) [23], Phrase-Discovering LDA [13], etc., all the conferences still use a manual approach to generate the topics of interest. There are many existing papers, such as [23,24], which have shown how one can use topic modeling to find topics of interest in bibliographic data. Although the topics returned by these algorithms can be very useful for text categorization, they are not as readable and organized like manually created topics of interest. In this paper, we present a novel algorithm based on frequent pattern mining and natural language processing to create topics of interest that are very similar to manually created topics.

[1] http://www.vldb.org/2017/cfp_research_track.php.

G. Cong et al. (Eds.): ADMA 2017, LNAI 10604, pp. 488–501, 2017.
https://doi.org/10.1007/978-3-319-69179-4_34

Topic modeling algorithms can be categorized into two broad categories namely, unigram based topic models [4,21] and phrase based topic models [13,22,23]. LDA is one of the most popular unigram based topic models that was developed based on 'bag-of-words' assumption. For the papers published in VLDB, the LDA algorithm generates topic words such as 'based', 'methods', 'data', etc. Many of these words do not convey complete information [12,19]. For example, the meaning of 'graph data management' cannot be completely captured by any one of the three words in isolation. Phrase based topic models generate longer phrases but many of the top phrases, as explained later on, are ambiguous, redundant, and less understandable such as 'case study', 'free data', 'large scale', etc.

Once we have an algorithm to create human-like topics, we can use it in various applications. For example, at present, conferences show year-wise list of accepted papers, such as "CIKM 2016 accepted papers". Similarly, one can show other useful information, such as, "key topics in CIKM 2016 accepted papers", "key topics in CIKM 2011–2016 accepted papers", "key topics from all Data Mining conferences in 2011–2016 accepted papers". We can use topic of interest information to compute various types of similarity, such as similarity between conferences, similarity between researchers and conferences, and similarity between researchers. All these above applications depend on our ability to generate topics in a principled manner, and these topics should match human generated topics, as the list of research topics of interest seen on homepages of researchers. In this paper, we use association mining to generate a large number of possible topics, and then use NLP to refine and select the best topics.

Apart from generating topics from research communities (conferences and research areas), another problem that we address in this paper is to group related topics. For example, from the VLDB 2017 conference, one can observe that the topics Graph Data Management, Social Networks, and Recommendation Systems are shown as a group of related topics. All these three topics address graph related problems. The existing topic modeling algorithms cannot be used to group such semantically related topics. In this paper, we use word-embeddings to group semantically related topics. Our key contributions are as follows:

- We show the limitation of existing probabilistic topic modeling (PTM) algorithms. These algorithms do not generate topics that are similar to manually generated topics.
- We present a novel topic modeling algorithm based on association mining and NLP. As compared to existing PTM algorithms, our algorithm with NLP refining generates topics that are almost twice more similar to manually created topics of interest and with 13.9% higher precision.
- We also present a novel algorithm to group similar topics using word-embeddings.

2 Related Work

Analysis of online bibliographies is one of active research directions in the field of network and text mining. While most of the works focus on the analysis of network property of the scientific community [2,3], there are also some related works on topic development and distribution [16,25]. Mei et al. [16] proposed a method that combines topic modeling and social network analysis to discover topical community and topical authors. Zaiane et al. [25] used DBLP collaboration network to compute relevance score between authors to discover communities and use them in recommendation system. However, our work focus on finding meaningful research topics of research communities such as conferences and research areas.

Many statistical methods [4,11,17] has been proposed to determine topics for text documents. One such topic model, Latent Dirichlet Allocation (LDA) [4] that relies on bag-of-words assumption has a great impact in the fields of machine learning and text mining. LDA considers the document as a mixture of topics, and the topics are multinomial distribution of words present in the document. Unlike PLSA [9], the LDA model is a well-defined generative model and can create topics without overfitting. However, LDA does not generate the meaningful phrases.

To identify phrases from text documents, several methods have been proposed [7,13,22,23]. Two such methods are Topical N-Gram (TNG) and PD-LDA that generate phrases. Although these methods generate phrases but often suffer from high complexity and poor scalability. In our experiments, these methods generate many less interpretable phrases such as 'empirical study', 'based malware', 'case study' which cannot be used to label the topics of interest of research communities. We propose a method based on association mining and natural language processing that generates more meaningful topics. Results of our evaluations show that the proposed method generates topics that are more interpretable and meaningful than those generated by existing methods.

3 Methodology

We perform the following five steps to determine the topics: (1) categorize publications based on the conferences and research areas; (2) generate candidate topics for the individual conference or research area; (3) prune topics that are redundant, ambiguous, or uninteresting; (4) refine candidate topics to get more readable topics; (5) group semantically related research topics.

3.1 Data Categorization

In DBLP publications are not categorized (grouped) by conference or research area. Since our goal is to show topics based on conference and research area, our first step is to create two types of groups, one based on conference and the other based on research area. As DBLP data contains the name of the conference, we group papers based on conference name. However, as conference names are not given in a uniform manner, we use standard entity resolution algorithms to clean our data and give a unique abbreviation to each conference.

To determine the topics of areas, we categorize the publications based on their areas. We first find all the conferences related to an area and then assign all the publications of those conferences to that area. We observe that information about the area of publication is not available in DBLP dataset. Although a paper is published in one conference, the conference may belong to multiple research areas. The information about the research areas that a conference belongs to is not available on the web. In this paper, we use WikiCFP[2] to get the research areas for the conference. WikiCFP includes almost all the areas and sub-areas of Computer Science. When a conference organizer posts a CFP in WikiCFP, the organizers tag the conference with one or more of these areas (categories). We extract this information from WikiCFP. Even in WikiCFP, more than 50% of the conferences do not have any category assigned to them. We use collaborative filtering algorithms from recommendation systems to find the possible areas for conferences that do not have any assigned category by using the category information from similar conferences with known categories. In WikiCFP, for any conference, they show the top-10 similar conferences. The similarity is determined based on the fact that users who are interested in this conference are also interested in these other conferences.

3.2 Candidate Topic Generation

In this section, we first describe existing techniques to find topics and then we propose our method to find the topics.

There are two techniques namely, LDA [4] and TNG [23], which have been widely used to find top topics from the text corpora. We use these techniques to find topics of interest of conferences and research areas from the publications. We apply LDA on titles of the publications that belong to conferences and areas. As titles are more precise compared to abstracts, we use titles of the publications to find topics [14]. LDA represents each document (conference or area) as a mixture of various topics with definite probabilities. The terms that often occur together are placed under the same topic with high probabilities.

However, LDA relies on the bag-of-words model and assumes that words are generated independently from each other. Therefore, it is not able to generate the meaningful phrases. For example, it generates the words like 'social', 'network' as two different words even if they frequently occur together in the corpus. Topical n-gram (TNG) is a probabilistic model that determines topics containing words as well as meaningful phrases. As phrases convey more precise meaning compared to a single word, we use TNG model to generate meaningful phrases. Although TNG generates better topics than LDA, we observe that it generates many phrases which are not so useful such as 'based malware', 'case study', 'solving linear system', etc. Therefore, we propose a novel method that generates the better collocations by taking care of both co-occurrences and phrases.

Now, we describe our method of finding topics based on association mining [1]. We use association mining to find co-occurring words and phrases present

[2] http://www.wikicfp.com/cfp/.

in titles of the papers. Abstract or full-text contain lots of trivial words and phrases. If we use full-text of the papers, we end up getting several unimportant words and phrases. Researchers often use the main underlying concept precisely in titles itself, so it is useful to apply association mining to find out these frequently occurring topic words or phrases [14]. The topics that are not frequent are likely to be rare or non-research topics. We use the FP-Growth [8] association mining algorithm as it is one of the most efficient and scalable method for mining frequent patterns [5]. The algorithm generates frequent topics by using the criteria of minimum support and confidence. We perform experiments to determine appropriate value of minimum support and confidence. We found that 0.1% minimum support and 60% confidence leads to the sufficient number of prominent topics. However, we observe that lots of distorted, redundant, ambiguous words or phrases are generated, and all of them are not interesting topics. We therefore apply pruning and refining to get well-formed topics.

3.3 Topic Pruning

Not all the frequent topics generated by association mining are useful; there are topics that are ambiguous, uninteresting, and redundant. We observe that some common words frequently occur in the titles of the papers. As a result, we get lots of uninteresting single words and phrases that contain these single words. Most of these words do not convey any useful topic information. Phrases are often more descriptive and carry a more precise meaning than single words. However, some candidate phrases are not interesting topics such as 'mining frequent', 'component analysis', 'using support vector', etc. Therefore, we perform compactness pruning and redundancy pruning to remove such uninteresting topics.

Compactness Pruning. Compactness pruning aims to remove those phrases whose words do not appear together in a specific order. It identifies the topics that contain at least two words and remove those that are meaningless or whose words are not in right order. We perform compactness pruning to maintain the right word-order within a phrase as association mining does not consider the order of words in the publications. We first find the sets of phrases in such a way that in each set, phrases are equivalent but their word-orders are different such as {mining frequent, frequent mining}, {wireless sensor network, sensor network wireless}, etc. We then use term frequency-inverse document frequency (tf-idf) to prune the disorder phrase(s) from these sets of phrases.

We consider all the publications (titles) of a conference or area as one document and generate the unigram, bigram and trigram phrases from each publication of the document. The reason for using unigram, bigram and trigram phrases rather than full titles or longer phrases is because most topics can be found based on local information. Using long titles or phrases tend to generate a large number of spurious results. We compute the tf-idf weight for each unique phrase which signifies the importance of the phrase in a document. We select top phrases from the tf-idf generated phrases. We compare all of these phrases with previously generated sets of equivalent phrases. If any of the phrases in the set matches with the tf-idf generated phrase, we consider that phrase as a potential topic and remove other phrases of the same set from the list of topics. In this step, we also perform an additional process of removing those topics which are common and do not convey any useful information. These topics have low idf score because they appear frequently in the titles of all areas and conferences. We prune the topics that have very low idf score.

Redundancy Pruning. Redundancy pruning removes redundant words and phrases from the selected list of topics. We observe that topic list contains many bigram phrases which are part of the trigram phrases such as ‘component analysis’ is part of ‘principal component analysis’. We remove these types of insignificant redundant bigrams which are the part of the trigrams. However, we cannot remove all the bigrams which are part of the trigrams. For example, we cannot remove ‘neural network’ which is part of ‘artificial neural network’ as both are the significant phrases with distinct meanings. Therefore, we inspect the titles of the publications to know if bigram appears significantly in the titles without its superset trigram(s). We prune those bigrams which are subsets of trigrams and do not appear independently significant number of times in the titles. Similarly, we prune unigram words that are part of some bigrams or trigrams topics and do not appear significantly in titles without its superset bigrams or trigrams.

3.4 Topic Refining

Existing topic modeling algorithms or the algorithms described above generate topics that are useful in applications where approximate or less understandable topics are sufficient. However, to generate topics that are similar to human labels, we present how to further refine the topics using NLP grammar rules.

We observe that some of the phrases appear in distorted forms such as ‘databases distributed’, ‘learning supervised’, ‘feature selection unsupervised’, ‘using support vector’, ‘programming genetic’, etc. We refine these kinds of topics to get cleaner topics using grammar rules from NLP. To apply grammar rules, we first need to tag the topics using Part-of-Speech (POS) tagger. POS Tagger assigns part-of-speech tag to each word of the topic, such as noun (‘NN’), verb (‘VB’), adjective (‘JJ’), etc. We use Stanford POS tagger [15] to do the tagging. We perform the following steps to refine the topics:

1. We observe that many phrases containing verbs appear in distorted forms such as ‘sensor networks distributed’, ‘data mining distributed’, ‘learning supervised’, ‘databases distributed’, ‘wireless network efficient’, etc. One common issue in all these phrases is that the verb does not appear at the beginning of the phrases. We notice that if the verb appears at the beginning of the phrase, it will lead to a better topic.

   Among all the verbs, the verbs associated with ‘VBD’, ‘VBN’, ‘VBP’ tag frequently appear at the end of the phrases that lead to distorted topics.

Therefore, we find the phrases (bigrams and trigrams) that contain the last words associated with 'VBD', 'VBN', 'VBP' tag. These tags indicate that the corresponding word is either past form of the verb ('VBD', 'VBN') or non-third person singular present verb ('VBP'). The last words of the phrases assigned with 'VBD', 'VBN', or 'VBP' tag are placed at the beginning of the phrases. By using this rule, we get the topics that are more interpretable than the actual candidate topics. For example, the phrases like 'data mining distributed', 'learning supervised' are transformed into 'distributed data mining', 'supervised learning' respectively.
2. We refine the bigram phrases that contain progressive verb (gerund form of the verb) such as 'programming genetic', 'scheduling sporadic', 'computing international', 'learning active', etc. These are the phrases whose first word is a progressive verb ('VBG') and the second word is an adjective ('JJ'). We observe that the verb appears after the adjective leads to form a better topic. Therefore, we swap the first and second word of the phrase. For example, phrases like 'scheduling sporadic', 'programming genetic' are transformed into 'sporadic scheduling', 'genetic programming' respectively which are well-formed phrases compared to actual candidate phrases.
3. We observe that there are many trigram phrases containing progressive verb appear frequently in the titles of the papers such as 'solving linear system', 'mining association rules', 'training neural network', 'neural network modeling', etc. These verbs do not convey any additional information while generating the topics. We improve the trigram phrases that contain the progressive verb at the first or last position of the phrases by removing the progressive verbs from the trigram phrases. By using this rule, phrases like 'neural network modeling', 'solving linear system' are transformed into 'neural network', 'linear system' respectively. These shorter phrases without progressive verb form better topics that can convey a more general concept.

3.5 Topic Grouping

To group similar topics, we find similarities among the topics by exploiting their co-occurrences in the papers. As titles rarely have more than one topic, we use abstracts [20] of the papers to find topic co-occurrences. We use Google's Word2vec model [18] to find the similarity among the topics. Word2vec model creates the word embeddings by generating vector space from the text corpus where each word in the corpus is assigned to a vector in the space. We train the Word2vec model using abstracts of the papers and then use k-medoid algorithm [10] to group the topics generated by the proposed method based on their Word2vec similarities. We use k-medoid algorithm instead of widely used k-means algorithm because of its robustness to outliers as compared to k-means.

4 Experimental Evaluations

In this section, we present our evaluation. Section 4.1 contains the experimental setup. In Sect. 4.2, we compare the performance of all the algorithms using precision and similarity measures. In Sect. 4.3, we show through empirical results that the topics generated by our proposed method are superior to existing popular topic modeling algorithms.

4.1 Experimental Setup

We use publicly available DBLP bibliographic dataset[3] for experiment. The dataset contains information from more than 5000 conferences, 1500 journals, and indexes over 3.3 million publications of Computer Science. We also extract data from WikiCFP to categorize the publications based on research areas. WikiCFP is a platform that lists conferences, scholarly events, meetings and allows for advertising information about workshops, conferences, seminars, meetings, etc. We extract the data from WikiCFP to know the conferences that belong to different areas of Computer Science, and then select 27 most popular areas, such as databases, machine learning, etc., for our analysis.

As the dataset contains many noisy and unimportant words, we do preprocessing to remove these words. We remove stop-words, such as ‘a’, ‘an’, ‘the’, etc., as these words do not contain significant information for our analysis. Stemming and lemmatization are two commonly used text pre-processing techniques. These techniques reduce inflected or derived words to their root forms. However, we found that these techniques do not generate readable topics. For example, if we use these pre-processing, we get topics as *distribut databas system* instead of *distributed database system*. We observed that paper titles, unlike paper abstracts, often contain good topics and they do not have inflected words. In this paper, we do very mild stemming to remove redundant topics. For example, we found redundant topics such as Database and Databases; Neural Network and Neural Networks. For such redundant topics, we chose the topic that was more frequent in the dataset.

4.2 Performance Evaluation

In this section, we compare the performance of different topic modeling algorithms. There are different metrics to evaluate the topic models such as perplexity, precision, similarity, etc. Chang et al. [6] showed that the perplexity metric is not well suited for topic model evaluation as it is not well correlated with human judgment. The topic models that achieve better perplexity have less human-interpretable topics. Therefore, we use precision and similarity metrics for evaluations. Later in Sect. 4.3, we will show the superiority of our generated topics using empirical results.

Precision Analysis. In topic modeling, precision is defined as the fraction of generated topics that are relevant to the topics of interest, which could either be of a conference or of a research area. Since there is no labeled data for this

[3] http://dblp.uni-trier.de/.

evaluation, we asked 10 PhD students from our CSE department to manually label the topics generated by the topic finding algorithms. We chose these students from different areas of Computer Science. We chose two researchers, with expertise in the same area, to label the topics generated from research area or conference. Topics of each conference and area are labeled by researchers independently without influencing each other. We consider a topic as a relevant topic if both the researchers labeled it as a relevant topic. We found that there was 94% agreement among the researchers while labeling the topics.

Table 1. MAP of different topic modeling algorithms

Techniques/MAP (%)	Baseline	With pruning	With refining	With pruning + refining
LDA	51.4	56.7	51.4	56.7
TNG	68.3	72.3	70.1	75.2
Proposed method	62.8	79.4	68.9	89.1

Our association mining based method is scalable to a large dataset. Due to a dearth of experts from different domains, it is difficult to find experts to judge the results. We therefore perform our experiments on 20 conferences and 10 areas. We compute the mean average precision (MAP) for each algorithm by averaging the precision values of the conferences and areas. As we discussed in Sect. 3, our proposed method consists of several NLP processing. We compare the performance of all the methods with and without NLP processing, namely the pruning and the refining step. We find the precision of these methods with pruning, with refining and with both pruning and refining. From the first row of Table 1, we observe that LDA has the lowest MAP value (51.4%). The reason for this poor result is that LDA generates single words and many of them do not convey any information as these words are part of topic phrases. LDA with refining does not improve the precision as refining does not apply to LDA single terms, while LDA with pruning performs better (56.7%). TNG performs better than LDA, it gives 75.2% MAP with both pruning and refining but it generates many irrelevant words and phrases that lower the performance of TNG. The performance of proposed method without any processing is less compared to TNG. The reasons for this is that many of the topics are disordered, redundant and incomplete. However, when topic pruning and topic refining are individually added to proposed method, there are notable improvements, but the largest improvement comes when topics generated by association mining are processed by both pruning and refining, yielding 89.1% mean average precision. The reason for this is that after processing the topics, proposed method generates relatively more meaningful as well as relevant topics compared to other methods. Further, applying pruning on the list of generated topics decreases recall of the proposed method. However, we set a fitting value of support such that proposed method generates adequate topics (as shown in Table 3).

Similarity Analysis. We next use similarity measures to evaluate the performance of topic finding algorithms. We want to compare how the topics generated by the algorithms compare with manually labeled topics. However, the challenge is that there is no existing gold-standard list of topics to compare against the generated topics. We created our baseline gold-standard topics for conferences and research areas by collecting topics from Wikipedia and WikiCFP.

Wikipedia is a publicly available encyclopedia which provides domain-specific information. We extract topics of conferences and areas using Wikipedia API[4]. However, Wikipedia offers much more information than required for the analysis of the topics. In order to avoid adding noise, we only consider anchor texts present in the infobox table and first two paragraphs from the searched web page as this information is most related. We also extract the list of the topics by crawling the WikiCFP with the name of conference and area which are provided by the conferences to call for papers. Conferences contain the topics of their interests but areas contain the conferences belong to the area. To get the topics of the area, we take the topics of top-20 conferences of that area. We then compute the cosine similarity between the collected topics and topics generated by the algorithms. We present the similarity score of few popular areas in Table 2.

Table 2. Similarity of topics with manually listed topics

Algorithms/Results	LDA	TNG	Proposed method
Machine learning	0.14	0.26	0.51
Computer networks	0.16	0.25	0.45
Compilers	0.13	0.16	0.38
Databases	0.10	0.21	0.36

As can be seen in Table 2, LDA has the lowest similarity for all the areas. Although TNG performs better than LDA, its similarity is also low. The reason for this low similarity is that most of the topics generated by these algorithms do not match with manually written topics as collected from WikiCFP and Wikipedia. However, the proposed algorithm with pruning and refining performs the best, with almost twice higher similarity compared to TNG. Although the absolute values of similarity appear small, they account for a large number of topics, and many of them are related but do not match exactly. The cosine similarity is incapable of matching the topics if they are related but have different terms. Further, we observe that similarity varies across the areas for all the methods as it is highly dependent on the quality of the baseline topics generated through Wikipedia and WikiCFP. We therefore collect the topics of 20 conferences and 10 research areas of Computer Science and compute the average similarity score. We obtain the average similarity scores of the topics generated by LDA, TNG and proposed algorithm as 0.127, 0.228, 0.435 respectively.

[4] https://pypi.python.org/pypi/wikipedia.

4.3 Empirical Analysis

In this section, we compare different topic labeling algorithms using empirical evaluation. We then show groups of similar topics created by our algorithm.

Topic Comparison. In Table 3, we show the topics generated by LDA, TNG and our proposed for the *Machine Learning* research area.

Table 3. Key-topics of machine learning area

Groups	Topics
LDA	learning, based, data, neural, network, algorithm, model, analysis, system, approach, classification, detection, recognition, image, clustering, mining, control, genetic, method, optimization, information
TNG	neural approach, visualize high, automatic translation, logical foundation, based representability, based divisive, dimensional shape, investigating temporal, channel state, neural network, genetic programming, active learning, empirical study, large scale, support vector, data mining, big data, online learning, vectorial data, feature selection, case study
Proposed method	neural network, reinforcement learning, face recognition, swarm optimization, matrix factorization, semi-supervised learning, big data, recommender system, association rule, monte carlo, social media, k-means clustering, multi-label classification, logistic regression, sentiment analysis, support vector machine, artificial neural network, hidden markov model, principal component analysis, deep neural network, natural language processing

As can be seen in Table 3, LDA generates topics that are generic words such as ‘model’, ‘data’, ‘algorithm’, ‘approach’, ‘control’, etc. Many of them are not actual topics and some of them are part of topic phrases, such as ‘learning’, ‘data’, and ‘neural’ are the parts of ‘reinforcement learning’, ‘big data’, and ‘neural network’ respectively. Many topic words such as ‘based’, ‘method’, ‘control’ do not convey any meaningful information. Most of the manually created labels are phrases. TNG generates phrases but many top phrases of TNG are noisy and less interpretable such as ‘based divisive’, ‘based representability’, ‘case study’, ‘empirical study’, etc. Even after we remove the terms like ‘based’, ‘study’, ‘approach’ by pre-processing, TNG generates many not so useful topics such as ‘visualize high’, ‘large scale’, ‘logical foundation’, etc. Without the NLP pruning and refining, our proposed approach also generates many tedious and less interpretable topics such as ‘using support vector’, ‘based association rule’, ‘processing natural language’, ‘neural networks training’, etc. However, after performing the text processing, our proposed method generates topics which are quite similar to manually written topics.

Grouping of the Topics. To provide the comprehensive summary of topics of interest to conference or area, we create groups of similar topics. These groups provide the overall theme of the conference or area. We present the groups which are obtained from the Machine Learning area in Table 4:

Table 4. Topic groups of machine learning area

Groups	Topics
Group1	neural network, deep neural network, fuzzy neural network, genetic algorithm, handwritten recognition, artificial neural network
Group2	natural language, sentiment analysis, knowledge bases, data streams, social media, big data
Group3	support vector classification, support vector regression, active learning, face recognition, feature selection
Group4	hidden markov model, conditional random fields, decision making, ant colony, monte carlo, reinforcement learning
Group5	matrix factorization, recommender system, collaborative filtering, dimensionality reduction, principal component analysis

As can be seen in Table 4, topics, which are related, are placed under the same group. Group 1 consists of topics related to neural network such as deep neural network, artificial neural network, fuzzy neural network, handwritten recognition, etc. Similarly, Group 2 consists of topics related to natural language analysis such as sentiment analysis, knowledge bases, data streams, social media, and so on. Each group contains a set of semantically related topics.

5 Conclusion

In this paper, we proposed a novel topic finding algorithm that uses association mining and natural language processing. We apply our algorithm on bibliographic data to generate topics of interest for conferences and research areas. We show that our algorithm can generate topics which are very similar to manually created topics of interest. We implemented various NLP based pruning and refining techniques to get near-perfect topics. We have shown in our evaluation that the topics generated by our proposed method are more meaningful and human interpretable than the existing state-of-the-art methods.

References

1. Agrawal, R., Srikant, R., et al.: Fast algorithms for mining association rules. In: Proceedings of 20th International Conference on Very Large Data Bases, VLDB, vol. 1215, pp. 487–499 (1994)

2. Bird, C., Devanbu, P., Barr, E., Filkov, V., Nash, A., Su, Z.: Structure and dynamics of research collaboration in computer science. In: Proceedings of the 2009 SIAM International Conference on Data Mining, pp. 826–837. SIAM (2009)
3. Biryukov, M., Dong, C.: Analysis of computer science communities based on DBLP. In: Lalmas, M., Jose, J., Rauber, A., Sebastiani, F., Frommholz, I. (eds.) ECDL 2010. LNCS, vol. 6273, pp. 228–235. Springer, Heidelberg (2010). doi:10.1007/978-3-642-15464-5_24
4. Blei, D.M., Ng, A.Y., Jordan, M.I.: Latent Dirichlet allocation. J. Mach. Learn. Res. **3**, 993–1022 (2003)
5. Borgelt, C.: An implementation of the FP-growth algorithm. In: Proceedings of the 1st International Workshop on Open Source Data Mining: Frequent Pattern Mining Implementations, pp. 1–5. ACM (2005)
6. Chang, J., Boyd-Graber, J.L., Gerrish, S., Wang, C., Blei, D.M.: Reading tea leaves: how humans interpret topic models. In: NIPS, vol. 31, pp. 1–9 (2009)
7. El-Kishky, A., Song, Y., Wang, C., Voss, C.R., Han, J.: Scalable topical phrase mining from text corpora. VLDB **8**(3), 305–316 (2014)
8. Han, J., Pei, J., Yin, Y.: Mining frequent patterns without candidate generation. ACM Sigmod Rec. **29**, 1–12 (2000). ACM
9. Hofmann, T.: Probabilistic latent semantic indexing. In: ACM SIGIR, pp. 50–57. ACM (1999)
10. Kaufman, L., Rousseeuw, P.J.: Finding Groups in Data: An Introduction to Cluster Analysis, vol. 344. Wiley, London (2009)
11. Li, W., McCallum, A.: Pachinko allocation: dag-structured mixture models of topic correlations. In: ICML, pp. 577–584. ACM (2006)
12. Lim, K.W., Chen, C., Buntine, W.: Twitter-network topic model: a full Bayesian treatment for social network and text modeling. In: NIPS 2013 Topic Model Workshop, pp. 1–5 (2013)
13. Lindsey, R.V., Headden III, W.P., Stipicevic, M.J.: A phrase-discovering topic model using hierarchical Pitman-Yor processes. In: Proceedings of the 2012 Joint Conference on EMNLP and CoNLL, pp. 214–222. ACL (2012)
14. Liu, Z., Chen, X., Zheng, Y., Sun, M.: Automatic keyphrase extraction by bridging vocabulary gap. In: CoNLL, pp. 135–144. ACL (2011)
15. Manning, C.D., Surdeanu, M., Bauer, J., Finkel, J.R., Bethard, S., McClosky, D.: The stanford CoreNLP natural language processing toolkit. In: ACL (System Demonstrations), pp. 55–60 (2014)
16. Mei, Q., Cai, D., Zhang, D., Zhai, C.: Topic modeling with network regularization. In: WWW, pp. 101–110. ACM (2008)
17. Mei, Q., Zhai, C.: A mixture model for contextual text mining. In: SIGKDD, pp. 649–655. ACM (2006)
18. Mikolov, T., Sutskever, I., Chen, K., Corrado, G.S., Dean, J.: Distributed representations of words and phrases and their compositionality. In: Advances in Neural Information Processing Systems, pp. 3111–3119 (2013)
19. Paul, M.J., Dredze, M.: Discovering health topics in social media using topic models. PLoS ONE **9**(8), e103408 (2014)
20. Tang, J., Zhang, J., Yao, L., Li, J., Zhang, L., Su, Z.: Arnetminer: extraction and mining of academic social networks. In: SIGKDD, pp. 990–998. ACM (2008)
21. Teh, Y.W., Newman, D., Welling, M.: A collapsed variational Bayesian inference algorithm for latent Dirichlet allocation. In: NIPS, vol. 6, pp. 1378–1385 (2006)
22. Wallach, H.M.: Topic modeling: beyond bag-of-words. In: Proceedings of the 23rd International Conference on Machine Learning, pp. 977–984. ACM (2006)

23. Wang, X., McCallum, A., Wei, X.: Topical n-grams: phrase and topic discovery, with an application to information retrieval. In: ICDM, pp. 697–702. IEEE (2007)
24. Yin, Z., Cao, L., Gu, Q., Han, J.: Latent community topic analysis: integration of community discovery with topic modeling. ACM Trans. Intell. Syst. Technol. (TIST) **3**(4), 63 (2012)
25. Zaïane, O.R., Chen, J., Goebel, R.: Mining research communities in bibliographical data. In: Zhang, H., Spiliopoulou, M., Mobasher, B., Giles, C.L., McCallum, A., Nasraoui, O., Srivastava, J., Yen, J. (eds.) SNAKDD/WebKDD -2007. LNCS, vol. 5439, pp. 59–76. Springer, Heidelberg (2009). doi:10.1007/978-3-642-00528-2_4

An Evolutionary Approach for Learning Conditional Preference Networks from Inconsistent Examples

Mohammad Haqqani(✉) and Xiaodong Li

Computer Science and Software Engineering, School of Science,
RMIT University, Melbourne, Australia
mohammad.haqqani@rmit.edu.au

Abstract. Conditional Preference Networks (CP-nets) have been proposed for modeling and reasoning about combinatorial decision domains. However, the study of CP-nets learning has not advanced sufficiently for their widespread use in complex, real-world applications where the problem is large-scale and the data is not clean. In many real world applications, due to either the randomness of the users' behaviors or the observation errors, the data-set in hand could be inconsistent, i.e., there exists at least one outcome preferred over itself in the data-set. In this work, we present an evolutionary-based method for solving the CP-net learning problem from inconsistent examples. Here, we do not learn the CP-nets directly. Instead, we frame the problem of learning into an optimization problem and use the power of evolutionary algorithms to find the optimal CP-net. The experiments indicate that the proposed approach is able to find a good quality CP-net and outperforms the current state-of-the-art algorithms in terms of both sample agreement and graph similarity.

Keywords: User behavioral modeling · Preference learning · Conditional preference · CP-net · Genetic algorithm

1 Introduction

Preference learning (or preference elicitation) is a critical problem in many scientific fields, such as decision theory, economics, logistic and databases [8,13]. A good preference representation should capture statements that are natural for users to assess, or are easy to learn from data. When modeling user preference, preference learning can be regarded as an optimization problem which maximizes one or more utility functions. However, in practice we are not given a utility *a priori*. In fact, in most practical problems, we only have access to a finite history of user choice data. Therefore, the *preference learning problem*, that is, how to learn user preferences using her choice data, has gained a lot of attention in recent years [2].

One of the common assumptions in preference learning is that the user preferences over the values of outcome attributes are independent [2]. However, this

G. Cong et al. (Eds.): ADMA 2017, LNAI 10604, pp. 502–515, 2017.
https://doi.org/10.1007/978-3-319-69179-4_35

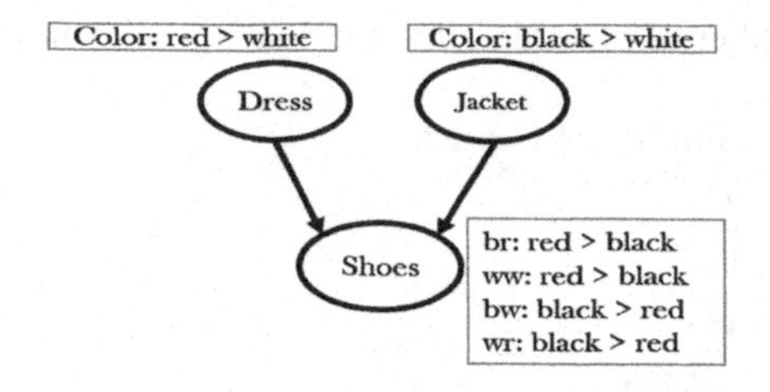

Fig. 1. A simple CP-net N, $o_1 \succ o_2$ indicates that the user strictly prefers o_1 over o_2.

assumption is not necessary true in many real world scenarios. For example, in a cloth shopping problem as shown in Fig. 1, a customer might choose the color of the shoes depending on the color of the dress she/he would buy. In other words, the preference over shoes' color is conditioned on the color of available dresses. Thus, we say the preferences induced by the user's behavior are intrinsically related to *conditional preferential independence*, a key notion in multi-attribute decision theory [19].

Conditional preference networks (CP-nets) was proposed for handling such problems [6], and have received a great deal of attention due to their compact and natural representation of ordinal preferences in multi-attribute domains [8–12, 17–19,22]. Strictly speaking, a CP-net, as shown in Fig. 1, is a *digraph*, with its nodes corresponding to alternative attributes, and edges corresponding to the dependency between nodes. Here, each node is annotated with a conditional preference table describing the preferences over that particular attribute (see Sect. 2).

Several CP-net learning algorithms have been developed depending on the users' choice data. Some algorithms work on the historical choice data [11,22,23], a process known as *passive learning*. Others actively offer solutions in an attempt to learn the users' preferences as they choose [9,11,14]. The work of this paper falls into the category of *passive learning*, where the learner uses the recorded users' choices and then fits a CP-net model to the observed data. Mathematically speaking, we collect the set of samples $S = \{o_i \succ o'_i\}$, where $o_i \succ o'_i$ means that the user strictly prefers outcome o_i over outcome o'_i and then we try to find a model N that best describes S. Such set of samples may be gathered, for instance, by observing online users' choices.

There are two major problems using CP-nets for real-world applications: the curse of dimensionality and noisy data. First, learning CP-nets is known to be NP-Complete even for small problems [1]. Table 1 shows the number of binary CP-nets up to 7 nodes, i.e., each outcome consists of 7 attributes with binary domains. From the values, it is evident that even for a small number of attributes, finding the best CP-net is not a trivial task. To the best of our knowledge, there is no existing approach that can perform well on problems with more than 10 attributes, which makes them impractical in real world situations, in which the alternatives usually consist of tens or even hundreds of attributes.

Table 1. Number of possible binary CP-nets with complete CPTs [3]

Nodes	Number of CP-nets
1	2
2	12
3	488
4	481776
5	157549032992
6	4059976627283664056256
7	524253448460177960474729517490503566696576

Second, a common problem that arises when dealing with human subjects is the possibility of noise or inconsistent information. The objective of most CP-net learning techniques is to learn (i.e., re-build) a CP-net that can capture the whole data-set [11]. However, since the S is not usually clean, there is no possibility of finding such a CP-net, which is consistent with every data-points in S. This fact motivated us to frame the CP-net learning problem as an optimization problem, that is to identify a model that maximizes some objective function, f, with respect to the choice data-set.

In this work, we harness the power of Genetic Algorithm (GA) as an optimization technique. GA is an optimization algorithm inspired from the mechanism of natural selection and natural genetics, which has received a growing interest in solving the complex combinatorial optimization problems, especially for its scalability as compared with the deterministic algorithms [5]. In this work, we investigate the possibility of applying the GA to solve the passive CP-net learning problem. The main contributions of this paper are as follows:

- Proposing a new formulation for CP-net learning as an optimization problem.
- Applying the GA with customized solution formulation and operators, to learn multi-valued CP-nets from inconsistent data.
- Carrying out experimental analysis on both state-of-the-art CP-net learning and learning-to-rank methods using real world data.

The rest of the paper is organized as follows. Section 2 gives the background information on CP-nets, and Sect. 3 reviews the related work. Section 4 describes our proposed GA-based learning algorithm. Section 5 shows the evaluation of the proposed method on simulated data and real data sets, and comparisons with state-of-the-art learning-to-rank methods as well as the CP-net learning methods. Finally, Sect. 6 concludes with some possible future research directions.

2 Background on CP-net

We begin with an outline of some relevant notions on CP-net. Let $V = \{X_1, X_2, ..., X_n\}$ be a set of attributes. Each attribute X_i is associated with a finite set of domain values $Dom(X_i)$. For set $U \subset V$ of attributes, $Dom(U) = \prod_{X_i \in U} Dom(X_i)$. The outcome space is denoted by $\Omega = Dom(V)$. Each $o \in \Omega$ is called an outcome.

Definition 1. *Preference: A strict preference relation $\succ_u$ is a partial order on a set of outcomes $O \in \Omega$ defined by a user u. $o_i \succ_u o_j$ indicates that the user strictly prefers o_i over o_j.*

Definition 2. *Conditional Preference Rule (CP-rule): A CP-rule on an attribute X_i is an expression of the form $t : p \succ \overline{p}$, where p is a literal of X_i and t is a term such that $t \in \{V \backslash X_i\}$.*

Such a rule means given that t holds, the value p is preferred to the value $\overline{p}$ for the attribute X_i.

Definition 3. *Conditional Preference Table (CPT): $CPT(X_i)$ is a table associated with each attribute consists of conditional preference rules (CP-rules) $t : p \succ_i \overline{p}$ specifying a linear order on $Dom(X_i)$ where t indicated to the parents of X_i in the dependency graph.*

Definition 4. *Conditional Preference Network (CP-net): A CP-net is a digraph on $V = \{X_1, ..., X_n\}$ in which each node is labeled with a CPT. An edge (X_i, X_j) indicates that the preferred value of X_j is conditioned by the value of its parent attribute X_i.*

Definition 5. *Dominance Testing: A dominance testing, defined by a triple (N, o_i, o_j), is a decision of whether o_j is dominated by o_i given the CP-net N and $o_i, o_j \in \Omega$. The answer is in the affirmative if and only if $N \models o_i \succ o_j$.*

3 Related Work

Lang and Mengin were [20] are among the first to study the complexity of the CP-net learning problem. To establish a lower bound, they proposed a simple class of so-called separable CP-nets (SCP-nets) for which the dependency graph is an anti-chain, i.e., a graph with no edges. Their later work [21] proved that, while it was possible to find the solution in polynomial time whether there exists a binary-valued SCP-net that entails all examples, the problem of finding such a network is NP-complete.

The earliest work on learning CP-nets was done by Dimopoulos et al. [4], which proposed a *passive learning* algorithm to find a CP-net that entails all examples in a data-set. However, as investigated by Lang and Mengin [20], fully entailment is an exceptionally strong requirement since the CP-net can only handle partial ordering. In other words, if a subject has a linear preference order on the outcome space arising from some utility function, then arguably there may be no CP-net such that the observed comparison data are consistent with the learned model. Therefore the algorithm would never terminate.

1	2		n
$Parent_1$	$Parent_2$	...	$Parent_n$
CPT_1	CPT_2	...	CPT_n

Fig. 2. Solution representation.

Later on, Dimopoulos et al. introduced an algorithm that passively learns an acyclic, binary-valued CP-net that was consistent with all preference orders in the data-set [11]. They proved that the problem of learning a CP-net consistent with the choice data is hard even for acyclic, binary CP-nets. Their algorithm attempts to categorize attributes into independents (those with 0 parents), then those who are dependent on 1 attribute, then 2, and so on until a node for each attribute had been added to the model. In order to determine whether a subset of nodes could be the parents of a particular node, the authors propose constructing a 2-SAT instance, which is solvable in linear time. Using this, they find a position in the network for the node that is consistent with all available preference order data. Note that the algorithm may output failure in some cases since there might be no such a position for a node in the preference graph. Additionally, in the worst case scenario, the algorithm could iterate an exponential number of times to the number of attributes.

As mentioned previously, one of the problems inherited in learning preferences from human subjects is the possibility of noise or inconsistent information in the data set. Liu et al. [22,23] are the first authors who tackled this problem. In [22], they proposed a method which is not restricted to binary-valued domains, that first attempts to find an optimal preference graph for the subject, then constructs a CP-net from the preference graph. They claim that their algorithm runs in time polynomial in the size of the preference graph. However, it has been shown that the size of the preference graph grows exponentially with the number of attributes [21]. Moreover, because the algorithm employs a branch-and-bound method, it seems unlikely that it is polynomial. Our experimental study support this claim as these methods did not perform well in the large problem instances.

The main difference between the proposed method in this paper and the existing passive CP-net learning methods is that for the first time (to the best of our knowledge), we treat the problem of learning CP-nets as an optimization problem. The privilege of doing so is that, unlike [11] we can find a CP-net that partially entails the data set and therefore can work over inconsistent data sets. On the other hand, since our proposed method is an evolutionary-based method, it does not depend on the domain knowledge, unlike other existing methods [22,23].

4 The Proposed Method

In this section, we provide the algorithmic details of the Evolutionary-based CP-net learning method used in this work. To identify the optimal CP-net, we use

Jacket	Shoes	Dress
Nil	{Jacket, Dress}	Nil
Color: black > white	br: red > black ww: red > black bw: black > red wr: black > red	Color: red > white

Fig. 3. Equivalent chromosome for the sample CP-net in Fig. 1.

the Genetic Algorithm and design a problem specific crossover, mutation and repair operators, apart from an objective function.

4.1 Solution Representation and Population Initialization

The chromosome that we used to represent each CP-net, i.e., solution, is shown in Fig. 2. The length of each chromosome is set to the number of attributes and is composed of two main parts: $Parent_i$ and CPT_i. $Parent_i$ denotes to the nodes $j \in \{N \backslash i\}$ in the dependency graph which the preference over the value of node i depends on them and CPT_i denotes to the conditional preference table associated with node i. Figure 3 represents the equivalent chromosome for the sample CP-net in Fig. 1.

For population initialization, we used the GenCPnet method presented in [3]. This method generates acyclic CP-nets uniformly at random with respect to a specified set. It is also possible to specify parameters such as the number of nodes, bound on in-degree, and the size of domains.

4.2 Genetic Operators

We make mutation by the means of local search to explore the neighborhood space of the selected solution. We implemented this by applying the mutation in either *parent* or *CPT* part of a gene. We randomly select a gene in a selected chromosome and then apply the mutation. Changing the parent section is equivalent to a local search in dependency graph of a CP-net while changing the CPT part explores the neighboring *CPRs*.

For crossover, we used a Fitness-based scanning multi-parent crossover (FB-Scan) between selected parents. FB-Scan, as proposed in [12], is a general mechanism that produces one child from $n > 1$ parents. This method traverses all the positions in the child from left to right, and for each position, it selects one of the parents and chooses the value of the corresponding gene for the child. This method uses roulette wheel selection when deciding from which parent a gene will be inherited. Specifically, if parent i has a fitness value of $f(i)$ the probability that a value for a position in the child is inherited from this parent is: $p(i) = \frac{f(i)}{\sum_j f(j)}$.

Repair function: The offspring resulted by mutation and crossover operators may suffer from the *degeneracy* problem. That is, when one or more dependencies in the graph are not reflected in the conditional preference rules (CPRs). Let us consider the CP-net in Fig. 4. The edge (B, A) indicates that the preference over the values of A depends on the value of B. However, if we examine the CPT of A closely, we realize that the preference over A does not in fact depend on B. The preferences can thus be represented by the simpler CP-net shown in Fig. 4(b). When degeneracy happens in a CP-net, not only some fictional dependencies are added to the model, which in reality the user preference is not dependent on them, but also multiple, different CP-net models can map to the same induced preference order.

In [2] the authors described the procedure to detect the degeneracy in a CP-net. They showed that if the preference over X_i is the same for all values of parents of X_i then the CPT is vacuous in X_i hence it is degenerate.

4.3 Fitness Function

Many different notions of fitness could be considered for the objective function. In this work, we use a simple fitness function as follows: Let *agree* denotes the examples for which the learned CP-net, N_l results in the *same* ordering as in the original CP-net N_o and let *disagree* denote those for which the model results in the *opposite* ordering as follows:

$$agree = \{(o_i, o_j) | (o_i \succ_{N_o} o_j) \, and \, (o_i \succ_{N_l} o_j)\} \tag{1}$$

$$disagree = \{(o_i, o_j) | (o_i \succ_{N_o} o_j) \, and \, (o_j \succ_{N_l} o_i)\} \tag{2}$$

Using these metrics, and S as the choice data, we define the fitness score of the learned CP-net as:

$$f(N_l, N_o, S) = \frac{|agree| - |disagree|}{|S|} \tag{3}$$

Note that the fitness value can range between -1 and 1 and for the pairs (o_i, o_j) that do not fall into neither *agree* nor *disagree* categories, i.e., the pairs that the N_l model cannot decide about preference, the fitness score of the model reduces as well. By using f as a fitness function, the learning problem can be stated as:

$$N^* = argmax_{N_l} f(N_l, N_o, S) \tag{4}$$

5 Experimental Results

In order to evaluate the correctness and accuracy of our algorithm, we applied our proposed method on both synthetic and real data. For synthetic data, we manually generated pairwise comparisons data-sets, with different levels of noise, using a random CP-net. For real data, users' preferences collected by Kamishima [16] are used to generate the learning data set. The Kamishima data set contains 100 kinds of sushi and 5000 users' preferences orders on them. We compare the

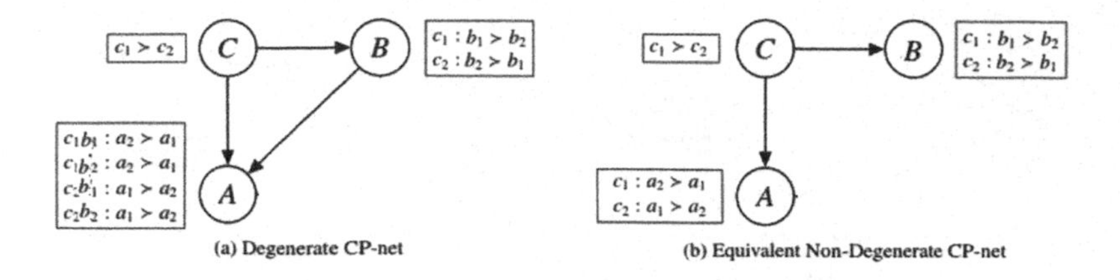

Fig. 4. An example of degeneracy in CP-nets.

Table 2. GA setup used in experiments

Selection mechanism	Ranked bias = 1.2
Nr. of parents	Nr. of attributes
Xover rate	0.8
Mut. rate	0.4
Pool size	200
Max. nr. of evaluation	20000
Results average over	30

proposed method with two categories of preference learning techniques: passive CP-net learning methods and learning-to-rank methods. For the former, we chose [22,23], two state-of-the-art algorithms to learn CP-net from noisy data and for latter, we compare our method with the most popular learning-to-rank methods, RankNet [7], AdaRank [24], OSVM [18] and SVOR [15].

In all the experiments, we used the proposed GA configuration with the setup described in Table 2. We have chosen a non-parametric test, Wilcoxon Signed Rank Test [10] as the statistical significant testing. This test allows us to judge the difference between paired scores when we cannot make an assumption such that the population is normally distributed, as required by the t-test. As a null hypothesis, it is assumed that there is no significant difference between the mean values of the two methods. Whereas the alternative hypothesis is that there is significant difference in the mean fitness values of the two methods. The testing is performed at the 5% significance level.

5.1 Results on Synthetic Data

An obvious idea to evaluate a CP-net learning method is to start with a random CP-net N_o, and then generate a set of pairwise comparison $S = \{(o_i \succ_{N_o} o_j)\}$ entailed by N_o and then use this dataset to estimated a CP-net. Note that the N_o entails all the elements of S, i.e. $N_o \models (o_i \succ_{N_o} o_j) \forall i, j \in S$. In the next step, in order to evaluate the robustness of the learning method, we add some noise to the data set S. Formally, in the data set S, we change the preference relation between two outcomes at a probability of ρ, which is called noise level. Finally, we apply the learning algorithm to S in order to learn a CP-net model N_l.

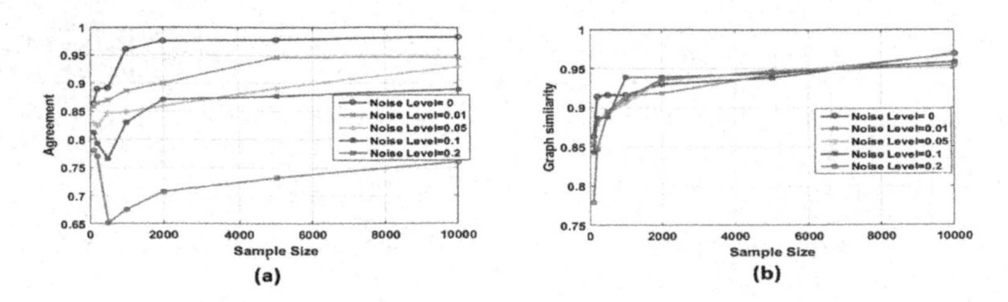

Fig. 5. The average sample agreement (a) and the average CP-net similarity (b) at different noise level on synthetic data.

In this case, we generated a binary-valued CP-net N_o with n = 10 attributes. For the choice data S, we generated 50, 100, 1000, 2000, 5000 and 10000 pairwise comparisons. Then different level of noise, 0, 0.01, 0.05, 0.1 and 0.2, is applied to each dataset. For each configuration, we repeat the algorithms 30 times, and calculated the average evaluation metrics between original CP-net and learned CP-net.

The performance of each algorithm is evaluated in terms of both *sample agreement* and *graph similarity* measures. The *sample agreement* is the proportion of samples entailed by both learned and original CP-nets defined as:

$$agreement = \frac{|\{(o_i, o_j)_{\in S} | o_i \succ_{N_l} o_j, o_i \succ_{N_o} o_j\}|}{|\{(o_i, o_j)_{\in S} | o_i \succ_{N_o} o_j\}|} \tag{5}$$

We use Eq. 6 to calculate the *similarity* between the preference graphs of two CP-nets. The numerator compute the number of edges that two CP-net have in common and the denominator is the maximum number of possible edges in the preference graphs. Note that since the two preference graphs are over the same outcome space, the maximum number of edges in them are the same.

$$similarity(G_1, G_2) = \frac{|\{(o_i, o_j) | (o_i, o_j) \in E_1, (o_i, o_j) \in E_2\}|}{k} \tag{6}$$

where G_1 and G_2 are the preference graphs of CP-nets, E_1 and E_2 are the sets of edges in G_1 and G_2 respectively.

Figure 5(a) represents the average sample agreement between original CP-net and learned CP-net at different noise level and training set size. As expected, we observed better performance when the sample size increases. We also observed that, for larger noise level ρ, at first we have a very good sample agreement for small data-set and suddenly it drops and then starts to climb to $1 - \rho$. The reason is that for small data-sets, the noisy data cause less conflicts in the data-set and it is easier to find a CP-net that satisfies the examples. However, as the number of examples increases, the conflicting examples become distinguishable to our algorithm. The convergence to $1 - \rho$ indicates that the conflicting affect of inconsistent examples are detected and thus removed by our method. Figure 5(b) represents the average similarity between learned and original CP-net. As the number of training example increases, so does the similarity measure even with high level of noise. The convergence of similarity measure to 1 indicates that both the learned and original CP-nets contain the same set of edges in their preference graphs.

Table 3 shows the evaluation results of our algorithm against two CP-net learning algorithm proposed in [22,23] on synthetic data. Similar to our method, these methods learn CP-nets passively from inconsistent examples. For every setting, we gave every algorithm 2000 s of processing time. If the algorithm does not return in 2000 s, it will be stopped and the intermediate result will be reported. As we can see, for smaller problems, e.g., 5 attributes, all algorithms performs similarly, but as the number of attributes increases the performance of [22,23] drops significantly. Note that for larger problems (e.g., with 20 or 50 attributes) these algorithms need a large training set in order to prove their hypothesis. We also tested the robustness of these methods in noisy condition by adding 10% of noise to the data set. We observed that all methods have handled the noisy data and could find similar preference graphs as the noise-free setting, however, we again observed a significant gap between our learned CP-net model and theirs with respect to their performance.

Regarding the processing time, not surprisingly, the proposed method is slower than the ones presented in [22,23] for small number of attributes. This is due the natural disadvantage of Genetic Algorithm which includes a significant overhead during the optimization process. Although, for small number of attributes, there is a big gap in processing time between the proposed method and others (ours is almost 1000 times slower on average) however, this gap decreases as the number of attributes increases. As we discuss earlier, we chose GA as the optimization algorithm due to it's ability to work well with NP-hard problems. As we can see, other algorithms practically fail in large-scale problems (i.e. more that 15 attributes) but the proposed method gives acceptable results even for problems with 100 attributes. For instance, for 100 attributes in noiseless setting, the output CP-nets of the other algorithms had less than %2 similarity with the original CP-net while the CP-nets returned by the proposed algorithm had around %58 similarity, on average, with the original CP-net.

Table 4 shows the comparison between our algorithm with the learning-to-rank methods, namely RankNet [7], AdaRank [24], OSVM [18] and SVOR [15], on synthetic data. These methods are among the most popular methods for learning-to-rank in recent years, and can perform under noisy training samples. The experiment shows that our method significantly outperforms all the learning-to-rank methods on synthetic data at different noise levels. However, we should mention that the results could be biased in our favor, because the experiment on synthetic data suffers from a significant problem, that is, it assumes that all comparisons are entailed by a CP-net. Therefore, in order to further examine the correctness of the method, in the next section we evaluate our algorithm against real-world preference data obtained from human subjects.

Table 3. Comparison between the proposed method and two CP-net learning methods on synthetic data (sample size = 1000, 30 independent runs for each algorithm).

ρ	Node	[23]			[22]			Proposed method		
		Similarity	Agreement	Time (s)	Similarity	Agreement	Time (s)	Similarity	Agreement	Time (s)
0	5	0.9767	0.9834	<0.01	0.9812	0.9870	<0.01	**0.9912**	**0.9965**	35
	10	0.5448	0.5429	<0.1	0.5941	0.5087	<0.1	**0.9155**	**0.9411**	51
	15	0.3393	0.4832	552	0.3983	0.4010	836	**0.7769**	**0.8261**	351
	20	0.2711	0.3011	1776	0.2861	0.3154	2075	**0.6124**	**0.7088**	571
	50	0.2181	0.1919	>2000	0.1803	0.2209	>2000	**0.6110**	**0.6747**	792
	100	0.0714	0.1452	>2000	0.1006	0.1713	>2000	**0.5793**	**0.5808**	1098
0.1	5	0.9543	0.8996	<0.01	0.9551	0.8717	<0.01	**0.9955**	**0.8993**	41
	10	0.5292	0.2932	<0.1	0.5845	0.3549	<0.1	**0.9169**	**0.8669**	67
	15	0.4393	0.2976	617	0.3862	0.2528	799	**0.7798**	**0.7331**	373
	20	0.2666	0.2386	1971	0.2038	0.2310	2101	**0.6008**	**0.6310**	656
	50	0.2176	0.1709	>2000	0.2104	0.2217	>2000	**0.6159**	**0.6318**	910
	100	0.0814	0.1912	>2000	0.0709	0.1117	>2000	**0.5814**	**0.5880**	1333

Table 4. Comparison between the proposed method and the learning-to-rank methods on synthetic data.

$\lvert S\rvert$	ρ	0	0.01	0.05	0.1	0.2
	Method	Sample agreement				
500	AdaRank	0.8585	0.8570	0.7826	0.7127	0.5315
	RankNet	0.8251	0.8100	0.7896	0.7773	0.5195
	OSVM	0.8831	0.8779	0.8163	0.6054	0.4103
	SVOR	0.8568	0.8236	0.8030	0.6717	0.4561
	Our method	**0.9722**	**0.9482**	**0.9163**	**0.8550**	**0.7817**
1000	AdaRank	0.8953	0.8683	0.8235	0.8167	0.6629
	RankNet	0.8147	0.8149	0.7939	0.7939	0.6265
	OSVM	0.8938	0.8736	0.7939	0.6225	0.4291
	SVOR	0.8868	0.8424	0.7684	0.7277	0.4514
	Our method	**0.9948**	**0.9801**	**0.9352**	**0.8821**	**0.7869**

5.2 Results on Real Data

Sushi data-set [17] collected by Kamishima et al. has been adapted by several authors for their CP-net learning algorithms [22,23]. This data set contains 100 kinds of sushi and 5000 users' preferences on them, with each sushi represented by 3 categorical and 6 numerical attributes. Each user was asked to rank ten types of sushi. Knowing the preference orders of these categories, for each user we generated 50, 100, 200, 500, and 1000 pairwise comparisons at 0, 0.01, 0.1, 0.2 noise levels respectively. For each configuration we chose 500 users randomly to repeat the experiment. With respect to the CP-net, we considered all 7 attributes of the sushi data set (ID and name attributes are excluded). Categorical attributes are applied directly while numerical attributes are converted into binary attributes: all data lower than the median are set to 0, and to 1 otherwise.

Table 5. Comparing the proposed method with two CP-net learning methods on sushi data.

$\|S\|$	500				1000			
ρ	0	0.01	0.05	0.1	0	0.01	0.05	0.1
Method	Sample agreement				Sample agreement			
[22]	0.8080	0.8160	0.7921	0.7628	0.8240	0.7917	0.7660	0.7520
[23]	0.7921	0.7970	0.7496	0.7311	0.8125	0.8133	0.7998	0.7852
Our method	**0.8417**	**0.8431**	**0.8189**	**0.7967**	**0.8697**	**0.8749**	**0.8402**	**0.8308**

Table 6. Comparing the proposed method with learning to rank methods on sushi dataset.

$\|S\|$	500				1000			
ρ	0	0.01	0.05	0.1	0	0.01	0.05	0.1
Method	Sample agreement				Sample agreement			
AdaRank	0.7653	0.7682	0.7405	0.7331	0.7895	0.7917	0.7660	0.7495
RankNet	0.6626	0.6626	0.6425	0.6160	0.6999	0.6992	0.6768	0.6765
OSVM	0.7270	0.7212	0.6792	0.6441	0.7572	0.7482	0.7201	0.6893
SVOR	0.7301	0.7324	0.6615	0.6366	0.7784	0.7704	0.6424	0.6311
Our method	**0.8417**	**0.8431**	**0.8189**	**0.7967**	**0.8697**	**0.8749**	**0.8402**	**0.8308**

Tables 5 and 6 provide the comparison result of the preference learning methods on sushi data-set. With respect to the CP-net learning techniques [22,23], like the results of synthetic data-set, our method significantly outperforms others (Table 5). Also, like the first experiment, here we observe that the proposed method clearly outperforms all the learning-to-rank methods with respect to sample agreement (Table 6). This is due to the fact that learning-to-rank methods do not take into account the conditional dependency of the attributes.

6 Conclusions

In this paper, we have proposed an evolutionary optimization based model of learning CP-nets that has scalability advantages over exiting passive preference learning methods, providing leverage with respect to inconsistent examples. Our preference learning method does not learn the CP-nets directly. Instead, we framed the problem of learning into an optimization problem and harness the power of evolutionary algorithms to find an optimal CP-net. Our experiment results have demonstrated that the proposed method is able to find a good quality CP-net and outperforms the current state-of-the-art preference learning algorithms.

Our future work is to further improve the performance of preference learning methods. We also plan to improve the initialization method used in this paper.

Since the problem of learning CP-net from inconsistent examples is NP-complete, having good quality initial solutions may play an important role in scaling up the algorithm to large-scale preference learning problems.

References

1. Alanazi, E., Mouhoub, M., Zilles, S.: The complexity of learning acyclic CP-nets. In: IJCAI, pp. 1361–1367 (2016)
2. Allen, T.E.: CP-nets: from theory to practice. In: ADT, pp. 555–560 (2015)
3. Allen, T.E., Goldsmith, J., Mattei, N.: Counting, ranking, and randomly generating CP-nets. In: MPREF (2014)
4. Athienitou, F., Dimopoulos, Y.: Learning CP-networks: a preliminary investigation. In: MPREF (2007)
5. Baok, T.: Evolutionary Algorithm in Theory and Practice. Oxford University Press, Oxford (1998)
6. Boutilier, C., Brafman, R.I., Hoos, H.H., Poole, D.: Reasoning with conditional ceteris paribus preference statements. In: UAI, pp. 71–80 (1999)
7. Burges, C., Shaked, T., Renshaw, E., Lazier, A., Deeds, M., Hamilton, N., Hullender, G.: Learning to rank using gradient descent. In: ICML, pp. 89–96 (2005)
8. Chen, H., Zhou, L., Han, B.: On compatibility of uncertain additive linguistic preference relations and its application in the group decision making. Knowl. Based Syst. **24**(6), 816–823 (2011)
9. Chevaleyre, Y., Koriche, F., Lang, J., Mengin, J., Zanuttini, B.: Learning ordinal preferences on multiattribute domains: the case of CP-nets. In: Preference Learning, pp. 273–296 (2010)
10. Corder, G.W., Foreman, D.I.: Nonparametric statistics: a step-by-step approach (2014)
11. Dimopoulos, Y., Michael, L., Athienitou, F.: Ceteris paribus preference elicitation with predictive guarantees. In: IJCAI 2009, pp. 1–6 (2009)
12. Eiben, A.E.: A method for designing decision support systems for operational planning. Ph.D. thesis, Technische Universiteit Eindhoven (1991)
13. Emrouznejad, A., Mustafa, A., Al-Eraqi, A.S., et al.: Aggregating preference ranking with fuzzy data envelopment analysis. Knowl. Based Syst. **23**(6), 512–519 (2010)
14. Guerin, J.T., Allen, T.E., Goldsmith, J.: Learning CP-net preferences online from user queries. In: ADT, pp. 208–220 (2013)
15. Herbrich, R., Graepel, T., Obermayer, K.: Support vector learning for ordinal regression. In: ICANN, vol. 1, pp. 97–102 (1999)
16. Kamishima, T.: Nantonac collaborative filtering: recommendation based on order responses. In: ACM SIGKDD, pp. 583–588 (2003)
17. Kamishima, T., Akaho, S.: Nantonac collaborative filtering: a model-based approach. In: Proceedings of the Fourth ACM Conference on Recommender Systems, pp. 273–276 (2010)
18. Kazawa, H., Hirao, T., Maeda, E.: Order SVM: a kernel method for order learning based on generalized order statistics. Syst. Comput. Jpn. **36**(1), 35–43 (2005)
19. Keeney, R.L., Raiffa, H.: Decision with multiple objectives (1976)
20. Lang, J., Mengin, J.: Learning preference relations over combinatorial domains. In: NMR, pp. 207–214 (2008)

21. Lang, J., Mengin, J.: The complexity of learning separable ceteris paribus preferences. In: IJCAI, pp. 848–853 (2009)
22. Liu, J., Xiong, Y., Caihua, W., Yao, Z., Liu, W.: Learning conditional preference networks from inconsistent examples. IEEE TKDE **26**(2), 376–390 (2014)
23. Liu, J., Yao, Z., Xiong, Y., Liu, W., Caihua, W.: Learning conditional preference network from noisy samples using hypothesis testing. Knowl. Based Syst. **40**, 7–16 (2013)
24. Xu, J., Li, H.: AdaRank: a boosting algorithm for information retrieval. In: ACM SIGIR, pp. 391–398 (2007)

Bioinformatic and Medical Data Analysis

Predicting Clinical Outcomes of Alzheimer's Disease from Complex Brain Networks

Xingjuan Li, Yu Li[✉], and Xue Li

School of Information Technology and Electrical Engineering,
The University of Queensland, Brisbane 4067, Australia
x.li4@uq.edu.au, {yuli,xueli}@itee.uq.edu.au

Abstract. Brain network modelling has been shown effective to study the brain connectivity in Alzheimer's disease (AD). Although the topological features of AD affected brain networks have been widely investigated, combining hierarchical networks features for predicting AD receives little attention. In this study, we propose a spectral convolutional neural network (SCNN) framework to learn combinations of hierarchical network features for a reliable AD prediction outcomes. Due to the complex high-dimensional structure of brain networks, conventional convolutional neural networks (CNN) are not able to learn the complete geometrical information of brain networks. To address this limitation, our SCNN is spectrally designed to learn a complete set of network topological features. Specifically, we construct structural brain networks using magnetic resonance images (MRI) from 288 ADs, 272 mild cognitive impairments (MCI) and 272 normal controls (NC). Then, we deploy SCNN to classify ADs from MCIs and NCs. Experiment results show that SCNN is able to achieve the accuracy of 91.07% in AD/NC classification, 87.72 in AD/MCI classification and 85.45% in MCI/HC classification. In addition, we show that SCNN is able to predict clinical scores associated with AD with high precision.

Keywords: Alzheimer's disease · Structural brain networks · Deep learning · Prediction

1 Introduction

Alzheimer's disease (AD) is a type of brain disorders and the most common cause of dementia, which is characterized by memory loss and cognitive decline. Worldwide, over 46.8 million people are living with AD [1]. Caring for patients with AD causes a huge social and economic impact on both the government and family members. Promote detection of AD is critical for early intervention, which can prevent the permanent damage to the brain. However, predicting AD in the early stage is challenging because the symptoms of AD are not fully expressed and often misdiagnosed with other types of dementia [2].

Brain network has been shown effective to analyze AD by modelling the human brain as a complex network consisting of a set of nodes connected by edges. From this perspective, AD is often regarded as "disconnection syndrome" [3]. Some studies focus on analyzing the topological characteristics of brain networks affected by AD [4–7].

G. Cong et al. (Eds.): ADMA 2017, LNAI 10604, pp. 519–525, 2017.
https://doi.org/10.1007/978-3-319-69179-4_36

Compared with the normal human brain network, they have found alterations in AD affected brain networks, such as reduced clustering coefficients and local efficiency. Other studies investigate changes of network patterns in the progression of AD [8, 9]. Only a limited number of recent studies attempt to use brain network for AD prediction [10, 11]. These work employ pattern recognition method and the support vector machine (SVM) to identify diseased brain networks from the normal. However, the hidden network features underlying AD are still underexplored.

In this study, we attempt to predict the AD progression and severity though combining multilevel network features derived from magnetic resonance images (MRI). To perform the prediction task, we employ the convolutional neural network (CNN). CNN is one of the most successful deep neural networks. It has achieved desired performance on many real world tasks, such as medical image analysis [12]. However, traditional CNN is unable to learn the geometrical features from brain networks due to its complexity. More recently, BrainNetCNN has been proposed to exploit hidden network features for predicting the neurodevelopment outcomes in infants [13]. Although BrainNetCNN is able to learn the topology features of brain networks using specially designed convolutional filters, the geometric features is still underexplored due the nature of convolution in Euclidean space. To solve this limitation, we proposed Spectral Convolutional Neural Networks (SCNN) framework to predict AD progression. SCNN is spectrally designed to be independent on the input network dimensions, leading to improved feature representation.

The paper is organized as follows. Section 2 introduces the formal framework of SCNN. In Sect. 3, we show our experiment result, including how structural brain network is constructed and the prediction results. Section 4 concludes with a brief summary.

1.1 Contributions

Our main contributions are summarized as follows:

- We show that SCNN is able to represent hierarchical brain networks features for the prediction of AD.
- Compared with classical CNNs, deploying SCNN in the spectral domain reduces the computation complexity.

2 Method

Here, we present our novel SCNN architecture, the dataset used in the study, and evaluation metrics.

2.1 SCNN Architecture

The architecture of SCNN is based on a common CNN, which is made up of convolutional layers, subsampling layers and fully-connected layers. Figure 1 gives a schematic representation of SCNN.

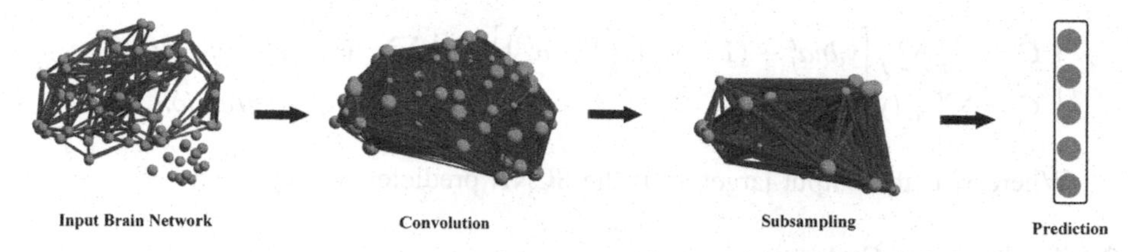

Fig. 1. SCNN architecture. Input layer holds the raw values about the brain networks. Convolutional layer extracts informative network elements for AD prediction, followed by the ReLU activation. Subsampling layer performs the dimension reduction. Fully-connected layer computes the prediction scores.

2.1.1 SCNN Layers

A anatomical MRI-derived brain network, $G = \{N, W\}$, is a compact representation of the grey matter (GM) connections in a person's brain, where N is a set of nodes representing region of interests (ROI) in the brain and W is a weighted connectivity matrix represent connection strength between region pairs. Let $\{g_1, g_2, \ldots, g_N\}$ be the grey matter volumes of ROIs, the weighted connectivity matrix is measured by

$$W(g_i, g_j) = \frac{\sum_{i=1}^{N}(g_i - \bar{g}_i)(g_j - \bar{g}_j)}{\sqrt{\sum_{i=1}^{N}(g_i - \bar{g}_i)^2}\sqrt{\sum_{i=1}^{N} g_j - \bar{g}_j^2}} \tag{1}$$

Where g_i is the grey matter volume of brain region i, $\bar{g}_i$ is the mean of all brain regions, i and j represent brain regions from left and right hemispheres.

The input layer of SCNN is the spectral graph representation of brain networks, where the connections between region pairs and locations of nodes have been represented by a set of eigenvalues.

Instead of directly learn the topological features from complex brain networks, SCNN learn their corresponding eigenvalues graph Laplacian L, resulting a compact and complete feature representation.

$$G * f = U^T(UG \odot Uf). \tag{2}$$

Where U is the unitary matrix, f is the filters.

All features learned from the layer have been activated by the ReLU function before feeding into next layer.

The subsampling layer in SCNN is summarize learned features from previous layer and reduce the spatial size of representation, resulting in reduced number of features and computation complexity.

Finally, a fully-connected layer is connected to compute the prediction scores.

Cost function of SCNN is designed as:

$$\begin{cases} C = -\frac{1}{n}\sum_{xj}\left[y_i ln a_j^L + (1-y_i)\ln\left(1-a_j^L\right)\right] + \frac{\lambda}{2n}\sum_w w^2, & classification \\ C = \sum_{i=0}^{n}(y_i - a_i)^2, & regression \end{cases}. \quad (3)$$

Where y_i is the output target, a_i is the SCNN predicted value.

2.1.2 Program Code

```
Algorithm: Training SCNN
  Given input network G.
  for i = 1:n:
      Fetch the input G and the target y.
      Compute interpolated weights w.
      Compute activated output a.
      Compute error signal e = Σ_{i=0}^{n}(y − a)^2 .
      Compute gradient of weights de/dw.
      Adjusting weights w = w + de/dw.
  end.
```

2.2 Dataset

We collect all the MRI data from Alzheimer's Disease Neuroimaging Initiative (ADNI) database (http://adni.loni.usc.edu/), including 288 ADs, 272 mild cognitive impairments (MCI), and 272 normal controls (NC). The demographic information of the dataset has been described in Table 1.

Table 1. Demographic information about participants

Attributes	AD	MCI	NC
Number	288	272	272
Gender(Male/Female)	141/147	179/93	126/146
Age	74.28 ± 6.97	75.42 ± 6.37	75.43 ± 4.27
MMSE	18.60 ± 7.37	24.36 ± 7.12	41.02 ± 10.67
CDRSB	20.41 ± 5.94	13.29 ± 3.80	6.22 ± 2.74

Values represent mean ± standard deviation. Abbreviations: MMSE = mini-mental state examination; CDRSB = clinical dementia rating sum of box.

For all MRI brain images, the whole brain is segmented into GM, white matter, and cerebrospinal fluid tissues. Then, we extract ROIs of GM using ICBM452 template [14].

2.3 Evaluation Metrics

In the group classification task, we report accuracy, sensitivity and specificity. While sensitivity reflects the probability of a test to correctly identify individuals with the disease, specificity reflects the probability of test to correctly identify those without disease. In the regression task, we report mean absolute error (MAE) and R2 score to evaluate the performance of SCNN.

3 Experiments

A 10-fold cross validation strategy has been employed in our experiments to split the dataset into the training data, the validation data and the test data.

3.1 Structural Brain Network Construction

We constructed structural brain networks from MRI images. Nodes were defined using ROIs extracted from MRI images, edges are computed using Pearson correlation. Figure 2 showed how brain network is constructed from MRI images.

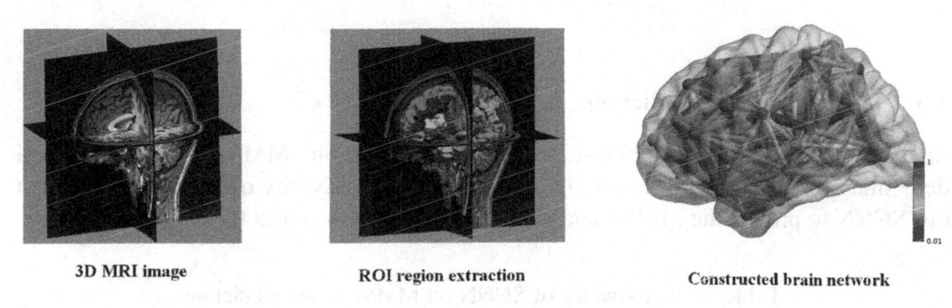

Fig. 2. The process to construct structural brain networks start from whole brain extraction from MRI images, ROI regions extraction, followed by edges estimation.

3.2 Group Classification

We deploy our SCNN to classify AD from MCI and NC. Table 1 gives the classification results compared with SVM and random forest (RF). Experiment results show that SCNN is able to classify AD from other with high accuracy. Although Sensitivity reported by SCNN is relatively lower than SVM and RF in AD/MCI classification, it is still higher than the ideal biomarker sensitivity of 80% [15]. Table 2 gives the comparison of our SCNN with similar work using graph constructed from MRI to predict AD (Table 3).

Table 2. Comparison of the performance of SVM, RF and the proposed SNN methods in the classification task

Methods	AD vs. NC (%)			MCI vs. NC (%)			AD vs. MCI (%)		
	ACC	SEN	SPE	ACC	SEN	SPE	ACC	SEN	SPE
SVM	78.57	79.31	77.77	74.54	80.00	70.00	74.54	92.59	57.14
RF	87.50	86.20	88.88	83.63	88.00	80.00	80.00	92.59	67.85
SCNN	**91.07**	**88.24**	**95.45**	**85.45**	**92.86**	**77.78**	**87.72**	**84.38**	**92.00**

Abbreviations: ACC = accuracy, SEN = sensitivity, SPE = specificity

Table 3. Comparison of the accuracy of different classification methods using MRI-constructed graph

Methods	Subjects	Modalities	AD vs. NC (%)	MCI vs. NC (%)
Zhang et al. in NeuroImage (2011)	51 AD, 99MCI, 52 NC	MRI	86.2	72.0
Tong et al. in PatternRecognition (2017)	37 AD, 75 MCI, 35 NC	MRI	82.6	73.3
SCNN	288 AD, 284 MCI, 272 NC	MRI	**91.07**	**85.45**

3.3 Clinical Scores Prediction

In the clinical setting, the mini-mental state examination (MMSE) and the clinical dementia rating (CDR) scores are often used to staging severity of AD. Here, we train our SCNN to predict the MMSE and CDR scores. Table 4 shows the prediction results.

Table 4. Performance of SCNN on MMSE score prediction

SCNN	MAE	R^2-score
MMSE	6.11	0.34
CDR	4.72	0.12

Abbreviations: MAE = mean absolute error.

4 Conclusion

In this study, we presented SCNN to predict the clinical outcomes associated with AD from structural brain networks. We first introduced spectral designed neural network architecture to learn the geometric information from brain networks. Our experiment results show that SCNN is able to learn all possible combinations of network features for the prediction of AD. Classification results of SCNN is higher than SVM and RF using MRI data only. In addition, MMSE and CDR scores predicted by SCNN are highly correlated with ground truth scores.

References

1. Prince, M.J.: World Alzheimer Report 2015: the global impact of dementia: an analysis of prevalence, incidence, cost and trends. Alzheimer's Disease International (2015)
2. Lisa, M., Berti, V., Glodzik, L., Pupi, A., De Santi, S., de Leon, M.J.: Pre-clinical detection of Alzheimer's disease using FDG-PET, with or without amyloid imaging. J. Alzheimer's Dis. **20**(3), 843–854 (2010)
3. Delbeuck, X., Van der Linden, M., Collette, F.: Alzheimer'disease as a disconnection syndrome? Neuropsychol. Rev. **13**(2), 79–92 (2003)
4. Sanz-Arigita, E.J., Schoonheim, M.M., Damoiseaux, J.S., Rombouts, S.A., Maris, E., Barkhof, F., Scheltens, P., Stam, C.J.: Loss of 'small-world'networks in Alzheimer's disease: graph analysis of FMRI resting-state functional connectivity. PLoS ONE **5**(11), e13788 (2010)
5. Daianu, M., Jahanshad, N., Nir, T.M., Toga, A.W., Jack Jr., C.R., Weiner, M.W., Thompson, P.M.: Breakdown of brain connectivity between normal aging and Alzheimer's disease: a structural k-core network analysis. Brain Connect. **3**(4), 407–422 (2013). For the Alzheimer's Disease Neuroimaging Initiative
6. Vecchio, F., Miraglia, F., Piludu, F., Granata, G., Romanello, R., Caulo, M., Onofrj, V., Bramanti, P., Colosimo, C., Rossini, P.M.: "Small World" architecture in brain connectivity and hippocampal volume in Alzheimer's disease: a study via graph theory from EEG data. Brain Imag. Behav. **11**(2), 473–485 (2017)
7. Gomez-Ramirez, J., Wu, J.: Network-based biomarkers in Alzheimer's disease: review and future directions. Frontiers Aging Neurosci. **6** (2014)
8. Zhou, J., Greicius, M.D., Gennatas, E.D., Growdon, M.E., Jang, J.Y., Rabinovici, G.D., Kramer, J.H., Weiner, M., Miller, B.L., Seeley, W.W.: Divergent network connectivity changes in behavioural variant frontotemporal dementia and Alzheimer's disease. Brain **133** (5), 1352–1367 (2010)
9. Zhang, H.-Y., Wang, S.-J., Liu, B., Ma, Z.-L., Yang, M., Zhang, Z.-J., Teng, G.-J.: Resting brain connectivity: changes during the progress of Alzheimer disease. Radiology **256**(2), 598–606 (2010)
10. Zeng, L.-L., Shen, H., Liu, L., Wang, L., Li, B., Fang, P., Zhou, Z., Li, Y., Dewen, H.: Identifying major depression using whole-brain functional connectivity: a multivariate pattern analysis. Brain **135**(5), 1498–1507 (2012)
11. Zhang, Y., Dong, Z., Wang, S., Ji, G., Phillips, P.: Prediction of MCI to Alzheimer's conversion based on tensor-based morphometry and kernel support vector machine. Alzheimer's Dement. J. Alzheimer's Assoc. **11**(7), P702 (2015)
12. Greenspan, H., van Ginneken, B., Summers, R.M.: Guest editorial deep learning in medical imaging: overview and future promise of an exciting new technique. IEEE Trans. Med. Imag. **35**(5), 1153–1159 (2016)
13. Kawahara, J., Brown, C.J., Miller, S.P., Booth, B.G., Chau, V., Grunau, R.E., Zwicker, J.G., Hamarneh, G.: BrainNetCNN: convolutional neural networks for brain networks; towards predicting neurodevelopment. NeuroImage **146**, 1038–1049 (2017)
14. Pantazis, D., Joshi, A., Jiang, J., Shattuck, D.W., Bernstein, L.E., Damasio, H., Leahy, R.M.: Comparison of landmark-based and automatic methods for cortical surface registration. Neuroimage **49**(3), 2479–2493 (2010)
15. Weiner, M.W., Veitch, D.P., Aisen, P.S., Beckett, L.A., Cairns, N.J., Green, R.C., Harvey, D., et al.: Recent publications from the Alzheimer's Disease neuroimaging initiative: reviewing progress toward improved AD clinical trials. Alzheimer's Dement. **13**, e1–e85 (2017)

Doctoral Advisor or Medical Condition: Towards Entity-Specific Rankings of Knowledge Base Properties

Simon Razniewski[1,2](✉), Vevake Balaraman[3], and Werner Nutt[1]

[1] Free University of Bozen-Bolzano, Bolzano, Italy
{razniewski,nutt}@inf.unibz.it
[2] Max-Planck-Institute for Informatics, Saarbrücken, Germany
[3] University of Trento, Trento, Italy
vvek.9291@gmail.com

Abstract. In knowledge bases such as Wikidata, it is possible to assert a large set of properties for entities, ranging from generic ones such as name and place of birth to highly profession-specific or background-specific ones such as doctoral advisor or medical condition. Determining a preference or ranking in this large set is a challenge in tasks such as prioritisation of edits or natural-language generation. Most previous approaches to ranking knowledge base properties are purely data-driven, that is, as we show, mistake frequency for interestingness. In this work, we have developed a human-annotated dataset of 350 preference judgments among pairs of knowledge base properties for fixed entities. From this set, we isolate a subset of pairs for which humans show a high level of agreement (87.5% on average). We show, however, that baseline and state-of-the-art techniques achieve only 61.3% precision in predicting human preferences for this subset. We then develop a technique based on a combination of general frequency, applicability to similar entities and semantic similarity that achieves 74% precision. The preference dataset is available at https://www.kaggle.com/srazniewski/wikidatapropertyranking.

1 Introduction

General-purpose knowledge bases such as Wikidata [23], YAGO [22] or DBpedia [3] are becoming increasingly popular, and are used for a variety of tasks such as structured search, entity recognition or question answering. These knowledge bases can store a large number of entity types, and for each entity type a large number of properties. For instance, for the class of *human* alone, more than 100 properties are used in Wikidata at least 1000 times, among which are the following:

1: sex or gender	70: doctoral advisor
2: occupation	71: pseudonym
3: date of birth	72: medical condition
...	...
39: height	78: convicted of
40: instrument	79: singles record
...	...

G. Cong et al. (Eds.): ADMA 2017, LNAI 10604, pp. 526–540, 2017.
https://doi.org/10.1007/978-3-319-69179-4_37

An issue with these properties is that it is not known how interesting they are for specific entities. For instance, while 90% of the data in Wikidata is created by bots [23], it is not clear whether the entered data captures actually what is of interest to humans. As a consequence, the large number of properties and their unclear interestingness severely hinder the usability of knowledge bases, and make many data analytics tasks difficult.

A way to better structure these properties would be rankings by interestingness. Such rankings would be useful for at least three tasks:

1. *Recommendations to authors:* Rankings by interestingness could help human authors in focusing their work [1,16,18]. For Wikidata, there exists a tool called *Wikidata property suggester*[1] for that purpose. However, the current instance is association-rule-based, which, as we show below, does not well approximate the human perception of interestingness.
2. *Automatically generating descriptions:* One of the major motivations for the Wikidata project is to automatically generate article stubs, which is especially relevant for low-resource languages. As a 2015 report of the Wikimedia Foundation found, "[the] lack of any clear identifier for importance or primacy in Wikidata items"[2] is one of the primary obstacles to this goal.
3. The lack of ordering also makes comparing the relative completeness of entities [21], as for instance attempted by the Recoin tool [2], difficult.

Predicting the interestingness of properties is difficult for at least three reasons: (i) Looking at the knowledge base alone is not sufficient: just because a property is very frequent in a knowledge base, one cannot conclude that the property is also very important. For instance, there are about 27k people with a blood type, but only 2k people with a hair color in Wikidata, but nevertheless, the latter is generally more interesting than the former. (ii) The interestingness of properties is very dependent on the person. For a politician, for instance, the political party is generally much more important than music instruments played, while for musicians, it is usually the other way around. (iii) There is a lack of datasets for this task, as most previous work used ablation studies, i.e., assessed performance on randomly removed portions of the data.

Previous work on property recommendation has mostly focused on data-driven approaches [1,12,16,24], which does not approximate human judgment too well. For instance, the Wikidata Property Suggester recommends to add *date of death* and *place of death* as most important missing properties to nearly all persons still alive. Similarly, it appears that frequent properties such as *gender* and *nationality* are overrated. Closest to ours, work by Atzori and Dessi [10] has investigated how to predict what human annotators actually find important, ignoring however the characteristics of individual entities, and using listwise learning-to-rank approaches that are not scalable.

---

[1] https://github.com/Wikidata-lib/PropertySuggester.

[2] https://meta.wikimedia.org/wiki/Research:Wikidata_gap_analysis#Conclusion.

Contribution. Our technical contributions are: (i) We introduce the problem of property ranking and discuss its significance in Sect. 3. (ii) We develop a human-annotated gold-standard dataset containing 350 sets of an entity and two properties, each annotated with 10 preference judgments in Sect. 4. (iii) We evaluate baseline approaches and the state-of-the-art against our dataset, showing that these only achieve 61.3% precision on records where humans have 87.5% agreement (Sect. 5). (iv) We develop techniques based on regression, LSI, LDA and ensembles that are able to achieve 74% precision in Sect. 6.

2 Background

Learning to rank (L2R). Learning to rank is a classic machine learning problem, where one aims to learn how to optimally rank given items. There are three main approaches to L2R, the so-called pointwise, pairwise, and listwise ranking [6,17]. The pointwise approach, which is usually the easiest to implement, is based on the idea that each item has a score, which can be learned. Items can then be ranked by their score. Issues with the pointwise approach are mainly that the individual scores can be hard to interpret, and are not stable wrt. framing.

The pointwise and listwise approach aim to overcome this limitation of the pointwise approach by learning from ranked pairs and ranked lists, respectively. They can lead to more stable and better rankings, however, potentially require more effort during training data creation.

Wikidata. Wikidata is a crowd-sourced knowledge base that maintains information about entities of human knowledge, called *items* in Wikidata parlance, which can be topics of Wikipedia articles (people, cities, movies, etc.) or anything else deemed of interest. Information about an entity is structured as a collection of *statements*, which are pairs consisting of a key, called, *property*, and a value, which can be an atomic data value, an item, a property, or some possibly complex structure. Currently, Wikidata contains roughly 25 mio. entities, and 2719 properties, whose usage follows roughly an exponential distribution. This has two implications: First, it confirms the perception that many properties are quite specific, and apply only to few people. Second, it indicates that solely frequency-based rankings of properties tend to become imprecise in the long tail.

Ranking of Knowledge Base Properties. There have been various works on knowledge base property ranking. Most prominently, editors of Wikidata items are supported by the Property Suggester facility, which, given an entity, produces a list of typically 3 to 10 properties for which no statement exists as yet. It implements an approach by Abedjan and Naumann [1] that leverages techniques from association rule mining, and ranks rules according to squared confidence. On the one hand, this allows a few strong rules to outweigh many weaker ones, while on the other hand inapplicable properties may be suggested if they are highly correlated with some existing properties.

Atzori and Dessi [10] addressed the problem to rank the existing properties of individual items in a knowledge base, like Wikidata or DBpedia. They identified three parameters for automating such rankings: (i) algorithms for machine learning to rank; (ii) possible features of properties; and (iii) methods to create training sets. In a study, they chose eight algorithms, nine features, and six training sets and combined them in all possible ways. To test these combinations, they let a group of students pointwise rank the properties of 50 random Wikipedia entities. It turned out that the best combinations beat other state-of-the art techniques by improvements of precision and recall of 5 to 10%. Like the authors of the present paper, Atzori and Dessi aim at creating automated methods that approximate human judgment about property ranks. However, while they want to rank the properties that are already present for an item, we want to find out which properties of an item humans would find important or interesting, regardless of whether or not they are mentioned. Also, we aim to include information specific to the entity, not just use information on the level of the whole class.

Fact Ranking. Ranking knowledge base facts by importance, interestingness or unexpectedness is a very related topic [11,16,20]. Recent work by Bast et al. [4], for instance, investigates how to predict the relevance of attribute values on a scale from 0 to 1 for the multi-valued attributes profession and nationality. In their work, they show that methods that are based on the Wikipedia articles of persons and use a generative model can achieve reasonable accuracies on this task, i.e., less than 28% numerical error in 80% of cases. The problem was subsequently posed as challenge at the WSDM 2017 conference [13]. However, having a ranking for facts does not help in the three applications above, as for the recommendation as to what to add, and the completeness comparison task, the properties that do not yet have facts are the ones that should be ranked, while for the natural language generation task, it is generally desired that values of multivalued properties appear together, thus, a ranking of individual facts will not do.

3 Problem Definition and Challenges

We define our problem as follows:
Problem: Given an entity and a set of knowledge base properties, rank the properties according to their interestingness for the entity.

The notion of *interestingness* is hereby left somewhat vague, which however is intentional as our ranking is not intended to serve only one specific purpose. We identify the following technical challenges for this task:

1. *Lack of datasets*: Previous approaches [1,12,16,24] rely on ablation studies, i.e., they randomly remove a portion of knowledge base facts, then evaluate how well they can predict removed facts or properties. This however does not say anything about their ability to rank properties by interestingness. The only dataset available is that of [10], which contains however only pointwise annotations for properties of 50 entities, and is of unknown quality.

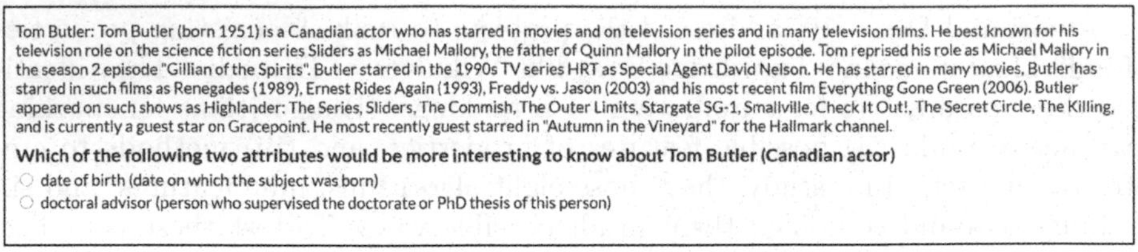

Tom Butler: Tom Butler (born 1951) is a Canadian actor who has starred in movies and on television series and in many television films. He best known for his television role on the science fiction series Sliders as Michael Mallory, the father of Quinn Mallory in the pilot episode. Tom reprised his role as Michael Mallory in the season 2 episode "Gillian of the Spirits". Butler starred in the 1990s TV series HRT as Special Agent David Nelson. He has starred in many movies, Butler has starred in such films as Renegades (1989), Ernest Rides Again (1993), Freddy vs. Jason (2003) and his most recent film Everything Gone Green (2006). Butler appeared on such shows as Highlander: The Series, Sliders, The Commish, The Outer Limits, Stargate SG-1, Smallville, Check It Out!, The Secret Circle, The Killing, and is currently a guest star on Gracepoint. He most recently guest starred in "Autumn in the Vineyard" for the Hallmark channel.

Which of the following two attributes would be more interesting to know about Tom Butler (Canadian actor)

- date of birth (date on which the subject was born)
- doctoral advisor (person who supervised the doctorate or PhD thesis of this person)

Fig. 1. Interface of the crowdsourcing task.

2. *Inapplicability of pointwise and listwise annotations:* While pointwise annotations are easy to solicit, the resulting scores can only be interpreted within the context in which they were generated [14,15]. Using the annotation scheme from [4], for instance, we found that the 0–1 interestingness score of properties of medium interestingness was 0.43 when preceded by 7 questions about more interesting properties, but 0.62 if preceded by 7 less interesting ones. As the set of properties in Wikidata is constantly growing,[3] this would mean that pointwise scores collected now could not be interpreted well at later development stages of Wikidata. Likewise, listwise approaches are not applicable, as it is not possible to elicit meaningful rankings for large sets of items.
3. *No supervised learning possible:* Given that there are more than 3 million *humans* in Wikidata, and that we rely on pairwise annotations, it is clear that it is impossible to generate enough training data for supervised learning.

We next address Issue (1), the generation of a suitable dataset.

4 Dataset Preparation

Records. We generated 350 random records consisting of a human and two properties, like (*Trump, doctoral advisor, medical condition*). As sampling humans at random from Wikidata would give mostly unknown persons, we decided to sample humans whose Wikidata pages had been edited within the month of November, 2016. As the pages of famous people tend to get edited more often than the pages of non-famous ones, this gave a better mix of humans of different fame. As Wikidata items contain a large fraction of properties that are identifiers, with many stemming from national libraries and directories that can only be understood by experts of the respective domain, we did not consider such ID properties. Of the properties that were not IDs, we considered all that were assigned to humans at least 1000 times, which resulted in 101 as of November 14, 2016.

Annotation. We used the CrowdFlower platform[4] for obtaining preference judgments. In the annotation task, a short biographical sketch and the two properties

[3] For instance, as of March 21st, 2016, there were 2202 properties, while as of February 7, 2017, there are 2719 according to https://tools.wmflabs.org/hay/propbrowse/.
[4] https://www.crowdflower.com.

Table 1. Sample records from our gold dataset.

Name	Description	Property 1	Property 2	Preferred	Agrmt
Albert Johnson	Canadian soccer player	Military conflict	Drafted by	Prop. 2	1
Andrew Collins	British actor	Field of work	Sister	Prop. 1	0.9
Svetlana Navasardyan	Armenian musician	Member of political party	Place of detention	-	0.5
Filip Stanislaw Dubiski	Polish officer	Residence	Sports discipline	Prop. 1	1
Dipankar Bhattacharjee	Indian badminton player	Roman praenomen	Bowling style	Prop. 2	0.6
David Ball	Electronic music producer	Doubles record	Military branch	Prop. 1	0.8
Kalim Kashani	17th century Persian poet	Languages spoken/written	Sexual orientation	Prop. 1	1

were presented to the annotators, and they were asked, knowing about which of the two properties would be more interesting. The core part of the interface is shown in Fig. 1. Quality was ensured via an entrance test and hidden test questions, based on questions unanimously answered in previous runs. For each record, 10 opinions were collected. At 2 ct. per annotation, the platform cost (including fees) to generate the whole dataset was $100. Six sample records are shown in Table 1.

Annotator Agreement. The agreement of the annotators is shown in Fig. 2 (solid bars). The dashed bars also show the agreement distribution that would be expected if annotators would answer at random. As one can see, annotator agreement is significantly different from random answers, especially evident for the high agreement cases (e.g., if annotators were to answer at random, only 0.2% instead of 8% of records would have an agreement of 1). The average agreement is 73%, and Fleiss' Kappa is 0.40. We also had two authors of this paper annotate a subset of the records, finding that they had 78% agreement with 16 records where annotators had 80% agreement, and 100% agreement with 16 records where annotators had 100% agreement. In turn, a manual inspection of low-agreement records showed that many of them correspond to cases where both properties appear unrelated, like *goalsScored* and *militaryRank* for *Pope Francis*, on which agreement is difficult.

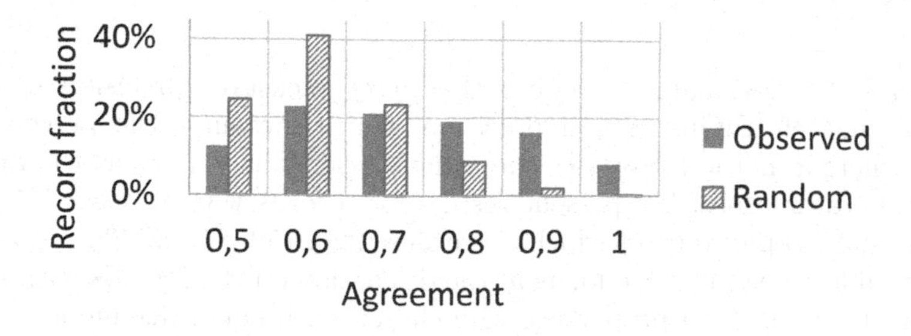

Fig. 2. Agreement distribution in our gold dataset.

Table 2. Performance of baseline approaches for property ranking.

Method	ppref on records with agreement			
	≥70% (n=223)	≥80% (n=150)	≥90% (n=85)	=100% (n=28)
Random	50%	50%	50 %	50%
Annotators	81.8%	87.5%	93.3%	100%
Human frequency	57.4%	60.6%	62.3%	50%
Occupation frequency	57.4%	58.6%	61.2%	53.6%
Google count	58%	58.3%	61.2%	53.6%
Property suggester	58.7%	61.3%	62.3%	50%

5 Baselines

Techniques. We evaluate four baselines, the first two being simple counts, while the latter two use the state of the art in textual information retrieval and property ranking, respectively:

1. *Human frequency:* This baseline always chooses the property that is more frequently used for *humans* as winner.
2. *Occupation frequency:* A modification of the previous that only looks at people having the same profession, aiming to capture the observation that professions are similar to classes.
3. *Google count:* This method chooses the property with more search results for Google queries concatenating entity name and property as winner. For instance, for *Pope Francis*, *goals scored* and *military rank*, the queries would be "Pope Francis goals scored" (470,000 results) and "Pope Francis military rank" (3,870,000 results), thus, *military rank* would be chosen as winner.
4. *Wikidata property suggester:* This baseline uses the suggestions of the Wikidata property suggester, and represents the state of the art in property ranking [24]. The version available online gives natively only few properties, so we modified the code by removing thresholds, in order to obtain further properties. Given an entity-property-property record from our dataset, the winning property according to this method was the one that was ranked higher by the property suggester.

Evaluation. For evaluation, we use the *ppref* measure (precision of preference) [7], henceforth just called precision, which measures the percentage of records where a method proposes the same property as winner as the majority of the annotators does. We present results for records with at least 70%, 80%, 90% and 100% separately, of which there were 226, 152, 85 and 28, respectively. Where trends are similar, we focus in the discussion on the records with at least 80% agreement. If both properties were chosen with equal likelihood, a record would have a probability of 11.2% to fall into this group, i.e., it is unlikely that for many of the records in this group, the property with more votes has been voted that way only by chance.

Results and Analysis. As Table 2 shows, all four baselines perform comparably bad, agreeing only in about 60% of the answers with the majority of the annotators. For Baselines (1), (2), and (4), we believe their main weakness is that they rely on describing the data that is present (remember *blood type* vs. *hair color*, where the former exists 14 times as often as the latter). While association rules (Baseline 4) are more sophisticated than simple counts (Baselines 1 and 2), apparently, better capturing correlations does not improve predictions on interestingness. It may be noteworthy that association rules were originally developed for discovering patterns in applications where data is complete, not for making statements about absent data. For Baseline (3), Google count, we trace the low performance to the fact that text search is not able to sufficiently capture the connection between entities and predicates. For instance, for *Pope Francis* and *military rank*, all top ranked results talk about his relation to the Argentinian dictatorship or the Swiss Guard, none about his *own* military rank.

6 Improving Property Ranking

6.1 Transfer Learning via Property Pivoting

We have seen that statistical approaches that learn patterns over the whole dataset do not yield a high precision in predicting pairwise interestingness preferences. We also discussed that it is virtually impossible to obtain enough training data for supervised learning. One approach often taken if supervised learning is not possible is *transfer learning.* Transfer learning refers to the training of models to solve a Problem A, for which enough training data is available, then applying them to a related Problem B [19]. An idea adapted from [4] is to predict, which of two properties is asserted for an entity, and which one is not.

Consider the case of *position played on team* (P413) and *religious order* (P611). There are 225,821 humans in Wikidata that have the former property but not the latter, and 7,976 humans that have the latter but not the former. Are there chances to accurately decide, for a person picked from either of these sets, to which of the two sets it belongs? We call this the *property pivoting problem.*

Deciding Property Pivoting via Regression. In the following, we use a logistic regression classifier trained on bags of words taken from person descriptions from Wikipedia to decide the property pivoting problem.

Wikipedia articles provide a messier, but considerably larger source of information about a person than Wikidata. By considering Wikipedia articles as bags of words, we can use the number of occurrences of each word as feature on which to train a classifier. In particular, for each pair of properties, we trained a logistic regression classifier on up to 20,000 entities, if available: 10,000 entities that had the first property but not the second one, and 10,000 entities that had the second but not the first property.

As an example of what these classifiers learned, the box below shows the most distinctive weights learned by the TF-IDF-based regression classifier that was trained for *position played on team* versus *religious order*:

-3.09: footballer	-2.39: season	2.67: jesuit	1.88: work
-2.85: football	-2.21: career	2.43: catholic	1.85: life
-2.75: played	-2.16: league	2.41: died	1.77: order
-2.72: team	-2.08: cup	2.04: priest	1.64: church
-2.67: player	-2.02: club	1.99: works	1.50: death

Negative weights hereby indicate that the occurrences of the word appear frequently in articles of entities with *position played on team* being present instead of *religious order*, while positive weights indicate the opposite. For instance, *season* (weight -2.39) is a word in the former category, while *priest* (weight 2.04) belongs to the latter. Interestingly, also some rather general words like *works* and *died* appear in the latter category. We conjecture that soccer players are mostly recent figures still alive, while monks are more frequently from the past, thus, *died* is more relevant for them, and that monks are known for more diverse activities than sports players, thus the term *work*.

Property Pivoting Quality. Evaluated each over 200 entities that had either the one or the other property, the regression classifiers achieved a respectable average precision of 94.8%. For *position played on team* versus *religious order*, for instance, the precision is even 100%, while difficult cases are for instance *field of work* versus *member of* (84% precision), or *child* versus *sister* (72% precision).

Transfer Learning. Our hope was that characteristics that describe whether a person has one property, but not another also relate to how interesting the one property is over the other. That is, for people that have a *position played on team* but no *religious order*, maybe knowing about the former is indeed more interesting than the latter. The results of transferring our regression classifiers are shown in Table 5 (third and fourth row). As we can see, the precision on records with at least 80% annotator agreement is 69.3% and 72%, depending on whether TF-IDF is used or not. These precisions are remarkably better than those of the baselines, though still leaving a considerable gap to the 95% precision on the pivoting task, indicating that property pivoting and property interestingness are only moderately related problems. For instance, although all annotators agree that for the soccer player *Albert Johnson*, *drafted by* is more interesting than *military conflict* (Table 1 first row), property pivoting still chooses the latter property, presumably, because *drafted by* is used in Wikidata only in very specific contexts of baseball and ice hockey, not for soccer. Similarly, for Kalim Kashani, a 17th century Persian poet, property pivoting chooses *sexual orientation* over *languages spoken or written*, although crowd agreement is 100% on *languages spoken or written* (Table 1 last row). Presumably the reason is that many people that are not poets have information about languages as well, while sexual orientation is especially frequently asserted for artists.

6.2 Semantic Approaches

As exemplified above, while regression is very well able to decide the property pivoting problem, existence of a property is still only a moderate indicator for interestingness. In particular, there are several cases where it is intuitive that one property does not apply to a person at all, while another is relevant, but regression is not able to discover that. In the following we thus propose to use semantic similarity as alternative proxy for interestingness. We conjecture that if a property bears some semantic similarity to an entity, like *goals scored* for *Ronaldo*, where humans can easily see an association of Ronaldo scoring goals, then it is more likely that property is also interesting.

Concretely, we propose to look at the semantic similarity of the textual descriptions of entities and properties. For entities, we use their English Wikipedia articles as text sources, while for properties we use their textual label and description on Wikidata. To compute semantic similarity, we rely on standard latent topic models, in particular Latent Semantic Indexing (LSI) [9] and Latent Dirichlet Allocation (LDA) [5]. We proceed in three steps:

1. In the first step, we train topic models on Wikipedia.
2. In the second step, we represent each entity and each property as distribution over the learned topics.
3. In the third step, for each (entity, property, property) record in our gold dataset, we compute the similarity between the topics of the entity and the two properties. We then assert that the more similar property is the more interesting one.

We further detail each step below.

Learning Topic Models. In the first step, we used LSI and LDA to learn 400 and 100 distinct topics over the English Wikipedia text corpus (12.5 GB). We used the *gensim* Python library, with which training could be done on a standard laptop within hours. LDA has a parameter α, which is a prior asserting whether texts are preferentially assigned to more or to fewer topics. This parameter is important for our application as assignment to fewer topics leads to sparser vectors. We report the results for the default value (1/#topics=0.01). We also tested a higher value, 0.05, and a setting called auto-optimization, where α is dynamically set for each topic, but both performed worse. Notably, we found in this setting that too high values of α lead to properties being assigned all to the same topics, resulting in entity-property distances that were indistinguishable. In Table 3 we show some of the most frequent words in four topics as learned by LDA.

Describing Entities and Properties using Topic Models. In the next step we used the learned topic models to describe entities and properties. To that end, given a set of words, LSI and LDA are able to compute a distribution of topics that is the most likely one to generate the given set of words.

Table 3. Sample topics as learned by LDA over Wikipedia

Topic	Terms
Topic 6:	0.011*league + 0.011*championships + 0.009*tournament + 0.008*cup + 0.008*club + 0.007*football + 0.007*women + 0.007*rank + 0.006*championship + 0.006*round + 0.006*games + 0.005*player + 0.005*goals + 0.005*men + 0.005*teams + 0.005*competed + 0.004*apps + 0.004*division + 0.004*event
Topic 26:	0.005*court + 0.004*law + 0.004*police + 0.003*rights + 0.003*women + 0.003*act + 0.003*sarpanch + 0.003*administrated + 0.002*prison + 0.002*case + 0.002*political + 0.002*party + 0.002*president + 0.002*legal + 0.002*justice + 0.002*arrested + 0.002*security + 0.002*said + 0.002*trump + 0.002*supreme
Topic 18:	0.017*brazil + 0.016*brazilian + 0.013*da + 0.012*paulo + 0.012*portuguese + 0.011*rio + 0.008*do + 0.007*portugal + 0.007*janeiro + 0.006*joão + 0.006*silva + 0.005*porto + 0.004*dos
Topic 41:	0.005*episode + 0.005*films + 0.004*cast + 0.004*directed + 0.004*television + 0.004*actor + 0.004*tv + 0.004*festival + 0.004*role + 0.004*awards + 0.003*actress + 0.003*drama + 0.003*award + 0.003*director + 0.003*filmography + 0.003*comedy

For the soccer player *Ronaldo*, for instance, LDA states that his Wikipedia article can be described using 52% of Topic 6, 12% of Topic 18, 7% of Topic 41, 6% of Topic 26 (all shown in Table 3), and low fractions of a few others. This distribution appears sensible, as he is most importantly known for playing soccer in leagues and tournaments (Topic 6), comes from Portugal (Topic 18, note that LDA has merged Brazil and Portugal into one topic), is featured frequently in the media (Topic 41) and has been under legal investigation (Topic 26). Similarly, the article of the former US president *Barack Obama* can be generated by combining 48% of Topic 26 (law and politics), 18% of a topic concerned with parties and elections, 12% of a topic concerned with business and industry, and various others.

In the same way, also properties can be described as combinations of topics. The property *height*, for instance, is composed of Topic 14 (geometry), 36 (abstraction), 84 (biology) and an unclear topic 88, whereas *member of sports team* is composed entirely of Topic 6.

Computing Similarities. For computing similarities between entities and properties, we use cosine similarity between vectors, a standard approach in vector-space-modelling and word embedding. The idea is to interpret topic distributions as vectors in a high-dimensional space, then compute the distance using the cosine of the angle between these vectors. In the case of *Ronaldo* and *goals scored* versus *military rank*, for instance, we find a cosine similarity of 0.987 versus 0.611. Thus, *goals scored* is the semantically more similar property, and hence we propose this to be the more interesting one.

Analysis. The performance of semantic similarity as a proxy for interestingness is shown in Table 5. As we can see, LDA does not outperform the baselines at 60% precision for records with at least 80% annotator agreement. In contrast, LSI performs considerably better at 65.3% precision, though still not achieving the performance of regression (72%).

We find that semantic similarity is better able to capture when one property does not make sense at all, as evidenced by the increase (LDA) or smaller drop

Table 4. Pearson correlation coefficients on records with at least 80% agreement

	Human freq.	Occupation freq.	Google count	Property Suggester	Regression (plain)	Regression (TF-IDF)	LDA	LSI
Human frequency	-	0.37	0.11	0.99	0.29	0.33	-0.07	0.07
Occupation frequency	0.37	-	-0.02	0.36	0.33	0.25	0.08	0.00
Google count	0.13	-0.02	-	0.11	0.01	0.03	-0.10	-0.01
Property Suggester	0.99	0.36	0.11	-	0.28	0.33	-0.07	0.05
Regression (unweighted)	0.26	0.33	0.01	0.28	-	0.87	0.14	0.29
Regression (TF-IDF)	0.32	0.25	0.03	0.33	0.87	-	0.09	0.26
LDA	-0.09	0.08	-0.10	-0.07	0.14	0.09	-	0.16
LSI	0.04	0.00	-0.01	0.05	0.29	0.26	0.16	-

(LSI) towards the records with 100% human agreement than regression. For instance, from the records with at least 80% agreement, the precision of LDA increases by 11.4%, the precision of LSI decreases by 1.1%, but the precision of regression drops by 6.1/7.5%.

But there are also various spectacular failures: For *Gabriel Kicsid*, a handball player, for instance, both LSI and LDA believe that *religious order* is more similar than *follows*, even though all annotators agree that the second is more interesting. A possible reason is that the description of *follows* is quite abstract and hard to match (*"immediately prior item in some series of which the subject is part"*[5]), even though human annotators correctly understand the usage, which is about succession for instance on a position in a team. Similarly, for the Polish officer *Filip Stanislaw Dubitzki* (Table 1, 4th row), unlike all annotators, LSI believes that *sports discipline* is more interesting than *residence*.

6.3 Ensembles

Considering the methods discussed so far along with their strong and weak points, the question arises whether it is possible to combine them and achieve a better performance. By Condorcet's jury theorem [8], it is beneficial to combine weak predictors whenever these show a sufficient level of statistical independence, and have each more than 50% accuracy. To see whether our methods exhibit sufficient statistical independence, we computed pairwise Pearson correlation coefficients, which are shown in Table 4.

There are two surprising insights. The first is the near-perfect correlation between human frequency and Property Suggester (0.99). In other words, even though the Property Suggester uses sophisticated ways for computing association rules and combining predictions, it does essentially nothing different from simply counting how often a property occurs. The second surprising insight is that apart from human frequency/property suggester and the two variants of regression, the pairwise correlation between the methods is very low. This even holds for similar techniques such as human frequency compared with occupation frequency

[5] https://www.wikidata.org/wiki/Property:P155.

(correlation 0.37) or LSI compared with LDA (correlation 0.16). Two methods, Google count and LDA, exhibit almost no correlation to any other method.

The results are in itself remarkable, and suggest that ensembles predictors[6] can give better performances than the individual methods. We tested to take the majority vote from various permutations of three and five of our presented methods. It turned out that the best performing ensemble was not only a combination of three advanced methods, but that even adding some of the baselines improved precision. In particular, the best performing combination used five methods that showed the biggest pairwise difference in Pearson correlation, namely the Google count, LSI, LDA, Occupation frequency, and regression (TF-IDF). This ensemble performed 2% and 4.6% better than the best single method, regression (TF-IDF) on records with at least 80% and 90% agreement, respectively.

6.4 Analysis

Results on the performance of the baselines are shown in Table 2, while the performance of the advanced methods is shown in Table 5. In both cases, we can see random agreement (50%) as a lower bound that any method should outperform, and annotator agreement as an upper bound. As one can see, regression trained on property pivoting as the best single advanced method beats the baselines by a margin of 10% on records with at least 80% agreement, with LSI performing 5% worse, and LDA being on par with the baselines. The best ensembles then add a further 2% precision on top of the regression. We draw the following conclusions:

1. *The state of the art methods alone are inadequate for property ranking.* The state of the art in property suggestion (Property Suggester) and document retrieval (Google count) achieved only 58.3 and 61.3% precision on records where annotators had 87.5% agreement, not significantly different from an approach that simply counts how often a property appears (60.6% precision).
2. *Regression is well-suited for property pivoting, but has still limitations, as it is data-driven.* Regression based on bags-of-words from Wikipedia articles achieves an accuracy of 94.8% for property pivoting on records with at least 80% agreement, i.e., deciding whether an entity has one property but not another. And while it is an expensive method, requiring to train $O(n^2)$ many classifiers for n properties, it is worth its price also for property ranking, as it outperforms the baselines by more than 10%. It has still limitations as it is data-driven, though, i.e., it predicts interestingness of properties based on their presence, which in some cases is not a good indicator.
3. *Semantic approaches are great at discovering applicability of properties, but struggle with short property descriptions.* Semantic similarity based on latent topic modeling turned out to be better able to capture cases where certain properties did not at all make sense. Nevertheless, there are problems with description shortness.

[6] Not to be mixed with *ensemble learning*, a machine learning approach where consecutive instances of the same classifier are trained especially on records that previous instances predicted wrongly. Ensemble learning requires a sufficient amount of labeled training data, which is not available in our case.

Table 5. Performance of advanced methods for property ranking.

Method	ppref on records with agreement			
	≥70% (n=223)	≥80% (n=150)	≥90% (n=85)	=100% (n=28)
Random	50%	50%	50%	50%
Annotators	81.8%	87.5%	93.3%	100%
Regression (unweighted)	67.7%	69.3%	70.4%	64.3%
Regression (TF-IDF)	70.4%	72%	71.8%	64.3%
LDA	57%	60%	61.2%	71.4%
LSI	59%	65.3%	67%	64.3%
Ensemble of Google count, LSI, LDA, Occupation frequency, regression (TF-IDF)	69.1%	74%	76.4%	67.9%

4. *Ensembles work best.* Taking the majority vote among methods based on counting (Occupation frequency, Google count), correlation (regression) and semantic similarity (LSI, LDA) approximated human judgment best.

7 Conclusion

We have introduced the problem of property ranking, shown the limitations of the state-of-the-art, and developed approaches that combine classical frequency-based approaches, transfer learning and semantic similarity. Our methods outperform the state of the art by over 10% precision, though still being inferior to human agreement by 11.5%. We hope that the dataset developed in this paper can stimulate research that can further approach human agreement.

We see two interesting avenues to extend this work: One is to improve the methods presented in this paper, for instance, by using other learning algorithms for the property pivoting problem, or by extending the short descriptions from which the semantic methods currently learn. The other is to find completely new approaches to the problem, which, even if they do not individually outperform the existing methods, might add information to ensembles. The challenge would be here to find related problems that can be used for transfer learning.

References

1. Abedjan, Z., Naumann, F.: Improving RDF data through association rule mining. Datenbank-Spektrum **13**(2), 111–120 (2013)

2. Ahmeti, A., Razniewski, S., Polleres, A.: Assessing the completeness of entities in knowledge bases. In: ESWC P&D (2017)
3. Auer, S., Bizer, C., Kobilarov, G., Lehmann, J., Cyganiak, R., Ives, Z.: DBpedia: a nucleus for a web of open data (2007)
4. Bast, H., Buchhold, B., Haussmann, E.: Relevance scores for triples from type-like relations. In: SIGIR, pp. 243–252. New York (2015)
5. Blei, D.M., Ng, Y.M., Jordan, M.I.: Latent Dirichlet allocation. J. Mach. Learn. Res. **3**, 993–1022 (2003)
6. Cao, Z., Qin, T., Liu, T.-Y., Tsai, M.-F., Li, H.: Learning to rank: from pairwise approach to listwise approach. In: ICML, pp. 129–136 (2007)
7. Carterette, B., Bennett, P.N., Chickering, D.M., Dumais, S.T.: Here or there. In: Macdonald, C., Ounis, I., Plachouras, V., Ruthven, I., White, R.W. (eds.) ECIR 2008. LNCS, vol. 4956, pp. 16–27. Springer, Heidelberg (2008). doi:10.1007/978-3-540-78646-7_5
8. de Condorcet, M.: Essai sur l'application de l'analyse à la probabilité des décisions rendues à la pluralité des voix. Imprimerie Royale, Paris (1785)
9. Deerwester, S.: Improving information retrieval with latent semantic indexing (1988)
10. Dessi, A., Atzori, M.: A machine-learning approach to ranking RDF properties. FGCS **54**, 366–377 (2016)
11. Fatma, N., Chinnakotla, M., Shrivastava, M.: The unusual suspects: deep learning based mining of interesting entity trivia from knowledge graphs. In: AAAI 2017 (2017)
12. Gassler, W., Zangerle, E., Specht, G.: Guided curation of semistructured data in collaboratively-built knowledge bases. FGCS **31**, 111–119 (2014)
13. Heindorf, S., Potthast, M., Bast, H., Buchhold, Haussmann, E.: WSDM cup 2017: vandalism detection and triple scoring (2017)
14. Jones, N., Brun, A., Boyer, A.: Comparisons instead of ratings: towards more stable preferences. In: WI-IAT, pp. 451–456 (2011)
15. Kalloori, S., Ricci, F., Tkalcic, M.: Pairwise preferences based matrix factorization and nearest neighbor recommendation techniques (2016)
16. Langer, P., Schulze, P., George, S., Kohnen, M., Metzke, T., Abedjan, Z., Kasneci, G.: Assigning global relevance scores to dbpedia facts. In: ICDE Workshops, pp. 248–253 (2014)
17. Li, H.: A short introduction to learning to rank. In: IEICE Transactions (2011)
18. Mousavi, H., Gao, S., Zaniolo, C.: IBminer: a text mining tool for constructing and populating infobox databases and knowledge bases. In: VLDB (2013)
19. Pan, S.J., Yang, Q.: A survey on transfer learning. In: TKDE (2010)
20. Prakash, A., Chinnakotla, M.K., Patel, D., Garg, P.: Did you know?-mining interesting trivia for entities from wikipedia (2015)
21. Razniewski, S., Suchanek, F.M., Nutt, W.: But what do we actually know. In: AKBC, pp. 40–44 (2016)
22. Suchanek, F.M., Kasneci, G., Weikum, G.: YAGO: a core of semantic knowledge. In: WWW, pp. 697–706 (2007)
23. Vrandečić, D., Krötzsch, M.: Wikidata: a free collaborative knowledge base. CACM **57**(10), 78–85 (2014)
24. Zangerle, E., Gassler, W., Pichl, M., Steinhauser, S., Specht, G.: An empirical evaluation of property recommender systems for Wikidata and collaborative knowledge bases. In: Opensym (2016)

Multiclass Lung Cancer Diagnosis by Gene Expression Programming and Microarray Datasets

Hasseeb Azzawi[1(✉)], Jingyu Hou[1], Russul Alanni[1], Yong Xiang[1], Rana Abdu-Aljabar[2], and Ali Azzawi[3]

[1] School of Information Technology, Deakin University, Burwood, VIC, Australia
{hazzawi,jingyu.hou,ralanni,yong.xiang}@deakin.edu.au
[2] Information Engineering College, Al-Nahrain University, Baghdad, Iraq
rdhiaa@yahoo.com
[3] Iraqi Ministry of Education, Baghdad, Iraq
ali_iraq82@yahoo.com

Abstract. There are various types of lung cancer and they can be differentiated by the cell size as well as the growth pattern. They are all treated differently. Classification of the various types of lung cancer assists in determining the specified treatments to decrease the fatality rates. In this paper, we broaden the analysis of lung by using gene expression data, binary decomposition strategies and Gene Expression Programming (GEP) technique, aiming at achieving better classification performance. Classification performance was assessed and compared between our GEP models and three representative machine learning techniques, SVM, NNW and C4.5 on real microarray Lung tumor datasets. Dependability was evaluated by the cross-informational collection validation. The evaluation results demonstrate that our technique can achieve better classification performance in terms of Accuracy, standard deviation and range under the recipient working trademark bend. The proposed technique in this paper provides a helpful tool for Lung cancer classification.

Keywords: Multiclass classification · Lung cancer diagnosis · Gene expression analysis · Gene expression programming

1 Introduction

Lung cancer growth is considered as a hereditary issue with obscure causes among different types [1, 2]. The rate of death by Lung cancer is recorded as around 25% of the demise by disease on the planet. This rate is higher than that of other most common cancers together, for example, breast, colorectal, and prostate cancers [3]. Lung cancer has two fundamental types: small cell Lung cancer (SCLC) and non-small cell Lung cancer (NSCLC). The most common type is NSCLC, which accounts ~80% of patients, while SCLC accounts 20%. Patients with non-small cell Lung tumors are usually treated uniquely in contrast to those with small cell Lung cancer. Therefore, precise classification for these two types of Lung cancer is exceptionally important to

G. Cong et al. (Eds.): ADMA 2017, LNAI 10604, pp. 541–553, 2017.
https://doi.org/10.1007/978-3-319-69179-4_38

the treatment effectiveness and the poisonous quality minimization on patients [4]. The World Health Organization (WHO) classifies the Lung cancer into two primary types: non-small cell Lung cancer (NSCLC) and small cell Lung cancer (SCLC), SCLC can be sub- divided into three histological subtypes: squamous cell carcinoma, adenocarcinoma and large cell carcinoma. SCLC is subdivided into small cell carcinoma (SCC) or oat cell cancer and combined small cell carcinoma [5].

Microarray technology is a standout in finding and visualizing distinctive tumors on a genome-wide scale. Cancer classification is the most promising application of this technology and has been studied extensively all around the world [6]. The conventional diagnostic techniques are hard to classify the tumors with comparable histo-pathological appearance (phenotype), because these techniques relies upon subjective assessment of the morphological appearance of the tissue test, which requires clear phenotype and prepared pathologist who can translate the vision [7]. With the development and quick progression of microarray technologies, analysts utilized as a part of their examinations the expression array analysis as a quantitative phenotyping instrument. The reason is the microarray registers at the same time the activities of a few thousand genes, and some of these genes are probably going to have infection relevance. This capacity makes the microarray a good tool for diagnosis, exact class prediction and the recognizable proof of subclasses [8].

In cancer diagnosis, the classification is the most noteworthy procedure to recognize various tumor types. The issues of muti-class are increasing, because of clearness of cancer heterogeneity in lately studies [9], and new subtypes of tumor would be recognized. Clinical testing can be done during cancer tumor testing in terms of drug sensitivity grade, stage and survival time [10, 11]. These developments need us to develop methods for multi-class classification.

A lot of research has been done for binary classification and a few studies have taken into consideration the direct multiclass classification. However, direct multiclass classification is more difficult than binary classification and the accuracy of classification may decrease when the number of classes increases [12–14].

The shortcomings of the direct multiclass classification was usually overcome by using decomposition strategies that break a multiclass classification problem into several binary classification problems. Some of the decomposition strategies have been reviewed in study [15]. The most common strategies are "one-vs-all" (OVA) [16, 17] and "one–vs-one" (OVO) [18]. OVA strategy is working to learn a classifier for each individual class, to distinguish the class from other classes and for class prediction made from the base classifier. Whereas, OVO the second strategy is working to learn all classifiers, each classifier can be distinguished between two pairs of classes and the prediction result can be made by combining all the results of the base classifiers. Biological multiclass problems can be analysed by these strategies, which have been applied with other classification algorithms such as support vector machine, neutral works and random forest but due to insufficient classification performance these approaches are still marginal [19, 20].

A novel evolutionary algorithm for data analysis named Gene Expression Programming (GEP) was introduced by Ferreira [21] in recent years. GEP was developed from the

Gene Expression Programming (GEPs) and genetic programming (GP), combining the strengths of the two algorithms and overcoming individual limitations. GEP represents various shapes and sizes of expressions trees, and finds the best expression tree by performing GA because of the high evolution efficiency of GA [22–24]. Weinert and Lopes [25] worked on classification by employing logical and rational functions in place of arithmetical functions. Jedrzejowicz and jedrzejowicz [26] used Gene Expression Programming (GEP) to induce ensemble classifiers with accurate classification. Wang et al. [27] presented GEP decision tree (GEPDT) system that is globally used in searching of gene expression programming.

The conventional classification design of GEP algorithm is for binary decisions. Many GEP classifiers solve multi class problems by building a multiclass classifier directly using multiclass base classifiers [25, 27–31] in practice. OVA strategy are used to convert multi-class problem into multiple binary classification problems [32, 33]. Previous studies have two main issues: complicity and disproportionate classes. GEP suffered some issues especially the computation efficiency and direct multi-classification can increase the computational complicity. Moreover, disproportionate classes in GEP can occur when the number of sample positive class is unbalanced in comparison to the merged superclass.

A few methods that use multiclass for lung cancer subtypes classification (e.g. more than two classes) have been proposed. All these previous studies assumed that no similarities between classes and ignored that maybe some classes have simple disparities and others have very clear disparities. For instance, lung cancer types NSCLC and SCLC have many disparities between one another in terms of growth pattern and cell size which translates to different treatment. A mix up in subtypes leads to increased error in classification thus wrong diagnosis.

Many studies have shown that GEP provides a very promising approach to cancer prediction diagnosis and prognosis [34–38]. In this paper we propose a new GEP based classifier with OVA and OVO strategies for multiclass classification of lung cancer subtypes to find which strategy is best. GEP-OVA and GEP-OVO were compared to three representative classifiers: SVM, MLP AND C4.5 classifiers in terms of accuracy standard deviation and AUC ROC. For reliability of evaluation the tenfold cross validation and average results are used.

The main contribution of this paper is as follows:

- GEP algorithm for lung cancer subtypes was developed. To our knowledge, there is no research on using the GEP model for multiclass purposes to classify lung cancers subtype from microarray data.
- Popular decomposition binary strategies were investigated in the context of multi-class classification.

The rest of this paper is organized as follows. Section 2 provides a brief overview of GEP. In Sect. 3, strategies of multi-class decomposition are described. In Sect. 4 experiment results are presented and discussed. Conclusions are given in Sect. 5.

2 Gene Expression Programming

Gene Expression Programming (GEP) is proposed by Ferreira, it's a type of evolutionary algorithm. In GEP, five components are used to solve the problem: population which represents chromosomes, fitness function to evaluate the chromosomes, control parameters of stop conditions and genetic operations to enhance the individual's chromosomes for next generation.

The first component is the population. The population includes several individuals (chromosomes). GEP chromosomes consist of predefined number of genes. These genes are linked by one arithmetical function or Boolean function. Each gene contains a head and a tail. The head consists of both functions and terminals symbols (including problem specific variables and preselected constants). The head consists of both functions like {+ , −, *, /} and terminals symbols (including problem specific variables and preselected constants), while the tail consists of only terminal symbols. Tail size can be calculated by t = h (n − 1) + 1, where h and n represent the size of head and maximum number of parameters respectively by the functions in the function set. For example, one chromosome can be constructed as follow where the tail is shown in bold. This notation is also known as the genotype.

01234567890
+Q-abc**bcaac**

The individual GEP include two representations the genotype and phenotype. The genotypes is a fixed length strings whereas phenotype represent as expression Trees (ETs) that is a result of conversion process from genotype. The ET (phenotype) of the above example genotypes is shown in Fig. 1 below:

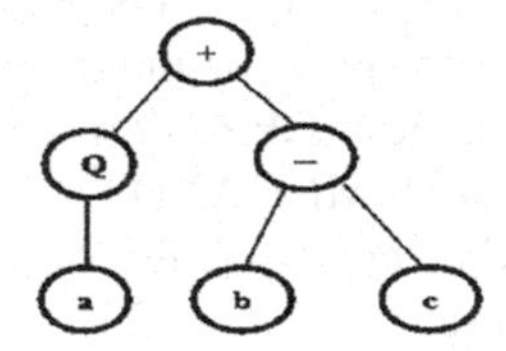

Fig. 1. Expression tree (phenotype)

The fitness function being the second component is used to evaluate each individual in the population. In this paper we used SSPN fitness function:

$$SSPN\text{i} = SN\text{i} \times SP\text{i} \times PPV\text{i} \times NPV\text{i} \tag{1}$$

Where $SN\text{i}, SP\text{i}, PPV\text{i}$, and $SN\text{i}, SP\text{i}, PPV\text{i}$, are calculated by the following formulas for chromosome i (1 $\leq$ i $\leq$ population size) over the whole training dataset.

$$SNi = TPi/(TPi + F\text{N}i) \tag{2}$$

$$SPi = TNi/(TNi + FPi) \tag{3}$$

$$PPVi = TPi/(TPi + FPi) \tag{4}$$

$$NPVi = TNi/(TNi + FNi) \tag{5}$$

Where *TNi*, *TPi*, *FNi* and *FP*i are the numbers of true negatives, true positives, false negatives, and false positives of classification/prediction respectively for chromosome i over the whole training dataset. This evaluation process has been repeated for each chromosome in the population.

The third component is control parameters. GEP is flexible algorithm which contains several parameters that control the algorithm process. These parameters are shown in Sect. 3.4.

The fourth component is the condition. GEP algorithm will repeat the entire process until the condition is met. Ideal condition is that the result of the fitness function is 100, which means all predictions are correct.

Genetic operations are the last component. GEP as an evaluation algorithm contains several genetic operations such as Mutation, IS Transposition, RIS Transposition, Gene Transposition, One-Point Recombination, Two-Point Recombination and Gene Recombination. Genetic operations are used to enhance the individuals and guide the solution towards the optical solution. Genetic operations will be applied to create the next generation if the condition is not satisfied and the whole process should be repeated. Figure 2 illustrates the flow chart of the GEP process.

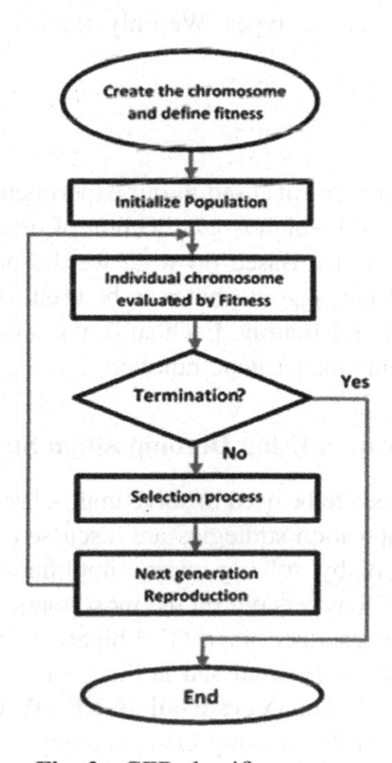

Fig. 2. GEP classifier process

3 Materials and Methods

As discussed earlier for non-structural classification, merging classes in multiclass classification leads to information loss. Thus, in this article, we implement Lung cancer subtypes tree structure with selective class merging (SBC) at each splitting node.

3.1 Datasets and Preparation

Evaluation of GEP classification model was conducted on three publicly available gene microarray datasets. Characteristics of the data sets are shown in Table 1. The first two datasets GSE2109 and GSE6044 were downloaded from the Gene Expression Omnibus (GEO, http://www.ncbi.nlm.nih.gov/pubmed), and Third dataset Harvard (Dana-Farber Cancer Institute, Harvard Medical School) was downloaded from (http://datam.i2r.a-star.edu.sg/datasets/krbd/LungCancer/LungCancer-Harvard1.html).

Table 1. Characteristics of microarray datasets

Dataset	Gene	Sample	Class
GSE2109	54675	103	5
GSE6044	8793	47	4
Harvard	12600	203	5

GEO series GSE2109 contains more than 2000 gene expression samples that are related to numerous various cancer types. We only extracted samples relevant to lung cancer types.

3.2 Attribute Selection

Initially evaluator relief Attribute was used in our experiments [39–41]. This technique is given by weka software [42] which is a collection of open access machine learning algorithms for data mining tasks. Based on what we did previously [35], top ranked informative genes were selected e.g. attributes to be used for creation of sub data sets for each original lung cancer microarray. Each sub dataset had equal number of patient (samples) as the original but smaller gene number.

3.3 GEP Multi Classification Using Decomposition Strategies

Decomposition strategies need to be used to solve multi-classification problem by using GEP classification. Decomposition strategies are discussed in Sect. 1. They deal with original multi-class problem by solving more simplified binary problems that are suitable to GEP classifier. Focus was put on the most popular decomposition strategies in our paper which will be described next. GEP binary classification for dealing with the multi-classification problem is discussed in this section.

GEP Classification with One-Versus-all (GEP-OVA). GEP classification for solving multi-classification problem using OVA strategy is elaborated in this section.

OVA strategy was proposed independently by several authors [16, 17], which is known as one-against-all or one-vs-rest and is a popular choice for ensemble solution of multi-class classification. OVA strategy divides the classes into two groups. The first includes positive class and the second group includes samples in all the other negative classes.

In other words, to use GEP classification to solve multi-classification problem using this strategy, several GEP binary classifier models are built. GEP models are equal to the number of classes. If we have c classes then GEP-OVA will build c GEP models, each model will take one class i (i = 1, 2….c) to be the positive class and the other classes will be the negative class. The class prediction result can be made by combining all the results of these classifier models. For example, if we find the classifier GEP from a dataset with four classes, as in Fig. 3, we let all instances in Class 1 be the positive set, and all instances in the remaining classes (2, 3 and 4 be the negative set, as in Fig. 4. Then, by combining all classifiers GEPi(i = 1, 2, 3, 4), we derive the function:

$$\text{GEP(x)} = \arg\max_{i} \text{GEPi (x)} \tag{6}$$

To classify test data x as class i, with the index giving the largest value GEPi, ∀ i.

GEP Classification with One-Versus-One (OVO). In this section, we explain how to use GEP classification to solve multi-classification problem with OVO strategy.

OVO strategy proposed by Knerr et al. (1990), is also known as all-pairs (AP), "pairwise coupling" or "round robin". It is commonly used to solve problems of multi-class classification because it is guaranteed that required class is contrasted with other classes one by one. In this strategy, to solve c-class problems, we need to construct (c(c – 1))/2 GEP classification models and train the GEP classifiers between each pair of the classes. Because of the complexity (n_classes^2) this strategy performs slower than OVA strategy. The class prediction result can be made by combining all the results of the GEP models. For example, if we find the GEP classifier GEP12 to identify Class 1 over Class 2 from a dataset with four classes, as in Fig. 5, we let Class 1 be the positive set and Class 2 be the negative set, as in Fig. 5. Then, by combining all the GEP classifiers GEPij(i, j = 1, 2, 3, 4, i ≠ j), we derive the function

$$\arg\max_{i} \left(\sum\nolimits_{j} GEPij\,(x)\right) \tag{7}$$

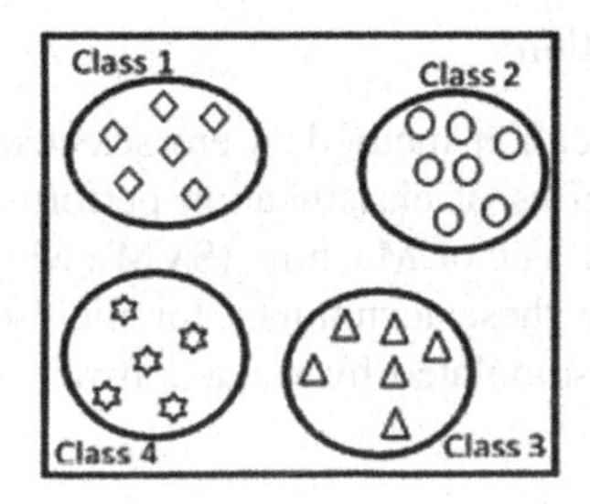

Fig. 3. Example of a dataset containing four classes.

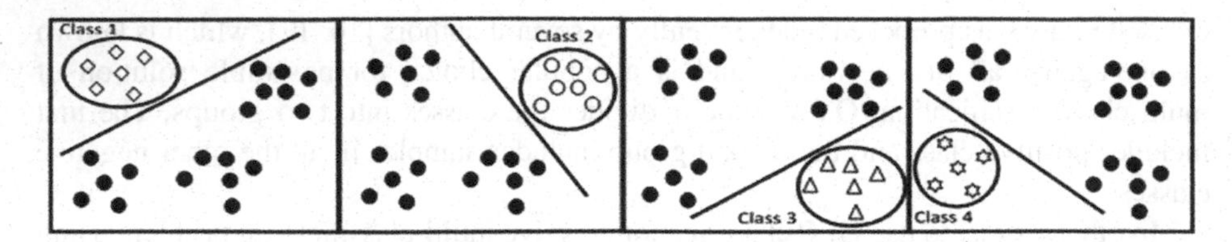

Fig. 4. GEP with One Versus All (OVA) strategy.

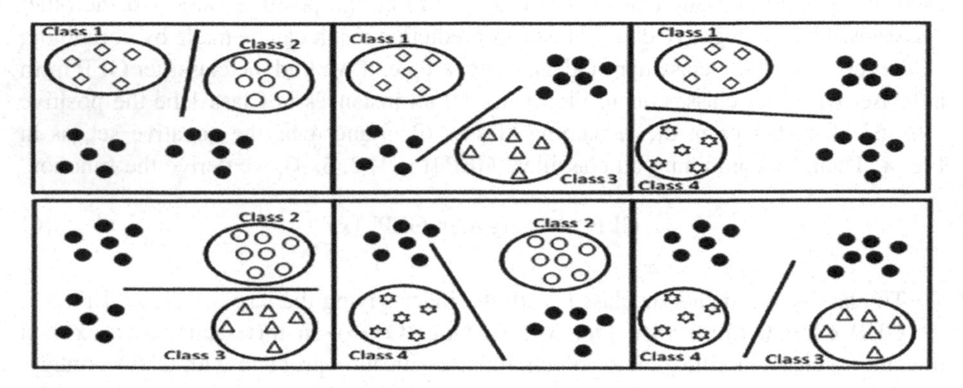

Fig. 5. GEP with One Versus One (OVO) strategy

to classify test data x as class i, corresponding to the index giving the largest value $\sum\_(i \neq j)GEP\_i\ (x), \forall\ i$

3.4 GEP Based Classifier

An open-source implementation of Gene Expression Programming (GEP4J) programmed in java in the early phases by Jason Thomas [43] was used to implement GEP Algorithm. Table 2 shows the configuration parameters of GEP. The genetic operations were selected based on what Ferreira recommended [21]. The stopping condition is either fitness function has reached 100% e.g. there is no misclassification or the number of generations has reached the maximum (1000) which will be considered the mean highest fitness value.

3.5 Method for Cooperation

Representative multi-classification methods were selected to compare with our GEP models based classifier in terms of classification performance using GEP algorithm.. These methods were Support Vector Machine (SVM), Multi-Layer Perceptron (MLP), and C4.5. Many studies use these techniques for multi-classification purposes (48). SVM, MLP and C4.5 were stimulated by weka software [42].

Table 2. Configuration parameters of GEP

Parameters	Value
Chromosome length	21
Genes number	4
Head size	10
Tail size	11
Population size	500
Generations number	1000
Function set	+, −, ∗, /, sqrt
Mutation rate	0.044
Transposition rate	0.1

4 Results and Discussion

Performance of our proposed modules (GEP-OVA and GEP-OVO) for multi-class cancer diagnosis is evaluated in this section. Three benchmark microarray data sets are used in this study. To get a fair assessment of the proposed strategy extensive comparisons with other machine learning methods are performed: Support Vector Machines, Multi-Layer Perceptron and C4.5. Weka platform for implementations is used for comparison with default settings provided by the software.

Reliability was assessed by cross data validation, datasets were randomly divided into ten equal subsets using the ten-fold cross validation. Nine subsets were used as a training data set to construct the model whereas the remaining subset was used as a testing dataset for prediction for each run. The average of the ten iterations was recorded as the final measurement.

Two GEP models were set up to investigate their performance in diagnosis. We first analyse their performance in diagnosis of lung cancer subtypes and pick the one that obtains the highest prediction accuracy rate as the optimum GEP model. Then comparison is conducted between it and other machine learning methods (SVM, MLP and C4.5).

4.1 Investigation of GEP Models and Their Performance in Diagnosis

The results of the evaluations in terms of Accuracy, standard deviation and AUC ROC are shown in Table 3. It can be noticed that GEP-OVA achieved highest average accuracy 91.61, and GEP-OVO achieved 91.29. For the standard deviation average, the best result was achieved by GEP-OVA which was 0.26 and GEP-OVO achieved 0.27.

For the AUC ROC average, it can be noticed that also GEP-OVA achieved highest results 0.89.

4.2 Comparison with Other Existing Methods

The comparison outputs of classification performance among GEP classifiers, SVM, MLP and C4.5 classifiers in terms of Accuracy, standard deviation and AUC ROC are

Table 3. Accuracy, standard deviation and AUC ROC for GEP modules for each dataset with average of all datasets.

	GEMS dataset	GSE2109 dataset	GSE6044 dataset	Average
Accuracy				
GEP-OVA	97.25	88.63	88.96	91.61
GEP-OVO	97.01	87.92	88.96	91.29
Standard deviation				
GEP-OVA	0.26	0.26	0.26	0.26
GEP-OVO	0.27	0.52	0.02	0.27
AUC ROC				
GEP-OVA	0.96	0.86	0.86	0.89
GEP-OVO	0.96	0.8	0.86	0.87

shown in Table 4. It can be noticed that GEP-OVA achieved the highest average accuracy 91.61 than other existing methods. SVM has achieved 87.35, which is slightly better than MLP (86.47), and C4.5 achieved lowest average accuracy 82.58. For the standard deviation average, the best result was achieved by GEP-OVA with 0.26, while the other methods SVM, MLP and C4.5 achieved 0.60, 0.64 and 0.59 respectively. Regarding the AUC ROC average the best result was achieved by our strategy GEP-OVA (0.89), while the AUC for SVM, MLP and C4.5 was 0.84, 0.84 and 0.76 respectively.

For all three data sets, the experimental results showed that the performance of GEP-OVA strategy was better than the strategy GEP-OVO and other existing methods. Also, the results were more efficient for lung cancer multiclass diagnosis.

Table 4. Accuracy, standard deviation and AUC ROC with average for all classifiers and all datasets

	Datasets	GEP-OVA	GEP-OVO	SVM	MLP	C4.5
Accuracy	GEMS	97.25	97.01	95.51	94.21	80.7
	GSE2109	88.63	87.92	80.63	80.01	79.98
	GSE6044	88.96	88.96	85.93	85.21	87.08
Average	All	91.61	91.29	87.35	86.47	82.58
Standard deviation	GEMS	0.26	0.27	0.41	0.51	0.59
	GSE2109	0.26	0.52	0.41	0.51	0.59
	GSE6044	0.26	0.02	1	0.92	0.59
Average	All	0.26	0.27	0.60	0.64	0.59
AUC ROC	GEMS	0.96	0.96	0.96	0.95	0.76
	GSE2109	0.86	0.8	0.76	0.76	0.72
	GSE6044	0.86	0.86	0.82	0.82	0.8
Average	All	0.89	0.87	0.84	0.84	0.76

5 Conclusions

The proposed method GEP-OVA in this paper can effectively solve the multi-class classification problem for lung cancer microarray data. The evaluation results on three real lung cancer datasets have shown that GEP-OVA has improved classification performance for lung cancer subtypes. We plan to explore other types of cancer with many subclasses in the future.

References

1. American Cancer Society: Cancer facts & figures 2011, vol. 1, no. 34. American Cancer Society INC. (2011)
2. Laureen, W., Goh, B.C.: An overview of cancer trends in Asia. Innovationmagazine.com (2012)
3. Balgkouranidou, I., Liloglou, T., Lianidou, E.S.: Lung cancer epigenetics: emerging biomarkers. Biomark. Med. **7**(1), 49–58 (2013)
4. Hosseinzadeh, F., Ebrahimi, M., Goliaei, B., Shamabadi, N.: Classification of lung cancer tumors based on structural and physicochemical properties of proteins by bioinformatics models. PLoS ONE **7**(7), e40017 (2012)
5. Beasley, M.B., Brambilla, E., Travis, W.D.: The 2004 World Health Organization classification of lung tumors. In: Seminars in Roentgenology, vol. 40, no. 2, pp. 90–97. WB Saunders (2005)
6. Pham, T.D., Wells, C., Crane, D.I.: Analysis of microarray gene expression data. Current Bioinform. **1**(1), 37–53 (2006)
7. Golub, T.R., et al.: Molecular classification of cancer: class discovery and class prediction by gene expression monitoring. Science **286**(5439), 531–537 (1999)
8. Joseph, S.J., Robbins, K.R., Zhang, W., Rekaya, R.: Comparison of two output-coding strategies for multi-class tumor classification using gene expression data and latent variable model as binary classifier. Cancer Inform. **9**, 39 (2010)
9. Burgess, D.J.: Cancer genetics: initially complex, always heterogeneous. Nat. Rev. Genet. **12**(3), 154–155 (2011)
10. Dyrskjøt, L., et al.: Gene expression signatures predict outcome in non–muscle-invasive bladder carcinoma: a multicenter validation study. Clin. Cancer Res. **13**(12), 3545–3551 (2007)
11. Shah, M.A., et al.: Molecular classification of gastric cancer: a new paradigm. Clin. Cancer Res. **17**(9), 2693–2701 (2011)
12. Li, T., Zhang, C., Ogihara, M.: A comparative study of feature selection and multiclass classification methods for tissue classification based on gene expression. Bioinformatics **20** (15), 2429–2437 (2004)
13. Mukherjee, S.: Classifying microarray data using support vector machines. In: Berrar, D.P., Dubitzky, W., Granzow, M. (eds.) A Practical Approach to Microarray Data Analysis, pp. 166–185. Springer, Boston (2003)
14. Ghorai, S., Mukherjee, A., Sengupta, S., Dutta, P.K.: Multicategory cancer classification from gene expression data by multiclass NPPC ensemble. In: 2010 International Conference on Systems in Medicine and Biology (ICSMB), pp. 41–48. IEEE (2010)
15. Lorena, A.C., De Carvalho, A.C., Gama, J.M.: A review on the combination of binary classifiers in multiclass problems. Artif. Intell. Rev. **30**(1–4), 19–37 (2008)

16. Clark, P., Boswell, R.: Rule induction with CN2: some recent improvements. In: Kodratoff, Y. (ed.) EWSL 1991. LNCS, vol. 482, pp. 151–163. Springer, Heidelberg (1991). doi:10.1007/BFb0017011
17. Anand, R., Mehrotra, K., Mohan, C.K., Ranka, S.: Efficient classification for multiclass problems using modular neural networks. IEEE Trans. Neural Netw. **6**(1), 117–124 (1995)
18. Knerr, S., Personnaz, L., Dreyfus, G.: Single-layer learning revisited: a stepwise procedure for building and training a neural network. In: Soulié, F.F., Hérault, J. (eds.) Neurocomputing. NATO ASI Series (Series F: Computer and Systems Sciences), vol. 68, pp. 41–50. Springer, Heidelberg (1990)
19. Ramaswamy, S., et al.: Multiclass cancer diagnosis using tumor gene expression signatures. Proc. Natl. Acad. Sci. **98**(26), 15149–15154 (2001)
20. Vlahou, A., Schorge, J.O., Gregory, B.W., Coleman, R.L.: Diagnosis of ovarian cancer using decision tree classification of mass spectral data. Biomed. Res. Int. **2003**(5), 308–314 (2003)
21. Ferreira, C.: Gene expression programming: a new adaptive algorithm for solving problems. Complex Syst. **13**(2), 87–129 (2001)
22. Teodorescu, L., Sherwood, D.: High energy physics event selection with gene expression programming. Comput. Phys. Commun. **178**(6), 409–419 (2008)
23. Shi, W., Zhang, X., Shen, Q.: Quantitative structure-activity relationships studies of CCR5 inhibitors and toxicity of aromatic compounds using gene expression programming. Eur. J. Med. Chemistry **45**(1), 49–54 (2010)
24. Nazari, A.: Prediction performance of PEM fuel cells by gene expression programming. Int. J. Hydrogen Energy **37**(24), 18972–18980 (2012)
25. Weinert, W.R., Lopes, H.S.: GEPCLASS: a classification rule discovery tool using gene expression programming. In: Li, X., Zaïane, O.R., Li, Z. (eds.) ADMA 2006. LNCS, vol. 4093, pp. 871–880. Springer, Heidelberg (2006). doi:10.1007/11811305_95
26. Jedrzejowicz, J., Jedrzejowicz, P.: Experimental evaluation of two new GEP-based ensemble classifiers. Expert Syst. Appl. **38**(9), 10932–10939 (2011)
27. Wang, W., Li, Q., Han, S., Lin, H.: A preliminary study on constructing decision tree with gene expression programming. In: First International Conference on Innovative Computing, Information and Control (ICICIC 2006), vol. 1, pp. 222–225. IEEE (2006)
28. Ávila, J.L., Gibaja, E.L., Ventura, S.: Multi-label classification with gene expression programming. In: Corchado, E., Wu, X., Oja, E., Herrero, Á., Baruque, B. (eds.) HAIS 2009. LNCS, vol. 5572, pp. 629–637. Springer, Heidelberg (2009). doi:10.1007/978-3-642-02319-4_76
29. Ávila, J.L., Gibaja, E., Zafra, A., Ventura, S.: A gene expression programming algorithm for multi-label classification. J. Multiple Valued Logic Soft Comput. **17**, 255–287 (2011)
30. Shi, W., Liu, Y., Kong, W., Shen, Q.: Tea classification by near infrared spectroscopy with projection discriminant analysis and gene expression programming. Anal. Lett. **48**(18), 2833–2842 (2015)
31. Huang, J., Deng, C.: A novel multiclass classification method with gene expression programming. In: International Conference on Web Information Systems and Mining, WISM 2009, pp. 139–143. IEEE (2009)
32. Zhou, C., Xiao, W., Tirpak, T.M., Nelson, P.C.: Evolving accurate and compact classification rules with gene expression programming. IEEE Trans. Evol. Comput. **7**(6), 519–531 (2003)
33. Khattab, H., Abdelaziz, A., Mekhamer, S., Badr, M., El-Saadany, E.: Gene expression programming for static security assessment of power systems. In: 2012 IEEE Power and Energy Society General Meeting, pp. 1–8. IEEE (2012)

34. Al-Anni, R., Hou, J., Abdu-aljabar, R.D.A., Xiang, Y.: Prediction of NSCLC recurrence from microarray data with GEP. IET Syst. Biol. **11**(3), 77–85 (2017)
35. Azzawi, H., Hou, J., Xiang, Y., Alanni, R.: Lung cancer prediction from microarray data by gene expression programming. IET Syst. Biol. **10**, 1–11 (2016)
36. Yu, Z., et al.: A highly efficient Gene Expression Programming (GEP) model for auxiliary diagnosis of small cell lung cancer. PLoS ONE **10**(5), 1–19 (2015)
37. Yu, Z., Chen, X.Z., Cui, L.H., Si, H.Z., Lu, H.J., Liu, S.H.: Prediction of lung cancer based on serum biomarkers by gene expression programming methods. Asian Pac. J. Cancer Prev. **15**(21), 9367–9373 (2014)
38. Kusy, M., Obrzut, B., Kluska, J.: Application of gene expression programming and neural networks to predict adverse events of radical hysterectomy in cervical cancer patients. Med. Biol. Eng. Comput. **51**(12), 1357–1365 (2013)
39. Kira, K., Rendell, L.A.: A practical approach to feature selection. In: Proceedings of the Ninth International Workshop on Machine Learning, pp. 249–256 (1992)
40. Kononenko, I.: Estimating attributes: analysis and extensions of RELIEF. In: Bergadano, F., De Raedt, L. (eds.) ECML 1994. LNCS, vol. 784, pp. 171–182. Springer, Heidelberg (1994). doi:10.1007/3-540-57868-4_57
41. Robnik-Šikonja, M., Kononenko, I.: An adaptation of relief for attribute estimation in regression. In: Proceedings of the Fourteenth International Conference on Machine Learning (ICML 1997), pp. 296–304 (1997)
42. Witten, I.H., Frank, E., Hall, M.A., Pal, C.J.: Data Mining: Practical Machine Learning Tools and Techniques. Morgan Kaufmann, Burlington (2016)
43. Gene Expression Programming for Java. https://code.google.com/archive/p/gep4j/. Accessed 26 Aug 2010

Drug-Drug Interaction Extraction via Recurrent Neural Network with Multiple Attention Layers

Zibo Yi[1(✉)], Shasha Li[1], Jie Yu[1], Yusong Tan[1], Qingbo Wu[1], Hong Yuan[2], and Ting Wang[1]

[1] National University of Defense Technology, Changsha, Hunan Province, China
{yizibo14,shashali,yj,yusong.tan,qingbo.wu,wangting}@nudt.edu.cn

[2] The Center of Clinical Pharmacology, The Third Xiangya Hospital of Central South University, Changsha, Hunan Province, China
yuanhongxy3@163.com

Abstract. Drug-drug interaction (DDI) is a vital information when physicians and pharmacists intend to co-administer two or more drugs. Thus, several DDI databases are constructed to avoid mistakenly drug combined use. In recent years, automatically extracting DDIs from biomedical text has drawn researchers' attention. However, the existing work utilize either complex feature engineering or NLP tools, both of which are insufficient for sentence comprehension. Inspired by the deep learning approaches in natural language processing, we propose a recurrent neural network model with multiple attention layers for DDI classification. We evaluate our model on 2013 SemEval DDIExtraction dataset. The experiments show that our model classifies most of the drug pairs into correct DDI categories, which outperforms the existing NLP or deep learning methods.

Keywords: Drug-drug interaction · Natural language processing · Recurrent neural network · Attention layer

1 Introduction

Drug-drug interaction (DDI) is a situation when one drug increases or decreases the effect of another drug [18]. Adverse drug reactions may cause severe side effect, if two or more medicines were taken and their DDI were not investigated in detail. DDI is a common cause of illness, even a cause of death [8]. Thus, DDI databases for clinical medication decisions are proposed by some researchers. These databases such as SFINX [2], KEGG [17], DDI corpus [6] help physicians and pharmacists avoid most adverse drug reactions.

Traditional DDI databases are manually constructed according to clinical records, scientific research and drug specifications. For instance, The sentence "With combined use, clinicians should be aware, when **phenytoin** is added, of the potential for reexacerbation of pulmonary symptomatology due to lowered serum **theophylline** concentrations [16]", which is from a pharmacotherapy

G. Cong et al. (Eds.): ADMA 2017, LNAI 10604, pp. 554–566, 2017.
https://doi.org/10.1007/978-3-319-69179-4_39

report, describe the side effect of phenytoin and theophylline's combined use. Then this information on specific medicines will be added to DDI databases.

As biomedical researches have being increasingly published, manually extract DDIs from biomedical text are unrealistic. In the bibliographic database MedLine, 863,022 English biomedical research articles' abstract have been added in year 2015–2016 and the total number of English abstracts in MedLine is 14,561,362[1]. Fortunately, progresses on NLP techniques and deep learning offer promising prospects for automatically DDI extraction.

There have been many efforts to automatically extract DDIs from biomedical text [4,10–12,15,19]. Among them deep learning based approaches [10,11,15] show the state of the art performance. These approaches capture the semantic features through well designed neural networks. Another advantage of deep learning based approach is that it avoids complex feature engineering and NLP toolkits' usage, both of which will propagate errors if improper features or NLP tools are selected.

We employ deep learning approaches for sentence comprehension as a whole. As for the choice of neural networks, recurrent neural network (RNN) is considered a better performance than CNN in text comprehension task for the reason that CNN's slide window split the sentence into segments of 3–5 words and can not make connections between the distant but relevant segments. To make more precise DDI predictions, the attention mechanism instead of max pooling are used in our model.

We train our language comprehension model with labeled instances. Figure 1 shows partial records in DDI corpus [6]. We extract the sentence and drug pairs in the records (See Sect. 3.1). The DDI corpus annotate each drug pair in the sentence with a DDI type. The DDI type, which is the most concerned information, is described in Table 1. The details about how we train our model and extract the DDI type from text are described in the remaining sections. In summary, this work makes the following contributions:

- We propose a model that takes in a sentence from biomedical literature which contains a drug pair and outputs what kind of DDI this drug pair belongs. This assists physicians refrain from improper combined use of drugs.
- We introduce word level attention and sentence level attention to our model, which outperforms the state-of-the-art systems on DDI Extraction dataset.
- We present two variants of our model and evaluate these models so that the attention layers and other optimizations are demonstrated to be effective.

2 Related Work

In 2013, Herrero *et al.* [6] proposed an annotated DDI corpus to address the lack of well annotated pharmacological substances and DDIs. This DDI corpus was

[1] https://www.nlm.nih.gov/bsd/medline_lang_distr.html, accessed May 22nd, 2017.

```
<sentence id="DDI-DrugBank.d353.s8" text="Methotrexate: An increased risk
of hepatitis has been reported to result from combined use of methotrexate
and etretinate.">
        <entity id="DDI-DrugBank.d353.s8.e0" charOffset="0-11"
            type="drug" text="Methotrexate"/>
        <entity id="DDI-DrugBank.d353.s8.e1" charOffset="94-105"
            type="drug" text="methotrexate"/>
        <entity id="DDI-DrugBank.d353.s8.e2" charOffset="111-120"
            type="drug" text="etretinate"/>
        <pair id="DDI-DrugBank.d353.s8.p0" e1="DDI-DrugBank.d353.s8.e0"
            e2="DDI-DrugBank.d353.s8.e1" ddi="false"/>
        <pair id="DDI-DrugBank.d353.s8.p1" e1="DDI-DrugBank.d353.s8.e0"
            e2="DDI-DrugBank.d353.s8.e2" ddi="false"/>
        <pair id="DDI-DrugBank.d353.s8.p2" e1="DDI-DrugBank.d353.s8.e1"
            e2="DDI-DrugBank.d353.s8.e2" ddi="true" type="effect"/>
</sentence>
```


Fig. 1. Partial records in DDI corpus.

Table 1. The DDI types and corresponding examples

DDI types	Definition	Example sentence	Drug pair
False	An interaction between the two drugs is not shown in the sentence.	Concomitantly given thiazide diuretics did not interfere with the absorption of a tablet of digoxin.	thiazide diuretics, digoxin
Mechanism	An pharmacokinetic mechanism is shown in the sentence.	Additional iron significantly inhibited the absorption of cobalt.	iron, cobalt
Effect	The effect of two drugs' combination use is shown in the sentence.	Methotrexate: an increased risk of hepatitis has been report to result from combined use of methotrexate and etretinate.	methotrexate, etretinate
Advise	An advise about two drugs is given in the sentence.	UROXATRAL should NOT be used in combination with other alpha-blockers.	UROXATRAL, alpha-blockers
Int	A drug interaction without any further information is mentioned in the sentence.	Clinical implications of warfarin interactions with five sedatives.	warfarin, sedatives

also used in semeval 2013 task 9[2] as a stand dataset for drug recognition and DDI classification.

In DDI extraction task, NLP methods or machine learning approaches are proposed by most of the work. Chowdhury [3] utilize negation (a linguistic phenomenon) to determine whether the drugs have interactions or not. Then various of features are extracted to train a linear SVM and classify DDI to specific category. Thomas *et al.* [19] also proposed a two step approach, in which the ensemble technique in machine learning is introduced and multiple classifiers are trained for a better performance. FBK-irst [4] ranks first in task 9 of semeval 2013 challenge. A hybrid kernel method is proposed in FBK-irst. Exploiting multiple linguistic phenomenon and heterogeneous set of features, it has a well performed DDI classification result.

Neural network based approaches have been proposed by several works. Zhao *et al.* [20] employ CNN for DDI extraction for the first time which outperforms

[2] https://www.cs.york.ac.uk/semeval-2013/task9.html.

the traditional machine learning based methods. Words are represented by vectors in this method, then convolutional kernels slide along the word sequence to capture feature vectors. Liu *et al.* [10] also employ CNN, which drops features generated by NLP tools so that only word embedding and position embedding are retained. However, limited by the convolutional kernel size, the CNN can only extracted features of continuous 3 to 5 words rather than distant words. Liu *et al.* [11] proposed dependency-based CNN to handle distant but relevant words. Sahu *et al.* [15] proposed LSTM based DDI extraction approach and outperforms CNN based approach, since LSTM handles sentence as a sequence instead of using slide windows. To conclude, Neural network based approaches have advantages of (1) less reliance on extra NLP toolkits, (2) simpler preprocessing procedure, (3) have better performance than text analysis and machine learning methods.

3 The Proposed Model

In this section, we present our bidirectional recurrent neural network with multiple attention layer model. The overview of our architecture is shown in Fig. 2. For a given sentence, which describes the details about two or more drugs, the model represents it as a feature vector and classifies it as specific DDI using a softmax classifier. The remaining of this section describe will describe this in detail.

3.1 Preprocessing

The DDI corpus contains thousands of XML files, each of which are constructed by several records. For a sentence containing n drugs, there are C_n^2 drug pairs. We replace the interested two drugs with "drug1" and "drug2" while the other drugs are replaced by "durg0", as in [10] did. This step is called drug blinding. For example, the sentence in Fig. 1 generates 3 instances after drug blinding: "drug1: an increased risk of hepatitis has been reported to result from combined use of drug2 and drug0", "drug1: an increased risk of hepatitis has been reported to result from combined use of drug0 and drug2", "drug0: an increased risk of hepatitis has been reported to result from combined use of drug1 and drug2". The drug blinded sentences are the instances that are fed to our model.

We put the sentences with the same drug pairs together as a set, since the sentence level attention layer (will be described in Sect. 3.5) will use the sentences which contain the same drugs.

3.2 Embedding Layer

Given an instance $S = (w_1, w_2, ...w_u, ..., w_v, ..., w_t)$ which contains specified two drugs $w_u =$ "drug1", $w_v =$ "drug2", each word is embedded in a $d = d_{WE} + 2d_{PE}$ dimensional space (d_{WE}, d_{PE} are the dimension of word embedding and position embedding). The look up table function $LT.(\cdot)$ maps a word or a relative position

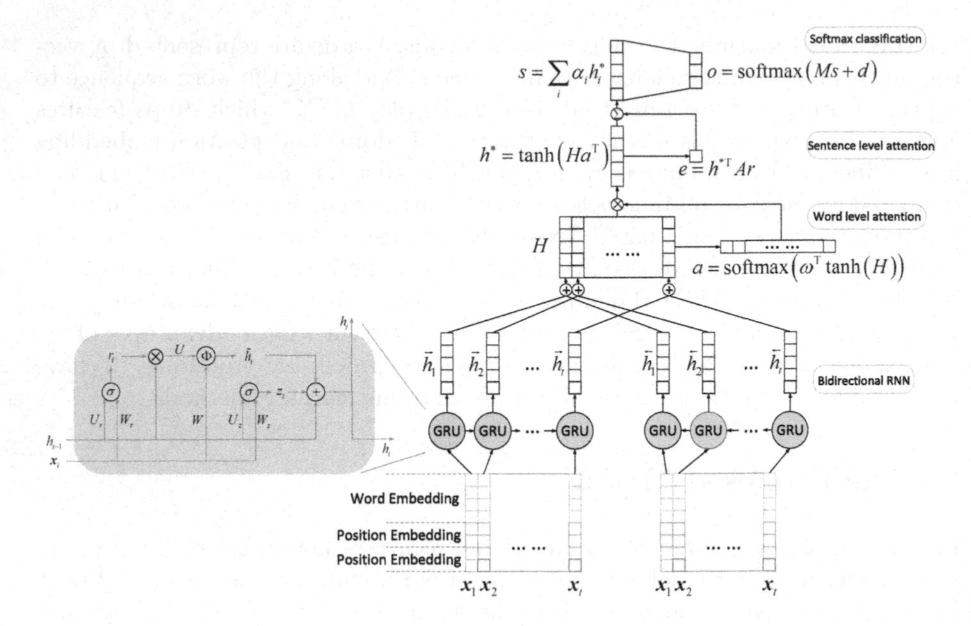

Fig. 2. The bidirectional recurrent neural network with multiple attentions.

to a column vector. After embedding layer the sentence is represented by $S = (\boldsymbol{x}_1, \boldsymbol{x}_2, ..., \boldsymbol{x}_t)$, where

$$\boldsymbol{x}_i = (LT_W(w_i)^{\mathrm{T}}, (LT_P(i-u)^{\mathrm{T}}, (LT_P(i-v)^{\mathrm{T}})^{\mathrm{T}} \tag{1}$$

The $LT.(\cdot)$ function is usually implemented by matrix-vector product. Let $\overline{w_i}$, $\overline{k}$ denote the one-hot representation (column vector) of word and relative distance. E_w, E_p are word and position embedding query matrix. The look up functions are implemented by

$$LT_W(w_i) = E_w\overline{w_i}, LT_P(k) = E_p\overline{k} \tag{2}$$

Then the word sequence $S = (\boldsymbol{x}_1, \boldsymbol{x}_2, ..., \boldsymbol{x}_t)$ is fed to the RNN layer. Note that the sentence will be filled with $\mathbf{0}$ if its length is less than t.

3.3 Bidirectional RNN Encoding Layer

The words in the sequence $S = (\boldsymbol{x}_1, \boldsymbol{x}_2, ..., \boldsymbol{x}_t)$ are read by RNN's gated recurrent unit (GRU) one by one. The GRU takes the current word $\boldsymbol{x}_i$ and the previous GRU's hidden state h_{i-1} as input. The current GRU encodes h_{i-1} and $\boldsymbol{x}_i$ into a new hidden state h_i (its dimension is d_h, a hyperparameter), which can be regarded as informations the GRU remembered.

Figure 2 shows the details in GRU. The reset gate r_i selectively forgets informations delivered by previous GRU. Then the hidden state becomes $\tilde{h}_i$. The update gate z_i updates the informations according to $\tilde{h}_i$ and h_{i-1}. The equations below describe these procedures. Note that $\otimes$ stands for element wise multiplication.

$$r_i = \sigma(W_r \boldsymbol{x}_i + U_r h_{i-1}) \tag{3}$$

$$\tilde{h}_i = \Phi(W \boldsymbol{x}_i + U(r_i \otimes h_{i-1})) \tag{4}$$

$$z_i = \sigma(W_z \boldsymbol{x}_i + U_z h_{i-1}) \tag{5}$$

$$h_i = z_i \otimes h_{i-1} + ((1, 1, ..., 1)^{\mathrm{T}} - z_i) \otimes \tilde{h}_i \tag{6}$$

The bidirectional RNN contains forward RNN and backward RNN. Forward RNN reads sentence from $\boldsymbol{x}_1$ to $\boldsymbol{x}_t$, generating $\overrightarrow{h}_1$, $\overrightarrow{h}_2$, ..., $\overrightarrow{h}_t$. Backward RNN reads sentence from $\boldsymbol{x}_t$ to $\boldsymbol{x}_1$, generating $\overleftarrow{h}_t$, $\overleftarrow{h}_{t-1}$, ..., $\overleftarrow{h}_1$. Then the encode result of this layer is

$$H = (\overrightarrow{h}_1 + \overleftarrow{h}_1, \overrightarrow{h}_2 + \overleftarrow{h}_2, ..., \overrightarrow{h}_t + \overleftarrow{h}_t) \tag{7}$$

We apply dropout technique in RNN layer to avoid overfitting. Each GRU have a probability (denoted by Pr_{dp}, also a hyperparameter) of being dropped. The dropped GRU has no output and will not affect the subsequent GRUs. With bidirectional RNN and dropout technique, the input $S = (\boldsymbol{x}_1, \boldsymbol{x}_2, ..., \boldsymbol{x}_t)$ is encoded into sentence matrix H.

3.4 Word Level Attention

The purpose of word level attention layer is to extract sentence representation (also known as feature vector) from encoded matrix. We use word level attention instead of max pooling, since attention mechanism can determine the importance of individual encoded word in each row of H. Let ω denotes the attention vector (ω is a randomly initialized column vector and will be revised during training), Eq. 8 calculates a, which is a filter that gives each element in each row of H a weight. The following equations shows the attention operation, which is also illustrated in Fig. 2.

$$a = \mathrm{softmax}(\omega^{\mathrm{T}} \tanh(H)) \tag{8}$$

$$h^* = \tanh(H a^{\mathrm{T}}) \tag{9}$$

h^* denotes the feature vector captured by this layer. Several approaches [15,21] also use this vector and softmax classifier for classification. Inspired by [9] we propose the sentence level attention to combine the information of other sentences for an improved DDI classification performance.

3.5 Sentence Level Attention

The previous layers captures the features only from the given sentence. However, other sentences may contains informations that contribute to the understanding of this sentence. It is reasonable to look over other relevant instances when determine two drugs' interaction from the given sentence. In our implementation, the instances that have the same drug pair are believed to be relevant. The relevant instances set is denoted by $\mathcal{L} = \{h_1^*, h_2^*, ..., h_N^*\}$, where h_i^* is the sentence feature vector. e_i stands for how well the instance h_i^* matches its DDI r (Vector representation of a specific DDI). A is a diagonal attention matrix, multiplied by which the feature vector h_i^* can concentrate on those most representative features.

$$e_i = h_i^{*\mathrm{T}} A r \tag{10}$$

$$\alpha_i = \frac{\exp(e_i)}{\sum_{k=1}^{N} \exp(e_k)} \tag{11}$$

α_i is the softmax result of e_i. The final sentence representation is decided by all of the relevant sentences' feature vector, as Eq. 12 shows.

$$s = \sum_{i=1}^{N} \alpha_i h_i^* \tag{12}$$

3.6 Training and Prediction

A given sentence $S = (w_1, w_2, ..., w_t)$ is finally represented by the feature vector s. Then we feed it to a softmax classifier. Let C denotes the set of all kinds of DDI. The output $o \in R^{|C|}$ is the probabilities of each class S belongs.

$$o = \mathrm{softmax}(Ms + d) \tag{13}$$

We use cross entropy cost function and L^2 regularization as the optimization objective. For i-th instance, Y_i denotes the one-hot representation of it's label, where the model outputs o_i. The cross entropy cost is:

$$l_i = -Y_i^{\mathrm{T}} \ln o_i \tag{14}$$

For a mini-batch $\mathcal{M} = \{S_1, S_2, ..., S_M\}$, the optimization objective is:

$$J(\theta) = -\frac{1}{|\mathcal{M}|} \sum_{i=1}^{|\mathcal{M}|} Y_i^{\mathrm{T}} \ln o_i + \lambda ||\theta||_2^2 \tag{15}$$

All parameters in this model is:

$$\theta = \{E_w, E_p, W_r, U_r, W, U, W_z, U_z, \omega, A, r, M, d\} \tag{16}$$

We optimize the parameters of objective function $J(\theta)$ with Adam [7], which is a variant of mini-batch stochastic gradient descent. During each train step, the gradient of $J(\theta)$ is calculated. Then θ is adjusted according to the gradient. After the end of training, we have a model that is able to predict two drugs' interactions when a sentence about these drugs is given.

After training, the parameters in list θ are fixed. Given a new sentence with two drugs, we can use this model to predict the DDI type. The DDI prediction follows the procedure described in Sects. 3.1–3.6. The given sentence is eventually represented by feature vector s. Then s is classified to a specific DDI type with a softmax classifier. In next section, we will evaluate our model's DDI prediction performance and see the advantages and shortcomings of our model.

3.7 The Variants of This Model

We name the proposed model "**dynamic + 2ATT**", since the dynamic word embedding and two layers of attention have been used. To inspect the effect of dynamic word embedding and sentence level attention, we also propose two variants of this model.

Static + 2ATT. There exists some approaches that use the static word embedding – a word embedding query matrix which stay constant during training. Except word embedding, this model are the same as "dynamic + 2ATT". The implementation of this model is to optimize the objective function $J(\theta')$. The parameters list θ' becomes

$$\theta' = \{E_p, W_r, U_r, W, U, W_z, U_z, \omega, A, r, M, d\} \tag{17}$$

Dynamic + ATT. The "dynamic + ATT" model drops the sentence level attention layer and use the word level attention only, as most of other approaches do. We slightly modify the "dynamic + 2ATT" model to get the "dynamic + ATT" model. The softmax classification layer omits the sentence level attention layer and takes h^* as input.

$$o = \text{softmax}(Mh^* + d) \tag{18}$$

The objective function still use cross entropy cost and L^2 regularization, while the parameters become

$$\theta'' = \{E_w, E_p, W_r, U_r, W, U, W_z, U_z, \omega, M, d\} \tag{19}$$

4 Experiments

4.1 Datasets and Evaluation Metrics

We use the DDI corpus of the 2013 DDIExtraction challenge [6] to train and test our model. The DDIs in this corpus are classified as five types. This standard dataset is made up of training set and testing set. We use the overall precision,

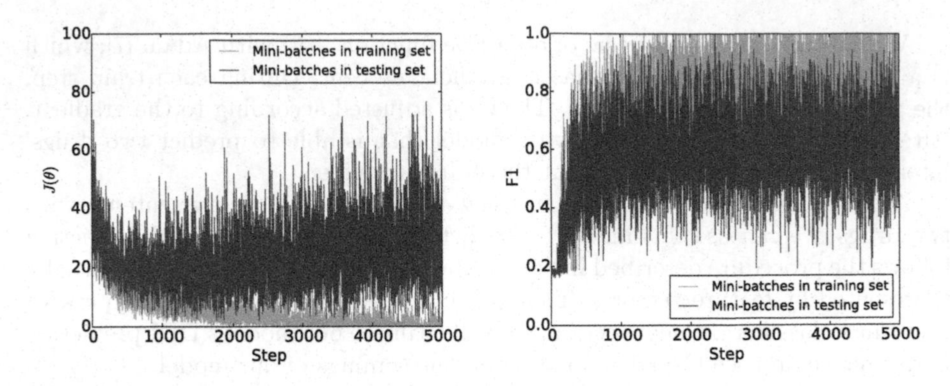

Fig. 3. The objective function and F1 in the train process

recall, and F1 score on testing set to evaluate our model. C denotes the set of {False, Mechanism, Effect, Advise, Int}. The precision and recall of each $c \in C$ are calculated by

$$P_c = \frac{\# \ DDI \ is \ c \ and \ is \ classified \ as \ c}{\# \ Classified \ as \ c} \tag{20}$$

$$R_c = \frac{\# \ DDI \ is \ c \ and \ is \ classified \ as \ c}{\# \ DDI \ is \ c} \tag{21}$$

Then the overall precision, recall, and F1 score are calculated by

$$P = \frac{1}{|C|}\sum_{c \in C} P_c, \ R = \frac{1}{|C|}\sum_{c \in C} R_c, \ F1 = \frac{2PR}{P+R} \tag{22}$$

Besides, we evaluate the captured feature vectors with t-SNE [5], a visualizing and intuitive way to map a high dimensional vector into a 2 or 3-dimensional space. If the points in a low dimensional space are easy to be split, the feature vectors are believed to be more distinguishable.

Table 2. Performance comparison with other approaches

Systems	Methods	Performance		
		P	R	F1
WBI [19]	Two stage SVM classification	0.6420	0.5790	0.6090
FBK-ist [4]	Hand crafted features + SVM	0.6460	0.6560	0.6510
SCNN [20]	Two stage syntax CNN	0.725	0.651	0.686
Liu *et al.* [10]	CNN + Pre-trained WE	0.7572	0.6466	0.6975
DCNN [11]	Dependency-based CNN + Pretrained WE	**0.7721**	0.6435	0.7019
Sahu *et al.* [15]	Bidirectional LSTM + ATT	0.7341	0.6966	0.7148
This paper	RNN + dynamic WE + 2ATT	0.7367	**0.7079**	**0.7220**

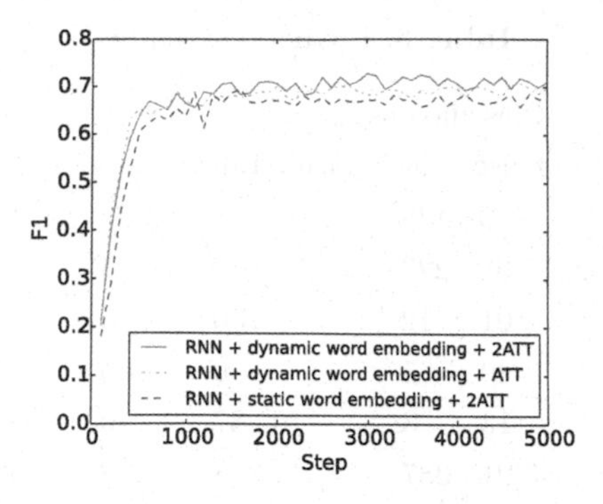

Fig. 4. The F1 scores on the whole testing set.

4.2 Hyperparameter Settings and Training

We use TensorFlow [1] r0.11 to implement the proposed model. The input of each word is an ordered triple (*word, relative distance from drug1, relative distance from drug2*). The sentence, which is represented as a matrix, is fed to the model. The output of the model is a $|C|$-dimensional vector representing the probabilities of being corresponding DDI. It is the network, parameters, and hyperparameters which decides the output vector. The network's parameters are adjusted during training, where the hyperparameters are tuned by hand. The hyperparameters after tuning are as follows. The word embedding's dimension $d_{WE} = 100$, the position embedding's dimension $d_{PE} = 10$, the hidden state's dimension $d_h = 230$, the probability of dropout $Pr_d = 0.5$, other hyperparameters which are not shown here are set to TensorFlow's default values.

The word embedding is initialized by pre-trained word vectors using GloVe [14], while other parameters are initialized randomly. During each training step, a mini-batch (the mini-batch size $|\mathcal{M}| = 60$ in our implementation) of sentences is selected from training set. The gradient of objective function is calculated for parameters updating (See Sect. 3.6).

Figure 3 shows the training process. The objective function $J(\theta)$ is declining as the training mini-batches continuously sent to the model. As the testing mini-batches, the $J(\theta)$ function is fluctuating while its overall trend is descending. The instances in testing set are not participated in training so that $J(\theta)$ function is not descending so fast. However, training and testing instances have similar distribution in sample space, causing that testing instances' $J(\theta)$ tends to be smaller along with the training process. $J(\theta)$ has inverse relationship with the performance measurement. The F1 score is getting fluctuating around a specific value after enough training steps. The reason why fluctuating range is considerable is that only a tiny part of the whole training or testing set has been calculated the F1 score. Testing the whole set during every step is time consuming and not necessary. We will evaluate the model on the whole testing set in Sect. 4.3.

Table 3. Prediction results

	Classified as					Sum
	False	Mechanism	Effect	Advise	Int	
False	4490	138	49	45	15	4737
Mechanism	68	229	2	3	0	302
Effect	101	12	230	15	2	360
Advise	49	5	0	165	2	221
Int	13	3	37	0	43	96
Sum	4721	387	318	228	62	5716

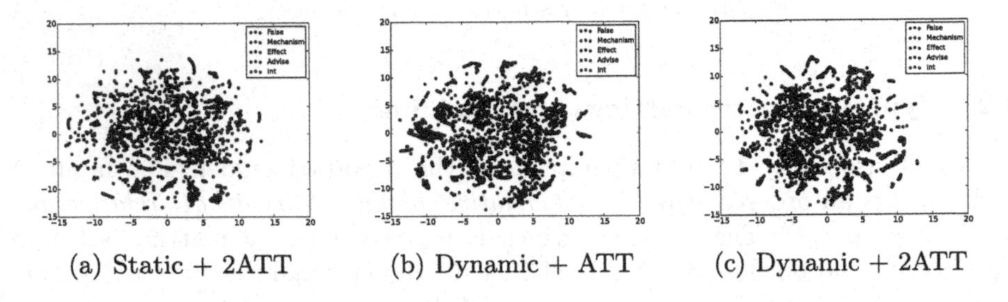

(a) Static + 2ATT (b) Dynamic + ATT (c) Dynamic + 2ATT

Fig. 5. The features that are captured by the three model.

4.3 Experimental Results

We save our model every 100 step and predict all the DDIs of the instances in the testing set. These predictions' F1 score is shown in Fig. 4. To demonstrate the sentence level attention layer is effective, we evaluate Dynamic + ATT model (See Sect. 3.7). The result is shown with "RNN + dynamic word embedding + ATT" curve, which illustrates that the sentence level attention layer contributes to a more accurate model.

Whether a dynamic or static word embedding is better for a DDI extraction task is under consideration. We let the embedding be static when training, while other conditions are all the same. The "RNN + static word embedding + 2ATT" curve shows this case. We can draw a conclusion that updating the initialized word embedding trains more suitable word vectors for the task, which promotes the performance.

We compare our best F1 score with other state-of-the-art approaches in Table 2, which shows our model has advantage in dealing with drug-drug interaction extraction. The predictions confusion matrix is shown in Table 3. The DDIs other than "False" being classified as "False" makes most of the classification error. It may perform better if a classifier which can tells "True" and "False" DDI apart is trained. We leave this two-stage classifier to our future work. Another phenomenon is that the "Int" type is often classified as "Effect". The "Int" sentence describes there exists interaction between two drugs and this information implies the two drugs' combination will have good or bad effect. That's the reason why "Int" and "Effect" are often obfuscated.

To evaluate the features our model captured, we employ scikit-learn [13]'s t-SNE class[3] to map high dimensional feature vectors to 2-dimensional vectors, which can be depicted on a plane. We depict all the features of the instances in testing set, as shown in Fig. 5. The "Dynamic + 2ATT" model is the most distinguishable one. Comparing Table 3 with Fig. 5(c), both of which are from the best performed model, we can observe some phenomena. The "Int" DDIs are often misclassified as "Effect", for the reason that some of the "Int" points are in the "Effect" cluster. The "Effect" points are too scattered so that plenty of "Effect" DDIs are classified to other types. The "Mechanism" points are gathered around two clusters, causing that most of the "Mechanism" DDIs are classified to two types: "False" and "Mechanism". In short, the visualizability of feature mapping gives better explanations for the prediction results and the quality of captured features.

5 Conclusion

To conclude, we propose a recurrent neural network with multiple attention layers to extract DDIs from biomedical text. The sentence level attention layer, which combines other sentences containing the same drugs, has been added to our model. The experiments shows that our model outperforms the state-of-the-art DDI extraction systems. Task relevant word embedding and two attention layers improved the performance to some extent.

Acknowledgments. This work is supported by the NSFC under Grant 61303190.

References

1. Abadi, M., Agarwal, A., Barham, P., Brevdo, E., Chen, Z., Citro, C., Corrado, G.S., Davis, A., Dean, J., Devin, M., et al.: Tensorflow: large-scale machine learning on heterogeneous distributed systems. arXiv preprint arXiv:1603.04467 (2016)
2. Böttiger, Y., Laine, K., Andersson, M.L., Korhonen, T., Molin, B., Ovesjö, M.L., Tirkkonen, T., Rane, A., Gustafsson, L.L., Eiermann, B.: Sfinx: a drug-drug interaction database designed for clinical decision support systems. Eur. J. Clin. Pharmacol. **65**(6), 627–633 (2009)
3. Chowdhury, M.F.M., Lavelli, A.: Exploiting the scope of negations and heterogeneous features for relation extraction: a case study for drug-drug interaction extraction. In: HLT-NAACL, pp. 765–771 (2013)
4. Chowdhury, M.F.M., Lavelli, A.: FBK-irst: a multi-phase kernel based approach for drug-drug interaction detection and classification that exploits linguistic information. Atlanta, Georgia, USA 351, 53 (2013)
5. Der Maaten, L.V., Hinton, G.E.: Visualizing data using t-SNE. J. Mach. Learn. Res. **9**, 2579–2605 (2008)

[3] http://scikit-learn.org/stable/modules/generated/sklearn.manifold.TSNE.html.

6. Herrero-Zazo, M., Segura-Bedmar, I., Martinez, P., Declerck, T.: The DDI corpus: an annotated corpus with pharmacological substances and drug-drug interactions. J. Biomed. Inform. **46**(5), 914 (2013)
7. Kingma, D., Ba, J.: Adam: a method for stochastic optimization. arXiv preprint arXiv:1412.6980 (2014)
8. Lazarou, J., Pomeranz, B.H., Corey, P.N.: Incidence of adverse drug reactions in hospitalized patients: a meta-analysis of prospective studies. JAMA **279**(15), 1200–1205 (1998)
9. Lin, Y., Shen, S., Liu, Z., Luan, H., Sun, M.: Neural relation extraction with selective attention over instances. In: Meeting of the Association for Computational Linguistics, pp. 2124–2133 (2016)
10. Liu, S., Tang, B., Chen, Q., Wang, X.: Drug-drug interaction extraction via convolutional neural networks. Comput. Math. Methods Med. **2016**, 1–8 (2016)
11. Liu, S., Chen, K., Chen, Q., Tang, B.: Dependency-based convolutional neural network for drug-drug interaction extraction. In: IEEE International Conference on Bioinformatics and Biomedicine, pp. 1074–1080 (2016)
12. Melnikov, M.P., Vorobkalov, P.N.: Retrieval of drug-drug interactions information from biomedical texts: use of TF-IDF for classification. In: Kravets, A., Shcherbakov, M., Kultsova, M., Iijima, T. (eds.) JCKBSE 2014. CCIS, vol. 466, pp. 593–602. Springer, Cham (2014). doi:10.1007/978-3-319-11854-3_52
13. Pedregosa, F., Varoquaux, G., Gramfort, A., Michel, V., Thirion, B., Grisel, O., Blondel, M., Prettenhofer, P., Weiss, R., Dubourg, V., Vanderplas, J., Passos, A., Cournapeau, D., Brucher, M., Perrot, M., Duchesnay, E.: Scikit-learn: machine learning in Python. J. Mach. Learn. Res. **12**, 2825–2830 (2011)
14. Pennington, J., Socher, R., Manning, C.: Glove: global vectors for word representation. In: Conference on Empirical Methods in Natural Language Processing, pp. 1532–1543 (2014)
15. Sahu, S.K., Anand, A.: Drug-drug interaction extraction from biomedical text using long short term memory network. arXiv preprint arXiv:1701.08303 (2017)
16. Sklar, S.J., Wagner, J.C.: Enhanced theophylline clearance secondary to phenytoin therapy. Ann. Pharmacother. **19**(1), 34 (1985)
17. Takarabe, M., Shigemizu, D., Kotera, M., Goto, S., Kanehisa, M.: Network-based analysis and characterization of adverse drug-drug interactions. J. Chem. Inf. Model. **51**(11), 2977–2985 (2011)
18. Tari, L., Anwar, S., Liang, S., Cai, J., Baral, C.: Discovering drug-drug interactions: a text-mining and reasoning approach based on properties of drug metabolism. Bioinformatics **26**(18), 547–53 (2010)
19. Thomas, P., Neves, M., Rocktschel, T., Leser, U.: WBI-DDI: drug-drug interaction extraction using majority voting. In: DDI Challenge at Semeval (2013)
20. Zhao, Z., Yang, Z., Luo, L., Lin, H., Wang, J.: Drug drug interaction extraction from biomedical literature using syntax convolutional neural network. Bioinformatics **32**(22), 3444–3453 (2016)
21. Zhou, P., Shi, W., Tian, J., Qi, Z., Li, B., Hao, H., Xu, B.: Attention-based bidirectional long short-term memory networks for relation classification. In: Meeting of the Association for Computational Linguistics, pp. 207–212 (2016)

Spatio-Temporal Data

People-Centric Mobile Crowdsensing Platform for Urban Design

Shili Xiang(✉), Lu Li, Si Min Lo, and Xiaoli Li

Institute for Infocomm Research A*STAR, #21-01, 1 Fusionopolis Way,
Singapore 138632, Singapore
{sxiang,lilu,losm,xlli}@i2r.a-star.edu.sg

Abstract. With the inevitability of urbanization, it is of critical importance to understand how effective the urban spaces are planned and designed to build comfortable and lively smart cities. Our approach is to develop a people-centric mobile crowdsensing platform to provide insights for urban designers, by leveraging on the proliferation of mobile phones and recent advancements in mobile sensing and data analytics technologies. More specifically, we have designed and developed a smartphone based platform to collect both user-generated data and data from multiple sensors contributed by various demographic groups, especially the aged, to understand how they perceive and utilize public spaces. The data collection is also conducted in a privacy-aware manner. Based on the collected data, we then develop advanced and dedicated analytics tools to derive insights about users' opinions towards public spaces in their neighborhood, utilization of public spaces and mobility patterns of the different demographic groups, etc. These insights will be utilized to enhance urban design of future smart towns.

Keywords: Crowdsensing · Urban design · Mobile data analytics

1 Introduction

It has been forecasted that more and more of the world population will live in urban areas and this will result in an increasing demand for space and resources. Recent works have estimated that 70% of the world population will live in cities, and consume about 75% of the world's total daily energy expenditure while releasing about 80% of total daily greenhouse gas emissions in the year 2050. In addition, ageing societies with a growing percentage of the elderly is an issue of increasing concern for cities. For example, in Singapore, those over-60s are expected to form 38% of Singapore population by 2050. Such a prospect will pose significant challenges in urban planning and monitoring, high-density living, sharing of public spaces and sharing of elder care resources, etc. It is of critical importance to understand how effective urban spaces are planned, and how they contribute to the livability and liveliness of densely populated cities.

G. Cong et al. (Eds.): ADMA 2017, LNAI 10604, pp. 569–581, 2017.
https://doi.org/10.1007/978-3-319-69179-4_40

Meanwhile, smartphones have become an integral part of every citizen's life. Besides traditional functions such as calling and messaging, modern smartphones can be used for a countless number of other activities, such as social networking, navigation, gaming, consumption of multimedia content, etc. Many high-level needs that cover various aspects of our daily lives have been met by a wide number of mobile applications, and this trend is still continuing. The intelligence of these Apps is mainly derived from modeling and analyzing the rich data from embedded sensors in the smartphone. Examples of these sensors are GPS sensor, cell tower scanner, WiFi scanner, accelerometer, gyrometer, sound sensor, light sensor etc.

Smartphones are ideal devices for us to conduct crowd sourcing and sensing to collect useful data for facilitating urban design. Users can conveniently use their mobile phones to complete surveys and provide opinions and feedback on various public space, anywhere and anytime. Moreover, when users move around with their mobile phones, the sensors will continue to capture data, which enables the sensing of the ambient environment, understanding of crowd behavior and dynamics as well as the tracking of activities by individuals. These insights can then be incorporated as an input into urban design to make the process bottom-up and more intelligent.

Therefore, we design and develop an innovative and easy to use mobile crowdsensing platform, to gather various datapoints from residents, and understand how they perceive and utilize public spaces. This will in turn enhance the design of public spaces for future smart towns. More specifically, a smartphone based platform is developed to collect three generic types of data from participants: (1) demographics data; (2) user-generated data such as opinions, feelings and activities; (3). data from multiple sensors in the smartphones that reveals clues on activities of users, their environment and location. Based on the collected data, we develop advanced and dedicated analytics tools to derive insights about users' opinions towards public spaces in their neighborhood, utilization of public spaces and mobility patterns of the different demographic groups, etc. The mobile crowdsensing platform has been deployed in a testbed site located in Singapore, consisting of four clusters with a total of 38 HDB blocks and a commercial subarea with shopping malls near an MRT station and bus interchange.

Overall, our approach leverages on the proliferation of mobile phones and recent advancements in mobile sensing and data analytics technologies, to gain insights from a variety of data. The user-generated data explicitly tell us opinions of users towards facilities in public spaces and what they were doing there, and at what time of the day. It enables us to analyze how comfortable and lively targeted *places of interests* (POIs) are, in the viewpoint of the residents. On the other hand, the strength of getting data from multiple sensors lies in its wide coverage and truthfulness (sensor data are objective and patterns are to be discovered instead of being told subjectively). We mine the sensor readings and location updates, to complement the limited number of submissions from our App users. Both types of information coupled with the demographics data provided jointly provide a great opportunity to understand how individuals or groups of people perceive public spaces, their mobility patterns and the utilization patterns of public spaces.

The rest of this paper is organized as follows. We present related works in Sect. 2, and give an overview of the platform in Sect. 3. In Sect. 4, we describe the implementation of our platform, including the developed App with its design rationale, functionalities and features, and backend data management. Data preprocessing methodologies are described in Sect. 5. Section 6 includes the description of various types of analysis with the collected data, together with some preliminary analysis results. In Sect. 7, we briefly introduce the integration with system components. We finally conclude our work in Sect. 8.

2 Related Work

In this section, we present a literature review of methodologies used in the study of urban planning and human mobility pattern analysis.

2.1 Urban Planning

Calabrese et al. [1] provide a survey on ideas and techniques that apply mobile phone data for urban sensing, by focusing on using mobile phone data to understand human mobility. Recently, most existing works (e.g., [2–4]) utilize CDR data to derive human mobility in cities. In general, there are three different CDR data analysis methods: (1) *trip-based analysis* (e.g., [2]) which is to convert CDR data into node-to-node transient origin-destination (OD) matrices in the city road network, (2) *activity-based analysis* (e.g., [3]) which is to conduct activities from human daily travels by considering travel demand, and (3) *system-based analysis* (e.g., [4–6]) which is to synthesize methods of estimating travel demand, deriving estimated traffic on road networks and understanding road usage patterns from CDR data. Due to the low quality (sparse in space and time, low location precision) of CDR spatiotemporal data, existing works mostly target on the urban transportation planning, but the single source of CDR data is not enough to derive the utilization analysis of urban public space. Furthermore, due to a lack of social demographic information, the anonymous spatiotemporal CDR data can not be directly used to analyze the human behavior of different user groups (e.g., by age, by gender) and the mobility patterns of users with close relationship (e.g., family members, good friends). Even though the analysis [6] uses a separate source of travel survey data, it is still limited due to the unclear linkage between CDR data and the survey data.

2.2 Human Mobility Pattern Analysis

Recently, some existing works (e.g., [7,8]) focus on understanding human mobility patterns, and some others (e.g., [9–11]) study frequent pattern mining of human movement, based on frequent patterns (e.g., [9]), association rules (e.g., [10]) or predictive models (e.g., [11]).

Based on human mobility patterns, some existing works (e.g., [12]) study the detection of home and work places. Rather than considering home and work places, our research focuses on other public spaces within the residential area.

Papandrea et al. [13] analyze human mobility patterns to derive utilization of commonly visited places, by taking into consideration the semantics of these visited places. Compared with the proposed method [13], our analysis takes into account not only the semantics of visited places but also the semantics of users.

3 Platform Description

In this section, let us briefly describe the people centric mobile crowdsensing platform. Figure 1 shows the platform diagram. As can be seen in Fig. 1, our platform mainly contains of five parts: (1) mobile App development, (2) backend data management, (3) data cleaning and pre-processing, (4) data analysis and (5) data integration with other system components.

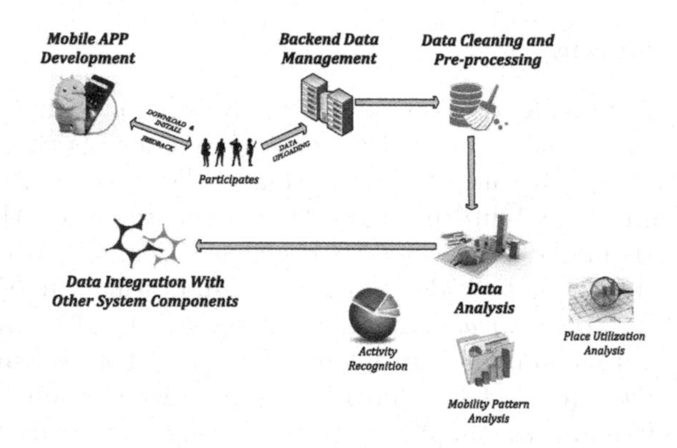

Fig. 1. The people-centric mobile crowdsensing platform

More specifically, an Android mobile App was developed to collect the opinions and feelings of participants about public places in the testbed area, together with phone sensor data. An incentive scheme was designed to encourage users to actively contribute their mobility data. All collected data in the phone will be uploaded periodically into our cloud server when the phone is connected to WiFi. Data management infrastructure has been established to coordinate and store streaming data to enable real-time processing, answer queries from the mobile App, and facilitate progress monitoring and future data analysis work. Privacy preserving features and lightweight stream mining are included to make the system safe and ensure the entire data collection process is manageable. After pre-processing and intelligently cleaning the collected people-centric data, we develop advanced and dedicated analytics tools to derive insights from the crowdsourced and crowd-sensed people-centric data. Examples of these analyses are public opinion analysis, place utilization analysis, activity recognition and mobility pattern analysis. The pre-processed data and analytics results are also uploaded to the Informed Design Platform [14–16] for integrated visualization and analysis with data from other sources (e.g. sensing data, survey data, CDR spatiotemporal data and so on), to provide a holistic view and turn the collected data into insights and actions.

4 Platform Implementation

Let us now introduce the implementation of our platform. In Sect. 4.1, we present the development of our Android mobile App, followed by the description of our backend data management in Sect. 4.2.

4.1 Mobile App Development

Figure 2 shows the UI of our App, which includes the menu, registration page, rewards page, notifications panel, visited places and ratings submission page.

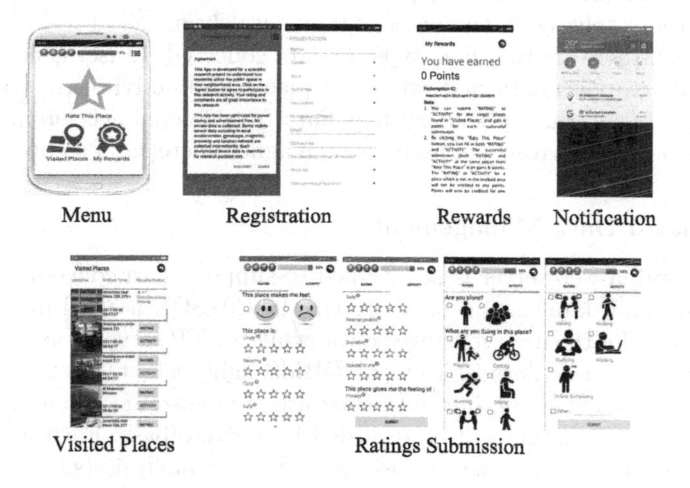

Fig. 2. UI of our mobile App

Around 280 residents in the testbed area were gradually recruited to participate in the study through an incentive scheme. With the App installed, users can provide their opinions and feedback about public spaces in the testbed area at any time by submitting their ratings through the "Rating" page, as well as what they were doing at that place through the "Activity" page. To encourage residents to actively contribute their data, reward points are credited after filling in and submitting the "Rating" and "Activity" pages. These reward points can be used to redeem for shopping vouchers.

Ratings given are used to determine how closely users associate a place with certain attributes, identified by social science experts. A short explanation for the terminology used is given by clicking on the superscript 'i' button. Examples are lively (full of animated ambience and excitement), relaxing (the place facilitates your physical or mental rest making you feel relaxed), cosy (the place makes you feel intimate, comfortable and relaxed), etc.

For targeted data collection, we have designated a specific list of places within the testbed area to collect feedback on. To automatically detect whether the user passes any of these places of interest (POIs), the App runs in the background and alerts the user via a notification when the user passes a POI. The user can then choose to respond immediately by clicking on the notification, which will take him/her into the App to rate the place. Alternatively, the user can also complete the submission at a later time from the "Visited Places" page in the App, which holds a history of the places visited at today. For added flexibility, the App also has the functionality to submit ratings for the user's current location within the testbed area even if it is not included in the list of POIs.

All this while, data from multiple sensors in the phone will be captured continuously in the background mode without affecting the user's regular interactions with his/her phone. From these phone sensor data, we could derive users' activities and locations, and infer public space utilization and mobility patterns of users without relying on submissions they actively make.

In general, there are two main types of data collected: 1. user generated data, such as demographics data and ratings of places and activities; 2. background data captured from smartphone, such as data from 3-axial accelerometer, gyroscope, geo-location, gyroscope, barometer, magnetometer and so on.

4.2 Backend Data Management

In the backend, a web server is maintained to support data collection, incentive management and data management. A DBMS (MySQL is used in the current version) is used for the user-generated data, while a FTP server is used to manage the background sensor data to keep the DBMS light-weight.

Once the resident living in the testbed area installs our App and completes registration, a user profile will be recorded in our database. Each user's profile includes demographic information necessary for our analysis (such as a unique userID assigned by our App, gender, age-group etc.), and essential personal information required to check their eligibility and engage them for reward redemption (such as the user's name, residential block, mobile number). Similarly, whenever a user successfully submits ratings or reports activities in a location, it would be recorded in the database and our server will check whether it is inside the testbed area. If yes, the correct number of reward points to be credited will be calculated. Reward points are deducted and exchanged for vouchers monthly. The DBMS can also process received queries. For example, a participant can check his/her reward points in his/her phone through our App by sending a SQL query which has been embedded in our App. Our analysts can also issue specific SQL queries to extract data for analysis.

To avoid consuming too much memory and bandwidth on user devices, background data are kept in an efficient manner and uploaded in batches. Our App automatically zips all background data when the total size is larger than a predefined threshold, and uploads the zipped files when the phone is connected to an available WiFi network. In addition, the App only stores the time and the sensor readings, while the userID and date information are conveyed separately to the server through the folder structure and the naming format for the uploaded files.

5 Data Cleaning and Pre-processing

To facilitate data analysis, we apply several strategies to clean and pre-process the collected data. In our platform, we focus on three different parts: trajectory noise filtering, user generated data cleaning, and stay point detection.

5.1 Trajectory Noise Filtering and Reduction

Spatiotemporal data are collected from users through our App, but it is known that spatiotemporal data are never perfectly accurate, due to noise from the sensor and other factors, such as satellite errors and atmospheric effects. Unfortunately, noise tolerance is limited in residential areas. For example, consider a collected GPS location for a user when he/she visited one of two nearby POIs in the testbed area with the pair-wise distance being 50 m. Assuming that the GPS error is bounded within 100 m, it would be dramatically challenging to determine the exact POI which the current user visited.

To filter trajectory noise, we apply outlier detection algorithms [17] to remove all detected outlier/noisy points in a trajectory. In a trajectory, the travel speed of each point is calculated based on the time interval and distance between the current point and its successor, and the point is considered an outlier if its speed is larger than a given threshold.

Besides filtering out GPS noises, we also apply two strategies of limiting the GPS error boundary, and avoiding effects between nearby POIs. We simply encourage users to turn on the WiFi in their phones even if there is no available WiFi network that they can connect to. With a large number of sensors installed in the testbed area, the GPS error would be bounded within the comparatively more limited boundary of around 30 m if WiFi had been turned on. Furthermore, instead of analyzing individual POIs, we cluster them into different *regions of interests* (ROIs) by grouping nearby POIs into the same ROI.

5.2 User Generated Data Cleaning

In general, the user-generated data contains two main problems. Firstly, some redundant data are recorded in the database due to system or network errors. Regarding this issue, we can simply remove the duplicates based on a spatiotemporal constraint.

Secondly, it is observed that not all the user generated data are reliable. For example, consider a user who after visiting a coffee shop in the testbed area, reports his/her activities to be the following: "Alone", "Cycling", "Studying" and "Talking". From the submitted activities, being "Cycling" rules out any "Studying", while "Cycling" is also obviously impossible within the coffee shop POI. To remove such conflicting data, we build two conflict tables shown in Table 1: (a) activity-activity conflict table and (b) POI-activity conflict table. Based on the two conflict tables, we can filter out unreliable user-generated records if the submitted activities are inconsistent with each other or with the relevant POI. Reconsider the previous example, the record can simply be filtered out, since "Cycling" is contradicted by "Studying" based on the activity-activity conflict table shown in Table 1(a), and "Cycling" is also not plausible within the coffee shop POI based on the POI-activity conflict table shown in Table 1(b).

Table 1. Activity conflict tables

ACTIVITY	CONFLICTED ACTIVITIES
Alone	Group, Talking
Group	Alone
Playing	Studying, Working
Cycling	Running, Sitting, Walking, Studying, Working Online Socializing
...	...

(a) Activity-Activity

POI	CONFLICTED ACTIVITIES
POI_1 (coffee shop)	Cycling, Running, Walking
POI_2 (community club)	Cycling, Running, Walking
POI_3 (play ground)	Studying, Working
...	...

(b) POI-Activity

5.3 Stay Point Detection

In the mobility patterns of a user, not all spatial points are equally important. Some points denote locations where residents have stayed for a long time, while some other points denote locations where residents have merely passed. We are much more interested in the "Stay Points" POIs where participants have stayed for a while, since it is very useful in understanding public space utilization by further analyzing the duration and period of stay. In our platform, we apply a density clustering based stay point detection algorithm [18].

6 Data Analysis

Before introducing the analytics models, we briefly describe the demographic information (shown in Fig. 3) of the participants in our study. As can be seen in Fig. 3, the number of female participants (at 63%) is much larger than the number of male participants. Also, elderly residents above 60 years old form the largest group of recruited participants.

In order to analyze the utilization of public spaces in the testbed area, we build several different models using the collected heterogeneous data, including

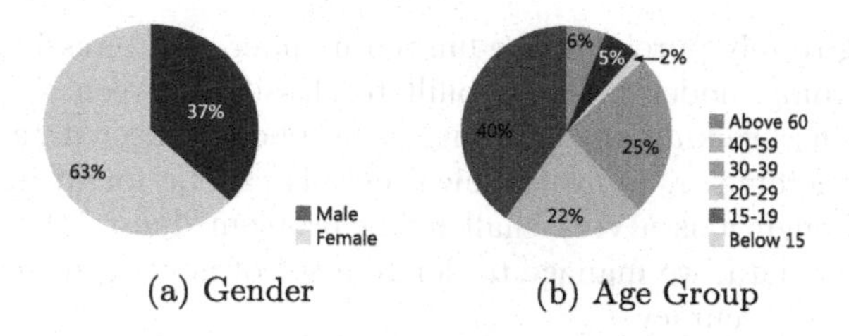

Fig. 3. Participants' demographic profile

the user-generated data, phone sensor data, and spatiotemporal data. Based on these collected data, the models provide a data-driven way to guide urban designers in (re)designing public spaces in future. Let us now briefly introduce the models used to analyze the different types of data in the following sections.

6.1 User Generated Data Analysis

To analyze user opinions towards the public spaces as well as utilization, we first build a statistical model on the user generated data.

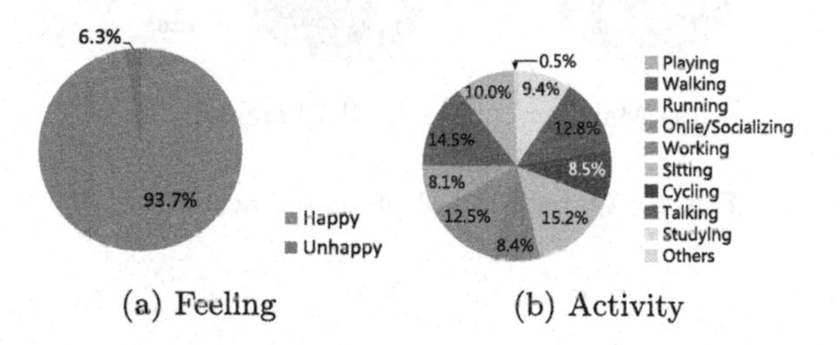

Fig. 4. Summary of feeling and activities

Figure 4 shows a summary of feelings App users have towards public spaces in the testbed area, the distribution of activities they engaged in. As shown, residents are generally happy with existing public spaces in the testbed area.

Furthermore, we can also drill down into different dimensions by age group, gender, time and location to detect patterns and understand segments where the unhappiness arises from. This statistical based analysis of user-generated data can be used to derive insights about public space utilization by different demographic groups (age group, gender), by time of the day, by day of the week, and by location.

6.2 Activity Recognition from Phone Sensor Data

Human activity recognition is important in allowing us to understand the utilization of public places and the activity levels of App users in the testbed area, without having to rely purely on the limited number of submissions from users. A machine learning model has been built to classify between several activities still (stand or sit), walking and running, using phone sensor data such as from the 3-axial accelerometer. More technical details can be found in our previous work [19]. Although it is a very challenging problem due to the size and heterogeneity of the data, we manage to derive a set of novel features and achieve good classification accuracy.

Having derived the activities, a wide range of analysis could be conducted, (for example, activities by gender, by age-group, by time of the day, by day of the week, by location), to answer the questions of when and where users do which type of activities.

Figure 5 shows the aggregated activity of residents grouped by their gender. As can be seen in Fig. 5, the activity "still" dominates both participant groups, and men are generally more active than their female counterparts, with more engaging in the "walking" activity.

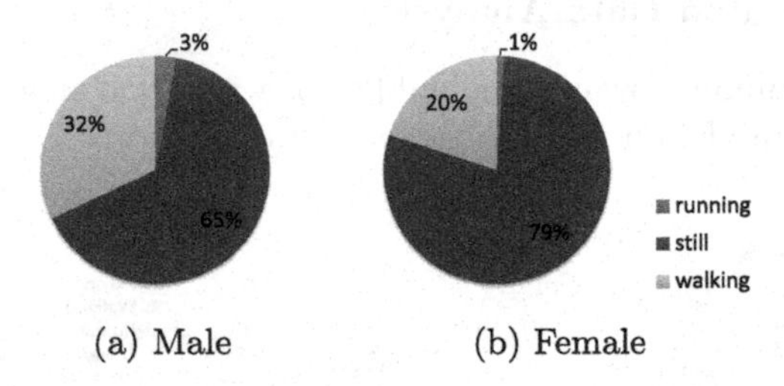

Fig. 5. Aggregation of predicted activities

6.3 Mobility Pattern Analysis from Spatiotemporal Data

Mobility Pattern Analysis is very important towards understanding the mobility behaviour of residents and the usage of public facilities in the testbed area. Using the background data captured about location and time, and after data cleaning and pre-processing to filter out noise in the trajectory and detect stay points, a set of trajectory analysis algorithms can be applied to derive insights on the mobility patterns. Example questions that can be answered with the data are categorized into:

- Duration Patterns. How long and how often do users stay within the public space? How many participants stayed within the public space during a given period of time? This is regarding the popularity and utilization patterns of various public spaces.
- Movement Patterns. How do participants move in and out of the testbed area? How do they move from one public space to another within the testbed area? Do they travel-together? This is regarding the mobility patterns of different demographic groups and which type of urban design would suit them best.

In the following, we show two figures comparing trend lines of males and females inside and outside of the testbed area throughout a day.

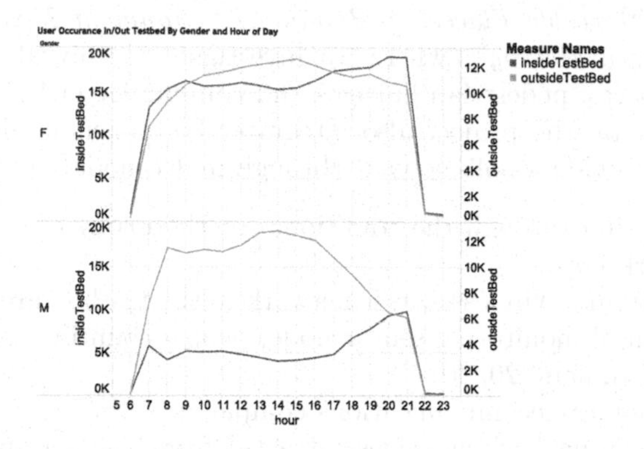

Fig. 6. User occurence in/out testbed by gender and hour of day

Figure 6 shows the trend comparison grouped by their gender. As can be seen, the two trend lines for female residents are quite similar, but the trend line representing occurences outside the testbed area is significantly higher than the other trend line representing occurrences inside the testbed area. The reason could be that most of the male residents are working outside during the day.

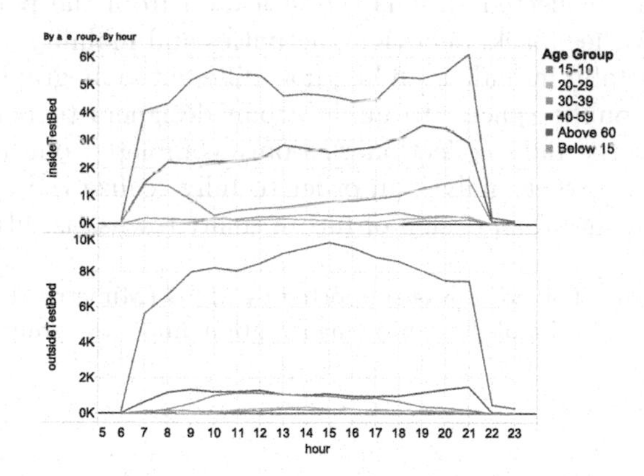

Fig. 7. User occurence in/out testbed by age group and hour of day

Figure 7 shows the same analysis but grouped by age instead. As shown, both trends are quite comparable for most groups. However, the trend of staying within the testbed area for age-group (40–59) is much higher than the others. After we further break down into gender, we found that this age-group is dominated by female residents. Furthermore, it can also be seen that residents above 60 years old are more likely to leave the testbed area during the afternoon period.

7 Data Integration with Other System Components

Our people-centric mobile crowdsensing platform is one part of the multidisciplinary project "*Liveable Places: A Building Environment Modeling Approach for Dynamic Place Making*", where we investigate the liveability and liveliness of public spaces, pedestrian linkages and community facilities. Besides our mobile sensing data, the project also integrates heterogenous data from other data sources to provide a holistic view through multi-modal data analysis:

- feedback collected through the traditional methodology of surveys and participatory workshops;
- sensing data from a wireless sensor network in the testbed area, consisting of an environmental monitoring sensor node, people counting sensor node, and passive Wi-Fi sniffers [20,21];
- CDR data from a telecommunications company;
- geo-tagged social network messages extracted from Twitter and Instagram to understand public sentiment as well as utilisation of the places.

For more details of the project, please refer to [14–16,20,21].

8 Conclusion and Future Works

In this paper, we have introduced our platform of people-centric mobile crowdsensing for urban design applications. Through the Android mobile App we developed, we have collected various types of data from the participants, and have studied crowd feedback, behaviors, activities and mobility patterns. These findings will be helpful in understanding how different demographic groups perceive and utilize public spaces, to guide urban designers to better (re)design public spaces. As the data collection was only completed one month ago, we will continue with further analysis in order to fully realize the potential of the datasets in enhancing urban design of future smart towns, as future work.

Acknowledgement. This work was supported by MND (Ministry of National Development) Singapore, Sustainable Urban Living Program, under the grant no. SUL2013-5.

References

1. Calabrese, F., Ferrari, L., Blondel, V.D.: Urban sensing using mobile phone network data: a survey of research. ACM Comput. Surv. **47**(2), 25:1–25:20 (2014)
2. Wang, P., Hunter, T., Bayen, A.M., Schechtner, K., González, M.C.: Understanding road usage patterns in urban areas. Scientific Reports, 2:1001, 47 p, December 2012. arXiv:1212.5327
3. Schneider, C.M., Belik, V., Couronné, T., Smoreda, Z., González, M.C.: Unravelling daily human mobility motifs. J. Roy. Soc. Interface **10**(84), 20130246 (2013)
4. Toole, J.L., Colak, S., Sturt, B., Alexander, L.P., Evsukoff, A., González, M.C.: The path most traveled: travel demand estimation using big data resources. Transp. Res. Part C Emerg. Technol. **58**, 162–177 (2015)

5. Çolak, S., Alexander, L.P., Alvim, B.G., Mehndiratta, S.R., González, M.C.: Analyzing cell phone location data for urban travel: current methods, limitations, and opportunities. Transp. Res. Rec. **2526**, 126–135 (2015)
6. Jiang, S., Ferreira, J., Gonzalez, M.C.: Activity-based human mobility patterns inferred from mobile phone data: a case study of Singapore. TBD **3**(2), 208–219 (2017)
7. Brockmann, D., Hufnagel, L., Geisel, T.: The scaling laws of human travel. Nature **439**(7075), 462–465 (2006)
8. Gonzalez, M.C., Hidalgo, C.A., Barabasi, A.-L.: Understanding individual human mobility patterns. Nature **453**(7196), 779–782 (2008)
9. Giannotti, F., Nanni, M., Pedreschi, D.: Efficient mining of temporally annotated sequences. In: ICDM, pp. 348–359. SIAM (2006)
10. Morzy, M.: Prediction of moving object location based on frequent trajectories. In: Levi, A., Savaş, E., Yenigün, H., Balcısoy, S., Saygın, Y. (eds.) ISCIS 2006. LNCS, vol. 4263, pp. 583–592. Springer, Heidelberg (2006). doi:10.1007/11902140_62
11. Yavaş, G., Katsaros, D., Ulusoy, Ö., Manolopoulos, Y.: A data mining approach for location prediction in mobile environments. DKE **54**(2), 121–146 (2005)
12. Isaacman, S., Becker, R., Cáceres, R., Kobourov, S., Martonosi, M., Rowland, J., Varshavsky, A.: Identifying important places in people's lives from cellular network data. In: Lyons, K., Hightower, J., Huang, E.M. (eds.) Pervasive 2011. LNCS, vol. 6696, pp. 133–151. Springer, Heidelberg (2011). doi:10.1007/978-3-642-21726-5_9
13. Papandrea, M., Jahromi, K.K., Zignani, M., Gaito, S., Giordano, S., Rossi, G.P.: On the properties of human mobility. INFOCOM **87**, 19–36 (2016)
14. You, L., Tunçer, B.: Exploring the utilization of places through a scalable "activities in places" analysis mechanism. In: IEEE BigData, pp. 3563–3572. IEEE (2016)
15. You, L., Tunçer, B.: Exploring public sentiments for livable places based on a crowd-calibrated sentiment analysis mechanism. In: ASONAM, pp. 693–700 (2016)
16. You, L., Tunçer, B.: SAPAM: a scalable activities in places analysis mechanism for informed place design. In: BDCAT, pp. 158–167. ACM (2016)
17. Zheng, Y., Chen, Y., Xie, X., Ma, W.-Y.: Geolife2. 0: a location-based social networking service. In: MDM, pp. 357–358 (2009)
18. Yuan, J., Zheng, Y., Zhang, L., Xie, X., Sun, G.: Where to find my next passenger. In: UbiComp, pp. 109–118 (2011)
19. Liao, L., Xue, F., Lin, M., Li, X., Krishnaswamy, S.P.: Human activity classification in people centric sensing exploiting sparseness measurement. In: ICICS (2015)
20. Lau, B.P.L., Chaturvedi, T., Ng, B.K.K., Li, K., Hasala, M.S., Yuen, C.: Spatial and temporal analysis of urban space utilization with renewable wireless sensor network. In: BDCAT, pp. 133–142. ACM (2016)
21. Li, K., Yuen, C., Kanhere, S.: Senseflow: an experimental study of people tracking. In: RealWSN, pp. 31–34. ACM (2015)

Long-Term User Location Prediction Using Deep Learning and Periodic Pattern Mining

Mun Hou Wong[1], Vincent S. Tseng[1(✉)], Jerry C.C. Tseng[2], Sun-Wei Liu[3], and Cheng-Hung Tsai[3]

[1] National Chiao Tung University, Hsinchu, Taiwan, Republic of China
vtseng@cs.nctu.edu.tw
[2] National Cheng Kung University, Tainan, Taiwan, Republic of China
jerry.cc.tseng@gmail.com
[3] Institute for Information Industry, Taipei, Taiwan, Republic of China
{SunwayLiu, jasontsai}@iii.org.tw

Abstract. In recent years, with the advances in mobile communication and growing popularity of the fourth-generation mobile network along with the enhancement in location positioning techniques, mobile devices have generated extensive spatial trajectory data, which represent the mobility of moving objects. New services are emerged to serve mobile users based on their predicted locations. Most of the existing studies on location prediction were focused on predicting the next location of a user, which is regarded as short-term next location prediction. While more advanced location-based services could be enabled for the users if long-term location prediction could be achieved, the existing methods constrained in next-location prediction are not applicable for long-term prediction scenario. In this paper, we propose a novel prediction framework named LSTM-PPM that utilises deep learning and periodic pattern mining for long-term prediction of user locations. Our framework devises the ideology from natural language model and uses multi-step recursive strategy to perform long-term prediction. Furthermore, the periodic pattern mining technique is utilized to reduce the accumulated loss in the multi-step strategy. Through empirical evaluation on a real-life trajectory dataset, our proposed approach is shown to provide effective performance in long-term location prediction. To the best of our knowledge, this is the first work addressing the research topic on long-term user location prediction.

Keywords: Long-Term prediction · Location prediction · Trajectory pattern mining

1 Introduction

With the fast development of mobile network techniques and the enhancement in location positioning techniques, mobile devices have generated extensive spatial trajectory data, which represent the mobility of moving objects. The ability to predict the future location of a moving object allows for a rich set of innovative services becoming feasible. As a result, predicting the next location of a user given the history spatial trajectory has increasingly gained significance in recent years [1–7].

G. Cong et al. (Eds.): ADMA 2017, LNAI 10604, pp. 582–594, 2017.
https://doi.org/10.1007/978-3-319-69179-4_41

Next location prediction can enhance the effectiveness of advertisement publishing scheme. While integration of location in advertising has demonstrated that it generates considerably higher return than traditional mobile advertising, location based advertisement scheme only utilise the real-time location information of the target customer. This is where the next location prediction can play a role. We believe that if ones can know the likely places where a person will visit, the more valuable context they can get.

Due to the applicability of next location prediction, research on this area has attracted much attention [1–5]. However, most of the existing studies on location prediction were focused on predicting the next location of a user, which is regarded as short-term next location prediction. While more advanced location-based services could be enabled for the users if long-term location prediction could be achieved, the existing methods constrained in next-location prediction are not applicable for long-term prediction scenario. In this paper, we proposed *LSTM-PPM (Long Short Term Memory with Periodic Pattern Mining)*, a new prediction framework based on deep learning and periodic pattern mining that can perform long-term location prediction. We devise the ideology underlying the natural language model and apply it into the location prediction problem. Furthermore, the periodic pattern mining technique is utilised to reduce the accumulated loss in a multi-step strategy we designed. The proposed prediction framework consists of two major steps. Firstly, we pre-process the data and map it into language model. Secondly, we design a hybrid model for predicting user's long-term location at a given time *t* by means of techniques drawn from deep learning and periodic pattern mining. The contributions of this paper can be summarised as follows:

- We propose *LSTM-PPM*, a new prediction framework that performs long-term location prediction based on deep learning and periodic pattern mining. A multi-step recursive prediction strategy is used in prediction and its accumulated loss is reduced with periodic pattern mining. To the best of our knowledge, this is the first work addressing the research topic on long-term user location prediction.
- We devise the ideology of natural language model and apply it into location prediction. Several data pre-processing techniques were deployed to map the location traces to sentences in language model.
- We evaluate LSTM-PPM by comparing it with Markov predictors on a real-life dataset. We report an overall performance increment over the Markov-based predictor on long-term location prediction.

2 Related Works

Mobility models are a set of well-studied algorithms for next location prediction tasks. Over the course of the last few decades, many mobility model approaches have been developed [1–7]. The mobility models can be grouped into different categories.

Markov Chain (MC) model for next location prediction has been presented in [1, 2, 6]. Markov Chain model is a mobility model that based on probabilistic reasoning to predict the future location of a user using sequences of past observation [8]. The Markov assumption implies that the future predictions are independent of all but the n most recent observations. Markov model can be used to predict a user's next location by computing the transition probability. However, a Markov model with order n can only discover the patterns of length n.

Similarly, [3] employed hidden Markov model to infer user's next location. As described in [8], the Hidden Markov model is a state space model where each observation x_n is attached by a corresponding latent variable z_n. At any time-step n, the states of the latent variable of a hidden Markov model represent a mixture distribution given by the probability $p(x_n|z_n)$, which has generated the observation x_n. A hidden Markov model is used to predict a user's next prediction due to its ability to consider the location characteristics as an unobservable parameter.

[4, 7] proposed a rule-based approach that discovers spatial and temporal patterns from users' trajectory data. After all the frequent patterns have been discovered, they predict users' next location using pattern matching technique.

Recently, some of the studies leverage Recurrent Neural Network (RNN) to model people's mobility [5]. The authors presented that the RNN model archived good results on next location prediction compared to the state-of-the-art methods.

3 The Proposed Framework

Figure 1 shows the proposed framework, namely *LSTM-PPM* (Long Short Term Memory with Periodic Pattern Mining), which consists of three parts, namely the input, process, and output. The input is a set of user's history spatial trajectory and a specified future time t. The process consists of two major parts: the data pre-processing module and the LSTM training. Finally, the output is the predicted location or place semantic of an user at the given time t.

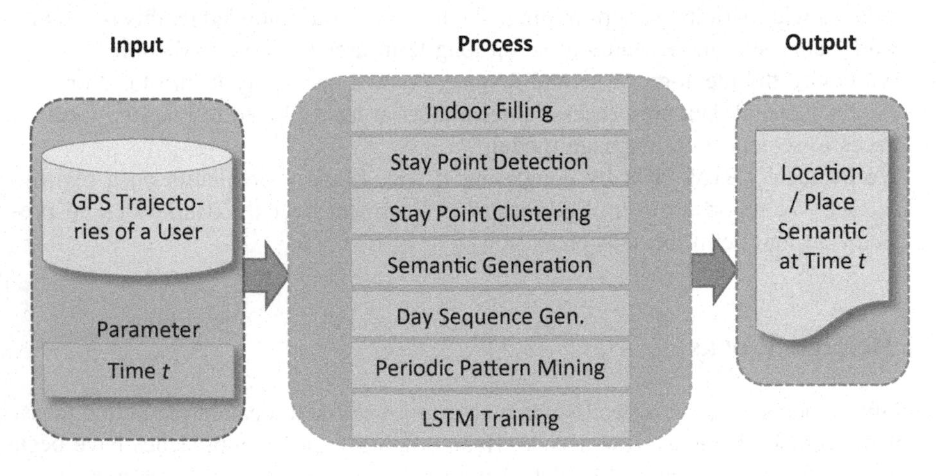

Fig. 1. The proposed framework.

In this section, we first introduce the data pre-processing methods. Next, we will present the whole framework in details.

3.1 Dataset Pre-processing

Indoor Filling. The reliability of GPS data depends on many factors. Most of the time, the GPS track logs collected using a GPS logger exist gaps. This is because GPS signals are often heavily attenuated when users are inside buildings. To overcome this problem, we apply a simple heuristic rule originally from [6]. When the gap between two consecutive GPS records are within a distance of 35 m and the gap duration is greater than 5 min, we consider the user was staying at the same location during that time. Thus, we reconstruct the trajectory by adding as many GPS points equal to the starting point of the gap as the duration in second of the gap.

Stay Point Detection. In a trajectory, not all GPS points are equally important. Some points denote the locations where people have stayed for a while, the other points represent the transition from one place to another. Therefore, we should extract all of his visited places from the raw GPS trajectories, which can be regarded as the locations where the user has stayed. We call these places as stay points. Formally, the data collected by the GPS logger are of the GPS form, which is a sequence of GPS point $P = \{p_1, p_2, \ldots, p_n\}$. Each point $p_i \in P$ contains the longitude, latitude, and time stamp.

A single stay point s can be considered as a group of consecutive GPS points $G = \{p_m, p_{m+1}, \ldots, p_n\}$ such that $distance(p_m, p_i) \leq \varepsilon$ and $time\ difference(p_m, p_n) \geq \tau$, where ε is distance threshold, τ is time threshold and $\forall m < i < n$. As illustrated in, p1→p2→...→p9 forms a GPS trajectory and a stay point can be constructed by p5→p6→p7→p8. We follow the algorithm proposed in [9] to extract the stay points of a user.

Stay Point Clustering. Occasionally, the detected stay points are too shattered and may not reflect the region where the user stays. Therefore, the detected stay points should be clustered into several groups to represent the possible places where a user has stayed. Thus, we apply the DBSCAN algorithm with these stay points to form stay locations. Each cluster generated by DBSCAN is given a cluster id and the location history of each user is then formulated using these cluster ids.

Place Semantic Inferring. Since a stay location is a cluster of stay points and represented with only geographic coordinates, to retrieve a richer and more meaningful information, we use Google Places API [10] to infer the semantic meaning of each stay location. We search the nearest place to the centroid of each cluster through the Google Places API and associate them with the places type of the nearest place.

Day Sequence Generation. Intuitively, the raw trajectory can be transformed to a sequence of detected stay locations. Hence, we use a predefined time interval length to divide each day into several numbers of equal length time intervals. For example, if the time interval length is set to 30 min, each day can be discretised into 48 windows. Each window is filled with the stay location where it was visited within that time interval (Table 1).

Table 1. An example of day sequence with 30 min time interval.

x^{th} minutes of the day	0th	30th	60th	90th	…	1350th	1380th	1410th
Cluster ID	0	0	0	0	…	1	1	1

It is possible that more than one stay location exists for the same time interval. For such cases, that window is filled with the last visited stay location during that time interval.

Periodic Pattern Mining. Discovering periodic mobility patterns of user can be useful for location prediction task as it unveils repeated activities at regular time intervals. To discover those cyclic patterns, we apply PFPM algorithm [11]. PFPM aims to discover sets of items that periodically appear in transactions. Hence, we treat each location label in the day sequences as a transaction with only one item.

3.2 Design Logic and Implementation Details

[12] demonstrates the power of RNN in language modelling and generating sequences. In language modelling, the input is a sequence of words and the output is the sequence of predicted words. A language model measures how likely a sentence is and predicts the probability of each word given the previous words. An obvious way to generate a sequence is to repeatedly predict what will happen next.

This is my cat. I love my cat.

Fig. 2. Text generation example.

We use Fig. 2 to explain the philosophy behind the text generator. Given a sequence of words "This is my cat." as the input, the text generator tries to generate the next word "I". To generate a word sequence, we append the new generated word to the input and re-run the text generator (Fig. 3).

Sentence	This	is	my	cat.	I	love	my	cat.
Location Trace	1	1	1	2	2	2	3	3

Fig. 3. Mapping from location trace to sentence.

We hypothesise that LSTM could be used in long-term location prediction due to its ability to infer the rich contextual information of the input locations. It can learn the hidden contextual meaning of the location labels in the location traces. We model the location traces of each user as sentences and each location label as a word. The location labels correspond to words in the language model. The entire location trace can be mapped into sentences, where the prediction of the next location is the same as the prediction of next word.

Figure 4 depicts our proposed LSTM architecture. In our LSTM model, each trajectory is reformed as a day sequence and represented as a sequence of tuple $(\mathbf{x}_\tau, \mathbf{h}_\tau, \mathbf{d}_\tau)$, where $\mathbf{x}$ is the centroid ID of the stay location visited at time τ, while $\mathbf{h}$ and $\mathbf{d}$ are the associated beginning time of the interval and day of week. Its task is to predict the future location of a user during the next time interval.

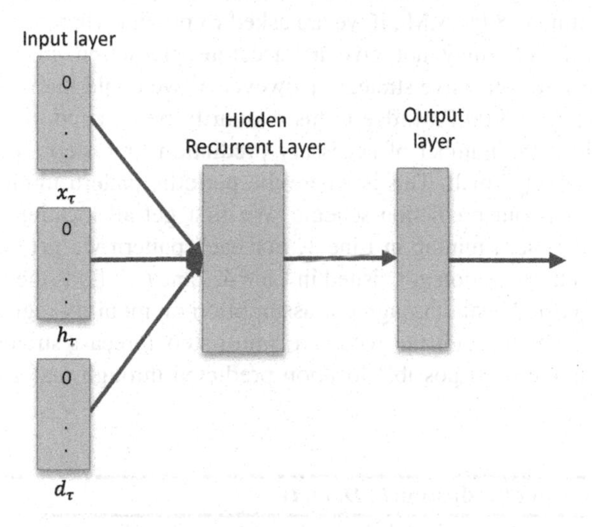

Fig. 4. Proposed LSTM architecture.

Our proposed LSTM model consists of three layers: input layer, hidden recurrent layer and output layer. The input layer consists of three vectors. The first one is $\mathbf{x}_\tau \in R^N$ which represents the centroid ID of the stay location at time τ, where N is the number of all stay location. The second vector represents the beginning time of the interval at time t, denoted as $\mathbf{h}_\tau \in R^M$, where M is the number of time intervals in day sequence. Finally, the third vector, denoted as $d_\tau \in R^L$ represents the associated day of week of time τ. L is the number of days in a week. Each vector in the input layer is encoded using one-hot encoding.

We use LSTM recurrent unit in hidden layer to learn and capture the latent information of user mobility behaviour. As mentioned before, we apply LSTM in modelling the sequence and use its ability to connect previous locations to present location. At last, the output layer $\mathbf{y}_\tau \in R^N$ is a categorical classification layer, produces the probability of all the locations and it has the same dimensionality as the input vector $\mathbf{x}_\tau$.

Since the day sequence we put into the LSTM model is a sequence with fixed time interval and our model always outputs the next location where the user may visit for the next equal time interval, to predict a location at a given time t, we use a recursive multi-step prediction strategy. The recursive strategy uses the prediction for the prior time step as an input for making a prediction on the following time step. Specifically, we first calculate the number of time steps the model needs to predict, denoted as K. Then, for each prediction, the previous output is treated as the new input for the model, until K predictions have been done. The last output is considered as the prediction result for the given time t.

However, since the predictions are used as observations, the recursive strategy accumulates prediction errors and performance can quickly degrade as the time-step increases. We argue that human mobility patterns are regular. Hence, we combine the periodic pattern mining and LSTM model to overcome the shortfall. For instance, given that the current time is 8:00 A.M., if we are asked to predict where the user might be at 4:00 P.M., our LSTM may not give an accurate prediction since the number of time-steps is large for recursive strategy. However, if we could know that the user will visit a restaurant A at 3:00 P.M. due to his regularity beforehand, the prediction error can be lower since the number of necessary prediction time-steps from 3:00 P.M. to 4:00 P.M. is relatively small. This is where the periodic pattern mining plays its role.

Figure 5 depicts our prediction scheme. We first get all location and their period through periodic pattern mining in Line 1. For each pattern we get, we find the most recent time when that location got visited in Line 4. Line 6–7 finds the furthest time that location will be visited again through our assumption on mobility regularity. Line 8–16 predicts the location through the recursive multi-step forecast strategy. Finally, our algorithm returns the most possible location predicted through majority voting.

```
Algorithm MakePrediction(L, D, ct, t)
Input:    An LSTM model L, all user's day sequences D, current time ct,
          expected time t
Output:   Possible location at t
1.    patterns = PPM(D) // get periodic patterns
2.    possible_locations = []
3.    for pattern in patterns:
4.        last_occur_time = get_most_recent_occur(D, ct, pattern.location)
5.        possible_occur_time = last_occur_time
6.        while possible_occur_time < t:
7.            possible_occur_time += pattern.period
8.        require_time_step = calculate_time_step(possible_occur_time, t)
9.        h = possible_occur_time.h
10.       d = possible_occur_time.d
11.       while k < require_time_step:
12.           predict_location = L.predict(x, h, d)
13.           x = predict_location
14.           h = update_h(h)
15.           d = update_day_of_week(d)
16.           k += 1
17.       possible_locations.append(x)
18.   return majority_voting(possible_locations)
```

Fig. 5. LSTM-PPM prediction scheme.

4 Experiment Evaluation

4.1 Data Description

We evaluate our framework using Geolife dataset [13], a real-life GPS trajectories dataset. This GPS trajectory dataset was collected in Geolife project initiated by Microsoft Research Asia. It collected trajectories of 182 users in a period of over five years, beginning from April 2007 to August 2012. Each GPS trajectory is represented by a sequence of time-stamped points, containing absolute latitude, longitude, and latitude in fine granularity. These trajectories were logged in a dense representation by different GPS loggers and GPS phones.

4.2 Experiment Settings

Geolife dataset is a dataset built for transportation prediction task. Consequently, not all trajectories contain stay locations. Hence, we selected users under two considerations: the period a trajectory spans and the number of days which all trajectories of a single user cover. In particular, for each user, we only consider the daily trajectories that are recorded for more than 3 h. Under this premise, we consider only the users with more than 90 days of data. The resulting number of users is 11. In addition, since visited locations, mobility, and moving trajectories are different among users, we built one prediction model for each user.

We use Hyperopt [14] to find the optimal hyper-parameters of the recurrent model. Hyperopt is a Python library that use both random search and Tree of Parzen Estimators (TPE) algorithms to search for a set of optimal hyper-parameters in a search space with real-valued, discrete, and conditional dimensions. Finally, we use the first 60 days of data as training dataset and evaluate the model performance with the remaining 30 days of data.

4.3 Comparison Targets and Metrics

We compare our proposed framework with Markov Chain model, which was introduced in [1] and built based on the contextual co-occurrences between sequences of locations.

To assess the performance of our proposed framework, we use the Recall score as an evaluation metric in all experiments. The Recall@K is defined as the ratio between the number of correct predictions over the total number of prediction. We first ranked a list of all potential locations arranged in descending order according to their probabilities. Then the Recall score is calculated as the percentage of times in which the real visited location was found in the top K most likely location in the ranked list:

$$Recall@K(\%) = \frac{Number\ of\ instances\ predicted\ correctly\ at\ TOP\ K}{Number\ of\ instances}$$

4.4 Performance Evaluation

We evaluate the performance of our proposed method by performing, long-term location prediction, in which we predict the user's location for the forthcoming 100 to 500 h. Meanwhile, each group of experiments predicts both the location label and location semantic.

4.4.1 Long-Term Prediction Experiments

Figures 6, 7, 8, 9, 10 and 11 report the performance of the LSTM-PPM on long-term prediction. For long-term prediction, the LSTM-PPM prediction scheme significantly reveals the advantages of periodicity of human mobility. Our prediction scheme generally performs better than the LSTM-only and Markov Chain prediction scheme. On the other hands, the LSTM-only prediction scheme performs better than the Markov Chain prediction scheme for every prediction hour in long-term prediction experiments. This is due to the incapability of Markov Chain to handle the unseen combination of location as input.

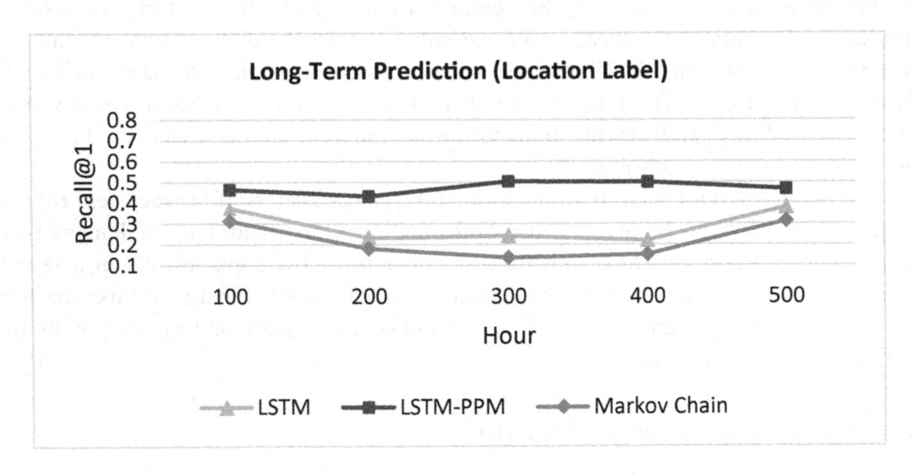

Fig. 6. Long-term prediction (label) Recall@1.

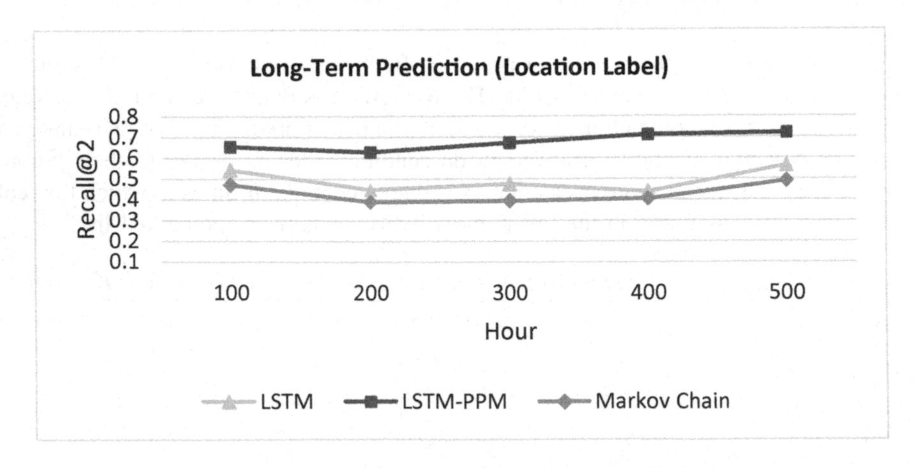

Fig. 7. Long-term prediction (label) Recall@2.

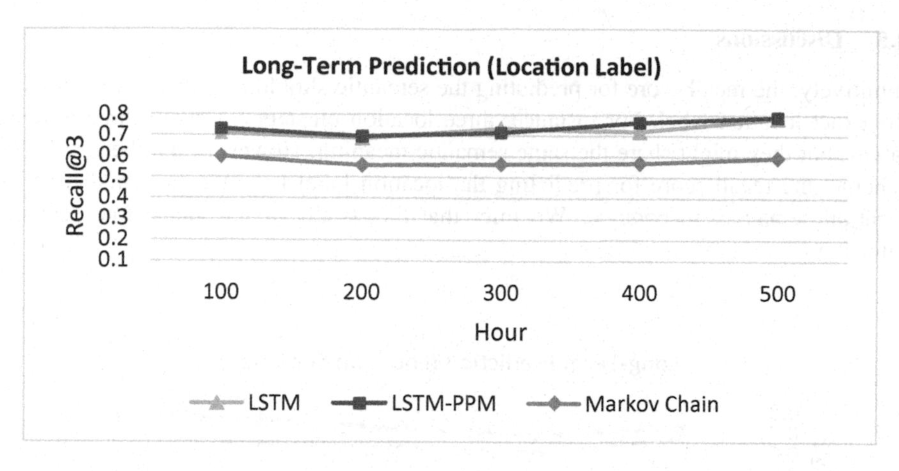

Fig. 8. Long-term prediction (label) Recall@3.

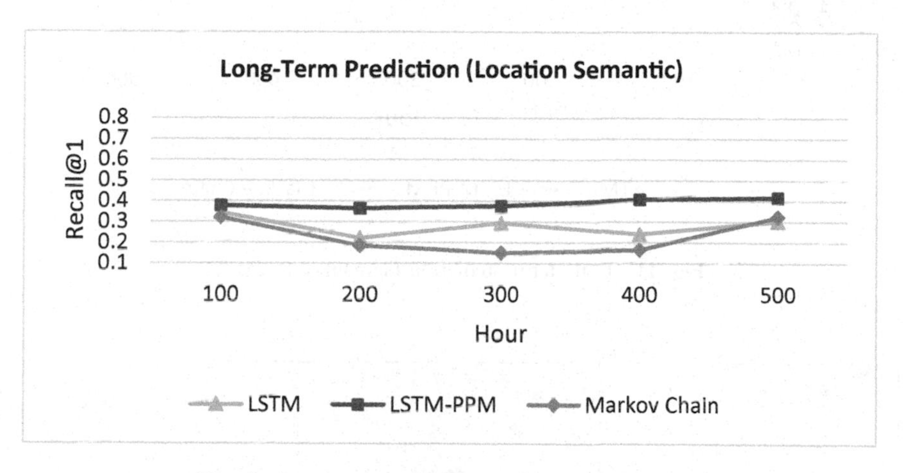

Fig. 9. Long-term prediction (semantic) Recall@1.

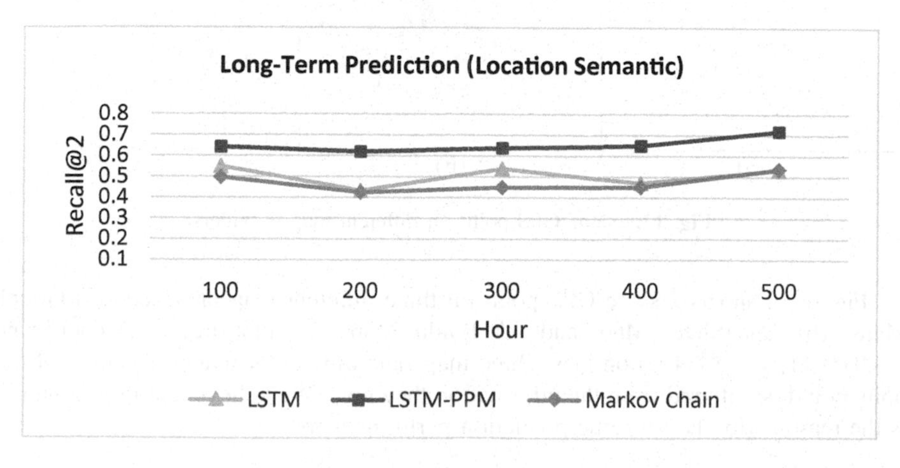

Fig. 10. Long-term prediction (semantic) Recall@2.

4.5 Discussions

Intuitively, the recall score for predicting the semantic should be better than predicting the exact location label. For instance, three location clusters are given three different labels, but they might share the same semantic meaning. However, in either prediction scheme, the recall score for predicting the location label is better than predicting the location semantic, in contrast. We infer that this is due to the inaccurate semantic inferring.

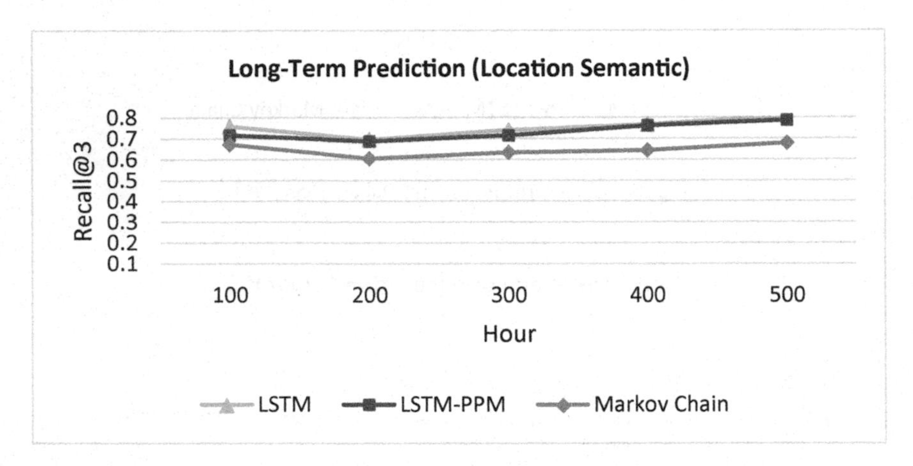

Fig. 11. Long-term prediction (semantic) Recall@3.

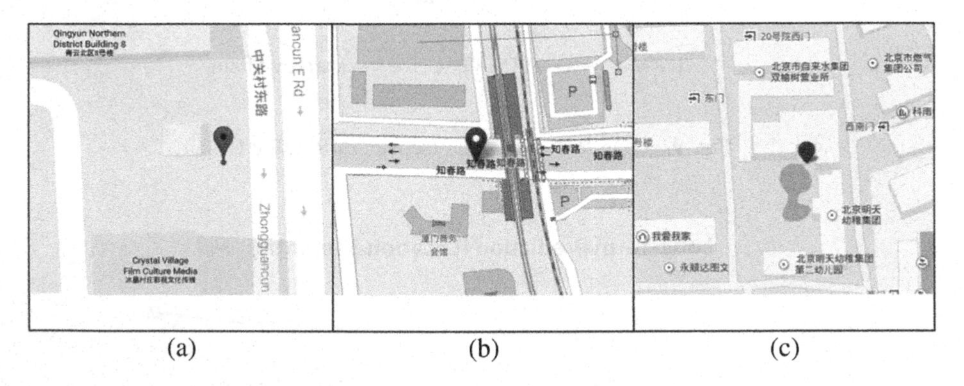

Fig. 12. Same GPS point on different map providers.

Figure 12 shows a same GPS point on three different map providers: (a) Google Maps, (b) OpenStreet Map, and (c) Baidu Map. We plot the GPS coordinate, (39.975011, 116.333481) on these three maps and different semantic meaning of that point could be inferred from the information they give. We believe that this ambiguity is the reason why the semantic prediction performs worse.

5 Conclusion

In this paper, we addressed the topic of long-term user location prediction and investigate the applicability of Long Short-Term Memory Network built upon the analogy between human mobility and natural language models. We have proposed a novel prediction framework with several core ideas: First, to utilise the LSTM network, we apply several data pre-processing techniques to extract the significant locations and transform the trajectories into day sequences to match the ideology of language model. Second, we devised a multi-step recursive prediction strategy based on the idea of text generation to perform prediction. Third, to conquer the loss issue in multi-step recursive prediction strategy, we utilise the periodic pattern mining technique to reduce the number of required time steps for prediction and thus reduce the accumulated loss.

Through experimental evaluation on a real dataset, our proposed framework was shown to deliver good performance compared to other representative methods. To sum up, this paper achieves several contributions: First, we devise a data pre-processing method to make the trajectories fit into the architecture of LSTM. Second, we proposed a multi-step recursive strategy that enables our prediction scheme for long-term prediction. Finally, we combine the periodic pattern mining technique to reduce the accumulated loss in multi-step recursive strategy and make the whole approach appealing in terms of the accuracy. To the best of our knowledge, this is the first work addressing the research topic of long-term user location prediction with providing an appealing approach. We believe that many innovative location-based applications can be enabled through the proposed approach.

Acknowledgement. This study is partially supported under the "System-of-systems Driven Emerging Service Business Development Project (2/4)" of the Institute for Information Industry which is subsidized by the Ministry of Economy Affairs of the Republic of China.

References

1. Asahara, A., Maruyama, K., Sato, A., Seto, K.: Pedestrian-movement prediction based on mixed Markov-Chain model. In: Proceedings of the 19th ACM SIGSPATIAL International Conference on Advances in Geographic Information Systems, pp. 25–33. ACM (2011)
2. Gambs, S., Killijian, M.-O., del Prado Cortez, M.N.: Next place prediction using mobility Markov Chains. In: Proceedings of the First Workshop on Measurement, Privacy, and Mobility, p. 3. ACM (2012)
3. Mathew, W., Raposo, R., Martins, B.: Predicting future locations with hidden Markov models. In: Proceedings of the 2012 ACM Conference on Ubiquitous Computing, pp. 911–918. ACM (2012)
4. Lee, S., Lim, J., Park, J., Kim, K.: Next place prediction based on spatiotemporal pattern mining of mobile device logs. Sensors **16**, 145 (2016)
5. Liu, Q., Wu, S., Wang, L., Tan, T.: Predicting the next location: a recurrent model with spatial and temporal contexts. In: AAAI, pp. 194–200 (2016)
6. Ashbrook, D., Starner, T.: Using GPS to learn significant locations and predict movement across multiple users. Pers. Ubiquit. Comput. **7**, 275–286 (2003)

7. Ozer, M., Keles, I., Toroslu, H., Karagoz, P., Davulcu, H.: Predicting the location and time of mobile phone users by using sequential pattern mining techniques. Comput. J. **59**, 908–922 (2016)
8. Bishop, C.M.: Pattern Recognition and Machine Learning. Springer, New York (2006)
9. Ye, Y., Zheng, Y., Chen, Y., Feng, J., Xie, X.: Mining individual life pattern based on location history. In: International Conference on Mobile Data Management: Systems, Services and Middleware (MDM), pp. 1–10. IEEE (2009)
10. Google. https://developers.google.com/places/?hl=en-gb
11. Fournier-Viger, P., Lin, C.-W., Duong, Q.-H., Dam, T.-L., Ševčík, L., Uhrin, D., Voznak, M.: PFPM: discovering periodic frequent patterns with novel periodicity measures. In: Proceedings of the 2nd Czech-China Scientific Conference 2016. InTech (2017)
12. Graves, A.: Generating Sequences with Recurrent Neural Networks. Arxiv Preprint arXiv:1308.0850 (2013)
13. Zheng, Y., Xie, X., Ma, W.-Y.: Geolife: a collaborative social networking service among user, location and trajectory. IEEE Data(base) Eng. Bull. **33**, 32–39 (2010)
14. Bergstra, J., Yamins, D., Cox, D.: Making a science of model search: hyperparameter optimization in hundreds of dimensions for vision architectures. In: International Conference on Machine Learning (ICML), pp. 115–123 (2013)

An Intelligent Weighted Fuzzy Time Series Model Based on a Sine-Cosine Adaptive Human Learning Optimization Algorithm and Its Application to Financial Markets Forecasting

Ruixin Yang[1], Mingyang Xu[1], Junyi He[3], Stephen Ranshous[1], and Nagiza F. Samatova[1,2](✉)

[1] North Carolina State University, Raleigh, NC, USA
ryang9@ncsu.edu, samatova@csc.ncsu.edu
[2] Oak Ridge National Laboratory, Oak Ridge, TN, USA
[3] Shanghai University, Shanghai, China

Abstract. Financial forecasting is an extremely challenging task given the complex, nonlinear nature of financial market systems. To overcome this challenge, we present an intelligent weighted fuzzy time series model for financial forecasting, which uses a sine-cosine adaptive human learning optimization (SCHLO) algorithm to search for the optimal parameters for forecasting. New weighted operators that consider frequency based chronological order and stock volume are analyzed, and SCHLO is integrated to determine the effective intervals and weighting factors. Furthermore, a novel short-term trend repair operation is developed to complement the final forecasting process. Finally, the proposed model is applied to four world major trading markets: the Dow Jones Index (DJI), the German Stock Index (DAX), the Japanese Stock Index (NIKKEI), and Taiwan Stock Index (TAIEX). Experimental results show that our model is consistently more accurate than the state-of-the-art baseline methods. The easy implementation and effective forecasting performance suggest our proposed model could be a favorable market application prospect.

Keywords: Weighted fuzzy time series · Human learning optimization algorithm · Financial markets forecasting

1 Introduction

During the last decade, the world stock market cap has soared by 133% (from 28 trillion to 65 trillion), especially in emerging markets, e.g., the market cap of China and India has exploded by 1479% and 639%, respectively [12]. Thus, driven by the market power, stock market prediction plays an increasingly important and even crucial role in economic decisions [10]. However, since the financial markets are complex and nonlinear systems which can be influenced by various factors, such as economic cycle and government policies, it is

G. Cong et al. (Eds.): ADMA 2017, LNAI 10604, pp. 595–607, 2017.
https://doi.org/10.1007/978-3-319-69179-4_42

extremely challenging to do an accurate stock forecasting, and thus has attracted considerable worldwide attention, in both the research and financial community. Subsequently, a variety of forecasting approaches have been developed [4,11,13,15,21,23,25,30,31]. Among these approaches, researchers have recently shown a renewed interest in using Fuzzy Time Series (FTS) models for stock forecasting [4,7,17,29], as FTS possesses the universal approximation property in nature and has thus been successfully used in many financial applications in the real world [1,9,14,16]. The concept of FTS was first proposed by Song and Chissom to forecast university enrollment. In a financial context, Teoh et al. [22] presented a model that incorporated trend-weighting into the FTS models, and applied their model to the forecasting of empirical stock markets. Chen and Chen [7] proposed a method for forecasting the Taiwan Stock Index (TAIEX) based on FTS and fuzzy variation groups. By using high-order fuzzy logical relationships, Chen et al. [6] also presented an approach to forecast the TAIEX and inventory demand based on FTS. Zhou et al. [33] developed a portfolio optimization model combining information entropy and FTS to forecast stock exchange in the Chinese financial market. Uslu et al. [24] considered the recurrence number of the fuzzy relations in the defuzzification stage of FTS, and applied their method to spot gold forecast. Rubio et al. [17] proposed weighted FTS model based on the weights of chronological-order and trend-order to forecast the future performance of stock market indices.

Although these approaches show reasonable success for stock data forecasting, they have several drawbacks. On one hand, it is known that the length of intervals, as well as weighting factor, influence forecast accuracy in FTS, which leads to many models that are very sensitive of parameters settings in real world applications [17]. On the other hand, most models only depend on the trend indicated by the fuzzy logic group, but ignore the large influence of the short-term trend developed by neighbor series. In addition, few methods consider the stock volume, one of the most important metrics in stock analysis, which may also weaken the forecast accuracy, since stock volume is closely related with the trend.

In this research, the initial goal is to address the above weaknesses of existing FTS models. To this end, we first develop and deploy a novel evolutionary algorithm, Sine-Cosine adaptive Human Learning Optimization (SCHLO), to optimize the FTS and required parameters automatically and globally. Human Learning Optimization (HLO), which was presented recently by [26], is an evolutionary computation method, and has been successfully used to resolve optimization problems in different applications [3,27,28]. Thanks to the simple but effective structure of HLO, it does not need the gradient information in its optimization procedure, which is very suitable for the FTS optimization. Second, new weighted operators that consider the frequency based chronological order and stock volume are analyzed and integrated with SCHLO for optimization. Finally, a novel short-term trend repair operation is developed to complement the final forecasting process.

The rest of this paper is organized as follows. In Sect. 2, we briefly review the basic concepts of a fuzzy time series forecasting model [5]. In Sect. 3, we introduce the concepts of standard HLO techniques proposed by Wang et al. [26] and present the proposed SCHLO. In Sect. 4, we propose a new FTS forecasting approach based on optimal partitions of intervals and hybrid weighting factors, obtained concurrently by SCHLO. In Sect. 5, we analyze the experimental results of the proposed FTS forecasting method and several state-of-the-art weighted fuzzy time series methods, when applied to forecasting several stock indices (Dow Jones Index (DJI), German Stock Index (DAX), Japanese Stock Index (NIKKEI) and Taiwan Stock Index (TAIEX)). Finally, the conclusions are discussed in Sect. 6.

2 Fuzzy Time Series Forecasting Model

Over the past decade, many fuzzy time-series models have been proposed by following Song and Chissom's definitions [18–20]. Among these models, Chen [5] proposed a model by applying simplified arithmetic operations in forecasting algorithms, replacing the complicated max-min composition operation introduced by Song and Chissom, and thus is more effective. Since we will modify Chen's model to a new weighted FTS, we first illustrate its procedure, as follows:

Step 1 Partition the universe of discourse. First, according to the min and max values in the dataset, define the D_{min} and D_{max} variables and choose two arbitrary positive numbers, D_1 and D_2, to partition the universe of discourse, i.e., $U = \{D_{\min} - D_1, D_{\max} + D_2\}$. Then divide this universe into equal length intervals, i.e., $u_1, u_2, ..., u_m$.

Step 2 Define the fuzzy sets and fuzzify the historical data. Using the defined sub intervals in former step, the fuzzy sets are defined as Eq. (1) and each historical datum in time series is fuzzified its corresponding fuzzy set accordingly.

$$A_i = \frac{0}{u_1} + \frac{0}{u_2} + ... + \frac{0.5}{u_{i-1}} + \frac{1}{u_i} + \frac{0.5}{u_{i+1}} + ... + \frac{0}{u_m}, i = 1, 2, 3, ...m. \quad (1)$$

Step 3 Establish fuzzy logic relationships (FLRs) and fuzzy logic relationship groups (FLRGs). FLRs are grouped based on the current states of the data according to [5].

Step 4 Calculate the forecast values. Let $F(t) = A_i$. If there is only one fuzzy logical relationship in the sequence, and $A_i \rightarrow A_j$, then $F(t+1)$, the forecast output, equals A_j. If $A_i \rightarrow A_1, A_2, ..., A_k$, then $F(t+1)$ equals $A_1, A_2, ..., A_k$. If there are no fuzzy relationship groups, then the forecast output equals A_i.

Step 5 Defuzzify. If the forecast $F(t+1) = A_{i1}, A_{i2}, ..., A_{ik}$, the forecast values at time t+1 are calculated as

$$Final(t+1) = \frac{\sum_{j=1}^{k} M_{ij}}{k} \quad (2)$$

where $M_{i1}, M_{i2}, ..., M_{ij}$ are the defuzzified values of $A_{i1}, A_{i2}, ..., A_{ik}$, respectively, and $Final(t+1)$ is the final forecast.

3 Sine-Cosine Adaptive Human Learning Optimization Algorithm

Recently, the human learning optimization algorithm [26], inspired by human learning mechanisms, has been successfully applied to real world applications, in large part due to its excellent global search ability and robustness to various problems [3,27,28]. In this section, we first introduce the basic techniques of HLO, and then propose a sine-cosine adaptive mechanism to further improve the performance of HLO. In HLO, three learning operators, i.e., the random learning operator, individual learning operator, and social learning operation, are used to yield new candidates to search for the optima, which simulates the human learning process. The detailed processes can be found in [26].

In summary, HLO emulates three human learning operators (random, individual, and social) to yield new solutions and search for the optima. These learning operators are based on the knowledge stored in the individual knowledge data (IKD) and individual knowledge data (SKD), and can be further integrated and operated to improve learning as shown in Eq. (3).

$$x_{ij} = \begin{cases} Rand(0,1), 0 \leq rand() \leq pr \\ ik_{ipj}, pr < rand() \leq pi \\ sk_{qj}, else \end{cases} \tag{3}$$

where pr is the probability of random learning, and the values of $(pi - pr)$ and $(1 - pi)$ represents the probabilities of performing individual learning and social learning, respectively.

Sine-Cosine Adaptive Mechanism. In this paper, we observe that the individual and social learning parameter pi as well as random learning parameter pr are extraordinarily important, since they directly determine the balance between exploration and exploitation, and consequently influence the performance of the algorithm. However, it is not easy to set the optimal parameters of meta-heuristics, as they usually depend on the problems. Moreover, it is very hard to get rid of local optima in some types of complex optimization problems. Thus, it is very critical to determine when to increase (decrease) pi and pr for the purpose of increasing (decreasing) the exploration/exploitation ability. As a result, the monotonous linear adaptive mechanisms are not that effective. Therefore, we propose a new adaptive mechanism based on sine-cosine to dynamically strengthen the search efficiency and relieve the effort of the parameter setting, as follows

$$pr = pr_{\text{mid}} + pr_{\text{mid}} \times \cos\,(Ite + r) \tag{4}$$

$$pi = pi_{\text{mid}} + pr_{\text{mid}} \times \sin\,(Ite + r) \tag{5}$$

$$r = \begin{cases} 0, 0 \leq rand() \leq 0.5 \\ 1, else \end{cases} \tag{6}$$

where pr_{mid} and pi_{mid} are the middle point of fluctuation of pr and pi, respectively, and Ite is the current iteration number. Figure 1 shows the change of the parameters. In this way, various combinations of pr and pi are generated, so that the SCHLO is able to intelligently handle the complex optimization cases.

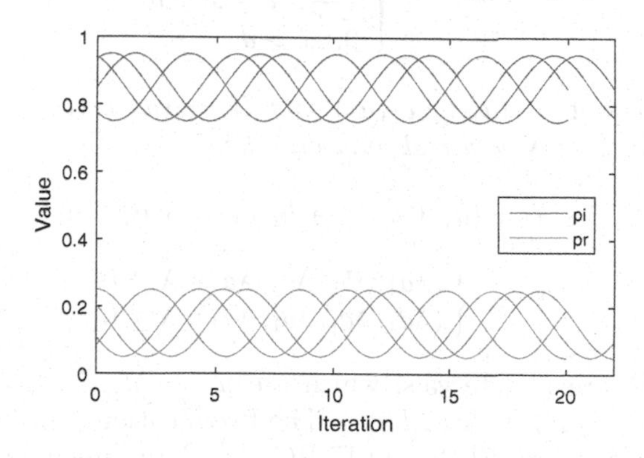

Fig. 1. Adaptive mechanism for *pi* and *pr*.

4 A Novel Weighted Fuzzy Time Series Method Based on SCHLO

In this section we propose a novel weighted FTS forecasting method based on SCHLO (WFTS-SCHLO). Specifically, we first propose several modifications for the basic FTS method, by introducing three types of weights. These weights not only consider the frequency based chronological order, but also take the stock volume into consideration. In addition, based on our observation that there is a big influence of the short-term trend developed by neighbor series, we further propose a novel short-term trend repair operation to complement the forecasting process. Then, SCHLO is utilized to find the optimal partitions of intervals in the universe of discourse and the optimal weight factors simultaneously, based on the historical training data. Next, using the optimal settings obtained by SCHLO, the proposed model fuzzifies the historical data on each trading day into fuzzy sets, and establishes fuzzy logic relationship groups. Finally, based on the fuzzified historical testing data, the model performs defuzzification and uses the obtained optimal weight factors to calculate the forecast outputs.

4.1 The Proposed Weighted FTS Model

In our model, the trapezoidal fuzzy numbers [32] with midpoints of intervals [5] are used to analyze and derive the forecast values.

Definition 1. *A fuzzy number A is said to be a trapezoidal fuzzy number,* $A = (a, b, c, d)$*, if its membership function has the following form:*

$$\mu_{\widetilde{A}}(x) = \begin{cases} 0, & x < a \\ \frac{x-a}{b-a}, & a \leq x \leq b \\ 1, & b \leq x \leq c \\ \frac{d-x}{d-c}, & c \leq x \leq d \\ 0, & x > d \end{cases} \quad (7)$$

Definition 2. *Let* $A = (a_1, b_1, c_1, d_1)$ *and* $B = (a_2, b_2, c_2, d_2)$ *be trapezoidal fuzzy numbers, and let* λ *be a real number. Then,*

$$A \oplus B = (a_1 + a_2, b_1 + b_2, c_1 + c_2, d_1 + d_2) \quad (8)$$

$$\lambda A = \begin{cases} (\lambda a_1, \lambda b_1, \lambda c_1, \lambda d_1) & \lambda \geq 0 \\ (\lambda d_1, \lambda c_1, \lambda b_1, \lambda a_1) & \lambda \leq 0 \end{cases} \quad (9)$$

Assume there are m intervals, which are $u_1 = [d_1, d_2]$, $u_2 = [d_2, d_3]$, ... , $u_{m-1} = [d_{m-1}, d_{m-2}]$,$u_m = [d_m, d_{m+1}]$. The fuzzification process is as shown in Eq. (10) and the standard FLRs and FLRGs are determined according to [5].

$$\text{fuzzify}(F(t)) = A_i \ if \ u(A_i) = \max[\ u(A_z)] \ \ for \ all \ z \quad (10)$$

where where $z = F(1), F(2), ..., F(t)$ is the datum at time t; and $u(A_z)$ is the degree of membership of $F(t)$ under A_z.

Following the above preparations of FTS, we next turn to the proposed weighting rules that consider the frequency based chronological order and the stock volume. Generally, in our model, the forecast of stock is based on the trend of FTS in two aspects. One is pattern trend (PT), and the other is long-term trend (LT). Specifically, for PT, suppose we have observed the stock data $F(t) = s_t$ for $t = 1, 2, ..., N$, and they are all assigned to a fuzzified number A_i (e.g., $fuzzify(F(N)) = A_n$) Our task is to predict $F(N + 1)$. After prediction, we will check if the same fuzzified number exists in the historical data, if it is equal to A_n, and where the trend continues afterwards. As for LT, it means the model will not focus on $F(N)$ but on the whole history data since as economy, the stock has its own cycle [2]. The long-term trend, LT, will now focus on $F(N)$, but instead on the entirety of the historical data, as, similar to the economy, stocks have their own cycle. Thus, we scan all the $FLRs$ and determine what the current cycle is, and what follows. Since the frequency, chronological order, and stock volume all have a large influence over the trend in stock time series data, we propose the following weight factors for getting an accurate PT and LT.

PT Weight Factor. Let $F(t_0) \rightarrow A_p$ and $F(t_0 + 1) \rightarrow A_q$, with $V(t_0)$ and $V(t_0+1)$, where V stands for stock volume, have three relationships, $t_0 \rightarrow t_0+1$,

$V(t_0) \rightarrow V(t_0+1)$ and $A_p \rightarrow A_q$. The weight associated with this FLR, based on the two data points, is defined as follows:

$$w_d = V(t_0) * V(t_0+1) * sqrt[t_0 + (t_0+1)] \tag{11}$$

Considering there may be lots of data in a logical relationship, $A_p \rightarrow A_q$, the total weight associated with this FLR is calculated as

$$w_r = \sum_j w_d \tag{12}$$

where j is the number of data combinations that fall into the same FLR. On the other side, A_p can also constitute many $FLRs$, namely $A_p \rightarrow A_{k1}$, $A_p \rightarrow A_{k2}$,..., $A_p \rightarrow A_{ko}$, which forms PT. Therefore, we have the PT weight as:

$$w_{PT}^k = \frac{w_r^k}{\sum_o w_r} \tag{13}$$

where o is the number of $FLRs$ A_p constitutes.

LT Weight Factor. Inspired by the jump theory in [17], here we use a jump metric together with the proposed w_d to measure the LT. Let $\delta = p - q$ be the jump between a FLR. Obviously, δ can be positive, negative, and zero (representing a rise, fall, and square position in stock context). Similar to PT, the total weight associated with δ is calculated as

$$w_\Delta = \sum_c w_d \tag{14}$$

where c is the number of data combinations formed from the same jump. Accordingly, The LT weight is calculated as

$$w_{LT}^k = \frac{w_\Delta^k}{\sum_b w_\Delta} \tag{15}$$

where b is the number of deltas.

Based on the proposed PT and LT weight factors, we have a rough picture of the current trend and are able to do the forecast. However, we find it is not enough to only take PT and LT into account, since these two metrics are not closely related to the short-term trend. In other words, although they have considered the chronological order, there is still the possibility that the movement of a stock is largely influenced by a short period, only within a few days (e.g., the stock may continue to drop after a nose dive caused by "black swan event"). Therefore, the short-term trend should be carefully addressed. To this end, we propose a short-term trend repair operation to further improve the forecast performance.

Short-Term Trend Repair Operation. Let s_l be the length of a short-term period we observed before the last observed data. Thus, we have the sequence $F(t-s_l)$, $F(t-s_l+1)$,..., $F(t-1)$, $F(t)$ and the corresponding fuzzified numbers A. Here, we use a differential strategy to recognize the short-term trend as follows.

$$\begin{aligned} &Diff\,(s_l) = A_{(t-s_l+1)} - A_{(t-s_l)} \\ &Diff\,(s_{l-1}) = A_{(t-s_l+2)} - A_{(t-s_l+1)} \\ &\ldots\ldots \\ &Diff\,(2) = A_{(t-1)} - A_{(t-2)} \\ &Diff\,(1) = A_{(t)} - A_{(t-1)} \end{aligned} \tag{16}$$

Then, we have a differential sequence $DS = [Diff(s_l), Diff(s_l-1), ..., Diff(2), Diff(1)]$ for this short-term period, and to simulate three closing quotations (rise, fall, and square position), DS is simplified to the following form:

$$DS_c = \begin{bmatrix} cmp\,(Diff\,(s_l)\,,0)\,, cmp\,(Diff\,(s_l-1)\,,0) \\ ,\ldots, cmp\,(Diff\,(2)\,,0)\,, cmp\,(Diff\,(1)\,,0) \end{bmatrix} \tag{17}$$

where cmp is the compare operation with 0, and it only returns -1, 0 and 1. The short-term trend is now represented by DS_c, and the model will learn from historical data to output the result of this trend. Using a similar step, we have:

$$\begin{aligned} &DS_{c1} => cmp\,(Diff(0)_1, 0) \\ &DS_{c2} => cmp\,(Diff(0)_2, 0) \\ &\ldots \\ &DS_{cn} => cmp\,(Diff(0)_n, 0) \end{aligned} \tag{18}$$

where $Diff(0)$ is the differential result between the fuzzified numbers A of next days data and the last observed data in sequence. In other words, it is the output of the current differential sequence. Since some DSs in the historical data may be the same, the model groups all the same DSs by simply adding the corresponding output, and finally the model gets the comprehensive trend results.

4.2 Fuzzy Forecast Outputs

In the forecasting step, we propose to use a linear combination of the above weight strategies and repair operation, as shown in Eq. (19).

$$\widetilde{A}_{t+1} = \alpha\widetilde{A}_{PT} + \beta\widetilde{A}_{LT} + \gamma\widetilde{A}_{RO} \;\; (\alpha + \beta + \gamma = 1) \tag{19}$$

where

$$\widetilde{A}_{PT} = w_{PT}^1 A_{k1} \oplus w_{PT}^2 A_{k2} \ldots \oplus w_{PT}^o A_{ko} \tag{20}$$

$$\widetilde{A}_{LT} = w_{LT}^1 A_{t+\Delta 1} \oplus w_{LT}^2 A_{t+\Delta 2} \ldots \oplus w_{LT}^b A_{t+\Delta b} \tag{21}$$

$$\widetilde{A}_{RO} = A_{t+Diff} \tag{22}$$

Here, t means the time stamp of last observed data.

4.3 Algorithm of the Weighted Fuzzy-Trend Time Series Method Based on SCHLO

In this section, SCHLO is utilized to find the optimal partitions of intervals in the universe of discourse and the optimal weight factors simultaneously. The proposed weighted FTS forecasting method proceeds as follows:

Step 1 Let the universe of discourse U of the main factor be $[D_{min} - D_1, D_{max} + D_2]$, where D_{max} and D_{min} are the maximum value and the minimum value of the historical training data of the main factor, respectively; D_1 and D_2 are two proper positive real values to let the universe of discourse U cover the noise of the testing data of the main factor.

Step 2 Specify the control parameters of SCHLO, such as population size, pr_{mid}, and pi_{mid}. Randomly initialize the population, including interval length m and three weights α, β, γ for optimization. The fitness values are calculated and initial $IKDs$ and SKD are generated. Each individual does the following sub-steps to calculate the fitness value:
- (a) Based on the generated interval length, define the fuzzy sets on U and fuzzify the historical data as Eq. (10).
- (b) Establish $FLRs$ from the fuzzy time series, and $FLRs$ and $FLRGs$ according to [5].
- (c) Defuzzify and calculate the forecast outputs. Specifically, the algorithm first calculates PT and LT weight factors and derives the $\widetilde{A}_{PT}$ and $\widetilde{A}_{LT}$ according to Eqs. (20) and (21), respectively. Then, short-term trend repair operation is performed to get $\widetilde{A}_{RO}$. Based on the obtained $\widetilde{A}_{PT}$, $\widetilde{A}_{LT}$, and $\widetilde{A}_{Ro}$ SCHLO generates α, β, γ. The model can calculate $\widetilde{A}_{t+1}$ according to Eq. (19). Finally, the one-step forecast will be the middle point of the interval-valued mean of $\widetilde{A}_{t+1}$.
- (d) Calculate the fitness value, i.e. the root mean square error (RMSE), as follows:

$$RMSE = \sqrt{\frac{\sum_{t=1}^{t_{\max}} (F_t - R_t)^2}{t_{\max}}} \tag{23}$$

where t_{max} denotes the number of trading days of the historical training data, F_t, denotes the forecast value of the validation datum on trading day t, and R_t is the actual value of the historical validation datum on trading day t.

Step 3 Improvise new individuals. The new solutions are yielded by performing the adaptive pr and pi rule and the learning operators shown in Eqs. (3–6).

Step 4 Calculate the fitness of new candidates. The fitness value of new individuals is computed as steps 2.1–2.4.

Step 5 Update the $IKDs$ and SKD according to the fitness of the new individuals.

Step 6 Check the termination criterion. If the termination criterion is not met, steps 3–5 will be repeated to keep searching for the optimal parameters, otherwise go to the next step.

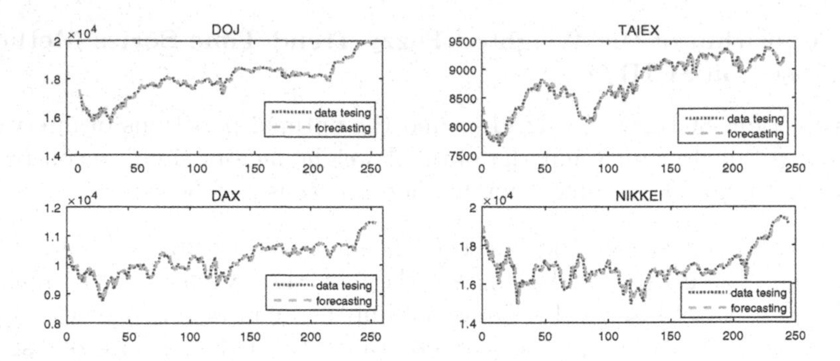

Fig. 2. Time series of the daily observations and the daily forecasts provided by WTFS-SCHLO for the different markets in year 2016.

Step 7 Based on the obtained optimal parameters, the model performs steps 2.1–2.4 to calculate the final forecast on the test datasets.

5 Real-World Experiments and Results

5.1 Stock Market Data and Experimental Settings

To evaluate the forecast accuracy of the proposed model, we analyze data sets from four major world trading markets (DJI, DAX, NIKKEI and TAIEX) obtained from Yahoo Finance (https://finance.yahoo.com/). For every stock market index, we work with daily values collected over three years, from January 2014 to December 2016. Data from 2014 and 2015 are used for training and validation, and data from 2016 is for testing. Similar to mainstream financial forecast methods, a daily rolling horizon strategy is applied. Specifically, this strategy preserves the size of each training set by eliminating the first observation and by including the last observed quotes. Thus, the FLRs and FLGs, as well as all weighting factors, are then re-evaluated. To compare the performance of the WFTS-SCHLO, four state-of-the-art fuzzy time series methods with various strategies [8,17,29,31] as well as a standard HLO based WFTS (WFTS-HLO) are used for comparison. The performance is measured by RMSE, Eq. (23). All of the parameters for the baseline models are set to those reported in the initial publications. For our model, WFTS-SCHLO, the population size is 30, pi_{mid} is set to 0.1, and pr_{mid} is set to 0.9. The number of iterations is fixed at 300. All implementations are in Python, and programs were run on a PC with an Intel Core CPU i7-4790 @3.60 GHz and 16 GB RAM.

5.2 Results and Analysis

Figure 2 shows the time series of the daily observations and the daily forecasts provided by WTFS-SCHLO for the year 2016. Table 1 shows that WTFS-SCHLO consistently outperforms the baseline methods, having the lowest RMSE for its

Table 1. The Forecast performance (RMSE) of four stock markets

Markets	Models					
	Yu model [31]	Cheng model [8]	Wang model [29]	Rubio model [17]	WTFS-HLO	WTFS-SCHLO
DOJ	174.81	172.51	468.36	141.59	139.06	136.53
DAX	137.23	138.74	335.29	132.92	130.09	127.53
NIKKEI	267.37	262.04	514.18	284.77	259.40	252.29
TAIEX	82.17	82.84	199.35	74.54	72.91	69.46

Table 2. Adjusted p-values of the pairwise comparison of the RMSE forecast errors between WTFS-SCHLO with different models

Markets	Models				
	Yu model [31]	Cheng model [8]	Wang model [29]	Rubio model [17]	WTFS-HLO
DOJ	6.41e−3	0.002	4.54e−12	0.021	0.038
DAX	0.008	1.84e−3	5.07e−10	0.017	0.029
NIKKEI	0.012	0.019	7.30e−11	5.25e−3	0.034
TAIEX	0.026	0.015	4.81e−10	0.031	0.042

predictions in every market, which means our model has the best forecasting accuracy. In order to analyze the forecast error achieved by each method, a statistical analysis was carried out. Table 2 shows the adjusted p-values of the pairwise statistical comparisons of the RMSE forecast errors, performed through the paired t-test at Holm's adjustment. The statistical analysis reveals that there are significant differences between our model and the other forecasting methods, in favor of the proposed model.

6 Conclusion

In this paper, an intelligent weighted fuzzy time series model is presented for financial market forecasting. The model utilizes a sine-cosine adaptive human learning optimization algorithm to search for the optimal parameters, improving forecasting performance. New weighted operators that consider frequency based chronological order and stock volume are analyzed and integrated with SCHLO to determine the effective universe discourse and intervals. Furthermore, a novel short-term trend repair operation is developed to complement the final forecasting process. Finally, the proposed model is applied to data from four major world trading markets, the Dow Jones Index, the German Stock Index, the Japanese Stock Index, and Taiwan Stock Index. The experimental results demonstrate that the proposed model consistently outperforms its counterparts, in terms of accuracy. The easy implementation and effective forecasting performance suggest our proposed model could be a favorable market application prospect.

Acknowledgements. This material is based upon work supported in whole or in part with funding from the Laboratory for Analytic Sciences (LAS). Any opinions, findings, conclusions, or recommendations expressed in this material are those of the author(s) and do not necessarily reflect the views of the LAS and/or any agency or entity of the United States Government.

References

1. Alfonso, G., de Hierro, A.R.L., Roldán, C.: A fuzzy regression model based on finite fuzzy numbers and its application to real-world financial data. J. Comput. Appl. Math. **318**, 47–58 (2017)
2. Balcilar, M., Gupta, R., Wohar, M.E.: Common cycles and common trends in the stock and oil markets: evidence from more than 150 years of data. Energy Econ. **61**, 72–86 (2017)
3. Cao, J., Yan, Z., He, G.: Application of multi-objective human learning optimization method to solve AC/DC multi-objective optimal power flow problem. Int. J. Emerg. Electr. Power Syst. **17**(3), 327–337 (2016)
4. Chen, M.Y., Chen, B.T.: A hybrid fuzzy time series model based on granular computing for stock price forecasting. Inf. Sci. **294**, 227–241 (2015)
5. Chen, S.M.: Forecasting enrollments based on fuzzy time series. Fuzzy Sets Syst. **81**(3), 311–319 (1996)
6. Chen, S.M., Chen, C.D.: Handling forecasting problems based on high-order fuzzy logical relationships. Expert Syst. Appl. **38**(4), 3857–3864 (2011)
7. Chen, S.M., Chen, C.D.: TAIEX forecasting based on fuzzy time series and fuzzy variation groups. IEEE Trans. Fuzzy Syst. **19**(1), 1–12 (2011)
8. Cheng, C.H., Chen, T.L., Teoh, H.J., Chiang, C.H.: Fuzzy time-series based on adaptive expectation model for TAIEX forecasting. Expert Syst. Appl. **34**(2), 1126–1132 (2008)
9. García-Crespo, Á., López-Cuadrado, J.L., González-Carrasco, I., Colomo-Palacios, R., Ruiz-Mezcua, B.: SINVLIO: Using semantics and fuzzy logic to provide individual investment portfolio recommendations. Knowl. Based Syst. **27**, 103–118 (2012)
10. Guresen, E., Kayakutlu, G., Daim, T.U.: Using artificial neural network models in stock market index prediction. Expert Syst. Appl. **38**(8), 10389–10397 (2011)
11. Hung, J.C.: Applying a combined fuzzy systems and garch model to adaptively forecast stock market volatility. Appl. Soft Comput. **11**(5), 3938–3945 (2011)
12. Iskyan, K.: China's stock markets have soared by 1,479% since 2003. Business Insider November 2016, http://www.businessinsider.com/world-stock-market-capitalizations-2016-11
13. Javedani Sadaei, H., Lee, M.H.: Multilayer stock forecasting model using fuzzy time series. Sci. World J. **2014** (2014)
14. Marszałek, A., Burczyński, T.: Modeling and forecasting financial time series with ordered fuzzy candlesticks. Inf. Sci. **273**, 144–155 (2014)
15. Merh, N.: Stock market forecasting. J. Inf. Technol. Appl. Manage. **19**(1), 1–12 (2012)
16. Ravi, K., Vadlamani, R., Prasad, P.: Fuzzy formal concept analysis based opinion mining for CRM in financial services. Appl. Soft Comput. **58**, 35–52 (2017)
17. Rubio, A., Bermúdez, J.D., Vercher, E.: Improving stock index forecasts by using a new weighted fuzzy-trend time series method. Expert Syst. Appl. **76**, 12–20 (2017)

18. Song, Q., Chissom, B.S.: Forecasting enrollments with fuzzy time series—part I. Fuzzy Sets Syst. **54**(1), 1–9 (1993)
19. Song, Q., Chissom, B.S.: Fuzzy time series and its models. Fuzzy Sets Syst. **54**(3), 269–277 (1993)
20. Song, Q., Chissom, B.S.: Forecasting enrollments with fuzzy time series–part II. Fuzzy Sets Syst. **62**(1), 1–8 (1994)
21. Su, C.H., Cheng, C.H.: A hybrid fuzzy time series model based on anfis and integrated nonlinear feature selection method for forecasting stock. Neurocomputing **205**, 264–273 (2016)
22. Teoh, H.J., Chen, T.L., Cheng, C.H., Chu, H.H.: A hybrid multi-order fuzzy time series for forecasting stock markets. Expert Syst. Appl. **36**(4), 7888–7897 (2009)
23. Ticknor, J.L.: A bayesian regularized artificial neural network for stock market forecasting. Expert Syst. Appl. **40**(14), 5501–5506 (2013)
24. Uslu, V.R., Bas, E., Yolcu, U., Egrioglu, E.: A fuzzy time series approach based on weights determined by the number of recurrences of fuzzy relations. Swarm Evol. Comput. **15**, 19–26 (2014)
25. Wang, J., Hou, R., Wang, C., Shen, L.: Improved v-support vector regression model based on variable selection and brain storm optimization for stock price forecasting. Appl. Soft Comput. **49**, 164–178 (2016)
26. Wang, L., Ni, H., Yang, R., Fei, M., Ye, W.: A simple human learning optimization algorithm. In: Fei, M., Peng, C., Su, Z., Song, Y., Han, Q. (eds.) LSMS/ICSEE 2014. CCIS, vol. 462, pp. 56–65. Springer, Heidelberg (2014). doi:10.1007/978-3-662-45261-5_7
27. Wang, L., Ni, H., Yang, R., Pardalos, P.M., Du, X., Fei, M.: An adaptive simplified human learning optimization algorithm. Inf. Sci. **320**, 126–139 (2015)
28. Wang, L., Yang, R., Ni, H., Ye, W., Fei, M., Pardalos, P.M.: A human learning optimization algorithm and its application to multi-dimensional knapsack problems. Appl. Soft Comput. **34**, 736–743 (2015)
29. Wang, L., Liu, X., Pedrycz, W.: Effective intervals determined by information granules to improve forecasting in fuzzy time series. Expert Syst. Appl. **40**(14), 5673–5679 (2013)
30. Wei, L.Y.: A hybrid ANFIS model based on empirical mode decomposition for stock time series forecasting. Appl. Soft Comput. **42**, 368–376 (2016)
31. Yu, H.K.: Weighted fuzzy time series models for taiex forecasting. Phys. A **349**(3), 609–624 (2005)
32. Zadeh, L.A.: Fuzzy sets. Inf. Control **8**(3), 338–353 (1965)
33. Zhou, R., Yang, Z., Yu, M., Ralescu, D.A.: A portfolio optimization model based on information entropy and fuzzy time series. Fuzzy Optim. Decis. Making **14**(4), 381 (2015)

Mobile Robot Scheduling with Multiple Trips and Time Windows

Shudong Liu(✉), Huayu Wu, Shili Xiang, and Xiaoli Li

Institute for Infocomm Research, A*STAR, 1 Fusionopolis Way, Singapore, Singapore
{liush,wuhu,sxiang,xlli}@i2r.a-star.edu.sg

Abstract. We consider a vehicle routing problem with multiple trips and time windows (VRPMTTW) in which a mobile robot transports materials from a central warehouse to multiple demanding places. The robot needs to strictly satisfy the time windows at demanding places and it can run multiple trips. How to effectively scheduling the robot is a key problem in operations of Smart Nations and intelligent automated manufacturing. In the literature three-index mixed integer programming models are developed. However, these three-index models are difficult to solve in reasonable time for real problems due to computational complexity of integer programming. We propose an innovative two-index mixed integer programming model. The numerical results show our model can successfully obtain optimal solutions fast for cases where the existing literature has not found the optimal solution yet. To our best knowledge, it is the first two-index model for this type of problems.

Keywords: Vehicle routing problem · Combinatorial optimization · Time window · Multiple trip · Two-index model

1 Introduction

In this work we consider a vehicle routing problem with multiple trips and time windows (VRPMTTW) in which vehicles or mobile robots can perform multiple trips/routes to satisfy customers' demands. Each demand of each customer has its own time window such that a vehicle needs to arrive in this window. This type of problems will become increasingly important in the contexts such as Smart Nations and Factory of Future. It is obvious that in smart nations and factories in the future, intelligent autonomous vehicles and mobile robots will be widely used to transport people, goods and materials. Effective scheduling of these mobile robots and vehicles is critical for implementing Smart Nations and intelligent manufacturing.

With the fast development of technologies, e.g. in artificial intelligence and computational power and communication, intelligent mobile robots/vehicles are becoming more and more matured, and more and more nations and companies are adopting them. Among other countries, Singapore is carrying out trials for self-driving vehicle technologies and mobility concepts along the many kilometer test route; The Centre for Healthcare Assistive and Robotics Technology

G. Cong et al. (Eds.): ADMA 2017, LNAI 10604, pp. 608–620, 2017.
https://doi.org/10.1007/978-3-319-69179-4_43

(CHART) at Changi General Hospital in Singapore is working with academia, industry and research institutions to develop healthcare solutions leveraging on mobile robots and assistive technology. In industries, some companies in Singapore have already used mobile robots to transport materials in the factories. Amazon is also a pioneer in adopting mobile robots in its warehouse.

A common characteristic of both intelligent vehicles and mobile robots is vehicle routing. In some applications, the time window is very important. For example, in the case of mobile robots transporting material to feeders of production lines, the robots need to strict respect to the time windows of feeders, otherwise the production lines may have to stop or generate wasted products due to missing some materials. During our engagement with industries, we encountered a very similar situation as Dang et al. [6]: a robot transports materials to multiple feeders of production lines. Another example is the transportation of materials such as operational tools in hospitals where the time windows are also very important. In addition, in modern city logistics, vehicles often need to satisfy customers' time windows, though they may not be so strict as in production and healthcare situations.

In order to save cost, it is natural that a vehicle/mobile robot may perform multiple trips only if it can satisfy the requirement of time windows. So, vehicle routing problems with multiple trips and time windows (VRPMTTW) arise in many real-life contexts and will become more and more important. In the classical literature for vehicle routing problem with time window (VRPTW), it is in general assumed that each vehicle runs only one trip/route. In the problem VRPMTTW, we need to explicitly consider the precedence of trips when a vehicle runs multiple trips, which makes the problem more complicated.

In spite of the importance of VRPMTTW in practice, currently there is no much literature. This problem is NP-hard and more complex than the traditional vehicle routing problems. Some researchers [6] developed three-index mixed integer programming (MIP) models which have huge number of integer variables and exponential-size of constraints. They are very difficult to solve in reasonable time for real problems. Hence some researchers developed heuristics for it. We develop an innovative model which uses two-index integer variables and has linear-size of constraints. In this way, both the searching space and computational time are significantly reduced. To our best knowledge, it is the first two-index model for this type of problems in the literature.

The remainder of this paper is organized as follows. The literature review is given in Sect. 2. In Sect. 3, the problem is described and in Sect. 4 we present the mathematical programming model. The numerical results are reported in Sect. 5. Finally, concluding remarks follow in Sect. 6.

2 Literature Review

Vehicle routing problem was first studied by George Dantzig and John Ramser [7] in 1959. Since then many researchers have studied it and a variety of variants and made many significant progresses in developing heuristics and exact algorithms. Some important variants are Vehicle Routing Problem with Backhaul

(VRPB), Vehicle Routing Problem with Time window (VRPTW), Pickup and Delivery Problem (VRP) and Dial-a-ride Problem. There are a few excellent comprehensive literature review, refer to [4,9,15].

Most papers in the above literature assume one vehicle performs only one route/trip. However, in practice people often use one vehicle for multiple trips to save cost. Nevertheless, only a few consider the Vehicle Routing Problem with Multiple Trip (VRPMT). Fleischmann [8] first considered this problem in 1990. He modified the well-known saving algorithm and used a bin-packing heuristic to assign routes to vehicles. Since then more people developed some heuristics using genetic algorithms, tabu search and so on (e.g. [5,12–14]). Mingozzi et al. [10] developed an exact algorithm for VRPMT using set-partition like formulations, which heavily depends on the initial upper bound.

The literature for vehicle routing problem considering both multiple trip and time window (VRPMTTW) is scarce. Azi et al. [1] first addressed this type of problem in 2007. They developed an exact method for the single vehicle case. This method consists of two phases: in the first phase, all non-dominated feasible routes are generated; in the second phase, some trips are selected and sequenced to form the vehicle workday. In 2010 Azi et al. [2] extended their previous work [1] to multiple vehicles cases. Note that in both papers, the vehicle is not forced to visit all customers, but serve them as many as possible to maximize profit. In addition, there is a maximum duration in each route. These two aspects are different from the problem considered in this paper. Battarra et al. [3] developed a heuristic for it. They decomposed the problem into two easier problems, and developed two heuristics for them: the first heuristic is to create routes and the second is for a bin packing problem to connect routes.

Dang et al. [6] considered VRPMTTW in 2014 in which a single mobile robot was used for transporting parts from a warehouse to a few feeders of machines. The time windows are hard constraints, i.e. needing to respect them strictly. They developed a three-index integer programming model with exponential-size constraints. As solving this model is very time consuming as shown in their numerical study, they developed a genetic algorithm for it. Nielsen et al. [11] extended the work of [6]. As mentioned in [11], genetic algorithms may not be able to find feasible solutions in such complex situations, hence they considered the soft time windows, i.e. allowing delay in delivery, and the objective was changed into weighted sum of traveling distance and delay.

In this paper, we consider the same problem as [6] in which a single robot transports materials/parts from a warehouse to feeders. We propose an innovative two-index integer programming model. This model has far less integer variables and constraints, compared with the three-index model in [6]. Hence it is much easier to solve using general purpose solvers as shown in Sect. 5.

3 Problem Description

During our industrial engagement, we encountered very similar problems as Dang et al. [6]. For simplicity, we describe the problem in [6].

In a flexible manufacturing system, there are a few production lines and each line has multiple machines. During production, machines consume materials/components and transform them into the final products. Later we just use material to represent both material and components when it is clear in the context. Some machines have its own feeders so that people or robots can feed material to it. Material is stored in a central warehouse. During the production, robots need to transport material from warehouse to the places near machines, and then put them into the feeders. Putting materials into feeders may be done by robots or by people, which depends on the capability of robots, but transporting material from warehouse to feeders will be done only by mobile robots. An example of layout of flexible manufacturing systems is shown in Fig. 1, which is adapted from [6].

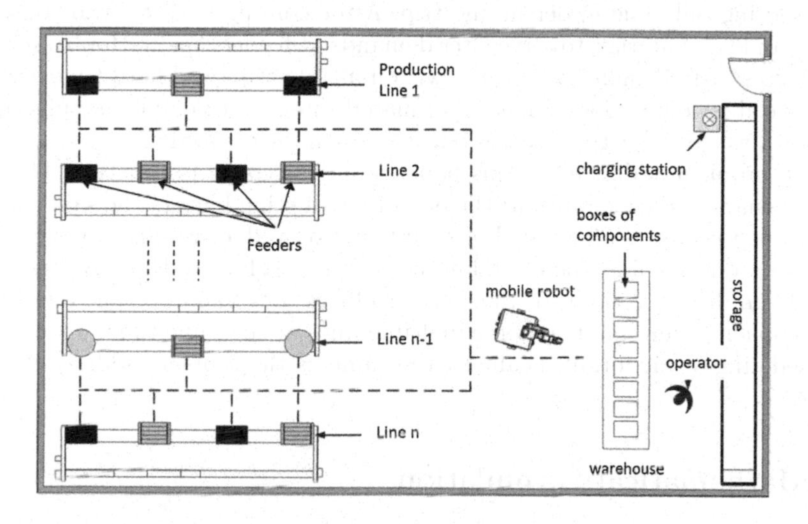

Fig. 1. Layout of a flexible manufacturing system with mobile robots

From the figure, we can see that the mobile robot transports materials from warehouse to feeders. Each robot has a carry capacity. It is possible for a robot to carry materials for multiple feeders in one trip (if the robot capacity allows it) and then come back to warehouse to start a new trip. The capacity of robots can be measured by boxes as in [6] where the boxes are called Small Load Carrier (SLC) and each SLC includes multiple components.

The times of feeding materials to feeders are controlled by a (s, Q) inventory policy. Each machine in general runs at a constant speed, i.e. the consumption rate of materials is constant. The (s, Q) policy is shown in Fig. 2 which shows how the inventory (material/components) at a feeder changes with time. At the beginning, there is an initial inventory. The inventory decreases with the time. When the inventory reaches the threshold level s, the system sends a signal to ask for replenishing inventory. The replenishing amount is a fixed value Q.

The replenishment must be done before running out of stock. Hence for each replenishment, there is a time window. This time window is a hard constraint, because if replenishment starts too early, i.e. before the release time, the inventory will be above the maximal level $(s + Q)$ which may be beyond the physical space of feeders. If the replenishment is too late, i.e. after the due time, then the machine has to stop or generate bad products due to missing materials. As each machine of production lines runs at its constant speed, the inventory decrease at a constant rate. Due to the constant machine speed, the release times of two consequential replenishment has a fixed gap, i.e. the period length p. Note that different machines can have different speeds/material consumption rates and different feeders can have different s and Q.

A robot may carry materials for multiple feeders in one trip (from departure from warehouse to coming back to warehouse). This should be more efficient than serving only one feeder in one trip. After coming back to warehouse, the robot can load materials to serve later demands at feeders again. How to schedule robots to satisfy demands at feeders with multiple trips and hard time windows is a critical problem to implement automated intelligent flexible manufacturing. As in [6], we consider the single robot case for multiple feeders.

The problem addressed in this paper is quite typical in practice. There are other scenarios. For example, at the end of production lines in the same factory, the finished products are needed to send back to product warehouse. At the end of each production line, there is a limited buffer area for products. An intelligent forklift (no driver) is used to transport products to warehouse. The forklift also has a capacity limit and may serve multiple lines at the same time. The problem of scheduling of the forklift is almost the same as the problem addressed in this paper.

4 Mathematical Formulation

In this section we present a two-index mixed integer programming model for scheduling the mobile robot with the objective of minimizing total traveling distance/time.

4.1 Assumptions and Notations

Assume there are n_f feeders. Let $V = \{1, ..., n_f\}$ be the set of feeders, and $V^+ = \{0\} \cup V$, where 0 denote the warehouse. A single mobile robot of capacity Q_m transports materials. Each element (feeder or warehouse) in V^+ has its own location. A distance d_{ij} and traveling time t_{ij} is associated with each pair of locations (i, j) where $i, j \in V^+$. Each feeder requests material replenishment by its own (s, Q) policy. Assume material consumption rates, initial inventory, parameters (s and Q) of inventory policies are known. Hence the time window (from release time to due time) of each request at each feeder is given. At each location, there is a working time. At the warehouse, it is the time of loading material up to robot, while at feeders it is the unloading time from robot to feeders. These working times are constants.

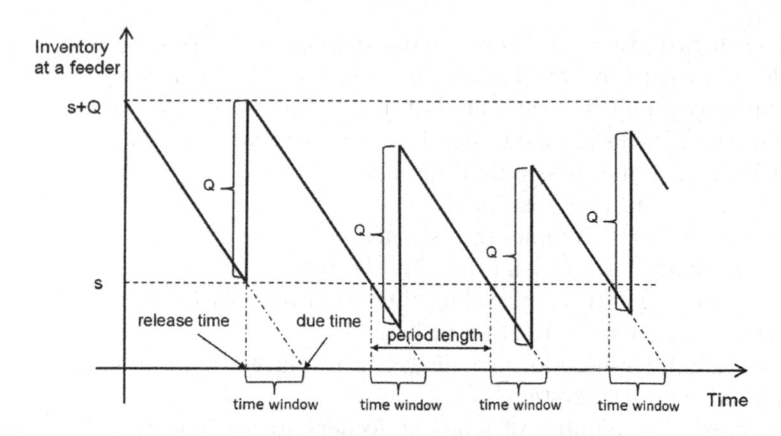

Fig. 2. (s,Q) inventory policy for feeding materials at feeders

Assume a single delivery/stop at a feeder can fulfill one replenishment of this feeder. When $Q_m = n$, the robot can carry materials to serve n feeders in a single trip. Assume at the beginning of planning horizon, the robot is at the warehouse.

Material replenishment at feeders and loading material at warehouse are regarded as different task types. Let $A_{type} = \{0, 1, ..., n_f\}$ denote the set of task types. Type $i \in V^+$ means the tasks at location i, e.g. type 0 is tasks of loading material to robot at the warehouse (plus possible unloading empty boxes from previous trip). Each task type can repeat many times. So, each task is identified by its type and the index in its own type. Following are more notations:

$A_{type} = \{0, 1, ..., n_f\}$, set of task types for production.

T, planning horizon.

$c_a, a \in A_{type} \backslash \{0\}$, material consumption rate at feeder a.

$N_A^a, a \in A_{type}$, number of times of repeating for task type a. $N_A^a, a \in A_{type} \backslash \{0\}$, is defined as $N_A^a = \lfloor T/c_a \rfloor$. N_A^0 is the number of tasks at warehouse, for which we will derive an upper and lower bound and will set a value for it.

$N_A = \sum_{a \in A_{type}} N_A^a$, total number of tasks at all places.

$N_A^- = N_A - N_A^0$, total number of tasks at feeders.

$I_A^a = \{1, ..., N_A^a\}, a \in A_{type}$, set of index of tasks of type a.

$I_A = \{1, ..., N_A\}$, set of index of tasks.

(a, i), $a \in A_{type}, i \in I_A^a$, the task which is the i_{th} task in the group of type a. So, each task is identified by two indexes: a and i.

$A^a = \{(a, i) | a \in A_{type}, i \in I_A^a\}$, set of tasks of type a.

$A = \underset{a}{\cup} A^a$, set of all tasks of all types.

$Pre = \{(a1, i1, a2, i2)\}$, $(a1, i1), (a2, i2) \in A$, set of precedence relation among tasks, which means task $(a2, i2)$ cannot start until task $(a1, i1)$ is finished.

For each task, there is a time window (from release time to due time) such that the task must be finished in this window. Given material consumption rates, inventory policies and initial state of inventories, we can calculate the time windows of tasks at each feeder. For each task, there is a working/processing time, e.g. loading and unloading time. Let

$TR_{a,i}$, release time of task (a, i).

$TD_{a,i}$, due time (deadline) of task (a, i).

TP_a, working time of task type a by the robot.

$TC_{a1,a2}$, $a1, a2 \in A_{type}$, traveling time from one place (after having finished task $a1$) to another place to start task $a2$.

M, a big number used for modeling, which is larger than any time (expressed in real number) in the system.

Q_m, maximum number of stops at feeders in a single trip, i.e. maximum number of feeders that the robot can carry material and serve in a trip due to its capacity.

We have following decision variables:

$x_{a1,i1}^{a2,i2} \in \{0, 1\}$, $(a1, i1), (a2, i2) \in A$. It is 1 if the robot is assigned to do the task $(a1, i1)$, followed by task $(a2, i2)$, 0 otherwise.

$s_{a,i}$, $(a, i) \in A$, starting time of task (a, i). $z_k^{a,i} \in \{0, 1\}$, $(a, i) \in A, k \in \{1, ..., N_A\}$. It is 1 if the task (a, i) is assigned to do as the k_{th} task in the all tasks, 0 otherwise.

Note that the above $x_{a1,i1}^{a2,i2}$ are two-index integer variables which shows the relation between one task (an index) to another task (an index). In the literature, people developed models using three-index variables $x_{a1,i1}^{a2,i2,k}$ where k is the index of trips. The number of integer variables in three-index formulation is many times of ours.

4.2 The Two-Index Mixed Integer Programming Model

As mentioned before, we need to set a value for number of tasks at warehouse, i.e. N_A^0. As there are N_A^- tasks at feeders, there are at most N_A^- trips to finish these tasks based on the assumption that a single delivery/stop at a feeder can fulfill one replenishment of this feeder, i.e. $Q_m \geq 1$. So, the number of tasks at warehouse $N_A^0 \leq N_A^- + 1$, where the last "1" is for returning back to warehouse after finishing all tasks at feeders. On the other hand, the robot also needs at least $\lceil N_A^-/Q_m \rceil$ trips by assuming each trip the robot can server Q_m feeders, hence $N_A^0 \geq \lceil N_A^-/Q_m \rceil + 1$. Again the last "1" is for returning back to warehouse at the end. There are two extreme cases. The real number of trips needed should be some value in the middle of these two extreme points. When we assign a smaller and feasible value to N_A^0, the computation time will be shorter because there will be smaller number of variables and constraints in the model. For safety, we set the maximal value, i.e. $N_A^0 = N_A^- + 1$, which means we add $N_A^- + 1$ tasks of type 0 to tasks at feeders. So, the total number of tasks $N_A = 2N_A^- + 1$. The robot will execute these tasks following a sequence. We will assign these tasks onto a sequence of length N_A.

Each trip starts from warehouse and ends at warehouse. The tasks from task $(0, i), i \in \{1, ..., N_A^0 - 1\}$ to task $(0, i+1)$ belong to the i_{th} trip. If there is no other tasks between $(0, i)$ and $(0, i+1)$, then this trip is empty, i.e. the robot does not server any feeders. Task $(0, i+1)$ is the end of i_{th}trip and also the beginning of $(i+1)_{th}$ trip. If task$(0, i)$ is executed as the m_{th}task in all tasks, and task $(0, i+1)$ is executed as the n_{th} task in all tasks, then $(n - m - 1)$ is the number of feeders served in the i_{th} trip. Due to robot's capacity, we have the constraint that $(n - m - 1) \leq Q_m$. In this way, we enforce the precedence relation between trips and the robot capacity limit.

We also need other constraints such as satisfying time windows. The objective is to minimize total traveling distance. The new compact two-index MIP model is as follows:

$$min \sum_{(a1,i1)\in A} \sum_{(a2,i2)\in A} TC_{a1,a2} \cdot x_{a1,i1}^{a2,i2} \tag{1}$$

$$s.t. \sum_{(a2,i2)\in A} x_{a1,i1}^{a2,i2} = 1, \ \forall (a1,i1) \in A \backslash \{(0, N_A^- + 1)\} \tag{2}$$

$$\sum_{(a2,i2)\in A} x_{a1,i1}^{a2,i2} = 0, \ \forall (a1,i1) \in \{(0, N_A^- + 1)\} \tag{3}$$

$$\sum_{(a1,i1)\in A} x_{a1,i1}^{a2,i2} = 1, \ \forall (a2,i2) \in A \backslash \{(0,1)\} \tag{4}$$

$$\sum_{(a1,i1)\in A} x_{a1,i1}^{a2,i2} = 0, \ \forall (a2,i2) \in \{(0,1)\} \tag{5}$$

$$x_{a1,i1}^{a1,i1} = 0, \ \forall (a1,i1) \in A \tag{6}$$

$$TR_{a,i} \leq s_{a,i}, \ \forall (a,i) \in A \tag{7}$$

$$s_{a,i} + TP_a \leq TD_{a,i}, \ \forall (a,i) \in A \tag{8}$$

$$s_{a1,i1} + TP_a + TC_{a1,a2} x_{a1,i1}^{a2,i2} - (1 - x_{a1,i1}^{a2,i2})M \leq s_{a2,i2},$$
$$\forall (a1,i1) \in A, (a2,i2) \in A \text{ such that } (a1,i1) \neq (a2,i2) \tag{9}$$

$$\sum_{k\in I_A} z_k^{a,i} = 1, \ \forall (a,i) \in A \tag{10}$$

$$\sum_{(a,i)\in A} z_k^{a,i} = 1, \ \forall k \in I_A \tag{11}$$

$$z_1^{0,1} = 1 \tag{12}$$

$$z_1^{0,i} = 0, \ \forall i \in \{2..N_A^0\} \tag{13}$$

$$z_{N_A}^{0,N_A^0} = 1 \tag{14}$$

$$z_{N_A}^{0,i} = 0, \ \forall i \in \{1..N_A^0 - 1\} \tag{15}$$

$$\sum_{k\in I_A} (k \cdot z_k^{a,i}) - \sum_{k\in I_A} (k \cdot z_k^{a,i-1}) \leq Q + 1, \ \forall (a,i) \in A^0 \backslash \{(0,1)\} \tag{16}$$

$$\sum_{k \in I_A} (k \cdot z_k^{a,i-1}) + 1 \leq \sum_{k \in I_A} (k \cdot z_k^{a,i}), \; \forall (a,i) \in A \backslash \{(a,1) | a \in A_{type}\} \quad (17)$$

$$s_{a,i-1} + TP_a \leq s_{a,i}, \; \forall (a,i) \in A \backslash \{(a,1) | a \in A_{type}\} \quad (18)$$

$$\sum_{k \in I_A} (k \cdot z_k^{a1,i1}) + 1 \leq \sum_{k \in I_A} (k \cdot z_k^{a2,i2}) + (1 - x_{a1,i1}^{a2,i2})M,$$

$$\forall (a1,i1) \in A, (a2,i2) \in A \text{ such that } (a1,i1) \neq (a2,i2) \quad (19)$$

$$x_{a1,i1}^{a2,i2} \in \{0,1\}, \; \forall (a1,i1), (a2,i2) \in A \quad (20)$$

$$s_{a,i}, \; \forall (a,i) \in A \quad (21)$$

$$z_k^{a,i} \in \{0,1\}, \; \forall (a,i) \in A, k \in \{1, ..., N_A\} \quad (22)$$

The objective function (1) is to minimize total traveling time of the robot. Constraint (2) means every task except the last task at warehouse (returning warehouse at the end) has one and only one immediate following task. Constraint (3) means the last task at warehouse has no following task. Constraint (4) ensures every task expect the first task at warehouse has one and only one immediate precedent task. Constraint (5) enforces the first task at warehouse has no immediate precedent task. Constraint (6) ensures no link from a task to itself. Constraint (7) ensures the starting time of each task is not earlier than its release time, and constraint (8) enforces the finishing time (starting time + working time) is before the due time. This is safer than only requiring the starting time is before the due time. In the latter it is possible the feeders has already no stock/materials when loading material from robot to feeders.

Constraint (9) ensures that if task $(a2, i2)$ is the immediately following task of $(a1, i1)$, then the starting time of task $(a2, i2)$ should be after the starting time of task $(a1, i1)$ plus its working time plus the traveling time from location $a1$ to location $a2$. All tasks are executed one by one in a sequence. Constraints (10–11) ensure that each task is assigned to an index number in the sequence and each index number is assigned from only one task. Constraints (12–15) enforce the first task at warehouse (loading material to robot) is the first task executed in the sequence of all tasks, and the last task at the warehouse (returning warehouse at the end of execution) is the last task in the sequence of all tasks. Constraint (16) ensures the capacity limit of robot. Constraint (17) makes sure that the index of execution for task (a, i) is after that of task $(a, i - 1)$ at least by one, and the starting time of task (a, i) is later than that of task $(a, i - 1)$ by the working time of task type a. Constraint (19) states that if task $(a2, i2)$ is the immediately following task of $(a1, i1)$, then the index of executing task $(a2, i2)$ in the sequence is after that of task $(a1, i1)$ by one. Constraints (20–21) define the variables.

5 Numerical Results

In this section we investigate the performance of the two-index MIP model, comparing with the three-index MIP model in [6].

We use the cases in [6] to run experiments. To make completeness, the input data are also described here. There are 4 feeders in the system. The traveling times are shown in Table 1. From the table, we can see that the traveling time from a to b may be different from b to a, i.e. it is not symmetric. The working times are: 90 s at warehouse and 42 s at each feeder.

Table 1. Traveling time of robot among feeders and warehouse (seconds)

From	To				
	Warehouse 0	Feeder 1	Feeder 2	Feeder 3	Feeder 4
0	0	34	37	34	40
1	39	0	17	34	50
2	35	17	0	35	49
3	34	33	35	0	47
4	36	47	48	46	0

The robot was initially designed to carry at most 3 boxes and each box contains a replenishment of a feeder. So it can serve at most three feeders in a single trip, i.e. $Q_m = 3$. In the experiment, a variety of values for Q_m are considered. For the cases D-1 and D-2 in [6], the planning horizon is 1 h and there are 10 tasks. The time windows of tasks are calculated and shown in Table 2. From the table, we can see that each of Feeders 1 and 4 has 4 tasks while each of Feeders 2 and 3 has 1 task.

Table 2. Time windows of tasks in cases D-1 and D-2 (1 h planning horizon)

Task index	Feeder 1	Feeder 2	Feeder 3	Feeder 4
1	[562.5, 1125.0]	[1650.0, 3000.0]	[1650.0, 3000.0]	[562.5, 1125.0]
2	[1125.0, 1687.5]	—	—	[1125.0, 1687.5]
3	[1687.5, 2250.0]	—	—	[1687.5, 2250.0]
4	[2250.0, 2812.5]	—	—	[2250.0, 2812.5]

The MIP models are solved using solver CPLEX. Experiments are run on a notebook with Intel Core i7-6500U CPU @2.50 GHz and 16 GB RAM. The results for cases D-1 and D-2 and a comparison with [6] are shown in Tables 2 and 3 and Fig. 3. Note that [6] run the experiments on a PC with Intel Core i5 CPU @2.67 GHz and 4 GB RAM.

Table 3 shows the objective values and computation times under different ways: two-index model of this paper, three-index MIP model and Genetic Algorithm (GA) in [6]. Note that for both cases D-1 and D-2, we found the optimal

Table 3. Comparison of results (cases D-1 and D-2)

Case	Q_m	3-Index MIP (Dang et al.)		GA (Dang et al.)		2-Index MIP	
		Objective	Time(s)	Objective	Time(s)	Objective	Time(s)
D-1	2	488	21589	504	1	452	1152
D-2	3	384	8377	396	1	384	199

solutions fast (in minutes) while the three-index model cannot obtain optimal solution after 6 h for Case D-1. For Case D-1, the computation time 1152 of our method is the time of finally proving that 452 is optimal objective. In fact the solver obtained the optimal solution much earlier (in 82 s). The solution progress for D-1 is shown in Fig. 3.

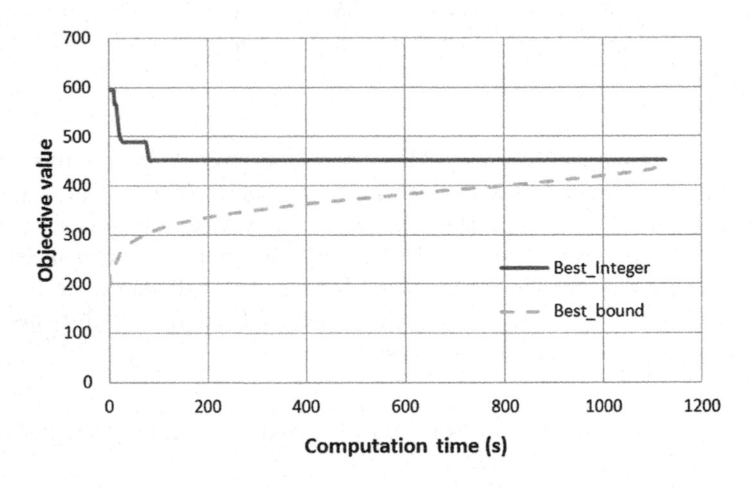

Fig. 3. Solution progress with time (Case D-1)

From Fig. 3, we can see that the objective value of integer solutions decreases with time and it reaches 452 at about 82 s while the lower bound of the solutions increases with time, and finally at time 1152 (second) the lower bound is equal to the integer feasible solution, proving 452 is the optimal objective. For Case D-2, it is similar: the solver finds optimal solutions much earlier than proving optimality.

The effectiveness of two-index model can be explained by number of integer variables and constraints. In three-index models, Case D-1 has 4040 variables and the number of constraints increase exponentially with number of tasks. While in two-index model, there are only 903 integer variables and the number of constraints increase linearly with number of tasks. Increasing by only one binary integer variable, the searching space will be double. So our two-index model can significantly reduce the searching space and hence find optimal solutions fast. In addition, the usage of computer memory of our model is small. The searching tree needs less than 100 M.

As there are 10 tasks at feeders, there are at most 10 trips. In the optimal solutions there are some empty trips, i.e. the robot departs the warehouse and return back without serving any feeders. The non-empty serving trips for Case D-1 are as follows: Trip 1: (0,4) → (1,1) → (0,5); Trip 2: (0,5) → (4,1) → (4,2) → (0,6); Trip 3: (0,6) → (1,2) → (1,3) → (0,7); Trip 4: (0,7) → (4,3) → (4,4) → (0,8); Trip 5: (0,9) → (1,4) → (2,1) → (0,10); Trip 6: (0,10) → (3,1) → (0,11). So there are 6 non-empty trips in which 4 trips each serve 2 feeders and 2 trips each serve only one feeder.

As for Case D-2 (can serve 3 feeders in one trip), the non-empty trips are as follows: Trip 1: (0,5) → (1,1) → (4,1) → (4,2) → (0,6); Trip 2: (0,6) → (1,2) → (1,3) → (3,1) → (0,7); Trip 3: (0,9) → (4,3) → (4,4) → (0,10); Trip 4: (0,10) → (1,4) → (2,1) → (0,11). So, there are only 4 non-empty trips in which 2 of them each serve 3 feeders and others each serve 2 feeders.

From the above, when we increase the capacity of robot from 2 (Case D-1) to 3 (Case D-2), the optimal total traveling time decreases from 452 to 384, and the number of trips decreases from 6 to 4. It is intuitive.

It is desirable to compare the models for more cases. However, [6] provided results of MIP model for only two cases, as it cannot solve larger size problems. Nevertheless, the results of above two cases have already shown the benefit of the two-index MIP model in some degree (found optimal solution in mins VS not found optimal solutions in 6 h), which confirms the theoretical analysis for the reason why the two-index model can significantly save computational time.

6 Conclusions

We have considered the vehicle routing problem with multiple trips and time windows and proposed an innovative two-index MIP model. To our best knowledge, it is the first two-index MIP model for this type of problem. This model has significant advantage in terms of computation time due to its concise modeling which significantly reduced number of integer variables and constraints, compared with the three-index model. Numeral results show this two-index model can obtain optimal solutions fast for cases while the three-index model cannot solve in many hours.

Due to the wide applications of this type of problem in smart nations and intelligent automated manufacturing, this type of problem is worth to further study. The two-index model still cannot solve larger size problems in short time. It is interesting to develop high quality heuristic for them by combining this two-index model with other techniques such as rolling horizon. In addition, the models considering stochastic characteristics in the systems are also very useful in real applications. Finally, it is natural to extend to cases of a fleet of robots. Though it is feasible to classify feeders/demands/customers into groups and each group is served by a single mobile robot using the method in this paper, considering multiple robots simultaneously still have much benefits in cost saving, improving service level and increasing system robustness.

References

1. Azi, N., Gendreau, M., Potvin, J.Y.: An exact algorithm for a single-vehicle routing problem with time windows and multiple routes. Eur. J. Oper. Res. **178**(3), 755–766 (2007)
2. Azi, N., Gendreau, M., Potvin, J.Y.: An exact algorithm for a vehicle routing problem with time windows and multiple use of vehicles. Eur. J. Oper. Res. **202**(3), 756–763 (2010)
3. Battarra, M., Monaci, M., Vigo, D.: An adaptive guidance approach for the heuristic solution of a minimum multiple trip vehicle routing problem. Comput. Oper. Res. **36**(11), 3041–3050 (2009)
4. Braekers, K., Ramaekers, K., Nieuwenhuyse, I.V.: The vehicle routing problem: state of the art classification and review. Comput. Ind. Eng. **99**, 300–313 (2016)
5. Brandão, J.C.S., Mercer, A.: The multi-trip vehicle routing problem. J. Oper. Res. Soc. **49**(8), 799–805 (1998)
6. Dang, Q.V., Nielsen, I., Steger-Jensen, K., Madsen, O.: Scheduling a single mobile robot for part-feeding tasks of production lines. J. Intell. Manuf. **25**(6), 1271–1287 (2014)
7. Dantzig, G.B., Ramser, J.H.: The truck dispatching problem. Manage. Sci. **6**(1), 80–91 (1959)
8. Fleischmann, B.: The vehicle routing problem with multiple use of vehicles (1990). Facbereich Wirtschaftswissenschafte Universitat Hamburg
9. Laporte, G.: Fifty years of vehicle routing. Transp. Sci. **43**(4), 408–416 (2009)
10. Mingozzi, A., Roberti, R., Toth, P.: An exact algorithm for the multitrip vehicle routing problem. INFORMS J. Comput. **25**(2), 193–207 (2013)
11. Nielsen, I., Dang, Q.V., Bocewicz, G., Banaszak, Z.: A methodology for implementation of mobile robot in adaptive manufacturing environments. J. Intell. Manuf. **28**(5), 1171–1188 (2017)
12. Olivera, A., Viera, O.: Adaptive memory programming for the vehicle routing problem with multiple trips. Comput. Oper. Res. **34**(1), 28–47 (2007)
13. Salhi, S., Petch, R.J.: A GA based heuristic for the vehicle routing problem with multiple trips. J. Math. Model. Algorithms **6**(4), 591–613 (2007)
14. Taillard, E.D., Laporte, G., Gendreau, M.: Vehicle routeing with multiple use of vehicles. J. Oper. Res. Soc. **47**(8), 1065–1070 (1996)
15. Toth, P., Vigo, D., Toth, P., Vigo, D.: Vehicle Routing: Problems, Methods, and Applications, 2nd edn. Society for Industrial and Applied Mathematics, Philadelphia (2014)

Natural Language Processing and Text Mining

Feature Analysis for Duplicate Detection in Programming QA Communities

Wei Emma Zhang[1(✉)], Quan Z. Sheng[1], Yanjun Shu[2], and Vanh Khuyen Nguyen[1]

[1] Department of Computing, Macquarie University, Sydney, Australia
{w.zhang,michael.sheng}@mq.edu.au,
thi-vanh-khuyen.nguyen@students.mq.edu.au
[2] School of Computer Science and Technology, Harbin Institute of Technology, Harbin, China
yjshu@hit.edu.cn

Abstract. In community question answering (CQA), duplicate questions are questions that were previously created and answered but occur again. These questions produce noises in the CQA websites which impede users to find answers efficiently. Programming CQA (PCQA), a branch of CQA that holds questions related to programming, also suffers from this problem. Existing works on duplicate detection in PCQA websites framed the task as a supervised learning task on the question pairs, and relied on a number of extracted features of the question pairs. But they extracted only textual features and did not consider the source code in the questions, which are linguistically very different to natural languages. Our work focuses on developing novel features for PCQA duplicate detection. We leverage continuous word vectors from the deep learning literature, probabilistic models in information retrieval and association pairs mined from duplicate questions using machine translation. We provide extensive empirical analysis on the performance of these features and their various combinations using a range of learning models. Our work could be helpful for both research works and practical applications that require extracting features from texts that are not all natural languages.

Keywords: Feature analysis · Question answering · Duplicate detection

1 Introduction

Community question answering (CQA) websites are considered as exhaustive knowledge bases to get expert opinions. Therefore, they are gaining increasing popularity in recent years and becoming a promising alternative to the search engines. There are two types of CQA sites that hold general questions and answers (e.g., Quora[1] and Yahoo! Answers[2]) or focus on a particular topic

[1] https://www.quora.com/.
[2] https://answers.yahoo.com/.

G. Cong et al. (Eds.): ADMA 2017, LNAI 10604, pp. 623–638, 2017.
https://doi.org/10.1007/978-3-319-69179-4_44

(e.g., Stack Overflow[3] for programming questions and TripAdvisor[4] for travel information). However, question duplication is a pervasive issue in CQA. Duplicate questions are questions that were previously created and answered but occur again. They produce noises in the CQA websites, leading to the users having to take long time to browse the websites and find answers for their questions. Therefore, duplicate detection is required to automatically detect the duplicate questions and suggest further actions. Existing works tackle this problem or similar problems by framing the task as a classification task on the question pairs [5,20,22,28]. A question pair consists of a historical question and a question that needs to be examined. A number of features are extracted from the question pairs and be fed into the classification models (i.e., classifiers), which help identify that the questions in a pair are duplicate/similar or not.

Programming CQA (PCQA) is a branch of CQA that holds questions related to programming. Very limited works have studied duplication detection for PCQA. Existing works followed the CQA solution to turn the problem into a classification task [1,27] and relied on the features extracted from the question pairs. However, they considered only syntactical and lexical features that are not necessarily able to reveal the latent semantics of questions. Moreover, they eliminated the source code contained in questions, which could be indicative.

In this paper, we focus on developing novel features that address the mentioned issues and aim to provide a good reference for researchers that are required to extract features from texts that are not all natural languages. Following the works in [1,27], we target the question duplication in Stack Overflow. Stack Overflow contains questions from a range of programming languages, tools and frameworks, enabling programmers to find working solutions to their questions and projects. Thus, it allows for minimal "noise" among its posts. However, duplicate questions occur frequently despite detailed posting guidelines. To tackle this issue, Stack Overflow provides a mechanism for reputable users (or moderators) to manually mark duplicate questions and take further actions. But this requires laborious effort, yet leads to many duplicate questions remain undetected. Our goal is to extract features that are able to capture the characteristics of Stack Overflow questions and facilitate the duplicate detection process. Given a question pair, we generate three types of features. *Vector similarity feature* represents questions as continuous vectors in a high-dimensional space by adopting doc2vec [14]. This feature effectively captures semantics of questions. *Relevance feature* adapts the query-document relevance measurements used in information retrieval. We turn the query likelihood to question likelihood and obtain the relevance (similarity) score for the two questions. Five types of relevance scores are computed. *Association feature* is generated upon mined association phrases (i.e., pairs of phrases that co-occur frequently in known duplicate questions) and lexical features. After obtaining these features, we perform extensive empirical analysis of their performance on the duplicate detection.

[3] https://stackoverflow.com/.
[4] https://www.tripadvisor.com/.

Our contributions include: (i) developing novel features for question pairs in Stack Overflow; (ii) mining domain-specific association pairs from known duplicate questions; (iii) evaluating extensively on the performance of features and their combinations. The rest of paper is organised as follows. In Sect. 2, we describe features we have developed. We report experimental results and analysis in Sect. 3. In Sect. 4, we review some representative related works. Finally, the paper is concluded in Sect. 5.

2 Feature Modelling

We develop three types of features for a question pair (m, t) that contains master question m and target t. These features are both latent features (Sect. 2.1) and surface textual features (Sects. 2.2 and 2.3).

2.1 Vector Similarity Feature

Vector similarity feature is computed on the vector representation of m and t. A conventional approach is to vectorise text using term frequency-inverse document frequency (tf-idf) scores for documents. Each question is considered as a document and we generate a tf-idf vector for a question. Given the question pair, we compute the cosine similarity of the two tf-idf vectors, which is considered as the baseline in this work.

Neural methods for learning word embeddings/vectors have seen many of successes for a range of NLP tasks. word2vec [15] is an efficient neural architecture to learn word embeddings via negative sampling using large corpora of text. Its extension doc2vec, was then introduced to extend word2vec to learn embeddings for word sequences [14] and is able to learn embeddings for a sentence, paragraph or document. We adopt doc2vec to learn vectors for questions.

Given the question pair (m, t), we apply doc2vec on the title, body content, tags, and the concatenation of title, body and tags (title+body+tag) on both master question m and target question t. Thus we train four doc2vec models, one for each type of vector and obtain eight vectors for each question pair, namely t_t, t_m, b_t, b_m, ta_t, ta_m, $tbta_t$ and $tbta_m$ in Fig. 1. Cosine similarities on (t_t, t_m), (b_t, b_m), (ta_t, ta_m) and ($tbta_t$, $tbta_m$) constitute the vector similarity features.

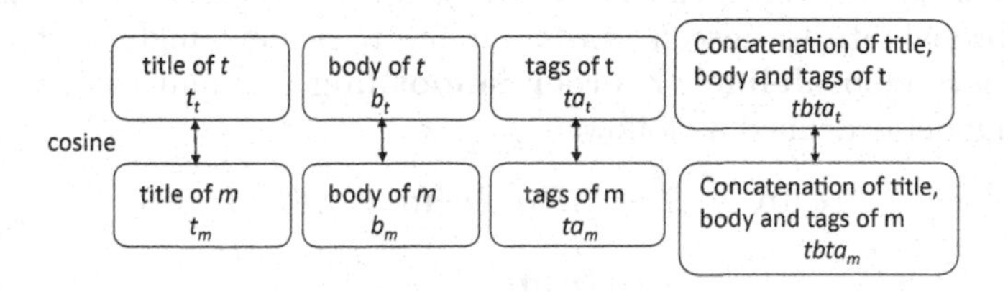

Fig. 1. Vector Similarities Computation. t_t: title vector of t, t_m: title vector of m, b_t: body vector of t, b_m: body vector of m, ta_t: tag vector of t, ta_m: tag vector of m.

2.2 Relevance Feature

Relevance feature reflects the relevance between question m and t in a question pair (m, t). We measure the relevance leveraging the query-document similarity measurement which are widely used in information retrieval. To apply these probability model based methods, we consider each question as a document.

2.2.1 Relevance Feature Using BM25

BM25 [19] is an empirically well performed ranking algorithm [1]. It is a bag-of-words retrieval function that ranks a set of documents based on the query terms appearing in each document. To adapt BM25 in our task, we leverage the scoring part that produces the similarity score between document and query to generate similarity score for the question pair (m, t). Following equation defines the BM25 score for (m, t):

$$BM25(t,m) = \sum_{w \in (\mathbf{t} \cap \mathbf{m})} tf(w,\mathbf{t}) \frac{(k+1)tf(w,\mathbf{m})}{tf(w,\mathbf{m}) + k(1 - b + \frac{b|m|}{avgl})} log \frac{n+1}{df(w)} \tag{1}$$

where $tf(w, \mathbf{m})$ is the frequency of word w in the master question $\mathbf{m}$, $avgl$ is the average length of questions, $df(w)$ is the number of questions word w appear, n is the total number of questions and b and k are free parameters.

2.2.2 Relevance Feature Using Query Likelihood

We adopt the query likelihood to measure the question likelihood, which is the similarity between m and t. The basic idea of the query likelihood in search engines is to estimate a language model for each document in a collection, and then rank them by the likelihood of the query according to the estimated language model [24]. In our work, the question likelihood is defined using log likelihood as follows by adapting equations in [24]:

$$\log P(\mathbf{t}|\mathbf{m}) = \sum_{w \in \mathbf{t}} \log \frac{P(w|\mathbf{m})}{\alpha P(w|Q)} + n \log \alpha + \sum_{w \in \mathbf{t}} \log P(w|Q) \tag{2}$$

where w is a word in the new question t, n is the length of the query, α is related to the smoothing parameter and Q is the collection of the questions.

As mentioned previously, query likelihood model depends on the language model estimation, in which the *smoothing* is a core problem. *Smoothing* assigns non-zero probability to unseen words, aiming to achieve higher retrieval accuracy. We first adopt **Jelinek-Mercer smoothing** [12] and the corresponding language model is defined as follows:

$$\begin{aligned} P(w|\mathbf{m}) &= (1-\lambda)P_{ML}(w|\mathbf{m}) + \lambda P_{ML}(w|Q), \\ P_{ML}(w|\mathbf{m}) &= \frac{tf(w,\mathbf{m})}{\sum_{w' \in \mathbf{m}} tf(w',\mathbf{m})}, \\ P_{ML}(w|Q) &= \frac{tf(w,Q)}{\sum_{w' \in Q} tf(w',Q)}, \end{aligned} \tag{3}$$

where $P_{ML}(w|\mathbf{m})$ is the *Maximum Likelihood* estimate of word w in existing question $\mathbf{m}$, $P_{ML}(w|Q)$ is the *Maximum Likelihood* estimate of word w in the question collection Q, $tf(w, \mathbf{m})$ is the frequency of word w in $\mathbf{m}$ and λ is the smoothing parameter ($\alpha = \lambda$).

We also apply the **Bayesian smoothing using Dirichlet priors** [24] and the language model is accordingly defined as follows:

$$P(w|\mathbf{m}) = \frac{tf(w, \mathbf{m}) + \mu P(w|Q)}{\sum_{w' \in \mathbf{m}} tf(w', \mathbf{m}) + \mu}, \tag{4}$$

where the Dirichlet parameters are: $\mu P(w_1|Q), \mu P(w_2|Q), ..., \mu P(w_n|Q)$, n is the total number of unique words in Q, μ is the smoothing parameter and $\alpha = \frac{\mu}{\sum_{w' \in \mathbf{m}} tf(w', \mathbf{m}) + \mu}$.

2.2.3 Relevance Feature Using Probability Models

There are other probability models that can be used to measure the similarity between texts. Here we use two frameworks that provide the combinations of multiple models.

Divergence From Randomness Similarity (DFRS). Amati et al. [2] proposed a framework for deriving probabilistic models for information retrieval. In their method, a query is assumed to be a set of independent terms, whose weights are computed by measuring the divergence between a term distribution produced by a random process and the actual term distribution. Then the term weights are tuned via normalization methods to measure the similarity between document and query. Specifically, their framework builds the weighting algorithm in three steps: (i) the first step is to measure the informative content of the term in the document and they applied seven models for this task, namely *Limiting form of Bose-Einstein, Geometric approximation of Bose-Einstein, Poisson approximation of the Binomial, Divergence approximation of the Binomial, Inverse document frequency, Inverse expected document frequency* and *Inverse term frequency*; (ii) then they apply two normalization methods *Laplace's law of succession* and *Ratio of two Bernoulli processes* to compute the information gain when accepting the term in the document as a good document descriptor; (iii) finally, they resize the term frequency in light of the length of the document by using two hypothesis: H_1 and H_2. We further discuss the combinations of these models in the experiment (Sect. 3.3.2).

Information Based Similarity (IBS). Another framework that combines different probability models is the work in [7]. Similar to language models, BM25 and DFR framework, their work based on the idea that the respective behaviours of terms in documents bring information on the word. Differ with the mentioned works, information based framework use information models, especially the Shannon information is used to capture whenever a term deviates from its average behaviour. Same as DFR, IB utilises the term's informativeness to measure the query-document relevance and applies two probabilistic distribution

Table 1. Association feature. (m, t) is a pair of questions. s_m, s_t are spans in m and t respectively.

Association feature [4,23].
▷ count of $\langle lemma(s_m), lemma(s_t)\rangle$ if $\langle lemma(s_m), lemma(s_t)\rangle \in \mathcal{A}$, 0 otherwise.
▷ $lemma(s_m) \wedge lemma(s_t)$. $lemma(w)$ is the lemmatised word of w.
▷ $pos(s_m) \wedge pos(s_t)$. $pos(w)$ is the POS tag of w.
▷ $lemma(s_m)$ and $lemma(s_t)$ are synonyms?
▷ $lemma(s_m)$ and $lemma(s_t)$ are WordNet derivations?

to model term occurrence: *Log-logistic* and *Smoothed power-law*. We adopt this framework to measure the relevance between two questions.

2.3 Association Feature

Association pair refers to the pair of phrases that co-occurs frequently in duplicate question pairs. They are strong indicators for identifying duplicate questions. For example, question "*Managing several EditTexts in Android*" is the duplicate of question "*android: how to elegantly set many button IDs*", in which the "*EditTexts*" and "*button IDs*" are association pair, because "*EditTexts*" are used to set "*button IDs*". In other words, they are semantically related. Therefore, strong association between phrases in (m, t) could suggest a high similarity between these two questions. We first mine association pairs from existing duplicate question pairs. Then we generate two types of features based on the mined association pairs and denote them as *association feature* and *association score feature*. Note that we use only question titles to generate association pairs.

2.3.1 Association Pair Mining

We use existing duplicate questions (marked as "Duplicate" in Stack Overflow) and their master questions to form question pairs. For a pair of question (m, t), we learn alignment of words between t and m via machine translation [16]. The word alignment is performed in each direction of (m, t) and (t, m) and then combined. Given the word alignments, we then extract associated phrase pairs based on 3-gram heuristics developed in [17] and prune the ones that occur less than 10 times, producing over 130 K association pairs from 25 K duplicate questions. To cover a wider range of general phrase pairs, we further include a complementary set of 1.3 million association pairs [4] mined from 18 million pairs of questions from WikiAnswers.com. We denote this set of association pairs as $\mathcal{A}$ and examples from $\mathcal{A}$ are: ("command prompt", "console") and ("compiled executable", "exe") etc.

2.3.2 Association Feature Generation

Given target question t and master question m, we iterate through all spans of text $s_t \in t$ and $s_m \in m$ and check if they are associated phrases in $\mathcal{A}$. If

$\langle s_t, s_m \rangle \in \mathcal{A}$, we retrieve its counts from $\mathcal{A}$ as the feature value, otherwise it is set to zero.

We also consider lexical features not only for association pairs, but also for other phrase pairs. Lexical features reflect that whether the word pairs of in t and m share the same lemma, POS tag or are linked through a *derivation* link on WordNet [4,10]. Lexical features are only generated from the titles of m and t. For each (m, t), we iterate through spans of text and generate lexical features according to Table 1. For example, for question pair ("*Managing several EditTexts in Android*", "*android: how to elegantly set many button IDs*"), an association feature ("*EditTexts*" $\in t$, "*button IDs*" $\in m$) is generated for the span ("*EditTexts*", "*button IDs*"). Take Java related duplicate pairs for example, we generate association features with over 80 K dimensions in total using 5 K randomly selected duplicate pairs based on Table 1.

2.3.3 Association Score Feature Generation

The association feature is high dimensional feature which introduces high computational cost. This inspires us to reduce the dimension of the association feature. One way is to utilise traditional dimension reduction algorithms such as Principal Component Analysis (PCA). The other way is to compute a score from the 80K-dimensional association feature and regard this score as a one-dimensional feature, which we refer to as association score feature. We will discuss and evaluate the first way in the experiment section and discuss how to implement the idea of second way here.

We propose to use the weighted sum of the 80 K features as the score. To this end, we need to first learn the weights of the 80 K features. In our work, the weights learnt by a multilayer perceptron with one hidden layer [8] using 5 K duplicates and 5 K non-duplicates for duplicate classification task. The weights indicate the predictive power of the features. Features with zero weight are pruned from the feature space. This reduces the number of features to 16K. Accordingly, we obtained weights for the 16 K features respectively. After obtaining weights for the features, we compute a weighted combination of the features for a given question pair to generate the association score feature.

3 Implementation and Experiment

In this section, we aim to showcase the effectiveness of different features given the classification task in the duplicate detection scenario. We first introduce the dataset we used and how we set up the experimental environment. After that, we report the experiment results and provide analysis.

3.1 Datasets and Pre-processing

Datasets. We used the data dump of Stack Overflow posts available online[5]. The dataset consists of 28,793,722 questions posted from April 2010 to June 2016.

[5] https://archive.org/details/stackexchange.

After pruning questions without answers and considering the "Duplicate" marks, we obtained 250,710 duplicate question pairs, among which 28.6K (28,656) question pairs have "Java" tag (case-insensitive). Accordingly, we randomly sampled 28.6K non-duplicate question pairs to avoid the imbalance class issue. Our dataset thus has 57.2 K question pairs or 114.4 K questions. To generate vector similarity feature, we trained the doc2vec model using Java questions in our dataset. For relevance feature, we used all these questions as the document collection. Association pairs were mined from all existing duplicate pairs (250,710). We randomly sampled 5K Java duplicate pairs to generate association feature for Java questions and used another 5 K duplicate and 5 K non-duplicate Java question pairs to learn feature weights and compute the association score feature. The rest of the Java question pairs were used for training and test the features' performances and we split them in the ratio of 4:1.

Pre-Processing. As the data dump provides texts in the HTML form, we first parsed and cleaned the data, extracting the question title, body and tags. We also used the "RelatedPostId" and "PostTypeId" information to identify the duplicate questions. Then we performed a special mapping from symbols to texts tailed for the programming related questions. Specifically, we mapped all symbols used in programming languages to their symbol names (i.e., "$" to "dollar"). The set of symbols used is: {!, @, #, $, %, ^, &, *, (,), (),+, {, }, {}, >>, .*, _}.[6] Note that we only map symbols that are tokenised as a single token, so e.g., termdiv[class=] will not be converted. The mapping was performed only on question titles, as question bodies may contain source code where symbol conversion might not be sensible. We then did general text processing including stop words pruning, tokenisation and lemmatisation.

3.2 Implementation and Evaluation Metrics

We used gensim[7] implementation of doc2vec and the hyper-parameter settings adopted from [13]. We implemented the relevance features by leveraging the lucene library[8] and developing our own Python wrapper. The parameters were set according to the suggestion in [24]. For generating association feature, we used the GiZA++[9] to get word alignment based phrases pairs and developed the association miner based on SEMPRE [3].

In terms of classifiers, we chose three offline classifiers (logistic regression [21], naive Bayes [6] and adaptive boosting (AdaBoost) [11]) and three incremental/online classifiers (Stochastic Gradient Descent (SGD) learning [25],

[6] Symbols are collected from: https://www.tutorialspoint.com/computer_programming/computer_programming_characters.htm.
[7] https://radimrehurek.com/gensim/.
[8] https://lucene.apache.org/.
[9] http://www.statmt.org/moses/giza/GIZA++.html.

perceptron and multi-layer perceptron [8]) and adopted the scikit-learn[10] implementations of them. For SGD learning, we chose log loss function, which gives SGD via logistic regression (SGD-LR), and for multi-layer perceptron (MLP), we used $\alpha = 1$ and the number of layers equals to 50. All other parameters were set using the default settings in scikit-learn.

The metrics we used to evaluate the features' performances are: (i) *Recall* rate, which reflects the ability to identify duplicate pairs among the true duplicate pairs; (ii) F_1 score, which is the harmonic mean of precision and recall, and is a measure of accuracy; (iii) *Area under the Receiver Operating Characteristic (ROC) curve (AUC)*, which computes the probability that our model will rank a duplicate higher than a non-duplicate question pair.

3.3 Results and Analysis

In this section, we first report the behaviors of features in terms of recall and F_1 score within each category of features (Sects. 3.3.1, 3.3.2 and 3.3.3). Next we analyse classification performance using various combinations of the three categories of features (Sect. 3.3.4).

3.3.1 Vector Similarity Feature Analysis

As described in Sect. 2.1, we trained four doc2vec models, hence we obtained eight vectors for each question pair. Cosine similarities on the four pairs of vectors were computed. In Table 2 recall rate and F_1 score of multiple combinations of these five vector similarities given the classification task are detailed. We also compared the performance of baseline tf-idf document vectors (VSM) with our proposed vector similarity features. *title*, *body*, *tags* denote the title vector similarity, body vector similarity, tags vector similarity respectively, and we used their short form t, b and ta henceforth. $t + b + ta$ is the concatenation vector similarity. Same as t, b and ta, $t+b+ta$ is a one-dimensional feature, namely for each question pair, only one value is used for classification. $(t, b, ta, t + b + ta)$ is a four-dimensional feature that concatenates the vectors mentioned previously.

Results in Table 2 show that $t + b + ta$ performs the best among the four one-dimensional features, giving the highest recall rate and F_1 score for all three classifiers. Also $t + b + ta$ is better than the baseline VSM, which is better than b. Following b and t, ta performs the worst, indicating vectors generated from longer texts could produce better performance. Combining the four one-dimensional features, the four-dimensional feature $(t, b, ta, t{+}b{+}ta)$ gives the best performance of all among the features, no matter what classifiers were tested. Thus we used $(t, b, ta, t + b + ta)$ to represent the vector similarity feature in the following experiments. AdaBoost on $t, b, ta, t + b + ta$ gives 83.0% recall rate and 0.859 F_1 score, followed by logistic regression, then the naive Bayes. The classifiers have different performances on different features. For example, logistic regression is the best classifier for t, ta and $t{+}b{+}ta$, while naive Bayes is best for b. AdaBoost contributes the best overall recall rate and F_1, for $(t, b, ta, t{+}b{+}ta)$.

[10] http://scikit-learn.org/stable/.

Table 2. Performance of different combinations of vector similarity features and VSM. **Bold** value indicate the best result among all features with certain classifier. **Bold**$^{\triangle}$ refers to the best of all.

Features	Recall			F_1		
	NaiveBayes	LogisticRgr	AdaBoost	NaiveBayes	LogisticRgr	AdaBoost
VSM	67.8%	73.6%	69.6%	0.784	0.803	0.790
title (t)	40.9%	48.4%	44.2%	0.328	0.467	0.540
body (b)	69.4%	68.6%	56.6%	0.708	0.706	0.658
tags (ta)	40.8%	47.6%	41.5%	0.493	0.529	0.507
t+b+ta	75.4%	75.6%	68.7%	0.782	0.785	0.767
(t, b, ta, t+b+ta)	**75.7%**	**82.8%**	**83.0%**$^{\triangle}$	**0.785**	**0.849**	**0.859**$^{\triangle}$

It is important to note that the dimension of vectors learned by doc2vec will affect the effectiveness of the vector similarity feature: the higher dimension gives the better classification performance. However, higher dimensional vectors induce higher computational cost. As a balance between accuracy and efficiency, we empirically set the dimension of doc2vec vectors as 100 in this paper.

3.3.2 Relevance Feature Analysis

The relevance feature considers multiple probability models to produce relevance scores between questions. We denote the language model using Jelinek-Mercer smoothing as lm-$_{JM}$ and using Bayesian smoothing with Dirichlet priors as lm-$_{DR}$. As described in Sect. 2.2.3, DFR provides multiple models. It supports seven basic models and two normalization methods, producing 14 combinations. Due to the limited space, we only chose the combinations that performed well in [2], which are B_eB_2, GB_2 and $I(F)B_2$, in which B_e is *Limiting form of Bose-Einstein*, G refers to *Geometric approximation of Bose-Einstein* and $I(F)$ represents Inverse term frequency. We denote these three solutions as $dfrs$-$_{B_eB_2}$, $dfrs$-$_{GB_2}$ and $dfrs$-$_{I(F)B_2}$ respectively. In the IB framework, two probability models are provided and we denote the two solutions as ibs-$_{SPL}$ for smoothed power-law and ibs-$_{LL}$ for log-logistic. For relevance feature computed via BM25, we denoted this feature as $bm25$.

Table 3 presents the evaluation results on these features with the three offline classifiers. For all the three classifiers, $bm25$ gives the best recall and F_1 score among the one-dimensional features. lm-$_{JM}$ has better performance than lm-$_{JM}$ when using naive Bayes and logistic regression, but generates lower recall rate and F_1 score when using AdaBoost. The three features derived from DFR show similar performances, indicating they are similar. The two features computed from IB perform slightly different and in most cases, ibs-$_{LL}$ gives better results compared to ibs-$_{SPL}$. From the results we can see that IB features are better than DFR features in general and language model features are the worst. In order to achieve better result, we chose the best feature from each group (LM, DFR and IB) and concatenate them with $bm25$, generating the *combined* feature. Except for naive Bayes, *combined* achieves the best performance overall: 75.2%

Table 3. Performance of different combinations of relevance features. **Bold** value indicate the best result among all features with certain classifier. **Bold**$^{\triangle}$ refers to the best of all.

Features	Recall			F_1		
	NaiveBayes	LogisticRgr	AdaBoost	NaiveBayes	LogisticRgr	AdaBoost
$lm\text{-}_{JM}$	63.8%	72.5%	71.3%	0.760	0.797	0.798
$lm\text{-}_{DR}$	55.1%	70.5%	72.8%	0.706	0.813	0.826
$dfrs\text{-}_{B_eB_2}$	65.9%	74.2%	74.1%	0.778	0.817	0.816
$dfrs\text{-}_{GB_2}$	66.0%	74.2%	74.0%	0.779	0.817	0.815
$dfrs\text{-}_{I(F)B_2}$	66.4%	75.1%	74.0%	0.783	0.823	0.819
$ibs\text{-}_{SPL}$	67.3%	73.5%	71.4%	0.788	0.807	0.806
$ibs\text{-}_{LL}$	67.9%	75.4%	74.1%	0.793	0.827	0.823
$bm25$	**69.0%**	75.4%	75.1%	**0.800**	0.829	0.830
combined[a]	68.1%	**76.1%**$^{\triangle}$	**75.2%**	0.793	**0.839**$^{\triangle}$	**0.831**

[a] *combined* is four-dimensional combining $lm\text{-}_{JM}$, $dfrs\text{-}_{I(F)B_2}$, $ibs\text{-}_{LL}$ and $bm25$

recall rate and 0.831 F_1 score when using AdaBoost. Interestingly, when using naive Bayes, $bm25$ generates the highest recall and F_1 score, but still worse than the best results achieved by AdaBoost using *combined*. Therefore, we chose *comibined* to represent the relevance feature in the following evaluations.

From the evaluation in this section and Sect. 3.3.1, we found that AdaBoost is the best classifier for vector similarity feature and relevance feature. We will further evaluate it on association features.

3.3.3 Association Feature Analysis

We developed two types of association related features: association feature and association score feature to showcase the different effectiveness of these features. As the association feature is a high dimensional feature with more than 80 K dimensions, we intuitively tried to reduce the computation cost without losing information by using PCA. ass_{R2000} denotes the association with 2,000 features after performing PCA on the original association feature ass. Similarity, ass_{R100} and ass_{R2} are 100-dimensional and 2-dimensional features respectively.

In this evaluation, we additionally chose some incremental learning models as association is high dimensional. Table 4 details the classification performance of association feature on both the offline and incremental classifiers. MLP refers to multi-layer perceptron. The features after dimensional reduction do not perform as well as the original feature. The reason should be the dimensions of these after-reduction features are still not high enough to capture all the characteristics of ass. In other words, ass contains high dimensional information that the dimension reduction would possibly cause the information lost. *ass score* is better than after-reduction features but still worse than ass, showcasing ass is the most effective feature among the five listed in Table 4. Working with logistic regression, ass achieves the best recall rate 86.1% and F_1 score 0.872. The second

Table 4. Performance of association features. **Bold** value indicate the best result among all features with certain classifier. **Bold**$^{\triangle}$ refers to the best of all. MLP: Multilayer Percetpron. ass_{R*}: *-dimensional association feature after dimension reduction.

Recall						
Features	NaiveBayes	LogisticRgr	AdaBoost	SGD-LR	Perceptron	MLP
ass	**83.1%**	**86.1%**$^{\triangle}$	**84.5%**	**85.5%**	**83.7%**	**85.8%**
ass_{R2000}	46.2%	56.5%	46.4%	58.0%	55.6%	54.7%
ass_{R100}	43.0%	53.7%	49.0%	60.0%	51.6%	55.5%
ass_{R2}	38.1%	50.7%	67.2%	50.8%	51.4%	68.3%
$ass\ score$	82.8%	78.6%	76.9%	82.7%	2.40%	78.4%
F_1						
Features	NaiveBayes	LogisticRgr	AdaBoost	SGD-LR	Perceptron	MLP
ass	**0.826**	**0.872**$^{\triangle}$	**0.854**	**0.863**	**0.846**	**0.870**
ass_{R2000}	0.538	0.587	0.504	0.602	0.590	0.572
ass_{R100}	0.513	0.579	0.521	0.622	0.571	0.576
ass_{R2}	0.483	0.561	0.628	0.564	0.466	0.646
$ass\ score$	0.804	0.828	0.827	0.838	0.034	0.829

best performance is produced by MLP, which gives recall 85.8% and F_1 score 0.870. Therefore, we used *ass* to represent the association feature for the following evaluations. The results show that incremental learning is not necessarily better than offline learning algorithms. One other interesting observation is that perceptron gives very low recall (2.40%) and F_1 (0.034) for *ass score*. This is because perceptron is very sensitive to the dimension of features and quite unreliable for very low dimensional features, especially the one-dimensional feature.

3.3.4 Feature Combination Analysis

We report the analysis of performances of different combinations of the three features (VS: vector similarity, RE: relevance, and AS: association). In Table 5, classification recall and F_1 score using different combinations of features over the selected six classifiers are summarised. The combination of any two of the features outperforms single feature, suggesting that these three features complement each other (recall the results from Tables 2, 3 and 4). RE+AS always gives better performance than VS+RE and VS+AS when using the six classifiers, suggesting RE and AS are better complementary features. VS+RE and VS+AS interchangebly performs better. For example, VS+RE produces higher recall than VS+AS when using AdaBoost, but lower recall when using naive Bayes. When combining all the individual features (VS+AS+RE), it yields the best performance on all the tested six classifiers, among which AdaBoost achieves 96.1% for recall and 0.953 for F_1 score. Recall that for VS working indepen-

Table 5. Performance of different combinations of three categories of features. **Bold** value indicate the best result among all features with certain classifier. **Bold**$^{\Delta}$ refers to the best of all. MLP: Multi-layer Percetpron. VS: vector similarity feature, RE: relevance feature, AS: association feature.

Recall						
Features	NaiveBayes	LogisticRgr	AdaBoost	SGD-LR	Perceptron	MLP
$VS + RE$	81.3%	93.8%	92.7%	83.7%	72.0%	92.7%
$VS + AS$	83.1%	90.2%	91.2%	81.4%	85.9%	90.8%
$RE + AS$	83.2%	94.2%	94.5%	86.6%	90.0%	91.4%
$VS + AS + RE$	**83.3%**	**95.7%**	**96.1%**$^{\Delta}$	**90.5%**	**92.9%**	**92.8%**
F_1						
Features	NaiveBayes	LogisticRgr	AdaBoost	SGD-LR	Perceptron	MLP
$VS + RE$	0.827	0.915	0.921	0.884	0.792	0.893
$VS + AS$	0.826	0.920	0.928	0.882	0.892	0.913
$RE + AS$	0.827	0.925	0.919	0.892	0.892	0.914
$VS + AS + RE$	**0.871**	**0.950**	**0.953**$^{\Delta}$	**0.898**	**0.922**	**0.938**

dently, AdaBoost also gives the best performance. But for RE and AS, logistic regression is the best classifier. This indicates that VS has strong impact on the overall performance of VS+AS+RE.

Figure 2 illustrates the ROC curve and AUC score for various feature combinations using AdaBoost. The results are consistent with the recall and F_1 score: VS+AS+RE always gives the best performance.

4 Related Works

Very limited research efforts have been devoted to question duplication in PCQA. Zhang et al. [27] proposed the first work to tackle this issue for Stack Overflow.

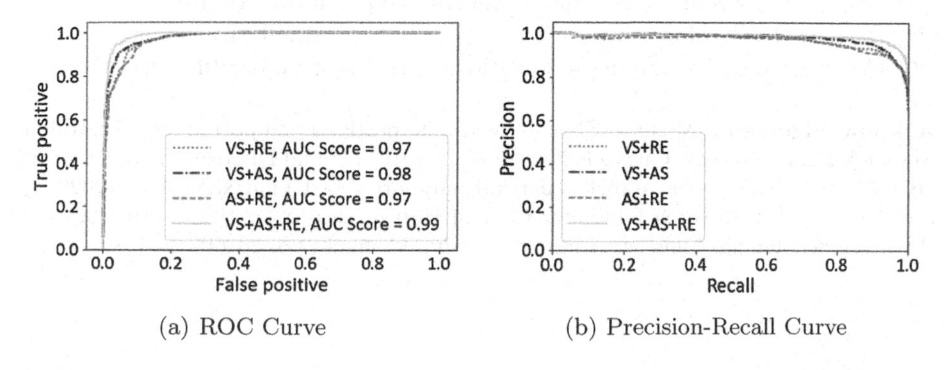

(a) ROC Curve

(b) Precision-Recall Curve

Fig. 2. ROC and PR curve on different feature combinations using AdaBoost

They developed textual features using question title, description, topic and tags. Ahasanuzzaman et al. [1] improved their work and proposed both textural and semantic features for the same task. Moreover, they conducted extensive analysis to understand the reason of duplicate questions on Stack Overflow. Very recently, Zhang et al. [26] extracted features for Stack Overflow question pairs leveraging latent semantics learned through word2vec, frequently co-occurred phrases pairs mined from existing duplicate question pairs and topic models. These features produces strong performance for duplicate detection from Stack Overflow posts. However, these works lack the analysis of the developed features.

In a broader CQA domain, similar researches were proposed. Correa et al. [9] developed four categories of features to predict the possibility of deletion of a newly issued question. The 47 proposed features are all textural features considering issuer profile, issuer community history, question content and syntactic statistics. Shtok et al. [20] treated the question-answering task as a similarity identification problem, and retrieved questions that have similar titles as candidates. Yang et al. [22] classified questions based on heuristics and topical information to predict whether they will be answered. Qin et al. [18] studied the learning to rank problem and developed a range of features. The 64 features consider the language models, probability models and statistic information.

5 Conclusion

In this paper, we developed three categories of features for the PCQA duplicate detection problem. We performed extensive evaluation and analysis on the features and their combinations. We found the combination of vector similarity, relevance and association features gives the best performance, achieving more than 95% recall rate. We also observed that online learning algorithms do not necessarily perform better than offline algorithms. One more result is that the dimensional reduction algorithm are not effective for the association feature. Our work could be a helpful reference for research works that require extracting features from texts that are not all natural languages.

In the future, we would further develop features from communities, e.g., the question issuer's profile as auxiliary. Another research direction could be investigating how to develop features on questions from small and domain-specific PCQA, where data for mining association pairs might be insufficient.

Acknowledgement. Michael Sheng's work is partially supported by Australian Research Council (ARC) Future Fellowship FT140101247 and Discovery Project Grant DP140100104. Yanjun Shu's work is partially supported by China NSF (No. 61202091), the Fundamental Research Funds for Central Universities (No. NSRIF. 2016050) and the State Scholarship Fund of China Scholarship Council (No. 201606125073).

References

1. Ahasanuzzaman, M., Asaduzzaman, M., Roy, C.K., Schneider, K.A.: Mining duplicate questions in stack overflow. In: Proceedings of MSR 2016, pp. 402–412 (2016)
2. Amati, G., Van Rijsbergen, C.J.: Probabilistic models of information retrieval based on measuring the divergence from randomness. ACM Trans. Inf. Syst. **20**(4), 357–389 (2002)
3. Berant, J., Chou, A., Frostig, R., Liang, P.: Semantic parsing on freebase from question-answer pairs. In: Proceedings of EMNLP 2013, pp. 1533–1544 (2013)
4. Berant, J., Liang, P.: Semantic parsing via paraphrasing. In: Proceedings of ACL 2014, pp. 1415–1425 (2014)
5. Cao, X., Cong, G., Cui, B., Jensen, C.S., Yuan, Q.: Approaches to exploring category information for question retrieval in community question-answer archives. ACM Trans. Inf. Syst. **30**(2), 7 (2012)
6. Chan, T.F., Golub, G.H., LeVeque, R.J.: Updating formulae and a pairwise algorithm for computing sample variances. In: Proceedings of COMPSTAT 1982, pp. 30–41 (1982)
7. Clinchant, S., Gaussier, É.: Information-based models for ad hoc IR. In: Proceedings of SIGIR 2010, pp. 234–241 (2010)
8. Collins, M.: Discriminative training methods for hidden markov models: theory and experiments with perceptron algorithms. In: Proceedings of EMNLP 2002, pp. 1–8 (2002)
9. Correa, D., Sureka, A.: Chaff from the wheat: characterization and modeling of deleted questions on stack overflow. In: Proceedings of WWW 2014, pp. 631–642 (2014)
10. Fellbaum, C.: WordNet: An Electronic Lexical Database. MIT Press, Cambridge (1998)
11. Freund, Y., Schapire, R.E.: A desicion-theoretic generalization of on-line learning and an application to boosting. In: Vitányi, P. (ed.) EuroCOLT 1995. LNCS, vol. 904, pp. 23–37. Springer, Heidelberg (1995). doi:10.1007/3-540-59119-2_166
12. Jelinek, F., Mercer, R.L.: Interpolated estimation of markov source parameters from sparse data. In: Proceedings of PRNI 1980, pp. 381–397 (1980)
13. Lau, J.H., Baldwin, T.: An empirical evaluation of doc2vec with practical insights into document embedding generation. In: Proceedings of RepL4NLP 2016, pp. 78–86 (2016)
14. Le, Q.V., Mikolov, T.: Distributed representations of sentences and documents. In: Proceedings of ICML 2014, pp. 1188–1196 (2014)
15. Mikolov, T., Sutskever, I., Chen, K., Corrado, G.S., Dean, J.: Distributed representations of words and phrases and their compositionality. In: Proceedings of NIPS 2013, pp. 3111–3119 (2013)
16. Och, F.J., Ney, H.: A systematic comparison of various statistical alignment models. Comput. Linguist. **29**(1), 19–51 (2003)
17. Och, F.J., Ney, H.: The alignment template approach to statistical machine translation. Comput. Linguist. **30**(4), 417–449 (2004)
18. Qin, T., Liu, T., Xu, J., Li, H.: LETOR: a benchmark collection for research on learning to rank for information retrieval. Inf. Retrieval **13**(4), 346–374 (2010)
19. Robertson, S.E., Walker, S., Jones, S., Hancock-Beaulieu, M.M., Gatford, M.: Okapi at TREC-3. In: Proceedings of TREC-3, pp. 109–126 (1996)
20. Shtok, A., Dror, G., Maarek, Y., Szpektor, I.: Learning from the past: answering new questions with past answers. In: Proceedings of WWW 2012, pp. 759–768 (2012)

21. Walker, S.H., Duncan, D.B.: Estimation of the probability of an event as a function of several independent variables. Biometrika **54**(1–2), 167–179 (1967)
22. Yang, L., Bao, S., Lin, Q., Wu, X., Han, D., Su, Z., Yu, Y.: Analyzing and predicting not-answered questions in community-based question answering services. In: Proceedings of AAAI 2011, pp. 1273–1278 (2011)
23. Yin, P., Duan, N., Kao, B., Bao, J., Zhou, M.: Answering questions with complex semantic constraints on open knowledge bases. In: Proceedings of CIKM 2015, pp. 1301–1310 (2015)
24. Zhai, C., Lafferty, J.D.: A study of smoothing methods for language models applied to information retrieval. ACM Trans. Inf. Syst. **22**(2), 179–214 (2004)
25. Zhang, T.: Solving large scale linear prediction problems using stochastic gradient descent algorithms. In: Proceedings of ICML 2004, pp. 919–926 (2004)
26. Zhang, W.E., Sheng, Q.Z., Lau, J.H., Abebe, E.: Detecting duplicate posts in programming QA communities via latent semantics and association rules. In: Proceedings of WWW 2017, pp. 1221–1229 (2017)
27. Zhang, Y., Lo, D., Xia, X., Sun, J.: Multi-factor duplicate question detection in stack overflow. J. Comput. Sci. Technol. **30**(5), 981–997 (2015)
28. Zhou, G., Liu, Y., Liu, F., Zeng, D., Zhao, J.: Improving question retrieval in community question answering using world knowledge. In: Proceedings of IJCAI 2013, pp. 2239–2245 (2013)

A Joint Human/Machine Process for Coding Events and Conflict Drivers

Bradford Heap[1(✉)], Alfred Krzywicki[1], Susanne Schmeidl[2], Wayne Wobcke[1], and Michael Bain[1]

[1] School of Computer Science and Engineering, University of New South Wales, Sydney, NSW 2052, Australia
{b.heap,alfredk,w.wobcke,m.bain}@unsw.edu.au
[2] School of Social Sciences, University of New South Wales, Sydney, NSW 2052, Australia
s.schmeidl@unsw.edu.au

Abstract. Constructing datasets to analyse the progression of conflicts has been a longstanding objective of peace and conflict studies research. In essence, the problem is to reliably *extract* relevant text snippets and *code* (annotate) them using an ontology that is meaningful to social scientists. Such an ontology usually characterizes either types of violent events (killing, bombing, etc.), and/or the underlying drivers of conflict, themselves hierarchically structured, for example security, governance and economics, subdivided into conflict-specific indicators. Numerous coding approaches have been proposed in the social science literature, ranging from fully automated "machine" coding to human coding. Machine coding is highly error prone, especially for labelling complex drivers, and suffers from extraction of duplicated events, but human coding is expensive, and suffers from inconsistency between annotators; thus hybrid approaches are required. In this paper, we analyse experimentally how human input can most effectively be used in a hybrid system to complement machine coding. Using two newly created real-world datasets, we show that machine learning methods improve on rule-based automated coding for filtering large volumes of input, while human verification of relevant/irrelevant text leads to improved performance of machine learning for predicting multiple labels in the ontology.

1 Introduction

Identifying and tracking drivers of conflict in order to anticipate the outbreak of violence has been an elusive challenge for social science. The field of peace and conflict studies suffers greatly from the lack of reliable quantitative data on societal and political factors and events which are more abstract than the basic information typically collected for armed conflicts, such as individual battle statistics. This limits the ability of analysts to develop effective and general conflict analyses and early warning models [3].

G. Cong et al. (Eds.): ADMA 2017, LNAI 10604, pp. 639–654, 2017.
https://doi.org/10.1007/978-3-319-69179-4_45

A serious problem is that, even when data is collected, it needs to be stored in a form that analysts can later search and use to analyse the long-term progression of a conflict. The idea is to *code* the data by annotating *relevant* information with concepts from a pre-defined ontology [10,15]. Abstract concepts in the ontology are designed to capture what analysts consider to be important for making sense of the many individual events or factors involved in an extended conflict. Moreover, useful information can originate from a variety of sources and be of a variety of types. At one extreme, long and complicated formal analyst reports can provide historical context and in-depth analysis, often focusing on underlying *conflict drivers* (structural and causal factors contributing to the progression of a conflict). At another extreme, news and social media can provide timely and useful information (and also misinformation) on a daily basis, typically reporting many isolated events (such as individual battles, attacks, deaths, gains/losses of territory) that need to be classified for future analysis.

During the past two decades, much progress has been made in automating event coding through the development of systems that apply term dictionaries and syntactic rules to automatically filter text content and extract actors, actions, places and times related to an event [3,4,7]. However, while this machine extracted information is more suited for studies that involve the consolidation of event statistics, the coding is typically less sophisticated than human analysts require for conflict analysis [10]. Automated event coding methods are error-prone and suffer from the problem of extracting the same event multiple times (duplicated events). On the other hand, human coding is expensive and time-consuming, which means information is not up to date, and datasets suffer from disagreement between coders as to how best to characterize an event or fact (this disagreement is sometimes legitimate, as "coding" is subject to interpretation and made on the basis of background knowledge that may differ amongst experts). Thus hybrids of human and machine coding systems are required to balance the accuracy and complexity of coding with the timeliness and coverage of the events and factors involved in a conflict.

In this paper we empirically analyse a proposed hybrid human/maching coding process. We study two different conflict domains, which, while different in the type of document sources and the information to be extracted and coded, nevertheless are similar in the requirements to: (i) identify the small amount of *relevant* text from a large volume of input, and (ii) *code* (annotate) the relevant text using concepts from a (possibly) domain-specific ontology. As part of our work, we have developed two new datasets that may be of independent interest to social scientists studying those conflicts. The specific conflicts are the long and ongoing "cycles" of violence in the Democratic Republic of the Congo (DRC) during the period 2002–2006 (before the outbreak of violence surrounding the presidential elections), and the long-running war in Afghanistan, focusing on events reported in news sources in 2016 (which we have called the AfPak dataset, following common usage of this term to denote Afghanistan/Pakistan). The basic approach to the experiments is that, given a "ground truth" dataset constructed by human expert coders, we mimic the performance of a hypothetical joint human/machine coding process, to determine where, in the future, human input is best utilized. Considering t two-step process of determining relevance and coding, we simulate the effect o using human input at each step to refine the output of the system at that stage. This enables us to determine the specific strengths and weaknesses of a variety of machine learning methods, on the individual steps and in combination. Our results show that human input at the stage of identifying relevance can greatly improve the overall performance of the system (in terms of precision and recall), and that machine learning is most effective in identifying a small number of concepts from the ontology for using in coding, from which a human can select the best one(s).

We begin the paper with a more detailed description of coding, including the construction of our ontologies and datasets, then present a formalization of document coding as a machine learning problem, and finally describe our proposed process for joint human/machine coding and the experimental results forming the evaluation of the process.

2 Coding of Events and Conflict Drivers

In essence, *coding* requires both the development of a coding scheme or ontology, and a systematic coding process specifying how to apply coding rules to extracted data for inclusion in a dataset [15]. Note here that the "coding rules" are typically meant for human use, so may be incomplete or open to interpretation.

Historically, the ontologies of the World Event/Interaction Survey (WEIS) [8] and the Conflict and Peace Databank (COPDAB) [1] have been used for large scale human coding in developing conflict datasets. While the largest coding projects, such as the Global Database of Events, Language, and Tone (GDELT) [7] have now become fully automated there are still some projects which are entirely human coder based [6,11].

2.1 Ontologies for Events and Conflict Drivers

The development of any coding scheme requires expert domain knowledge and careful consideration of what data to code to ensure the coding process results in a high quality and accurate dataset. Numerous coding schemes have been developed, originally focused on international relations [1,8], and later expanded to include domestic relations and local events [3,5,11,15].

Generally, coding ontologies are hierarchical and information can be classified at different levels of the hierarchy. Ontologies for events are simpler than for conflict drivers (see below) because the ontology takes the form of a type hierarchy. As our objective is to code events relating to the conflict in Afghanistan, we adapted the basic CAMEO ontology [5], focusing on violent events (attacks, killings, etc.) and statements (public announcements, claims of responsibility, etc.). Figure 1 shows part of our event type ontology. Note that with this coding scheme, events can be classified at the "top level" only, e.g. if an event is an attack but not one of the subtypes of attack specified in the hierarchy. Note also that some of the concepts are domain specific, due to the nature of the conflict

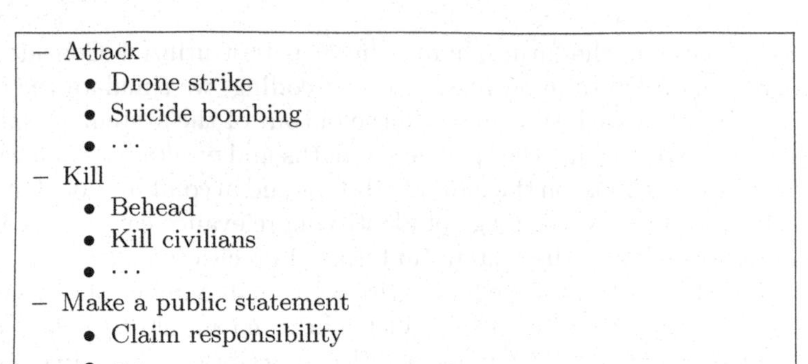

Fig. 1. AfPak event type ontology

in Afghanistan (such as suicide bombing), though the aim is make the ontology as domain independent as possible.

The ontology for conflict drivers focuses on factors (which could include events) that contribute causally to an ongoing conflict. One way to characterize conflict drivers is in terms of *structural causes* or *root causes* (pervasive factors or grievances that have become entrenched in a society and create the preconditions for violent conflict), *proximate conditions* or *intervening factors* (factors contributing to a climate conducive to violent conflict or its further escalation that are under more direct control), and *triggers* (single key acts or events that set off or escalate violent conflict).

Many existing machine-based coding ontologies consider only the extraction of events and ignore structural causes and proximate conditions, which, even for an expert human coder, can be difficult to extract [3]. But by coding only events, the resulting datasets may have inherent biases [14]. In contrast, our ontology includes drivers at multiple layers of abstraction.

The drivers for the Democratic Republic of the Congo (DRC) dataset are characterized as a three-level hierarchy of *pillars*, *categories* and *indicators*. Pillars capture the basic objectives of peacebuilding, including *economics*, *governance*, *rule of law* and *security*. The *indicators* cover dynamic conditions such as *economic decline* and *external influence*. Indicators are grouped into categories, such as *human rights* and *internal stability*, which are aspects of the associated pillar. Thus the hierarchy is not a simple type or part-whole hierarchy but a collection of abstract concepts some of which involve causal relations (e.g. *cross border aggression* causes (a decrease in) *internal security* which in turn is an aspect of *security*). Nonetheless, each indicator is associated with exactly one category and each category with exactly one pillar.

2.2 Datasets

In our work we have developed two new datasets. We describe first a dataset of events reported in news sources on Afghanistan and Pakistan (AfPak), then describe that based on conflict drivers extracted from analyst reports on th Democratic Republic of the Congo (DRC).

AfPak Events Dataset. This dataset focuses purely on single events of the form "who did what to whom and where". The ontology extends CAMEO [5] to include not only event types, as described above, but Afghanistan-specific individuals, organizations, locations, and types of equipment. In total, the ontology contains 441 individuals, 155 organizations, 708 locations and 7 types of equipment. The ontology includes 119 event types, making event coding a difficult problem for human and machine. The experiments in this paper use online news articles in English from local and international media, and NGO and extremist group sources; data is from August, October and November 2016.

To develop the dataset, human coders extracted events that could map to the ontology, and with each event, where possible, identified actors, targets and locations, and a snippet of text specifically expressing the event type. In total, human coders read over 6,500 webpages containing more than 112,000 sentences, and extracted a total of 1,478 events which were mapped to 72 top-level event types (lower level event types are not considered in this paper, due to the lack of instances). The low ratio of extracted events to the number of sentences reflects the amount of filtering required to determine the relevant sentences.

ICG DRC Dataset. This dataset contains "text snippets" (short fragments of text) extracted from 15 International Crisis Group (ICG) reports on the DRC during the period 2002–2006, annotated with indicators, categories and pillars from the ontology. Social science domain experts had full control over the creation of the ontology, coding rules and extraction of driver related text snippets included in the dataset. An ontology was defined before coding commenced, with minor adjustments made during the coding process. The final ontology contains 70 indicators, 17 categories and the 4 pillars. To construct the dataset, a domain expert read 8,836 sentences across the 15 reports, extracted 2,541 text snippets, and used 68 of the 70 indicators. The analysis in this paper is at the level of categories, as many indicators have very few examples in the data.

Figure 2 shows the distribution of assigned categories in the ICG DRC dataset, showing (as typical in this research field) the highly imbalanced nature of the dataset. Here the top 4 categories are all related to the *security* pillar, as

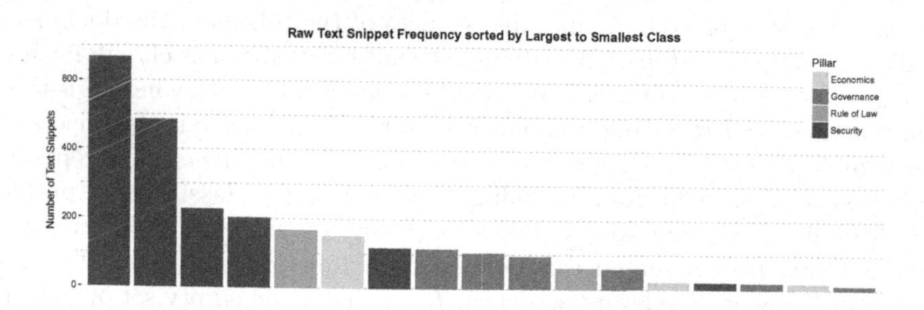

Fig. 2. Frequency distribution by category of text snippets in the ICG DRC dataset

.e data includes much information on fighting between militia groups in various parts of the country over the period.

3 Document Coding as a Machine Learning Problem

As outlined above, document coding is a two step process: (i) identifying relevant information (events or driver related text, for now assumed to be sentences), and (ii) coding the extracted information by annotating it with concepts from the ontology. An overview of an automated coding process is shown in Fig. 3, where the process uses two models, a sentence filtering model for determining relevant information, and a sentence classification model for the coding.

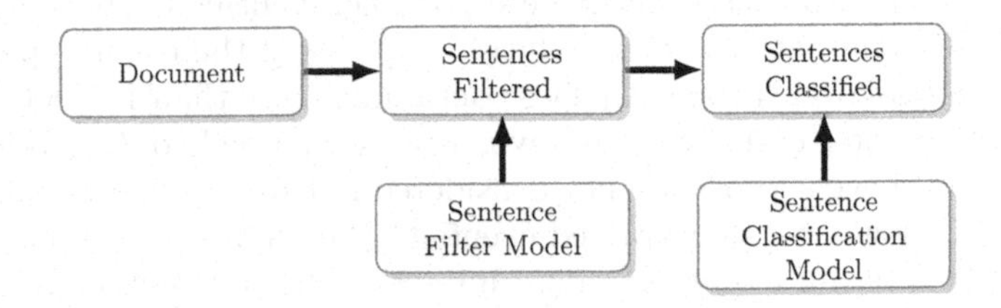

Fig. 3. Automated machine coding process

Formally, we define a *document* D in its simplest form as simply a sequence of tokens $D = [t_0, t_1, \ldots]$, where a *token* t is defined to be a word (individual or compound) or punctuation symbol. We then define a *text snippet* S as a (not necessarily contiguous) subsequence of tokens $S \sqsubseteq D$, and a *sentence* to be a maximal text snippet that is a contiguous subsequence of D, ends with a punctuation symbol indicating the end of a sentence, such as '.' or '?', and which, apart from this token, is grammatically correct. We can then reasonably assume that a text document D consists of a sequence of sentences (though also contains headings, footnotes, image captions, etc.).

Thus each text snippet S is a subsequence of the document's token sequence $S = [t_0, t_1, \ldots]$, however there is no guarantee that a text snippet forms a fully parsable sentence, and moreover, text snippets can cross sentence boundaries, and may not even be contiguous subsequences of the tokens in the document.

We now define the step of identifying relevant information as classifying a sentence as *relevant* by use of a classification function $f_r : \mathcal{S} \rightarrow R$, where $\mathcal{S}$ is the set of all sentences and $R = \{\text{relevant}, \text{not relevant}\}$. If a sentence is classified as relevant, the second step of the process is to assign to it one *or more* concepts from the ontology. Thus importantly, coding is a *multi-label* classification problem. More formally, if the ontology is taken as the set of concepts $C = \{c_0, c_1, \ldots\}$, the classification of a sentence is defined by a function $f_c : \mathcal{S} \rightarrow 2^C$, where obviously, if S is not a relevant sentence, f_c assigns S the empty set of concepts.

3.1 Automated Sentence Extraction and Classification

As with the construction of a human coding scheme, an automated text extraction and classification system (Fig. 3) requires information about relevant sentences and how to extract them. There is commonality with the human process, since the same classification labels are applied to the extracted sentences. However, where the human process requires the creation of a codebook and minimal set of examples, the machine process either requires a set of structural rules (c.f. [14]) or many examples per class to learn a model (c.f. [10]). This requirement of many training examples is problematic for rare events and events whose interpretation depends on context or background knowledge.

Once a coding scheme has been developed, models can be built to classify sentences. In most existing machine-based text extraction and classification systems for conflict analysis, there is a reliance on the direct matching of the text to the concepts in the coding ontology.

Machine-based sentence extraction and classification approaches are much quicker and cheaper than human systems. Once a model is developed, it can run continuously and will be consistent in its performance [14]. However, these systems are much less flexible than human coding systems. In particular, special cases are hard to handle and classification errors are often quite "far" from the correct classification [15]. Furthermore, many machine-based coding systems are unable to recognise new terms and phenomena [14], and models which are built based on assumptions about the distribution of events may perform poorly if that distribution changes.

The continued reliance on rule-based pattern matching in these systems is contrary to most trends in classification systems. In other domains, the supervised machine learning approaches of Multinomial Naive Bayes (MNB) and Support Vector Machines (SVM) have largely superseded rule-based systems [16].

4 A Joint Human/Machine Coding Process

Human and machine coding processes have different strengths and weaknesses. While machine coding processes are always consistent in their rule and pattern matching, this also forms part of their Achilles' heel. In contrast, a human coder can easily adapt to changes in language expression, use and terminology. A joint human/machine coding process should be designed to take advantage of the consistency of machine-based coding and also allow a human coder to correct errors or add information missed by the automated process. Although this joint process will be many times slower than a fully automated process, the overall quality of the data extracted should be higher, allowing for much richer analysis. In summary, the key benefit of a hybrid approach is to enable a machine to perform the mundane tasks of identifying possible sentences containing events, but with human verification. This prevents the human from missing events, and also allows the human to help the system classify rare events, or correct misclassifications.

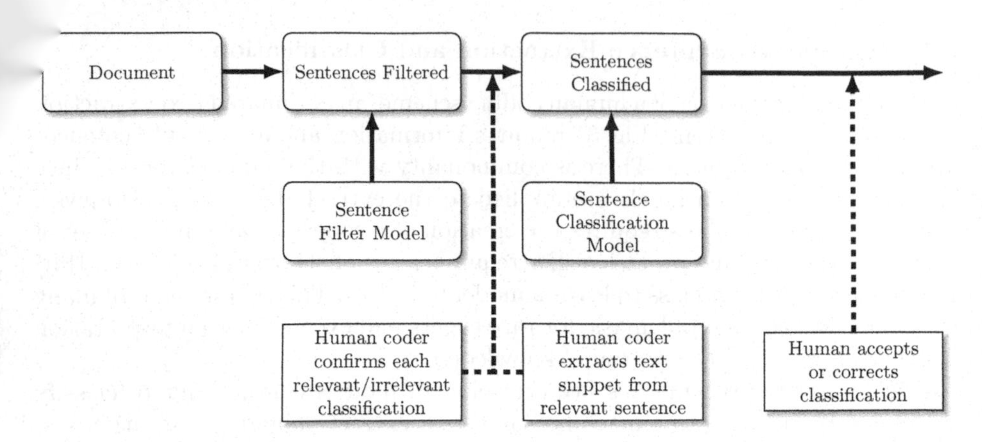

Fig. 4. A joint human/machine coding process

Figure 4 outlines the steps in our joint human/machine process. The key difference between this joint process and the fully automated machine-based process is the inclusion of the human coder after the extraction of relevant sentences. This allows the human coder to discard any incorrectly identified sentences, and to select a shorter text snippet from the sentence containing the tokens that the human coder judges to be sufficient to determine the correct classification. Finally, after the machine classifies the sentence (possibly using only the text snippet), the human coder can accept or change the classification. This optional step allows the system to present to the human coder a list of the most relevant potential classification labels, from which the human selects the correct labels.

4.1 Development and Evaluation of Sentence Extraction Models

Both the automated and joint coding processes involve a common step of extracting the relevant sentences. Although all the above-mentioned event extraction systems approach this problem using patterns based on NLP parsing, we propose using supervised machine learning for this task.

The two human-annotated datasets described in Sect. 2.2 give us a way to evaluate approaches for the extraction of relevant sentences. Our first evaluation involves identifying if a sentence is relevant in the AfPak dataset, and our second on the ICG DRC dataset. As the AfPak dataset is primarily based on news reports and is coded according to an extension of the CAMEO coding scheme, we are also able to compare supervised machine learning models to the PETRARCH Coding System.[1]

In comparing supervised machine learning approaches to PETRARCH, we expect some differences in performance. First, we expect similar or better levels of recall in the supervised machine learning models compared to PETRARCH,

[1] PETRARCH2, the most recent release, was used in our experiments (http://github.com/openeventdata/petrarch2).

because the supervised machine learning models operate independently of parsing rules and, given that the data were coded by human coders, we expect that the human coders did not consciously follow a subject-verb-object pattern of text extraction. Second, we expect that PETRARCH will identify many non-relevant events, since it is designed to extract events related to many areas of the world, not specifically Afghanistan/Pakistan.

Evaluation Methodology. In our analysis, we use the standard metrics of recall and precision to measure model performance. These metrics are defined as:

$$\text{recall} = \frac{tp}{tp + fn} \qquad \text{precision} = \frac{tp}{tp + fp}$$

where tp is the number of true positives, i.e., the number of sentences correctly classified as relevant, fn the number of misclassifications of relevant sentences as irrelevant, fp the number of irrelevant sentences incorrectly classified as relevant, and tn the number of irrelevant sentences correctly classified as irrelevant.

Ideally, a sentence extraction system should produce results which have both high recall and high precision. However, in practice models with high recall are also likely to produce many irrelevant sentences; for instance, a model could achieve perfect recall if it marks every sentence as relevant. In contrast, models with high precision are likely to have lower recall, since they only suggest relevant sentences in which they have high confidence.

For the joint human/machine coding system, we focus primarily on obtaining good recall, with a secondary focus on precision. This is warranted since, in validating the output of sentence extraction, when a human is shown an incorrect label for a sentence they can easily reject it, but when shown a sentence missing a correct label, they are likely to take longer to identify the relevant content and determine its correct classification.[2] Additionally, to capture variation between methods in the balance of the number of irrelevant sentences classified as relevant (false positives) and the number of relevant sentences not marked as relevant (false negatives), we also calculate the F1 score (the harmonic mean of recall and precision).

For evaluation, we split the AfPak dataset into a training set containing 65% of the articles and a test set the remaining 35%. Articles were presented to our human coders in chronological order, so the training/test split followed the same ordering. The training set contains the first 4,892 articles annotated by our human coders, of which 1,004 sentences (1.26%) are marked as relevant and 78,503 sentences as irrelevant. The test set contains 2,625 articles of which 362 sentences (0.84%) are relevant and 42,640 sentences are irrelevant. We followed the approach of Bagozzi and Schrodt [2] and reduced our dataset to contain only the first 6 sentences of each article. After this reduction, the training set contained 931 relevant sentences (3.95%) and 22,657 irrelevant sentences, and the test set 352 relevant sentences (2.92%) and 12,075 irrelevant sentences.

[2] This appears in timings in our log files and was explicitly stated by one of our coders.

We compare four approaches for identifying relevant sentences. The first, as a baseline, is Schrodt's PETRARCH system in its default form. The second and third are variants on Multinomial Naive Bayes (MNB). The fourth is a widely-used implementation of the Support Vector Machine (SVM) algorithm. For the ICG DRC dataset, we cannot apply PETRARCH, but we used the same three learning algorithms, and applied 10-fold cross validation.

Multinomial Naive Bayes. The MNB classifier [9] is a simple probabilistic classifier in which each token in the text is treated as conditionally independent, given the class. The conditional probability of a given token for a particular class is calculated using Laplace smoothing. We also use a version of MNB where we assume uniform priors (MNB-UP). This allows us to account for the heavy skew towards sentences being marked as irrelevant (c.f. [12,13]). In both models, before training and testing we apply the common pre-processing steps of removing stop words, stemming words using the Porter stemmer and removing words which only occur once in the training set.

Support Vector Machines. SVM classifiers are widely-used as an alternative to Naive Bayes for classifying text documents [16]. We build SVM models using Weka's[3] implementation of the Sequential Minimal Optimization (SMO) algorithm and our best models were produced without any text pre-processing.

AfPak Dataset Evaluation. Table 1 shows the results of our comparison of the models at identifying relevant sentences. The results show the limitation of the rule and pattern based approach as used by PETRARCH compared to machine learning. More than half the relevant sentences are not extracted by the PETRARCH system, and the best machine learning method showed a more than 3-fold improvement on its F1 score. Since we are using PETRARCH in its default form, there are several possible reasons for this. First, it may be discarding potentially relevant sentences as they do not match to known actors and locations in its dictionaries. Second, the form of the human annotated sentences may not match the forms it is configured to detect. Third, it may be discarding sentences which it is not able to classify according to the expanded form of the CAMEO ontology we used for annotatation. Although these issues could potentially be addressed by adding more rules and knowledge to the system, this illustrates the limitations of applying PETRARCH in domains differing from its "who did what to whom" definition of events.

In comparison, the supervised machine learning methods obtained higher levels of recall and precision. The MNB models had the best recall, and the SVM achieved highest precision. This is interesting as their performance in other domains is generally very evenly matched [12,16]. Furthermore, despite the low precision obtained by the MNB-UP classifier, it still correctly eliminated 89% of all irrelevant sentences which is a large aid to a human analyst.

[3] http://www.cs.waikato.ac.nz/ml/weka/.

Table 1. Sentence extraction - afpak dataset (Time-ordered train/test split)

	tp	*fn*	*fp*	*tn*	Recall	Precision	F1
PETRARCH	141	211	1,559	10,498	0.401	0.083	0.138
MNB	**213**	139	766	11,309	0.605	0.218	0.321
MNB-UP	**252**	100	1,303	10,772	**0.716**	0.162	0.264
SVM	156	196	172	11,903	0.443	**0.476**	**0.459**

Table 2. Sentence extraction - ICG DRC dataset (Mean 10-fold cross validation)

	tp	*fn*	*fp*	*tn*	Recall	Precision	F1
MNB	124.8	92.4	113.0	553.4	0.575	0.525	0.549
MNB-UP	**155.0**	62.2	188.3	477.7	**0.714**	0.452	**0.554**
SVM	98.4	118.8	93.2	572.8	0.453	**0.514**	0.482

ICG DRC Dataset Evaluation. Table 2 presents the results of our evaluation of the various models for identifying relevant sentences in the ICG DRC dataset. In this dataset, we used the models to classify *all* sentences, as relevant sentences were spread throughout the reports. However, we do not compare the machine learning models to the PETRARCH system as this dataset is not coded according to a CAMEO based ontology. These results show that recall for each of the classifiers in identifying relevant sentences is very similar to the results on the AfPak dataset. For the MNB models, precision is much higher than the AfPak dataset, which is possibly a consequence of the dataset containing a much higher proportion of relevant sentences.

4.2 Human Filtering of Relevant Sentences

After sentences have been classified as relevant or irrelevant, as in Fig. 4, a human coder is able to validate the output. To evaluate the relative contribution of a "human-in-the-loop" versus the automated process in removing irrelevant sentences, we simply assume the human coder eliminates any false positive classifications, resulting in maximum precision. Furthermore, the human coder may be able to select an important text snippet, that is, a specific portion of the sentence that more precisely expresses the event type or driver, and which is judged sufficient to determine the classification of the sentence. This text snippet could be a single word (such as 'attack') or a phrase (such as 'killed in a drone strike'). Again, in our evaluation of machine learning for sentence classification, we focus on recall and matching the classifications made by the human coder over precision, as this avoids the assumption that the human made a deliberate decision not to label a particular sentence in a particular manner. We note that if a human coder did not filter out the false positives, these would be classified in the next stage of the process which produces ontology labels for each sentence, resulting in a higher number of incorrectly labelled sentences.

4.3 Ontology Classification

The classification of sentences can be made at either the sentence level or the text snippet level. If a human in the process of filtering relevant sentences only accepts or rejects the sentences and provides no more filtering then the system can only operate at the sentence level. However, if a user is able to filter the sentence to the relevant text snippet then our classifier should have a higher recall as irrelevant tokens are manually filtered out.

To evaluate sentence classification, we construct models based on the two MNB approaches and the SVM approach. We then input into each model its corresponding true positive classifications from the previous stage of the process, assuming false positives are removed by a human coder. As each sentence may have multiple labels, our ontology classifiers are configured to produce the 3 most relevant classification labels, and use a modified definition of recall more suited to the multi-label setting. For each model, we define tc to be the number of correct labels within these top 3 labels and fc to be the number of correct labels that were not predicted by the model to be within the top 3 labels, summing over all sentences. We define the *relevant recall* of a model as the overall proportion of the correct labels that are found by the model:

$$\text{relevant recall} = \frac{tc}{tc + fc}$$

Let fs be the number of sentences for which the model produces no correct labels within the top 3. We define the *full sentence misclassification rate* as:

$$\text{full sentence misclassification rate} = \frac{fs}{|\text{Sentences Input}|}$$

The aim is high relevant recall and low full sentence misclassification rate.

Sentence Classification. Table 3 shows the results of this evaluation applied to the AfPak dataset in classifying the relevant sentences into our enhanced CAMEO ontology. These results show that the MNB-UP model produces the highest raw number of correct label classifications, although it has the lowest relevant recall. This first result is due to the model having the largest number of true positive relevant sentences supplied to it from the previous stage and the latter result suggests that the MNB-UP classifier is not as good in this

Table 3. Sentence classification - AfPak dataset

	Sentences input		Relevant recall				Fully misclassified sentences				
	Machine	Joint	Correct labels		Missed labels		Machine		Joint		Error reduction
MNB	979	213	260	72.2%	100	27.8%	811	82.8%	45	21.1%	74.5%
MNB-UP	1,555	252	**291**	71.5%	116	28.5%	1,362	87.6%	59	23.4%	73.3%
SVM	328	156	210	**78.1%**	59	21.9%	196	59.8%	24	15.4%	74.2%
MNB-UP + SVM	1,555	252	**323**	**79.4%**	84	20.6%	1,342	86.3%	39	15.5%	82.0%

Table 4. Sentence classification - ICG DRC dataset (Mean 10-fold cross validatior

	Sentences input		Relevant recall				Fully misclassified sentences				
	Machine	Joint	Correct labels		Missed labels		Machine		Joint		Error reduction
MNB	237.8	124.8	87.8	54.0%	74.6	46.0%	159.9	67.2%	46.9	37.6%	44.0%
MNB-UP	343.3	155.0	**109.1**	**56.0%**	85.8	44.0%	244.4	71.2%	56.1	36.2%	49.2%
SVM	191.6	98.4	71.0	53.9%	60.8	46.1%	129.4	67.5%	36.2	36.8%	45.5%

second stage. In contrast, the SVM model has the highest relevant recall and the lowest number of full sentence misclassifications. Using this result we form the hypothesis that the MNB-UP classifier is the best at identifying possible relevant sentences in the first stage of the process and the SVM classifier is the best performer at classifying relevant sentences into the ontology (on the AfPak dataset). To test this hypothesis we feed the MNB-UP's true positive result from the first stage into the SVM ontology classification model. This result is in the last row of Table 3 and shows that this approach produces the highest raw and relative number of correct labels. Importantly, we can see the effect of the human coder in filtering out irrelevant sentences prior to machine learning, which for MNB-UP + SVM gives an 82% reduction in full sentence misclassifications.

However, these results are not as pronounced on the ICG DRC dataset (shown in Table 4). On this dataset the MNB-UP classifier is the best performer in both stages of the classification process. Furthermore, the relevant recall rate in this dataset is much lower than the AfPak dataset evaluation; there is also a reduction in full sentence misclassifications, but it is not as large.

Text Snippet Classification. Our final evaluation considered whether the relevant recall rate would improve if a human annotator was able to extract only the relevant text snippet for classification into the ontology. Table 5 shows this evaluation on the AfPak dataset. This shows that for all models there is an increase in the number of correct labels predicted, with the largest increase in performance in the MNB-UP classifier, but at the expense of an increase in the full misclassified sentences rate. This suggests that although the relevant recall increases, the process by which the text snippet is selected can eliminate information from other sentences which were previously classified correctly. A similar but smaller increase in relevant recall is seen in the evaluation on the ICG DRC dataset in Table 6. In this dataset the number of fully misclassified

Table 5. Text snippet classification - AfPak dataset

	Sentences input	Relevant recall					Fully misclassified sentences	
	Joint	Correct labels		Gain	Missed labels		Joint	
MNB	213	279	77.5%	5.3%	81	22.5%	54	25.4%
MNB-UP	252	**333**	**81.8%**	**10.3%**	74	18.2%	60	23.8%
SVM	156	214	79.5%	1.4%	55	20.4%	39	25.0%

Table 6. Text snippet classification - ICG DRC dataset (Mean 10-fold cross validation)

	Sentences input	Relevant recall					Fully misclassified sentences	
	Joint	Correct labels		Gain	Missed labels		Joint	
MNB	124.8	90.8	57.2%	3.2%	68	42.8%	44.2	34.5%
MNB-UP	155.0	**114.5**	**58.7%**	2.7%	80.4	41.3%	49.4	31.8%
SVM	98.4	74.5	56.5%	2.6%	57.3	43.5%	31.4	31.9%

sentences decreases across all models. We conclude that with text snippets, classification is improved, but selecting only very specific words can result in a loss of contextual information and increase the number of fully misclassified sentences.

5 Related Work

With respect to existing approaches for this type of application, the Social, Political and Economic Event Database (SPEED) system [10] is the most similar. In this system human coders are presented with input data (documents) that has been automatically pre-processed and classified as relevant. It is then claimed that humans "perform only the most difficult coding decisions". The SPEED system is developed with a Naive Bayes classifier trained initially on 33,000 training documents. Relevant documents are then passed through a NLP pipeline which extracts people, locations and organisations. Human coders then check all the machine outputs. One of the key arguments of Nardulli et al. [10] for their approach is that menial work is handled by the machine and the cognitively challenging tasks are handled by the human. In developing their Naive Bayes model for selecting relevant documents their original document level true positive rate was 33% and was improved to 87% after an additional 60,000 training documents were added to the model. In our datasets, which trained relevant/irrelevant classification models at the sentence level we achieved a recall of 71% for both datasets with a MNB variant trained on a much smaller dataset. The finding that MNB is the best classifier for deciding relevance is consistent with the resuits of Nardulli et al. [10].

6 Conclusion

We have demonstrated that standard machine learning techniques can be applied to the problem extracting and classifying events and conflict drivers from news and NGO reports. This approach differs from previous work on event extraction in the social sciences that has focused on the use of rules for matching large dictionaries of actors, locations and specific verb phrases.

Recognizing the importance of human input to the coding process, we proposed a two-step "joint" process and showed experimentally that human input is effective when used to: (i) filter out irrelevant sentences from amongst those classified as relevant by an automated method, and (ii) select the correct classification(s) from a small number of suggestions given by a learning model. The models were tested using event data focusing on violent events in Afghanistan, and a dataset of conflict drivers in the Democratic Republic of the Congo.

Future work involves incorporating the process into a complete "pipeline" for ingestion of news, social media feeds and NGO reports, and storing events and drivers in a searchable database. Research will also address extracting the components of events (actors, targets, etc.), and the use of stream mining methods to extract information in real time, exploiting the temporal nature of the data.

Acknowledgements. This work was supported by Data to Decisions Cooperative Research Centre. We are grateful to Josie Gardner for labelling the ICG DRC dataset, and to Michael Burnside and Kaitlyn Hedditch for coding the AfPak event data.

References

1. Azar, E.E.: The conflict and peace data bank (COPDAB) project. J. Confl. Resolut. **24**, 143–152 (1980)
2. Bagozzi, B.E., Schrodt, P.A.: The dimensionality of political news reports. Paper Presented at the Second Annual General Conference of the European Political Science Association, Berlin (2012)
3. Bond, D., Bond, J., Oh, C., Jenkins, J.C., Taylor, C.L.: Integrated data for events analysis (IDEA): an event typology for automated events data development. J. Peace Res. **40**, 733–745 (2003)
4. Bond, D., Jenkins, J.C., Taylor, C.L., Schock, K.: Mapping mass political conflict and civil society: issues and prospects for the automated development of event data. J. Confl. Resolut. **41**, 553–579 (1997)
5. Gerner, D.J., Schrodt, P.A., Yilmaz, O., Abu-Jabr, R.: Conflict and mediation event observations (CAMEO): a new event data framework for the analysis of foreign policy interactions. Paper Presented at the Annual Meetings of the International Studies Association, New Orleans, LA (2002)
6. LaFree, G., Dugan, L.: Introducing the global terrorism database. Terrorism Political Violence **19**, 181–204 (2007)
7. Leetaru, K., Schrodt, P.A.: GDELT: global data on events, location, and tone, 1979–2012. Paper Presented at the Annual Meetings of the International Studies Association, San Francisco, CA (2013)
8. McClelland, C.: World Event/Interaction Survey (WEIS) Project 1966–1978. Inter-University Consortium for Political and Social Research (1978)
9. Murphy, K.: Machine Learning: A Probabilistic Perspective. MIT Press, Cambridge, MA (2012)
10. Nardulli, P.F., Althaus, S.L., Hayes, M.: A progressive supervised-learning approach to generating rich civil strife data. Sociol. Methodol. **45**, 148–183 (2015)
11. Raleigh, C., Linke, A., Hegre, H., Karlsen, J.: Introducing ACLED: an armed conflict location and event dataset special data feature. J. Peace Res. **47**, 651–660 (2010)
12. Rennie, J.D., Shih, L., Teevan, J., Karger, D.R.: Tackling the poor assumptions of Naive Bayes text classifiers. In: Proceedings of the Twentieth International Conference on Machine Learning, pp. 616–623 (2003)

13. Schneider, K.-M.: Techniques for improving the performance of Naive Bayes for text classification. In: Gelbukh, A. (ed.) CICLing 2005. LNCS, vol. 3406, pp. 682–693. Springer, Heidelberg (2005). doi:10.1007/978-3-540-30586-6_76
14. Schrodt, P.A., Davis, S.G., Weddle, J.L.: Political science: KEDS—a program for the machine coding of event data. Soc. Sci. Comput. Rev. **12**, 561–587 (1994)
15. Schrodt, P.A., Yonamine, J.E.: A guide to event data: past, present, and future. All Azimuth **2**(2), 5–22 (2013)
16. Wang, S., Manning, C.D.: Baselines and bigrams: simple, good sentiment and topic classification. In: Proceedings of the 50th Annual Meeting of the Association for Computational Linguistics: Short Papers, vol. 2, pp. 90–94 (2012)

Quality Prediction of Newly Proposed Questions in CQA by Leveraging Weakly Supervised Learning

Yuanhao Zheng[1(✉)], Bifan Wei[1], Jun Liu[1], Meng Wang[1], Weitong Chen[2], Bei Wu[1], and Yihe Chen[3]

[1] SPKLSTN Lab, Department of Computer Science, Xi'an Jiaotong University, Xi'an, China
yuanhaozheng521@gmail.com
[2] The University of Queensland, Brisbane, Australia
[3] The University of Toronto, Toronto, Canada

Abstract. Community Question Answering (CQA) websites provide a platform to ask questions and share their knowledge. Good questions in CQA websites can improve user experiences and attract more users. To the best of our knowledge, a few researches have been studied on the question quality, especially the quality of newly proposed questions. In this work, we consider that a good question is popular and answerable in CQA websites. The community features of questions are extracted automatically and utilized to acquire massive good questions. The text features and asker features of good questions are utilized to train our weakly supervised model based on Convolutional Neural Network to recognize good newly proposed questions. We conduct extensive experiments on the publicly available dataset from StackExchange and our best result achieves F1-score at 91.5%, outperforming the baselines.

Keywords: Question quality · Weakly supervised learning · CQA · CNN

1 Introduction

Community question answering (CQA) websites have attracted millions of users to share their knowledge by asking questions or providing answers. Popular CQA websites such as StackExchange[1], Yahoo Answer[2], Quora[3] and Zhihu[4] have become important knowledge sharing platforms and play an important role in new knowledge acquisition. The questions in CQA websites show a high variance in quality. The questions with high quality can improve the user experience and

[1] https://stackexchange.com/.
[2] answers.yahoo.com.
[3] www.quora.com.
[4] www.zhihu.com.

G. Cong et al. (Eds.): ADMA 2017, LNAI 10604, pp. 655–667, 2017.
https://doi.org/10.1007/978-3-319-69179-4_46

attract more users, even domain experts such as Yoshua Bengio[5]. Users are more willing to answer good questions and good questions are more likely to attract good answers in the future. In turn, good questions and answers attract more users. It is very important for CQA websites to recommend good questions to more users as soon as possible.

Many researchers have analyzed the answer quality [1,2] and recommend high quality answers for questions [3] in recent years. However, little attention has so far been paid to predicting the question quality, especially the newly proposed questions. In the paper, ***newly proposed questions*** refers the questions just been posted in a short time period (like an hour) which have not been answered by any users. The quality prediction of newly proposed questions is a key task for the development of CQA websites to attract more users. It is a challenge to discover the quality of newly proposed questions which are characterized as text features and asker features without community features, because the newly proposed questions have no answers, followers and other community activities.

In this work, we propose a novel model to predict the quality of newly proposed questions by leveraging weakly supervised learning with massive labeled questions. Based on the quality definition which is self-adapted to various domains, the text features and asker features are both utilized to train the proposed classification model which be applied for the quality prediction of newly proposed questions. **Our specific contributions include**:

(1) We propose a formalized quality definition for questions by community features, which can be self-adapted to domains and auto-trained in the model.
(2) We develop a weakly supervised learning model to identify high quality questions as well as predict the quality of newly proposed questions based on the text features and asker features.
(3) We conduct extensive experiments on the publicly available dataset and our best result achieves F1-score at 91.5%, outperforming the baselines.

For other parts of the paper, we first review the related work in Sect. 2. Then we introduce our methodology detailedly in Sect. 3. Next, the dataset and the experiment results are discussed in Sect. 4. Finally, we draw our conclusion in Sect. 5.

2 Related Work

The question quality and answer quality are two main aspects of quality research in CQA websites. However, to the best of our knowledge, a few researches have been done on question quality compared to answer quality [4–12].

Recent years, some researches have been engaged in predicting question quality. Some early researchers [3,13,14] focused on the quality of content in Yahoo! Answers. They asked domain experts to label the question quality on their datasets which contain 5,000 questions. Those researchers applied three different

[5] https://www.quora.com/profile/Yoshua-Bengio.

types of features to their classification models and finally achieved good classification results. However, models in those work may not be suitable to predict the quality of newly proposed questions which do not have any community features such as *Score*, *ViewCount* and *AnswerCount*. It may also be difficult to label numerous questions by human.

Therefore, some researchers [15,16] proposed a novel method to define and formalize the question quality with community features. They labeled the question quality based on the formalized definition. Meanwhile, the text features and asker features that are used for classification models have been proved effective by experimental results. For example, Ravi et al. [15] formalized the question quality with community features (*Score* and *ViewCount*) and employed models that capture the latent topical aspects of questions at three levels to train a classifier for quality prediction. However, the formalized definition of question quality may not be appropriate when the dataset contains questions from different domains since the evaluation criteria of question quality differs from domains.

3 Methodology

In this section, we propose a novel weakly supervised learning model to predict the quality of newly proposed questions in Fig. 1. During the training process of our model, we introduce the quality definition which is self-adapted to domains, as well as represent the text features and asker features for the existed questions. Based on the existed questions, we train the weakly supervised learning model, which can be employed to predict the quality of newly proposed questions.

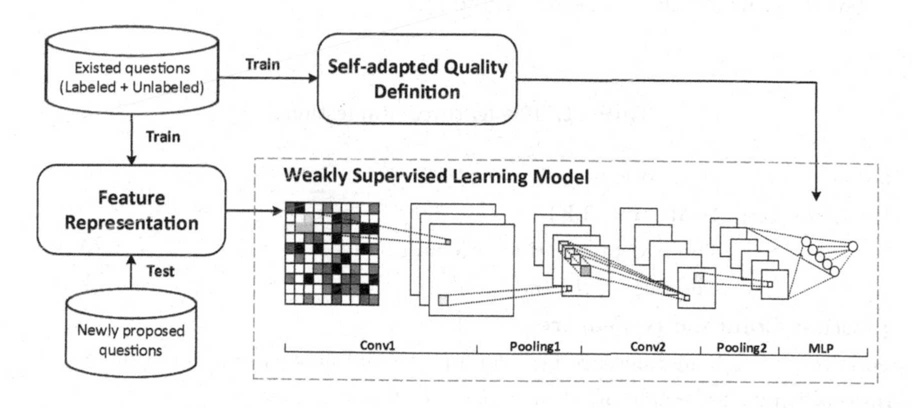

Fig. 1. The weakly supervised learning model in our work

3.1 Problem Definition

This work is to predict the quality of newly proposed questions in CQA websites based on the weakly supervised learning method. We denote the training set by $Q = \{q_1, q_2, \cdots, q_n\}$ where n is the total number of questions. The first l questions $Q_l = \{q_1, q_2, \cdots, q_l\}$ are labeled and the remaining ones, *i.e.*, $Q_u = \{q_{l+1}, q_{l+2}, \cdots, q_n\}$, are unlabeled questions whose labels are not given. Let $Y_l = \{y_1, y_2, \cdots, y_l\}$ be the label set of labeled questions Q_l where $y_i = 1$ when q_i is of high quality whereas $y_i = 0$ otherwise. We also denote the quality definition by $P = \{p_1, p_2, \cdots, p_l, p_{l+1}, \cdots, p_n\}$ for both Q_l and Q_u. Based on the Q and P, we train our weakly supervised learning model $\boldsymbol{M}$ as shown in Fig. 1. We also denote the newly proposed questions by $Q^+ = \{q_1^+, q_2^+, \cdots, q_m^+\}$ where m is the total number of newly proposed questions. The final quality label set for Q^+ is $Y^+ = \{y_1^+, y_2^+, \cdots, y_m^+\}$, where $y_i^+ = \boldsymbol{M}(q_i^+)$ refers to the predicted quality label for each newly proposed question $q_i^+ \in Q^+$.

3.2 Self-adapted Quality Definition

The features of questions in CQA websites can be broadly divided into question text features, question community features and asker features:

- *Question text features:* the *Content* and *Topic* of questions. The *Content* refers the natural language text of question body and question title while the *Topic* means the natural language tags of questions.
- *Question community features:* the *Score*, *AnswerCount* and *ViewCount* of questions. The *Score* can be divided into upvote and downvote of questions. The amount of answers under the question forms the *AnswerCount.*
- *Asker features:* the *Reputation* and *AnswerNumber* of askers. The *Reputation* denotes the reputation scores of askers which are built on the participation of askers in CQA websites. The *AnswerNumber* refers the total number of answers provided by the asker (Table 1).

Table 1. The features of questions

Name	Description	Symbol
Question Text Features (TF)		F_T
Content	The text of question title and body	X_i
Topic	The tags of the question	Y_i
Question Community Features (CF)		F_C
Score	The difference between upvote and downvote of question	s_i
AnswerCount	The amount of answer under the question	a_i
ViewCount	The page views of the question	v_i
Asker Features (AF)		F_A
Reputation	The reputation of the asker	ur_i
AnswerNumber	The answer count of the asker	ua_i

Based on the empirical analysis in StackExchange, we discover that the question quality is related to the question text features and question community features. It is time consuming to label high quality questions by reading all the question text. However, the community features can be acquired by programs easily. A question is defined as ***high quality*** if the question have more scores and answers, otherwise the question is defined as ***low quality***.

Because of the activity of CQA websites, *Score* and *AnswerCount* of questions are not only related to the quality but also related to the *ViewCount* of the question. For example, for some reason of CQA websites, if the question is recommended to be shown on the home page, the question will have more *Socre*, *AnswerCount* and *ViewCount* regardless of the quality of the question.

Therefore, for each question $q_i \in Q$, we introduce the quality definition

$$\begin{aligned} p_i &= S(\frac{\lambda \times s_i + \theta \times a_i}{v_i}) \\ &= \frac{1}{1 + e^{-(\lambda \times \frac{s_i}{v_i} + \theta \times \frac{a_i}{v_i})}} \end{aligned} \tag{1}$$

where p_i refers the quality score for question q_i and $S(x)$ means the sigmoid function which can be represented as $S(x) = \frac{1}{1+e^{-x}}$. The s_i, a_i and v_i are *Score*, *AnswerCount* and *ViewCount* of question q_i separately. For each domain, if users consider the question q_i as high quality question, they would upvote the question by n_i^+. Otherwise, they downvote the question by n_i^-. The *Score* of each question is then defined as $s_i = n_i^+ - n_i^-$. Meanwhile, domain users are more likely to answer good questions where a_i denotes whether the question is answerable.

λ and θ are alterable between domains indicating that question quality p_i should be varied between domains. For example, question q_1[6] with 2,437 scores, 26 answers and 2,688,565 views is of high quality in *StackOverflow*, while another good question q_2[7] in *Movie* has only 16 scores, 2 answers and 5,528 views. They have great differences in *Score*, *AnswerCount* and *ViewCount*. If we apply the same p_i to q_1 and q_2, q_2 might be a bad question compared to q_1. Therefore, the quality definition is different between domains.

However, the newly proposed questions do not have community features which means p_i is not available for them. We consider the question text features and asker features of newly proposed questions for quality prediction based on the trained model.

3.3 Feature Representation

Since community features such as the number of views would be unavailable for newly proposed questions, what we can acquire is the question text features (*TF*) and asker features (*AF*) such as question content and asker reputation. Therefore, we select *TF* and *AF* of each question as the input of our model.

[6] https://stackoverflow.com/questions/2334712/how-do-i-update-from-a-select-in-sql-server.

[7] https://movies.stackexchange.com/questions/72110/simpsons-episode-with-1000.

Question text features **(F_T)** refer to the text of the question title, the question body and the question topic tags. Questions are more likely to remain unanswered if they lack important information. In most cases, readable and comprehensible questions tend to attract users and answers. For example, question q_3[8] is a good question with 6,505 scores which is well expressed with a code snippet example. However, question q_4[9] is a bad question with -6 scores, which is too lengthy and complex to be understood by users.

In order to take full advantage of the semantic information in question content, we select the *Word2vec* model to produce word embeddings instead of topic model [15]. The *Word2vec* model is a two-layer neural network that is trained to reconstruct linguistic contexts of words. *Word2vec* takes a large corpus of text as its input and produces a vector space, with each unique word in the corpus assigned a corresponding vector in the space. We can then represent the question content or topics by word vectors.

Therefore, for each domain d, we use all questions within d as a corpus to train the vector space. The word is then presented as a vector of z (value is 200) dimension. For question $q_i \in Q$, we can represent the *Content* and the *Topic* as follows

$$X_i = \begin{bmatrix} vc_{11} & \cdots vc_{1z} \\ \vdots & \ddots \vdots \\ vc_{m_i 1} & \cdots vc_{m_i z} \end{bmatrix}, Y_i = \begin{bmatrix} vt_{11} & \cdots vt_{1z} \\ \vdots & \ddots \vdots \\ vt_{n_i 1} & \cdots vc_{n_i z} \end{bmatrix} \tag{2}$$

where m_i and n_i represent the word count and the topic count of q_i respectively. The k-th row of X_i denotes the z dimension vector $(vc_{k1}, vc_{k2}, \dots, vc_{kz})$ of the k-th word in question q_i. Since different q_i have different m_i, we unify m_i of each q_i to m. Similarly, we unify n_i of each q_i to n. Therefore, we apply

$$F_T = \begin{bmatrix} v_{11} & \cdots v_{1z} \\ \vdots & \ddots \vdots \\ v_{(m+n)1} & \cdots v_{(m+n)z} \end{bmatrix} \tag{3}$$

to represent the text features affecting the question quality. F_T is a $(m+n) \times z$ matrix which can combine the information of question content and topics.

Asker Features (F_A). For each question q_i, asker features including *Reputation* and *AnswerNumber* are also vital for quality prediction. *Reputation* denotes the reputation scores of askers which are built on the participation of askers in CQA websites. Askers with high reputations provide not only an essential contribution to CQA websites in general, but also the most helpful answers. For example, asker u_1[10] with 125,476 reputations has provided more good questions than asker u_2[11] who has only 83 reputations.

[8] stackoverflow.com/questions/231767/what-does-the-yield-keyword-do-in-python.
[9] stackoverflow.com/questions/37302912/command-not-working-in-an-interpreter-i-made.
https://stackoverflow.com/users/2901002/jezrael?tab=profile.
https://stackoverflw.com/users/5198106/m654?tab=profile.

Based on the analysis of asker features on the dataset, we use

$$F_A = ur_i + ua_i \tag{4}$$

to represent the asker features where ur_i and ua_i are normalized and range from 0 and 1. To combine TF and AF, we put forward the matrix T

$$T = F_T \times F_A = \begin{bmatrix} v'_{11} & \cdots v'_{1z} \\ \vdots & \ddots \vdots \\ v'_{(m+n)1} & \cdots v'_{(m+n)z} \end{bmatrix} \tag{5}$$

to represent the features of question q_i. Finally, for each question $q_i \in Q$ or $q_i^+ \in Q^+$, T refers to the $(m+n) \times z$ matrix of question text features and asker features. The newly proposed questions can also be represented by T whose quality could be predicted by the full trained model.

3.4 Weakly Supervised Learning Model

As we can see from our framework Fig. 1, we apply the convolutional neural network (CNN) (LeCun et al. 1998) to train a weakly supervised learning model which can predict the quality of newly proposed questions. Our CNN model is a classical structure containing two convolutional layers and two pooling layers. We set the convolutional window size as 5×5. The weights and the biases of two convolutional layers are W_i and b_i $(i = 1, 2)$ respectively. The pooling layers perform a downsampling operation along the spatial dimensions (width, height). We set the pooling window size as 2×2. The feature matrix T is the input of the CNN model for each question $q_i \in Q$ or $q_i^+ \in Q^+$. We can optimize the feature T of question q_i by the two convolutional and pooling layers. Finally, we acquire the feature matrix T' which is applied to the following fully connected layer.

The *MLP* is following the two convolutional layers and pooling layers in Fig. 1, which is a feedforward artificial neural network that maps sets of input data onto a set of appropriate outputs. The weights and the biases of *MLP* are W_j and b_j which are needed to be trained in the model. The sets $\boldsymbol{W}$ and $\boldsymbol{b}$ separately denote the weights and biases in the convolutional layers and the fully connected layers, which are iterated during the batch training of our CNN model.

For each question $q \in Q$, we can acquire its quality definition p and feature matrix T. If we assume that y_i refers to the quality of the labeled question, we can define each labeled question by $q = \{T_i, p_i, y_i\}$ as well as the unlabeled question by $q = \{T_j, p_j\}$. We assume the output of the *MLP* layer for each question $q \in Q$ in our CNN model is $r = MP(q)$ where r refers to the possibility of question q predicted as a *good* question or a *bad* question. Meanwhile, we define the target function of the model

$$Loss = \sum_{i=1}^{l}[f(r_i, p_i) + f(r_i, y_i)] + \sum_{j=1}^{n-l} f(r_j, p_j) \tag{6}$$

Algorithm 1. Quality Prediction Algorithm

Input: Q_d
Output: $\boldsymbol{M}(\boldsymbol{W}, \boldsymbol{b})$, λ, θ
  $Q_d = Q_l \cup Q_u, Q_l = \bigcup_{i=1}^{l} q_i, Q_u = \bigcup_{j=1}^{n-l} q_j$
  for each question $q \in Q_d$ **do**
    $p = S(\frac{\lambda \times s_i + \theta \times a_i}{v_i})$, by formula (1)
    $T = F_T \times F_A$, by formula (5)
    if q has label **then**
      $q = \{T_i, p_i, y_i\}$
    else
      $q = \{T_j, p_j\}$
    $r = MP(q)$, model output
  $loss = \sum_{i=1}^{l}[f(r_i, p_i) + f(r_i, y_i)] + \sum_{j=1}^{n-l} f(r_j, p_j)$, minimize target function
  optimize $(\boldsymbol{W}, \boldsymbol{b})$ during the batch training
  return $\boldsymbol{M}(\boldsymbol{W}, \boldsymbol{b})$, λ, θ

where p_i refers to the quality definition of the labeled question q_i and y_i represents the quality label. p_j refers to the quality definition of the unlabeled question. The $f(logits, labels)$ computes the softmax cross entropy between *logits* and *labels* which contains two steps. The first step is to compute the softmax for r_i which can acquire the probability of label as y_i'. The next step is to computes the cross entropy of y_i' and y_i. We summarize the two steps as follows.

$$\begin{aligned} softmax(r)_i &= \frac{e^{r_i}}{\sum_{j=1}^{K} e^{r_j}} \qquad for \quad i = 1, ..., K. \\ H(y', y) &= -\sum_{i}^{K} y_i log(y_i') \end{aligned} \tag{7}$$

As we can see, two aspects in our target function are optimized. $f(r_i, p_i)$ or $f(r_j, p_j)$ computes the prediction difference between our model and quality definition for labeled or unlabeled questions. $f(r_i, y_i)$ computes the prediction difference between our model and the human assessment. The target function is to enforce the quality definition and prediction result of the model to be close to human assessment. Meanwhile, we train our model with Q_l and Q_u by the weakly supervised learning method. The λ and θ in quality definition p_i can also be auto-trained during the optimization of the target function.

Finally, we can summarize our model for the prediction of question quality by the Algorithm 1. For the newly proposed questions Q^+, the model can predict their quality as $Y^+ = \{y_1^+, y_2^+, \cdots, y_m^+\}$, where y_i^+ refers to the predicted quality label for each newly proposed question $q_i^+ \in Q^+$.

4 Experiment

To verify the effectiveness of our model in predicting the quality of newly proposed questions, we conduct experiments on the dataset from *StackExchange*. For the 5 domains on the dataset, we also design comparative experiments on baselines to verify the effectiveness of the methods and the features we proposed.

4.1 Dataset

StackExchange is a prevalent network of CQA websites that contains more than 150 CQA websites involving various domains such as *Sports, Movies, Music* and so on. *StackOverflow* is one of those websites which is very popular among programmers. We select questions of 5 different domains as our dataset from *StackExchange*'s public data sets[12]. *Android*[13] and *StackOverflow* are related to science/technology, while *Movies*[14], *Music*[15] and *Sports*[16] are related to life/art.

Considering the difficulty of labeling the quality for all questions in five domains, we ask three experts to label small part of questions in each domain. Therefore, we define the dataset Q_d of each domain d

$$Q_d = Q_{tr} \cup Q_{te} = (\gamma Q_l \cup Q_u) \cup (1-\gamma)Q_l \tag{8}$$

where Q_{tr} is the training dataset, consisting of all the unlabeled questions Q_u and γ (for example 50%) of the labeled questions Q_l. Meanwhile, Q_{te} is the testing dataset which denotes the remaining $1-\gamma$ of the labeled questions. γ is a parameter referring the rate of labeled questions on the training dataset, which is changeable in our experiments. Table 2 shows the distribution of the labeled questions and the unlabeled questions within 5 domains.

Table 2. The distribution of labeled and unlabeled questions in 5 domains

Dataset	Labeled			Unlabeled	Labeled + Unlabeled
	Good	Bad	Good + Bad		
Android	3,232	7,375	10,607	30,816	41,423
StackOverflow	4,056	9,842	13,898	51,637	65,535
Movies	3,966	4,553	8,519	5,053	13,572
Music	1,218	1,725	2,943	6,222	9,165
Sports	96	443	539	2,678	3,217

[12] https://archive.org/details/stackexchange.
[13] https://android.stackexchange.com/.
[14] https://movies.stackexchange.com/.
[15] https://music.stackexchange.com/.
[16] https://sports.stackexchange.com/.

4.2 Baselines

We compare our weakly supervised learning model with the following methods:

- **Mutual Reinforcement Label Propagation (MRLP):** Li et al. [13] applied MRLP model to predict question quality by text features and user features in CQA websites. Here we adopt the same approach to predict question quality with *TF* and *AF*.
- **Topic Model:** Ravi et al. [15] employed three advanced topic models to predict question quality by considering the text, the length and the topics of questions in *StackOverflow*. We also conduct the topic model on our dataset to predict question quality with *TF*.
- **Stochastic Gradient Boosted Tree (SGBT):** Agichtein et al. [14] discovered that the stochastic gradient boosted trees (SGBT) outperform several classification models, such as SVM, to evaluate the content quality in CQA websites. Therefore, we apply the SGBT to predict question quality with *TF* and *AF* on our dataset.

Furthermore, to verify the necessity of considering *TF* and *AF* together, we also compare the results of our model by various features.

4.3 Performance Comparison

Table 3 shows the experiment results of our model compared with baselines on the dataset. Comparing the results of our model within different domains with various labeling rate γ (%) on the training dataset, we can summarize the following conclusions: (1) The model achieves the best F1-score at 91.5% in *StackOverflow* when γ is 80%. (2) For *Android*, *StackOverflow*, *Movies* and *Sports*

Table 3. F1-score of classification models compared in 5 domains

F1-score under labeling rate (%)		Domain				
		Android	StackOverflow	Movies	Music	Sports
20	Our model	0.775	0.762	0.743	0.725	0.701
	MRLP	0.601	0.637	0.574	0.608	0.559
	Topic model	0.613	0.679	0.657	0.625	0.586
	SGBT	0.565	0.594	0.0.603	0.542	0.531
50	Our model	0.857	0.864	0.834	**0.849**	0.769
	MRLP	0.652	0.686	0.623	0.654	0.601
	Topic model	0.667	0.724	0.702	0.677	0.624
	SGBT	0.621	0.638	0.645	0.603	0.586
80	Our model	**0.905**	**0.915**	**0.845**	0.801	**0.854**
	MRLP	0.673	0.696	0.643	0.664	0.609
	Topic model	0.682	0.758	0.721	0.702	0.658
	SGBT	0.655	0.668	0.679	0.631	0.621

domain, the best F1-score arises when $\gamma = 80\%$. *Music* domain achieves the best performance when $\gamma = 50\%$. (3) For each domain, the F1-score is gradually increasing with the increase of labeling rate γ of the training dataset.

Comparing the result of MRLP, Topic Model, SGBT and our model on our dataset, we can draw the following conclusions: (1) The F1-score of our model outperforms baselines obviously within each domain by a significant amount. (2) For MRLP, Topic Model and our model, the F1-score achieves the best results within *StackOverflow* domain, while SGBT achieves the best classification result within *Movies* domain.

Table 4. Assessment criteria of classification models in *StackOverflow*

Assessment criteria	Model			
	Our model	MRLP	Topic model	SGBT
Precision	0.988	0.823	0.921	0.604
Recall	0.852	0.588	0.644	0.722
F1-score	0.915	0.696	0.758	0.658

Table 4 shows the precision, recall and F1-score of four models in *StackOverflow* domain when the labeling rate is 80%. The precision is higher than recall in our model, MRLP and Topic Model indicating that those models are better at predicting quality of the good questions which can help websites recommend good questions to users.

4.4 Feature Analysis

In order to analyze the importance of *TF* and *AF* employed in our model, we conduct our quality prediction model on *TF*, *AF* as well as both *TF* and *AF* separately. Figure 2 shows the F1-score of our model considering various features, which can imply the three conclusions: (1) For each domain, the combination of *TF* and *AF* performs better in our model than just considering *TF* or *AF* only. (2) The F1-score of our model based on *TF* is higher than that on *AF* within each domain, indicating that *TF* can be more vital for quality prediction than *AF*. (3) We can achieve the best classification result of our model within *StackOverflow* domain in three cases comparing with the other four domains.

All in all, our model can achieve better result than baselines since our quality definition is self-adapted to domains which can be auto-trained in our model. The combination of *TF* and *AF* can also improve the F1-score of our model than applying only one of them. Furthermore, we can get λ and θ in quality definition for each domain, which can give a quality score to the question. Table 5 also shows the value of λ and θ, different between domains, after our model is trained.

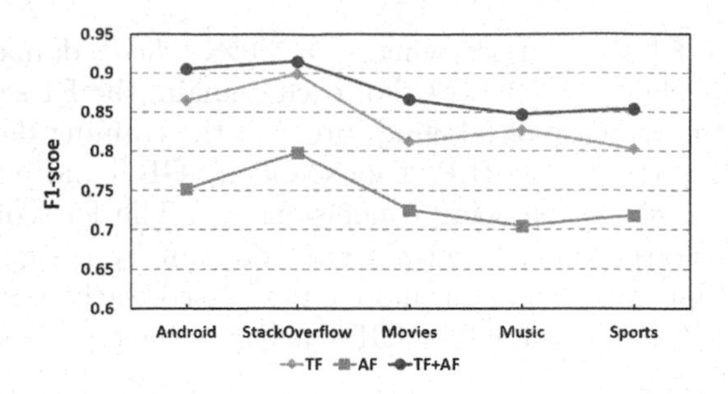

Fig. 2. F1-score of our model with various features

Table 5. The value of λ and θ in quality definition

Parameters	Android	StackOverflow	Movies	Music	Sports
λ	1.00	1.38	1.24	0.68	0.77
θ	2.15	3.43	2.85	1.16	1.68

5 Conclusion

In this paper, we focus on the quality prediction of newly proposed questions based on the weakly supervised learning model. We define and formalize the question quality, which is self-adapted to domains, by question community features. Meanwhile, based on acquired question text features and asker features, we analyze and represent those features by a feature matrix for each question. We propose our quality prediction model based on CNN and train the model on labeled and unlabeled datasets by weakly supervised learning.

We experiment with the StackExchange dataset and the results demonstrate that our model is more effective than MRLP, Topic Model and SGBT within each domain. We also compared the F1-score of our model by considering different features and the results indicate that the combination of *TF* and *AF* is necessary and vital for quality prediction. Furthermore, *TF* is more useful for quality prediction than *AF* according to the results. All in all, our model is capable of performing well on the quality prediction of newly proposed questions.

In future work, we will continue to modify our CNN model to improve the F1-score of our model. Then, we want to consider the answer quality and question quality together in the quality prediction model.

Acknowledgments. This work is sponsored by The Fundamental Theory and Applications of Big Data with Knowledge Engineering under the National Key Research and Development Program of China with grant number 2016YFB1000903, Ministry of Education Innovation Research Team No. IRT 17R86, Innovative Research Group of the National Natural Science Foundation of China (61721002); National Science Foundation of China under Grant Nos. 61672419, 61532004, 61532015, the MOE Research Program for Online Education under Grant No. 2016YB166.

References

1. Jeon, J., Croft, W.B., Lee, J.H., Park, S.: A framework to predict the quality of answers with non-textual features. In: Proceedings of the 29th Annual International ACM SIGIR Conference on Research and Development in Information Retrieval, pp. 228–235. ACM (2006)
2. Shah, C., Pomerantz, J.: Evaluating and predicting answer quality in community QA. In: Proceedings of the 33rd International ACM SIGIR Conference on Research and Development in Information Retrieval, pp. 411–418. ACM (2010)
3. Bian, J., Liu, Y., Zhou, D., Agichtein, E., Zha, H.: Learning to recognize reliable users and content in social media with coupled mutual reinforcement. In: Proceedings of the 18th International Conference on World Wide Web, pp. 51–60. ACM (2009)
4. Ko, J., Nyberg, E., Si, L.: A probabilistic graphical model for joint answer ranking in question answering. In: Proceedings of the 30th Annual International ACM SIGIR Conference on Research and Development in Information Retrieval, pp. 343–350. ACM (2007)
5. Blooma, M.J., Chua, A.Y., Goh, D.H.-L.: A predictive framework for retrieving the best answer. In: Proceedings of the 2008 ACM Symposium on Applied Computing, pp. 1107–1111. ACM (2008)
6. Harper, F.M., Raban, D., Rafaeli, S., Konstan, J.A.: Predictors of answer quality in online Q&A sites. In: Proceedings of the SIGCHI Conference on Human Factors in Computing Systems, pp. 865–874. ACM (2008)
7. Suryanto, M.A., Lim, E.P., Sun, A., Chiang, R.H.: Quality-aware collaborative question answering: methods and evaluation. In: Proceedings of the Second ACM International Conference on Web Search and Data Mining, pp. 142–151. ACM (2009)
8. Le, L.T., Shah, C., Choi, E.: Evaluating the quality of educational answers in community question-answering. In: 2016 IEEE/ACM Joint Conference on Digital Libraries (JCDL), pp. 129–138. IEEE (2016)
9. Liu, H., Huang, J., An, C., Fu, X.: Answer quality prediction joint textual and non-textual features. In: 13th Web Information Systems and Applications Conference, 2016, pp. 144–148. IEEE (2016)
10. Suggu, S.P., Goutham, K.N., Chinnakotla, M.K., Shrivastava, M.: Deep feature fusion network for answer quality prediction in community question answering. arXiv preprint arXiv:1606.07103 (2016)
11. Luo, M., Nie, F., Chang, X., Yang, Y., Hauptmann, A.G., Zheng, Q.: Adaptive unsupervised feature selection with structure regularization. IEEE Trans. Neural Netw. Learn. Syst. **PP**(99), 1–13 (2017)
12. Luo, M., Chang, X., Yang, Y., Nie, L., Hauptmann, A.G., Zheng, Q.: Simple to complex cross-modal learning to rank, arXiv preprint arXiv:1702.01229 (2017)
13. Li, B., Jin, T., Lyu, M.R., King, I., Mak, B.: Analyzing and predicting question quality in community question answering services. In: Proceedings of the 21st International Conference on World Wide Web, pp. 775–782. ACM (2012)
14. Agichtein, E., Castillo, C., Donato, D., Gionis, A., Mishne, G.: Finding high-quality content in social media. In: Proceedings of the 2008 International Conference on Web Search and Data Mining, pp. 183–194. ACM (2008)
15. Ravi, S., Pang, B., Rastogi, V., Kumar, R.: Great question! question quality in community Q&A. In: ICWSM, vol. 14, pp. 426–435 (2014)
16. Baltadzhieva, A., Chrupala, G., Angelova, G., Bontcheva, K., Mitkov, R.: Predicting the quality of questions on stackoverflow. In: RANLP, 2015, pp. 32–40 (2015)

Improving Chinese Sentiment Analysis via Segmentation-Based Representation Using Parallel CNN

Yazhou Hao[1], Qinghua Zheng[1], Yangyang Lan[1], Yufei Li[1], Meng Wang[1], Sen Wang[2], and Chen Li[1](✉)

[1] SPKLSTN Lab, Department of Computer Science and Technology, Xi'an Jiaotong University, No. 28, Xianning West Road, Xi'an 710049, Shaanxi, People's Republic of China
yazhouhao@gmail.com, {qhzheng,cli}@xjtu.edu.cn, {lanyangyang,vermouth,wangmengsd}@stu.xjtu.edu.cn

[2] Griffith University Gold Coast Campus, Gold Coast, Australia
sen.wang@griffith.edu.au

Abstract. Automatically analyzing sentimental implications in texts relies on well-designed models utilizing linguistic features. Therefore, the models are mostly language-dependent and designed for English texts. Chinese is with the largest users in the world and has a tremendous amount of texts daily generated from the social media, etc. However, it has seldom been studied. On another hand, a general observation, which is valid in many languages, is that different segments of a piece of text, e.g. a clause, having different sentimental polarities. The existing deep learning models neglect the imbalanced sentiment distribution and only take the entire piece of the text. This paper proposes a novel sentiment-analysis model, which is capable of sentiment analysis task in Chinese. Firstly, the model segments a text into smaller units according to the punctuations to obtain the preliminary text representation, and this step is so-called segmentation-based representation. Meanwhile, its new framework parallel-CNN (convolutional neural network) simultaneously use all segments. This model, we call SBR-PCNN, concatenate the representation of each segment to obtain the final representation of the text which does not only contain the semantic and syntactic features but also retains the essential sequential information. The proposed method has been evaluated on two Chinese sentiment classification datasets and compared with a broad range of baselines. Experimental results show that the proposed approach achieves the state of the art results on two benchmarking datasets. Meanwhile, they demonstrate that our model may improve the performance of Chinese sentiment analysis.

Keywords: Sentiment analysis · Deep learning · CNN · Chinese

yazhouhao@gmail.com (Y. Hao)—Contact email address.

G. Cong et al. (Eds.): ADMA 2017, LNAI 10604, pp. 668–680, 2017.
https://doi.org/10.1007/978-3-319-69179-4_47

1 Introduction

Sentiment analysis is an active research area in natural language processing in recent years, which studies people's opinions, sentiments and emotions toward entities or events and their subjective attributes expressed in text [1]. In the past few years, with the rapid development of internet technology, billions of people around the world use the Internet services like microblogging and e-commerce daily, e.g. Twitter, Facebook, and Amazon. These activities generate a tremendous volume of valuable data across different domains such as biomedical, sports and finance. The sentiment analysis based on these user-generated data is beneficial to many domain-specific tasks such as market analysis, decision making and it has attracted more and more attention from both academic and industrial community. One of the main research lines of sentiment analysis is to identify the polarity of a whole sentence or document such as positive, negative and neutral. Since early 2002, Pang et al. [2] and Turney [3] have applied machine learning methods to this field that combine both linguistic and statistic features of textual content with shallow classifiers such as support vector machine (SVM) or naive Bayes (NB). They treat this problem as a classification task. This type of methods is based on the linguistic features extracted from the textual content of sentences or documents and is time and labor consuming. Many existing works following the research line have focused on utilizing hand designed features from text [4–6]. In particular, Mohammad et al. [6] exploited this kind of strategy and built the top-performing system in the Twitter sentiment classification track of SemEval 2013 [7]. With the revitalization of deep learning, people apply more and more deep learning models [8–10] to this field. Exploiting the distributed representation of words and the compositionality of language to solve sentiment classification problem is another promising approach [11,12]. Convolutional neural network (CNN) and recurrent neural network (RNN) or their variants are fundamental components in deep models which can exploit supervised or unsupervised strategy to learn discriminative features (also known as representation) and then classify the polarity of text. Deep models have achieved the state of the art performance. Meanwhile, more and more competitive models are springing up. There are fewer research works which focused on Chinese sentiment analysis than sentiment analysis in general language (i.e., English), but the main direction of research in this field is just like case mentioned above.

Although deep learning methods have achieved remarkable performances, some problems still exist in this kind of models. The first one is that most of the existing works treat a text, e.g. a sentence or a document, as a whole unit, i.e. considering each segment in a text equally while disregarding the difference between different segments in the text. The above approach is a relatively coarse-grained approach which ignores the characteristics of each segment in some aspects, e.g. semantic, syntactic, and expressed sentiment polarities by each segment. In most cases, different segments in a text reveal different polarities, along the sequence of text, the different polarities interact with each other and compose the final sentiment polarity of a text. The second one comes from the architecture of CNN which consists of many cross convolutional layers and pooling operations, these cross operations can not make sure that critical information included in each segment of text would be transmitted to the final representation layer, i.e. they treat the text as a whole and then CNN can not learn the discriminative enough representation of the text for sentiment classification. The problem could be demonstrated by the following sentences:

Example 1. 苹果6屏幕和音质很好，外形也好看。可以作为一种选择，但是它性价比不高。看来我的信用卡额度已经强迫我做出了选择。
(The screen and sound quality of iPhone 6 are nice, appearance is also stylish. It could be a choice, but it is low cost-effective. The limitation of my credit card has forced me to make a choice.)

Example 2. 家庭作业很难, 我周围每个人都很不开心的样子.当然, 其中不包括我。
(The homework is very challenging, everyone around me seems not happy. Of course, except me.)

The term segment is referred to a text segment according to the punctuations. The examples mentioned above clearly show that different segments of a text express sentiment polarity differently. In *Example 1*, sentiment polarities of the segments could be: "positive, positive, positive, negative, negative", and the global polarity is negative. In *Example 2*, sentiment polarities can be labeled as: "negative, negative, negative", and the global polarity of this sentence is negative. This phenomenon is more significant in Chinese sentiment analysis because that Chinese is a character-based language which is ambiguous and has flexible compositionality. Another observation is that almost every single segment of a text has a relatively local, self-contained and independent information about sentiment. Information in a segment is self-contain to some degree, and different information of these segments influence each other. Thus, treating a text based on a view of segmentation instead of treating a text as a whole is intuitive.

Based on the observations, we propose a novel way to deal with this case in this paper. Particularly, segmentation based on punctuations generates several segments of a text, and we order these segments sequentially as they were in the original text, then feed each segment parallelly to multiple CNN simultaneously. After learning features of every segment of the text simultaneously, the feature vectors are concatenated while respecting the original order to obtain the final representation of the text. The final representation is taken to the fully connected network and the softmax layer output the classification results. The final representation may contains semantic and syntactic features like what existing methods do, but also make sure that the information in each text segment can be embedded in the final representation. Sequential information of the original text has been embedded because of the sequential concatenation which plays an important role seems like a RNN. Thus, through the procedure mentioned above, we can obtain a better representation than some conventional methods for sentiment classification.

We evaluate the effectiveness of our approach empirically on two benchmarking datasets. The first one is *ChnSentiCorp-4000* dataset introduced by Zhai et al. [13]. The second one is *IT168TEST* dataset consist of product reviews presented by Carroll and Zagibalov [14]. We compare our method with baselines including CNN with multi-channel [8], radical-embedding based methods [15] and self-training [16]. Experimental results show that the proposed approach achieves state of the art results. This show that segmentation of text (sentence or document) can improve the performance of Chinese sentiment analysis.

The main contributions of our method have two folds:

- We propose a novel two-step framework for Chinese sentiment classification by dividing a text into several segments via segmentation based on punctuations. Through the first process, we get a preliminary representation of the text, in which every word is represented as the word vector. The Word vectors that were used here is so-called pre-trained word vectors obtained by word2vec[1]. There can be two settings in this setup: (1) First setting is the whole original text itself isn't a part of the preliminary representation of input text, i.e. the original input text itself won't be fed to parallel CNN and only each segment draw from it will be. (2) We combine both the input text and its segments to obtain the prime representation of the text. Results draw from above process will be feed to parallel CNN to learn the final representation of text for sentiment classification.
- While most conventional deep learning methods treat input text as a whole, especially for sentences, we demonstrate that every single segment in a text plays a local, relatively complete and critical role on sentiment, not only we should make sure that information in every single text segment should be transmitted to the final representation layer, but also we should treat them separately in stead of taking them as a whole. We have validated in our experiments that segmentation-based parallel CNN would result in performance gains in Chinese sentiment classification.

The rest of this paper is organized as follows. In Sect. 2, we discuss the related works about text representation on different levels such as word embedding, sentence and document representation, the convolutional neural network for sentiment classification and some particular works for Chinese sentiment classification. In Sect. 3, we describe our segmentation-based approach in detail. Section 4 presents our datasets, experiment results, and some discussion. Finally, in Sect. 5, we conclude our work and outline the future research directions from our view.

2 Related Work

Sentiment analysis is a "suitcase" research problem which requires many NLP sub-tasks, such as word embedding and convolutional neural network.

2.1 Word Embedding and Text Representation

Word embedding is a vector-based distributed representation of words according to distributional assumption [17] which consist of low dimensional, continuous and dense vectors. Bengio et al. [18] firstly introduced a neural language model

[1] https://code.google.com/archive/p/word2vec/.

that can generate word embedding as a side effect. Ever since then, there have been many works that focus on topics related to word embedding such as [19–23]. Many works in sentiment analysis have exploited word embedding as pre-trained word vectors in the input of their model [8,9,24].

Generally, in most cases, text representation means sentence or document representation. There are three main directions in this research field. The first one is composing the word embeddings of words to obtain text representation based on the compositionality of natural language. The second one is directly through an unsupervised task based on a tremendous amount of unlabeled data. The third one is by a supervised task which utilizing a fine-tuned deep learning model such as CNN or RNN. In this paper, we chose the first way to obtain a preliminary representation, then choose the third way to learn the final one for sentiment classification.

2.2 Convolutional Neural Network

Convolutional neural network [25] has been widely evaluated in many works about sentiment analysis [8,9,26]. The structure of a convolutional neural network in different research works varies slightly. The basic structure of CNN utilized in sentiment analysis is shown in Fig. 1. The context of the following content based on segmentation and regard text segment as the core unit of processing, case in sentence or document is the same with here.

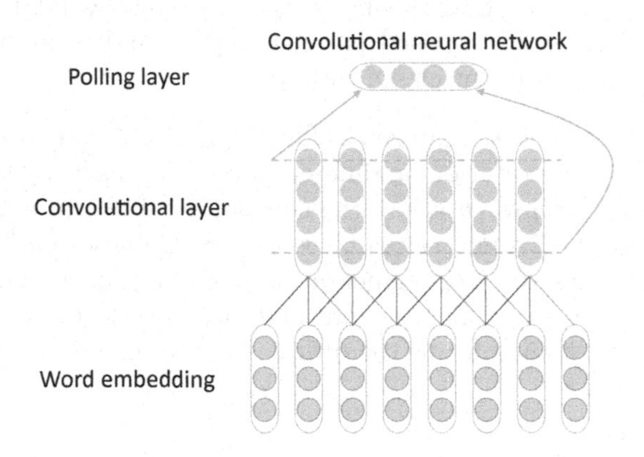

Fig. 1. The basic structure of CNN. There are *word embedding* layer, *convolutional* layer and *pooling* layer from bottom to top.

Convolutional Layer. Convolution can be regarded as a feature extractor which can extract local features from the text. It has some advantages than fully connected such as fewer parameters because of sharing weights. Its performance in sentiment analysis has already been evaluated in works as mentioned earlier. Let l and d be the length of a sentence and word vector respectively. Let $\boldsymbol{x}_i \in \mathbb{R}^d$

be the word vector with $d - dimensional$ corresponding to the $i - th$ word $\boldsymbol{w}_i$ in the sentence. Then a text segment of length n can be represented as

$$\boldsymbol{x}_1^n = \boldsymbol{x}_1 \oplus \boldsymbol{x}_2 \cdots \oplus \boldsymbol{x}_n, \tag{1}$$

in which $\oplus$ is the concatenation operator, $\boldsymbol{x}_1^n \in \mathbb{R}^{hd}$. Generally, we refer to $\boldsymbol{x}_i^j$ as the concatenation of word vectors $\boldsymbol{x}_i, \boldsymbol{x}_{i+1}, \cdots, \boldsymbol{x}_{i+j}$. Convolution operation can be viewed as a feature extraction process involves a convolutional kernel $\boldsymbol{W} \in \mathbb{R}^{hd}$ with size of h, which is applied to a window of h words to produce a new feature. For instance, a feature c_i is generated from a window of words w_i^{i+h-1} by

$$\boldsymbol{c}_i = \sigma\left(\boldsymbol{W} \odot \boldsymbol{x}_i^{i+h-1} + \boldsymbol{b}\right) \tag{2}$$

where $\boldsymbol{b} \in \mathbb{R}$ is a bias term and σ is a non-linear activation function such as sigmoid function, ReLU [27]. $\odot$ is element-wise product of matrices. The concolutional kernel is applied to each possible window of words in a segment to produce a *feature map*: $\boldsymbol{c} = [\boldsymbol{c}_1, \boldsymbol{c}_2, \cdots, \boldsymbol{c}_{l-h+1}]$, $\boldsymbol{c} \in \mathbb{R}^{l-h+1}$

Pooling Layer. After the convolution operation, we apply a pooling process over the feature map to capture the most salient feature. There are four strategies: max pooling, average pooling, k-max pooling and dynamic k-max pooling [9]. In this paper, we adopt max pooling strategy. Pooling can be regarded as a feature selection in natural language processing. The operation is as follows:

$$\hat{c} = max[\boldsymbol{c}_1, \boldsymbol{c}_2, \cdots, \boldsymbol{c}_{l-h+1}] \tag{3}$$

2.3 Chinese Sentiment Classification

Chinese is a character-based language which is very ambiguous and has flexible compositionality. There is no specific space for segmentation in Chinese text, and researchers firstly adopt a segmentation tool of Chinese, then process and analysis the result of segmentation as English text. There have been many works which exploited hand-designed features for sentiment classification [13,28–30]. Some other researchers have developed novel approaches by combining the compositional characteristic of Chinese with deep learning models [15,31,32]. To our best knowledge, the approach proposed in this paper firstly combines the segmentation-based representation of text and parallel CNN for Chinese sentiment classification.

3 Model

The overall architecture of our approach is shown in Fig. 2. We first describe the SBR[2] of text and two settings corresponding to it (Sect. 3.1), then we describe the PCNN[3] and the sequential concatenation layer (Sect. 3.2).

[2] Abbreviation of segmentation-based representation.

[3] Abbreviation of the parallel convolutional neural network.

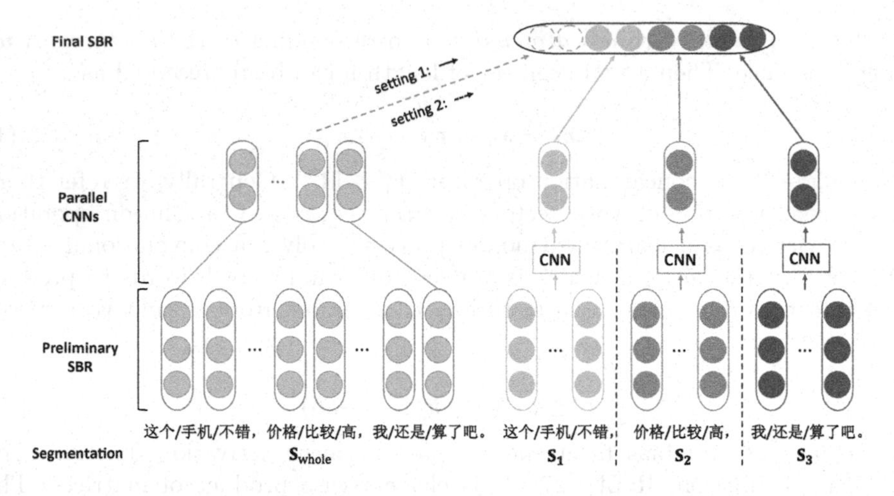

Fig. 2. The overall architecture of proposed model.

3.1 Segmentation-Based Representation

The illustration of SBR is shown in Fig. 3. We divide each text into several segments according to the punctuations in the text as we have stated before. Every single segment draws from the text has relatively complete and local sentiment information and interact with each other. There are two reasons for tackling sentiment classification via the segmentation-based model. The first one is that in many cases, the basic unit of expressing sentiment polarity is text segment rather than a word or several words, especially for long text such document or a long sentence. Only a word or several words can't supply enough context information for extracting informative features. It means we should compose the informative features of a segment to obtain the final representation of the whole text instead of just composing the n-gram features. Another reason comes from the convolutional neural network itself. Every convolutional kernel has a fixed size and can only handle a limited region of text, then these features extracted

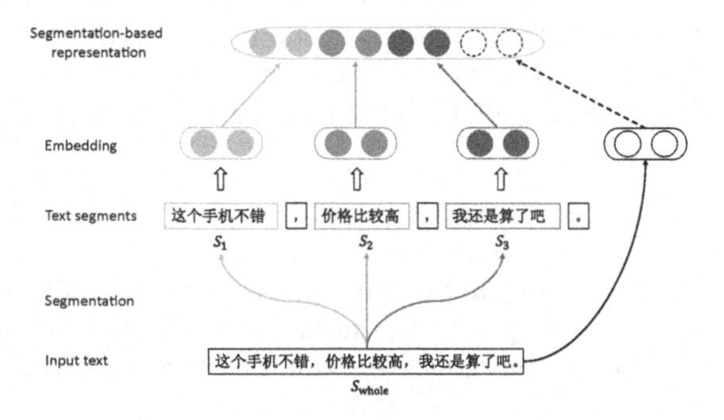

Fig. 3. The illustration of SBR.

by many kernels go through several interlaced convolutional layers and pooling layers. This process will directly get the final text representation which lost the sequential information, nevertheless, what involved in the final text representation is the composition of n-gram features extracted by kernels with a fixed size rather than the segment features. According to the mentioned above, it is intuitive that segmentation-based method may be a better choice than the existing methods which treating the text as a whole.

In addition, there are two settings in SBR. The first is combine the whole text and text segments. The second is only utilize text segments.

3.2 Parallel Convolutional Neural Network

PCNN means that all the representations of text segments are fed to convolutional neural networks corresponding to them parallelly and simultaneously. One convolutional neural network is applied to a text segment to extract the informative features, and before the concatenation layer, all of the CNNs are independent of each other. This architecture is flexible and could have more capacity. In the concatenation layer, we concatenate all the learned representations of text segments in their original order so that we can maintain the sequential information of the text. Many research works that apply CNN to text for sentiment classification can't obtain long dependency sequential information which parallel CNN can capture in concatenation layer.

4 Data and Experimental Setup

We evaluate the proposed model on two benchmarking datasets as follows:

- IT168TEST
  It contains more than 2000 reviews of mobile phones on IT168[4] which is a professional website for shopping guide for IT products.
- ChnSentiCorp-4000
  It contains 4000 hotel reviews on Ctrip[5] which is one of the most popular sites for booking hotel.

More statistics information is shown in Tables 1 and 2.

Table 1. Statistics of sentiment polarity.

Dataset	Positive reviews	Negative reviews
IT1687TEST	1159	1158
ChnSentiCorp-4000	2000	2000

[4] http://www.it168.com/.
[5] https://www.ctrip.com.

Table 2. Summary statistics of the two datasets.

Dataset	TC	Len	N	$\lvert V\rvert$	$\lvert V_{pre}\rvert$	$\lvert N_{test}\rvert$	Min_{len}	Max_{len}
IT168TEST	2	67	2317	10553	7577	CV	1	678
ChnSentiCorp-4000	2	91	4000	15499	12609	CV	2	1372

Here is the detailed description of Table 2. TC: Number of the target class. Len: Average text length. N: Number of text in the dataset. $\lvert V\rvert$: Number of words in the dataset. $\lvert V_{pre}\rvert$: Number of words presented in the pre-trained word vectors. $\lvert N_{test}\rvert$: Test set size. (CV means 10-fold CV was used). Min_{len}: Minimum text length. Max_{len}: Maximum text length.

4.1 Pre-trained Word Vectors

Initializing word vectors with those obtained from an unsupervised task has been proved that can improve the performance on sentiment classification task [8,9]. But different from the English, before training word vectors on Chinese corpus, we also need some extra preprocessing, including TC/SC[6], filtering non-UTF8 characters, word segmentation, etc. Then, we trained word2vec model (Skip-gram architecture) on Chinese wiki corpus[7] which has a size of 1.34 GB. The dimension of word vectors we set in the experiment is [50, 100, 150, 200, 250, 300, 350, 400, 450, 500] for an empirical analysis, window size equals 8. The number of word vectors we learned is 4,611,475. Words not present in the set of pre-trained words are initialized randomly.

4.2 Hyper Parameters and Training Settings

For all datasets we use: rectified linear units, size of convolutional kernel (h) is $3, 4, 5$ with 100 feature maps each, dropout rate (p) of 0.5, l_2 norm constraint of 3, batch size is 20, learning rate is 0.8, dimension of word vectors is 300 and epochs for iteration is 25. We didn't perform any tuning for a specific dataset. Training is done with the Adadelta update rule [33].

We utilized the punctuations in a text to divide the text into several segments. The punctuations list is [， 。 ： ； ！ ？] and the statistics of punctuation in datasets are shown in Fig. 4. According to the statistic information of punctuations, we know that the number of punctuations included in a text is between 4 and 12. Thus we divided each text into 5 to 13 segments. We achieved the best results when the text was divided into 9 segments.

[6] Translate simplified Chinese to traditional Chinese.

[7] https://dumps.wikimedia.org/zhwiki/latest/zhwiki-latest-pages-articles.xml.bz2.

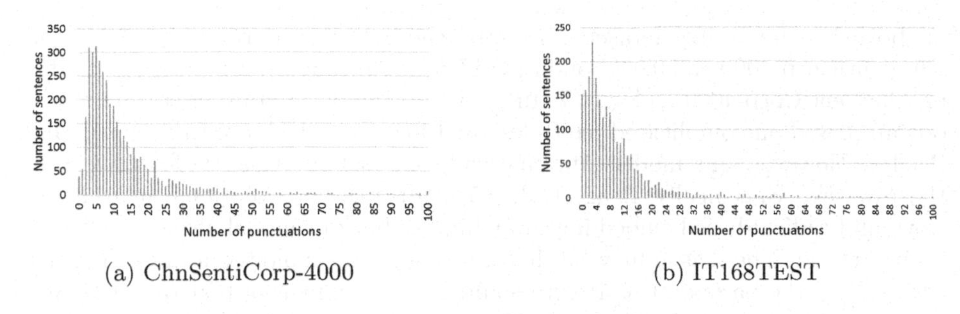

(a) ChnSentiCorp-4000 (b) IT168TEST

Fig. 4. Statistics of punctuations in datasets.

4.3 Model Variations

We experiment with several variations of the SBR-PCNN[8] according to different settings of SBR.

- SBR-PCNN-S: This model builds on the second setting of SBR, i.e. we only utilize the text segments to obtain the SBR.
- SBR-PCNN-H: This model builds on the first setting of SBR, i.e. we combine the input text and its segments simultaneously to obtain a hybrid SBR.

We trained two variants with the same experimental setup.

5 Results Analysis and Discussion

Results of our models against the other methods are listed in Table 3. Our SBR-PCNN-S model outperforms most of the other feature-based models on two benchmarking datasets. SBR-PCNN-H model achieves the best results

Table 3. Results of our SBR-PCNN models against other methods.

Models	ChnSentiCorp-4000		IT168TEST	
	Macro-F1	Accuracy	Macro-F1	Accuracy
Tan and Zhang [28]	88.58	-	-	-
Zagibalov and Carroll [14]	-	-	88.86	-
Zhai et al. [13]	**88.60**	**88.60**	80.90	81.30
Zhang and He [16]	-	-	**94.02**	**95.0**
Peng et al. [15]	87.02	-	84.33	-
SBR-PCNN-S	94.15	94.33	94.60	94.95
SBR-PCNN-H	**94.21**	**94.54**	**95.16**	**95.54**

[8] Abbreviation of segmentation-based representation and parallel convolutional neural network.

on both benchmarking datasets. Notably, the accuracy is raised by 5.94% on ChnSentiCorp-4000 and 0.54% on IT168TEST. The macro-F1 is raised by 5.61% on ChnSentiCorp-4000 and 1.14%. In addition, the other state of the art methods are based on complicated hand-designed features which are time-consuming [13,16]. However, our models automatically extract informative features from the raw text. Specifically, Peng et al. [15] utilize the convolutional neural network and radical-based embeddings of Chinese, but our model also outperforms their method. The reason may be that although they exploited a more granular embedding, the basic unit of a text should be the segment of text rather than a word or several words for this task. Though more granular embedding such as radical-based embedding can capture more morphological features, they might not be helpful for sentiment classification.

Intuitively, the SBR-PCNN-H model would capture more complete features and thus expected work better than the SBR-PCNN-S model. However, only limited progress was made. The investigation on regularization has been planned as the future work to reveal the reason. Comparing with the other feature-based and CNN-based methods, our model also benefits from the ability of capturing the sequential information by concatenating the text segments representations sequentially. The concatenation process is inspired by sequence learning models.

6 Conclusion

In this work, we propose a model named SBR-PCNN for Chinese sentiment analysis. The segmentation-based representation and the parallel convolutional neural network are developed respectively to determine the global sentiment of a sentence having the imbalanced sentiment distribution among the segments of a text. The segmentation-based representation are more informative and may overcome the limitation of the existing works which neglect the divergence of sentiment in different units of text. The parallel convolutional neural network may extract richer features for each text segment. We have evaluated the SBR-PCNN model and its variants on two benchmarking datasets. Experimental results have suggested that our model has achieved the state of the art results without any hand-crafted features. Meanwhile, our data indicated that segmentation-based representation is a better choice than treating the text as a whole. In the future, we would continue the study in two directions. Firstly, we will study the way to exploit the sequence model after the concatenation layer, which is capable of utilizing more sequential information. Secondly, we will investigate a new unsupervised method to learn informative text features more efficiently.

Acknowledgments. This work was supported by the Fundamental Theory and Applications of Big Data with Knowledge engineering under the National Key Research and Development Program of China with Grant No. 2016YFB1000903, Project of China Knowledge Center for Engineering Science and Technology, Ministry of Education Innovation Research Team No. IRT_17R86. The authors would like to thank all the reviewers and the area chairs for their constructive comments and helpful suggestions.

References

1. Liu, B.: Sentiment Analysis: Mining Opinions, Sentiments, and Emotions. Cambridge University Press, Cambridge (2015)
2. Pang, B., Lee, L., Vaithyanathan, S.: Thumbs up? Sentiment classification using machine learning techniques. In: Proceedings of the ACL-02 Conference on Empirical Methods in Natural Language Processing, vol. 10, pp. 79–86. Association for Computational Linguistics (2002)
3. Turney, P.D.: Thumbs up or thumbs down? Semantic orientation applied to unsupervised classification of reviews. In: Proceedings of the 40th Annual Meeting on Association for Computational Linguistics, pp. 417–424. Association for Computational Linguistics (2002)
4. Pang, B., Lee, L.: Seeing stars: exploiting class relationships for sentiment categorization with respect to rating scales. In: Proceedings of the ACL (2005)
5. Owoputi, O., O'Connor, B., Dyer, C., Gimpel, K., Schneider, N.: Part-of-speech tagging for twitter: word clusters and other advances. School of Computer Science (2012)
6. Mohammad, S.M., Kiritchenko, S., Zhu, X.: NRC-Canada: building the state-of-the-art in sentiment analysis of tweets. arXiv preprint arXiv:1308.6242 (2013)
7. Hltcoe, J.: Semeval-2013 task 2: Sentiment analysis in Twitter, Atlanta, Georgia, USA, p. 312 (2013)
8. Kim, Y.: Convolutional neural networks for sentence classification. arXiv preprint arXiv:1408.5882 (2014)
9. Kalchbrenner, N., Grefenstette, E., Blunsom, P.: A convolutional neural network for modelling sentences. arXiv preprint arXiv:1404.2188 (2014)
10. Ren, Y., Zhang, Y., Zhang, M., Ji, D.: Context-sensitive twitter sentiment classification using neural network. In: AAAI, pp. 215–221 (2016)
11. Maas, A.L., Daly, R.E., Pham, P.T., Huang, D., Ng, A.Y., Potts, C.: Learning word vectors for sentiment analysis. In: Proceedings of the 49th Annual Meeting of the Association for Computational Linguistics: Human Language Technologies, vol. 1, pp. 142–150. Association for Computational Linguistics (2011)
12. Labutov, I., Lipson, H.: Re-embedding words. In: ACL (2), pp. 489–493 (2013)
13. Zhai, Z., Xu, H., Kang, B., Jia, P.: Exploiting effective features for chinese sentiment classification. Expert Syst. Appl. **38**(8), 9139–9146 (2011)
14. Zagibalov, T., Carroll, J.A.: Unsupervised classification of sentiment and objectivity in Chinese text. In: Third International Joint Conference on Natural Language Processing, p. 304 (2008)
15. Peng, H., Cambria, E., Zou, X.: Radical-based hierarchical embeddings for Chinese sentiment analysis at sentence level. In: The 30th International FLAIRS Conference, Marco Island (2017)
16. Zhang, P., He, Z.: A weakly supervised approach to chinese sentiment classification using partitioned self-training. J. Inf. Sci. **39**(6), 815–831 (2013)
17. Harris, Z.S.: Distributional structure. Word **10**(2–3), 146–162 (1954)
18. Bengio, Y., Ducharme, R., Vincent, P., Jauvin, C.: A neural probabilistic language model. J. Mach. Learn. Res. **3**, 1137–1155 (2003)
19. Collobert, R., Weston, J.: A unified architecture for natural language processing: deep neural networks with multitask learning. In: Proceedings of the 25th International Conference on Machine Learning, pp. 160–167. ACM (2008)
20. Collobert, R., Weston, J., Bottou, L., Karlen, M., Kavukcuoglu, K., Kuksa, P.: Natural language processing (almost) from scratch. J. Mach. Learn. Res. **12**, 2493–2537 (2011)

21. Mikolov, T., Chen, K., Corrado, G., Dean, J.: Efficient estimation of word representations in vector space. arXiv preprint arXiv:1301.3781 (2013)
22. Mikolov, T., Sutskever, I., Chen, K., Corrado, G.S., Dean, J.: Distributed representations of words and phrases and their compositionality. In: Advances in Neural Information Processing Systems, pp. 3111–3119 (2013)
23. Pennington, J., Socher, R., Manning, C.D.: GloVe: global vectors for word representation. In: EMNLP, vol. 14, pp. 1532–1543 (2014)
24. Tang, D., Wei, F., Yang, N., Zhou, M., Liu, T., Qin, B.: Learning sentiment-specific word embedding for Twitter sentiment classification. In: ACL (1), pp. 1555–1565 (2014)
25. LeCun, Y., Bottou, L., Bengio, Y., Haffner, P.: Gradient-based learning applied to document recognition. Proc. IEEE **86**(11), 2278–2324 (1998)
26. Dos Santos, C.N., Gatti, M.: Deep convolutional neural networks for sentiment analysis of short texts. In: COLING, pp. 69–78 (2014)
27. Nair, V., Hinton, G.E.: Rectified linear units improve restricted Boltzmann machines. In: ICML (2010)
28. Tan, S., Zhang, J.: An empirical study of sentiment analysis for chinese documents. Exp. Syst. Appl. **34**(4), 2622–2629 (2008)
29. Zhang, C., Zeng, D., Li, J., Wang, F.Y., Zuo, W.: Sentiment analysis of chinese documents: from sentence to document level. J. Assoc. Inf. Sci. Technol. **60**(12), 2474–2487 (2009)
30. Liu, L., Lei, M., Wang, H.: Combining domain-specific sentiment lexicon with hownet for Chinese sentiment analysis. J. Comput. **8**(4), 878–883 (2013)
31. Chen, X., Xu, L., Liu, Z., Sun, M., Luan, H.B.: Joint learning of character and word embeddings. In: IJCAI, pp. 1236–1242 (2015)
32. Sun, Y., Lin, L., Tang, D., Yang, N., Ji, Z., Wang, X.: Radical-enhanced chinese character embedding. arXiv preprint arXiv:1404.4714 (2014)
33. Zeiler, M.D.: Adadelta: an adaptive learning rate method. arXiv preprint arXiv:1212.5701 (2012)

Entity Recognition by Distant Supervision with Soft List Constraint

Hongkui Tu[1(✉)], Zongyang Ma[2], Aixin Sun[2], Zhiqiang Xu[3], and Xiaodong Wang[1]

[1] National Laboratory of Parallel and Distributed Processing, National University of Defense Technology, Changsha, China
tuhkjet@foxmail.com, xdwang@nudt.edu.cn

[2] School of Computer Science and Engineering, Nanyang Technological University, Singapore, Singapore
{zyma,axsun}@ntu.edu.sg

[3] Institute for Infocomm Research A*STAR, Singapore, Singapore
xuzq@i2r.a-star.edg.sg

Abstract. Supervised named entity recognition systems often suffer from training data inadequacy when deal with domain specific corpora, *e.g.,* documents in medical and healthcare. For these domains, obtaining some seed words or phrases is not very difficult. Then, some positive instances obtained through distant supervision based on the seeds can be used to learn recognition models. However, with the limited size of training samples and no negative ones, the classifying results may not be satisfying. In this paper, we leverage the conjunction and comma writing style as the list constraint to enlarge the set of training instances. Different from earlier studies, we formulate two kinds of constraints, namely, soft list constraint and mention constraint, as regularizers. We then incorporate the constraints to a unified discriminative learning framework and propose a joint optimization algorithm. The experimental results show that our model is superior than state-of-the-art baselines on a large collection of documents about drugs.

Keywords: Distant supervision · Biomedical information extraction

1 Introduction

Named Entity Recognition (NER) is a fundamental task in Natural Language Processing (NLP). Named entities (*e.g.,* person, location, organization) identified and extracted from textual content are beneficial for the understanding of key concepts of the documents. Knowledge Base (KB) population is another typical application of NER where the named entities extracted from documents are added to knowledge bases to support other applications. To build a NER system

H. Tu—This work was done when the first author visiting School of Computer Science and Engineering, Nanyang Technological University.

G. Cong et al. (Eds.): ADMA 2017, LNAI 10604, pp. 681–694, 2017.
https://doi.org/10.1007/978-3-319-69179-4_48

with high accuracy, a large number of labeled instances are often required for training the classifier. However, it is very time consuming and costly to manually label a large number of instances.

The issue of labeling becomes more critical when building NER system for documents in a new domain, *e.g.,* healthcare and medical domain. More specifically, NER in this domain aims to identify and extract entities like drug, disease, and symptom from textual documents. Though a large number of documents in healthcare and medical are emerging with the explosion of the Internet, most of these documents are unlabeled due to the lack of professional knowledge for most users. Therefore, it is more challenging for NER on healthcare and medical documents with very limited labeled instances.

To minimize human annotation effort, there are typically two methods for NER in emerging domains: *semi-supervision* and *distant supervision*. The former starts with a few seed labeled instances and learns patterns on the whole corpus, then iteratively discovers new entity instances. However, semi-supervision methods often suffer from low precision and semantic drift [2]. Given a knowledge base with the type schema of entities, distant supervision heuristically labels entities. A critical challenge of distant supervision is the lack of negative samples.

1. These symptoms may include: anxiety, sweating, insomnia, rigors, **pain**, nausea, tremors, diarrhea, upper respiratory symptoms, piloerection, and rarely hallucinations.
2. The development of addiction to opioid analgesics in properly managed patients with **pain** has been reported to be rare.
3. They are also indicated in chronic anterior uveitis and corneal injury from **chemical, radiation** or **thermal burns**; or penetration of foreign bodies.

Fig. 1. Example sentences with lists (Sentences 1 and 3), and different labels for word "pain" in Sentences 1 and 2.

In this paper, we propose a novel model for NER in medical domain, which is an extension of the distant supervision model. To deal with the issue of limited labeled instances, we exploit the writing style in corpus for supplement. Illustrated in Fig. 1 Sentence 1, the entity candidates separated by commas and conjunction are tend to be of the same type with highly probability (*i.e., Symptom* type in this example). In this case, even with limited seed instances, we are able to obtain more training instances with high confidence. This list constraint has show its effectiveness in earlier studies [1,7]. Accordingly, we introduce this list constraint in our proposed distant supervision model, but with a new objective function, for an effective NER solution in medical domain.

As mentioned above, our model assumes that the entities mentioned in a list tend to be of the same conceptual type with high probability (*e.g.,* drug, disease, symptom). However, different from earlier studies, we do not assume a *hard list constraint*. In [1], the model assumes that entities in the list must belong to the same type, *i.e.,* hard list constraint. Such a strong assumption may not always hold. For instance, in Sentence 3 of Fig. 1, though the entity candidates "chemical", "radiation" and "thermal burns" are connected through a list clue "or" and ",", these three candidates do not belong to the same type. We therefore design a *soft list constraint* to deal with such exception cases. Note that, as in most studies, we utilize the standard parser tool and linguistic rules (*e.g.,* the list style with comma and conjunction) to obtain lists and entity candidates. Lists in different writing styles (*e.g.,* Sentences 1 and 3 in Fig. 1) cannot be distinguished by the parser and linguistic rules. We therefore argue the need of soft list constraint in distant supervision.

To the best of our knowledge, we are the first to formulate NER by distant supervision as a *PU learning problem* (*i.e.,* learning with positive and unlabeled examples) with *soft list constraint.* We then propose a novel and effective algorithm to address the learning problem. Through extensive experiments, we show that our proposed model outperforms several state-of-the-art baselines, evaluated by Precision, Recall, F_1, and Coverage.

2 Related Work

In this section, we survey the related work on *Supervised Entity Recognition, Nested and Overlapping Entity Recognition,* and *Supervised Entity Recognition with Constraints* followed by *Distant Supervised Entity Recognition.*

Supervised Entity Recognition: Traditional supervised entity recognition methods usually train a sequence model with effective learning algorithms(*e.g.* HMM, MaxEnt, CRF) and linguistic features (*e.g.* POS tagger, neighbor words etc.). They turn the labeled corpus into training data with BIO (*Begin, Inside, Outside*) or BILOU (*Begin, Inside, Last, Outside, Unit*) schema. The most famous one is the Stanford NER system [14]. It try to recognize some major kinds of entity with linear-chain CRF model. However, as mentioned before, it always lacks sufficient training data to train these sequence classifier models for emerging domain specific corpora.

Nested and Overlapping Entity Recognition: As there are many entities contain other entities inside them, Finkel et al. [4] propose a model to tackle the nested named entity recognition problem. Each sentence is represented as a constituency tree with each named entity corresponding to a phrase in it. Then they train a discriminative constituency parser. Lu and Roth [8] presented a model to handle overlapping entities. Each sentence is represented as a hypergraph to indicating entity types and boundaries information. In [9], the authors extend this model to recognize discontiguous entities. However, this kind of work also needs sufficient training data to achieve satisfying performance.

Supervised Entity Recognition with Constraints: Studies in this category usually use a CRF model to detect the entity boundaries. Then the probability of each entity is calculated by a classifier. Finally, the methods maximize the objective function with the proposed constraints. In [11,12], hand-coded hard constraints are exploited for supervised entity recognition. The authors use Integer Linear Programming (ILP) to solve the optimization function. The ILP-based method is extended to Integer Quadratic Programming (IQP) to better incorporate soft constraints, which can bear some exceptions [7]. However, the methods can only be used with *labeled training data*. Moreover, the inference algorithm runs at sentence level. It cannot be directly adapted in our proposed distant supervised framework. Besides, some other case-by-case patterns utilized in these works are difficult to generalize.

Distant Supervised Entity Recognition: Most related to ours, distant supervision methods usually suffer from lack of confident training data, especially in some specific domains. The authors in [1] propose a bipartite graph model and run label propagation algorithm on the graph, to get more confident training data for entity recognition. In this model, all the items in a list must have the same type (*i.e.,* hard list constraint), which cannot bear exceptions. Further, the bipartite graph model is likely to propagate noisy labels among the edges. Illustrated in Fig. 1, word "pain" in Sentence 1 is recognized as *Symptom* together with the other items in the same list. When the word propagates its entity type to Sentence 2, it will bring a noise training instance (*i.e.,* labeling "pain" with *Symptom* instead of *Disease*). In our study, we attempt to address this issue by leveraging the contextual information. In [1], there are no negative samples. Binary SVM classifiers are trained with one-vs-all schema on all positive instances of different types, one classifier for each type. A test instance might therefore be assigned to multiple types. If a test instance does not belong to any type, it will be assigned to *NIL* type.

In [10], the authors generate entity mention candidates from an extension of [3]. In their study, they distinguish the relation phrases and the entity phrases. An objective function with some graph constraints (*e.g.,* mention graph and relation graph) is proposed. The authors generate positive instances with DBpedia service, to cover the ambiguity problem and multi surface names. Negative instances are the ones that are confidently linked to *other type*. However, in specific domains like medical, it is very unlikely to get many accurate training data through DBpedia service. Different from [10], we use exact string match to label training instances. We also use bag-of-words and dependence features from a parser to represent an entity mention, which brings in more information for entity type classification. The authors in [5] formulate the distant supervision problem as a PU learning problem. They use the distant labeled instances as positive ones, and the other candidates as unlabeled ones. To be detailed shortly, the method in [5] is a special case of our proposed method.

3 Preliminaries

We first introduce the notations used in our study and present the problem definition. Then we detail our proposed model including the objective function and the constraints.

Knowledge Base: A knowledge base (KB), denoted by φ, consists of a set of types and entities that are instances of the types. The set of types is denoted by $\mathcal{T}$, and each $t \in \mathcal{T}$ is a type. Example types are *Drug* and *Disease* in medical domain.

Entity Mention: An entity mention candidate is a continuous word sequence (*i.e.,* phrase). We use a simple POS Tagging based noun phrase (NP) chunker to approximate the entity mentions. The regex expression[1] of the chunker is as follows:

< JJ. > * < NN. > +

where <JJ.> (resp., <NN.>) indicates the POS Tagging of the word starts with JJ (resp., NN).

List: A list is a series of items in a sentence connected with commas and conjunctions.

Shown in Fig. 2, we first chunk the parsed sentence with the above NP chunker. Then the conjunction word whose POS tag is <CC> is extracted (word "and" in the example). The NP which is connected with the conjunction with <nmod> modifier is collected into a list. All the NPs connected with any item in the list with <nmod> modifier are collected, until there is no new member. In the given example sentence, the resultant list collects: "skull hypoplasia", "anuria", "hypotension", "renal failure", and "death".

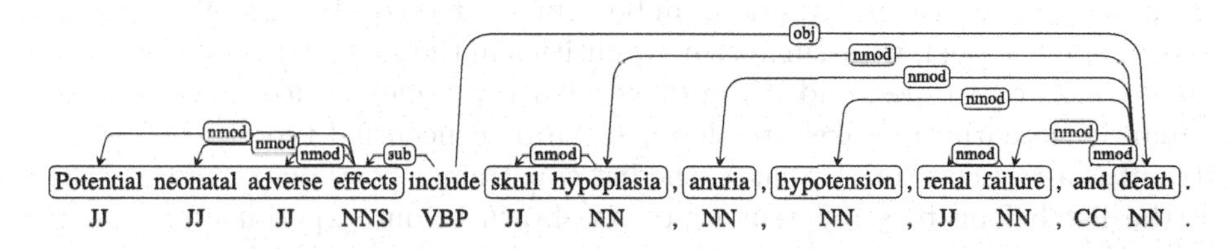

Fig. 2. An example sentence with POS tagging and parsing for list collection.

3.1 Problem Formulation

Given a document collection $\mathcal{D}$ and a knowledge base φ with its type schema $\mathcal{T}$, our entity recognition task is to recognize the entity mentions $\{m\}$ in $\mathcal{D}$ and label each mention with a type $t \in \mathcal{T}$. Note that, the same word may appear in multiple mentions (*e.g.,* word "pain" in Sentences 1 and 2 in Fig. 1) and be assigned to different types depending on the context of the mentions.

We design a pipeline architecture to fulfill this goal. First, we extract all entity mention candidates from the document collection $\mathcal{D}$. We denote the N extracted candidates by $\mathcal{M} = \{m_1, ..., m_N\}$, also represented by their feature vectors $(\mathbf{x}_i)_{1 \le i \le N}$. Second, we distantly label $\mathcal{M}$ with the knowledge base φ and get a labeled subset $\mathcal{M}_{\mathcal{P}} \subset \mathcal{M}$. Third, for a candidate $m_i \in \mathcal{M}_{\mathcal{Q}}$, we aim to label

[1] We adopt the Python style regex expression.

m_i with a vector $\mathbf{y}_i \in \{0,1\}^{(K+1)}$ as its type indicator, where $\mathcal{M}_{\mathcal{Q}} = \mathcal{M} \setminus \mathcal{M}_{\mathcal{P}}$ and $K = |\mathcal{T}|$. The $(K+1)$ dimension indicates that if an entity mention candidate does not belong to any of the K types, it is assigned to the *NIL* type. Finally, for each $m_i \in \mathcal{M}_{\mathcal{Q}}$, we are able to get its type k with $argmax_{1 \leq k \leq (K+1)} Y_{ik}$, assuming each mention belongs to exactly one type.

We use a binary matrix $\mathbf{Y} = [\mathbf{y}_1, ..., \mathbf{y}_N]^T \in \{0,1\}^{N \times (K+1)}$ as the type indicator for the N entity mention candidates. Each entry in the matrix is defined as follows:

$$Y_{ik} = \begin{cases} 1, \, m_i \text{ belongs to type } k \\ 0, \text{ otherwise} \end{cases}$$

Following [5], we use the discriminative clustering framework to perform the recognition task. Given a multiclass loss function ℓ, a multi classifier f, and regularizers Ω, the problem can be formulated as follows:

$$\begin{aligned} \min_{\mathbf{Y}, f} \quad & \sum_{i=1}^{N} \ell(\mathbf{y}_i, f(\mathbf{x}_i)) + \Omega \\ \text{s.t.} \quad & \mathbf{Y} \in \mathcal{Y} \end{aligned}$$

where the constraints $\mathbf{Y} \in \mathcal{Y}$ and regularizers Ω will be detailed next.

3.2 Constraints and Regularizers

We now show how the information can be expressed as constraints. As mentioned above, in our model, we assume that (i) entities in the same list tend to have the same conceptual types, and (ii) entities with the same surface name and high semantic similarity are likely to share the same conceptual types. The list constraint is a *soft* constraint, that is, the list constraint allows one or more entities in the list belong to a different type. As shown in our experimental analysis, more than 40% lists contain entities with multiple types, which evidences our assumption. The mention constraint aims to assign entities with same surface name and high semantic similarity to the same type. Intuitively, it is able to reduce noisy labeling. Next, we detail these two constraints.

We assume that each entity mention candidate belongs to exactly one type (including NIL). That is, there is one and only one dimension set to 1 in each row of matrix $\mathbf{Y}$, formally:

$$\forall i \in \{1, ..., N\}, \sum_{k=1}^{K+1} Y_{ik} = 1$$

The constraint can be re-written in matrix form as follows:

$$\mathbf{Y1} = \mathbf{1}$$

where $\mathbf{1}$ is a vector with full ones. For the positive examples, we impose the matrix $\mathbf{Y}$ to agree with the labels obtained through distant supervision:

$$\forall m_i \in \mathcal{M}_{\mathcal{P}}, Y_{ic_i} = 1$$

where c_i is the type indicator for m_i. In order to avoid semantic drift, we restrict that the percentage of the candidates to be classified as NIL to be at least p. This is equal to:

$$\sum_{m_i \in \mathcal{M}_Q} Y_{i(K+1)} \geq pN$$

Other than that, we use a graph G^{list} to model the list constraint. Each entity mention candidate is a node in the graph, and if entity mentions m_i and m_j are in the same list, then there is an edge from m_i to m_j. The weight matrix of the graph $\mathbf{S}^{list} \in \{0,1\}^{N \times N}$ is defined as follows:

$$S_{ij}^{list} = \begin{cases} 1, & m_i \text{ and } m_j \text{ are in the same list} \\ 0, & \text{otherwise} \end{cases}$$

Then we can formulate the list constraint related to the Laplacian regularization as follows:

$$\frac{1}{2} \sum_{i=1}^{N} \sum_{j=1}^{N} S_{ij}^{list} \times \|\mathbf{y}_i - \mathbf{y}_j\|^2 = \mathrm{Tr}(\mathbf{W}^T \mathbf{X}^T \mathbf{L}^{list} \mathbf{X} \mathbf{W})$$

where $\mathrm{Tr}(\cdot)$ denotes the trace of a matrix and $\|\cdot\|$ denotes the Euclidean norm of a vector. $\mathbf{L}^{list}$ is the Laplacian matrix of the graph G^{list}, which is defined as follows:

$$\mathbf{L}^{list} = \mathbf{D}^{list} - \mathbf{S}^{list}$$

where $\mathbf{D}^{list}$ is a diagonal matrix, $D_{ii}^{list} = \sum_{j=1}^{N} S_{ij}^{list}$. The purpose of this Lalacian regularization is to minimize the type differences among the entity mention candidates in the same list. In this paper, we use linear classifiers $\mathbf{W} \in \mathbb{R}^{L \times (K+1)}$, where L is the dimensionality of the feature vector $\mathbf{x}$. Because $\mathbf{XW}$ is expected to agree with $\mathbf{Y}$, we directly impose this constraint on $\mathbf{XW}$ to regularize the classifiers.

Though there are some words with ambiguity meanings, we argue that two candidates tend to be of same type if they have the same surface name, and are with similar context words. We use $G^{mention}$ to model the mention constraint, as in [10]. The corresponding weight matrix $\mathbf{S}^{mention}$ is defined as follows:

$$S_{ij}^{mention} = \begin{cases} sim(m_i, m_j), & m_i \in \mathcal{N}_j \text{ or } m_j \in \mathcal{N}_i \\ 0, & \text{otherwise} \end{cases}$$

where $sim(m_i, m_j)$ is the heat kernel similarity function [6] between the TF-IDF representation of the entity mentions' contexts; $\mathcal{N}_i$ is the set of nearest n neighbor candidates of m_i based on the similarity function.

By treating the list and mention constraints as regularizers, we reformulate the problem as:

$$\begin{aligned} \min_{\mathbf{Y}, f} \quad & \sum_{i=1}^{N} \ell(\mathbf{y}_i, f(\mathbf{x}_i)) + \Omega(f, list, mention) \\ \text{s.t.} \quad & \mathbf{Y} \in \mathcal{Y} \end{aligned}$$

Next, we detail this objective function.

3.3 Objective Function

The squared loss ℓ_2-norm is used as the regularizer of classifiers. Our objective function can be formulated as follows:

$$\begin{aligned}\min_{\mathbf{Y},\mathbf{W}} \quad & \frac{1}{2}\|\mathbf{Y}-\mathbf{XW}\|_F^2 + \frac{\alpha}{2}\|\mathbf{W}\|_F^2 \\ & + \frac{\beta}{2}\mathrm{Tr}(\mathbf{W}^T\mathbf{X}^T\mathbf{L}^{list}\mathbf{XW}) \\ & + \frac{\gamma}{2}\mathrm{Tr}(\mathbf{W}^T\mathbf{X}^T\mathbf{L}^{mention}\mathbf{XW}) \\ \text{s.t.} \quad & \mathbf{Y} \subseteq \{0,1\}^{N\times(K+1)} \\ & \mathbf{Y1} = \mathbf{1} \\ & Y_{ic_i} = 1, m_i \in \mathcal{M}_\mathcal{P} \\ & \sum_{m_i\in\mathcal{M}_\mathcal{Q}} Y_{i(K+1)} \geq pN \end{aligned} \tag{1}$$

where $\mathbf{X} = [\mathbf{x}_1, ..., \mathbf{x}_N]^T$ is the feature matrix and $\|\cdot\|_F$ indicates the Frobenius norm of a matrix.

4 Joint Optimization

The optimization problem to the above objective function is NP hard. We use a greedy strategy to get a local optimum solution. The problem is solved with joint optimization (see Algorithm 1):

Step 1: Optimize $\mathbf{Y}$ while keeping $\mathbf{W}$ fixed. Let the optimal $\mathbf{Y}$ be $\mathbf{Y}^*$ given $\mathbf{W}$, then $\mathbf{Y}^* = \pi(\mathbf{XW})$ where π represents an operator defined as follows.

- Keep Y_{ik} unchanged, for $m_i \in \mathcal{M}_\mathcal{P}$ and $k \in \{1, ..., K\}$.
- Set $Y_{ik} = 0, k \neq K+1$ and $Y_{i(K+1)} = 1$ for $m_i \in \mathcal{M}_{\mathcal{Q}_1}$ such that: $|\mathcal{M}_{\mathcal{Q}_1}| = \lceil pN \rceil$ and $r(Z_{i(K+1)}) \leq r(Z_{j(K+1)})$ for any $m_i \in \mathcal{M}_{\mathcal{Q}_1}$ and any $m_j \in \mathcal{M}_\mathcal{Q} \setminus \mathcal{M}_{\mathcal{Q}_1}$, where $\mathbf{Z} = \mathbf{XW}$ and $r(Z_{i(K+1)})$ represents that $Z_{i(K+1)}$ is the r-th largest entry in the i-th row of $\mathbf{Z}$.
- Set $Y_{ik} = \delta(k, \mathrm{argmax}_l Z_{il})$, $m_i \in \mathcal{M} \setminus (\mathcal{M}_\mathcal{P} \bigcup \mathcal{M}_{\mathcal{Q}_1})$, where δ is an indicator function:

$$\delta(k_1, k_2) = \begin{cases} 1, & k_1 = k_2 \\ 0, & \text{otherwise} \end{cases}$$

Step 2: Optimize $\mathbf{W}$ while keeping $\mathbf{Y}$ fixed. The subproblem is

$$\min_{\mathbf{W}} g(\mathbf{W}) = \frac{1}{2}\mathrm{Tr}(\mathbf{W}^T\mathbf{HW}) - \mathrm{Tr}(\mathbf{Y}^T\mathbf{XW}) \tag{2}$$

where $\mathbf{H} = \alpha\mathbf{I} + \mathbf{X}^T(\mathbf{I} + \beta\mathbf{L}^{list} + \gamma\mathbf{L}^{mention})\mathbf{X}$. This subproblem can be solved by gradient descent method. Specifically, the update is written as:

$$\mathbf{W}^{(t+1)} = \mathbf{W}^{(t)} - \tau_t \nabla g(\mathbf{W}^{(t)})$$

where $\nabla g(\mathbf{W}) = \frac{1}{2}(\mathbf{H} + \mathbf{H}^T)\mathbf{W} - \mathbf{X}^T\mathbf{Y}$ and τ_t is the step size at t-th iteration.

Algorithm 1. Joint Optimization Algorithm

Require: feature matrix: $\mathbf{X}$, positive labeled set: $\mathcal{M}_{\mathcal{P}}$, Laplatian matrices of list graph and mention graph: $\{\mathbf{L}^{list}, \mathbf{L}^{mention}\}$, parameters: $\{\alpha, \beta, \gamma, p\}$, max iterator times: $\{T_{outer}, T_{inner}\}$
Ensure: $\mathbf{Y}$
1: Random initialize $\mathbf{Y}, \mathbf{W}$
2: Revise $\mathbf{Y}$ according to $\mathcal{M}_{\mathcal{P}}$
3: $t_{outer} = 0$
4: **repeat**
5: $t_{inner} = 0$
6: Keeping $\mathbf{W}$ fixed.
7: Optimize $\mathbf{Y}$ according to **Step 1**.
8: **repeat**
9: Choose the step size $\tau_{t_{inner}}$ by line search.
10: Keeping $\mathbf{Y}$ unchanged.
11: Optimize $\mathbf{W}$ according to **Step 2**.
12: $t_{inner} += 1$
13: **until** $t_{inner} \geq T_{inner}$ or Equation 2 convergence.
14: $t_{outer} += 1$
15: **until** $t_{outer} \geq T_{outer}$ or Equation 1 convergence.

5 Experiments

5.1 Dataset Description

Seeds in KB: We take the seeds from [1]. There are four types of seeds in the dataset, namely *Disease*, *Drug*, *Ingredient*, and *Symptom*. All the seeds are extracted from Freebase. The number of instances in the 4 types are 4,605, 4,383, 4,066 and 1,244 respectively. The number of single-typed instances are 3,960, 2,133, 1,823, and 620 respectively.

Corpus: We downloaded a drug dataset from DailyMed.[2] It contains 30,563 XML documents and each details a drug which can be legally used in the United States. We split the corpus into sentences with NLTK[3] and get 1,268,557 sentences in total. Then we use the GDep parser [13,14], which was trained on the GENIA Treebank, to parse this corpus. The NPs and lists are extracted according to the definitions. Finally, there are 6,861,592 NPs in total. The data statistics are shown in Table 1.

Noun Phrases Filtering: We observed that the extracted NPs contain lots of general meaning phrases such as "patient", "hour", "well-controlled studies", etc. These NPs appear many times in the corpus and are very unlikely to be entities. In this paper, we use several simple rules to filter the NPs that are not related to our target domain. First, we remove the NPs which contain more than 6 words. Second, we calculate the inverse document frequency (IDF) score for

[2] http://www.daily.med.com.
[3] http://www.nltk.org.

Table 1. Dataset statistics of noun phrases (NP) and unique noun phrases (UNP)

	NP Length	1	2	3	4	5	≥6
Corpus	#NP	3,954,197	2,228,430	571,104	95,581	10,888	1,392
	#UNP	17,804	66,279	35,586	8,913	1,540	297
Corpus (after filtering)	#NP	1,365,080	1,044,651	433,879	93,407	10,793	1,215
	#UNP	15,802	45,933	31,383	8,835	1,518	232
Testing Data	#Positive NP	1762	858	317	58	6	0
	#Positive UNP	764	636	253	52	6	0

every word in the dataset. For each NP, we get its IDF score by averaging the IDFs of the words in it. Then we filter all the candidate NPs whose IDF score is lower than a threshold (set to 1.0 in our experiments), similar to [16]. We also utilize Google Ngram[4] to filter some general domain phrases. More specifically, we remove the NPs which appear more than 3,000,000 times in Google Ngram. Table 1 also reports the number of NPs in our dataset after filtering.

Testing Data: We randomly select 2,000 sentences from the corpus and *manually label* them to get the gold standard testing data. The number of instances in the four types *Disease*, *Drug*, *Ingredient*, and *Symptom*, are 376, 1,645, 181 and 799 respectively. The last row in Table 1 shows their length distribution.

After parsing the 2,000 sentences, there are 1,667 conjunction words, forming 895 lists. Each list contains at least two NPs. Among the 895 lists, there are 410 lists containing one or more positive candidates. We take the 410 lists for further analysis. The lists contain 1,121 NPs in total, which include 219 negative ones (*i.e., NIL*). Among the 410 lists, 186 lists have negative instances, and 2 lists have positive instances of different types. The 410 lists result in 1,764 NP pairs. Among these pairs, 1,307 ones satisfy the same-type assumption, which means that the two NPs in each pair have the same type. The above analysis shows that, in our manually labeled dataset, the above assumption holds for 74.10% $(1,307/1,764)$ of the NP pairs, while the exception rate of hard list constraint is 45.85% (188/410). This confirms the necessity of soft list constraint.

Feature Extraction: Each NP is treated as an entity mention candidate and we extract its features for classification. We show features extracted for an example mention in Table 2. The features are similar to that in [1]. However, [1] performs classification on the list level. We perform classification on the NP level. The most frequent 1% features are removed as stop-word-liked features. Besides, we ignore the singleton features.

5.2 Experiment Task 1: Classification

In this task, we aim to test the effectiveness of the proposed model when applied to NER problem. In order to avoid ambiguity, we use the single-type seeds in KB to distantly label positive instances, and the manually labeled 2,000 sentences

[4] https://books.google.com/ngrams.

Table 2. Features extracted for "**skull hypoplasia**" in the sentence "Potential neonatal adverse effects include skull hypoplasia, anuria, hypotension, renal failure, and death."

Feature	Example	Type
Words in the NP	skull hypoplasia	Shallow
Prefix/Suffix for each word in the NP	pf=sku pf=skul pf=hyp pf=hypo sf=ull sf=kull sf=sia sf=asia	Shallow
Other words in the sentence	potential neonatal adverse effects include anuria hypotension renal failure and death	Shallow
Left and right ngrams ($n = 1,2,3$) in a given window size (set 3)	l1gram=adverse l1gram=effects l1gram=include l2gram=adverse-effects l2gram=effects-include l3gram=adverse-effects-include r1gram=, r1gram=anuria r2gram=,-anuria r2gram=anuria-, r3gram=,-anuria-,	Shallow
Closest verb ancestor, the path to this verb and all the modifiers of the verb	v→include nmod→nmod→obj nmod→effect nmod→death	Dependence

as testing data (see Table 1). We use three recent methods as baselines, namely **DIEL** [1], **WNEC** [5] and **ClusType** [10].

We adopt ProPPR[5] [15] for label propagation for implementing the DIEL method, as in [1]. The WNEC method is a special case of our proposed method with $\beta = 0$ and $\gamma = 0$. The open source code[6] released by the authors are used for ClusType with modification to type schema for extracting the positive and negative samples from DBpedia entity linking service.[7] For DIEL method, classification results on NPs are computed based on the labels of the lists. For our model, we choose the parameters $\alpha, \beta, \gamma \in \{0.1, 0.5, 1.0, 2.0, 5.0, 10.0\}$ and $p \in \{0.2, 0.3, ..., 0.8\}$. Due to page limit, we only report the results obtained with the following parameter setting: $\alpha = 1.0$, $\beta = 5.0$, $\gamma = 1.0$ and $p = 0.3$. As for WNEC, we set $\alpha = 1.0$ and $p = 0.2$ for achieving the best F_1 in this task.

The classification results are reported in Table 3. ClusType reports the worst results, mainly because of the poor coverage of concepts in medical domain in DBpedia, particularly the *Ingredient* type. Recall that ClusType uses the DBpedia entity linking services to get some positive and negative samples. Because of the poor coverage in DBpedia, the few positive samples further affect the training algorithm. Other than that, in our dataset, neighbor relation phrase may be less representative than dependence features. Both DIEL and our model are better than WNEC method. It's understandable that both models utilize the list constraint. As discussed before, one NP may be assigned to two or more types in DIEL. As the result, the method reports higher recall score, with the cost of poorer precision.

[5] https://github.com/TeamCohen/ProPPR.
[6] http://shanzhenren.github.io/ClusType/.
[7] https://github.com/dbpedia-spotlight.

Table 3. Results by *P*recision, *R*ecall, and F_1 (%)

Type		DIEL	WNEC	ClusType	Ours
Disease	P	25.05	15.86	8.84	34.29
	R	31.38	39.89	16.48	28.72
	F_1	27.86	22.69	11.50	31.26
Drug	P	37.27	34.94	26.13	37.08
	R	8.92	13.63	7.22	8.29
	F_1	14.39	19.61	11.31	13.55
Ingredient	P	19.34	4.62	1.15	29.15
	R	42.22	18.33	3.33	36.11
	F_1	26.53	7.38	1.70	32.27
Symptom	P	52.62	19.58	9.46	54.43
	R	36.51	18.57	2.01	39.27
	F_1	43.11	19.06	3.31	45.63
Overall	P	34.87	18.04	10.88	**42.06**
	R	**21.29**	18.61	6.75	20.98
	F_1	26.44	18.32	8.33	**28.00**

Table 4. Coverage (%)

Runs	DIEL	WNEC	Ours	Upper bound
0	31.99	35.68	30.83	52.02
1	32.83	32.73	31.67	51.83
2	25.69	32.36	29.51	51.79
3	33.14	31.31	30.23	52.18
4	32.20	34.29	31.15	52.15
5	32.35	31.81	30.39	51.57
6	33.21	32.85	31.32	51.95
7	32.78	32.72	31.84	51.95
8	31.09	34.11	32.20	51.63
9	31.46	32.90	30.53	51.97
Average	31.67	**33.08**	30.97	51.90

5.3 Experiment Task 2: Recovering KB

As stated in [1], Freebase has a relative low coverage of medical concepts. Populating KB is also of significance for other tasks. In this experiment, we aim to find out the capability of our model in recovering the type instances in KB. We adopt the DIEL and WNEC methods as baselines. ClusType method cannot be directly applied to this task because it depends on the entity linking service. There is no change to parameter settings for all methods.

We randomly take 50% of the single-type seeds as training set. The remaining single-type seeds and the polysemous ones are used as heldout set. The result is reported in Table 4. We conduct the experiment for 10 times, each run with its own randomly selected training and heldout set. We adopt the same parameter settings as in the former task. The coverage score is computed with:

$$coverage = \frac{\sum_{t \in \mathcal{T}} |\text{Predict}(t) \cap \text{Seed}(t)|}{\sum_{t \in \mathcal{T}} |\text{Seed}(t)|}$$

where Predict(t) denotes the set of surface names that have been classified to type t; Seed(t) is the set of seeds belonging to type t. The upper bound of coverage score is computed with all entity candidates as positive ones for all $t \in \mathcal{T}$.

From Table 4, the method WNEC achieves the best coverage score. As stated before, it achieve the score with $p = 0.2$, which means that only a small proportion of the candidates will be classified to *NIL* type. As a result, the lower p setting hurts the precision in the first task.

6 Conclusion

In this paper, we explore the usage of comma and conjunction writing style in distant supervised learning framework. We propose a unified model to incorporate the discriminative learning algorithm with soft constraints. The experimental results demonstrate the effectiveness of our model. As part of our future work, we aim to utilize the embedding approaches as supplement features to further improve the performance.

Acknowledgment. This research was supported by Singapore Ministry of Education Academic Research Fund Tier-1 Grant RG142/14, National Natural Science Foundation of China (No. 61070203, No. 61202484, No. 61472434 and No. 61572512) and a grand from the National Key Lab. of High Performance Computing (No. 20124307120033).

References

1. Bing, L., Chaudhari, S., Wang, R.C., Cohen, W.W.: Improving distant supervision for information extraction using label propagation through lists. In: Proceedings of the 2015 Conference on Empirical Methods in Natural Language Processing, EMNLP 2015, Lisbon, Portugal, September 2015, pp. 524–529 (2015)
2. Curran, J., Murphy, T., Scholz, B.: Minimising semantic drift with mutual exclusion bootstrapping. In: 10th Conference of the Pacific Association for Computational Linguistics, Melbourne, Australia, pp. 172–180, September 2007
3. El-Kishky, A., Song, Y., Wang, C., Voss, C.R., Han, J.: Scalable topical phrase mining from text corpora. PVLDB **8**(3), 305–316 (2014)
4. Finkel, J.R., Manning, C.D.: Nested named entity recognition. In: Proceedings of the 2009 Conference on Empirical Methods in Natural Language Processing, EMNLP 2009, Singapore, August 2009, pp. 141–150 (2009)
5. Grave, E.: Weakly supervised named entity classification. In: Workshop on Automated Knowledge Base Construction (AKBC) (2014)
6. He, X., Niyogi, P.: Locality preserving projections. In: Neural Information Processing Systems, NIPS 2003, Canada, December 2003, pp. 153–160 (2003)
7. Jindal, P., Roth, D.: Using soft constraints in joint inference for clinical concept recognition. In: Proceedings of the 2013 Conference on Empirical Methods in Natural Language Processing, EMNLP 2013, October 2013, pp. 1808–1814 (2013)
8. Lu, W., Roth, D.: Joint mention extraction and classification with mention hypergraphs. In: Proceedings of the 2015 Conference on Empirical Methods in Natural Language Processing, EMNLP 2015, Lisbon, Portugal, September 2015, pp. 857–867 (2015)
9. Muis, A.O., Lu, W.: Learning to recognize discontiguous entities. In: Proceedings of the 2016 Conference on Empirical Methods in Natural Language Processing, EMNLP 2016, Austin, Texas, USA, November 2016, pp. 75–84 (2016)
10. Ren, X., El-Kishky, A., Wang, C., Tao, F., Voss, C.R., Han, J.: Clustype: effective entity recognition and typing by relation phrase-based clustering. In: Proceedings of the 21th ACM SIGKDD International Conference on Knowledge Discovery and Data Mining, Sydney, NSW, Australia, August 2015, pp. 995–1004 (2015)

11. Roth, D., Yih, W.: A linear programming formulation for global inference in natural language tasks. In: Proceedings of the Eighth Conference on Computational Natural Language Learning, CoNLL 2004, Boston, Massachusetts, USA, May 2004, pp. 1–8 (2004)
12. Roth, D., Yih, W.: Global inference for entity and relation identification via a linear programming formulation. In: Introduction to Statistical Relational Learning, pp. 553–580. The MIT press (2007)
13. Sagae, K., Tsujii, J.: Dependency parsing and domain adaptation with LR models and parser ensembles. In: Proceedings of the 2007 Joint Conference on Empirical Methods in Natural Language Processing and Computational Natural Language Learning, EMNLP-CoNLL 2007, Prague, Czech Republic, June 2007, pp. 1044–1050 (2007)
14. Tsuruoka, Y., Tateishi, Y., Kim, J.-D., Ohta, T., McNaught, J., Ananiadou, S., Tsujii, J.: Developing a robust part-of-speech tagger for biomedical text. In: Bozanis, P., Houstis, E.N. (eds.) PCI 2005. LNCS, vol. 3746, pp. 382–392. Springer, Heidelberg (2005). doi:10.1007/11573036_36
15. Wang, W.Y., Mazaitis, K., Cohen, W.W.: Programming with personalized pagerank: a locally groundable first-order probabilistic logic. In: 22nd ACM International Conference on Information and Knowledge Management, CIKM 2013, San Francisco, CA, USA, October 2013, pp. 2129–2138 (2013)
16. Zhang, S., Elhadad, N.: Unsupervised biomedical named entity recognition: experiments with clinical and biological texts. J. Biomed. Inf. **46**(6), 1088–1098 (2013)

Structured Sentiment Analysis

Abdulqader Almars[1(✉)], Xue Li[1], Xin Zhao[1], Ibrahim A. Ibrahim[1], Weiwei Yuan[2], and Bohan Li[2]

[1] The University of Queensland, Brisbane, QLD, Australia
{a.almars,xueli,x.zhao,i.ibrahim}@uq.edu.au
[2] Nanjing University of Aeronautics and Astronautics, Nanjing, China
{yuanweiwei,bhli}@nuaa.edu.cn

Abstract. Extracting the latent structure of the aspects and the sentiment polarities is important as it helps customers to understand people' preference to a certain product and show the reasons why they prefer this product. However, insufficient studies have been done to effectively reveal the structure sentiment of the aspects from short texts due to the shortness and sparsity. In this paper, we propose a structured sentiment analysis (SSA) approach to understand the sentiments and opinions expressed by people in short texts. The proposed SSA approach has three advantages: (1) automatically extracts a hierarchical tree of a product's hot aspects from short texts; (2) hierarchically analyses people's opinions on those aspects; and (3) generates a summary and evidences of the results. We evaluate our approach on popular products. The experimental results show that the proposed approach can effectively extract a sentiment tree from short texts.

Keywords: Hierarchical structure · Sentiment analysis · Sentiment tree · Topic model

1 Introduction

Discovering the latent structure of the aspects and their cosponsoring sentiments is significantly important from two points of view - individuals and business intelligence. From the individual's view point, a sentiment tree organises aspects from general to specific. Therefore, it allows individual to find people's attitudes on various aspects represented by the tree at different granularities. For example, some may be interested in people's opinions on the product in general, while others may look for people's opinions on specific aspects, such as the quality of the camera. From the point view of business, structured sentiment tree would allow them to trace public opinion on aspects of a product and services, and provide them with important information to help them improve future plans and strategies.

Recentely, researchers have proposed new approaches to effectively extract the hierarchical structure from text [4,5,12]. For example, Kim [5] and Titov [12] studied the problem by proposing a model that discovers a hierarchy from

G. Cong et al. (Eds.): ADMA 2017, LNAI 10604, pp. 695–707, 2017.
https://doi.org/10.1007/978-3-319-69179-4_49

review data. However, no sufficient studies have been done to effectively reveal the hierarchical tree of the hot aspects and their corresponding polarities form short texts. In fact, the existing approaches have only been designed to deal with traditionally long texts, such as online reviews and blogs. In general, their performance is less effective when these methods are applied to short texts [8], due to both the shortness and the sparsity of the texts.

There are three major challenges when discovering hierarchical sentiment tree from short texts. Firstly, compared with traditionally long texts, short texts suffer from sparsity, and this issue may result in an incomprehensible and incorrect concept hierarchy. Secondly, most existing methods perform a flat sentiment analysis on each extracted aspects independently, and ignore the concept hierarchy. In fact, the sentiment polarity for an aspect should also include the polarity of its offspring. Otherwise, the polarity of this aspect may not cover all people's genuine attitudes on it. Thirdly, generating understandable and convincing summaries is challenging. People prefer to visualise the results of the structured sentiment tree in a concise and comprehensible way. More importantly, people want to know the reasons why people like and dislike those aspects represented in the tree.

In this paper, we study the problem of extracting a sentiment tree from opinions expressed by people in short texts. We present a structured sentiment analysis (SSA) approach which automatically extracts the hierarchical structure of hot aspects as well as the people's opinions towards those aspects. *Hot aspects* can be defined as the most mentioned aspects people talk about. The input for the SSA is a collection of short messages about a particular product. A hierarchical process based on a topic model is proposed to capture the hidden relationships between aspects and extract the *Hot aspects*. The outcome of the SSA is a sentiment tree where the root is the most general aspects of a product, and as the depth increases, the aspects become more specific. Each node in the tree represents the name of an aspect, along with a set of messages relevant to this aspect and its polarity.

The three challenges mentioned above can then be dealt with by using the proposed new SSA as follows.

- First, we propose a hierarchical approach to extract hot aspects and identify relationships between aspects simultaneously. The aspects on $(i-1)^{th}$ level are used to extract the aspects on i^{th} level. In this way, the weak semantic relationship between aspects preserved from the short messages can be identified.
- Second, we propose a hierarchical sentiment approach to attach people' attitudes for each nodes in the tree. To identify people' opinions, our approach performs a polarity classification for each message, followed by hierarchical statistics. On other words, the polarity of an aspect is determined by including the sentiment polarity for the aspect itself and its children in the hierarchical tree.
- Third, we proposed a summarisation approach to effectively provide a comprehensive summary and explanation for the extracted results.

– Fourth, the experiment results show that the proposed approach is effective for analysing short texts and extracting the sentiment tree.

The rest of paper is organised as follows. Section 2 describes the related words. In Sect. 3, we illustrate the proposed methodology. Section 4 describes the experimental result. Finally, Sect. 5 concludes this paper.

2 Related Work

Aspect-based sntiment analysis and topic modeling are becoming a popular research area among the research community. Several approaches have been proposed to address the problem of feature extractions [3,9]. For example, Hu and Liu [3] used part-of-speech (POS) tagging to extract nouns and noun phrases as aspects, since nouns often represent aspects of a product.Then, they applied association rules to capture highly frequent feature words. Topic model tools have also shown great results in identifying the hidden patterns in texts in different domains [6,10,14]. However, the main problem with all of the models mentioned above is that the natural hierarchical structure of the aspects and their polarity are not considered.

Hierarchical topic modelling approaches have been proposed to address the problem of the current flat topic models. Titov and McDonald [12] approached the problem by proposing a multi-grain topic model that extracts the hierarchical structure of the topic at different granularities. Other works have been conducted to determine the topic hierarchy in review data, such as [1,4,7]. Kim et al. [5], for example, applied a more advanced model, namely, a hierarchical aspect-sentiment model (HASM), which automatically constructs the hierarchical representation of aspects from online reviews. Moreover, Wang [13] suggested a recursive approach for constructing a topical hierarchy from a collection of content-representative documents. However, the existing approaches have only been designed to deal with traditionally long texts. Applying this model to short texts produce incomprehensible and incorrect tree.

To the best of our knowledge, the only work that constructed a hierarchical structure from short texts was one conducted by Zhao and Li [15]. They used term frequency-inverse document frequency (TFIDF) and formal concept analysis (FCA) to discover a hierarchical tree of aspects of a particular product. In contrast to their approach, which relies on TFIDF, our approach can capture the semantics and the hidden patterns in texts and construct a much more meaningful tree. Another limitation of their work is that the evolution of the tree's quality and the usefulness of its output were not studied.

3 Methodology

In this section, we first formalise the problem definitions. We then describe our System Architecture.

3.1 Problem Definition

Given a set of messages $M = \{m_1, m_2, ..., m_n\}$ about a specific product that a user is interested in, where n is the number of messages, our task is to extract hot aspects $A = \{a_1, a_2, ...\}$ from M, where a_i contains a subset of messages M_i from M talking about the ith aspect, and the most frequent words $TW_i = \{tw_{i1}, tw_{i2}, ...\}$ within M_i. The top-1 word tw_{i1} is used as the name for the ith aspect. *Root* is one special aspect to represent the whole product. *Root* contains all messages M. Then, we construct a tree $T = \{t_1, t_2, ...\}$ where $t = \{i, j\}$ is a 2-tuple to indicate that aspect a_i is the parent of aspect a_j, where $a_i, a_j \in A$. Our second task is to analyse people's opinions on those aspects discovered by tree T. The output is $O = \{o_1, o_2, ..., \}$, where $o_i \in [0, 1]$ is the score for the people's opinions towards aspect a_i. 0 means the absolute negative attitude while 1 means the absolute positive attitude.

3.2 System Architecture

At the high level, our framework constructs a hierarchical tree of the most frequently mentioned aspects of a product with the corresponding sentiment polarity of those aspects. Figure 1 illustrates an architectural overview of the proposed system. The proposed system has four main components: (1) data pre-processing; (2) hierarchical extraction; (3) sentiment analysis; and (4) summary generation. The following sub-sections explain the four components in detail.

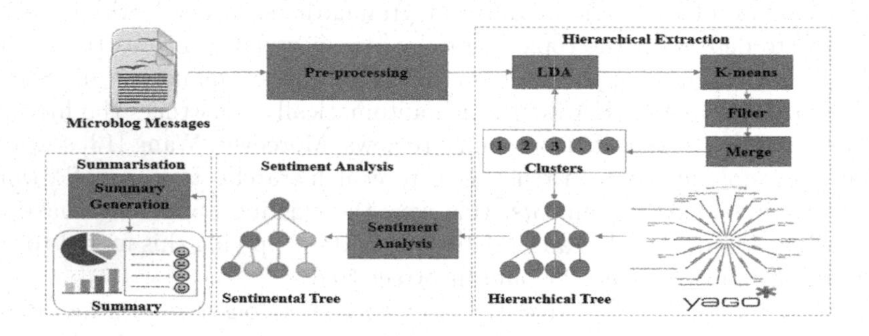

Fig. 1. System architecture of SSA.

Data Pre-processing. Data pre-processing is an important step as the quality of the hierarchy depends on the output of this step. To reduce the noise and improve the result of the SSA, we first pre-process the data to ignore common words that carry less important meaning. In this step, stop words, non-English characters and URLs are removed from the texts. Based on our observation, we noticed that most messages containing URLs are either spam or advertisements, and including them would produce irreverent information and noise to the tree. Finally, to construct the structured tree, we use the *part-of-speech tagging (POS)*[1] to extract *proper nouns*. We use only nouns and nouns phrase to

[1] http://www.cs.cmu.edu/~ark/TweetNLP/.

extract the hot aspects since people often use *nouns* to refer to aspects of a product.

Hierarchical Extraction. The problem that we address in this section is how to construct a tree-structured representation of the *hot aspects* that most people care about from short texts. The hierarchical tree shows the most frequent and general aspects close to the root, while the specific ones appear nearer the leaf nodes. It is important to mention that our hierarchical component can extract a hierarchical tree of hot aspects with any number of depth. The input of this component is a set of messages about specific product. Our aim to find the relationships between nouns that often appear together in the same context and to extract a tree of *hot aspects*.

Our hierarchical extraction function consists of two main components: the LDA model and the k-means clustering algorithm [2]. First, the LDA is a Bayesian probabilistic model, which views each message as a mixture of underlying topics where each message is assigned to a set of topics via LDA. A topic model such as LDA is useful in our task to discover the hidden patterns in a text. On other words, it allows us to find terms that often appear together and are put similar words (e.g., synonyms) in the same topic. The input of the LDA are the messages, and the number of topics is k specified by the user. The output of the LDA is $D = \{d_1, d_2, ..., d_n\}$ to represent the messages M_i as a mixture of topics, where d_i is a feature representation for message m_i.

The second component of hierarchical extraction is the k-means clustering algorithm. Though LDA can be used for clustering, the clusters split by LDA are imbalanced. So in this work, LDA is used for feature representation and k-means is used for clustering. Given a set of messages M_i and its feature representation D, and the number of cluster K, the output of k-means is a set of clusters $C = \{c_1, c_2, ..., c_k\}$. We group each message to one of the clusters based on its feature representation. A cluster c_i is a candidate of hot aspects A; the same as our definition for aspect a_i, a cluster c_i contains messages M_i belonging to this cluster and the most frequent words TW_i from M_i.

To explain the algorithm in more detail, our algorithm (i.e., Algorithm 1) starts by first receiving fourth inputs: (1) messages M; (2) array includes number of topics (clusters) K in each level Lev; (3) array includes threshold percentages to filter irrelevant clusters in each level Lev; and (4) the taxonomy of a product from YAGO. At the beginning, the hot aspects A only contain the *Root* and the T is empty. In order to create the aspects on the tree's first level, the algorithm begins by using the LDA model to create a K number of topics (Line 8). Then, the result will then be passed to the k-mean component to automatically group all similar messages together. Noise will be added to the result of our approach if all words in each cluster are included. Therefore, only the top five nouns for each cluster are kept for sentiment analysis (Sect. 3.2). The name of the cluster is represented by the top-1 noun. The two examples below show the top five nouns for each cluster.

Camera: *"camera, selfie, pic, picture, quality"*.

Audio: *"audio, headphone, adapter, earphone, headset"*.

Second, not all clusters generated by k-means are useful and relevant. To tackle this problem, our algorithm (Line 14) can filter those outliers which are not related as hot aspects based on the term frequency. In other words, the cluster will be eliminated if its top word is lower than a specified threshold. In our experiment, we set the threshold to 0.01 on the first level. The threshold means that the frequency of its top-1 word should appear in the whole message above one percent. Additionally, the k-mean component may produce duplicate clusters. In order to reduce the number of duplicate clusters, in line 12, we add a merging step which combines the redundant clusters into the same cluster if they have the same name. Third, our system performs the same process again for each cluster generated on level *Lev* to create aspects in the $Lev + 1$ level of the tree.

Algorithm 1: Hierarchical Extraction

```
Input:
M = {m_1, m_2, ..., m_n} #Crawled and pre-processed microblog messages.
K = [25, 2] #Number of topics for each cluster on level Lev.
ThPercentage = [0.01, 0.05] #Threshold to filter irrelevant cluster for
level Lev.
YAGO #The Taxonomy of product from Wikipedia.
Output:
T: Concept hierarchy of product aspects.
1  A = {Root}
2  T = ∅
3  for (Lev = 1 : length(K)) do
4  |   A_Lev = getNodes(A, T, Lev − 1) #Get all nodes from tree T on level
   |     Lev − 1, Root is on level 0.
5  |   foreach c_i ∈ A_Lev do
6  |   |   Threshold = length(M_i) ∗ ThPercentage_Lev #Threshold to filter
   |   |     irrelevant cluster for level Lev.
7  |   |   D = LDA(M_i,K_Lev) #Apply LDA model on messages, only nouns
   |   |     are considered.
8  |   |   C = Kmeans(D,M_i,K_Lev) #Clustering messages based on LDA
   |   |     representations.
9  |   |   foreach c_j ∈ C do
10 |   |   | TW_j = GetTopWords(M_j) #Set Top5 words for each cluster.
11 |   |   end
12 |   |   C = MergeDuplicateClusters(C) #Merge the cluster with the
   |   |     others if they share same name.
13 |   |   foreach c_j ∈ C do
14 |   |   |   if The frequency of tw_j1 in all messages M_i > Threshold then
15 |   |   |   |   A.add(c_j) #Add cluster to the list of hot aspects.
16 |   |   |   |   T.add(c_i, c_j) #Add cluster to level Lev of the output tree.
17 |   |   |   end
18 |   |   end
19 |   end
20 end
21 T = Enhance(T, YAGO) #We use Yago to enhance the tree structure.
22 return T;
```

Finally, the results of the previous steps may produce an incomplete or incorrect tree. We use a YAGO ontology [11] to enhance the hierarchical representation of the aspects by providing another level if necessary. YAGO is an available public resource for all products as long as the product has a Wikipedia page. An example of an incomplete tree is when our system might produce two children, namely *jet* and *matte* under the node *black*. In this case, we use the ontology to improve the structure by adding another level to represent the node *black* under *colour*. YAGO is also useful for reorganising nodes that are incorrectly placed on the tree. In other words, if the results of our system shows *gold* under *black*, the ontology can help put the node on the correct branch.

It is important to mention that our tree differs from YAGO from three perspectives. First, it is easy to obtain the physical aspects of a product from YAGO or other resources; however, some of aspects of the product are not important to people. Therefore, our system extracts only the hot aspects that people care about based on the microblog messages. Another difference in our system is that some emerging aspects about the product are mentioned by people in the microblog, but do not exist in YAGO. Third, our system provides users with people's feelings towards these aspects represented on the tree, which is not included in the YAGO ontology.

Sentiment Analysis. This section hierarchically analyses and classifies people's opinions about those extracted aspects. Our sentiment method differs from others as it hierarchically extract the sentiment of aspects. To express an opinion on an aspect of a product, people often use opinion words *adjectives* and *verbs*. Consider the following messages *"I love the quality of the camera"* and *"The new cell phone battery is amazing"*. The user uses the verb *love* as an opinion word to express their feeling about the *quality of the camera*. On the second example, the adjective *amazing* is used to express the user's opinion towards the aspect *battery*. In our research we use opinion words to identify the polarity of aspects.

Our method extracts the semantic orientation of hot aspects in a hierarchical way using three distinct steps. The input to our algorithm is the hierarchical tree T created from the previous stage. For sentiment analysis, we first retrieve the original messages M_i for each aspect a_i. Then, we remove the noise, irrelevant information, from the messages as we did in Sect. 3.2. After that, we tokenise the message and then perform the POS processing to assign parts of speech to words in each message. Next, all the words are stemmed to the original form by using *Lucense java API*[2].

After annotating the retrieved messages for each aspect a_i, the sentiment analysis phase is conducted by finding the opinion words in each message in M_i that are closest to any top word in TW_i. Then, we use the opinion lexicon from[3] and a swear list to identify the polarity of aspects. The polarity of the message is positive or negative based on the results returned from the opinion lexicon. If the result returned from the lexicon is empty, then the swear list will be used. If the closet opinion word is found in the swear list, it will be identified as negative; otherwise, the message is classified as neutral. To deal with negations, we fillip

[2] https://lucene.apache.org/.
[3] https://www.cs.uic.edu/~liub/.

the polarity from the opinion lexicon. For instance, the polarity of "is not good" is turned into a *negative*.

Once the sentiment polarity for each message in M_i for aspect a_i is extracted, our algorithm takes the sentiment analysis result to hierarchically draw the final polarity for each aspect a_i in T. It is clear that each aspect a_i is, in fact, a node in a tree. The polarity of a node is determined by including sentiment polarity for the node itself and its children. Because we split messages into aspects on each level in a hierarchical way, the direct children are enough to cover the whole branch rooted by the aspect. The polarity score o_i of the aspect a_i in T is calculated as follows:

$$\tilde{P}_i = \sum_j P_j, j = i | j \in Children_i \quad (1)$$

$$\tilde{N}_i = \sum_j N_j, j = i | j \in Children_i \quad (2)$$

$$o_i = \tilde{P}_i / (\tilde{P}_i + \tilde{N}_i) \quad (3)$$

where P_i is the number of positive messages from M_i for aspect a_i, $\tilde{P}_i$ is the number of all positive messages for the aspect a_i itself and all its children defined by $Children_i = \{j\}, \forall t \in T, t = \{i, j\}$. N_i is the number of negative message from M_i and $\tilde{N}_i$ is the number of all negative messages from itself and its children.

The final output of SSA is a tree of hot aspects of a product as well as the people's opinions about these aspects. Figure 1 shows the results of the tree construction and sentiment analysis.

Summarisation. Once we construct a structured sentiment tree, generating a structured summary of the sentiment tree is critical to help people better understand and interpret the sentiments about the product and its aspects. More specifically, a structured summary can help answer three questions: (1) What is the overall polarity of the product? (2) What are the most favourable and unfavourable aspects of the product? and (3) Why do people like or dislike those aspects?. For summary generation, the input of our algorithm is the sentiment tree. The output is three visualisation forms of the sentiment tree. First of all, our summary component generates a chart to show the final polarity of a product using the results of the sentiment tree. The polarity of the product is the polarity of all *Root* aspects. At any level of the tree, our system also provides an evidence of why people like or dislike certain aspects of a product by providing additional details from each message related to the aspect such as (e.g., message id, message date, text and polarity). Finally, our system discovers the top aspects that people like and dislike about a product. To achieve this, the system extracts the X top a_i which received the most positive and negative orientations from people.

4 Experiments and Evaluation

In this section, we first describe the settings of experiments and then demonstrate the experimental results.

4.1 Dataset and Experimental Stetting

In order to evaluate our SSA model, we crawled Twitter for three brands of cell phone by specifying the *hashtag*. The products are the *IPhone*, the *Galaxy* and the *HTC*. We selected these smartphones because they are the most talked about products on Twitter. Our collection spans from the release data of the smartphone to January 2017. See Table 1. To extract the hierarchical tree, we set the LDA model hyperparameters to $iteration = 2000$, $alpha = 0.1$, $eta = 0.01$, the number of topics to $k = [25, 2]$, and the threshold $ThPercentage = [0.01, 0.05]$. Figure 2 shows the result of our model. For the limitation of the space, the summary result is not given in this paper.

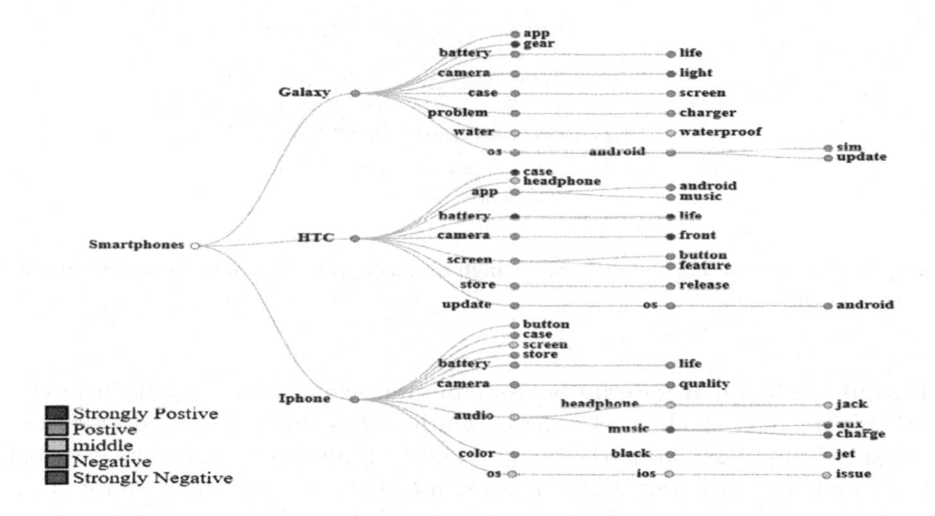

Fig. 2. A structured sentiment tree of the three products.

Table 1. Statistics used in the experiments

Product name	No. tweets	No. aspects (nouns)
IPhone	68004	6234
Galaxy	190494	6069
HTC	60895	2451

4.2 Hierarchy Analysis

The purpose of the evaluation is to measure the consistency and the quality of the SSA output. Since there is no prior work has been done to revele the strucuture from short text, a comprehensive comparison is difficult. In order to quantitatively evaluate the SSA result, we use parent-children relatedness and an online survey. First, we followed the prior work on hierarchical topic models to evaluate parent-children relatedness [5]. Additionally, to measure the quality of the tree, we conducted an online survey. The goal of the survey was to use people's experience to evaluate three major characteristics of the hierarchical tree: node specialisation, uselessness and aspect-sentiment accuracy. We recruited 115 participants who had experience with smartphones. In this experiment, 66 were IPhone users, 34 were Galaxy users, and only 15 were HTC users, due to the differing popularities of the three brands (Fig. 3).

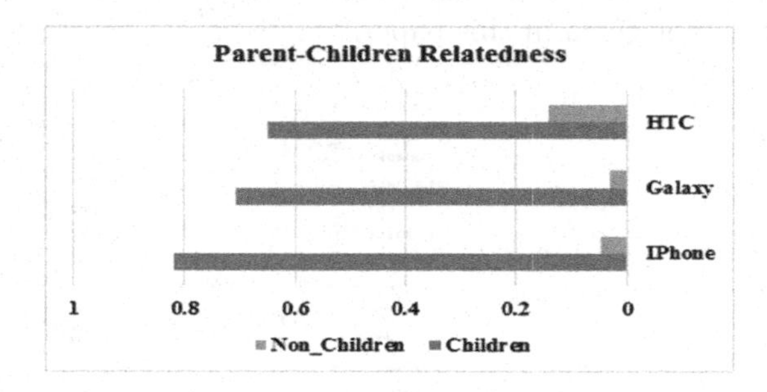

Fig. 3. Parent-Children Relatedness. A high distance indicates that the parent is similar to its children.

Parent-Children Relatedness. An important characteristic of the hierarchical tree is parent-children relatedness, which means that parent nodes are supposed to be more similar to their direct children than others. Therefore, our goal in this section is to evaluate the relationships between the parent and its children. We use cosine similarity to compute the distance between the two aspects a_i and a_j:

$$consin(\phi_i, \phi_j) = \frac{\phi_i \cdot \phi_j}{|\phi_i||\phi_j|} \tag{4}$$

where ϕ_i is the distribution of the word tw_{i1} over all k topics discovered via the LDA. The distance of aspect a_i and its direct children are calculated with:

$$\triangle(i) = \frac{\sum_j consin(\phi_i, \phi_j)}{|Children_i|}, j \in Children_i \tag{5}$$

$$\nabla(i) = \frac{\sum_j consin(\phi_i, \phi_j)}{|A| - |Children_i| - 1}, j \neq i, \notin Children_i \tag{6}$$

For each parent node ϕ_i, we compute the average cosine distance to its direct children, and then compare the average distance to non-children nodes. We average the result from children and non-children to all parent nodes for level 1. Figure 4 shows the parent-children relatedness score for all three phones.

Hierarchy Quality. We designed the SSA to construct a structured sentiment tree of hot aspects of a product. One important feature of our model is to hierarchically organise the product aspects from general to specific. To quantitatively evaluate node specialisation, we used the survey to ask the participants if the aspects were organised in a hierarchical way in the tree's structure. Figure 5 shows the percentage of people who agreed that the product's aspects were organised from general to specific on the tree. Overall, for all products, the results indicate that the participants were extremely satisfied with the tree's organisation.

Another important characteristic we aimed to measure was the usefulness of our automatically extracted tree, which consisted of product aspects. In our surveys, smartphone users were asked how relevant the discovered aspects were to the product on a scale of 1–5. The rating scale was as follows: 1 (totally not relevant aspects of the given product); 2 (slightly not relevant aspects of the given product); 3 (middle); 4 (slightly relevant aspects of the given product); 5 (totally relevant aspects of the given product). Figure 4 shows the score for each product. For IPhone users, the results illustrate that approximately 82% agreed that the product aspects were relevant and made sense. However, for the Galaxy and HTC, about 75% of the participants felt the quality of the structure was acceptable.

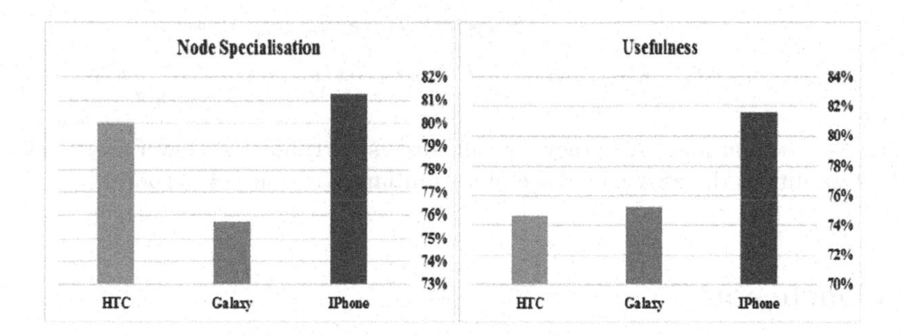

Fig. 4. Hierarchy quality.

Aspect-Sentiment Accuracy. In addition to extracting the concept hierarchy of the hot aspects, we designed our system to show people's opinions on those aspects. To evaluate the accuracy of the sentiment analysis results, we conducted a survey to ask the participants two questions: (1) What aspects are positive about the smartphone? and (2) What aspects are negative about the smartphone? We assumed that the participants and Twitter users shared the same opinions about the hot aspects of the products given in the survey.

In this experiment, we compared the score of the respondents with the score of our model with:

$$Accuracy = \sum_{i=1} |(p_i - q_i)| \frac{l_i}{L} \tag{7}$$

where o_i is the polarity score from our model for aspect a_i, and q_i is the polarity score from the respondents for aspect a_i. q_i is a ratio between the number of respondents who selected the aspect a_i as positive and the number who selected a_i as positive or negative. Since some aspects receive more responses than others for sentiment analysis, we believe the more responses an aspect receives, the higher the confidence level of people's attitudes towards this aspect. Thus, we added a weight for each aspect to calculate the final sentiment accuracy. The more responses for an aspect, the higher the weight of the aspect. L is the total number of respondents for all aspects, and l_i is the number of respondents who selected a_i as positive or negative. Figure 5 shows the aspect sentiment accuracy of our model for all products. It is obvious that for all smartphones, the results indicate consistency between the sentiment result of our model and the participants' opinions.

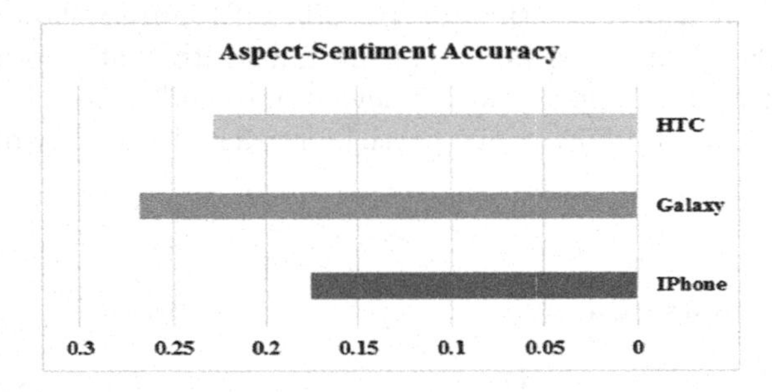

Fig. 5. Aspect-Sentiment Accuracy. For all three smartphones, a lower score indicates that the results of the SSA model are more similar to the survey responses.

5 Conclusions

We present in this paper a structured sentiment analysis approach (SSA) to analyse the opinions that people express about aspects of a particular product in short texts. The proposed approach first discovers the structured tree of the hot aspects of a product in a hierarchical way. Then, the corresponding sentiment analysis on those aspects identified in the tree is performed. Finally, our approach summarises people's attitudes. The results confirm the effectiveness of our proposed approach on analysing short texts. In future work, we will improved our methodology to automatically discover the optimal number of k and generate a tree with different shapes.

References

1. Blei, D.M., Griffiths, T.L., Jordan, M.I.: The nested chinese restaurant process and bayesian nonparametric inference of topic hierarchies. arXiv preprint arXiv:0710.0845 (2007)
2. Hartigan, J.A., Wong, M.A.: Algorithm as 136: a k-means clustering algorithm. J. Roy. Stat. Soc. Ser. C (Appl. Stat.) **28**(1), 100–108 (1979)
3. Hu, M., Liu, B.: Mining and summarizing customer reviews. In: Proceedings of the Tenth ACM SIGKDD International Conference on Knowledge Discovery and Data Mining, pp. 168–177. ACM (2004)
4. Kim, J.H., Kim, D., Kim, S., Oh, A.: Modeling topic hierarchies with the recursive Chinese restaurant process. In: Proceedings of the 21st ACM International Conference on Information and Knowledge Management, pp. 783–792. ACM (2012)
5. Kim, S., Zhang, J., Chen, Z., Oh, A.H., Liu, S.: A hierarchical aspect-sentiment model for online reviews. In: AAAI (2013)
6. Lin, C., He, Y.: Joint sentiment/topic model for sentiment analysis. In: Proceedings of the 18th ACM Conference on Information and Knowledge Management, pp. 375–384. ACM (2009)
7. Paisley, J., Wang, C., Blei, D.M., Jordan, M.I.: Nested hierarchical dirichlet processes. IEEE Trans. Pattern Anal. Mach. Intell. **37**(2), 256–270 (2015)
8. Phan, X.H., Nguyen, C.T., Le, D.T., Nguyen, L.M., Horiguchi, S., Ha, Q.T.: A hidden topic-based framework toward building applications with short web documents. IEEE Trans. Knowl. Data Eng. **23**(7), 961–976 (2011)
9. Popescu, A.M., Etzioni, O.: Extracting product features and opinions from reviews. In: Kao, A., Poteet, S.R. (eds.) Natural Language Processing and Text Mining, pp. 9–28. Springer, London (2007)
10. Ramage, D., Dumais, S.T., Liebling, D.J.: Characterizing microblogs with topic models. In: ICWSM, vol. 10, pp. 1–1 (2010)
11. Suchanek, F.M., Kasneci, G., Weikum, G.: Yago: a large ontology from Wikipedia and WordNet. Web Semant. Sci. Serv. Agents World Wide Web **6**(3), 203–217 (2008)
12. Titov, I., McDonald, R.: Modeling online reviews with multi-grain topic models. In: Proceedings of the 17th International Conference on World Wide Web, pp. 111–120. ACM (2008)
13. Wang, C., Danilevsky, M., Desai, N., Zhang, Y., Nguyen, P., Taula, T., Han, J.: A phrase mining framework for recursive construction of a topical hierarchy. In: Proceedings of the 19th ACM SIGKDD International Conference on Knowledge Discovery and Data Mining, pp. 437–445. ACM (2013)
14. Weng, J., Lim, E.P., Jiang, J., He, Q.: TwitterRank: finding topic-sensitive influential Twitterers. In: Proceedings of the third ACM International Conference on Web Search and Data Mining, pp. 261–270. ACM (2010)
15. Zhao, P., Li, X., Wang, K.: Feature extraction from micro-blogs for comparison of products and services. In: Lin, X., Manolopoulos, Y., Srivastava, D., Huang, G. (eds.) WISE 2013. LNCS, vol. 8180, pp. 82–91. Springer, Heidelberg (2013). doi:10.1007/978-3-642-41230-1_7

Data Mining Applications

Improving Real-Time Bidding Using a Constrained Markov Decision Process

Manxing Du[1(✉)], Redouane Sassioui[1], Georgios Varisteas[1], Radu State[1], Mats Brorsson[2], and Omar Cherkaoui[3]

[1] University of Luxembourg, Luxembourg City, Luxembourg
{manxing.du,redouane.sassioui,georgios.varisteas,radu.state}@uni.lu
[2] Royal Institute of Technology (KTH), Stockholm, Sweden
matsbror@kth.se
[3] University of Quebec in Montreal, Montreal, Canada
cherkaoui.omar@uqam.ca

Abstract. Online advertising is increasingly switching to real-time bidding on advertisement inventory, in which the ad slots are sold through real-time auctions upon users visiting websites or using mobile apps. To compete with unknown bidders in such a highly stochastic environment, each bidder is required to estimate the value of each impression and to set a competitive bid price. Previous bidding algorithms have done so without considering the constraint of budget limits, which we address in this paper. We model the bidding process as a Constrained Markov Decision Process based reinforcement learning framework. Our model uses the predicted click-through-rate as the state, bid price as the action, and ad clicks as the reward. We propose a bidding function, which outperforms the state-of-the-art bidding functions in terms of the number of clicks when the budget limit is low. We further simulate different bidding functions competing in the same environment and report the performances of the bidding strategies when required to adapt to a dynamic environment.

Keywords: Display Advertising · Real-time bidding · Markov Decision Process · Reinforcement Learning

1 Introduction

The share of digital ad spending in the global ad market has increased tremendously in the recent years and is expected to soar up to over 46% by 2020 as eMarketer forecasts [16]. Programmatic platforms like *Real-time bidding* (RTB) gradually takes over as the major tool for the digital ad trading [13]. Instead of bidding on keywords like in sponsored search [3], or on the context of the website as in contextual advertising [8], RTB targets the best match of users and campaigns at each ad impression level.

In an RTB system, the *demand-side platform* (DSP) plays the role of bidding for ad impressions on behalf of the advertisers. An ad exchange (ADX) receives bids

M. Brorsson—Work done while Mats Brorsson was at OLAmobile, Luxembourg.

G. Cong et al. (Eds.): ADMA 2017, LNAI 10604, pp. 711–726, 2017.
https://doi.org/10.1007/978-3-319-69179-4_50

from DSPs and holds second-price auctions; the DSP with the highest bid wins the auction but pays the second highest price, known as the *market price*. According to the Bayesian-Nash equilibrium in the auction theory [14], each bidder's optimal strategy in a second-price auction is to bid the value of each impression evaluated from its own perspective. This is known as truth-telling bidding.

However, in reality, truth-telling bidding may not be the optimal solution due to the budget limit for each ad campaign. Bidding constantly at the true value can lead to running out of budget quickly without having covered a wide range of users and impressions [20]. Consequently, the bidder fails to obtain potential profits and might even be subject to heavy losses since the payback of the impressions may be less than the total cost of winning the auction.

The optimization of bidding strategies has been widely studied in the computational advertising industry [9,21]. The goal of an optimal bidding strategy is to intelligently set the bid price for each ad auction in order to maximize the total number of clicks or profits [17] within a certain budget. This optimization problem fits perfectly into the framework of a *Constrained Markov Decision Process* (CMDP) [2], which allows to maximize one criterion while keeping another criterion below a given threshold.

In this paper, we cast the optimization of the sequential bid requests as a CMDP. This is done in order to find the optimal bid price under budget constraints for each auction. A CMDP is defined by the tuple $< S, A, P, R, C, V >$, which correspondingly represents state, action, state transition probability, reward, cost, and the value of the constrains. We consider the predicted *click-through-rate* (CTR[1]) as the *state*, the *number of clicks* as the *reward* to maximize, the *market price* as the *cost*, and the budget limit as the *constraint*. We integrate the optimization problem and the condition of budget limit into the model and use the linear programming method [11] to solve the CMDP. The policy derived from the solution gives an optimal bid price for each state.

Our contributions are summarized as follows:

- We formalize the bidding optimization problem as a CMDP which optimizes the bidding performance on the impression level. Instead of directly using the features from the impression space, our approach simplifies and limits the state as the discretized predicted CTR. This results in a significant decrease of the dimensionality of the state space. Another outcome is that we maximize the number of clicks within the constrained budget.
- We introduce the use of conditional market price distribution derived from the joint distribution of historical market price and the predicted CTR. This captures the correlation between the winning probability and the user level information.
- We show how the well-tuned bidding functions handle the dynamics of the market price, by simulating scenarios where different bidders compete with each other in the same environment. Previous studies compare the bid price of their proposed bidding strategies with only the historical winning price.

[1] The CTR can be seen as the probability of a user clicking on the ad being shown. The predicted CTR is a prediction of this probability based on features of the publisher site/app and the user visiting it.

2 Related Work

A bidding strategy is one of the key components of online advertising [3,12,21]. An optimal bidding strategy helps advertisers to target the valuable users and to set a competitive bid price in the ad auction for winning the ad impression and displaying their ads to the users. If the ads are clicked by the users or the users make purchases after clicking the ads, profits will be generated for the bidder.

The linear bidding strategy is widely used with real-world applications [17,21]. This strategy bids proportionally higher for bid requests with higher estimated CTR, failing however to deal with the budget constraints. In [21], a non-linear bidding function is proposed to adapt different budget constraints. It is shown to outperform the linear bidding function in terms of the number of clicks per ad campaign, however the winning probability function does not describe well the real winning price distribution. We are addressing this shortcoming with CMDP, since we derive the winning price distribution directly from the historical data and use it in the bid optimization process.

Reinforcement learning methods have been widely applied on solving decision making problems in online advertising applications. The models fall into two major frameworks, namely the Multi-Armed Bandits (MAB) [19] and the *Markov Decision Process* (MDP). In both models, the key components are the states, actions, and rewards. Several prior works have tried to formalize the online advertising problem as a reinforcement learning framework. In [11,18], the authors fit the banner delivery and the ad allocation problems into the MAB model while the rewards are the number of ad clicks and the profits. However, these prior works, assume no cost for showing the impressions and thus consider no constraints. This cost is highly important for an RTB system. Additional user-level information is also neglected in the previous works, which are of paramount importance for pricing the value of an ad impression, so that profitable customers are targeted.

In sponsored search, ad impressions are shown with certain costs, namely the market price, and the ad agent bids on keywords. The ad agent first needs to place a bid to win the auction, such that its ads can be displayed to the users. In [4], the authors proposed a bidding function for sequential bidding requests in sponsored search. That paper addressed the problem of right-censorship for the market price in the second-price auction scenario. The market price is right-censored because only the winner of the auction is informed; for lost auctions, the bidders only know that the market price is equal or higher than their own bid price. The authors formalized keyword bidding as a MDP, where the number of auctions and the budget limit are the states, the discretized bid price are the actions, and the total number of clicks are the rewards. With RTB, auctions are held for each single impression, thus the budget per auction needs to be constrained to optimize spending relative to profit. In our work, the CMDP model extends MDP by accounting for budget constraints directly and implicitly takes the impression level information in the predicted CTR to find the optimal bid price.

The CTR estimation reflects how well the user and the publisher match the targeting goal of each campaign. It directly impacts the bid price, which subsequently affects the winning price. The authors in [7] formulated a reinforcement learning based bidding function, by extending the concept in [4] and applying it into the RTB system. However, they implicitly correlate the user features to the winning rate approximation by multiplying the average CTR to the density function of the market price. In our work, we discuss the importance of correlating market price with the CTR and directly take the discretized CTR as the state for the bidding optimization. In addition, their bid price is set in two steps: state value lookup and action calculation in [7]. In contrast, our model solved the bidding optimization problem with linear programming which derives the optimal bid price for each state; thus the bid price can be set after a single lookup per bid request.

3 Background and Bidding Strategy Modeling

In an RTB system, whenever a user visits the publisher's website, the ad slots on the website are sold through real-time auctions. A bid request is sent from user's browser to an ad exchange, which contains the user profile, the publisher side information, and the description of the ad slot. The ADX distributes the bid requests to multiple DSPs which bid on behalf of advertisers. Each DSP derives the high dimensional feature vectors from the bid request and estimates the probability that the user clicks (or purchases) the ad campaign selected for bidding. The DSP integrates the CTR prediction, the budget, and the winning probability estimation to compute a bid price sending back to the ADX. An ADX holds a second-price auction, which selects the winner of the auction as the DSP with the highest bid and sends the URL of the corresponding ad back to the publisher. In a second-price auction, the second highest bid is denoted as the market price or the winning price. In this paper, we use market price and winning price interchangeably. The ad from the winner will be shown to the user. If the user clicks the ad, he/she will be redirected to the landing page of the ad. On the landing page, the user may complete subscription or purchase depending on the property of the ad. User's activity of ad clicks or purchase will be sent back to the DSP as feedback. DSPs correspondingly use the feedback to adjust their bidding strategies. Figure 1 shows these interactions graphically.

The interaction between the bidder and the ADX can be framed as an interaction between an agent and an environment, similar to the reinforcement learning framework [19]. As shown in Fig. 1, an agent (a DSP) receives a state (bid request) from the environment and takes an action (sets a bid price) which triggers the environment to respond with a reward (feedback per auction) and the next state (next bid request). The goal of the DSP is to learn an optimal mapping from a bid request to a bid price, which maximizes the reward it receives over a finite time period (an episodic task) or an infinite time period (a continuous task). In our work, the end of the time period is when the budget is exhausted.

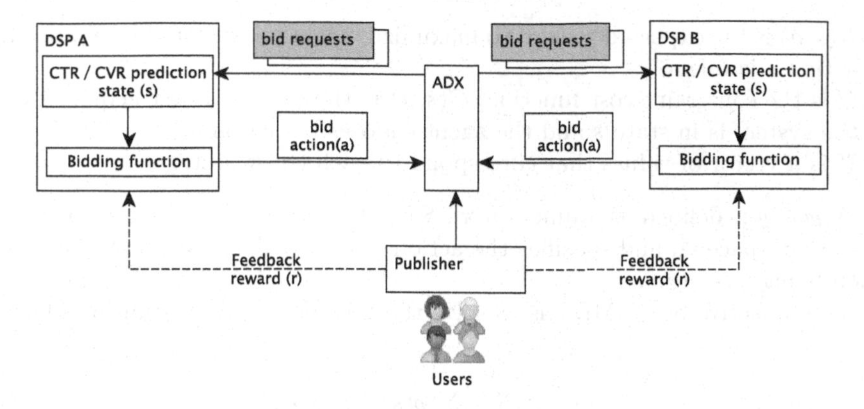

Fig. 1. A RTB system overview

3.1 Learning with Constraints

When no additional constraints exist, reinforcement learning is usually formalized as a Markov decision process (MDP) [19]. However, RTB requires to keep the budget under certain constraints and in the meantime maximize the total number of clicks. A Constrained Markov Decision Process (CMDP) is a class of MDP models which can set more than one conflicting objectives. A typical case of CMDP is the situation where we want to maximize one criterion while keeping another below a given threshold. Therefore we relied on such models to describe the bidding function.

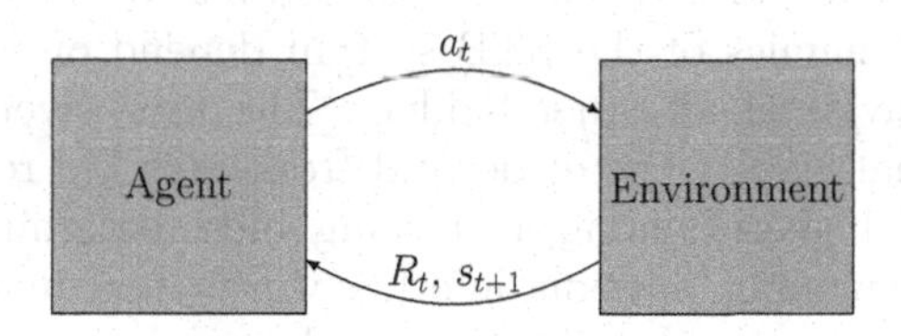

Fig. 2. Graphical representation of an MDP. At each time t the agent knows the environment state s_t and based on the transition probability model, it takes action a_t and receives the reward R_t and observe the next state s_{t+1}.

Figure 2 shows a graphical representation of a MDP at time t. A CMDP is defined by the tuple $< S, A, P, R, C, V >$.

- S is the state set.
- A is the action set.
- $P(s'|s, a)$ is the transition probability function, such that $P(s'|s, a)$ is the probability that the system moves to state s' given that it is in state s and the agent takes an action a.

- $R(s, a)$ is the expected reward to maximize, when the system is in state s and action a is taken.
- C is the constraint cost function. $C(s, a)$ is the expected cost acquired when the system is in state s and the agent chooses an action a.
- V is a vector of values that correspond to each constraint.

A *policy* is defined as a function $\pi : S \mapsto A$ which maps the state space S to the action space A, and specifies the action $a = \pi(s)$ that the agent will choose when being in state s.

The objective of a CMDP is to solve the following optimization problem

$$\begin{aligned} \max_{\rho} \quad & \overline{R} = \sum_{s,a} \rho(s, a) R(s, a) \\ \text{s.t} \quad & \sum_{s,a} \rho(s, a) C(s, a) \leq V \\ \text{and} \quad & \sum_{s \in S} \sum_{a \in A(s)} \rho(s, a) = 1 \end{aligned} \tag{1}$$

where ρ is a vector of length $|S| * |A|$ in which each element corresponds to the probability of being in state s and taking action a. Let $\tilde{\rho}$ be the optimal solution of Eq.(1), the optimal policy $\tilde{\pi}$ to apply in each state is the action a which is in the $\tilde{\rho}(s, a)$.

3.2 RTB as a Model-Based CMDP

As described above, an optimal bidding function combines the CTR estimation, the winning probability, and the budget constraint to set a bid price for each bid request. The dynamics of the RTB system depend on the diversity of the users and the behavior of all other bidders. The user diversity is reflected in the high dimensional feature vector derived from each bid request. The market price, which is the highest among all loosing bids, determines how much the winner pays for the winning auction, in other words, how much budget is spent. The historical market price distribution can be used to estimate the winning probability of bidding a certain price.

Directly using the high dimensional user feature vector $\mathbf{x}$ as the state in the Markov model is very difficult because of the sparsity of the data. However, mapping this feature vector into a lower dimensional space is possible through the CTR prediction $\theta(x)$. The latter takes the feature vector $\mathbf{x}$ as input and calculates the probability of a click. This method has been used to optimize a non-linear bidding strategy [21]. The underlying assumption is that the state dynamics of the RTB system can be completely captured by CTR. Obviously, both the bidding strategy and the winning rate estimation are dependent on the CTR.

We therefore also assume that user dynamics are described by the predicted CTR $\theta(x)$ and thus project the high dimensional feature space into an 1-dimensional space. The predicted CTR is the state of the RTB system, $S = \Theta$. The set of actions, A, consists of the set of permitted bids, i.e.,

$A = \{0, 1, 2, ..., a_{max}\}$, where a_{max} is the maximum bid that a bidder wants to pay for showing its ad. The transition probability function P equals the probability density function (pdf) of θ and is independent of the current state and the action taken. Formally:

$$P(\theta'|\theta, a) = p_{CTR}(\theta') \tag{2}$$

where p_{CTR} is the pdf of the predicted CTR. p_{CTR} can be approximated from historical data using a kernel density estimation.

The reward of an RTB system is usually defined by the advertisers. For branding purpose, the goal of the advertisers can be to maximize the number of ad impressions. However, more commonly, the advertisers are not satisfied by only displaying their ads. Thus, they set the goal as acquiring user interactions like clicks or even further, purchases. In this paper, the reward of an RTB system is the number of clicks. Since for example, in the iPinYou dataset, there are 5 out of 9 campaigns without any purchase in both training and test datasets. It is a chain process to calculate the expected reward. Firstly, the bidder needs to win an ad auction by placing a bid. The winning probability is derived from the market price distribution. After winning the auction, the expected reward is given by the estimated CTR. The cost is defined as the market price each bidder pays for a winning auction. If the bid price of a bidder is not the highest among all the bidders, the bidder loses the auction with no cost.

Hence, the system reward, R, and cost, C, are given by

$$R(\theta, a) = \theta \sum_{\delta=0}^{a} p_{MP}(\delta|\theta) \tag{3}$$

$$C(\theta, a) = \sum_{\delta=0}^{a} \delta p_{MP}(\delta|\theta) \tag{4}$$

where p_{MP} is the pdf of the market price that can be derived from historical data. Since CTR is a continuous value ranging from 0 to 1, it is discretized into bins and δ denotes the market price of a bin of CTR. The $R(\theta, a)$ represents the probability of winning an auction by bidding a multiplying the probability of getting a click after winning the auction. The $C(\theta, a)$ represents the expected cost of winning an auction by bidding a.

Our objective is to maximize the expected reward while keeping the expected cost below a certain threshold, V. We interpret V as the maximum of the average cost per impression each bidder is willing to spend. The derived policy from CMDP determines the bid price to set in each state.

3.3 Learning from Historical Data: Batch-CMDP

In the CMDP model, the correlation between the CTR and the real feedbacks (clicks of impressions) in the historical data is neglected. We argue that it should be utilized as valuable experience to learn from. We thus leverage *Batch Reinforcement Learning* (Batch-RL) to derive the best policy from a set of priori-known transition samples [15]. The objective of Batch-RL is to derive a model reflecting the reality learned from the historical data. The advantage of such approach is the efficiency in the learning process compared to the model free approaches, like the Q learning algorithm [19], which needs a huge amount of interactions with the environment to converge to the optimal solution, and which is often not possible in real life applications.

We modify the previous RTB model to derive the best policy from historical data. In the CMDP model, the only variable not derived from historical data is the probability for a click, θ, used in calculating the reward in Eq.(3). We adopt the reward function from the previous model to use only information from the historical data. For each bin of θ, we calculate the corresponding probability of a click using historical data. We denote $f(\theta)$ as the probability of a click given θ. We call this new model *Batch-CMDP*, formally defined as:

$$R(\theta, a) = f(\theta) \sum_{\delta=0}^{a} p_{MP}(\delta|\theta) \tag{5}$$

$$C(\theta, a) = \sum_{\delta=0}^{a} \delta p_{MP}(\delta|\theta) \tag{6}$$

3.4 Market Price Distribution

The market price can be seen as drawing from an unknown distribution generated from the online marketplace. In [7,10], the authors directly model the market price distribution. However, since the winning probability also relies on the CTR estimation, we introduce the correlation between the winning price and the CTR in the estimation of market price distribution. We estimate the probability distribution function of the market price p_{MP} using Eq.(7). This derives implicitly from the joint distribution of the winning price and corresponding CTR, as well as from the distribution of the predicted CTR according to the Bayesian theorem [6].

$$p_{MP}(\delta|\theta) = \frac{p(\delta,\theta)}{p(\theta)} \tag{7}$$

In order to validate our approach, we prove that a strong correlation exists between the market price and the CTR. A commonly used method for this purpose is to calculate the Pearson's correlation coefficient [1]. This technique is efficient in linear correlation cases, however it fails to capture non-linear relationships. *Mutual Information* (MI) [5] is one of the measures that captures any type of non-linear dependencies between two random variables. MI quantifies the amount of information obtained about one random variable given another random variable. In other words, it measures the degree of uncertainty of one variable knowing the other variable. Formally, the mutual information of two random variables X and Y is defined as

$$MI(X;Y) = \int_Y \int_X p(x,y) \log \frac{p(x,y)}{p(x)p(y)} dxdy \tag{8}$$

where $p(x,y)$ is the joint probability density of X and Y, $p(x)$ and $p(y)$ are the probability density function of X and Y respectively. In the following section, we present the mutual information between the market price and the CTR.

4 Experiment and Results

We have implemented a CMDP model for bidding trained on two real-world RTB datasets. The bidding results are compared with several state-of-the-art bidding algorithms. In this section, we elaborate the experiments and discuss the results.

4.1 Datasets and CTR Prediction

In our experiments, two real-world datasets are used. Due to privacy reasons, the public dataset of RTB bidding logs is very limited. A detailed RTB dataset was released by iPinYou, a leading RTB company in China, for a bidding competition in 2013. This is the only public dataset which contains the historical market price. It contains 19.5M impressions, ~15 K clicks and 1.2 K conversions over 9 ad campaigns. The training and test data are chronologically split into 7 days and 3 days, respectively. The other dataset is from OLAmobile, a global mobile advertising company in Luxembourg. The data are collected from 8 campaigns over 6 days, which include 800 K impressions and 6 K clicks.

The iPinYou dataset contains bid requests, winning impressions, ad clicks, and conversions. Each row in the log file represents a bid request at a certain time. The features can be categorized as user profile, publisher, and ad description. The user profile includes the *time stamp of the visit, user agent, IP address, region,* and *city.* The publisher is represented by *domain and ad exchange ID* and the ad slot is described by *slot size and format, advertiser ID, and creative ID.*

We applied the data pre-processing procedure[2] used in [22], which utilizes the one-hot-encoding method to convert the categorical features into binary features and we used the logistic regression training like in [21] to estimate the predicted CTR.

For the reproducibility, our code is available online[3]. We mainly report and publish the results on the iPinYou dataset. Due to the privacy reason, the OLAmobile dataset is not released, but the results are listed as supplementary.

---

[2] http://data.computational-advertising.org/.

[3] https://github.com/manxing-du/cmdp-rtb.

4.2 The Correlation Between Market Price and CTR

As introduced in Sect. 3.4, Table 1 shows the results of the normalized mutual information of δ and θ calculated in the iPinYou dataset. The normalization of the Mutual Information scales the results between 0 and 1 where 0 means no relationship and 1 means perfect correlation. It can be inferred from Table 1 that for all campaigns in the iPinYou, $MI(\delta, \theta)$ is significantly higher than 0. We conclude that δ and θ are strongly dependent on each other in the iPinYou data. This supports the rationale of our approach to model the relationship between δ and θ as a batch CMDP.

Table 1. Mutual information of the market price δ and CTR θ

iPinYou Camp	1458	2259	2261	2821	2997	3358	3386	3427	3476	OLA Camp	1	2	3	4	5	6	7	8
$MI(\delta, \theta)$	0.50	0.58	0.59	0.55	0.55	0.56	0.50	0.51	0.53	$MI(\delta, \theta)$	0.18	0.22	0.40	0.35	0.41	0.16	0.36	0.44

4.3 Evaluation Methods

The evaluation of the bidding functions is carried out on a per campaign basis. In our experiments we only focus on the total number of clicks as the KPI, due to the insufficient number of conversions. In addition, since every campaign has a limited budget, our goal is to maximize the number of clicks given the budget constraint. Thus, the *expected cost per click* (eCPC) is also used to measure how efficient the budget is spent.

4.4 Experiment 1: Compare Bid Prices to the Historical Data

In experiment 1, each bidding function computes a bid price for the same bid request and the price is compared with the historical market price. If the bid price is higher than the historical market price, then it wins the auction and the cost is the market price. The subsequent click will be accumulated. Otherwise we assume that the auction is lost with no additional cost. We used the source code available[4] for the work in [7] to generate results for the *Mcpc*, *Lin*, and *RLB* functions.

- **Mcpc**. Sets a maximum eCPC which is the goal of the bidding function. The bid price is calculated by multiplying the max eCPC from the training data with the predicted CTR.
- **Lin**. As proposed by [17], the bid price depends linearly on the predicted CTR as $b_0 \frac{\theta(x)}{\theta_{avg}}$,where b_0 is tuned as in [7] and θ_{avg} is the average CTR in the training set.
- **RLB**. One of the recent papers in [7] formalizes the bidding problem into a reinforcement learning framework. More details in this approach can be found in their paper [7].

[4] https://github.com/han-cai/rlb-dp.

- **CMDP**. Our proposed model of CMDP as described in Sect. 3.2
- **Batch-CMDP**. The second model we proposed in Sect. 3.3 where the policy is learned by using the real feedback (click or not) as the reward.

We first compare each bidding strategy with limited budget. We determine the budget $B = CPM_{train} * c0 * N_{test}$, where $c0 = 1/32, 1/16, 1/8$, and $1/4$. The $c0$ setting is as the same as in [7] to make our results comparable with theirs. In Table 2, the total number of clicks and the eCPC for $c0 = 1/32$ are listed. We find that (i) CMDP and batch-CMDP models outperforms all the other bidding strategies in terms of number of clicks when the CTR estimation has higher AUC, since the state only contains the CTR which directly impacts the performance of our model. (ii) In terms of eCPC, the CMDP solution does not always achieve the least cost. This is due to CMDP trying to keep the cost per impression (CPM) under the averaged value in the training set while obtaining the maximum number of clicks. We did not directly set the goal as the cost per click because before getting clicks, we need to win a certain amount of impressions first. As we can see in Table 2, for example, the *Lin* function has lower eCPC for campaign 2997 while the number of clicks is fewer than *CMDP*. We should note that even all the bidding strategies has the same budget setting, each of them spends different amount of the budget until the end of the test. In other words, within the same budget limit, different algorithms has won different number of auctions. The results suggests CMDP set the bid price efficiently to cover a wider range of impressions and also gets more clicks.

Table 2. Total number of clicks and (eCPC), c0 =1/32

iPinYou Camp	AUC	CTR	Mcpc	Lin	RLB	CMDP	Batch CMDP
1458	97.95%	0.084%	392(3.34)	464 (**1.09**)	424 (3.09)	**464** (2.71)	462 (2.8)
2259	67.12%	0.031%	10 (120.63)	7 (173.52)	12 (101.02)	**13(89.47)**	10 (119.16)
2261	62.69%	0.028%	7 (137.06)	9 (105.67)	**11 (87.39)**	8 (118.10)	7 (116.46)
2821	61.28%	0.057%	17 (107.63)	40 (40.26)	**47 (39)**	39 (45.32)	41 (45.05)
2997	60.79%	0.34%	62 (4.9)	64 (**2.73**)	**82** (3.7)	71 (2.95)	71 (2.98)
3358	97.48%	0.086%	180 (4.75)	189 (3.77)	199 (4.29)	**208 (3.38)**	203 (4.28)
3386	77.39%	0.082%	56 (23.12)	55 (**5.52**)	61 (21.21)	**92** (12.99)	91 (14.26)
3427	97.23%	0.068%	227 (5.91)	203 (6.55)	261 (5.14)	**292** (4.47)	292 (**4.36**)
3476	95.88%	0.055%	101 (12.76)	162 (**5.92**)	131 (9.87)	181 (7.16)	**188** (6.82)

Figure 3 illustrates the performance of the bidding functions with respect to different budget settings. The bidding functions are compared in terms of (i) number of clicks (ii) Winning rate (iii) eCPC and (iv) CPM

Without budget control, the *lin* and *mcpc* bidding wins fewer auctions and obtains fewer clicks than all the other bidding functions. Not surprisingly, with the same amount of budget, they win the auctions with high market price, so that the eCPC and CPM are both higher than the others. In general, *RLB*, *CMDP*, and *Batch-CMDP* perform better and especially with the low budget setting, *CMDP* outperforms all the other functions.

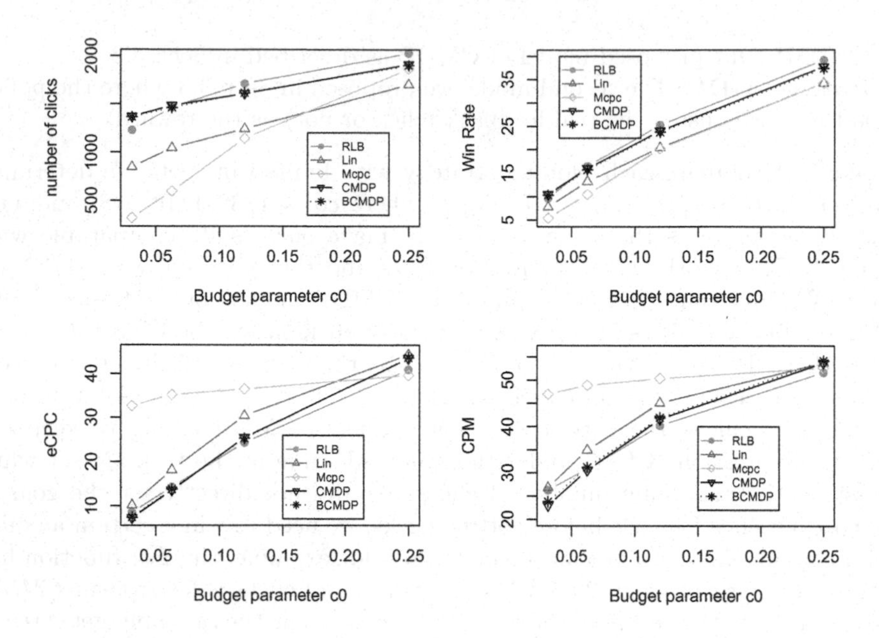

Fig. 3. Overall bidding performance on iPinYou Data.

In Table 3, the results of OLAmobile dataset show that *Batch CMDP* obtains the most clicks among all the bidding functions. In *Batch CMDP*, the reward is computed by Eq.(5) in which the probability of a click is derived from the historical clicking probability given the state θ (pCTR). Since the OLAmobile dataset spans 1–2 days, the conditional distribution of the winning probability given the predicted CTR is more reliable to be used as a factor in the reward function. Thus, it shows that if the model of the environment reflects the reality, *Batch-CMDP* provides the optimal policy for making bidding decisions. In the iPinYou dataset, the training data are from 7 days and the test data are from the

Table 3. Total number of clicks and (eCPC), c0 =1/32

OLA Camp	AUC	CTR	Mcpc	Lin	RLB	CMDP	Batch CMDP
1	69.96%	0.445%	1(46.41)	3(13.63)	3(15.42)	0 (NA)	**4**(30.59)
2	56.79%	0.466%	2(45.67)	2(39.56)	2(45.23)	3(29.84)	**4**(26.51)
3	73.22%	1.827%	**6**(2.74)	5(1.21)	6(2.51)	2(2.26)	3(1.53)
4	75.18%	0.938%	21(6.04)	22(4.34)	**26**(4.86)	14(8.94)	26(6.82)
5	71.35%	1.833%	3(3.4)	3(3.39)	4(2.54)	4(2.23)	**13**(2.64)
6	58.15%	0.465%	8(30.01)	16(14.28)	10(23.9)	6(39.55)	**28**(38.54)
7	67.69%	1.237%	4(60.95)	14(16.53)	5(48.42)	9(27.21)	**23**(23.83)
8	68.07%	0.554%	33(9.46)	51(5.78)	61(5.07)	71(4.37)	**88**(5.93)

following 3 days. Our interpretation is that the market price model changes over time, thus the model based on the long term history degrades the performance of *CMDP* and *Batch-CMDP*.

We should also note that in Eq. 1, the sum of $\rho(s, a)$ over the entire state and action is 1. In other words, the policy learned by CMDP also depends on the pCTR distribution in the training set. If the pCTR distribution in the test set changes dramatically, the policy may lead to budget overspending or underspending. The dynamics of the pCTR distribution is a strong focus of our future work.

4.5 Experiment 2: Compare Bidding Functions in the Same Environment

In the previous experiment, the performance of the bidding functions is independently compared with the historical winning prices. However, in a real world scenario, every bidder will try to improve his/her bidding functions at any time. Thus, we present the impact of the fluctuation of the market price distribution on the bidding strategies. We simulate the scenario by assuming that the historical winning prices come from a single virtual bidder and let the other bidding functions compete with each other as well as with the virtual bidder. The winner is the one which bids the highest and the winning price is the second highest price. If more than one bidders set the same price, all of them win the auction, which produces the maximum number of auctions and clicks each function can win in this setting.

If more than one functions bid the same price, all of them are considered as winners. The corresponding clicks and impressions are denoted as *Dual_win_clk* and *Dual_win_imp* respectively in Table 4. Meanwhile, the single winner case is represented as *Sig_win_clk* and *Sig_win_imp*. The *RLB*, *CMDP*, and *Batch*

Table 4. Comparing bidding functions in the same environment, c0 = 1/32

Camp. 1458	mcpc	Lin	RLB	CMDP	Batch CMDP
Dual_win_clk	55	367	361	101	100
Sig_win_clk	9	46	28	2	14
Dual_win_imp	216	700	2978	3512	3350
Sig_win_imp	30991	84	13731	4755	41783
total_ecpc	23269	453	2608	4647	10059
Camp. 2997	mcpc	Lin	RLB	CMDP	Batch CMDP
Dual_win_clk	0	0	7	5	3
Sig_win_clk	45	0	48	4	10
Dual_win_imp	11	0	2753	2736	2369
Sig_win_imp	15560	0	25799	1051	3718
total_ecpc	7458	0	5441	3624	4077

CMDP models are trained using the historical market price and the experiment was running on the test data. In this setting, the market price in the test set shifts towards higher prices when more than one functions bid higher than the historical market price.

The result suggests that for the campaigns with high AUC (e.g. campaign 1458), the linear bidding function targets the right impressions to bid high. Other functions, for example, like *CMDP* wins 10 times more impressions but only get 1/3 of clicks as *Lin*, which significantly increase the eCPC. On the contrary, *Lin* loses its advantage when the predicted CTR is not accurate since it only relies on pCTR to calculate the bid price. One extreme case is campaign 2997 having the lowest AUC in the dataset. *Lin* sets the bid price too low comparing to other functions and it does not win any impression. The results also show that the eCPC should not be the only metric to evaluate how well the bidding function performs. For example, for campaign 2997, *CMDP* has a lower eCPC while having 6 times less number of clicks than *RLB*. In this case, *CMDP* bids more conservative than *RLB* since *CMDP* follows the policy learned from the pCTR density function in the training set.

5 Conclusions and Future Work

In this paper, we formalize the bidding problem in the RTB system as a Constrained Markov Decision Process. We use linear programming to maximize the total reward with a cost limit. The reward is either derived from the CTR estimation (in CMDP) or from the historical observations (in Batch-CMDP), in which case the best policy is learned given the training data. We use Bayesian inference to obtain the market price distribution, which not only considers the correlation between the market price and the state (pCTR) but also captures the dynamics of market price. Our model outperforms the state-of-art bidding functions in terms of the total number of clicks constrained to a limited budget. However, when the bidding functions compete with each other, linear bidding performs the best for campaigns with a high AUC while RLB obtains more clicks for campaigns with a low AUC. *CMDP* relies on the correlation of the historical market price distribution and the predicted CTR distribution, thus bids more conservative compared to the others.

For future work, we will model the time-dependent dynamics of RTB to improve on the use of a single fixed market price distribution. In addition, we will investigate a model-free approach which does not assume a modeling of the market price distribution but only learns from the rewards.

Acknowledgement. We sincerely thank Prof. Weinan Zhang and his research group from Shanghai Jiaotong University for the short visit. Manxing thanks the National Research Fund (FNR) of Luxembourg for the research support under the AFR PPP scheme and thanks Dr.Tigran Avanesov from OLAmobile for the feedback.

References

1. Aggarwal, C.C.: Data Mining: The Textbook. Springer, Cham (2015)
2. Altman, E.: Constrained Markov Decision Processes. CRC Press, Boca Raton (1999)
3. Amin, K., Kearns, M., Key, P., Schwaighofer, A.: Budget optimization for sponsored search: censored learning in MDPs. In: Proceedings of the Twenty-Eighth Conference on Uncertainty in Artificial Intelligence. AUAI Press (2012)
4. Amin, K., Kearns, M., Key, P., Schwaighofer, A.: Budget optimization for sponsored search: censored learning in MDPs. CoRR (2012)
5. Applebaum, D.: Probability and Information: An Integrated Approach, 2nd edn. Cambridge University Press, Cambridge (2008)
6. Barber, D.: Bayesian Reasoning and Machine Learning. Cambridge University Press, New York (2012)
7. Cai, H., Ren, K., Zhag, W., Malialis, K., Wang, J.: Real-time bidding by reinforcement learning in display advertising. In: Proceedings of the 10th ACM International Conference on Web Search and Data Mining (WSDM) (2017)
8. Chakrabarti, D., Agarwal, D., Josifovski, V.: Contextual advertising by combining relevance with click feedback. In: Proceedings of the 17th International Conference on World Wide Web (WWW) (2008)
9. Chen, Y., Berkhin, P., Anderson, B., Devanur, N.R.: Real-time bidding algorithms for performance-based display ad allocation. In: Proceedings of the 17th ACM SIGKDD International Conference on Knowledge Discovery and Data Mining (2011)
10. Cui, Y., Zhang, R., Li, W., Mao, J.: Bid landscape forecasting in online ad exchange marketplace. In: Proceedings of the 17th ACM SIGKDD International Conference on Knowledge Discovery and Data Mining (2011)
11. Geibel, P.: Reinforcement learning for MDPs with constraints. In: European Conference on Machine Learning (2006)
12. Ghosh, A., Rubinstein, B.I., Vassilvitskii, S., Zinkevich, M.: Adaptive bidding for display advertising. In: Proceedings of the 18th International Conference on World Wide Web, pp. 251–260. ACM (2009)
13. Hoelzel, M., Ballvé, M.: The programmatic-advertising report: mobile, video, and real-time bidding drive growth in programmatic. BI Intelligence (2015)
14. Krishna, V.: Auction Theory. Academic Press, San Diego (2009)
15. Lange, S., Gabel, T., Riedmiller, M.: Batch Reinforcement Learning. Springer, Heidelberg (2012)
16. Liu, C.: US Ad Spending: eMarketer's Updated Estimates and Forecast for 2015–2020. Industry report (2016)
17. Perlich, C., Dalessandro, B., Hook, R., Stitelman, O., Raeder, T., Provost, F.: Bid optimizing and inventory scoring in targeted online advertising. In: Proceedings of the 18th ACM SIGKDD International Conference on Knowledge Discovery and Data Mining (2012)
18. Schwartz, E.M., Bradlow, E., Fader, P.: Customer acquisition via display advertising using multi-armed bandit experiments. Ross School of Business Paper (2015)
19. Sutton, R.S., Barto, A.G.: Reinforcement Learning: An Introduction, vol. 1. MIT Press Cambridge, London (1998)
20. Xu, J., Lee, K.c., Li, W., Qi, H., Lu, Q.: Smart pacing for effective online ad campaign optimization. In: Proceedings of the 21th ACM SIGKDD International Conference on Knowledge Discovery and Data Mining (2015)

21. Zhang, W., Yuan, S., Wang, J.: Optimal real-time bidding for display advertising. In: Proceedings of the 20th ACM SIGKDD International Conference on Knowledge Discovery and Data Mining (2014)
22. Zhang, W., Yuan, S., Wang, J.: Real-time bidding benchmarking with iPinYou dataset. CoRR (2014)

PowerLSTM: Power Demand Forecasting Using Long Short-Term Memory Neural Network

Yao Cheng[1(✉)], Chang Xu[2], Daisuke Mashima[3], Vrizlynn L.L. Thing[1], and Yongdong Wu[1]

[1] Institute for Infocomm Research, A*STAR, Singapore, Singapore
{cheng_yao,vriz,wydong}@i2r.a-star.edu.sg
[2] School of Computing Engineering, Nanyang Technological University, Singapore, Singapore
xuch0007@e.ntu.edu.sg
[3] Advanced Digital Sciences Center, Singapore, Singapore
daisuke.m@adsc.com.sg

Abstract. Power demand forecasting is a critical task to achieve efficiency and reliability in the smart grid in terms of demand response and resource allocation. This paper proposes PowerLSTM, a power demand forecasting model based on Long Short-Term Memory (LSTM) neural network. We calculate the feature significance and compact our model by capturing the features with the most important weights. Based on our preliminary study using a public dataset, compared to two recent works based on Gradient Boosting Tree (GBT) and Support Vector Regression (SVR), PowerLSTM demonstrates a decrease of 21.80% and 28.57% in forecasting error, respectively. Our study also reveals that metering/forecasting granularity at once every 30 min can bring higher accuracy than other practical granularity options.

1 Introduction

Modern smart grid is an enhanced electrical grid that takes advantage of sensing and information communication technologies to improve the efficiency, reliability and security of the power grid. Smart metering is a major improvement brought by smart grids, which facilitates real-time metering. One resulting benefit is the *power demand forecasting* based on such meter measurement, which affects the power generation scheduling and power dispatching for a future period by predicting the power demand in that period using historical data in hand.

Power demand forecasting is important for both power companies and power consumers [22]. In general, the forecasting results have different interpretations when applied to the aggregation and the individual. The aggregation forecasting, which is to predict the power demand of a number of consumption units, e.g., the apartments within an area, is more meaningful to power utility companies. Based on the aggregation demand forecasting results, they can allocate proper resources to balance the supply and demand or adjust the demand response

G. Cong et al. (Eds.): ADMA 2017, LNAI 10604, pp. 727–740, 2017.
https://doi.org/10.1007/978-3-319-69179-4_51

strategy such as dynamic pricing to shape the load so as to avoid the infrastructure capacity strain. On the other hand, individual power demand forecasting assists in the anomaly detection task in the smart metering system. Anomaly detection detects the abnormal meter measurements caused either by the unexpected meter failure or the deliberate meter manipulation by identifying those measurements that do not present a conformation to the predicted/expected values. Moreover, under dynamic pricing strategy, individual power forecasting also provides power consumers with their expected power consumption and cost in a future period, so that they can optimise their usage schedule accordingly to achieve a lower cost.

Though demand forecasting has been widely studied for years, two challenges in making accurate forecasting are still in front of us. One challenge is that even though the power demand seems like a univariate time series [28], it is subject to various influential factors which may have discriminative capability in influencing the power demand. The second challenge is that it is not trivial to chase optimal forecasting settings so as to obtain a promising results. The time granularity of metering is flexible in modern smart grids. By investigating what kinds of metering/forecasting granularities can bring an accuracy gain, it can not only provide empirical guidelines for better forecasting accuracy but also evaluate whether a model can work well with typical granularities in today's smart grid.

With the above challenges in mind, this paper proposes a power demand forecasting model named *PowerLSTM*. Firstly, we identify a set of features derived from three categories, i.e., the historical consumption data, the weather information, and the calendar information. In each category, there are a series of features that potentially and reasonably have influence on the consumers' power demand. Then, we analyse the significance of each feature and select an appropriate set of features to be used later in our forecasting model. After that, we introduce our model PowerLSTM. PowerLSTM takes advantage of the Long Short-Term Memory (LSTM) network, which is a special form of Recurrent Neural Network (RNN) with certain memory capability. In order to evaluate the effectiveness of PowerLSTM, we compare it with two representative techniques based on Gradient Boosting Tree (GBT) [5] and Support Vector Regression (SVR) [26]. For the sake of fair comparison, we implement our model and theirs as well, and evaluate all three models using a public real-world dataset. Finally, we experiment with different metering/forecasting granularities to evaluate the accuracy over different granularities that are used in practical services.

In summary, the main contributions of this paper are as below.

- We propose PowerLSTM, which, to the best of our knowledge, is the first power demand forecasting model based on LSTM that incorporates time-series features, weather features, and calendar features.
- We compare PowerLSTM with two representative models adopted in recent research works, i.e., GBT [5] and SVR [26]. In our preliminary study, PowerLSTM outperforms both models by reducing the Mean Squared Error (MSE) by 21.80% and 28.57% compared to GBT and SVR, respectively.

- We evaluate the accuracy of our model with various granularities that are typical in today's smart grid systems. The results reveal that a moderate metering/forecasting granularity at once every 30 min performs better than other granularities.

2 Related Work

Power demand forecasting has been widely studied due to its significance in power industry. The existing works can be generally classified into two categories, i.e., classic statistical models and modern machine learning algorithms.

In terms of statistical models, time-series modeling is used to capture the time-series characteristics of power demand, e.g., ARMA [14,19], ARIMA [2,7]. Hong et al. [16] adopt multiple linear regression to model hourly energy demand using seasonality (regarding year, week, and day) and temperature information. Their results indicate that complex featuring of the same information results in a more accurate forecasting. Fan and Hyndman [8] use semi-parametric additive model to explore the non-linear relationship between energy usage data and variables, i.e., calendar variables, consumption observations, and temperatures, in the short-term time period. Their model demonstrates sensitivity towards the temperature. Recently, conditional kernel density estimation is applied to power demand forecasting area [4] which performs well on dataset with strong seasonality. Time-series models are based on the assumption that the future power demand has the same or similar trend and distribution as the observed history. However, the power demand in reality is influenced by many factors in various ways. Therefore, it is essential to take these influential factors into consideration.

There are three major machine-learning algorithms used in demand forecasting tasks, namely Decision Tree (DT) [5,11,27], Support Vector Machine (SVM) [9, 17,21,23,25,26], and Artificial Neural Network (ANN) [9,29]. DT is used to predict building energy demand levels [27] and analyse the electricity load level based on hourly observations of the electricity load and weather [11]. Differently, Bansal et al. [5] use an evolved version of decision tree, Boosted Decision Tree Regression (BDTR), to model and forecast energy consumption so as to create personalised electricity plans for residential consumers based on usage history. The regression based on SVM is named Support Vector Regression (SVR). There are works using SVR to forecast power consumption [25] or using it in combination with other techniques, such as fuzzy-rough feature selection [23], particle swarm optimization algorithms [21], and chaotic artificial bee colony algorithm [17]. Gajowniczek and Zabkowski choose SVM and ANN because they believe that time-series analysis is not suitable in their work since they observe high volatility in the data [9]. Yu et al. [26] uses SVM and Backward Propagation Neural Network (BPNN), whose results show that SVM offers smaller prediction errors than BPNN. Zufferey et al. [29] apply Time Delay Neural Network (TDNN) and find out that the individual consumer's consumption is harder to predict than an aggregation of multiple consumers. Very recently, Marino et al. [18] construct LSTM deep neural networks to forecast building energy load using historical consumption data. Despite the extensive research carried out in power demand forecasting area, to the best of our knowledge, there is no such work taking advantage of LSTM RNN based on features other than time series. It is promising to explore the effectiveness of such idea in power demand forecasting area, which has motivated this work.

3 Our Approach

3.1 Overview

Our approach is to forecast power demand by modeling the relationship between power demand and relevant features using the proposed PowerLSTM. Figure 1 illustrates the high-level pipeline of our approach. A recent publicly available dataset recording apartment power usage in a high frequency is used. From this dataset, we develop three categories of features that are considered relevant to the power demand. Then, we employ feature selection to remove features that are less important to reduce dimensionality and model complexity as features may not be equally effective. After that, we use the selected features to train PowerLSTM. The details of each process are explained in the subsequent subsections.

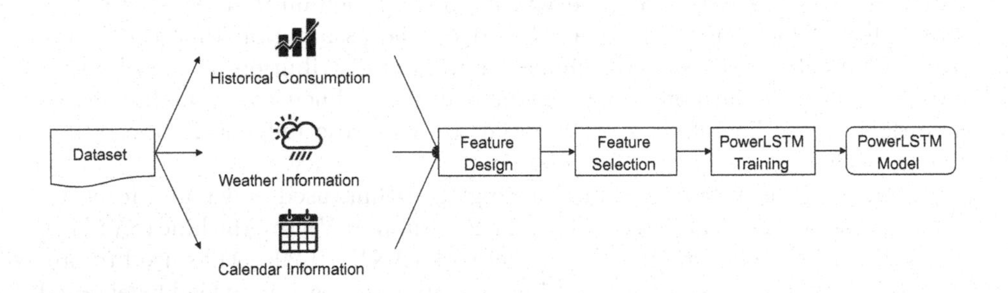

Fig. 1. Approach overview.

3.2 Power Usage Dataset

We use the publicly available power usage dataset provided by University of Massachusetts [1]. Three reasons for choosing this dataset are *(a)* when developing technology which reflects consumers' life styles and further the power consumption behaviours, a recent dataset would be beneficial to incorporate the latest power consumption characteristics; *(b)* power consumption data recorded at high frequency provides us with detailed information in finer time granularity and allows us to flexibly down-sample to explore lower granularities; and *(c)* as a public dataset, it would facilitate the further comparison with our work.

The dataset contains power usage data for 114 apartments located in Western Massachusetts for the period from year 2014 to 2016. The dataset records the power of every single apartment in fixed temporal frequency[1]. The metering frequency is once every 15 min for 2014 and 2015, and once every 1 min for 2016. Along with the power consumption data, hourly weather information, including various meteorological attributes, during the record period is available, a sample of which is shown in Table 1. In our experiment, we use the data of year 2016 because its finer granularity in recording provides us with more space for exploring influence of granularity on accuracy of power demand forecasting.

Table 1. Weather data sample.

time	**temperature**	**apparentTemperature**	**windBearing**	**dewPoint**
1451624400	36	29.75	278	24.54
summary	**humidity**	**precipIntensity**	**cloudCover**	**visibility**
Clear	0.63	0	0	10
icon	**windSpeed**	**precipProbability**	**pressure**	-
clear-night	7.94	0	1016.61	-

3.3 Feature Engineering

Feature Design. The features used by the existing forecasting models fall into three categories in terms of privacy, i.e., publicly available information (e.g., weather information), household private information (e.g., demography), and quasi-private information. The quasi-private information here is defined as privacy-related information which is known only to authorized entities. For example, the historical power consumption data acquired by a power utility company can be used to infer certain private household characteristics [3], but it is only available to the authorised personnel within the utility company.

Although household private information may have significant influence on the household power demand (e.g., more people living in the house leads to larger power demand), in this paper we limit the features to non-private information due to the following reasons. First of all, we would like to involve no household specific data in forecasting procedure other than power meter readings due to the privacy concern. Secondly, although utility companies may have access to some household private data such as locations, it is not common for them to have other private information, e.g., the number of occupants and their employment status. Thirdly, the forecasting model not based on the household specific data can be applied to larger scales easily, such as building level or area level.

We use the three categories of features in this paper, i.e., historical consumption data, weather information, and calendar information.

(a) Historical consumption data is the actual observation of the prediction target, which directly reflects the consumption pattern. Power utility companies can obtain this data by smart metering technology in smart grids.

[1] Given that the metering interval is fixed, the power is able to represent the power consumption.

(b) Weather information has influence on the power demand since some appliances (e.g., air conditions) are sensitive to weather conditions.
(c) Calendar information, such as weekday or weekend, shapes the consumers' power consumption behaviour in terms of different activities. It indicates the consumption pattern according to the calendar feature and cycle.

The features based on the above three categories are summarized in Table 2. There are $n + 18$ features in total, among which, n features are from historical consumption data, 13 are from weather information, and 5 are designed from calendar information. The historical data involves a huge number of data points which are not feasible to be fed to the model directly. Therefore, it is necessary to find out length of historical data points n that are most correlated with the target forecast value. To solve this problem, we use AutoCorrelation Function (ACF), which can quantify the correlation between time-series data points of various time lags, to find the appropriate n.

Table 2. Features for the power demand forecasting task.

Features category	Feature detail
Historical consumption data	Consumption data in past n time slots
Weather information	Summary, icon, temperature, apparent temperature, cloud cover, precip probability, precip intensity, visibility, wind speed, wind bearing, humidity, pressure, dew point
Calendar information	Day of the month, day of the week, hour of the day, period of the day (i.e., daytime and night time), is weekend (boolean value)

Feature Selection. In order to design a predictive and compact model, it is necessary to choose the features that have most significant influence on the power demand as some of the features may be redundant while some may be irrelevant. To investigate such discriminative power of features, we use feature selection to prune such redundant and irrelevant features and leave those important ones.

We use Random Forest-Recursive Feature Elimination (RF-RFE) to recursively select the optimal feature subset. It is to select a desired number of features by creating predictive models, weighing the importance of features, and eliminating those with least importance. Each recursive step is to consider a smaller set of features, and repeated till the desired number of features is reached.

3.4 Long Short-Term Memory Model

Long Short-Term Memory (LSTM) neural network [15] is a variant of RNN that is capable of learning long-term dependencies. Different from the traditional neural network that only relies on previous N histories when solving the problem, RNN allows unlimited history information to persist due to its internal loops. The network architecture of RNN makes it a prevailing choice for solving problems related to sequences. In theory, RNN should be able to learn long-term dependences, which, however, is demonstated to have practical difficulties [6]. Under this circumstance, LSTM is designed to solve the challenge of long-term dependences [13], which has demonstrated its practicality and sucess in tasks that are not solvable by other RNNs, such as continual prediction [10], speech recognition [12], language modeling [20], and translation [24]. Its capability in power demand forecasting is worth exploring due to the sequential nature of power readings.

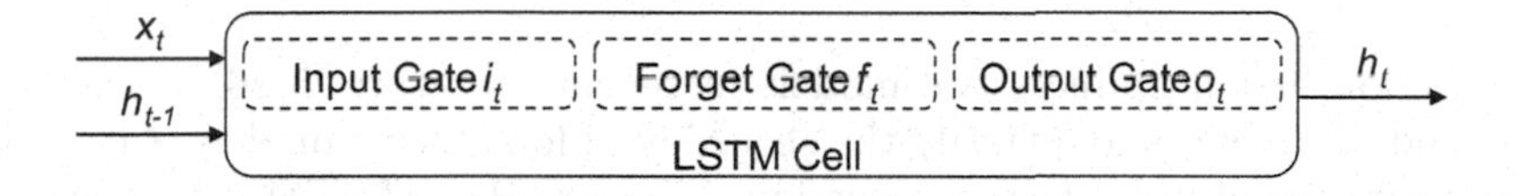

Fig. 2. LSTM cell.

The core idea of LSTM is a memory cell which can maintain the information over time controlled by various gate units. The LSTM cell as illustrated in Fig. 2 processes the information to maintain a cell status based on both current input x_t and previous output h_{t-1} (i.e., the recurrent input), then decides what information to be left and what to be passed on (i.e., h_t) by introducing gate units, i.e., "input gate", "output gate" and "forget gate". The input gate is used to control whether it allows the state in current cell to be overridden by outside information, as shown in Eq. (1),

$$i_t = \sigma_g(W_i x_t + U_i h_{t-1} + b_i) \tag{1}$$

where i_t is the input gate vector, σ_g the sigmoid function, x_t the input vector, W_i and U_i the parameter matrices, and b_i the bias vector. The output gate decides whether the status in the cell should affect other cells, whose formulation is shown in Eq. (2),

$$o_t = \sigma_g(W_o x_t + U_o h_{t-1} + b_o) \tag{2}$$

Another gate, forget gate, is introduced by Gers et al. [10] which allows the LSTM to reset its own state. It is formulated as below,

$$f_t = \sigma_g(W_f x_t + U_f h_{t-1} + b_f) \tag{3}$$

Finally, Eqs. (4) and (5) show how cell state c_t and output vector h_t are obtained from input gate, forget gate, and output gate,

$$c_t = f_t \odot c_{t-1} + i_t \odot \sigma_c(W_c x_t + U_c h_{t-1} + b_c) \tag{4}$$

$$h_t = o_t \odot \sigma_h(c_t) \tag{5}$$

where $\odot$ denotes the Hadamard product, and σ_c and σ_h are the hyperbolic tangent function.

LSTM can work in a multilayer manner, each layer of which composes of multiple cells. There is a trade-off between the modeling capability and the performance efficiency. The more complicated the model is, the better capability it may have. However, this may result in an over-fitting model which performs extremely well in training set but cannot adapt to the other data of the dataset. At the same time, over-complicate model would be an inefficient model. Due to the above considerations, PowerLSTM adopts a moderate structure with two LSTM layers, so as to prevent overfitting while allowing for reasonable generalization.

4 Evaluation

This section first introduces two models in recent literature [5,26] as the baselines, and two metrics to quantify the accuracy of forecasting models. After that, we evaluate the effect of feature selection, compare PowerLSTM with two baseline models, and investigate forecasting results in different metering/forecasting granularities for evaluating the accuracy in practical use cases.

4.1 Preparation

Baseline. We choose two recent works as the baseline models in this paper. One of them adopts GBT [5] and the other one adopts SVR [26].

GBT is adopted by Bansal et al. [5] to forecast power consumption. GBT is a supervised learning predictive model which can be used for classification and regression purposes. GBT builds the model, i.e., a series of trees, in a stepwise manner. In each step, it adds one tree, while maintaining the existing trees unchanged. The added tree is the optimal tree that minimizes a predefined loss function. Basically, GBT is an ensemble of weaker prediction models, which becomes a better model.

SVM is used in the work by Yu et al. [26] to forecast power usage. SVM is a supervised machine learning algorithm for solving both classification and regression problems. SVM does classification by seeking the hyper-plane that differentiates the two classes to the largest extent, i.e., maximizing the margin. Similarly, regression using SVM, that is SVR, is to seek and optimize the generation bounds by minimizing the predefined error function. SVR supports both linear and non-linear regression. For the non-linear SVR, it transforms the data into a higher dimensional space to perform the linear separation.

Evaluation Metric. In order to evaluate the accuracy of the forecasting model, we introduce Mean Squared Error (MSE) and Mean Absolute Percentage Error (MAPE). The closer the value is to zero, the more accurate the forecasting is.

MSE measures the average of the squared errors/deviations as directed by Eq. 6, where n is the total number of forecast values, A_t and F_t denote the actual and forecast value at time t, respectively.

$$MSE = \frac{1}{n}\sum_{t=1}^{n}(A_t - F_t)^2 \tag{6}$$

Different from MSE, MAPE measures the error proportion to the absolute value. It expresses the error as a percentage and can be calculated using Eq. 7.

$$MAPE = \frac{100\%}{n}\sum_{t=1}^{n}\left|\frac{A_t - F_t}{A_t}\right| \tag{7}$$

MSE is useful in comparison experiments with identical test dataset, as it is the absolute square error value that depends on the scale of actual values. On the other hand, MAPE is more indicative in comparison between different dataset since it represents the error in a percentage manner. However, MAPE, *(a)* is not defined when A_t is zero[2]; and *(b)* has a heavier penalty on negative errors when $A_t < F_t$. Therefore, we use both MSE and MAPE to provide complementary measurements on the model accuracy.

4.2 Effect of Feature Selection

As mentioned in Sect. 3.3, features may not positively contribute to the forecasting task. Redundant features may drag down the performance and irrelevant features may even disturb the prediction. This experiment investigates the contribution of each feature to the prediction, and the effect of feature selection.

We use RF-RFE to evaluate the importance weights of features in an hourly metering/forecasting granularity. Based on the ACF outcome which shows the most related number of lag is 49, we have 49 + 18 features in total. We run RF-RFE on these 67 features and obtain their importance weights. We select the top 12 important features since the importance weights after that are much less significant. Figure 3a presents the features with the top 12 importance weights. Energy-n denotes the hourly power consumption n hours prior to the target hour to be forecast. The feature with the most significant weight is the power consumption of the hour before the one to be forecast. Besides historical consumption features, three features from weather information category and calendar information category are selected into the top 12 important features list.

In order to evaluate the effect of feature selection, we separately train two models, one using all features and the other using selected features. Both models are trained on the hourly data of the first 28 days in September and tested on the following 2 days. Figure 3b shows the forecasting results of one apartment with ID 39. The results without feature selection are relatively more fluctuated than the results with feature selection. The MSE of forecasting with feature selection demonstrates an improvement by 5.44% compared to that with all features.

[2] In our experiments, we eliminate the undefined MAPE caused by a zero actual value. However, the actual power consumption values in our dataset are scarcely zero.

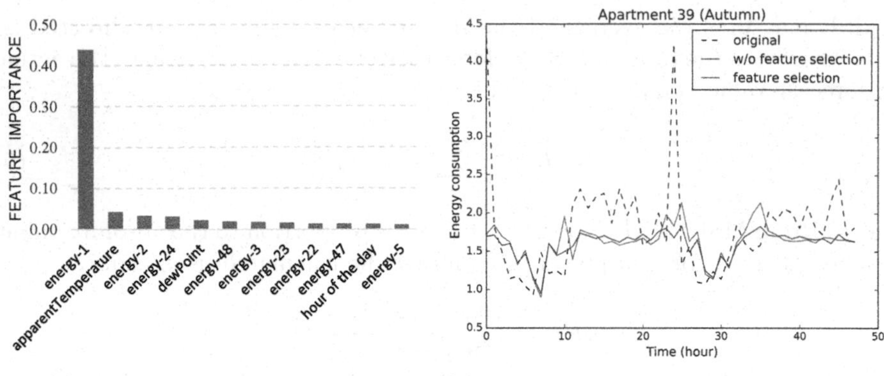

(a) Top 12 important features. (b) Forecasting results with and without feature selection.

Fig. 3. Feature selection.

4.3 Comparison with Baselines

In this experiment, we compare our model with two recent works, i.e., the works from Bansal et al. [5] and Yu et al. [26] with the same training and testing data.

PowerLSTM uses a two-layered LSTM network as discussed in Sect. 3.4. The cell memory size for each layer is tuned from 160 to 200 using grid search which can exhaustively search the optimal candidate from a grid of parameter values. Similarly, the parameters for baseline models are also automatically tuned using grid search. For GBT, three parameters are tuned, i.e., number of boosting stages to perform *n_estimators*, maximum depth of the individual regression estimators *max_depth*, and learning rate *learning_rate*. Its parameter grid is constructed using *n_estimators*: (50, 100, 150, 200, 250, 300, 350, 400, 450, 500), *max_depth*: (1, 2, 3, 4, 5), and *learning_rate*: (0.001, 0.01, 0.1, 1). For SVR, three parameters, C, *kernel*, and *gamma* are tuned. We construct the

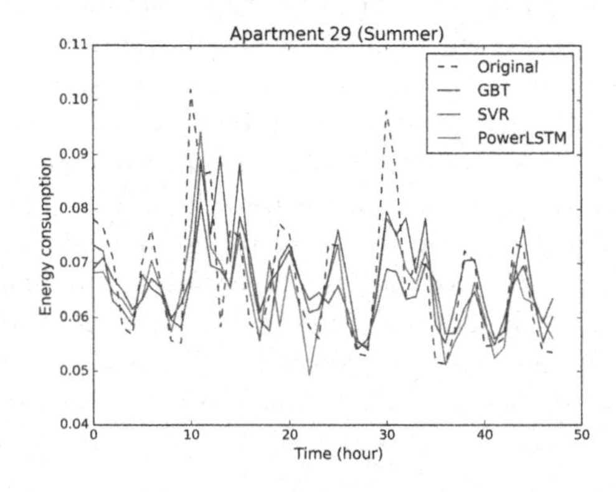

Fig. 4. Forecasting results from GBT [5], SVR [26] and PowerLSTM.

Table 3. Accuracy of GBT [5], SVR [26] and PowerLSTM.

Model	Error	
	MSE	MAPE
SVR	9.693E-05	10.391%
GBT	8.853E-05	9.512%
PowerLSTM	6.923E-05	8.935%

parameter grid using C: (0.001, 0.01, 0.1, 1), *kernel*: (rbf, linear, poly, sigmoid). *gamma* is automatically set corresponding to kernel coefficient or the reciprocal of number of features.

We use the consumption data of the first 28 days of July as the training set to train the three models, and forecast/test the expected demand for the next 2 days using the trained models. We show the forecasting results using data of apartment 29. As shown in Fig. 4, PowerLSTM is able to capture the trend as well as peaks and valleys better than both GBT [5] and SVR [26] do. Furthermore, according to Table 3, PowerLSTM brings an improvement in MSE by 21.80% and 28.58% comparing to GBT [5] and SVR [26], respectively.

4.4 Forecasting in Different Granularities

The intention of this experiment is to investigate the influence of different metering/forecasting granularities to forecasting tasks. In particular, we evaluate the forecasting accuracy under practical use cases, for instance., demand response services often require forecasting in half-hourly or hourly. In this direction, we use four different granularities when training the model, i.e., every 15 min, every 30 min, every 1 h and every 2 h. We prepare four training datasets by down-sampling the data points in the original dataset (1 min. granularity) with the four different granularities, respectively. The average value within the sample period is used in the down-sampled dataset. The model that is trained using the dataset with a lower sampling rate forecasts power demand using the same rate. To evaluate from the viewpoint of a power utility company, we show the results based on the aggregated power usage data of all 114 apartments. We use data from 1st February to 28th February as the training data and the data of the following 2 days as the testing data.

From the forecasting results shown in Fig. 5, all four models can capture the actual demand trend. Visually, the results from forecasting every 2 h are not as good as those from every 1 h and every 30 min. For quantitative understanding, we compare their MSE and MAPE in Table 4. The forecasting in 30 min. granularity demonstrates the best results in both MSE and MAPE. When the metering/forecasting granularity is low, the model may not be able to capture the consumption characteristics, as seen in the figure. On the other hand, when the granularity is high, the consumption may demonstrate more of its fluctuation and instantaneity, which may be a hindrance to the accurate forecasting task.

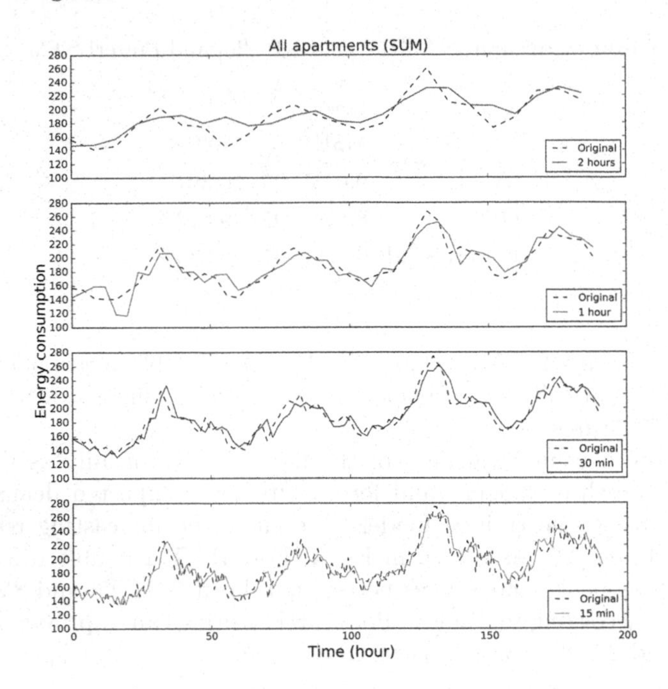

Fig. 5. Forecasting results in different granularities.

Table 4. Forecasting accuracy in different granularities.

Error	Granularity			
	15 mins	30 mins	1 h	2 h
MSE	193.218	130.982	199.767	254.400
MAPE	6.052%	4.880%	6.493%	6.773%

Having that said, PowerLSTM offers good performance when used with practically available smart meter data (e.g., in 30 min. granularity).

5 Conclusion

This paper proposes PowerLSTM, a power demand forecasting model based on LSTM, which shows an accuracy improvement comparing to two recent representative works. Further experiments in different metering/forecasting granularities reveal that the forecasting accuracy varies in different granularities and PowerLSTM can work well with typical granularities used in today's smart grid system.

Acknowledgement. This research is supported by the National Research Foundation, Prime Minister's Office, Singapore under the Energy Programme and administrated by the Energy Market Authority (EP Award No. NRF2014EWT-EIRP002-040).

References

1. Umass smart* dataset - 2017 release. http://traces.cs.umass.edu/index.php/Smart/Smart
2. Alberg, D., Last, M.: Short-term load forecasting in smart meters with sliding window-based ARIMA algorithms. In: Asian Conference on Intelligent Information and Database Systems, pp. 299–307 (2017)
3. Anderson, B., Lin, S., Newing, A., Bahaj, A., James, P.: Electricity consumption and household characteristics: Implications for census-taking in a smart metered future. Comput. Environ. Urban Syst. **63**, 58–67 (2017)
4. Arora, S., Taylor, J.W.: Forecasting electricity smart meter data using conditional kernel density estimation. Omega **59**, 47–59 (2016)
5. Bansal, A., Rompikuntla, S.K., Gopinadhan, J., Kaur, A., Kazi, Z.A.: Energy consumption forecasting for smart meters. arXiv preprint arXiv:1512.05979 (2015)
6. Bengio, Y., Simard, P., Frasconi, P.: Learning long-term dependencies with gradient descent is difficult. IEEE Trans. Neural Netw. **5**(2), 157–166 (1994)
7. Cho, M., Hwang, J., Chen, C.: Customer short term load forecasting by using ARIMA transfer function model. In: International Conference on Energy Management and Power Delivery, vol. 1, pp. 317–322 (1995)
8. Fan, S., Hyndman, R.J.: Short-term load forecasting based on a semi-parametric additive model. IEEE Trans. Power Syst. **27**(1), 134–141 (2012)
9. Gajowniczek, K., Zabkowski, T.: Short term electricity forecasting using individual smart meter data. Procedia Comput. Sci. **35**, 589–597 (2014)
10. Gers, F.A., Schmidhuber, J., Cummins, F.: Learning to forget: continual prediction with LSTM. Neural Comput. **12**(10), 2451–2471 (2000)
11. Gładysz, B., Kuchta, D.: Application of regression trees in the analysis of electricity load. Badania Operacyjne i Decyzje **4**, 19–28 (2008)
12. Graves, A., Mohamed, A.R., Hinton, G.: Speech recognition with deep recurrent neural networks. In: IEEE International Conference on Acoustics, Speech and Signal Processing (ICASSP), 2013, pp. 6645–6649 (2013)
13. Greff, K., Srivastava, R.K., Koutník, J., Steunebrink, B.R., Schmidhuber, J.: LSTM: a search space Odyssey. IEEE Trans. Neural Netw. Learn. Syst. **28**(10), 2222–2232 (2017)
14. Gross, G., Galiana, F.D.: Short-term load forecasting. Proc. IEEE **75**(12), 1558–1573 (1987)
15. Hochreiter, S., Schmidhuber, J.: Long short-term memory. Neural Comput. **9**(8), 1735–1780 (1997)
16. Hong, T., Gui, M., Baran, M.E., Willis, H.L.: Modeling and forecasting hourly electric load by multiple linear regression with interactions. In: IEEE Power and Energy Society General Meeting, pp. 1–8 (2010)
17. Hong, W.C.: Electric load forecasting by seasonal recurrent SVR (support vector regression) with chaotic artificial bee colony algorithm. Energy **36**(9), 5568–5578 (2011)
18. Marino, D.L., Amarasinghe, K., Manic, M.: Building energy load forecasting using deep neural networks. In: 42nd Annual Conference of the IEEE Industrial Electronics Society, IECON 2016, pp. 7046–7051 (2016)
19. Mashima, D., Cárdenas, A.A.: Evaluating electricity theft detectors in smart grid networks. In: International Workshop on Recent Advances in Intrusion Detection, pp. 210–229 (2012)

20. Mikolov, T., Karafiát, M., Burget, L., Cernocký, J., Khudanpur, S.: Recurrent neural network based language model. In: Interspeech, vol. 2, p. 3 (2010)
21. Qiu, Z.: Electricity consumption prediction based on data mining techniques with particle swarm optimization. Int. J. Database Theor. Appl. **6**(5), 153–164 (2013)
22. Siano, P.: Demand response and smart grids-a survey. Renew. Sustain. Energ. Rev. **30**, 461–478 (2014)
23. Son, H., Kim, C.: Forecasting short-term electricity demand in residential sector based on support vector regression and fuzzy-rough feature selection with particle swarm optimization. Procedia Eng. **118**, 1162–1168 (2015)
24. Sutskever, I., Vinyals, O., Le, Q.V.: Sequence to sequence learning with neural networks. In: Advances in Neural Information Processing Systems, pp. 3104–3112 (2014)
25. Wang, J., Zhu, W., Zhang, W., Sun, D.: A trend fixed on firstly and seasonal adjustment model combined with the ε-SVR for short-term forecasting of electricity demand. Energ. Policy **37**(11), 4901–4909 (2009)
26. Yu, W., An, D., Griffith, D., Yang, Q., Xu, G.: Towards statistical modeling and machine learning based energy usage forecasting in smart grid. ACM SIGAPP Appl. Comput. Rev. **15**(1), 6–16 (2015)
27. Yu, Z., Haghighat, F., Fung, B.C., Yoshino, H.: A decision tree method for building energy demand modeling. Energy Build. **42**(10), 1637–1646 (2010)
28. Zheng, J., Xu, C., Zhang, Z., Li, X.: Electric load forecasting in smart grids using long-short-term-memory based recurrent neural network. In: 51st Annual Conference on Information Sciences and Systems, pp. 1–6 (2017)
29. Zufferey, T., Ulbig, A., Koch, S., Hug, G.: Forecasting of smart meter time series based on neural networks. In: International Workshop on Data Analytics for Renewable Energy Integration, pp. 10–21 (2016)

Identifying Unreliable Sensors Without a Knowledge of the Ground Truth in Deceptive Environments

Anis Yazidi[1(✉)], B. John Oommen[2], and Morten Goodwin[3]

[1] Department of Computer Science,
Oslo and Akershus University College of Applied Sciences, Oslo, Norway
[2] School of Computer Science, Carleton University, Ottawa, Canada
anis.yazidi@hioa.no
[3] Department of Computer Science, University of Agder, Oslo, Norway

Abstract. This paper deals with the extremely fascinating area of "fusing" the outputs of sensors *without any knowledge of the ground truth.* In an earlier paper, the present authors had recently pioneered a solution, by mapping it onto the fascinating paradox of trying to identify *stochastic* liars without any additional information about the truth. Even though that work was significant, it was constrained by the model in which we are living in a world where "the truth prevails over lying". Couched in the terminology of Learning Automata (LA), this corresponds to the Environment (Since the Environment is treated as an *entity* in its own right, we choose to capitalize it, rather than refer to it as an "environment", i.e., as an abstract concept.) being "Stochastically Informative". However, as explained in the paper, solving the problem under the condition that the Environment is "Stochastically Deceptive", as opposed to informative, is far from trivial. In this paper, we provide a solution to the problem where the Environment is deceptive (We are not aware of any other solution to this problem (within this setting), and so we believe that our solution is both pioneering and novel.), i.e., when we are living in a world where "lying prevails over the truth".

Keywords: Sensor fusion · Unreliable sensors · Learning automata · Learning from Stochastic Liars

1 Introduction

We consider the problem of fusing the information obtained from a set of sensors where the knowledge of the "Ground Truth" is unavailable. However, unlike the problem that has been traditionally considered (i.e., whether the "Ground Truth" is available or not), we consider the intrinsically more complex model in which the sensors could be stochastically "truth telling" or "deceptive", and

B.J. Oommen—*Chancellor's Professor; Fellow: IEEE* and *Fellow: IAPR*. This author is also an *Adjunct Professor* with the University of Agder in Grimstad, Norway.

G. Cong et al. (Eds.): ADMA 2017, LNAI 10604, pp. 741–753, 2017.
https://doi.org/10.1007/978-3-319-69179-4_52

where the behavior of the sensor is not known *a priori*. This problem is, in and of itself, non-trivial, and as in the case when one deals with Stochastic Teachers and Stochastic Liars, there is no universal guaranteed solution to such puzzles. To place the field of sensor fusion in the right perspective, we mention that the aggregation of data obtained from sensors enables us to procure more reliable information about the underlying process, as opposed to utilizing the raw sensor information from the individual sensors themselves. However, the quality of the aggregated information is intricately dependent on the *reliability* of the individual sensors. In fact, understandably, unreliable sensors will tend to report erroneous values of the ground truth, and thus degrade the quality of the fused information. Finding strategies to identify unreliable sensors can assist in having a counter-effect on their respective detrimental influences on the fusion process, and this has been a focal concern in the literature. The body of the related work operate with the assumption of direct knowledge of the ground truth to assess the reliability of the sensors, or indirect knowledge using the concept of sensor accuracy that is deduced from historical data. The existing literature generally assumes that the reliability of the individual sensors can be inferred, whence one can invoke an efficient scheme to fuse their respective readings. Although the task of resolving this problem without the knowledge of the ground truth is apparently impossible, the authors of [4,5] (which are also the present authors) previously obtained conclusive results by utilizing the "agreement" between the sensors themselves and a set of Linear Reward-Inaction (L_{RI}) Learning Automata (LA) associated with the sensors. The results of [4,5] were constrained by the model in which "the truth prevails over lying", which, in the setting of LA corresponds to the Environment being "Stochastically Informative". Informally speaking, this is equivalent to the scenario where the proportion of truth-tellers in the society exceeds the proportion of liars. This paper considers the scenario in which the Environment is "Stochastically Deceptive", where "lying prevails over the truth", or if you like, where the proportion of liars exceeds the proportion of truth-tellers. This is not an unrealistic setting. Indeed, in cases of nuclear meltdowns, the majority of the sensors in the vicinity of the meltdown can be considered faulty and unreliable[1].

1.1 Survey of the Field

A myriad of pieces of literature can be cited that concentrate on using majority voting to faulty sensor fusion. The premise for invoking majority voting is that the decision of the group is better than the decision of the individual sensor.

The theory of sensor fusion has also found wide deployment in the field of "reputation systems" where users who want to promote a particular product or service can flood the domain (i.e., the social network) with sympathetic votes, while those who want to get a competitive edge over a specific product

[1] This being said, the content and goal of this paper is to present a solution within a theoretical and conceptual framework. Thus, we will not embark on the study of any real-life application domains here.

or service can "badmouth" it unfairly. Thus, although these systems can offer generic recommendations by aggregating user-provided opinions, unfair ratings may degrade the trustworthiness of such systems. This problem, of separating "fair" and "unfair" agents for a specific service, is called the Agent-Type Partitioning Problem ($ATPP$). Determining ways to solve the ($ATPP$) [3] and thus counter the detrimental influence of unreliable agents on a Reputation System, has been a focal concern of a number of very interesting studies.

The analogous sensor-related problem, of separating reliable and unreliable sensors, is called the Sensor-Type Partitioning Problem ($STPP$). We shall solve it in stochastically Deceptive Environments. Put in a nutshell, in this paper, we propose to solve the above-mentioned paradoxical $STTP$ using tools provided by LA, which have proven powerful potential in efficiently and quickly learning the optimal action when operating in unknown stochastic Environments. It adaptively, and in an on-line manner, gradually learns the identity and characteristics of the sensors that are reliable and those that are unreliable. In addition, we will provide two approaches for fusing the sensor readings which leverage the convergence result of our LA-based partitioning.

A recent work by the authors of the current paper, that was alluded to earlier, is found in [4,5]. This paper pioneered a solution by which it is feasible to solve the $STTP$ problem of identifying which sensors are unreliable *without any knowledge of the ground truth*, a claim that *is counter-intuitive*. The essence of the approach presented in [4,5] stems from the simple intuition that the "agreement" between the sensors themselves can give invaluable knowledge about their respective reliabilities. In a stochastic Environment where errors can take place according to some unknown underlying stochastic process, those sensors that tend to deviate from the decision of the majority are more likely to be unreliable than those that adhere to the decision of the majority. Such simple and intuitive remark works under the premise that the decision of the majority has some high likelihood of revealing the truth [4,5]. The main assumption of our legacy work was the fact that "the truth prevails over lying" which is translated into a condition that can be seen as an extension of the simple majority voting. In fact, the reader can observe in [4,5] that if the Environment is deterministic, i.e., the reliable sensors are deterministic (always report the ground truth with probability 1) and the unreliable sensors are deterministic too (always misreport the ground truth with probability 1), then the mild condition of the "the truth prevails over lying" translates to the simple and well-know majority vote in the setting that the number of reliable sensors forms the majority. Stochastically, the setting in which "truth prevails over lying" is tantamount to having more stochastically reliable sensors that stochastically unreliable ones.

In this paper, we consider a natural but non-obvious scenario where "lying prevails over the truth". Alluding to the terminology of LA (and more particularly the theory of the SPL [2]), such an Environment can be characterized as being "Deceptive" as opposed to "Informative"[2]. As a dual to the previous framework, stochastically, the setting in which "lying prevails over truth" is tantamount to having more stochastically unreliable sensors that stochastically reliable ones.

To justify the validity of the claims that we have made, rigorous theoretical results and a host of empirical results were presented in [4,5]. These have been extended and generalized in this paper for Deceptive Environments.

2 Modeling the Problem

We consider a population of N sensors, $\mathcal{S} = \{s_1, s_2, \ldots, s_N\}$. Let the real situation of the Environment at the time instant t be modeled by a binary variable $T(t)$, which can take one of two possible values, 0 and 1. The value of T is unknown and can only be inferred through measurements from sensors. The output from the sensor s_i is referred to as x_i. Let π be the probability of the state of the ground truth, i.e., $T = 0$ with probability π.

To formalize the scenario, we record four possibilities:

- $x_i = T$ (where $x_i = 0$ or 1): This is the case when the sensor correctly reports the ground truth.
- $x_i \neq T$ (where $x_i = 0$ or 1): This is the case when the sensor faultily reports the ground truth.

In our discussions, we make one simplifying assumption: The probability of the sensor reporting a value erroneously is symmetric. In other words, in terms of the binary detection problem, we assume that the probability of a false alarm and the so-called miss probability are both equal. Thus, presented formally, we assume that:

$$Prob(x_i = 0|T = 1) = Prob(x_i = 1|T = 0). \tag{1}$$

Further, let q_i denote the Fault Probability (FP) of sensor s_i, where:

$$q_i = Prob(x_i = 0|T = 1) = Prob(x_i = 1|T = 0).$$

Similarly, we define the Correctness Probability (CP) of sensor s_i as $p_i = 1 - q_i$.

It is easy to prove that the total probability $Prob(x_i = T)$ is, indeed, p_i, since, in fact:

$$\begin{aligned} Prob(x_i = T) &= Prob(T = 0)Prob(x_i = 0|T = 0) + Prob(T = 1)Prob(x_i = 1|T = 1) \\ &= \pi p_i + (1 - \pi)p_i \\ &= p_i. \end{aligned} \tag{2}$$

[2] In the case of a recommendation system, a Deceptive Environment can, for example, correspond to a compromised system where the integrity of the majority of the agents in the systems are compromised.

Thus, the quantity $p_i = Prob(x_i = T)$ can be re-rewritten as $p_i = Prob(I\{x_i = T\} = 1)$, where $I\{.\}$ is the Indicator function.

We refer to a sensor as being reliable when it has a FP $q_i < 0.5$. Conversely, the sensor is unreliable when it has a FP $q_i > 0.5$. Equivalently, a reliable sensor is one that has a CP $p_i > 0.5$, and an unreliable sensor as one that has a CP of $p_i < 0.5$.

Observe that as a result of this model, a reliable sensor will probabilistically tend to report 0 when the ground truth is 0, and 1 when the ground truth is 1. Otherwise, it is clearly, unreliable. Our aim, then, is to partition the sensors as being reliable or unreliable. Furthermore, once partitioned, our aim is to use the partitioning as a basis for better fusion.

To simplify the analysis[3], we assume that every p_i can assume one of two possible values from the set $\{p_R, p_U\}$, where $p_R > 0.5$ and $p_U < 0.5$. Then, a sensor s_i is said to be reliable if $p_i = p_R$, and is said be unreliable if $p_i = p_U$. To render the problem non-trivial and interesting, we assume that p_R and p_U are unknown to the algorithm.

Based on the above, the set of reliable sensors is $\mathcal{S}_R = \{s_i | p_i = p_R\}$, and the set of unreliable sensors is $\mathcal{S}_U = \{s_i | p_i = p_U\}$.

We now formalize the Sensor-Type Partitioning Problem (*STPP*). The *STPP* involves a set of N sensors[4], $\mathcal{S} = \{s_1, s_2, \ldots, s_N\}$, where each sensor s_i is characterized by a fixed but unknown probability p_i of it sensing the ground truth correctly. The *STPP* involves partitioning $\mathcal{S}$ into 2 mutually exclusive and exhaustive groups so as to obtain a 2-partition $\mathbb{G} = \{G_U, G_R\}$, such that each group, G_R, of size, N_R, and G_U, of size N_U, exclusively contains only the sensors of its own type, i.e., which are either reliable or unreliable respectively.

We define $P_{(N_R-1,N_U)}$ as the probability of a deterministic majority voting scheme, which involves the opinions of $N_R - 1$ reliable sensors and N_U unreliable ones, to yield the correct decision using the majority rule. In other words, this is the probability that a majority of more than $\frac{(N_R-1+N_U)}{2}$ of the sensors will advocate the ground truth. Similarly, we define $P_{(N_R,N_U-1)}$ as the probability of a deterministic majority voting scheme, which involves the opinions of N_R reliable sensors and $N_U - 1$ unreliable ones, to yield the correct decision using the majority rule. As one can see, this quantity is the same: It too is the probability that a majority of more than $\frac{(N_R+N_U-1)}{2}$ of the sensors will, in turn, advocate the ground truth.

In [4,5], we assumed that:

$$(N_R - 1)p_R + N_U p_U > \frac{(N_R + N_U)}{2}.$$

The latter condition is founded on a fundamental premise that has to hold in any sustainable society, where telling the "truth" is considered a virtue, while "lying"

[3] This assumption, however, does not simplify the problem. Indeed, p_R can be assigned to be the smallest value of all the values of p_i for the reliable sensors, and p_U can be assigned to be the largest value of all the values of p_i for the unreliable ones.

[4] Throughout this paper, since we will be invoking majority-like decisions, we assume that $N = N_R + N_U$ is an even number.

is considered detrimental and harmful to the society. In this paper, the task we undertake is to consider the non-intuitive complementary problem. Indeed, we will investigate the non-trivial case in which the phenomenon of "lying" is more prevalent than that of saying the "truth" exasperated by the case when the proportion of stochastic "lying" agents exceeds the number of stochastic "truth-telling" agents. We shall endeavor to state and prove the relevant theoretical results for the case where:

$$(N_R - 1)p_R + N_U p_U < \frac{(N_R + N_U)}{2} - 1.$$

The reader should observe that whenever the Environment is deterministic, i.e., $p_R = 1$ and $p_U = 0$, the above condition can be written as $N_R < N_R + N_U$, which simply means that the set of unreliable sensors form the Majority from among the sensors. Hence, in the special case of a deterministic Environment, the problem can be seen as resolving the problem using Majority voting.

3 The Solution

3.1 Overview of Our Solution

In this paper, we provide a novel solution to the *STTP* for the scenario where "lying prevails over the truth", and where this solution is based on the field of LA that was briefly surveyed above. It is appropriate to mention that we are not aware of any other solution to this problem (within this setting), and so we believe that our solution is both pioneering and novel. We intend to take advantage of the fact that LA combine rapid and accurate convergence with low computational complexity. In addition to its computational simplicity, unlike most reported approaches, as mentioned earlier, our scheme does not require prior knowledge of the ground truth. Rather, it adaptively, and in an on-line manner, gradually learns the identity and characteristics of the sensors which tend to provide reliable readings, and of those which tend to provide unreliable ones.

Our solution involves a team of *LA* where each *LA* is uniquely attached to (or rather, associated with) a specific sensor, on a one-to-one basis. Each automaton $\mathcal{A}^i$, attached to sensor s_i, has two actions.

By suitably modeling the agreement or disagreement of the opinions about the sensed ground truth between each sensor and the rest of the other sensors, we can appropriately model these as responses from the corresponding "Environment". Using these synthesized responses, our scheme will intelligently group the sensors according to the readings that they report about the ground truth. Since a sensor is reliable if it reports the ground truth correctly with a probability $p_i > 0.5$ (and unreliable otherwise), we will design our scheme so that it can infer the similar sensors and collect them into their respective groups. In other words, we will infer the crucial pieces of information, namely the identities of the sensors, from the random stream of sensor reports.

The fusion part of our scheme will be based on the result of a prior partitioning phase. Ultimately, the aim behind identifying the set of unreliable sensors, $\mathcal{S}_U$, is to improve the performance of the fusion process for inferring the ground truth. The result of the convergence of the team of LA, which results in a partitioning that infers the identity of the sensors, will serve as an input to the fusion process. In this vein, we present a simple approach for fusing the results, and study its performance in the section that describes the experimental result. The fusion approach only considers the measurements from the reliable sensors as being informative, and simultaneously discards measurements from the unreliable sensors. An alternate fusion scheme which considers the responses from all the sensors is also described. The first formal result concerning the performance of the LA is given below.

3.2 Theoretical Results for the Case Where: "Lying Prevails over Truth"

In this section, we provide theoretical results pertinent to the extremely interesting and fascinating case when "Lying Prevails over Truth-Telling", i.e., when it is more likely for the sensors to be unreliable than reliable, or if you like, the number of unreliable sensors is more than the number of reliable ones.

We analyze and provide the theoretical results for the case where $(N_R - 1)p_R + N_U p_U < \frac{(N_R+N_U)}{2} - 1$. The proofs of the following two theorems are quite involved and are omitted here for the sake of brevity. The proofs can be found in a unabridged version of this article [4].

Theorem 1. *Consider the scenario when* $N_R p_R + (N_U - 1)p_U < \frac{(N_R+N_U)}{2} - 1$ *and when* $N_R + N_U - 1 \geq 3$. *Let* $s_i \in \mathcal{S}_R$. *Consider now the agreement between the opinion of a reliable sensor* s_i *and the opinion of the majority formed by all the rest of the sensors* $S\backslash\{s_i\} = (\mathcal{S}_R\backslash\{s_i\}) \cup \mathcal{S}_U$. *Let* $y_{(N_R-1,N_U)}$ *be the decision of a majority voting scheme* $S\backslash\{s_i\}$, *based on the responses of* $N_R - 1$ *reliable and* N_U *unreliable sensors. Then, if* x_i *is the output of* s_i: $Prob(x_i = y_{(N_R-1,N_U)}) < 0.5$.

The next theorem, which deals with the analogous case of excluding an unreliable sensor, follows.

Theorem 2. *Consider the scenario when* $N_R p_R + (N_U - 1)p_U < \frac{(N_R+N_U)}{2} - 1$ *and when* $N_R + N_U - 1 \geq 3$. *Let* $s_i \in \mathcal{S}_U$. *Consider now the agreement between the opinion of an unreliable sensor* s_i *and the opinion of the majority formed by all the rest of the sensors,* $S\backslash\{s_i\} = \mathcal{S}_R \cup \mathcal{S}_U\backslash\{s_i\}$. *Let* $y_{(N_R,N_U-1)}$ *be the decision of a majority voting scheme based on the responses of* $S\backslash\{s_i\}$, *consisting of* N_R *reliable and* $N_U - 1$ *unreliable sensors. Then, if* x_i *is the output of* s_i: $Prob(x_i = y_{(N_R,N_U-1)}) > 0.5$

3.3 Construction of the Learning Automata

The results that we have presented in the previous section form the basis of our LA-based solution. We explain this below, including the strategy by which the majority vote is invoked.

In the partitioning strategy, with each sensor s_i we associate a 2-action L_{RI} automaton $\mathcal{A}^i$, $(\Sigma^i, \Pi^i, \Gamma^i, \Upsilon^i, \Omega^i)$, where Σ^i is the set of actions, Π^i is the set of action probabilities, Γ^i is the set of feedback inputs from the Environment, and Υ^i is the set of action probability updating rules. Each of these is explained below.

1. *The set of actions of the automaton:* (Σ^i)
   The two actions of the automaton are α_k^i, for $k \in \{0,1\}$, i.e., α_0^i and α_1^i.
2. *The action probabilities:* (Π^i)
   $P_k^i(n)$ represent the probabilities of selecting the action α_k^i, for $k \in \{0,1\}$, at step n. Initially, $P_k^i(0) = 0.5$, for $k = 0, 1$.
3. *The feedback inputs from the Environment to each automaton:* (Γ^i)
   Let the automaton select either the action α_0^i or α_1^i. Then, the responses from the Environment and the corresponding probabilities are tabulated below. For a chosen action, the Environment will respond by a "Reward", or a "Penalty". The conditional probabilities of the "Reward", and "Penalty" are also specified in the tables.
   A brief explanation about the equations in these tables could be beneficial.
   (a) The LA system is rewarded if it chooses action α_0^i, in which case the reading of the sensor s_i agrees with the opinion of the majority voting scheme associated with $S \backslash \{s_i\}$. This occurs with probability $Prob(x_i = y_{(N_R-1,N_U)})$ whenever $s_i \in \mathcal{S}_R$ and with probability $Prob(x_i = y_{(N_R,N_U-1)})$ whenever $s_i \in \mathcal{S}_U$.
   (b) Alternatively, the system is rewarded if it chooses action α_1^i, in which case the reading of the sensor s_i disagrees with the opinion of the majority voting scheme associated with $S \backslash \{s_i\}$. This occurs with probability $1 - Prob(x_i = y_{(N_R-1,N_U)})$ whenever $s_i \in \mathcal{S}_R$ and with probability $1 - Prob(x_i = y_{(N_R,N_U-1)})$ whenever $s_i \in \mathcal{S}_U$.
   (c) The penalty scenarios are the reversed ones.
4. *The action probability updating rules:* (Υ^i)
   First of all, since we are using the L_{RI} scheme, we ignore all the penalty responses. Upon reward, we obey the following updating rule:
   If α_k^i for $k \in \{0,1\}$ was rewarded then,

$$P_{1-k}^i(n+1) \leftarrow \theta \times P_{1-k}^i(n)$$
$$P_k^i(n+1) \leftarrow 1 - \theta \times P_{1-k}^i(n),$$

   where $0 \ll \theta < 1$ is the L_{RI} reward parameter.

Before we prove the properties of the overall system, we first state a fundamental result of the L_{RI} learning schemes which we will repeatedly allude to in the rest of the paper.

Lemma 1. *An L_{RI} learning scheme with parameter $0 \ll \theta < 1$ is ϵ-optimal, whenever an optimal action exists. In other words,* $\lim_{\theta \to 1} \lim_{n \to \infty} P_k^i(n) \to 1$.

The above result is well known [1]. By virtue of this property, we are guaranteed that for any L_{RI} scheme with the two actions $\{\alpha_0, \alpha_1\}$, if $\exists\ k \in \{0,1\}$ such that $c_k^i < c_{1-k}^i$, then the action α_k^i is optimal, and for this action $P_k^i(n) \to 1$ as $n \to \infty$ and $\theta \to 1$, where the $\{c_k^i\}$, are the penalty probabilities for the two actions of the automaton $\mathcal{A}^i$.

By invoking the property of the L_{RI} learning scheme, we state and prove the convergence property of the overall system.

Theorem 3. *Consider the scenario when* $(N_R - 1)p_R + N_U p_U < \frac{(N_R+N_U)}{2} - 1$ *and that* $N_R + N_U - 1 \geq 3$. *Given the* L_{RI} *scheme with a parameter* θ *which is arbitrarily close to unity, the following is true:*

$$\text{If } s_i \in \mathcal{S}_R, \text{ then } \lim_{\theta\to 1} \lim_{n\to\infty} P_0^i(n) \to 1;$$
$$\text{If } s_i \in \mathcal{S}_U, \text{ then } \lim_{\theta\to 1} \lim_{n\to\infty} P_1^i(n) \to 1.$$

Proof: To prove the theorem, we treat the two cases separately.

Case 1: $s_i \in \mathcal{S}_R$: Based on the result of Theorem 1, we can see that the inequality $Prob(x_i = y_{(N_R-1,N_U)}) < 0.5$ holds. We can thus deduce that:

$$Prob(x_i = y_{(N_R-1,N_U)}) < 1 - Prob(x_i = y_{(N_R-1,N_U)}). \tag{3}$$

If we now consider the entries of Table 1 that specify the penalty probabilities $s_i \in \mathcal{S}_R$, we see that:

$$c_1^i = Prob(x_i = y_{(N_R-1,N_U)}) < c_0^i = 1 - Prob(x_i = y_{(N_R-1,N_U)}),$$

implying that for this case, the action α_1^i is the optimal one. Consequently, by virtue of Lemma 1, for this action:

$$P_1^i(n) \to 1 \text{ as } n \to \infty \text{ and } \theta \to 1,$$

proving the result for this case.

Case 2: $s_i \in \mathcal{S}_U$: In this case, based on the result of Theorem 2, we see that the following inequality holds: $Prob(x_i = y_{(N_R,N_U-1)}) > 0.5$.

Therefore we can confirm that

$$Prob(x_i = y_{(N_R,N_U-1)}) > 1 - Prob(x_i = y_{(N_R,N_U-1)}). \tag{4}$$

Table 1. Reward and Penalty probabilities for sensor $s_i \in \mathcal{S}_R$

Action	Associated probability	
	Reward	Penalty
α_0^i	$Prob(x_i = y_{(N_R-1,N_U)})$	$1 - Prob(x_i = y_{(N_R-1,N_U)})$
α_1^i	$1 - Prob(x_i = y_{(N_R-1,N_U)})$	$Prob(x_i = y_{(N_R-1,N_U)})$

Table 2. Reward and Penalty probabilities for sensor $s_i \in \mathcal{S}_U$

Action	Associated probability	
	Reward	Penalty
α_0^i	$Prob(x_i = y_{(N_R, N_U - 1)})$	$1 - Prob(x_i = y_{(N_R, N_U - 1)})$
α_1^i	$1 - Prob(x_i = y_{(N_R, N_U - 1)})$	$Prob(x_i = y_{(N_R, N_U - 1)})$

From the entries of Table 2, that specify the penalty probabilities $s_i \in \mathcal{S}_U$, we obtain:

$$c_0^i = 1 - Prob(x_i = y_{(N_R, N_U - 1)}) > c_1^i = Prob(x_i = y_{(N_R, N_U - 1)}).$$

This implies that the action α_0^i is the optimal one, and for this action:

$$P_0^i(n) \to 1 \text{ as } n \to \infty \text{ and } \theta \to 1.$$

The theorem is thus proven. □

3.3.1 Remarks and Some Additional Notation

Based on what we have already seen, the following observations are in place:

1. Analogous to the above theorems, from Theorem 3, we see the similar result for the case when:

$$N_R p_R + (N_U - 1) p_U < \frac{(N_R + N_U)}{2} - 1.$$

   In fact, when $N_R p_R + (N_U - 1) p_U < \frac{(N_R + N_U)}{2} - 1$, the reliable sensors will converge to action α_0^i, while the unreliable ones to action α_1^i with an arbitrarily large probability. To summarize these results, let:
   - $G_R = \{s_i \in S \text{ such that } \lim_{n \to \infty} P_1^i(n) = 1\}$
   - $G_U = \{s_i \in S \text{ such that } \lim_{n \to \infty} P_0^i(n) = 1\}$.

   As the conclusions are ϵ-optimal results, if θ is arbitrarily close to unity, G_R will converge to $\mathcal{S}_R$ and G_U will converge to $\mathcal{S}_U$. On the other hand, if θ is not arbitrarily close to unity, some of the LA might fail to converge to the optimal action, and thus the set G_R may not necessarily be equivalent to $\mathcal{S}_R$, and G_U may not necessarily be equivalent to $\mathcal{S}_U$.
2. In our earlier work [4], we had dealt with a with a society where "truth prevails over lying" (i.e., where, effectively, the number of reliable sensors was more than the number of unreliable ones), characterized by the canonical equation:

$$(N_R - 1) p_R + N_U p_U > \frac{(N_R + N_U)}{2}.$$

   A naive way to *attempt* to obtain the condition for the opposite scenario involving a deceptive environment, i.e., one in which "lying prevails over truth", would be to invert the equations by exchanging N_R with N_U and p_R with p_U respectively. The inverted equation obtained by such a straightforward substitution is:

$$(N_U - 1)p_U + N_R p_R > \frac{(N_R + N_U)}{2}.$$

However, on performing a rigorous analysis, one observes that the above condition "does not lead anywhere". Further, the condition does not guarantee any form of convergence[5]. Rather, since reasoning by direct symmetry does not work, deducing the correct condition that is applicable for Deceptive Environments is far from being intuitive.

3. A more careful investigation reveals that the correct condition, $N_R p_R + (N_U - 1)p_U < \frac{(N_R+N_U)}{2} - 1$, is not symmetric. Indeed, it is *this* condition that is valid for the case where "lying prevails over truth". One will observe that the above condition reduces to $N_R < \frac{(N_R+N_U)}{2}$ for $(p_R, p_U) = (1, 0)$. In other words, whenever the Environment is deterministic, implying that a reliable sensor will always tells the truth ($p_R = 1$) and an unreliable sensor will always misreport the truth ($p_U = 0$), we will obtain a minority of reliable sensors since $N_R < \frac{(N_R+N_U)}{2}$, forcing the unreliable sensors to constitute the majority.

3.4 Fusion Schemes with Exclusion: Discarding the Opinions of the Unreliable Sensors

A possible strategy to increase the accuracy of the fusion process is to employ a simple majority voting strategy that excludes all the sensors whose LA converged to the action G_U during the partitioning phase. This means that the prediction of the ground truth will be exclusively based on the "accurate" sensors, i.e., those whose LA converged to the action G_R.

4 Experimental Results

The performance of the LA-based partitioning as well as the fusion schemes with exclusion (that makes use of the partitioning described in Sect. 3.4), have been rigorously tested by simulation in a variety of parameter settings, and the results that we have obtained are truly conclusive. In the interest of brevity, we merely report a few representative (and typical) experimental results, so that the power of our proposed methodology can be justified. In the experiments, the settings were chosen so that the condition $(N_R - 1)p_R + N_U p_U < \frac{(N_R+N_U)}{2} - 1$ was met, reflecting that the world possessed that the phenomenon in which "lying prevails over the truth".

[5] The absence of convergence was also supported by experimental results that are not reported here. This was, indeed, what motivated the present avenue of research.

4.1 Fusion Scheme with Exclusion

We now compare the "Fusion Scheme with Exclusion" with the deterministic Majority Voting (MV) strategy that incorporates all the sensors in S. As detailed earlier, the latter scheme relies exclusively on the decision of the vote of the majority of the sensors that converged to the G_R partition. Let $P(C_c)$ denote the probability of the consensus being correct, i.e., that the probability that the vote of the majority coincides with the ground truth. Table 3 reports the result of the comparison for the case when N_R and N_U are both equal to 10.

Table 3. Comparisons of the value of $P(C_C)$, the probabilities of the consensus being correct for different values of (p_R, p_U), and for the different approaches for $N_R = 10$ and $N_U = 10$.

(p_R, p_U)	$P(C_C)$ for Fusion Scheme with Exclusion	$P(C_C)$ for MV for all sensors
$(0.55, 0.25)$	0.738	0.234
$(0.6, 0.25)$	0.833	0.13
$(0.65, 0.25)$	0.905	0.401
$(0.7, 0.25)$	0.952	0.5
$(0.55, 0.2)$	0.738	0.16
$(0.6, 0.2)$	0.833	0.225
$(0.65, 0.2)$	0.905	0.426
$(0.7, 0.2)$	0.952	0.396

From this table, we observe:

1. The distribution of T does not play a role in determining the value of $P(C_c)$ for the Fusion Scheme with Exclusion because of the symmetry property of the fault. As one can see, the results we report are conclusive. In fact, we were able to increase the value of $P(C_c)$ quite remarkably. For example, for the case when $(p_R, p_U) = (0.7, 0.25)$, our scheme yielded a value of 0.952 for $P(C_C)$, while the scheme which operated with the MV involving all the sensors yielded the value of only 0.5.
2. The value of $P(C_C)$ for the simple MV involving all sensors gave a low accuracy (less than 0.5) as the Environment was Deceptive.
3. The value of $P(C_C)$ for our Fusion Scheme with Exclusion was immune to the variation of p_U. For example, for the entries corresponding to $p_R = 0.7$, we see that $P(C_C)$ was equal to 0.952 even if p_U changed, for example, by taking the values 0.25 or 0.2.

Consider now the case when the value N_U was doubled from 10 to 20 while the value of N_R was equal to 10. As expected, we see from Table 4, the value of $P(C_C)$ for our scheme was intact and independent of the value of N_U.

Table 4. Comparisons of $P(C_C)$, the probabilities of the consensus being correct for different values of (p_R, p_U), and for the different approaches for $N_R = 20$ and $N_U = 10$.

(p_R, p_U)	$P(C_C)$ for Fusion Scheme with Exclusion	$P(C_C)$ for MV for all sensors
$(0.55, 0.25)$	0.738	0.057
$(0.6, 0.25)$	0.833	0.081
$(0.65, 0.25)$	0.905	0.112
$(0.7, 0.25)$	0.952	0.15
$(0.55, 0.2)$	0.738	0.02
$(0.6, 0.2)$	0.833	0.03
$(0.65, 0.2)$	0.905	0.046
$(0.7, 0.2)$	0.952	0.066

5 Conclusion

The authors of the current articles have recently pioneered a solution to an extremely pertinent problem, namely, that of identifying which sensors are unreliable *without any knowledge of the ground truth.* This fascinating paradox can be formulated in simple terms as trying to identify *stochastic* liars without any additional information about the truth. In this paper, we provide a LA-based solution to the problem where the sensors operated in a world in which "lying prevails over truth telling", or informally speaking, where the number of unreliable sensors is stochastically more than the number of reliable ones.

References

1. Narendra, K.S., Thathachar, M.A.L.: Learning Automata: An Introduction. Prentice-Hall, New Jersey (1989)
2. Oommen, B.J.: Stochastic searching on the line and its applications to parameter learning in nonlinear optimization. IEEE Trans. Syst. Man Cybernet. B **27**, 733–739 (1997)
3. Yazidi, A., Granmo, O.C., Oommen, B.J.: Service selection in stochastic environments: a learning-automaton based solution. Appl. Intell. **36**(3), 617–637 (2012)
4. Yazidi, A., Oommen, B.J., Goodwin, M.: On solving the problem of identifying unreliable sensors without a knowledge of the ground truth: the case of stochastic environments. IEEE Trans. Cybernet. **47**, 1604–1617 (2017)
5. Yazidi, A., Oommen, B.J., Goodwin, M.: On distinguishing between reliable and unreliable sensors without a knowledge of the ground truth. In: 2015 IEEE/WIC/ACM International Conference on Web Intelligence and Intelligent Agent Technology (WI-IAT), vol. 2, pp. 104–111. IEEE (2015)

Color-Sketch Simulator: A Guide for Color-Based Visual Known-Item Search

Jakub Lokoč[1(✉)], Anh Nguyen Phuong[3], Marta Vomlelová[2], and Chong-Wah Ngo[3]

[1] SIRET Research Group, Department of Software Engineering, Faculty of Mathematics and Physics, Charles University, Prague, Czech Republic
lokoc@ksi.mff.cuni.cz

[2] Department of Theoretical Computer Science and Mathematical Logic, Faculty of Mathematics and Physics, Charles University, Prague, Czech Republic
marta@ktiml.mff.cuni.cz

[3] Department of Computer Science, City University of Hong Kong, Kowloon, Hong Kong
panguyen2-c@my.cityu.edu.hk, cscwngo@cityu.edu.hk

Abstract. In order to evaluate the effectiveness of a color-sketch retrieval system for a given multimedia database, tedious evaluations involving real users are required as users are in the center of query sketch formulation. However, without any prior knowledge about the bottlenecks of the underlying sketch-based retrieval model, the evaluations may focus on wrong settings and thus miss the desired effect. Furthermore, users have usually no clues or recommendations to draw color-sketches effectively. In this paper, we aim at a preliminary analysis to identify potential bottlenecks of a flexible color-sketch retrieval model. We present a formal framework based on position-color feature signatures, enabling comprehensive simulations of users drawing a color sketch.

1 Introduction

Known-item search (KIS) represents a multimedia retrieval scenario, where users know about an image (or scene) in a large collection, but do not know where it is located. The visual KIS task represents a special case, when users see and memorize some image/scene and try to find it in the collection. In order to prevent users from sequential browsing, modern multimedia retrieval systems offer query by sketch/concept/keyword options and additional browsing interfaces [14]. In this work, we aim at sketch based retrieval that has been intensively investigated during last decades, focusing on contours, shapes and/or colors [5,7,9,13]. Sketch-based retrieval has been also applied for interactive video retrieval [1,3,11].

Since the searched scene can be memorized only partially and also not all users are able to sufficiently paint (own experience), we focus on a query by color-sketch approach based on just simple low-level intuitive color features.

G. Cong et al. (Eds.): ADMA 2017, LNAI 10604, pp. 754–763, 2017.
https://doi.org/10.1007/978-3-319-69179-4_53

Furthermore, we focus on a very simple interface based on an interactive sketch drawing canvas where users place colored circles [4]. Despite its simplicity, the approach proved to be an effective option for visual known-item search tasks at the international Video Browser Showdown competition [6].

The effectiveness of color-sketch retrieval depends on many factors, including specific distributions of colors in the searched collections and also unpredictable user behavior. Therefore, any kind of optimization of the underlying color-based retrieval model represents a challenging difficult problem. The retrieval models have usually many parameters to finetune, the parameters depend also on user's focus, memorized color stimuli and the ability to reproduce colors at specific canvas positions. However, a thorough evaluation would require an enormous number of experiments involving real user interactions. In order to limit their number (i.e., to investigate just promising settings with real users), a simulation framework is of high importance. In this work, we design a formal simulation framework for a simple sketch drawing interface and a selected color-based retrieval model, focusing on the following two objectives:

- *Given a fixed retrieval model, guide the user to specify his query sketches for a database.*
- *Given a general idea of user's focus, enable preliminary inspection of the parameters of a retrieval model.*

The paper is structured as follows. Section 2 details the employed color-sketch retrieval model. Section 3 introduces the signature-sketch simulator and Sect. 4 presents our preliminary experimental case study. Section 5 concludes the paper and highlights the future work.

2 Color-Sketch Retrieval Model

In the following, a retrieval model based on position-color feature signatures is recapitulated. The model enables flexible image representation and at the same time provides a sound formal basis for sketch drawing simulations.

2.1 Image Representation

When searching for a known image using memorized colors, feature signatures represent a flexible model enabling an approximation of the color distribution of a particular image [2,12]. Given a feature space $\mathbb{F}$, a *feature signature* FS^o of a multimedia object o is defined as a finite set of tuples $\{\langle r_i^o, w_i^o \rangle\}_{i=1}^n$ from $\mathbb{F} \times \mathbb{R}^+$, consisting of representatives $r_i^o \in \mathbb{F}$ and their weights $w_i^o \in \mathbb{R}^+, \sum_{i=1}^n w_i^o = 1$. For color-sketch retrieval, the feature space $\mathbb{F}$ can be modeled as a subspace of $\mathbb{R}^5$, where the dimensions of the feature space correspond to position (x, y) and color (R, G, B) information present in each pixel. The color information is usually transformed to a perceptually uniform color space (in our work, CIE Lab color space is used). Note that the original image can be also considered as a feature signature if each pixel is assigned a prior weight. Instead of the

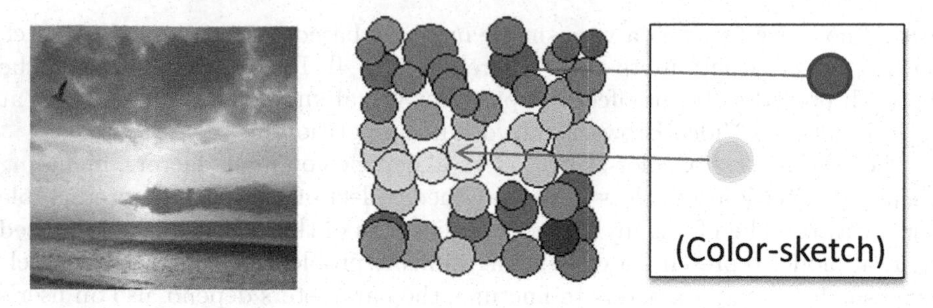

Fig. 1. From left to right, a database image, a corresponding position-color feature signature (the weight of each representative is depicted as the colored circle radius) and an interactive color-sketch drawing canvas, where users place colored circles to find the image. The red arrows depict the most similar tuples in the feature signature to tuples in the query sketch. (Color figure online)

original images, interpolation-based thumbnails in connection with an adaptive clustering can be used to flexibly compress the position-color information in the images [8].

2.2 Color-Sketch Ranking

Since users often memorize just few color stimuli, the sketch drawing tool can be implemented as a color circle positioning canvas (see Fig. 1). As presented in [4], such a user defined color sketch q can be directly interpreted as a feature signature $FS^q = \{\langle r_j^q, w_j^q \rangle\}_{j=1}^m$. Given a distance measure $\delta : (\mathbb{F} \times \mathbb{R}^+) \times (\mathbb{F} \times \mathbb{R}^+) \rightarrow \mathbb{R}_0^+$, a color-sketch ranking model can be generally defined as:

$$rank^{qo} = \underset{\forall t_j^q \in FS^q}{\text{avg}} f_j^q(\underset{\forall t_i^o \in FS^o}{\min} \delta(t_j^q, t_i^o)),$$

where FS^o is a feature signature of a database object o and $f_j^q : \mathbb{R}_0^+ \rightarrow \mathbb{R}$ is a monotonic decreasing transformation function, defined for each query tuple t_j^q separately. An example of such transformation is the *MinMax* function[1] $f_j^q(x) = \frac{\delta_{max} - x}{\delta_{max} - \delta_{min}}$, where real positive thresholds $\delta_{min} < \delta_{max}$ are selected from distances δ between the query tuple t_j^q and all tuples t_i^o from all database objects. As a distance δ for two tuples, in this work we consider the Euclidean distance for representatives, ignoring the weight of the tuples.

After each object o in the database receives its $rank^{qo}$ according to the query q, the objects are sorted in descending order and top k objects are returned. In order to speed up the evaluation for large datasets, the authors have proposed also a grid-based index that considers only tuples t_i^o in such grid cells, which intersect the query sphere with radius θ and centered in r_j^q. Note that θ represents an estimated threshold for a maximal acceptable user-error.

[1] In the original paper [4], the dual form $f_j^q(x) = \frac{x - \delta_{min}}{\delta_{max} - \delta_{min}}$ was defined, modelling similarities as distances.

2.3 Probabilistic Model

Let us denote p_i^q probability $P(t_i^q \in FS^o|FS^o \text{ is relevant})$ and $q_i^q = P(t_i^q \in FS^o|FS^o \text{ is not relevant})$. Then, presence of any color circle in an object increases the relevant/non–relevant ratio by $\frac{p_i^q}{q_i^q}$.

The p_i^q is modeled by user error described later. Basically, we model the user error in each of 5 coordinates by Gaussian distribution $\mathcal{N}(0,\sigma^2)$ independently. This leads to the product of distributions and after the logarithm transform to the negative quadratic Euclidean distance weighted by $1/\sigma^2$. We assume only a small number of objects to be relevant compared to the number of objects in the database. Therefore, we estimate q_i^q as observed frequencies ratio $\frac{|FS|_{t_i^q \in FS}}{|FS|}$, where $|FS|_{t_i^q \in FS}$ denotes the number of objects in a fixed radius around t_i^q. Putting it together, $log(\frac{p_i^q}{q_i^q}) = log(p_i^q) + log(\frac{1}{q_i^q}) \approx \frac{-\delta^2(t_i^q,t_i^o)}{\sigma^2} + log(\frac{|FS|}{|FS|_{t_i^q \in FS}})$, where the last term can be viewed as the inverse document frequency (IDF) in text-search domain [10]. The resulting expression is a monotonic decreasing transformation with respect to $x = \delta(t_i^q, t_i^o)$, $x \geq 0$. Hence it can be directly used as the transformation $f_j^q(x)$ in the ranking model presented in Sect. 2.2. Adding a (strong) assumption of independence of color-point presence in the object, these measures for all color-points in the query can be averaged. We do not include the absence of a color-point into the model since most color-points of the relevant object are not present in the query.

3 Signature-Sketch Simulator

An advanced formalization of user's behavior would require a complex model considering user's focus, perception, memory, position-color reproduction skills, environment conditions, etc. Furthermore, an extensive user behavior analysis would be necessary to set up all the parameters of the model. However, the users often search intuitively, without any clue about the effectiveness of their employed strategy. Therefore, the purpose of the presented signature-sketch simulator is not to perfectly mimic a user, but to identify and recommend potentially effective strategies or to provide a general benchmark framework for various parameters of the utilized retrieval models.

The signature-sketch simulator presented in this work is designed as a formal framework over a dataset of images represented by feature signatures. In order to model a user who draws a sketch to find an image o represented by feature signature FS^o, the framework modifies the reference feature signature FS^o to a query feature signature FS^q. Hence, the core of the framework is a feature signature transformation function determined by a tuple (Π, ϵ), where $\Pi : FS^o \rightarrow FS^{o'}, FS^{o'} \subseteq FS^o$ projects the original signature to a list of selected tuples (i.e., modelling a user focus), while $\epsilon : \mathbb{F} \rightarrow \mathbb{F}$ models a user error by shifting the projected centroids. Given a reference feature signature FS^o, the simulated query sketch is defined as:

$$FS^q = \{\langle \epsilon(r_j^o), w_j^o \rangle | \langle r_j^o, w_j^o \rangle \in \Pi(FS^o)\}$$

In this work, we employ a simplified user-error model to demonstrate the principles of the simulator. The mapping ϵ used in the experiments models the user error in each of 5 coordinates by Gaussian distribution $\mathcal{N}(0, \sigma^2)$ independently. The squared Euclidean distances $L_2^2(r_j^o, \epsilon(r_j^o))$ in the 5 dimensional space follow χ^2 distribution. This models the error as the white noise and resembles the results presented in Blazek et al. [4]. In the rest of the section, we will focus on projection strategies Π modeling the focus of users.

3.1 Projection Strategies

The designed simulator considers and investigates a whole family of various "artificial" yet intuitive color-sketch strategies for the users. In the following list, several examples of strategies are presented as projections of a reference feature signature FS^o.

- *Random* strategy Π^k_{random}. The strategy assumes that all tuples $\langle r_j^o, w_j^o \rangle \in FS^o$ have the same probability to be memorized, thus selects randomly k tuples from FS^o.
- *Color-based* strategies model a situation, where users focus on k tuples $\langle r_j^o, w_j^o \rangle \in FS^o$ based on specific colors. In this work we consider two color-based strategies – *dominant colors* and *most saturated colors*. The strategy $\Pi^k_{dominant}$ selects k representatives r_j^o with the highest sum of weights w_k^o of tuples $t_k^o \in X_j^o \subset FS^o$, where X_j^o represents the set of tuples close to r_j^o in the color space. The strategy $\Pi^k_{saturated}$ selects k representatives r_j^o with the most saturated colors.
- *Position-based* strategies. The selection of centroids in a given region represents a user friendly and intuitive strategy, where a user focuses just on a specific part of the canvas. As an example, in this work we consider a *center region strategy* $\Pi_{center}(FS^o)$ projecting a feature signature FS^o to tuples $\langle r_j^q, w_j^q \rangle \in FS^o$, where $r_j^q[x] \in [x_{min}, x_{max}] \wedge r_j^q[y] \in [y_{min}, y_{max}]\}$. We also consider a *border region strategy* defined as $\Pi_{border}(FS^o) = FS^o - \Pi_{center}(FS^q)$.
- Combinations of strategies can be used to extend the set of possible strategies. Since position-based strategies can return more than k tuples, they can be easily composed with Π^k_{random}, $\Pi^k_{dominant}$ and $\Pi^k_{saturated}$. For example, $\Pi^1_{random}(\Pi_{center}(FS^o))$ returns one randomly selected tuple from the center area of the feature signature FS^o.

4 Experiments

The objectives of the simulator framework are presented in several preliminary experiments using the IACC.3 video dataset from TRECVID AVS Task and the provided master shot reference with almost 335,944 selected keyframes. All the key-frames were resized to the size of 320×240 which is the proper size of videos in IACC.3 dataset. The feature signature extraction and reference retrieval model employing *MinMax* were taken from the Signature-based video browser [4] kindly provided by the authors of the tool. The overall number of representatives extracted from all keyframes was 8,124,854. We utilized the grid index to speed up query processing in the database of representatives, using the range $\theta = 40$ guaranteeing the requested cardinality of the results. We also compare the *MinMax* ranking with the probabilistic model labeled as *IDF*, where $|FS|_{t_i^q \in FS}$ was estimated using the number of returned images for the range θ.

We have investigated five types of user errors, modeled by $\mathcal{N}(\mu, \sigma^2), \sigma \in \{1, 2, 4, 8, 16\}$ to modify projected reference feature signatures. All the projection strategies from Sect. 3.1 were considered, focusing on color sketches comprising one up to four colored circles (i.e., $|FS^q| \in \{1, 2, 3, 4\}$). The investigated strategies are presented in Table 1:

Table 1. Labels of the tested strategies.

Projection strategy	Label
$\Pi^k_{random}(FS^o)$	$Random_k$
$\Pi^k_{dominant}(FS^o)$	$Dominant_k$
$\Pi^k_{saturated}(FS^o)$	$Saturated_k$
$\Pi^k_{random}(\Pi_{border}(FS^o))$	$Border_k$
$\Pi^k_{random}(\Pi_{center}(FS^o))$	$Center_k$
$\Pi^k_{dominant}(\Pi_{border}(FS^o))$	$BorDom_k$
$\Pi^k_{saturated}(\Pi_{border}(FS^o))$	$BorSat_k$
$\Pi^k_{dominant}(\Pi_{center}(FS^o))$	$CenDom_k$
$\Pi^k_{saturated}(\Pi_{center}(FS^o))$	$CenSat_k$
$Border_1 \cup Center_1$	$Bor\&Cen$
$Dominant_1 \cup Saturated_1$	$Dom\&Sat$
$Border_1 \cup Dominant_1$	$Bor\&Dom$
$Border_1 \cup Saturated_1$	$Bor\&Sat$
$Center_1 \cup Dominant_1$	$Cen\&Dom$
$Center_1 \cup Saturated_1$	$Cen\&Sat$

To generate the query sketches, 500 key-frames were randomly selected. Their corresponding feature signatures were transformed to simulated query sketches. For each-picked tuple t, 50 variations using Gaussian distribution with given σ were generated. Note that all types of considered user errors shared the same set of selected tuples. In the graphs, we present a score defined as $(1000 - pSI)/1000$, where pSI represents the position of the searched image in the top $k = 1000$ results. If the image was not in the top 1000 returned images, pSI was set to 1000.

Note that all the presented observations have to be taken with respect to the investigated dataset and also considered simulation framework.

In the left graph in Fig. 2, the effect of the user error was investigated in simulations of color-sketches with one query circle ($|FS^q| = 1$). Note that for one query circle, the results are the same for both *IDF* and *MinMax* ranking models. As expected, the score decreases with higher values of σ for all the strategies (*Bor&Dom*, *Bor&Sat* strategies were skipped as they had similar score as $Dominant_1, Saturated_1$). We may observe that for $\sigma \in \{1, 2, 4\}$ the $Center_1$ strategy provides the highest score for the investigated dataset. The strategy $CenSat_1$ seems to be most robust with respect to the user error, while $Saturated_1$ strategy represents a promising choice for $\sigma \in \{8, 16\}$. This could be explained by the properties of the TRECVID dataset, where highly saturated colors are rare. The good performance of the $Center_1$ strategy can be connected also to the utilized feature signature extraction function creating more tuples in the border area. Both observations highlight the subject of future investigation.

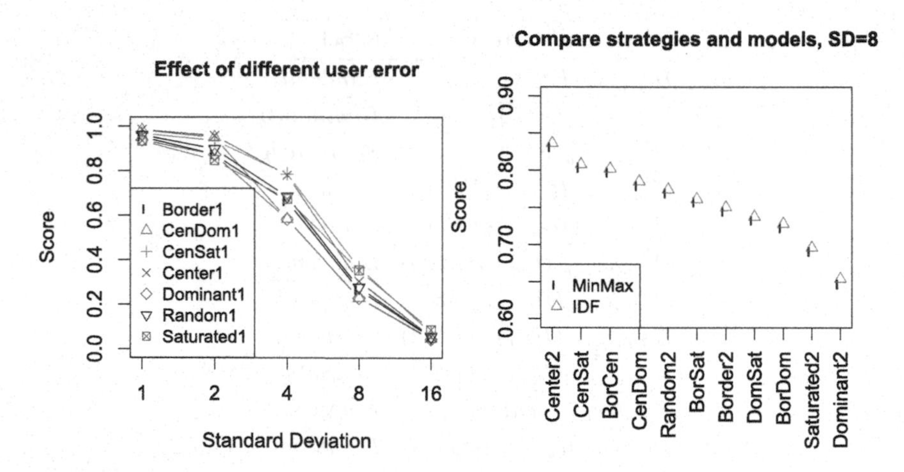

Fig. 2. On the left, the effect of user error on strategies in the simulated color-sketch query for $|FS^q| = 1$. On the right, the difference between strategies and ranking methods for $|FS^q| = 2$. (Color figure online)

In the right graph in Fig. 2, we investigated 11 different strategies for color sketches with $|FS^q| = 2$ and $\sigma = 8$. In all cases, the *IDF* ranking model slightly outperformed the *MinMax* ranking model. We may also observe that selecting two color circles randomly from the center area results in the highest score, while focusing on a dominant color does not seem to be an optimal strategy in average case. Another observation is that drawing two colored circles with $\sigma = 8$ results in a similar score as drawing one colored circle with $\sigma = 4$.

In Fig. 3, five types of color-sketch drawing strategies are compared for $|FS^q| \in \{1, 2, 3, 4\}$ using *IDF* ranking model. We may observe that for all tested strategies the additional colored circles in the query sketch improved the score for both tested σ values. The improvement between $|FS^q| = 1$ and $|FS^q| = 2$ is higher for $\sigma = 8$ than for $\sigma = 16$. Whereas the saturated colors are promising

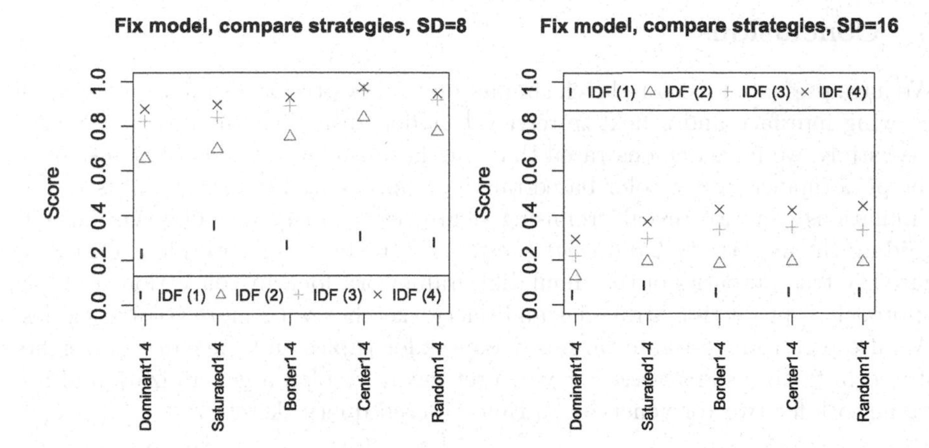

Fig. 3. The difference between strategies for $|FS^q| \in \{1, 2, 3, 4\}$ (distinguished by the numbers in the brackets). (Color figure online)

for $|FS^q| = 1$, for a higher number of query centroids the strategy performs not so well. This could be caused by a limited number of highly saturated colors in keyframes. The random and center strategies perform well for $|FS^q| \in \{2, 3, 4\}$.

4.1 Discussion

In our preliminary experiments, we have presented a case study that shows benefits of the simulation framework. Given some assumptions about user errors, the framework can help with the objectives presented in the introduction. The first objective is to guide the user, given a fixed retrieval model and a dataset. For example, Fig. 2 reveals that users drawing just one colored circle should focus on saturated colors in the center area as such strategy promises more effective retrieval in a given dataset. Users should also memorize and draw more colored circles, focusing on different colors. Such recommendations could help users to focus on specific colors and select more effective sketch-drawing strategies. In the future, we plan to investigate these findings in experiments involving two groups of real users – informed and not informed about the recommendation.

The second objective is to inspect clues to initialize parameters of a color-sketch retrieval model. Although our simulations are based on strong assumptions (known user error and strategy), the results can highlight promising initial settings, interesting trends and subjects for future investigation. For example, the *IDF* based ranking seems to consistently slightly outperform the *MinMax* based ranking in our settings for all considered types of users. Hence the *IDF* based ranking could be a preferred initial choice. The results of the comparison can also highlight promising topics for a sound formal analysis and explanations.

5 Conclusions

We have presented a color-sketch simulation framework for a simple color-sketch drawing interface and a flexible retrieval model. In a preliminary experimental case study, we have demonstrated that simulations can provide a first insight of the performance of two color-based ranking approaches for a given dataset. The simulations can also reveal promising strategies to query an unknown dataset, guiding the user to "*ask the right questions*". In the future, we plan to investigate the true potential of the simulation framework focusing on various ranking approaches, projection strategies and query sketches with more colored circles. We also plan to investigate various distances for tuples and the effect of weights stored in feature signatures. For video retrieval, we plan a generalization of the framework for two (or generally n) time-ordered query sketches.

Acknowledgments. This research has been supported by Czech Science Foundation project (GAČR) 15-08916S and the Research Grants Council of the Hong Kong Special Administrative Region, China (CityU 11210514).

References

1. Barthel, K.U., Hezel, N., Mackowiak, R.: Navigating a graph of scenes for exploring large video collections. In: Tian, Q., Sebe, N., Qi, G.-J., Huet, B., Hong, R., Liu, X. (eds.) MMM 2016. LNCS, vol. 9517, pp. 418–423. Springer, Cham (2016). doi:10.1007/978-3-319-27674-8_43
2. Beecks, C.: Distance based similarity models for content based multimedia retrieval. Ph.D. thesis, RWTH Aachen University (2013)
3. Blažek, A., Lokoč, J., Kuboň, D.: Video hunter at VBS 2017. In: Proceedings of 23rd International Conference MultiMedia Modeling, MMM 2017, Reykjavik, Iceland, 4–6 January 2017, Part II, pp. 493–498 (2017)
4. Blažek, A., Lokoč, J., Skopal, T.: Video retrieval with feature signature sketches. In: Traina, A.J.M., Traina, C., Cordeiro, R.L.F. (eds.) SISAP 2014. LNCS, vol. 8821, pp. 25–36. Springer, Cham (2014). doi:10.1007/978-3-319-11988-5_3
5. Bui, T., Collomosse, J.P.: Scalable sketch-based image retrieval using color gradient features. In: 2015 IEEE International Conference on Computer Vision Workshop, ICCV Workshops 2015, Santiago, Chile, 7–13 December 2015, pp. 1012–1019 (2015)
6. Cobârzan, C., Schoeffmann, K., Bailer, W., Hürst, W., Blazek, A., Lokoc, J., Vrochidis, S., Barthel, K.U., Rossetto, L.: Interactive video search tools: a detailed analysis of the video browser showdown 2015. Multimedia Tools Appl. **76**(4), 5539–5571 (2017)
7. Flickner, M., Sawhney, H.S., Ashley, J., Huang, Q., Dom, B., Gorkani, M., Hafner, J., Lee, D., Petkovic, D., Steele, D., Yanker, P.: Query by image and video content: the QBIC system. IEEE Comput. **28**(9), 23–32 (1995)
8. Krulis, M., Lokoc, J., Skopal, T.: Efficient extraction of clustering-based feature signatures using GPU architectures. Multimedia Tools Appl. **75**(13), 8071–8103 (2016)
9. Parui, S., Mittal, A.: Similarity-invariant sketch-based image retrieval in large databases. In: Fleet, D., Pajdla, T., Schiele, B., Tuytelaars, T. (eds.) ECCV 2014. LNCS, vol. 8694, pp. 398–414. Springer, Cham (2014). doi:10.1007/978-3-319-10599-4_26

10. Robertson, S.: Understanding inverse document frequency: on theoretical arguments for IDF. J. Documentation **60**(5), 503–520 (2004)
11. Rossetto, L., Giangreco, I., Tanase, C., Schuldt, H., Dupont, S., Seddati, O.: Enhanced retrieval and browsing in the IMOTION system. In: Proceedings of MultiMedia Modeling - 23rd International Conference, MMM 2017, Reykjavik, Iceland, 4–6 January 2017, Part II, pp. 469–474 (2017)
12. Rubner, Y., Tomasi, C., Guibas, L.J.: The earth mover's distance as a metric for image retrieval. Int. J. Comput. Vis. **40**(2), 99–121 (2000)
13. Saavedra, J.M., Barrios, J.M.: Sketch based image retrieval using learned keyshapes (LKS). In: Proceedings of the British Machine Vision Conference 2015, BMVC 2015, Swansea, UK, 7–10 September 2015, pp. 164.1–164.11 (2015)
14. Schoeffmann, K., Hudelist, M.A., Huber, J.: Video interaction tools: a survey of recent work. ACM Comput. Surv. **48**(1), 14:1–14:34 (2015)

Applications

Making Use of External Company Data to Improve the Classification of Bank Transactions

Erlend Vollset[1], Eirik Folkestad[1(✉)], Marius Rise Gallala[2(✉)], and Jon Atle Gulla[1(✉)]

[1] Department of Computer Science, Norwegian University of Science and Technology, Trondheim, Norway
eirik.ek.folkestad@gmail.com, jon.atle.gulla@ntnu.no
[2] Analytics, Sparebank1 SMN, Trondheim, Norway
marius.rise.gallala@smn.no

Abstract. This project aims to explore to what extent external semantic resources on companies can be used to improve the accuracy of a real bank transaction classification system. The goal is to identify which implementations are best suited to exploit the additional company data retrieved from the *Brønnøysund Registry* and the *Google Places API*, and accurately measure the effects they have. The classification system builds on a Bag-of-Words representation and uses Logistic Regression as classification algorithm. This study suggests that enriching bank transactions with external company data substantially improves the accuracy of the classification system. If we compare the results obtained from our research to the baseline, which has an accuracy of 89.22%, the *Brønnøysund Registry* and *Google Places API* yield increases of 2.79pp and 2.01pp respectively. In combination, they generate an increase of 3.75pp.

Keywords: Classification · Bank transactions · Logistic regression · Semantic resources

1 Introduction

This project has been carried out in collaboration with Sparebank1 in order to gain insight into the classification of bank transactions. Progress in the domain at the intersection of finance and machine learning is important as it has plenty of potential applications; accurate consumption statistics, financial trend predictions, and fraud detection to name a few. We wish to develop techniques to improve a baseline approach to bank transaction classification by enriching our feature set using external semantic resources.

We examine two external semantic resources; the *Brønnøysund Entity Registry*, containing information about Norwegian companies, and the *Google Places API*, containing information about businesses, companies, and establishments worldwide. Two main approaches to the problem are covered:

G. Cong et al. (Eds.): ADMA 2017, LNAI 10604, pp. 767–780, 2017.
https://doi.org/10.1007/978-3-319-69179-4_54

- Using extracted external data to extend the baseline feature set
- Using extracted external data to aid in the classification of transactions where the classifier is not sufficiently confident.

This paper gives a detailed description of the implementation of these two approaches. It also provides a thorough analysis of the results obtained from testing the system. We compare the results to a baseline in order to draw meaningful conclusions about the impact of the approaches studied. Due to the general nature of the techniques in this project, they can easily be transferred to other applications within text classification. Seeing as they have shown to improve the accuracy of the system, they introduce a new dimension to problem-solving in the classification domain.

The remainder of the paper is structured as follows. Section 2 describes the theoretical foundation upon which we have built our project. It explains in detail the techniques we have implemented, as well as giving a detailed description of the data we have used and how it is represented. Section 3 follows with a presentation of the experiments we conducted and the results they yielded. We also discuss our findings in this section. In Sect. 4 we present a few studies which are closely related to the work we are conducting in this project. The paper is summarized in Sect. 5 by summarizing our discussion and drawing our final conclusions.

2 Data and Methods

2.1 Data Set

The bank transaction data set consists of 220619 unstructured Norwegian transaction descriptions. These are actual bank transactions from a given time interval provided to us by Sparebank1 SMN, the central Norway branch of Sparebank1. SpareBank1 is a Norwegian alliance and brand name for a group of savings banks. The alliance is organized through the holding company SpareBank1 Gruppen AS that is owned by the participating banks. In total the alliance is Norway's second largest bank and the central Norway branch is the largest bank in its region.

Table 1. Transaction entry example

Description	Sub-category	Main category
Rema 1000 Norge AG 05.01	61	44
115603 EURO SKO Dikevn. 28	84	49
Mandal Kommune . Mandal	116	103
TAIGAEN AS . 2340 Løten	74	43
GOOGLE *AbZorba Games	91	48
Til: LM Strømko Betalt: 26.06.13	73	43
XL6000003445	120	181

Table 2. Main categories and their IDs

ID	Main category name	Category name English
42	Bil og transport	Automobile and transport
43	Bolig og eiendom	Housing and real-estate
44	Dagligvarer	Groceries
45	Opplevelse og fritid	Recreation and leisure
47	Helse og velvære	Health and well being
48	Hobby og kunnskap	Hobby and knowledge
49	Klær og utstyr	Clothes and equipment
103	Annet	Other
104	Kontanter og kredittkort	Cash and credit
181	Finansielle tjenester	Financial services

Each transaction description in the data set is labeled with a corresponding category and sub-category. There is a total of 10 main categories and 63 sub-categories. The main categories are shown in Table 2. A few examples of entries in the dataset are shown in Table 1.

We have also performed a human classifier experiment where we had two people manually classify random samples of 200 transactions. They achieved an average accuracy of **93%**, which indicates that the transaction descriptions are not always sufficiently descriptive. This limits the evaluation scores we should expect the system to yield.

2.2 Bag-of-Words Model

We continue this section by introducing a few concepts essential to understanding the approaches we have implemented. The Bag-of-Words Model is used to convert the transaction descriptions to a representation better suited for machine learning. This particular technique is commonly used in natural language processing and information retrieval. In our application of the model, it is used as a tool for feature generation. When generating features for a corpus of texts, each text is represented as a multiset (bag) of the terms contained in the text. Given a corpus of texts $X = x_1, x_2$ where x_1 = 'Alan has a chair' and x_2 = 'A chair is a chair', the bag-of-words representation produced is shown in Fig. 1a. The resulting matrix has a column for each term in the corpus and a row for each text. The value is the term frequency, i.e., the number of occurrences of the term in a given text. These features may then be used as input to a predictive model such as the one in this project.

X	Alan	has	a	chair	is
x1	1	1	1	1	0
x2	0	0	2	2	1

(a) Bag-of-Words

C1	1	0	0
C2	0	1	0
C3	0	0	1

(b) One-Hot Encoding

Fig. 1. Representation examples

2.3 One-Hot Encoding

One-Hot is a sequence of bits where a single bit is 1, and the rest are 0. One-Hot Encoding is a method for representing a set of features using One-Hot bit sequences. The length of the sequence of bits is equal to the size of the set of features. The bit which represents the given feature is 1 and all others 0. Assume three categories denoted as C_1, C_2, and C_3, their One-Hot encoded representation is shown in Fig. 1b.

The feature being represented is projected onto a plane, and all the produced planes are in equal distance of each other. This categorical representation ensures that there is no ordinal relationship between the features. This makes it ideal for representing non-numerical features. We have used this technique to represent certain external data elements.

2.4 Logistic Regression

In this project, we have used the Logistic Regression algorithm implemented in the Scikit-Learn machine learning library for Python. This is a linear algorithm and estimates the probability of a class A given a feature-vector B. It does this by applying a logistic function to find the relationship between the class and the feature vector. It assumes that the distribution P(A|B), where A is the class and B is the feature-vector, is on a parametric form and then estimates it using the training data. The probability P(A|B) of B belonging to class A is given by the sigmoid function (see Eqs. 1 and 2).

P(A|B) is estimated by creating linear combinations of the features of X and multiplying them by some weight w_i and applying a function $f_i(A|B)$ on the combinations. f_i returns a value denoting the relationship between a feature of a class and a feature in a feature-vector based on the probability exceeding a certain threshold. This value is either true or false. The weight w_i denotes the importance of the feature.

$$z(A,B) = \sum_{i=1}^{N} w_i f_i(A,B) \tag{1}$$

$$P(A|B) = \frac{1}{1 + exp(-z(A,B))} \tag{2}$$

This classifier uses a discriminative algorithm which means that it can compute $P(X|Y)$ directly, without having to compute the likelihood of $P(Y|X)$ first. From Logistic Regression's discriminative properties it can be assumed that it has a small asymptotic error compared to the generative approaches. However, it requires a larger set of training data to achieve such results.

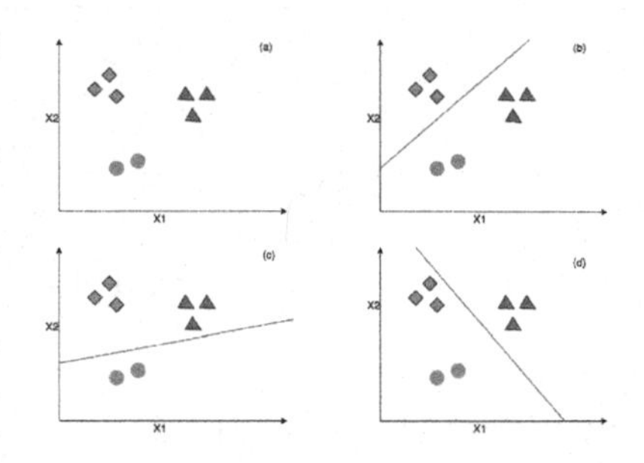

Fig. 2. Logistic Regression OvR example (a) feature-vectors | (b) classifier for diamonds | (c) classifier for circles | (d) classifier for triangles

In our implementation, we use the 'liblinear' solver provided by scikit-learn. This solver uses a coordinate descent algorithm and therefore does not learn a true multinomial model [1]. Instead, it uses a One-vs-Rest scheme, meaning that a binary classifier is trained for each class. These classifiers predict whether or not an observation belongs to the class. Then, to classify new observations, you pick the class whose classifier maximizes the probability of the observation belonging to it. In Figs. 2(a), (b) and (c), data from each individual class has been fit to their respective classifiers.

2.5 Baseline

A baseline refers to a set of techniques and configurations applied to our system intended to serve as a basis for defining change and measuring improvement. In our system, the baseline approach is a standard machine learning approach to text classification which involves using a Bag-of-Words representation and Logistic Regression. We have chosen to use this model because we believe our data to be linearly separable. Also, linear models are robust and tend to need much less hand holding than more sophisticated approaches [4]. In the research we previously conducted on this topic [7] we evaluated Naive Bayes and a Multi-Layer Perceptron. These algorithms were both outperformed by Logistic Regression and are therefore omitted in this paper.

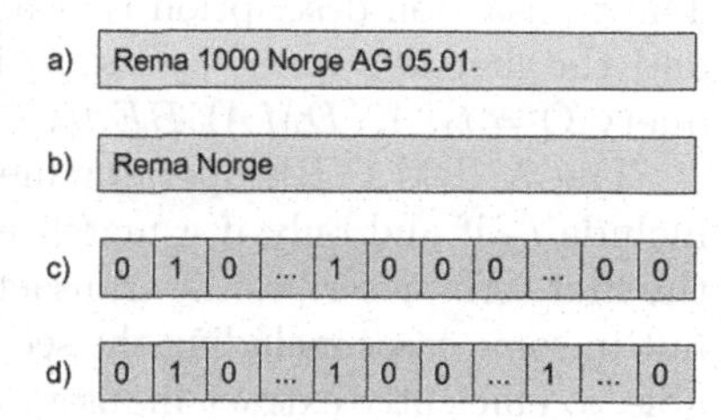

Fig. 3. Transaction representation example (a) Trans. text | (b) Trans.text cleaned | (c) Bag-of-Words w/o Brreg Code | (d) Bag-of-Words with One-Hot Brreg Code

A number of preprocessing steps are applied to the data in order to prepare it for the classification algorithm. First, the description string is cleaned to remove all punctuation, numbers, and words shorter than three letters (see Fig. 3b). The text is then converted to a vector representation using the Bag-of-Words Model (see Fig. 3c).

2.6 Brønnøysund Entity Registry

The *Brønnøysund Entity Registry* is a Norwegian governmental registry, accessible to the public, containing information about Norwegian companies. The registry includes information such as organization number, company address, business holder, and industry code. This industry code is likely to be correlated with the categories representing the transaction descriptions. Therefore it is desirable to be able to extract this industry code for every transaction and use this to extend the feature set used as input to the classification model. Seeing as the data is semantically defined, we can automate this lookup.

Trans. Description | Rema 1000 Norge AG 05.01.
Clean string
Input | Rema Norge
Use first two words as query
Query | 'Rema' ANDMAYBE 'Norge'
Send query to index
Search in registry index
Extract industry code
Output | 82.110
One-hot encode
One-hot encoded | [0,0,0,...,0,1,0,...,0,0,0]

Fig. 4. Industry code extraction example

The *Brønnøysund Entity Registry* has an API through which its data is accessible. However, seeing as our system can only make around 2–10 requests per second against a REST API, it is beneficial to download the entire registry and index it manually. In our system, the registry is indexed using Whoosh, a fast, pure Python search engine library. In order to formulate search queries which will return relevant data, it is necessary to identify which part of the transaction description contains company information and hence be used as search terms in the indexed entity registry. The transaction description is cleaned in the same way as described in Sect. 2.5 and the first two terms t_1 and t_2 in the resulting string are used to build the query $Q = t_1$ $ANDMAYBE$ t_2.

The ANDMAYBE operator means that we perform the query using t_1 and include t_2 if and only if a match is found while including it. Most of the time the first term describes the transaction well enough to make a successful lookup, but in some cases including the second term may be required. The system is now able to efficiently extract industry codes for transaction texts.

The industry code uses a representation which is not well suited as input to classification algorithms. It is a 2-part code represented as two numbers divided by a period. The first number represents the industry and the second part specifying the sub-category of said industry. These codes are therefore one-hot encoded and appended to the bag-of-words feature set produced for the baseline (see Fig. 3d). The transactions for which the system does not find a corresponding entry in the entity registry are assigned a default value of 0 (see Fig. 3c). This entire process for extracting industry codes is illustrated in Fig. 4.

2.7 Google Places API

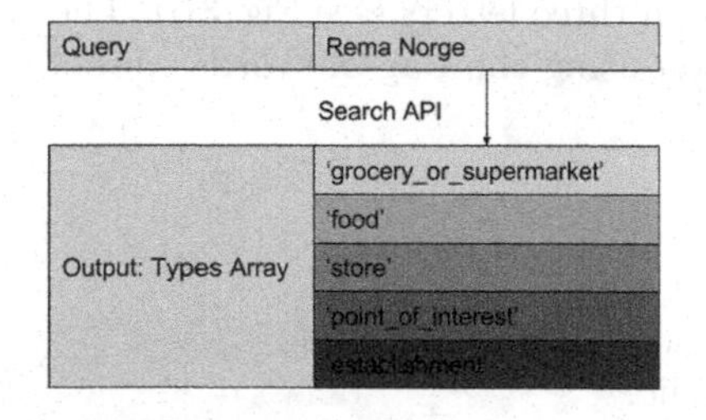

Fig. 5. Google Places API output example

The *Google Places API Web Service* is a service that returns information about places—defined within this API as establishments, geographic locations, or prominent points of interest—using HTTP requests [5]. This Web Service allows for a special type of query called Text Search Requests. This request service returns information about a set of places based on a string—for example, "pizza in New York" or "shoe stores near Ottawa" or "123 Main Street" [6]. The service responds with a list of places matching the text string, each of which contains a number of features. Among these features, there is a feature named 'types,' which is an array of feature types describing the given result.

The types in this array are ordered according to specificity, meaning that the first entry is the most descriptive. An example of a *Google Places* types array is shown in Fig. 5. These types are picked from a set of semantically defined types in the *Google Places* API. The first entry is extracted from this array and used as the type describing the transaction. There is likely to be some correlation between this type and the categories representing the transaction texts. It is therefore desirable to extract this data.

Seeing as this data is only accessible through the API and it costs a certain amount per request, it would not be financially or computationally sound to gather this information about every single transaction instance as done with the *Brønnyøsund Entity Registry*. Therefore we have chosen a different approach where we identify the subset of transactions which the classifier is not sufficiently confident about and collect *Google Places* data for these transactions only.

In order to identify this subset, the system evaluates the array of distances from the decision boundary of every class that the classifier produces for every transaction. If the distance measurement for a given class is positive, it means that the classifier predicts that the transaction belongs to this class. If it is negative, the classifier predicts it does not belong to the class. So, if there are multiple positive values in this array of distances, the classification model chooses the greatest one, but if there are none, the classification model is saying that the transaction doesn't belong to any of the classes. It is in this last case that we can conclude that the classifier is not sufficiently confident, and the *Google Places* approach is used.

Of course, we have not trained the classifier on the features gathered from the *Google Places* API so we cannot add them to the feature set to be used as input for the predictor. Therefore a direct mapping between *Google Places* type and transaction categories has been set up. Then, the system looks for a match for all of the non-confident classifications in the *Google Places* API. If there is a match, the mapping between *Google Places* Type and transaction category is used to decide the transaction's class. If there is no match, the system leaves the non-confident classification as it is.

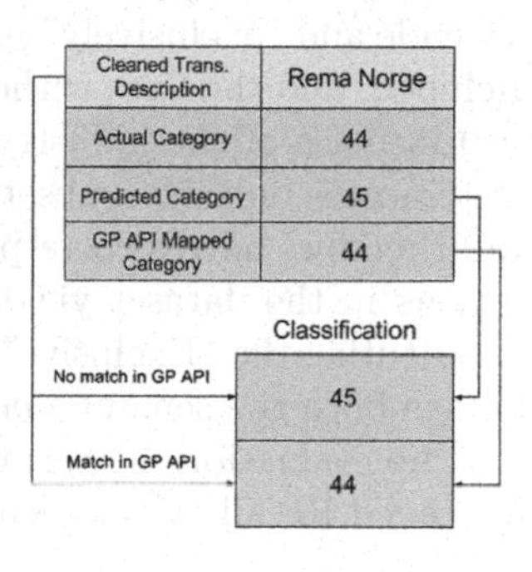

Fig. 6. Google Places API utilization example

This approach is exemplified in Fig. 6 where a transaction with the description "Rema Norge" has been classified by the model to category 45. This classification is deemed non-confident, and a lookup is therefore made in the *Google Places* API. If this lookup results in a match, the classification will be changed to the category mapped to by the GP type extracted, which in this case is 44. If the lookup doesn't result in a match, the classification uses the original prediction of category 45. The *Google Places* approach does not handle classification to sub-categories. This is because the types employed in the *Google Places* API are not sufficiently descriptive to be mapped directly to sub-categories.

3 Results and Discussion

3.1 Experiment Description

In this section, we describe the basis for which each experiment has been conducted. There is a total of 87199 distinct terms in the transaction texts. We plotted the accuracy of the baseline for Bag-of-Words sizes up to the 20,000 most frequently occurring terms as seen in Fig. 7. Here we can see that the accuracy begins to stabilize at size 4,000 making it a reasonable size to use.

For every experiment the data set is divided into a training and test set, respectively 80% and 20% of the data set. The results given are averages over 100 iterations, shuffling the training and test set each time. In the results obtained from the Baseline and *Brønnøysund Registry* approaches, we may differentiate between *Main Categories* and *Sub Categories*. This means that the target values used for training the model and performing the classifications are the main categories, of which there are 10, or the sub-categories, of which there are 63.

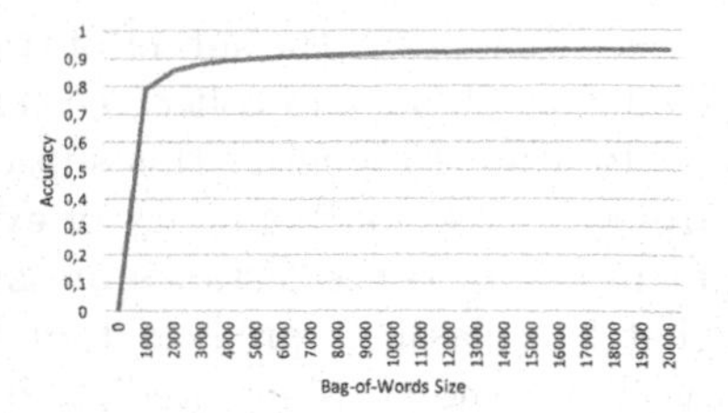

Fig. 7. Accuracy per 1000 increment in Bag-of-Words size

In the *Brønnøysund Registry* approach we differentiate between "with" industry code and "exclusively" industry code. "With" means that all transactions are included, and the ones without a match in the registry are given a dummy value of 0 in place of the industry code as shown in Fig. 3c. "Exclusively" means the system uses only the subset of transactions which have a match in the registry and therefore have a corresponding industry code. 192177 (87.13%) of the transactions in the dataset yield a match in the *Brønnøysund Entity Registry* thus constituting the "Exclusive" subset. In the "Combining Approaches" experiment we use both the semantic enrichment techniques.

The evaluation metrics used are Accuracy (Micro-Averaged Recall), Macro-Averaged Recall, Macro-Averaged Precision and F-Score [2].

3.2 Baseline

In Table 3 we observe that the performance measures (recall in particular) are affected by classifying to sub-categories rather than main categories (Table 4).

Table 3. Evaluation scores for the baseline

Target categories	Accuracy	Recall	Precision	F-Score
Main Categories	0,8922	0,8668	0,9322	0,8951
Sub Categories	0,8632	**0,7048**	0,8934	0,7707

Table 4. Percentage point improvements. Shows the improvement in evaluation scores each of the approaches made in relation to the baseline.

Approach	Accuracy	Recall	Precision	F-Score
Brønnøysund Registry	**2,79 %**	**3,25 %**	0,73 %	2,26 %
Google Places	**2,01 %**	**2,18 %**	0,47 %	1,49 %
Combination	**3,75 %**	**4,20 %**	1,04 %	2,92 %

Table 5. Baseline per class results. Shows the evaluation scores of each class.

Main category	Precision	Recall	F-Score
42	0.96	0.88	0.92
43	0.94	0.87	0.90
44	0.98	0.92	0.95
45	0.76	0.96	0.85
47	0.88	0.81	0.85
48	0.93	0.74	0.83
49	0.93	0.83	0.88
103	0.96	0.81	0.88
104	0.99	0.88	0.93
181	0.99	0.98	0.98

3.3 *Brønnøysund* Entity Registry

The intuition behind utilizing the industry codes extracted from the *Brønnøysund Entity Registry* was that they would be somewhat correlated to the target values for our transactions. This led to the hypothesis that using them to extend our feature set would lead to an increase in the accuracy of our classification model. Our results show an increase in accuracy of 4.58 and 2.79% points respectively for the exclusive and non-exclusive methods of evaluating the approach. Exclusive here referring to testing on the subset of our data for which we were able to extract industry codes.

The gap in accuracy between the exclusive and non-exclusive evaluations may have occurred for two possible reasons. The first is that the exclusive subset has a distribution of transactions which are more easily classified. The second reason could be that when using the exclusive subset, the classifier is not affected by the bias introduced by the 'dummy' value which is assigned to all transactions without a corresponding industry code.

The label distributions for the exclusive and non-exclusive transaction are approximately the same, which indicates that the baseline results should be the same in both cases. However, if we compare the per class results for the *Brønnøysund Registry* approach in Table 7 and the Baseline in Table 5, we see that the former performs better for the larger classes (43, 44, and 45). This could explain the gap in accuracy since the transactions without industry codes are not diminishing the effects of the *Brønnøysund Registry* approach in the exclusive subset. In other words, this indicates that replacing missing industry codes with a 'dummy'-value is the factor which causes this accuracy gap between the exclusive and non-exclusive transaction sets (Table 6).

The ideal situation would be to have industry codes for all transactions, but we are only able to retrieve industry codes for approximately 87% of all

Table 6. Brønnøysund Registry results. Shows the model's evaluation scores after the industry codes from the *Brønnøysund Registry* have been added to the feature set.

Target	Brreg	Accuracy	Recall	Precision	F-Score
Main Cat.	Exclusively	**0,9380**	0,9226	0,9466	0,9338
Main Cat.	With	**0,9201**	0,8993	0,9395	0,9177
Sub Cat.	Exclusively	0,9192	**0,7936**	0,8825	0,8253
Sub Cat.	With	0,8918	**0,7559**	0,8764	0,8011

Table 7. Brønnøysund Registry per class results. Shows the evaluation results of each class using the *Brønnøysund Registry* approach.

Main category	Precision	Recall	F-Score
42	0.96	0.92	0.94
43	0.93	0.93	0.93
44	0.97	0.94	0.95
45	0.87	0.97	0.92
47	0.94	0.91	0.93
48	0.93	0.80	0.86
49	0.94	0.91	0.92
103	0.93	0.84	0.88
104	0.98	0.92	0.95
181	0.98	0.99	0.99

transactions. We, therefore, decided to use the 'dummy'-values and accept the loss in contributed accuracy from the *Brønnøysund Registry* approach.

The *Brønnøysund Registry* approach adds very little overhead to the running time of the system. This is because it has been downloaded and indexed, and therefore can be queried locally. The downside to this approach is that the index is not kept up to date automatically. As we can see in both the Baseline and *Brønnøysund Registry* results, the evaluation scores fall significantly when classifying to the sub-categories. This is because the complexity of separating the data increases with the number classes.

3.4 *Google Places* API

This approach is a post-processing technique which aims to identify classifications which are believed to be incorrect and attempt to reclassify them to increase the accuracy of the system. The approach identifies 13.94% of the classifications as non-confident. These are the classifications which the system will try to reclassify by searching for a match in the *Google Places* API. Of these classification instances, we are able to find a match in the GP API for 65.6% of them, and 43.99% of these result in a correct classification. This means that as a stand-alone classifier it would achieve an accuracy score of approximately 28% (product of the number of matches and number of correct classifications), which is very poor.

If there is a match for a given transaction in the *Google Places* API, this approach can have four outcomes all of which are shown in Table 8. We refer to these outcomes as classification changes. It is desirable to maximize the False-to-Positive classification changes as these will increase accuracy, and minimize Positive-to False-classification changes as these will decrease accuracy. As we can see in Table 11, the class contributions, which are weighted normalized differences between negative and positive class changes, are positive for all classes. This means that positive classification changes outnumber the negative classification changes in all classes. If this were not the case, we could omit certain classes from the *Google Places* approach in order to increase its efficiency (Table 9).

Table 8. Possible outcomes for Google Places approach

False -> Positive	GP mapping changes incorrect prediction to correct
False -> False	GP mapping changes incorrect prediction to same or other incorrect prediction
Positive -> Positive	GP mapping leaves prediction unchanged
Positive -> False	GP mapping changes correct prediction to incorrect

Table 9. Google Places results. Shows the evaluation scores for the model after implementing the *Google Places* approach.

Accuracy	Recall	Precision	F-Score
0.9123	0.8886	0.9369	0.9100

Ultimately, the *Google Places* approach leads to a 2.01% point increase in accuracy compared to the baseline. It is, however, a time-consuming procedure as we are required to make requests to a REST API for all non-confident classifications (Table 10).

Table 10. Google Places per class results. Shows the evaluation results of each class using the *Google Places* approach.

Main category	Precision	Recall	F-Score
42	0.97	0.90	0.93
43	0.94	0.90	0.92
44	0.97	0.93	0.95
45	0.81	0.97	0.89
47	0.92	0.88	0.90
48	0.93	0.74	0.83
49	0.94	0.87	0.90
103	0.94	0.83	0.88
104	0.98	0.91	0.94
181	0.99	0.98	0.98

Table 11. Per class classification change contribution

Norm. positive class change	Norm. negative class change	Class contribution (Diff.)
3,50	0,24	3,26
4,63	0,15	4,48
0,35	0,24	0,11
3,16	0,67	2,50
6,22	0,25	6,00
0,95	0,14	0,81
4,13	0,26	3,87
0,15	0,02	0,13
0,31	0	0,31
0,27	0,03	0,24

3.5 Combining Approaches

When we combine the two approaches discussed in this paper, we would expect to reap the benefits of both approaches. This is almost the case, but there is a slight overlap between the two approaches when it comes to which transactions they improve the accuracy for. In the classes where there is no overlap, the contribution in accuracy from the two approaches separately should equal the contribution of the approaches in combination. If the combined contribution is smaller than the sum of individual contributions, then there is an overlap in the transactions they correctly classify.

If we look at Table 14 we can see the difference between combined contribution and sum of individual contributions defined as the overlap measure. If the overlap measure is 0, there is no overlap, if it is negative its magnitude determines the amount of overlap in the class. We observe that six of the ten of the classes are affected by this overlap (Tables 12 and 13).

Our combined approach yielded an accuracy of 92.97%, and seeing as our human classifier experiment resulted in an average accuracy of 93% we can argue that our data does not provide enough information for classification methods to achieve evaluation scores that are much higher than this.

Table 12. Combined approaches results. Shows the evaluation scores for the classification model when applying both the *Google Places* and the *Brønnøysund Entity Registry* approaches.

Accuracy	Recall	Precision	F-Score
0,9297	0,9088	0,9426	0,9243

Table 13. Combined approaches per class results. Shows the evaluation results of each class using a combination of the *Google* Places and *Brønnøysund Registry* approaches.

Main category	Precision	Recall	F-Score
42	0.96	0.92	0.94
43	0.93	0.93	0.93
44	0.97	0.94	0.95
45	0.87	0.97	0.92
47	0.94	0.91	0.93
48	0.93	0.80	0.86
49	0.94	0.91	0.92
103	0.93	0.84	0.88
104	0.98	0.92	0.95
181	0.98	0.99	0.99

Table 14. Per class overlap measure between approaches. The second column shows the sum of the improvements contributed by the two approaches individually. The third column shows the improvement contributed by the approaches in combination. The final column shows the overlap measure.

Main category	Sum indiv. approach	Combined approach	Overlap Measure
42	0,04	0,05	$-0,01$
43	0,06	0,08	$-0,02$
44	0,02	0,02	0
45	0,01	0,01	0
47	0,1	0,14	$-0,04$
48	0,06	0,06	0
49	0,08	0,09	$-0,01$
103	0,03	0,05	$-0,02$
104	0,04	0,06	$-0,02$
181	0,01	0,01	0

4 Related Work

A project conducted by Skeppe [3] attempts to improve on an already automatic process of classification of transactions using machine learning. No significant improvements were made using fusion of transaction information in either early or late fusion. The results do however show that bank transactions are well suited for machine learning, and that linear supervised approaches can yield acceptable scores.

In Gutiérrez et al. [8] they use an external semantic resource to supplement sentences designated for sentiment classification. The resource and methods they propose reach the level of state-of-the-art approaches.

In the study conducted by Albitar [9], classification of text is performed using a Bag-of-Words Model which is conceptualized and turned into a Bag-of-Concepts Model. This model is then enriched using related concepts extracted from external semantic resources. Two semantic enrichment strategies are employed, the first one is based on a semantic kernel method while the second one is based on a method of enriching vectors. Only the second strategy reported better results than those obtained without enrichment.

Iftene et al. [10] present a system designed to perform diversification in an image retrieval system, using semantic resources like YAGO, Wikipedia, and WordNet, in order to increase hit rates and relevance when matching text searches to image tags. Their results show an improvement in terms of relevance when there is more than one concept in the same query.

In the research conducted by Ye et al. [11] a novel feature space enriching (FSE) technique to address the problem of sparse and noisy feature space in email classification. The FSE technique employs two semantic knowledge bases to enrich the original sparse feature space. Experiments on an enterprise email dataset have shown that the FSE technique is effective for improving the email classification performance.

Poyraz et al. [12] perform an empirical analysis the effect of using Turkish Wikipedia (Vikipedi) as a semantic resource in the classification of Turkish documents. Their results demonstrate that the performance of classification algorithms can be improved by exploiting Vikipedi concepts. Additionally, they show that Vikipedi concepts have surprisingly large coverage in their datasets which mostly consist of Turkish newspaper articles.

In our research, we have combined feature enrichment using external semantic resources with the classification of real bank transactions. This is an important intersection that needs further research. We hope to have laid a foundation upon which others can continue research in the domain of classification of financial data.

5 Conclusion

Our results show that using external semantic resources to supplement the classification model provides a significant improvement to the overall accuracy of the system. The *Brønnøysund Registry* approach has proven to be the best contributor, both regarding the increase in accuracy, and the low running time as it requires minimal overhead compared to the *Google Places* approach. These approaches can be directly translated to other external semantic resources and therefore provide a robust method of extending classification models.

In order to further increase the accuracy of the system, we would propose to explore which other external resources could be used in combination with the approaches described in this project. We would also recommend exploring other representations than Bag-of-Words to see if this could have a positive impact on the accuracy of the system. A multi-label classification solution for this data could also be a potentially useful area to study.

References

1. Bishop, C.M.: Pattern Recognition and Machine Learning (Information Science and Statistics). Springer New York Inc., Secaucus (2006)
2. Van Asch, V.: Macro-and micro-averaged evaluation measures (2013). https://www.semanticscholar.org/. Accessed 23 Apr 2017
3. Skeppe, L.B.: Classifying Swedish bank transactions with early and late fusion techniques. Master thesis. KTH Royal Institute of Technology, Stockholm (2014)
4. Perlich, C.: Which is your favourite Machine Learning Algorithm? (2016). http://www.kdnuggets.com/2016/09/perlich-favorite-machine-learning-algorithm.html. Accessed 10 May 2017
5. The Google Places API Web Service. https://developers.google.com/places/web-service/intro. Accessed 15 June 2017
6. The Google Places API Text Search Requests. https://developers.google.com/places/web-service/search#TextSearchRequests. Accessed 15 June 2017
7. Vollset, E., Folkestad, E.: Automatic classification of bank transactions, Chap. 2. Master thesis. Norwegian University of Science and Technology, Trondheim (2017)
8. Gutiérrez, Y., Vázquez, S., Montoyo, A.: Sentiment classification using semantic features extracted from WordNet-based resources. In: Proceedings of the 2nd Workshop on Computational Approaches to Subjectivity and Sentiment Analysis, pp. 139–145 (2011)
9. Albitar, S., Espinasse, B., Fournier, S.: Semantic enrichments in text supervised classification: application to medical domain. In: Florida Artificial Intelligence Research Society Conference (2014)
10. Iftene, A., Baboi, A.M.: Using semantic resources in image retrieval. In: 20th International Conference on Knowledge Based and Intelligent Information and Engineering Systems, KES 2016, Vol. 96, pp. 436–445. Elsevier (2016)
11. Ye, Y., Ma, F., Rong, H., Huang, J.Z.: Improved email classification through enriched feature space. In: Li, Q., Wang, G., Feng, L. (eds.) AIM 2004. LNCS, vol. 3129, pp. 489–498. Springer, Heidelberg (2004)
12. Poyraz, M., Ganiz, M.C., Akyokus, S., Gorener, B., Kilimci, Z.H.: Exploiting Turkish wikipedia as a semantic resource for text classification. In: International Symposium on Innovations in Intelligent Systems and Applications (INISTA), pp. 1–5 (2013)

Mining Load Profile Patterns for Australian Electricity Consumers

Vanh Khuyen Nguyen[1(✉)], Wei Emma Zhang[1], Quan Z. Sheng[1], and Jason Merefield[2]

[1] Department of Computing, Macquarie University, Sydney, Australia
thi-vanh-khuyen.nguyen@students.mq.edu.au,
{w.zhang,michael.sheng}@mq.edu.au
[2] Mojo Power Company, Sydney, Australia
jmerefield@mojopower.com
https://www.mojopower.com.au

Abstract. The transformation from centralized and fossil-based electricity generation to distributed and renewable energy sources is an inevitable trend in the energy industry. One of the prime challenges in this transformation is the task of load/battery management, especially at the residential level. In solving this task, it is critical that a good strategy for analyzing and grouping residential electricity consumption patterns is in place so that further optimization strategies can be devised for different groups of consumers. Based on the real data from an Australian electricity retailer, we propose a clustering process to determine typical customer load profiles. It can be served as a standard framework for dealing with real-world unsupervised problems. In addition, some statistical techniques, including cumulative sum and calculation of the most frequent value in dataset by using *mode*, are integrated into our data preprocessing and analysis. CUSUM chart is a graphical method to clearly visualize as well as detect changes in time-series data and then using *mode* values is to replace missing values in the dataset. Furthermore, in our framework, more practical Elbow method is conducted to determine appropriated number of clusters for k-centers algorithm. We then apply multiple state-of-the-art clustering methods for time series data and benchmark their respective performance. We found that k-centers clustering techniques produces better results compared to exemplar-based methods. Additionally, choosing appropriated number of clusters for *k-means* can improve performance of clustering model. For example, *k-means++* with $k = 2$ has significantly outperformed other methods in our experiment.

Keywords: Time series clustering · Residential electricity consumption · Data mining

1 Introduction

According to Australian Energy Market Operator (AEMO), renewable energy resources, especially residential battery storage, have been significantly

G. Cong et al. (Eds.): ADMA 2017, LNAI 10604, pp. 781–793, 2017.
https://doi.org/10.1007/978-3-319-69179-4_55

increasing because of diverse driving factors such as improved technology in solar battery with affordable prices, increase in retail electricity prices, and environmental impacts [1]. Taking these opportunities, electricity retailers have attempted to build a new business model to minimize electricity costs for both industry and individual household [1]. Recently, there is significant development of micro solar management system for households, including smart meters and applications of demand-side management. Consequently, it is essential to keep track electricity consumption in order to maintain balance between demand side and supply side [1,3]. More importantly, segmenting consumer load profiles into separated groups has received more attention in research area [10]. Hino et al. also stated that determining energy consumption behaviors is useful for selecting and designing optimal tariff for different consumers groups [10].

In recent years, time-series clustering has received strong interest [8,14,23] due to its effectiveness for discovering data in many real-world applications [11], especially for clustering energy consumption patterns [10]. There are different types of clustering algorithms and some statistical techniques applied to determine typical load patterns as well as measure similarities between them [3,10,12]. For instance, the work of [12] segmented domestic electricity load profiles based on applying the most common methods included *k-means*, *k-medoid*, and Self Organizing Maps (*SOM*) whereas the study also carried out comparisons to investigate which algorithm is outperforming. On the other hand, Hino et al. proposed Gaussian mixture model for data representation before conducting hierarchical algorithm to cluster energy load profile patterns [10]. Similarly, Zakaria et al. [23] established another approach based on subsequent time-series clustering approach [11] to resolve unsupervised problems in real-world time series data.

However, most of the existing techniques focus more on technical or theoretical issues rather than practical aspect to resolve our realistic problems in real-world time series data. Yet, despite good performance of some complex algorithms, simple methods with less time consumption and cost effectiveness might be more invaluable and constructive in real applications of small business. Besides, how to combine all potential techniques going through various processes to obtain expected results for business purposes that is more challenging. Therefore, we propose a practical process to serve as a standard framework for resolving clustering problems in industries, especially for electricity industry. First of all, we utilize statistical techniques to analyze and visualize data to demonstrate the data characteristics. Based on our analysis, we found that missing or unknown values occur and they are often shown as `NaN` in the datasets or interruptions in time series chart. We then replace `NaN` with rational values by adopting *mode* method in statistics that indicates the highest frequent value in the data. After that, we can perform clustering on the user's load profiles by applying k-centroids approach. However, determining appropriated number of clusters in k-centers algorithms is typically challenging [3,22]. Therefore, we suggest to utilize a graphical and practical method, called Elbow method [5]. This technique is used by iterating *k-means* with the range of number of clusters

k from 1 to 10 and it effectively works for small range of number of clusters. Based on the Elbow chart, we can identify appropriated clusters number for our *k-means* model. In our work, we will consider original *k-means* and one of its variations (*k-means++*), and exemplar-based method (*affinity propagation*). As ground truth labels of data are often unknown in real world, Calinski-Harabaz and Silhouettes metrics are used for modeling evaluation. The more higher values of these metrics, the better quality of the clustering model.

There are significant findings in our experiment to prove that *k-means++* is outperforming compared to original *k-means* and *affinity propagation*, while the suitable selection of $k = 2$ also improves the performance of our approach. There are three main contributions in our work:

- Introducing a set of practical steps for clustering problems based on real-world dataset. It can be demonstrated as a standard framework for all steps involved in mining electricity load profile patterns.
- Suggesting more practical techniques in statistics that have been effectively applied in data preprocessing and data demonstration.
- Providing significant evidences on how different clustering approaches and methods of predefining number of clusters could impact on performance of clustering models.

The rest of the paper is organized as follows: Sect. 2 summarizes some studies related to time-series clustering problems. Then, Sect. 3 provides the fundamental theories applied in our research. In Sect. 4, we explain in more details of our experimental process as well as evaluating the application of clustering models. Finally, Sect. 5 concludes our study.

2 Related Work

Recently, the development of smart meters technology has provided the opportunity of collecting and storing consumer electricity load profiles in the form of time-series data [10]. Accordingly, there are many existing studies proposed to explore typical patterns of energy consumption of households.

One approach is to predefine typical load profiles (*TLPs*) for each group; and then cluster a specific consumer to a particular group by measuring and comparing individual consumer's load patterns with the predefined *TLPs*, namely pattern-recognition methods [9]. For instance, the research project of [9] applied FCM clustering algorithm in order to identify *TLPs* of each class and group consumers with similar load curves together. However, that approach might cause expensive costs and high time consumption due to *TLPs*-determination.

Very recently, it is claimed that subsequence time-series techniques has gained more interests in data mining area, namely *shapelets* [11]. Specifically, Zakaria et al. proposed a method based on shapelet-based time series classification to resolve unsupervised problems in real world [23]. In this study, it showed that subsequence time-series clustering technique does not only deal with unequal time series in length, but also improve accuracy of clustering results [23].

Our approach adopts similar ideas based on distances measurement to analyze the similarities between time series sequences, that has been widely used in both practice and literature, including *k-means*, *fuzzy k-means*, and hierarchical clustering [6, 10]. Those studies aim to investigate and identify consumer behaviors in using electricity and group them into similar classes. In the study of [10], they introduced the method for daily consumption data based on Gaussian Mixture Model and then applied hierarchical clustering to specify typical patterns of consumption. However, performing distance measurement method, including Euclidean or Dynamic Time Warping, might become difficult when there exists missing values or unequal time-series lengths [23]. There are some improved versions in *k-means* algorithm that has been established. For example, Wagstaff proposed improved version of *k-means* with soft constraints (KSC) to handle missing values in datasets without using any imputation techniques [21]; in addition, Mesquita added one more soft constraint into KSC to deal with imputed values [14].

3 The Methodology

The current clustering approaches has focused on improving existing clustering algorithms and then evaluating their modeling by using some common and public datasets. However, there are few studies proposed the completely clustering process to resolve the realistic problems based on real-world data collection. Our approach, which is illustrated in Fig. 1, serves as a framework for practical applications in industrial and scientific fields.

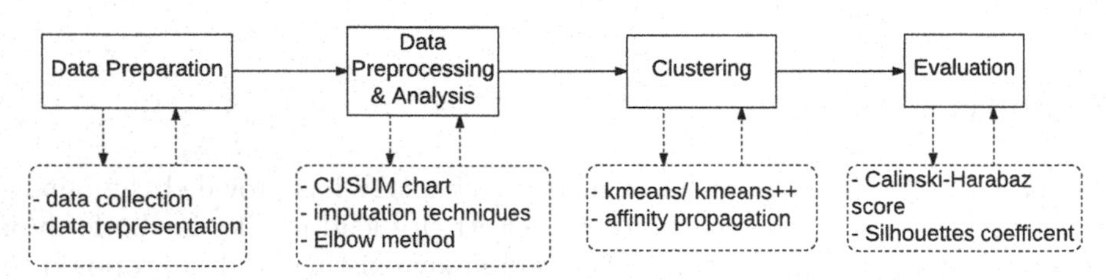

Fig. 1. The main clustering process steps

3.1 Data Preparation

In this work, we use the real data from an Australian electricity provider that contains 280 consumers records along with their total energy loads in 30-minute interval between September 2015 and October 2016. The data collection contains approximately 1% unknown values that produced automatically by some errors in system. Those values moreover are meaningless for our investigation, thereby removing them from our datasets.

Following the research of [10], we represent our data collection as a daily consumption data and then transform it to time series matrix $Q_{m \times n}$ defined as follows:

$$Q_{m \times n} = \begin{pmatrix} v_{1,1} & v_{1,2} & \cdots & v_{i,j} & \cdots & v_{1,n} \\ v_{2,1} & v_{2,2} & \cdots & v_{i,j} & \cdots & v_{2,n} \\ \vdots & \vdots & \ddots & \vdots & \ddots & \vdots \\ v_{m,1} & v_{m,2} & \cdots & v_{i,j} & \cdots & v_{m,n} \end{pmatrix}$$

where: $v_{i,j}$ is the daily consumption of a customer c_i at the time interval t_j; $i \in C$ and $j \in T$ with $C = \{c_1, c_2, \cdots, c_m\}$ is the list of account number and $T = \{t_1, t_2, \cdots, t_n\}$ is the list of time series by date, respectively.

Please note that the matrix might contain some `NaN` value as each record sequence does not often have the same length in real-world data [17]. Missing values is one of the most obstacles in data modeling since most of existing clustering algorithms do not allow any `NaN` in data inputs [21,23]. In our proposed approach, some imputation methods are applied to handle with this problem in the following sections.

3.2 Data Preprocessing and Analysis

Observing and analyzing data is an important step in order to have an overview and understanding data structure. In our clustering framework, we suggest to leverage *CUSUM* technique for detecting changes in time series data. This is one of the most popular statistical tool applied in various fields such as manufacturing process, signal anomaly detection in control system, and others [13].

Cumulative sum is defined as a sequence of partial sums of a given sequence $\{a_k\}_{k=1}^{n}$. The partial sum of the first N terms of the given sequence is defined by $S_N = \sum_{k=1}^{N} a_k$. For example, the cumulative sums of the sequence $\{a_1, a_2, a_3, ...\}$ are $\{a_1, a_1 + a_2, a_1 + a_2 + a_3, ...\}$. However, we excluded `NaN` values when implementing CUSUM chart so that we can effectively detect missing values. As seen in Fig. 2(b), it shows more clearly interruptions caused by missing values compared to time-series chart without using cumulative sum in Fig. 2(a). We then interpolated those missing values by computing the mean of the values before and after the `NaN` values. Furthermore, electricity data is consistently organized by time order; thereby using this method being more reasonable for missing values interpolation. The result is obtained as seen in Fig. 3(a).

However, another challenge in our existing data collection is unequal time series instances in length as seen in Fig. 3(a). In order to handle this issue, we proposed less costly imputation technique to replace those missing values by the values with the highest frequency in the specific time-series instances. As a result, dataset has obtained the same length (Fig. 3(b)) and that is well-prepared for our clustering models.

The next obstacle is to identify suitable number of clusters. In this case, the common Elbow method is applied to find the appropriated clusters for our model. In Fig. 4, sum of distances is significantly dropped down at k = 2 and it continues decreasing at k = 3 and k = 4. However, it is quite steady when $k > 4$. Therefore, the potential number of clusters k is the range between 2 and 4. In this work, we also discover how different k clusters chosen may affect on the quality of clustering model that will discuss further in the next section.

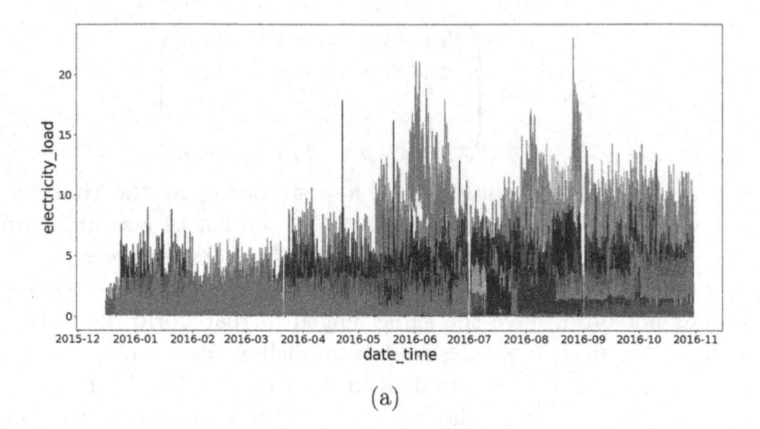

(a)

(b)

Fig. 2. Real-world data collection plotting

3.3 Clustering

In the literature, many existing or on-going developed clustering methods have been proposed in past decade [17]. In our application, we apply two different approaches, including *exemplar-based clustering* and *k-centers clustering* methods, which will be described in more detail in this section.

Clustering with K-means and K-means++. The classical *k-means* is one of the most well-known techniques in dealing with real-world clustering problems [4]. In this *k-means* approach, its simple idea is to select k clusters to minimize the total squared distance between each data point and its nearest centroids, defined by [4]:

$$\phi = \sum_{x \in X} min_{c \in C}(||x - c||)^2 \tag{1}$$

Another reason of utilizing *k-means* in this project is because of its less expensive computational cost and ease of use for our real-world problem [4].

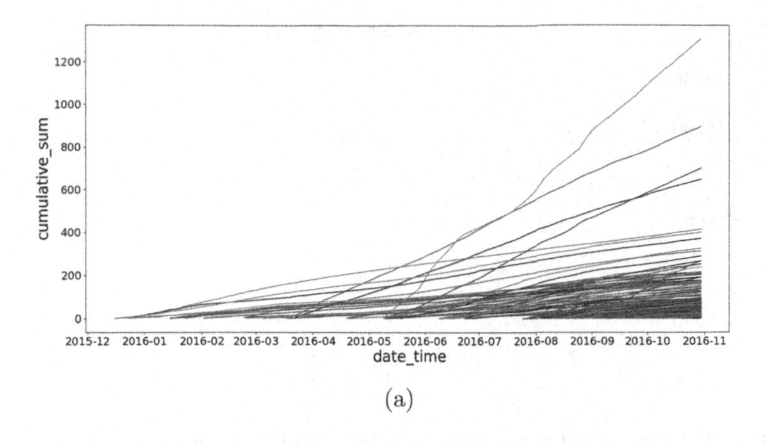

(a)

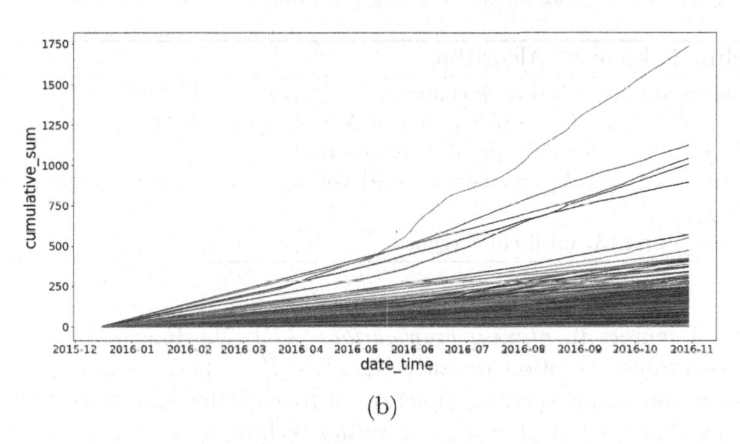

(b)

Fig. 3. CUSUM chart after interpolating missing values (a) and applying imputation technique (b)

However, the Algorithm 1 proposed by [4], we can not guarantee selected centers distributed optimally within data since those centers are chosen randomly. Furthermore, size of each cluster might not be equal in real-world data; thereby, leading to the largest clusters being dominated. Accordingly, Arthur and Vassilvitskii proposed improved version called *k-means++* in order to prevent these limitations in classical *k-means* [4]. The principal ideas of *k-means++* is to optimize the chosen centroids in k-means algorithm by calculating "D^2 weighting", given by: $P = \frac{D(x)^2}{\sum_{x \in X} D(x)^2}$. Here, $D(x)$ indicates the shortest distance from a specific data point to the nearest centroid that has been selected in prior step. Unlike random centroids selection in original *k-means*, new centroids in *k-means++* will be taken by measuring the probability P as above.

Clustering with Affinity Propagation. Unlike random initialization of centers selection in k-centers clustering techniques, all data points can be considered

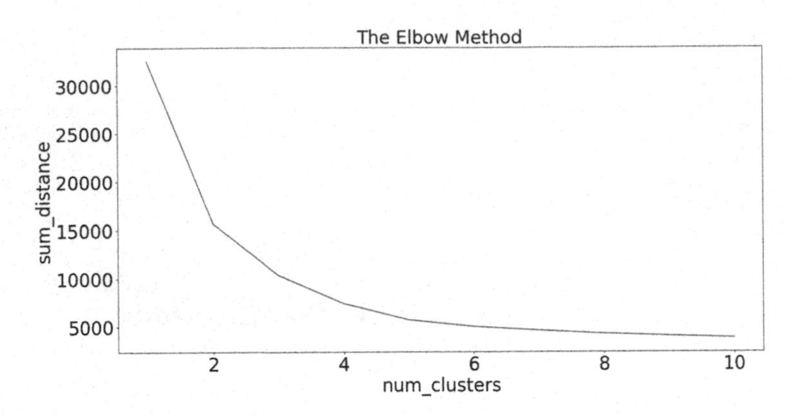

Fig. 4. Elbow chart for determining the number of clusters in *k-means*

Algorithm 1. k-means Algorithm

1: Choose randomly an initial k centers $C = \{c_1, c_2, ..., c_k\}$
2: For each $i \in \{1...k\}$, assign C_i to $x \in X$ if $D_{x \in X, c_i} < D_{x \in X, c_j}$, $\forall i \neq j$, $D_{x,c}$ is distance between data point x_i to centroid c_i
3: For each $i \in \{1...k\}$, recalculate and set new centroid for each group $c_i = \frac{1}{c_i} \sum_{x \in C_i} x$
4: Repeat (2) and (3) until convergence.

as potential centers in *affinity propagation (AP)* [7]. Hence, *AP* has received more considerable attention recently [22]. Let $X = \{x_1, x_2, ..., x_n\}$ be a set of data points and using $s(x_i, x_j)$ function is to measure similarity between two data points. The goal of *affinity propagation* technique is to minimize the negative squared distance [7] between x_i and x_j, given by:

$$s(i, j) = -||x_i - x_j||^2 \tag{2}$$

In other words, $s(i, j)$ is used to indicate how well-suited data point j can be an exemplar of data point i. An exemplar is defined as a center selected from actual data points. Then, *AP* take $s(i, i)$ as an input preference to determine how likely a particular input can be chosen as an exemplar [7].

The main process of *AP* algorithm is to exchange messages between two data points that belong to two different categories [7,22]. Firstly, the responsibility $r(i, k)$, which is accumulated evidence that indicates how well data point k should likely serve as exemplar of data point i. Secondly, the availability $a(i, k)$, which is accumulated evidence that reflects how appropriated data point i should take data point k as its exemplar.

4 Experimental Evaluations

The goal of this section is to express further details of our experimental implementation on the real-world data as well as evaluate performance of chosen clustering models. This section will first explain setting of our experiment and will then demonstrate metrics for model evaluation; finally, it will show results and comparisons between clustering models.

4.1 Experiment Setting

Recently, Python is a programming language in computer science which has been widely used in data mining and data analysis due to its clear and simple syntax. Moreover, it has gradually nominated in scientific field since a huge amount of extension libraries and packages developed for machine learning such as PyBrain [19], mlpy [2], and scikit-learn [16]. Taking advantages of scikit-learn library and pandas package[1], we effectively performed the clustering modeling to resolve our real-world problems in the electricity industry.

4.2 Evaluation Metrics

The ground truth labels in our dataset are unknown; thereby Calinski-Harabaz and Silhouettes metrics proposed to evaluate how well our models perform.

The Calinski-Harabaz score indicates how better clusters are defined by calculating ratio of within-cluster dispersion and between-cluster dispersion [18]. The higher Calinski-Harabaz score defines the better clustering model that the clusters are well separated.

Similarly, Silhouettes coefficient is conducted for dataset with unknown ground truth labels to evaluate model performance. The Silhouettes score s is simply computed [18] by $s = \frac{b-a}{max(a,b)}$, where: a is mean distance of a specific data point and other data points in same cluster, b is mean distance of a specific data point and other data points in neighboring clusters. Obviously, Silhouettes coefficient must belong to range $[-1, 1]$. When the score s is closer to 1, it means the clusters are well defined; otherwise, the clustering is incorrect. When the score s however equals to zero, it indicates that clusters might be overlapping [18].

Table 1. Clustering results of real world electricity data set.

Technique	k	Time(s)	Calinski-Harabaz(CH)	Silhouettes(S)
k-means++	$k = 4$	0.06	312.475	0.490
k-means++	$k = 3$	0.03	296.648	0.487
k-means++	$k = 2$	0.02	299.715	0.858
k-means	$k = 4$	0.07	253.400	0.356
MiniBatchKMeans	$k = 4$	0.02	250.855	0.317
Affinity propagation	*Automatic*	0.05	133.042	0.145

[1] https://pypi.python.org/pypi/pandas/.

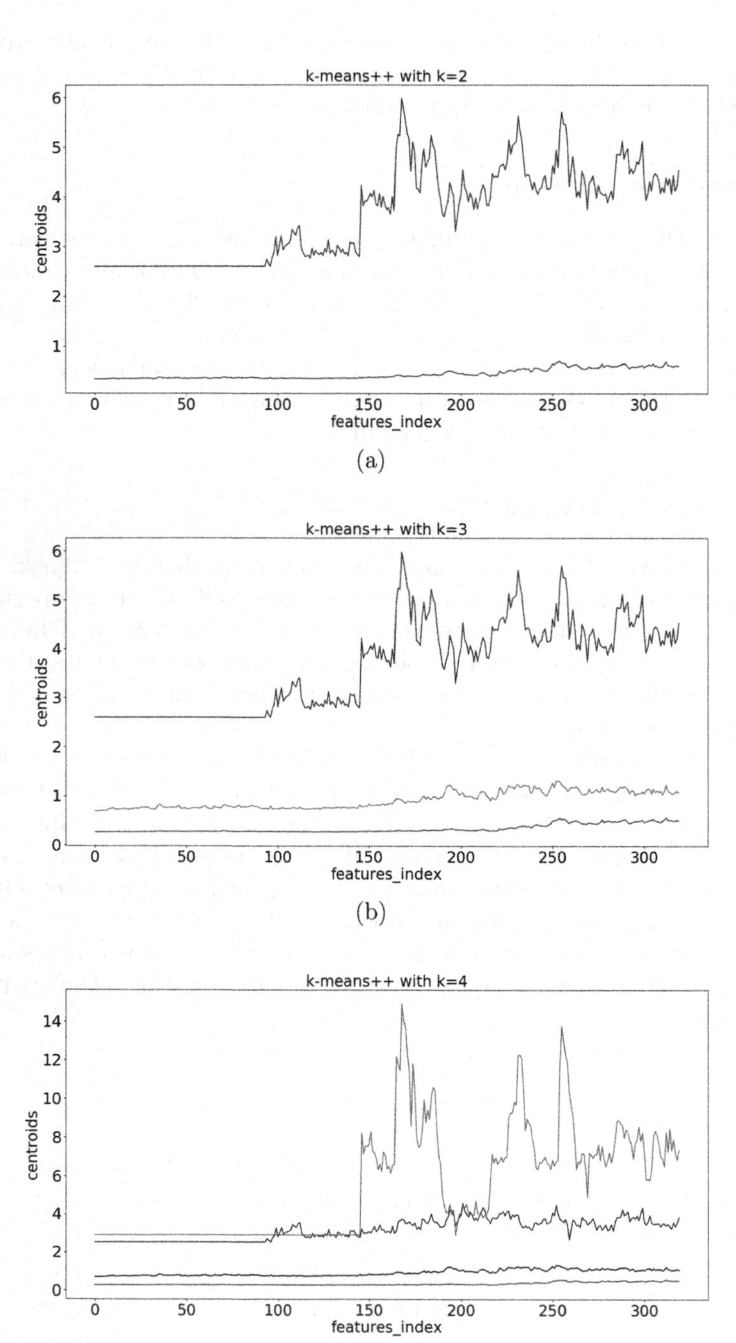

Fig. 5. Plots of *k-means++* results (Color figure online)

4.3 Results and Comparisons

In Table 1, it shows that the outperforming algorithm is *k-means++* with k = 2. In fact, its computing speed is shorter than others while the Silhouettes score is also double higher than other methods. In general, *k-means++* with $k = 2$ gains better results even though its Calinski-Harabaz score is lower approximately 13 points than *k-means++* with $k = 4$.

On the other hand, *Affinity Propagation* estimated automatically the number of clusters k shows lowest performance with lowest scores in Calinski-Harabaz and Silhouettes. The classical *k-means* by choosing random centers furthermore has lower score of Calinski-Harabaz (253.400) and Silhouettes (0.356) compared to the average scores of *k-means++* ($\bar{CH} = 302.946$ and $\bar{S} = 0.612$). In this study, we also attempt to test the computation time between *k-means++* and *Mini-batch k-means* proposed by [20]. As shown in Table 1, by choosing the same $k = 4$ for both *k-means++* and *Mini-batch k-means*, the computation time of *Mini-batch k-means* performed better than *k-means++*. However, when comparing between *k-means++* with $k = 2$ and *Mini-batch k-means*, both of them have the same computation time $t = 0.02s$ (Table 1).

Furthermore, by plotting centroids set of each cluster by time-series features, we can visibly recognize that the major difference in distance and pattern between clusters. As shown in Fig. 5, the two clusters in 5(a) are well separated with the average of centroids in the first cluster (orange line) that is double higher than another cluster (blue line). However, when choosing $k = 3$ in 5(b), the second and third clusters represented respectively by green line and blue line are very close in distance in spite of their slightly different patterns. On the other hand, 5(c) demonstrates the overlap between four clusters. It can be concluded that *k-means++* with $k = 2$ has provided outperforming results others in this study.

5 Discussion and Conclusion

The common challenge in time-series clustering problem is how to handle data with unequal length to improve the accuracy of the model [17]. Accordingly, there are many improved algorithms proposed in the literature such as *k-Shape* for shape-based clustering to replace classic clustering methods based on distance measurement [15], *k-means with soft constraint (KSC)* in [21] without requiring imputation for missing values, and *KSC-OI* algorithm proposed by [14] for the improvement of *KSC*. However, there is lack of practical proofs in these clustering algorithms.

Our current study might involve some limitations relevant to data bias due to imputation process for missing values and fill-in method for `NaN` values in data collection. However, the research project has been successfully implemented to segment consumption dataset provided by the Australian electricity retailer. The experiment has shown the significant performance of *k-means++* in time-computing cost and the quality of clustering groups compared to other methods like classical *k-means*, *Mini-batch k-means*, and *affinity propagation* for generating optimal number of clusters within itself. Furthermore, it has been proved that selecting the number of clusters k might also impact the quality of clusters. For example, applying *k-means++* with $k = 2$ obtained better results in our study. For our further research, we aim to design an appropriated algorithm to handle missing values as well as unequal time-series length based on current dataset in order to improve the accuracy of clustering model.

Acknowledgement. This study was funded by Capital Markets Cooperative Research Centre (CMCRC) (https://www.cmcrc.com) and supported for data collection by Mojo Power, Australia.

References

1. AEMO. Emerging Technologies Information Paper (2015)
2. Albanese, D., Visintainer, R., Merler, S., Riccadonna, S., Jurman, G., Furlanello, C.: mlpy: Machine Learning Python. CoRR (2012)
3. Anuar, N., Zakaria, Z.: Electricity load profile determination by using fuzzy C-means and probability neural network. Energ. Procedia **14**, 1861–1869 (2012)
4. Arthur, D., Vassilvitskii, S.: k-means++: the advantages of careful seeding (2007)
5. Bholowalia, P., Kumar, A.: EBK-means: a clustering technique based on elbow method and K-means in WSN. IJCA **105**(9), 17–24 (2014)
6. Chicco, G., Napoli, R., Piglione, F.: Comparisons among clustering techniques for electricity customer classification. IEEE Trans. Power Syst. **21**, 933–940 (2006)
7. Frey, B., Dueck, D.: Clustering by passing messages between data points. Science **315**(5814), 972–976 (2007). (Washington)
8. Fu, T.C.: A review on time series data mining. Eng. Appl. Artif. Intell. **24**(1), 164–181 (2011)
9. Gerbec, D., Gasperic, S., Smon, I., Gubina, F.: Allocation of the load profiles to consumers using probabilistic neural networks. IEEE Trans. Power Syst. **20**(2), 548–555 (2005)
10. Hino, H., Shen, H., Murata, N., Wakao, S., Hayashi, Y.: A versatile clustering method for electricity consumption pattern analysis in households. IEEE Trans. Smart Grid **4**(2), 1048–1057 (2013)
11. Hou, L., Kwok, J.T., Zurada, J.M.: Efficient learning of timeseries shapelets. In: Proceedings - 30th AAAI on Artificial Intelligence, pp. 1209–1215 (2016)
12. Mcloughlin, F., Duffy, A., Conlon, M.: A clustering approach to domestic electricity load profile characterisation using smart metering data. Appl. Energ. **141**, 190–199 (2015)
13. Mesnil, B., Petitgas, P.: Detection of changes in time-series of indicators using CUSUM control charts. Aquat. Living Res. **22**(2), 187–192 (2009)
14. Mesquita, D., Gomes, J., Rodrigues, L.: K-means for datasets with missing attributes: building soft constraints with observed and imputed values. In: 24th ESANN, pp. 27–29 (2016)
15. Paparrizos, J., Gravano, L.: k-shape. ACM SIGMOD Rec. **45**(1), 69–76 (2016)
16. Pedregosa, F., Varoquaux, G., Gramfort, A., Michel, V., Thirion, B., Grisel, O., Blondel, M., Prettenhofer, P., Weiss, R., Dubourg, V., Vanderplas, J., Passos, A., Cournapeau, D., Brucher, M., Perrot, M., Duchesnay, E.: Scikit-learn: machine learning in python. J. Mach. Learn. Res. **12**, 2825–2830 (2011)

17. Rani, S., Sikka, G., Liao, T.W.: Recent techniques of clustering of time series data: a survey. Pattern Recognit. **52**(15), 1–9 (2005)
18. Rousseeuw, P.J.: Silhouettes: a graphical aid to the interpretation and validation of cluster analysis. J. Comput. Appl. Math. **20**(C), 53–65 (1987)
19. Schaul, T., Bayer, J., Wierstra, D., Sun, Y., Felder, M., Sehnke, F., Ruckstiess, T., Schmidhuber, J.: PyBrain. J. Mach. Learn. Res. **11**, 743–746 (2010)
20. Sculley, D.: Web-scale k-means clustering. In: Proceedings - 19th WWW, p. 1177 (2010)
21. Wagstaff, K.: Clustering with missing values: no imputation required. In: Banks, D., McMorris, F.R., Arabie, P., Gaul, W. (eds.) Classification, Clustering, and Data Mining Applications. Studies in Classification, Data Analysis, and Knowledge Organisation, pp. 649–658. Springer, Heidelberg (2004)
22. Wang, C.D., Lai, J.H., Suen, C.Y., Zhu, J.Y.: Multi-exemplar affinity propagation. IEEE Trans. Pattern Anal. Mach. Intell. **35**(9), 2223–2237 (2013)
23. Zakaria, J., Mueen, A., Keogh, E.: Clustering time series using unsupervised-shapelets. In: Proceedings - IEEE ICDM, pp. 785–794 (2012)

STA: A Spatio-Temporal Thematic Analytics Framework for Urban Ground Sensing

Guizi Chen[1], Liang Yu[2], Wee Siong Ng[1(✉)], Huayu Wu[1], and Usha Nanthani Kunasegaran[3]

[1] Institute for Infocomm Research, A*STAR, Singapore, Singapore
{chengz, wsng, huwu}@i2r.a-star.edu.sg
[2] Alibaba Cloud, Hangzhou, China
liangyu.yl@alibaba-inc.com
[3] Urban Redevelopment Authority, Singapore, Singapore
Usha_NANTHANI@ura.gov.sg

Abstract. Urban planning has always involved getting feedback from various stakeholders and members of public, to inform plans and evaluation of proposals. A lot of rich information comes in textual forms, which traditionally have to be read manually. With advancements in machine learning capabilities, there is potential to tap on it to aid planners in synthesizing insights from large amount of textual feedback data more efficiently. In this paper, we developed a more general urban-centric feedback analysis framework, which encompasses the spatio-temporal thematic of ground sensing. Three essential methods: geotagging, topic modeling, and trend analysis are proposed and a prototype has been implemented. The results of experiments indicate that the proposed framework could not only accurately extract precise geospatial information, but also efficiently analyze the semantic themes based on a probabilistic topic modeling with Latent Dirichlet Allocation. Importantly, the spatial and temporal trends of detected topics indicate the effectiveness of our proposed algorithm and then benefit domain experts in their routine work and reveal many interesting insights on ground sensing matters.

Keywords: Geotagging · Topic modeling · Urban planning · Spatio-temporal analysis

1 Introduction

Singapore, a 710 km^2 island with more than 5 million people, is one of the most densely populated countries in Asia, even in the world. In order to build a high quality living environment, establishing a smart and integrated urban planning framework is one of the many important efforts by the government agencies and research communities in Singapore [1]. The development in artificial intelligence and big data analytics provides a pretty good opportunity for smart urban planning [2, 3]. In recent years, the Urban Redevelopment Authority of Singapore (URA) initiated several projects with the Institute for Infocomm Research (I2R) under Singapore's Agency for Science, Technology and Research on leveraging data analytics for better urban planning.

G. Cong et al. (Eds.): ADMA 2017, LNAI 10604, pp. 794–807, 2017.
https://doi.org/10.1007/978-3-319-69179-4_56

Urban planning has always involved getting feedback from various stakeholders and members of public, to inform plans and evaluation of proposals. A lot of rich information comes in textual forms, which traditionally have to be read manually. With advancements in machine learning capabilities, there is potential to tap on it to aid planners in synthesizing insights from large amount of textual feedback data more efficiently. Public feedback in the form of text are typically informative and helpful. However, a great deal of tedious manual work has been done to perform useful thematic analysis, such as detecting events or topics over a designated planning area or a period of time in practice [3]. Moreover, if planners need to investigate the ground sensing problem in different domains, similar efforts have to be made repeatedly. Thus, it is necessary and important to automate this process.

Driven by the business needs, the objective of this study is to develop a geo-tagging and theme modeling system, which not only infers locations of messages but also detects underlying events or topics and monitors their trends from user feedback data. The system can automate the process of learning about the ground concerns and thus improve the productivity of urban planners. For the past years, many researchers have been working on smart urban planning using artificial intelligence and data analytics techniques [2, 3, 4–6]. However, limited research has been done on mining unstructured textual user feedback data. In this paper, we design and develop a spatio-temporal thematic analytics (STA) system. Specifically, we have made the following contributions:

- Practical ground sensing solutions and the results are validated by domain experts.
- Extracting precise geospatial information by developing a geotagging tool which integrates machine learning techniques.
- Analyzing themes and providing a quick and comprehensive understanding of some of the ground concerns using a probabilistic topic modelling.
- Exploring the trend of the detected topics both spatially and temporally to analyze the changes of event or topic popularity over times at different locations.
- Using real-world urban planning data for experiments and effectiveness validation.

The rest of this paper is organized as follows. In Sect. 2, we describe the location identification and theme detection problems which we would address in this paper. The methodology for spatio-temporal thematic analytics (STA) engine is presented in details in Sect. 3. In Sect. 4, we present the implementation of STA system. The practical application and evaluation of our system on the real-life user feedback data are described in Sect. 5. After that, we review the related work in Sect. 6 and conclude this paper in Sect. 7.

2 Problem Statement

2.1 Location Identification

In fact, the analysis of the GS datasets shows that most of the textual data contain location information embedded within the feedback, *i.e.*, the issues are related to some certain geo-locations. The analytical results can be visualized clearly using a map. Figure 1 shows the planning area map in five regions in Singapore. The central region with a high population density is one of the major concerns in urban planning, and hence it is further divided into 3 sub-regions, i.e., central area, central west and central east. Thus, the urban planning subdivisions of Singapore include 7 regions. Each region can be divided into several planning areas. For example, Table 1 lists the corresponding planning areas for Central Area, Central East and Central West. By identifying locations, each textual feedback would be annotated with a location of concern. Syntactically, we need to identify all location names from the textual feedback data. It is similar to a geo-coding task, but the input is a full textual paragraph rather than pure address text. Semantically, we need to identify the most appropriate location especially when multiple locations co-occur in the data.

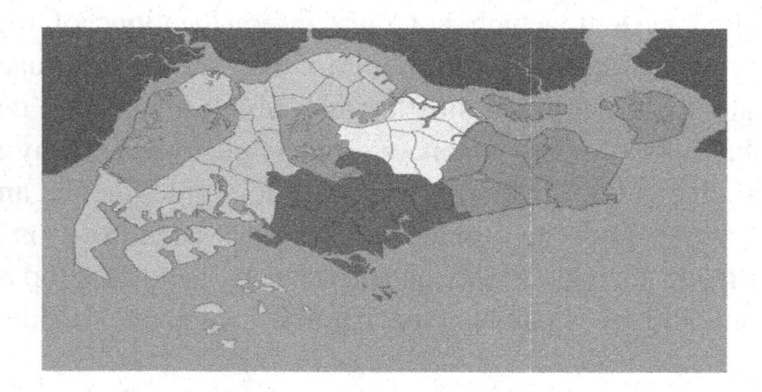

Fig. 1. Urban planning subdivisions of Singapore [7]

Table 1. Subdivisions and corresponding planning areas

Regions	Planning areas
Central Area	Orchard, Rochor, Museum, Singapore River, Downtown Core, Outram, Straits View, Marina South, Marina East
Central East	Marine Parade, Newton, Geylang, Kallang, Toa Payoh, Novena
Central West	Bishan, Bukit Timah, Queenstown, Bukit Merah, Tanglin, River Valley

2.2 Theme Detection

Considering the great amount of textual information, it would be difficult for urban planners to have a quick overview and insight into some of the rising concerns of the public. The thematic analytics module *via* probabilistic topic modeling provides an automatic way to understand and respond to public concerns timely. Combining with the detected location information above, the urban planning officers can quickly understand what the concerns are in a planned area/region, and offer the corresponding feedback in a timely manner. It will help to reduce the manual efforts needed to read through all the feedback data for gathering an overview of the key ground concerns. To achieve the objectives, a well-established topic modeling approach via Latent Dirichlet Allocation (LDA) [2] is introduced to infer a set of latent events/topics from given textual feedback data.

3 Methodology

3.1 STA Framework

In this section, an overview of the proposed spatio-temporal thematic analytics (STA) framework, including five major components in the framework, *i.e.*, data pre-processing, geo-tagging, thematic analysis, spatial analysis, and temporal analysis. Since the input data to the system are informal feedback emails, in the first step we clean the data and then extract the representative words with thematic indicator. Next, we analyze the specific geo-locations by using a Gazetteer based method followed by an information extraction method, which can discover and annotate the large archives of public feedback to explore what aspects of the key ground concerns are mentioned. As noted above, urban planners may have interests in the evolving trends of particular topics over certain time periods or locations, rather than merely focusing on detected list of topics and the feedbacks that are closely related to the topics. Therefore, we further analyze the trend of the detected particular topics over given timelines and geographic locations. The essential components will be described in details in the following section.

3.2 Geo-Tagging

Location extraction is one of the fundamental tasks of Named Entity Recognition (NER) [8] in Natural Language Processing (NLP). However, general NER method may suffer from two real issues related to user feedback data. One is that feedback data typically consists of short text or even grammatically incorrect content. The other is that many local location names are implicitly mentioned in the feedback text. In contrast, we import a number of maps shown in Table 2 as a gazetteer to look up the location names. All address names are indexed in a tree structure to speed up the searching. Since they are extracted from maps, each address name is coupled with coordinates. For those maps containing polygon and polyline shapes, such as planning area and road map, we use their internal center points as the locations.

Table 2. Imported map layers

Map name	Number of features	Granularity	Map name	Number of features	Granularity
Postal code	197214	1	Planning area	55	5
Cadastral parcel	143210	2	Map name	Number of features	Granularity
Road network	8413	3	Map name	Number of features	Granularity
Subzone	311	4			

If there is only one location extracted, we just treat it as the location for the feedback. However, in fact, there are often more than one addresses mentioned in the feedback. For example, one might complain about the noise around his office, but he may attach his residential address to the end of the feedback. To locate the appropriate location name from multiple candidates, a machine learning based method is developed in order to estimate the probability of location candidates.

3.2.1 Feature Engineering

Whether a location is predicted correctly depends on the context where it is mentioned. We model the context by the following attributes

- Surrounding words (uni-gram [5]). We use the words in the same sentence where the address is mentioned.
- Position of the address in the whole text. The position is denoted by the percentage, *i.e.,* beginning - 0% and ending - 100%.
- Layer granularity level. We use integers to denote the granularity values for each map layer. For example, postal map has higher granularity than planning area, using the central point of a planning area often introduces higher error range.
- Roles of the address words. Since all location names should be noun, we use Part-of-Speech (POS) [9] tag as an attribute and only the cases in which the address words are all noun are retained.

3.2.2 Training and Prediction

In reality, there are feedback already annotated with geo-locations by users who addressed the feedbacks, we use the feedback data as the training set and treat the known locations as the ground truth. If there are multiple locations identified from a feedback, the one near the true location is more appropriate, which are annotated 1 and others are annotated by 0

As well known, random forest is a bagging algorithm based on decision tree while it corrects for overfitting habit of decision trees. Additionally, the introduction of randomized node optimization and bootstrapping procedure leads to robust model performance in many practical applications [10]. In this paper, random forest is used as a classifier to predict the probability for location candidates.

3.3 Thematic Analysis Method

We employ a probabilistic thematic analysis method via latent Dirichlet allocation model (LDA) to infer the location-based topics/themes. LDA model is a generative probabilistic algorithm that discovers latent semantic structure of a given collection of text documents. And it assumes that each document is associated with a mixture of various underlying topics, and each word in a document is attributable to one of the

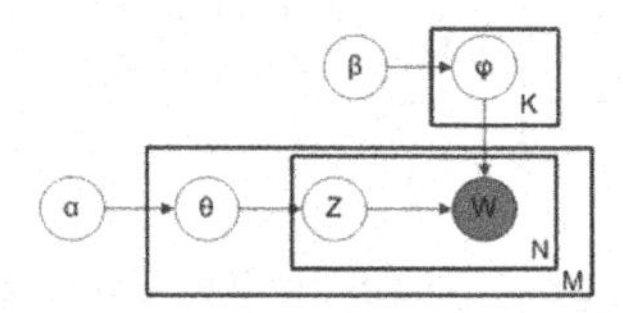

Fig. 2. Graphical representation of LDA model. The boxes refer to plates that indicate replicates. The outer plate refers to document, while the inner plate refers to the repeated selections for latent topics and words within each document.

document's topics [2]. Figure 2 show the graphical representation of LDA model, and Table 3 lists the meanings of the notations used in the model.

Table 3. Notations in LDA

Notations	Meanings	Notations	Meanings
M	Number of documents	θ_m	Topic distribution for document m
N_m	Number of words in a document m	φ_k	Word distribution for topic k
K	Number of hidden topics	z_{mn}	Topic for the nth word in document m
α	Parameter of Dirichlet prior for per-document topic distribution	w_{mn}	A specific word
β	Parameter of Dirichlet prior for per-topic word distribution		

Given a collection of text documents as training data, by using Gibbs sampling method [11], we can infer the model parameters of LDA based on the drawn samples. In particular, we can compute the per-document topic distribution θ, an $M \times K$ matrix, where each entry means the probability of the document m belonging to the topic k:

$$\vartheta_{m,k} = \frac{n_m^{(k)} + \alpha_k}{\sum_{k-1}^{K} n_m^{(k)} + \alpha_k} \tag{1}$$

where $n_m^{(k)}$ means the number of times that the words in a document m are allocated to a topic k [2, 3]. Then, we compute the per-topic word distribution φ, a $K \times V$ matrix, where each entry means the probability of clustering a word t into the topic k:

$$\varphi_{k,t} = \frac{n_k^{(t)} + \beta_t}{\sum_{t-1}^{V} n_k^{(t)} + \beta_t} \tag{2}$$

where V means the size of the vocabulary generated from the training data, and $n_k^{(t)}$ means the number of times that a term (word) in the vocabulary is allocated to a topic k across all the documents [2, 3].

4 Implementation of System

In this section, we present the implementation information of our proposed spatio-temporal thematic analytics (STA) system, as illustrated in Fig. 3.

From Fig. 3, it can be seen that the major modules of the STA systems, i.e., Input data, Content extraction, Preprocess, Geo-tagging, Thematic analysis, Result view, Visualization & Trend analysis. Each of the modules would be briefly described below.

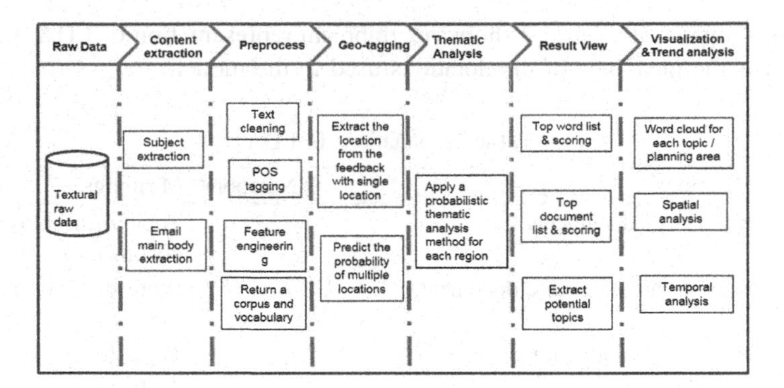

Fig. 3. Flow chart of STA system with main modules.

4.1 Email Content Extraction and Preprocessing

In the customer feedback collection system, the input data are 5596 emails from 55 planning areas of Singapore. Email is one of convenient and common means for communication *via* text, but it has many noisy words and needs to be in-depth cleaned before high quality email mining. Hence, a specially designed cascade information extraction method (CIEM) is proposed to extract the email subject and main body. The specific rule for subject extraction is that if a line begins with a pattern of "Subject:" and ends with line break, then extract the middle part of characters. For email main body extraction, the rule is that if a line begins with a pattern of "Dear sir", "Hi Officer", et al., remove these pattern characters, as well as the words ahead of them. After that, if a line begins with a pattern of "Regards", "Cheers", et al., remove these pattern characters and the words behind them. In this way, the signature, email disclaimer and confidentiality declaration can be removed and only the email main body is retained. As a consequence, the meaningful information could be extracted by combining the email subject and main body parts. Generally, only the content words that possess actual meanings, such as noun, will pose an important influence on semantics or meaning. Therefore, in the pre-process, the part-of-speech (POS) tagging technique [9] is also applied to label the cleaned email text. The meaningless words are filtered and the words with actual meaning are retained for the following process. Finally, normal text cleaning process is implemented to remove common and stop words, punctuation, numbers and non-English words.

4.2 Geo-Tagging and Thematic Analytics

We propose a meaningful list of features, and then develop a random forest classification method to identify location names from preprocessed feedback data. Section 3.2 presents the method in details. Also, we employ a probabilistic thematic analysis method via latent Dirichlet allocation to detect semantic events or themes from processed feedback data. Section 3.3 describes the detailed information. Moreover, the trends of the detected topics from the public's feedback/complain emails could be tracked over issue time and geographic locations. The demonstration form in STA system is described in details in Sect. 4.3.

4.3 User Interface

Our system provides efficient user interface for urban planners to upload data, perform analysis, view insights and save results. Fig. A in appendix shows how resident submit issues to the system. Geotagging of individual issue is shown in Fig. B, where top 3 possible locations are recommended. In Fig. C, urban planners can upload the issues and perform topic by specifying the number of topics. When the training of topic modeling is done, the top words list are shown automatically and the top documents list can be saved locally. The spatial and temporal trend analysis is illustrated in Fig. D, where the urban planners are free to choose any combination of locations and period of interests to see how the topic is changing over location or time.

5 Experimental Results

In this section, we use real-world feedback data to evaluate the major tasks in our spatio-temporal thematic analytics system.

5.1 Geo-Tagging

In the 5596 emails, 75% feedbacks have locations mentioned in the text. We extracted those which have the true location annotation to generate a training dataset, and ran a 10-fold cross validation to estimate the performance according the criteria below:

- Correct Recommendation. We use the Planning Area map (Table 2) to validate, *i.e.*, if the recommended location fall into the same planning area of the true location, it is considered correct.
- Wrong Recommendation. If the recommended location is not in the same planning area of the true location, but at least one candidate location is, it is considered wrong. We may try to improve the machine learning algorithms to reduce this percentage.
- Wrong Candidates. All candidates are not matched to the true locations. This part can be considered as "base error" which is very hard to improve.

Finally, we have achieved 78.6% for the correct recommendation, 10.7% for the wrong recommendation, and 12.4% for the wrong candidates.

5.2 Topic Detection

5.2.1 Probabilistic Topic Modeling Based Method

In this section, the topic modeling with Latent Dirichlet allocation (LDA) is applied in each region to detect the potential topics. As discussed with domain experts, the number of topics is set as 10, 8 common topics and 1 or 2 new topics, based on their domain knowledge and experience. As mentioned in Sect. 3, in the topic modeling, each document can be viewed as a mixture of various topics and each topic has a probability distribution over the vocabulary. Therefore, topic distribution per document, distribution over the vocabulary per topic and the per-document per-word topic assignment can be derived from hidden variables. Also, based on the distribution over the vocabulary per topic, we can get the top words those are assigned to every topic. Table 4 illustrates some partial results of top words, in decreasing order of the corresponding scores (as computed from Eq. (1)). As we can see, given this list of words, the potential topic is quite distinct from each other and it could be easily derived. The first entry in each column is a title suggested by domain experts from URA, *e.g.*, enquiries on sale sites, feedback on noise, sub-letting of apartment, enquiries on outdoor structure, which are issues of public's most concerned.

Table 4. Partial results of top words for the clustered topics (central west region).

Topic #1 Enquiries on Sale Sites	Topic #2 Feedback on Noise	Topic #3 Sub Letting of Apartment	Topic #4 Outdoor Structures
Ratio	Construction	Rooms	Roof
Plan	Fire	Owner	Structure
Tender	Noise	Agent	Height
Planning	Car	Condominium	Entrance
Masterplan	Activities	Apartments	Trellis
Check	Caller	Tenant	Glass
Land	Repair	Owners	Ceiling
Zone	Street	Lease	Staircase
Map	Residence	Airbnb	Door
Sale	Caveat	Occupants	Renovation

Also, from the topic modeling with LDA, we can get the top documents closely related to the topics. Partial results of top articles (index of documents for space saving) for the clustered topics are listed in Table 5, in decreasing order of the corresponding scores (as computed from Eq. (2)). Based on these documents, we could verify the above inferred topics and have a further understanding of these topics.

Table 5. Partial results of top documents for the clustered topics (central west region).

Topic #1 Enquiries on Sale Sites	Topic #2 Feedback on Noise	Topic #3 Sub Letting of Apartment	Topic #4 Outdoor Structures
Doc #1816	Doc #848	Doc #883	Doc #2303
Doc #2566	Doc #850	Doc #4970	Doc #1233
Doc #1056	Doc #945	Doc #4732	Doc #1920
Doc #3770	Doc #707	Doc #3838	Doc #1026

5.2.2 Topic Visualization

In order to have a direct and clear visualization of these inferred topics for each region, a very handy way is through a word cloud. Figure 4 provides a quick visualization for top words of 4 reprehensive topics in central west region. The size of the words in the word cloud represents the possibility of the word given the topic. We also named each topic with a title manually which help us gain an overview of the inferred topics.

From Fig. 4, we can see that, while visualizing the clustered words with a word cloud, it is clear for the major topic in the input text. For example, in Fig. 4(a), the words of "planning", "ratio", "masterplan", "building", "sales" and "development" automatically clustered together and the potential topic can be distinctly derived, which is enquiries on sale sites related. And we could summarize what the residents are talking about is sub-letting of apartment when the words of "occupants", "owner", "agent", "tenant" and so on appeared together in one cluster.

To facilitate the urban planning and management, the regions are further divided into 55 planning areas and thus the word clouds with highly frequent words are plotted based on the planning area for refining the urban event/topic. For instance, Fig. 5 shows the highly frequent words in Punggol and Changi, respectively. As we know, Punggol is one of residential eco-towns and provides a high-quality living environment. Hence, more words like HDB, outer door structure, and parking appear in Fig. 5 (a). Mention of Changi, however, the first one that probably pops into your head is the airport. Thus, in Fig. 5(b), there are a lot words about airport, aviation and dormitory/tenant. From Fig. 6, it can be seen the clear characteristics of a particular urbanized planning area.

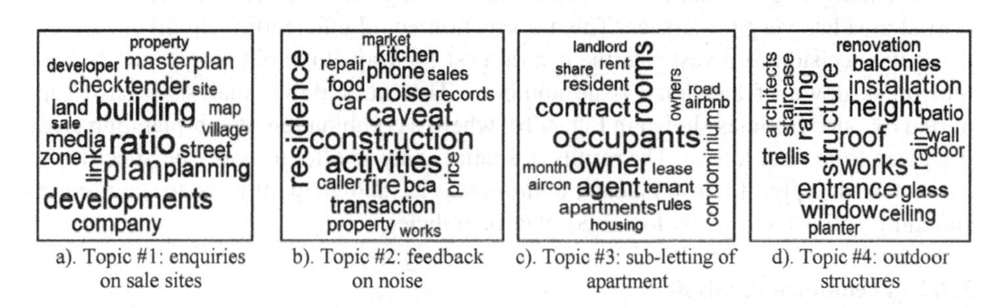

a). Topic #1: enquiries on sale sites b). Topic #2: feedback on noise c). Topic #3: sub-letting of apartment d). Topic #4: outdoor structures

Fig. 4. Thematic words with word cloud (central west)

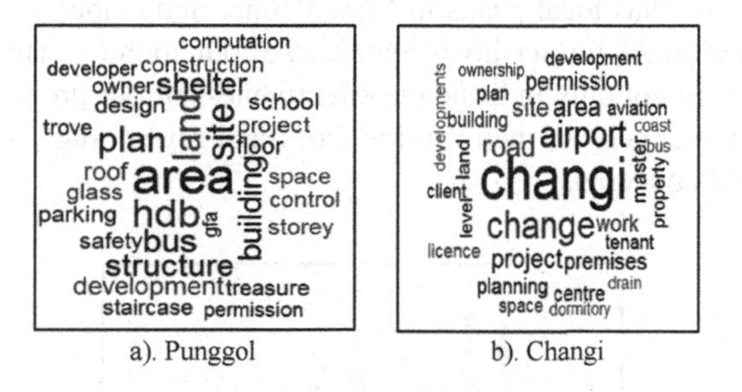

a). Punggol b). Changi

Fig. 5. Word cloud with highly frequent words in planning area.

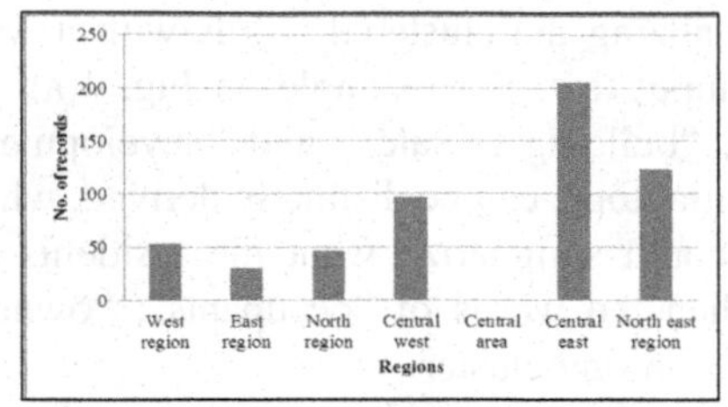

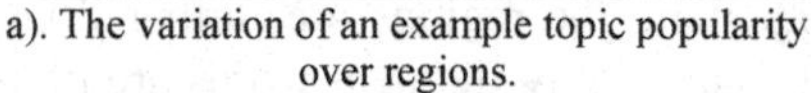
a). The variation of an example topic popularity over regions.

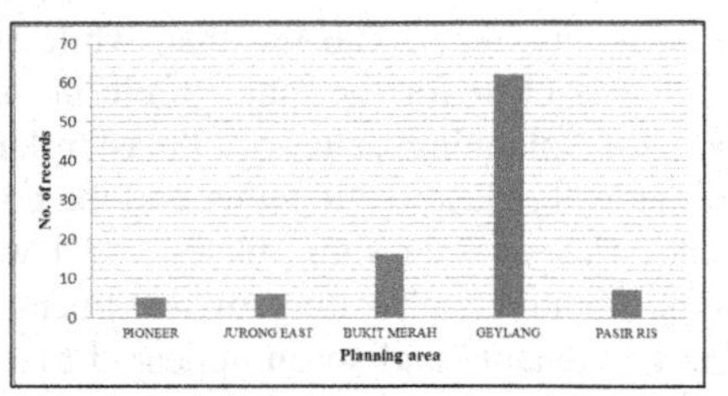

b). The variation of the example topic popularity over partial planning areas.

Fig. 6. Locational topic trend (Example topic: outdoor structures)

5.3 Trend Analysis

5.3.1 Spatial Analysis

A spatial analysis is done for displaying location-based topic popularity and thereby providing more efficient guidelines for urban policy or planning. For example, Fig. 6(a) shows the evolution of an example topic (outdoor structures) in these seven urbanized regions, indicating the central east region has the highest number of issues while the central area has very few issues. This information could efficiently help urban planner make the decision to investigate the central east for ways to avoid issues, and to look into break down of locational issue numbers. The break down analysis is also supported by our system as shown in Fig. 6(b), where a combination of sub-planning areas is chosen from west to east. The results of spatial analysis offer us wider perspective for the detected topics to understand public concerns and help officers to take corresponding actions and make localized plan or policies

5.3.2 Temporal Analysis

The detected topics are also analyzed with the issued date and the variation plot of the topic popularity is supported in our system. Figure 7 shows the temporal trend in Geylang from Jan 2015 to Dec 2015. As illustrated in Fig. 7, the topic of outdoor structures in Geylang has local peaks in March June, September and December 2015. The urban planner could further investigate these four months. These clear trends of detected topics could not only indicate the effectiveness of our proposed algorithm, but also benefit domain experts in their routine work and reveal many interesting insights on the key ground concerns.

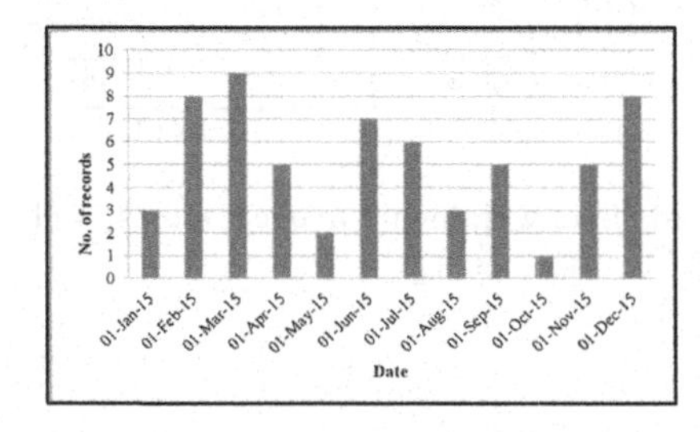

Fig. 7. Time series of detected topics. (topic: outdoor structures; planning area: Geylang)

6 Related Work

In recent years, the challenge of text-based geotagging has been receiving significant interest from research area due to the emergence of large amount of social media data such as tweets, posts and emails. Most existing studies of text-based geotagging aimed to identify the location where the text is talking about. For some social media with user profile and networks such as tweets, multi-indicator approach was proposed in Schulz et al. [12] to consolidate different user-profiled spatial indicators to identify the location of the tweet and the home location. Moreover, additional features from connections such as friends' location [6] can be incorporated to approximate the location of the text. Other than tweets, Flickr is another example of social media which is used to link photos with popular places where the photos were taken for the purpose of geotagging [13]. However, such techniques do not apply in our case because there is no user information. On the other hand, one advantage of the emails we have collected is that most of the texts contain words or phrases indicating the region. Therefore, the texts talking about the same region can be gathered to extract insights about this region. Along this direction, Quercia et al. [14] applied sentiment analysis to tweets in London to identify "well being" areas.

7 Conclusions

In addressing the requirements from urban planners on geotagging and analyzing extensive textural data on ground concerns, we propose a spatial-temporal thematic analytics (STA) framework to detect the specific locations of citizen's feedbacks and analyze the semantic themes. Importantly, a prototype implementation was tested with real data. The result shows that the geospatial information could be effectively extracted and urban planning subdivisions could be accurately geolocated. Furthermore, the topics extracted from the feedbacks have clear locational representation, and time trend with tremendous benefits to the procedure of locational and timely effective urban planning-making. With the output from our system, the urban planners can take corresponding actions more timely and make localized plans or policies based on the characteristics of the regions.

Acknowledgments. This work was partially supported by the A*STAR Science and Engineering Research Council (SERC) Grant No. 1524100032.

Appendix

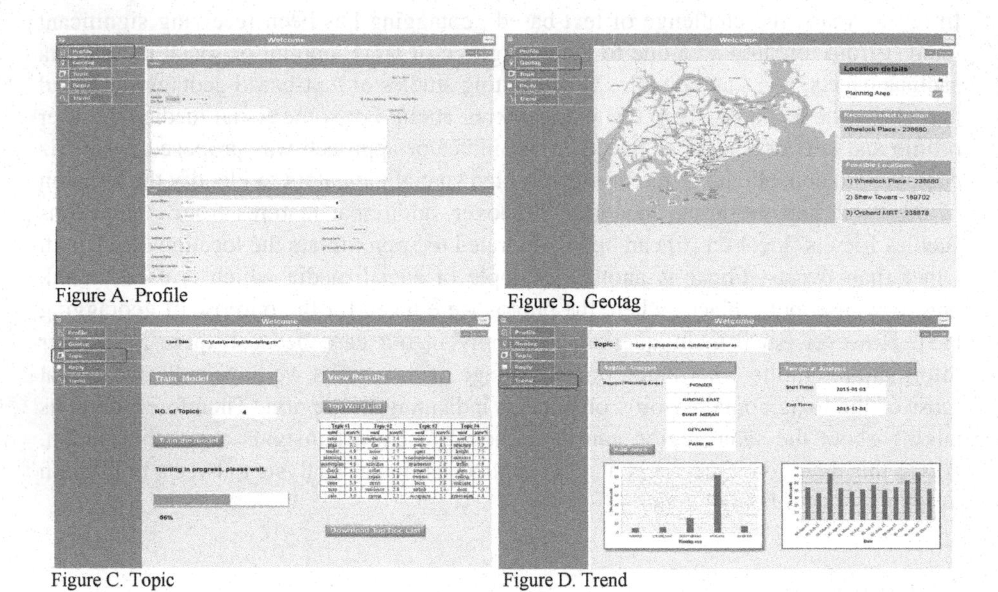

Figure A. Profile

Figure B. Geotag

Figure C. Topic

Figure D. Trend

References

1. Peter, Q.: Exploit Technology for Smart Urban Planning. Urban Redevelopment Authority, Singapore (2014)
2. Blei, D.M., Ng, A.Y., Jordan, M.I.: Latent dirichlet allocation. J. Mach. Learn. Res. **3**(Jan), 993–1022 (2003)
3. Chang, J.: Collapsed Gibbs sampling methods for topic models (2012)
4. Bolelli, L., Ertekin, Ş., Giles, C.L.: Topic and trend detection in text collections using latent dirichlet allocation. In: Boughanem, M., Berrut, C., Mothe, J., Soule-Dupuy, C. (eds.) ECIR 2009. LNCS, vol. 5478, pp. 776–780. Springer, Heidelberg (2009). doi:10.1007/978-3-642-00958-7_84
5. Broder, A.Z., Glassman, S.C., Manasse, M.S., Zweig, G.: Syntactic clustering of the web. Comput. Netw. ISDN Syst. **29**(8), 1157–1166 (1997)
6. Compton, R., Jurgens, D., Allen, D.: Geotagging one hundred million twitter accounts with total variation minimization. In: 2014 IEEE International Conference on Big Data (Big Data), pp. 393–401. IEEE (2014)
7. https://en.wikipedia.org/wiki/Regions_of_Singapore
8. Nadeau, D., Sekine, S.: A survey of named entity recognition and classification. Lingvisticae Investigationes **30**(1), 3–26 (2007)
9. Voutilainen, A.: Part-of-speech tagging. In: The Oxford Handbook of Computational Linguistics, pp. 219–232, Oxford University Press, New York (2003)
10. Liaw, A., Matthew, W.: Classification and regression by randomForest. R News **2**(3), 18–22 (2002)

11. Thijs, G., Marchal, K., Lescot, M., Rombauts, S., De Moor, B., Rouzé, P., Moreau, Y.: A Gibbs sampling method to detect overrepresented motifs in the upstream regions of coexpressed genes. J. Comput. Biol. **9**(2), 447–464 (2002)
12. Schulz, A., Hadjakos, A., Paulheim, H., Nachtwey, J., Mühlhäuser, M.: A multi-indicator approach for geolocalization of tweets. In: ICWSM (2013)
13. Crandall, D.J., Backstrom, L., Huttenlocher, D., Kleinberg, J.: Mapping the world's photos. In: Proceedings of the 18th International Conference on World Wide Web, pp. 761–770. ACM (2009)
14. Quercia, D., Ellis, J., Capra, L., Crowcroft, J.: Tracking gross community happiness from tweets. In: Proceedings of the ACM 2012 Conference on Computer Supported Cooperative Work, pp. 965–968. ACM (2012)

Privacy and Utility Preservation for Location Data Using Stay Region Analysis

Manoranjan Dash and Sin G. Teo(✉)

Institute for Infocomm Research, Singapore, Singapore
{dashm,teosg}@i2r.a-star.edu.sg

Abstract. Location data is very useful for providing location-based services to its users. But the problem in releasing this type of data is that sensitive and private information about users may be leaked. In [11] it is stated that even four spatio-temporal points are enough to uniquely identify 95% of the individuals. There are different approaches for privacy preservation of spatio-temporal data. But in most of these approaches, the utility is severely curtailed in order to ensure risk-free release of data. Our method made a few innovations to retain more utility while not compromising privacy. First of all, for each user we extracted stay regions which are places where a user spends significant amount of time. Then we extracted trajectories or trips between these stay regions. Now the whole data of very big trajectories is converted to trips where each trip has start and end times, and start and end lat-lons. We used these four dimensions in a round robin manner to k-anonymize each trip. We proposed two measures for estimating risk and utility. A nice feature of our method is visualization of k-anonymized trips which can give much better information about mass mobility within a city or area.

Keywords: Spatio-temporal data · Privacy-preserving · Utility · k-anonymization

1 Introduction

Location data is very useful for providing location-based services (LBS) to its users. Examples of such services include finding a place of interest given the current location of a user, guiding the user for a more efficient transportation including avoiding traffic jams. But the problem in releasing this type of data is that sensitive and private information about users may be leaked. For example, let us consider that there is a user whose trajectory is very unique. In [11] it is stated that even four spatio-temporal points is enough to uniquely identify 95% of the individuals. The released data may be used unscrupulously to know sensitive information. This is against the principle of privacy preservation. Compared to other types of data which are non-correlated, spatio-temporal data is correlated, i.e., each point of a trajectory is correlated to all other points by time and by location. This makes spatio-temporal data harder to preserve privacy.

G. Cong et al. (Eds.): ADMA 2017, LNAI 10604, pp. 808–820, 2017.
https://doi.org/10.1007/978-3-319-69179-4_57

In a typical mobile data, used for LBS, each record has an anonymized userID, a timestamp, and a lat-lon. So, any algorithm that can protect the privacy information of this data will be applicable for many LBS.

There are different approaches for privacy preservation of spatio-temporal data. In [2] authors first of all converted the spatio-temporal data to count data where, for each given lat-lon and for a given time interval, it simply counts the number of users present. Then they show, using differential privacy, how to preserve privacy for such count data. Several other methods in the literature are also based on this type of count data. We observed that such count information removes patterns of trajectories. By 'patterns of trajectories' we mean common spatio-temporal patterns found in multiple trajectories. Although these methods do not compromise privacy, they drastically reduce the utility of the data in extracting important trajectory patterns. In this paper we propose a method that can retain trajectory patterns while not compromising privacy.

First of all, we extract short yet meaningful trajectories for each user. Next, we apply k-anonymization over these trajectories to determine k-anonymized clusters of trajectories. We represent these clusters by representative trajectories which are privacy preserved and can be published. Our specific contributions include:

- Converting extremely long trajectories to short yet meaningful trajectories using stay region analysis.
- A unique framework for k-anonymizing the trajectories.
- Finally, representing each k-anonymized cluster by a representative using Markov model.

The rest of the paper is organized as follows. In the next section we discuss related work. Methodology is presented in Sect. 3. Section 4 describes the performance evaluation. The paper ends in Sect. 5.

2 Related Work

Many existing privacy-preserving techniques [8–10,13,15–17] have been proposed to anonymize microdata presented in statistical and tabular form by limiting their disclosure, e.g., k-anonymity [8,13,15,16] ensures quasi-identifiers of a record must be indistinguishable with at least other k-1 records in the dataset (i.e., at least k records in each equivalent class). However, k-anonymity can not guarantee above if all of the records in the class have less than k values for any sensitive attribute. The limitation of k-anonymity is addressed by ℓ-diversity [10,17]. It ensures that each equivalent class of the k-anonymity has at least ℓ values for the sensitive attributes. To further give protection of data privacy in ℓ-diversity, t-closeness [9] has been proposed to ensure that each equivalent class of the ℓ-diversity that has t-closeness, which is a value less than a user-defined threshold. t-closeness is measured by the distance between two distributions, i.e., the sensitive attribute distribution in the class and the non-sensitive attribute distribution in the dataset. The survey of above the techniques can be found in [3]. However, the techniques are not applicable in protecting privacy of spatio-temporal data.

Some of the important existing privacy preserving methods for LBS are as follows. In [5,7] authors proposed a method that fakes database results to a user's query. But the result is related to the query location. Ghinita et al. [4,6] used a space transforming method to convert the data and query but preserving their inter-relationship. In [18], instead of faking database results, it fakes the query location. The database server would continue to send resultant location until the user is satisfied.

Another set of methods use k-anonymity to achieve privacy while attempting to preserve utility. In [1], authors try to anonymize the spatio-temporal trajectories which are single trips made by vehicles. These trajectories are quite short in length. But in location data sets such as CDR (Call Detail Records) trajectories are very long. It is not possible to anonymize these trajectories using the existing methods.

In some existing methods, authors anonymize trajectories by first converting the spatio-temporal data to count data [2]. Number of users is partitioned by their spatio-temporal whereabouts. These spatio-temporal whereabouts are based on cell tower lat-lons. We argue that, by doing this, significant amount of utility is lost. Particularly, it loses information about the sequence of cell towers visited by a user, thus it loses the flow of mobility.

Our proposed method also uses k-anonymization. But, unlike the existing k-anonymization methods that experience heavy loss of utility, we argue that our proposed method is able to preserve utility much better while not compromising the privacy of the users.

3 Privacy-Preserving Spatio-Temporal Data

The general problem we try to solve is how to preserve spatio-temporal privacy of users. In particular we propose a novel algorithm to preserve anonymity of users in order to publish spatio-temporal data. Data consists of users' call detail records (CDR) where each record has $< id >< timestamp >< lat - lon >$ among possibly other information. Here $< lat - lon >$ is the location of a cell tower that renders required service. $< Timestamp >$ is the time when an event (a phone/sms call/receive) takes place. Our privacy-preserving spatio-temporal algorithm is composed of a few steps as depicted in Fig. 1. We skip to discuss

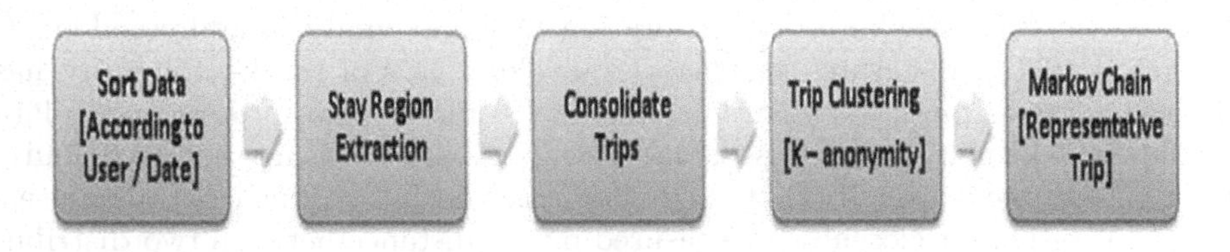

Fig. 1. Algorithm overview

the two steps of Fig. 1, sorting data based on user and date, and consolidating trips after the stay region extraction, which they are straightforward steps. This section is structured as follows: first, we show how to convert each user's CDR data to spatio-temporal trajectories; second, we describe our proposed method to k-anonymize the trajectories with the goal of publishing the resultant data; and finally, we show how to evaluate the outcome.

3.1 Convert CDR to Trajectories

It is not possible to treat the entire trajectory over several months or weeks or even days as one trajectory. We break each trajectory into days. This has an advantage. Typically a user repeats her trajectories over a week. So, by grouping these trajectories into each day of a week, or just weekdays and weekends, we can retain the important patterns. Examples of such patterns include going from home to office and returning from office to home on weekdays, whereas going to shopping mall and other places (except office) on weekends. Next, we observed that even a day is too long to preserve privacy [11]. It becomes very unique leading to difficulties in satisfying k-anonymization conditions.

Stay Regions and Trips. Note that in a single day a user makes one or more *trips*. A trip is between any two *stay regions*. A stay region is a place where the user spends significant amount of time, or in other words, it is not a transit place. Each stay region is expressed as a lat-lon. Examples are home, work place, friend's place, shopping mall, gym, etc. Some stay regions are visited regularly on a daily basis whereas others are visited sporadically or just once.

j^{th} stay region of a user u_i is denoted as r^i_j. It is defined by a spatial and another temporal thresholds. Spatial threshold $SpaThresh$ helps to cluster the cell towers in close proximity of each other. Temporal threshold $TimeThresh$ discriminates events within a stay region from those on transit. Both the two above thresholds are user-defined values in the proposed algorithm. $r^i_j.LatLon$ denotes the center point of a stay region. Any cell tower within a distance of $SpaThresh$ from $r^i_j.LatLon$ belongs to the stay region. A user spends at least $TimeThresh$ amount of time in a stay region. Figure 2 (scenario 1) depicts stay regions pictorially. A, B, C and D are cell towers. Towers A and D satisfy both thresholds whereas B and C do not. Circles around A and D represent the stay regions. Note that a stay region can have more than one cell tower.

The task of extracting stay regions (Algorithm 1) can be stated as follows: Given mobile phone records d^i_h, $h = 1 \dots n^i$ for a user u_i, extract all stay regions r^i_j such that both thresholds are met. As a pre-processing step all records for a user are sorted according to their timestamps. Note that consecutive records of a user with the same cell tower are replaced by their first and last records.

ED method computes Euclidean distance between the new record and the current centroid. *Centroid* method employs a weighted average technique to compute the new centroid of a stay region. For example, if three cell towers are already included in a stay region, to include a fourth cell tower, *Centroid*

Algorithm 1. Algorithm for Extracting Stay Regions

```
1: procedure ExtractStayRegions(LocationData)
2:   for each user u_i, i = 1...n do
3:     j = 1; h = 1;
4:     while not EOF for user u_i do
5:       Get record d^i_h;
6:       distance = 0; time = 0;
7:       r^i_j.LatLon = d^i_h.LatLon
8:       r^i_j.StartTime = d^i_h.TimeStamp
9:       h++;
10:      distance = ED(d^i_h.LatLon, r^i_j.LatLon);
11:      while distance < SpaThresh do
12:        r^i_j.LatLon = Centroid(r^i_j, d^i_h);
13:        time += d^i_h.timestamp − r^i_j.StartTime;
14:        h++;
15:        Get record d^i_h;
16:        distance = ED(d^i_h.LatLon, r^i_j.LatLon);
17:      if time > timeThresh then
18:        Store r^i_j as a stay region;
19:        j++;
```

method assigns a weight of 3 to the current centroid $r^i_j.LatLon$ and a weight of 1 to the fourth cell tower lat-lon ($d^i_h.LatLon$). After extracting stay regions for a user, extract trips which are nothing but trajectories between stay regions. These trips or trajectories are stored for further processing (the consolidating steps as depicted in Fig. 1).

Time Complexity of Algorithm 1. User trajectory u_i (for $i = 1 \ldots n$) is processed by the algorithm, where n is the number of the users. The algorithm finds stay region of the user trajectory u_i based on the distance threshold, *SpaThresh* and the time threshold, *timeThresh*. The distance and time difference between two locations in the stay region is less than the distance threshold, *SpaThresh*, and greater than the time threshold, *timeThresh*, respectively. Let m be the number of iterations needed in finding both of the distance and time thresholds of two locations to satisfying the above requirement. Therefore, the time complexity of Algorithm 1 is $O(n^2m)$.

3.2 k-Anonymization

Our goal in this project is to release the trips of users after ensuring that privacy is preserved. We extend the classical concept of k-anonymity [12] to deal with this particular form of data. We approach the k-anonymization problem from two angles.

1. Generalize using the pre-defined hierarchies of distance and time.

   Our goal is to generalize each trip so that it will be indistinguishable from $k-1$ other trips at least. A trip has information about locations (source and

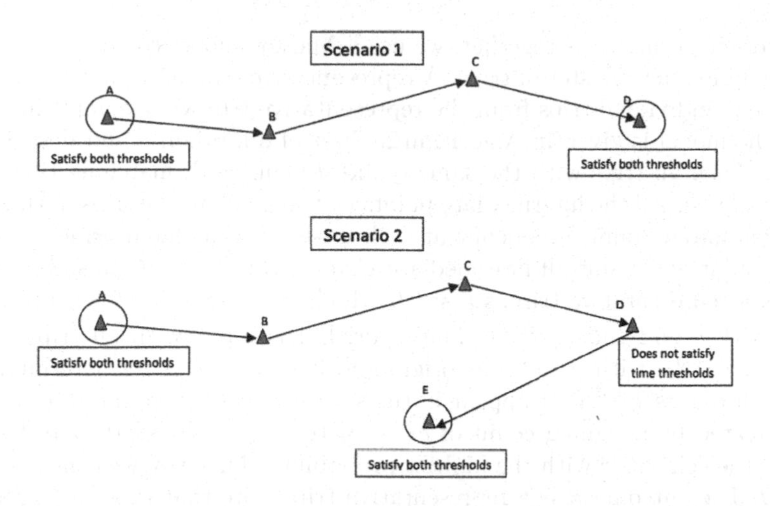

Fig. 2. Two scenarios of stay regions

destination) and time (start and end). We use two hierarchies, a temporal and another spatial, to generalize the trips. Temporal hierarchy is based on intervals. If the start time of a user's trip is 8 am (Monday), we can begin with an interval of 1 h, i.e., 7:30–8:30 am (Monday). All trips of all users that fall in this interval are grouped together. Similarly, we group the trips by their end times. Spatial hierarchy is based on increasing radius and/or specific geographical regions. If the source of a user's trip is in a given lat-lon, group all trips that have source lat-lon within the radius. Radius can start with 500 m, then 1 km, and so on. Hierarchies based on regions can start with subzones (there are 322 subzones in Singapore), then planning areas (there are 55 planning areas) and finally regions (there are five regions in Singapore). The four dimensions, i.e., start and end times, and start and end lat-lons, are selected in a round-robin manner to find at least $k-1$ number of trips. As soon as we achieve at least $k-1$ trips, the k-anonymization stops.

2. Generalize until exactly $k-1$ other trips are found.

   In the previous approach many times there may be significantly large number of trips in a single k-anonymized trips cluster. We start with the next available trip as origin. In order to stop exactly at $k-1$, we sort the trips by their time (start and end) and distance (start and end) from the origin. We use the round-robin approach here as well. We start with source lat-lon. After including the trip with the closest distance between its source lat-lon and lat-lon of the origin, we select the trip with the closest start time. Then we select the trip with the closest destination distance, and finally we select the trip with the closest end time. After selecting a trip, we remove it from the list of available trips. We continue in a round robin fashion until $k-1$ trips are selected.

After clustering trips together, we use a Markov model to create a representative trip for each cluster of trips. A representative trip helps in calculating the distance of individual trips from the representative trip while computing distortion. The model is given in Algorithm 2. First of all, origin o and destination d are set. Then all trips with the same o and d along with matching timestamps are considered. All the intermediate points (lat-lons) of all the trips in the cluster are taken into account. Frequency at each lat-lon is calculated using a radius of 500m, i.e., it will count all intermediate visits within 500 m radius. Algorithm 2 returns a representative trip as a set R which is a sequence of cell towers that starts with o and ends with d. The algorithm is input with all trips ($p_k^{(i,o,d)}$, $k = 1 \ldots n^{(i,o,d)}$) with o and d as origin and destination. After determining the set of cell towers $T^{o/d}$ that appear in the set of trips $P^{o/d}$ from o to d, a matrix M is created by assigning count of $c_1 \rightarrow c_2$ to M_{c_1,c_2}. We start at o. Using M we find the cell tower with the highest probability. This way we continue till we reach d. The outcome R is a representative trip. Note that these representative trips can be publicly released because they have preserved the privacy of users. See Fig. 3. The trips are in green color whereas the single representative trip is in red color.

Algorithm 2. Markov Chain Model to determine representative trip

1: **procedure** RepTrip($p_k^{(i,o,d)}$, $k = 1 \ldots n^{(i,o,d)}$)
2: Let R be the representative trip
3: $R = \Phi$; $R = R \cap \{o\}$
4: Set of trips $P^{o/d} = \{p_k^{(i,o,d)}\}$
5: Determine $T^{o/d}$, set of towers in all trips $p \in P^{o/d}$
6: Let $T' = \{o, T^{o/d}, d\}$
7: Create a matrix M of size $T'XT'$
8: Populate M: M_{c_1,c_2} = Count of $c_1 -> c_2$ in $P^{o/d}$
9: Start with $c_1 = o$;
10: $c_2 = argmax_{c2} M_{c_1,c_2}$; $R \cap \{c_2\}$
11: Go to Step 10 with $c_1 = c_2$ until $c_2 = d$
12: Return $R \cap \{d\}$

Time Complexity of Algorithm 2. The time complexity of creating representative trips using Markov chain model is $O(n)$.

Our overall proposed privacy-preserving spatio-temporal algorithm is given in Algorithm 3. At the end of the algorithm, the representative trips are based on Markov chain model are published while preserving spatio-temporal privacy of the users.

3.3 Measures for Evaluation

We introduce two measures, discernibility and distortion, to have a rough estimate of risk and utility. These measures are described in [1] in different contexts.

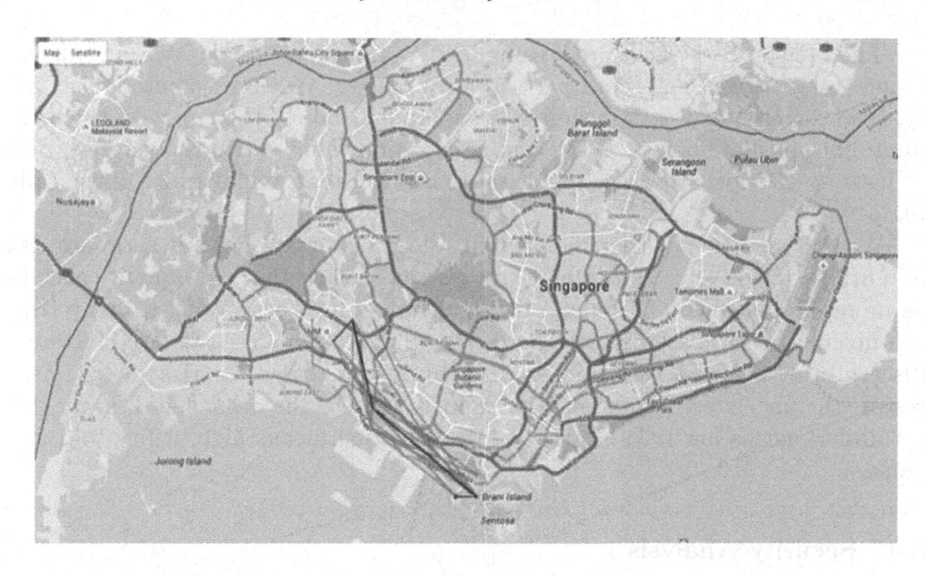

Fig. 3. Representative trip using Markov model (Color figure online)

Algorithm 3. Algorithm for privacy preservation of location data

1: **for** each user u_i, $i = 1 \ldots n$ **do**
2: $\quad R_i = ExtractStayRegions(u_i)$
3: $\quad T_i = ExtractTrips(u_i, R_i)$
4: Collate trips of all users into one set of trips T
5: $cluCnt = 0$
6: markTrips[] = False // initially no trip is clustered
7: **while** $notEmpty(T)$ **do**
8: $\quad t = first(T)$
9: $\quad clust[cluCnt] = kanonTrips(t, T, markTrips)$
10: $\quad reprTrip[cluCnt] = RepTrip(clust[cluCnt])$

We apply them to our methodology. Given a clustering $P = \{p_1, \ldots, p_n\}$ of D, where p_n represents the trash bin, the discernibility metric is defined as:

$$DM(D) = \sum_{i=1}^{n-1} \|{p_i}^2\| + \|p_n\|\|D\|, \tag{1}$$

where $\|D\|$ is data size, which in this case is the number of trips.

Another measurement, Information distortion (ID) is calculated as follows.

$$ID(D, D') = \sum_{t \in D} ID(t, t') \tag{2}$$

$$ID(t, t') = \left\{ \begin{array}{rl} DTWdist(t, t') & \text{if } t \text{ is in a cluster} \\ \Omega & \text{otherwise} \end{array} \right\}, \tag{3}$$

where distance between two trajectories (trips).

Their distance is measured using DTW (Dynamic Time Warping) technique [14]. t' is the representative trip for a cluster. We experimented with two types of representatives: (a) using Markov model, and (b) the trip with the maximum intermediate points. DTW dist is used only when a trip is clustered with, at least, $k-1$ trips, otherwise the distance is a constant weight which is typically high.

We will analyze whether discernibility and distortion help us estimate risk and utility. Intuitively, discernibility represents the fact that data quality shrinks as more data elements become indistinguishable. In other words, if many trips are not clustered, discernibility increases, whereas if many trips are clustered, discernibility decreases. So, higher discerniblity increases the risk factor. As a result, the unclustered trips may be suppressed. On the other hand, lower discernibility means low risk. Similarly, low distortion means high utility, and vice versa.

3.4 Security Analysis

Should we include the anonymized userid in the publicized or released data? Considering our design, it is possible to include anonymized userid. We can include the anonymized userids followed by information about the start and end and the common representative trip for an entire cluster. But, by doing so, there is a possibility that privacy is leaked. A single anonymized userid may appear in different clusters of trips. Although each cluster of trips is k-anonymized, by combining several clusters that a user participates in, it is possible to uniquely identify the trajectories of a single user. That user may be the only one present in the combination of clusters. This may lead to compromising the user's privacy. So, in our approach we do not release the anonymized userid.

4 Performance Evaluation and Discussions

4.1 Data

We use the location data provided by DataSpark (Singapore) published on the occasion of the 'IDA Personal Data Protection Challenge' held in 2016. There are 192,690 number of records where each record is of format (date-time, anonymized-id, lat, lon). These are location data of more than 900 people over a period of 15 days (1–15, September, 2015). Temporal resolution varies with maximum frequency of one record per 15 min. Spatial resolution is fixed to two decimal places of latitude and longitude coordinates. Data is not ordered.

We ran the Algorithm 3 over the data. Stay regions are extracted for each person, and using these stay regions trips are extracted. These trips are input to the k-anonymization function. In the following sections we show some of these results both pictorially and using figurative results.

4.2 Stay Regions

In the experiment, we used one hour time threshold (i.e., *TimeThresh*) and one km as distance threshold (i.e., *SpaThresh*), as given in Algorithm 1. For simplicity, we show the top five (i.e., most frequent) stay regions extracted for a person in Fig. 4. Darker color indicates higher frequency. The two most frequent stay regions are most probably home and office of the person.

4.3 Behavior of Discernibility and Distortion

As part of k-anonymization we varied k as 5, 10, 15, and 20. For each k we measured discernibility and distortion. Table 1 shows the results. Some observations are as follows. Number of valid clusters reduces as k increases. Here 'valid' means a cluster has at least k number of trips. Discernibility increases with k. When k increases, it becomes more difficult to satisfy and form a cluster. Thus, as k increases, size of the suppressed set (trips that could not be clustered) increases. According to Eq. 1, trash bin p_n is the suppressed set. Out of the two terms in the right hand side, $|p_n| * |D|$ contributes significantly more than the other term. Thus, as suppressed set size increases, so also discernibility.

Distortion increases with k for both types of representatives of clusters (representative trip using Markov model and the trip with the maximum number of intermediate points as the representative trip). As k increases, there are fewer clusters. This most probably increased the distance of each trip from the corresponding representative trip. Note that distortion is less for Markov model than for maximum intermediate points indicating the superiority of Markov model

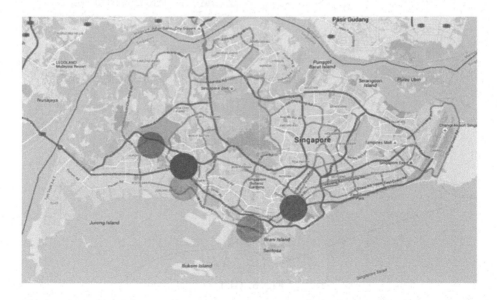

Fig. 4. Top five stay regions of a person (Color figure online)

Table 1. Study of discernibility and distortion with a varying k

	$k = 5$	$k = 10$	$k = 15$	$k = 20$
Number of valid clusters	2140	1100	758	594
Discernibility	12,044,063	28,100,581	39,338,127	48,223,101
Size of the largest cluster	74	76	101	101
Size of suppressed set	590	1387	1944	2385
Distortion (Markov model)	74,373	78,367	79,174	79,364
Distortion (Max intermediate points)	79,442	85,585	88,234	89,543

representative. We also reported the size of the largest cluster for each k. Ideally, it should be k. But, for the data in this challenge, each latitude and longitude has only two decimal digits. This rounding off increases the chance of having equal distance.

4.4 GUI

Figure 5 shows a gui developed as part of the proposed system. On the right a list of records is shown with details about k-anonymized clusters. Details include start and end times, and start and end lat-lon. DoW is also shown. The last column shows total number of trips in a cluster. On the left representative trip of a chosen cluster is shown pictorially.

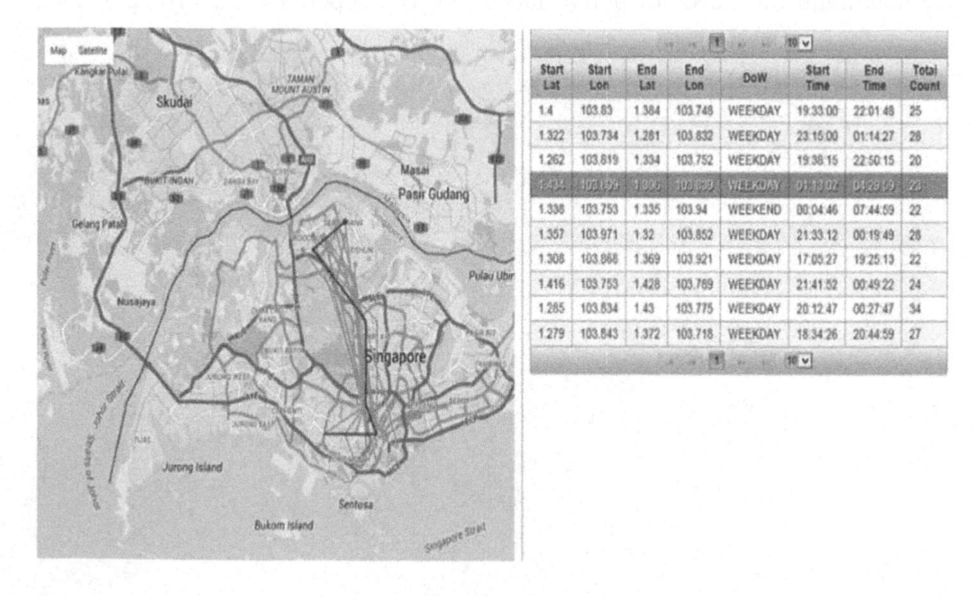

Start Lat	Start Lon	End Lat	End Lon	DoW	Start Time	End Time	Total Count
1.4	103.83	1.384	103.748	WEEKDAY	19:33:00	22:01:48	25
1.322	103.734	1.281	103.832	WEEKDAY	23:15:00	01:14:27	28
1.262	103.819	1.334	103.752	WEEKDAY	19:38:15	22:50:15	20
[illegible]	[illegible]	[illegible]	[illegible]	[illegible]	[illegible]	[illegible]	[illegible]
1.338	103.753	1.335	103.94	WEEKEND	00:04:46	07:44:59	22
1.357	103.971	1.32	103.852	WEEKDAY	21:33:12	00:19:49	28
1.308	103.868	1.369	103.921	WEEKDAY	17:05:27	19:25:13	22
1.416	103.753	1.428	103.769	WEEKDAY	21:41:52	00:49:22	24
1.285	103.834	1.43	103.775	WEEKDAY	20:12:47	00:27:47	34
1.279	103.843	1.372	103.718	WEEKDAY	18:34:26	20:44:59	27

Fig. 5. GUI

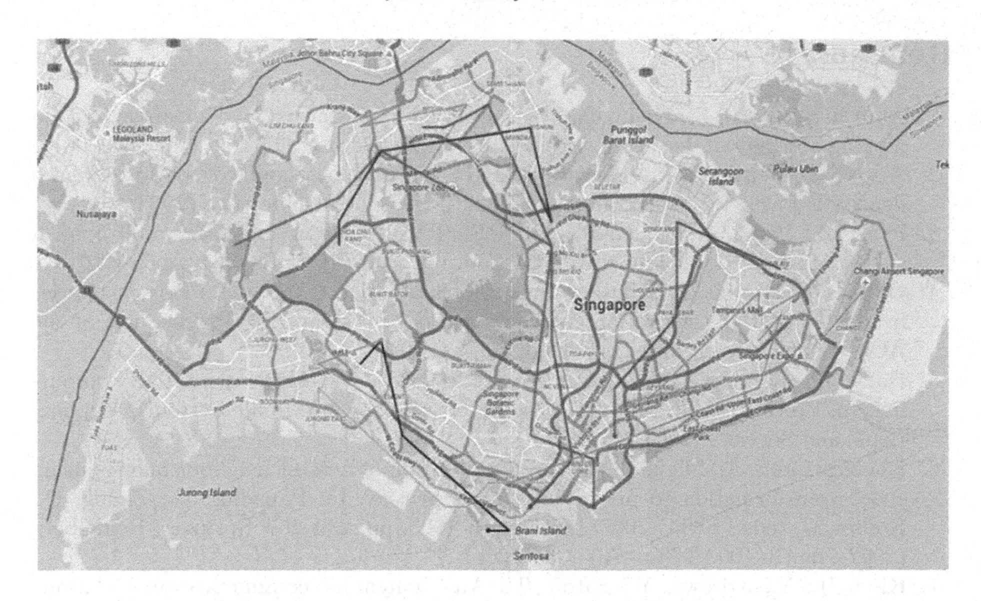

Fig. 6. Ten clusters and their representatives

4.5 Results of Privacy Preservation

Figure 6 pictorially shows the result of our privacy preservation method. It shows representatives of 10 clusters. Each representative trip has a start and end. Starting point has a time stamp (average over start times of all participating trips) that includes the day of the week or weekday/weekend. It also includes a lat-lon which is average over starting lat-lons of all participating trips. Similar information is also extracted for the end point. Note that this way of representing the trips is much more useful than the one using count data as in [2].

5 Conclusion

We proposed a method for privacy preservation of location data. Our method made a few innovations compared to the existing algorithms. We made use of stay regions and trips in order to make the trajectories privacy preservable and also to retain as much mobility pattern as possible. We implemented our method and computed discernibility and information distortion as rough estimates for risk and utility. Our evaluation shows that the proposed method is reasonable and can be used in practical scenarios.

References

1. Abul, O., Bonchi, F., Nanni, M.: Never walk alone: uncertainty for anonymity in moving objects databases. In: Proceedings of the 24th ICDE Conference (2008)
2. Acs, G., Castellucia, C.: A case study: privacy preserving release of spatio-temporal density is Paris. In: Proceedings of the 20th SIGKDD Conference (2014)
3. Fung, B., Wang, K., Chen, R., Yu, P.S.: Privacy-preserving data publishing: a survey of recent developments. ACM Comput. Surv. (CSUR) 14:1–14:53 (2010)
4. Ghinita, G., Kalnis, P., Khoshgozaran, A., Shahabi, C., Tan, K.L.: Private queries in location based services: anonymizers are not necessary. In: Proceedings of the ACM Conference on Management of Data (2008)
5. Hong, J.I., Landay, J.A.: An architecture for privacy-sensitive ubiquitous computing. In: Proceedings of the International Conference on Mobile Systems, Applications, and Services (2004)
6. Khoshgozaran, A., Shahabi, C.: Blind evaluation of nearest neighbor queries using space transformation to preserve location privacy. In: Papadias, D., Zhang, D., Kollios, G. (eds.) SSTD 2007. LNCS, vol. 4605, pp. 239–257. Springer, Heidelberg (2007). doi:10.1007/978-3-540-73540-3_14
7. Kido, H., Yanagisawa, Y., Satoh, T.: An anonymous communication technique using dummies for location based services. In: Proceedings of IEEE International Conference on Pervasive Services (2005)
8. LeFevre, K., DeWitt, D.J., Ramakrishnan, R.: Mondrian multidimensional k-anonymity. In: ICDE 2006, pp. 25–25. IEEE
9. Li, N., Li, T., Venkatasubramanian, S.: t-closeness: privacy beyond k-anonymity and l-diversity. In: ICDE 2007, pp. 106–115 (2007)
10. Machanavajjhala, A., Gehrke, J., Kifer, D., Venkitasubramaniam, M.: l-diversity: privacy beyond k-anonymity. In: ICDE 2006, pp. 24–24 (2006)
11. de Montjoye, Y.A., Hidalgo, C.A., Verleysen, M., Blondel, V.D.: Unique in the crowd: the privacy bounds of human mobility. Sci. Rep. Nat. (2013)
12. Samarati, P., Sweeney, L.: Generalizing data to provide anonymity when disclosing information. In: Proceedings of the 17th PODS Conference (1998)
13. Samarati, P.: Protecting respondents identities in microdata release. IEEE Trans. Knowl. Data Eng. **13**(6), 1010–1027 (2001)
14. Silva, D.F., Batista, G.E.: Speeding up all-pairwise dynamic time warping matrix calculation. In: Proceedings of the 2016 SIAM International Conference on Data Mining, pp. 837–845
15. Sweeney, L.: Achieving k-anonymity privacy protection using generalization and suppression. Int. J. Uncertain. Fuzziness Knowl. Based Syst. **10**(05), 571–588 (2002)
16. Sweeney, L.: k-anonymity: a model for protecting privacy. Int. J. Uncertain. Fuzziness Knowl. Based Syst. **10**(05), 557–570 (2002)
17. Xiao, X., Yi, K., Tao, Y.: The hardness and approximation algorithms for l-diversity. In: Proceedings of the 13th International Conference on Extending Database Technology, pp. 135–146 (2010)
18. Yiu, M.L., Jensen, C., Huang, X., Lu, H.: Managing the trade-offs among location privacy, query performance, and query accuracy in mobile services. In: Proceedings of IEEE International Conference on Data Engineering (2008)

Location-Aware Human Activity Recognition

Tam T. Nguyen[1(✉)], Daniel Fernandez[2], Quy T.K. Nguyen[2], and Ebrahim Bagheri[1]

[1] Ryerson University, Toronto, Canada
nthanhtam@gmail.com
[2] Lazada South East Asia, Singapore, Singapore

Abstract. In this paper, we present one of the winning solutions of an international human activity recognition challenge organized by DrivenData in conjunction with the European Conference on Machine Learning and Principles and Practice of Knowledge Discovery in Databases. The objective of the challenge was to predict activities of daily living and posture or ambulation based on wrist-worn accelerometer, RGB-D camera, and passive environmental sensor data, which was collected from a smart home in the UK. Most of the state of the art research focus on one type of data, e.g., wearable sensor data, for making predictions and overlook the usefulness of *user locations* for this purpose. In our work, we propose a novel approach that leverages heterogeneous data types as well as user locations for building predictive models. Note that while we do not have actual location information but we build models to predict location using machine learning models and use the predictions in user activity recognition. Compared to the state of the art, our proposed approach is able to achieve a 38% improvement with a Brier score of 0.1346. This means that roughly 9 out of 10 predictions matched the human-labeled descriptions.

1 Introduction

Human Activity Recognition (HAR) has been well explored in the recent years due to its potential applications in healthcare, public well-being, and public safety, just to name a few. HAR aims at categorizing user activities based on body-worn sensor data. In 2014, Bulling et al. [3] published an excellent survey paper in this field in which they reviewed how traditional pattern recognition approaches can be used for building machine learning models based on sensory data. They extensively discussed that such models often extract features from sensor data, apply feature selection, and train standard classification models [18] for activity recognition. The extracted features range from simple statistical metrics to physical, *e.g.*, speed, distance, entropy of acceleration data, and user behavioral features [10], *e.g.*, time span, activity frequency of time series data. Based on the extracted features, many different machine learning algorithms can be used for model training whose performance depends on the quality of the feature sets. For instance, with high-dimensional data, linear models such as

G. Cong et al. (Eds.): ADMA 2017, LNAI 10604, pp. 821–835, 2017.
https://doi.org/10.1007/978-3-319-69179-4_58

Support Vector Machines (SVM) and Logistic Regression [4] are highly recommended. However, using linear models, one implicitly assumes that the data is linearly separable. That may not be true in practice. Therefore, other machine learning algorithms such as k-Nearest Neighbor (KNN) [4,13] and Deep Belief Networks (DBN) [13] are also considered to solve the problem. All these models rely on the quality of the feature sets, which are time consuming to generate and require domain knowledge and skills from practitioners. Considering these issues, Yang et al. [17] have proposed an emerging deep learning method, known as Convolutional Neural Networks (CNNs/ConvNets), to tackle this problem. CNNs have been widely used for image classification but the work in [17] was the first to apply it for activity recognition.

While quite valuable and informative, user location information are often overlooked in activity recognition. To overcome this limitation, we propose a location-aware human activity recognition approach that utilizes location and leverages multimodal sensory data to boost the performance of classification models. The main contributions of our work are as follows:

- We perform extensive feature extraction, especially video features such feature engineering for depth camera data, which have not been thoroughly investigated in recent research work.
- We undertake large-scale feature selection for sensor and camera features, which work well with high-dimensional datasets.
- We propose and build accurate location prediction models for tracking participants' movements, which is not readily available in the sensor data.
- We build different activity recognition models for predicting daily life activities by leveraging various types of data including sensory and user location data.

The main objective of this paper is to show how systematic feature engineering and model learning on multimodal data can be performed for addressing downstream predictive analytics. The successful systematic approach presented in this paper can be easily applied to a host of similar application areas that consist of multimodal data.

2 Related Work

In this section, we review the related work in HAR. A running theme among the current methods is to generate features from sensor data and build predictive models. In [18], Zhang et al. generated many statistical and physical features from raw data. They then applied the filter method (Relief-F), single feature classification, and sequence forward selection to choose useful features. Finally, SVM [7] with linear kernel was used for classification. For combining different kinds of data, one may use multiview learning technique [12].

Similarly, Cao et al. [4] used SVM for activity recognition. Together with linear models, another popular machine learning algorithm, KNN [4,13], was applied. Moreover, sequential algorithms such as Hidden Markov Models (HMM) [14] and

Conditional Random Fields (CRF) [9] were used as the baselines. The experimental results showed that SVM outperforms sequential algorithms. However, these methods need domain knowledge to generate features from raw data.

In 2015, Yang et al. [17] and Jiang et al. [8] proposed to use deep learning to automatically extract useful features. Specifically, the authors treated multi-channel sensor data as time series and used CNN to learn temporal information from raw data. Similar to image classification, lag signals of time series are taken into consideration as neighborhood data for training CNN. Using this methods, manual feature extraction is no longer required.

Moreover, there is one earlier research work that takes location into consideration when predicting human activity. In order to do this, Lu and Fu [11] installed a pad with size of 30 × 30 cm to capture user locations.

3 Problem Setting

In this section, we introduce HAR in the DrivenData competition (SPHERE challenge) [16] where data collection was performed in a single SPHERE smart home. The goal of this challenge was to use multimodal data and advanced machine learning algorithms to help senior people live safely at home.

3.1 The Data

The following subsections present the summary of the whole dataset[1]. For more details, one may refer to [16].

Accelerometers. The acceleration data consists of eight columns as follows:

- t: this is the time of the recording (relative to the start of the sequence)
- x/y/z: these are the acceleration values recorded on the x/y/z axes of the accelerometer.
- Kitchen_AP/Lounge_AP/Upstairs_AP/Study_AP: these specify the received signal strength (RSSI) of the acceleration signal as received by the kitchen/lounge/upstairs access points. Empty values indicate that the access point did not receive any packets.

RGB-D Cameras. RGB-D cameras were located in the living room, hallway, and the kitchen. No cameras were located in the residence. The camera data consists of the following columns:

- t: the current time (relative to the start of the sequence)
- centre_2d_x/centre_2d_y: the x and y coordinates of the center of the 2D bounding box

[1] http://www.irc-sphere.ac.uk/sphere-challenge/home.

- bb_2d_br_x/bb_2d_br_y: the x and y coordinates of the bottom right (br) corner of the 2D bounding box
- bb_2d_tl_x/bb_2d_tl_y: the x and y coordinates of the top left (tl) corner of the 2D bounding box
- centre_3d_x/centre_3d_y/centre_3d_z: the x, y and z coordinates for the center of the 3D bounding box
- bb_3d_brb_x/bb_3d_brb_y/bb_3d_brb_z: the x, y, and z coordinates for the bottom right back corner of the 3D bounding box
- bb_3d_flt_x/bb_3d_flt_y/bb_3d_flt_z: the x, y, and z coordinates of the front left top corner of the 3D bounding box.

Environmental Sensors. The environmental sensing nodes were built on development platforms (Libelium, with CE marking [3]), powered by batteries and/or 5 V DC converted from mains. Passive Infra-Red (PIR) sensors were employed to detect presence. Values of 1 indicate that motion was detected, whereas values of 0 means that no motion was detected.

- start: the start time of the PIR sensor (relative to the start of the sequence)
- end: the end time of the PIR sensor (relative to the start of the sequence)
- name: the name of the PIR sensor being activated (from the above list)
- Index: the index of activated sensor from pir_locations list starting at 0.

Locations. This data point specifies the room or location that was occupied at that point in time by the recruited participant. The rooms were annotated as bathroom, bedroom 1, bedroom 2, hallway, kitchen, living room, stairs, study room, and the toilet.

Ground Truth. As the data included high inter-annotator disagreement for activity recognition labeling, the ground truth data contains the probabilistic targets of 20 activities that belong to three categories: ambulation, posture, and posture-to-posture.

4 Human Activity Recognition

This section presents our proposed framework as shown in Fig. 1 for human activity recognition, which consists of 5 major layers as follows:

- Feature extraction: In the first phase, we extract features from four data sources including accelerator, RSSI, PIR, and camera. The output of this layer is acceleration, RSSI, PIR, and camera feature sets, respectively.
- Meta-feature extraction: In order to take advantage of historical information, we extract previous activity or sensor signals of the user. We then use these lag meta-features in activity recognition models.

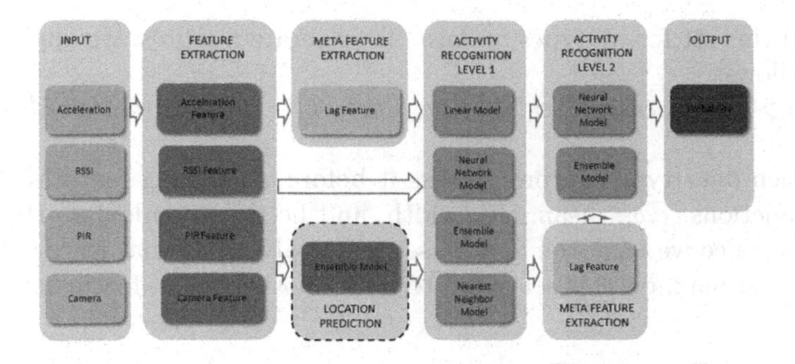

Fig. 1. Location-aware activity recognition framework

- Location prediction: We aim at predicting participants' locations in the smart home using predictive models and use the predictions as meta-features in the activity recognition models.
- First level activity recognition: After computing feature sets, we train various machine learning models using families of algorithms including linear, neural network, ensemble and nearest-neighbor models through cross validation and prediction.
- Second level activity recognition: In the final step, we use stacking based on neural network and ensemble algorithms to take advantage of the diversity of algorithms. We use the previous predictions as meta-features to train the second level models.

4.1 Data Preprocessing

Since sensor data is extremely noisy, we applied rolling mean by time series for preprocessing the data before extracting features. Specifically, the current record i is replaced by the average of $(i-t):(i+t)$ records. When $t = 10$, a given record will be valued as the average of the 10 previous records, the actual record, and the next 10 records. We experimented with different t values to choose the optimal values. We use infix M_t in the feature names to differentiate the preprocessed data from the raw signals.

4.2 Feature Design

In this section, we present our feature sets which were used for building the classification models. Given three major sources of data, we generate 4 features sets derived from accelerometer, Received Signal Strength Indications (RSSI), PIR sensors, and RGB-D cameras. These feature sets consist of acceleration feature, RSSI feature, PIR feature, and RGB-D camera feature whose names start with prefix *'accel_'*, *'rssi_'*, *'pir_'*, and *'video_'*, respectively. The simplest feature set is statistics features such as *mean*, *std*, *min*, *max*, and *median*. We

generated this set for all types of data. To generate features, we applied a chain rule as follows:
data type > [preprocessing] > [feature function] > [feature function]

For each data type, we pre-process it before generating features. We apply feature functions, *e.g.*, mean, std, width, and height, to calculate the features. After that, once we have the feature set, we apply additional feature functions, *e.g.*, min and max, on this set again to have another set of features.

Acceleration Feature. The accelerometer readings (units of g) are a continuous numerical stream for (x, y, z) axes. The accelerometers record data at 20 Hz, and the maximum accelerometer range is 8 g. So for a window size of 1 s, when no signal is lost, there are 20 (x, y, z) triples. Before extracting features, we apply the beforementioned pre-processing technique with $t \in \{1, 3, 6, 10\}$ to have 4 new datasets $M01$, $M03$, $M06$, and $M10$, respectively. For each dimension, we calculated statistical features using different time windows as shown in Table 1.

Table 1. Statistical feature set

Feature name	Description
dif	Difference between positions in which we find the maximum and the minimum values of the time series
slo	Difference between mean of the first 25% of the values and mean of the last 25% of the values
moment	1st central moment of signal values
iqr	Interquartile range of signal values
mad	Median absolute deviation
energy	Sum of the squares divided by the number of signal values
mag	The Frobenius norm of signal values

The feature functions such as mean and std are used as the suffix of the feature names. Besides, we also generate geometric features from the acceleration data as shown in Table 2.

RSSI Feature. The signal strength indicator (RSSI) of the acceleration signal specifies access to kitchen, lounge, upstairs, and study room locations. For preprocessing data, we used $t \in \{4, 16, 32\}$ to obtain $M04$, $M16$, and $M32$ datasets. To capture RSSI, we generated the following statistical features as shown in Table 3.

Table 2. Acceleration geometric feature set

Feature name	Feature calculation
comp	$sqrt(x^2 + y^2 + z^2)$
xy	$arctan(y/x)$
xz	$arctan(x/z)$
yz	$arctan(y/z)$
xyz	$arctan(sqrt(y^2 + z^2)/x)$
zxy	$arctan(sqrt(x^2 + y^2)/z)$
yzx	$arctan(sqrt(z^2 + x^2)/y)$

Table 3. RSSI feature set

Feature name	Description
nanmax	Indicator of which AP receives the nanmean max strength signal
nanmin	Indicator of which AP receives the nanmean min strength signal
meansdiff	The difference between nanmean and mean features
max_mean	Max of mean for each record of the time-window (20 for 1 s), calculate the nanmax, and after that calculate the mean value of nanmax for each AP
min_mean	Min of mean for each record of the time-window (20 for 1 s), calculate the nanmin, and after that calculate the mean value of nanmin for each AP

PIR Feature. PIR sensors are employed to detect presence of the participants at a certain location. These locations consist of bathroom, bedroom 1, bedroom 2, hall, kitchen, living room, stairs, study room, and toilet. Values of 1 indicate that a motion is detected, whereas value of 0 means that no motion was detected. Together with statistics features, we also engineered the following feature for PIR data: *sumON*: how many detectors are activated.

RGB-D Camera Feature. There are three cameras installed in the smart home in three locations including living room, hallway, and kitchen. The raw video data are not disclosed due to privacy concerns. Instead, the coordinates of 2D bounding boxes, 2D centers of mass, 3D bounding boxes, and 3D centers of mass are provided. Similar to acceleration and PIR data, we also preprocessed camera data with $t \in \{1, 3, 6, 10\}$ and extracted statistic features including the following feature: *asum*: sum of all absolute values of the series (Table 4).

Table 5 shows a list of camera features which capture participant's gesture. For 2D data, we have width, height, area, and aspect ratio features. For 3D data, we calculated the same 2D feature for 3 different dimensions. In addition, we also computed volume features. Similar to the raw data, given the bounding boxes, we extracted the statistical features for them. Since we have the same type of calculation for both raw and bounding box data, we used the infixes *'sta'* and *'fig'* in the feature names to differentiate between these two types of features.

Table 4. Camera centers of mass feature set

Feature name	Feature calculation
center_2d_xy	centre_2d_x/centre_2d_y
bb_2d_br_xy	bb_2d_br_x/bb_2d_br_y
bb_2d_tl_xy	bb_2d_tl_x/bb_2d_tl_y
center_3d_xyz	centre_3d_x/centre_3d_y/centre_3d_z
bb_3d_brb_xyz	bb_3d_brb_x/bb_3d_brb_y/bb_3d_brb_z
bb_3d_flt_xyz	bb_3d_flt_x/bb_3d_flt_y/bb_3d_flt_z

Table 5. Camera bounding box feature set

Feature name	Feature calculation
d2_width	bb_2d_br_x − bb_2d_tl_x
d2_height	bb_2d_br_y − bb_2d_tl_y
d2_area	d2_width * d2_height
d2_ratio	d2_height/d2_width
d3_width	bb_3d_brb_x − bb_3d_flt_x
d3_height	bb_3d_flt_y − bb_3d_brb_y
d3_depth	bb_3d_brb_z − bb_3d_flt_z
d3_wh_area	d3_width * d3_height
d3_wd_area	d3_width * d3_depth
d3_hd_area	d3_height * d3_depth
d3_wh_ratio	d3_width/d3_height
d3_wd_ratio	d3_width/d3_depth
d3_hd_ratio	d3_height/d3_depth
d3_vol	d3_width * d3_height * d3_depth

4.3 Feature Selection

In this section, we present our practical approach to feature selection. Given a feature set, recursive feature selection (RFS) starts with a feature and incrementally selects a new one that improves the performance of a classifier. This method is widely used in practice because it is easy to implement. However, if the training data is very large and the number of features is extremely high, this method is impractical. Hence, we propose a tractable approach by adapting RFS on a feature subset level instead of an individual feature. It means that we split our feature set into smaller subsets and carry out feature selection on these subsets.

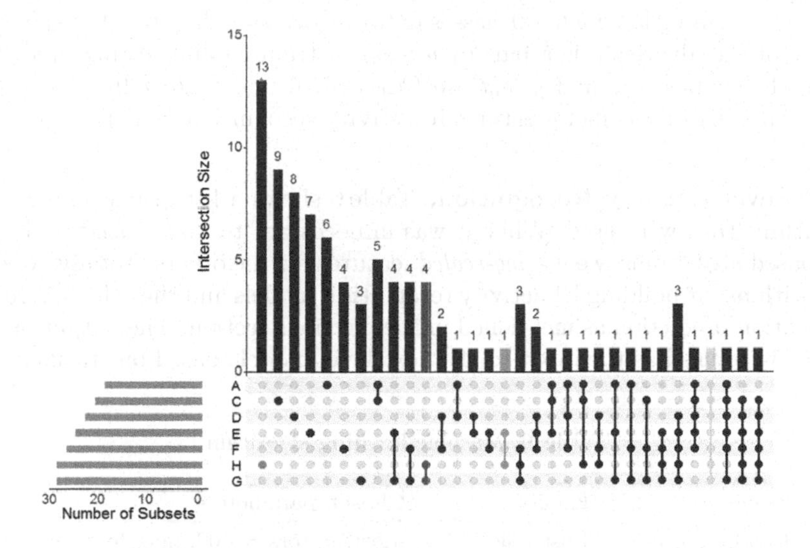

Fig. 2. Feature set selection (best view in color) (Color figure online)

We sample the feature set mentioned in the previous section to have 9 subsets. Then we apply feature selection on all of them to have new features A, B, C, D, E, F, G, and H as shown in Fig. 2 where, for instance, set B is the combination of set H, location features, and physical features calculated from acceleration data. The left bar chart shows the number of subsets in each set were G and H are the largest sets with 30 subsets. The grid in the middle shows the relationship between these sets. If they share the sample subsets, there should be a link between them. Correspondingly, the bar chart on the top shows how many times these subsets have been shared. For instance, there are 3 subsets that are shared by both G and H (blue color). At the same time, there is only one subset that A, C, D, G, and H have in common (orange color).

4.4 Modeling Methodology

In this section, we present our modeling approach for human activity recognition.

Location Prediction. There are 9 locations in this dataset. They include bathroom, bedroom 1, bedroom 2, hall, kitchen, living room, stairs, study room, and toilet. Although location data was provided in the training data, we did not have any location in the testing data. In order to take advantage of location information to improve the predictive power in the testing phase, we needed to predict participants' location in both training and testing data. We tackled the location prediction problem by using a single label multi-class classification model. Specifically, we passed the location of both training and testing data; and an ensemble model (e.g. Extra Trees) as the input of the master algorithm where the training label y has 9 classes in total corresponding to 9 locations. The output of the algorithm is a pair $(\hat{y}, y\_test)$ of training and testing predictions where the shapes of $\hat{y}$ and y_test are $(n\_train, 9)$ and $(n\_test, 9)$, respectively. We use predictions as meta-features in activity recognition models.

First Level Activity Recognition. Table 6 shows a list of machine learning algorithms that were used. While it was unnecessary to *normalize* the data for tree-based algorithms, we use *log-scaled* features for the others. Totally, we chose 6 algorithms for building L1 activity recognition models and the others were used for location prediction as mentioned in the previous section. The output of these models were used as the input to the next level models based on stacking.

Table 6. Machine learning algorithm

	Name	Family	Chosen parameters
RFC	Random forest classifier [1]	Ensemble method	n_estimators = 500; max_features = 0.12; min_samples_leaf = 5
ETC	Extra trees classifier [2]	Ensemble method	n_estimators = 250; max_features = 0.75; min_samples_leaf = 3
XGB	Extreme boosting machine [5]	Ensemble method	n_estimators = 200; max_depth = 6; learning_rate = 0.04; colsample_bytree = 0.2; subsample = 0.9
ANN	Artificial Neural network [6]	Neural network method	layer1 = (1000 neurons, dropout = 0.90); layer2 = (100 neurons, dropout = 0.60); loss = 'categorical_crossentropy'; epoch = 20; batch_size = 64
LoR	Logistic regression [7]	Linear method	penalty = l2; C = 1.0
LiR	Linear regression	Linear method	default
KNN	K-Nearest neighbor	Nearest neighbor	n_neighbors = 10
RNN	Bidirectional recurrent neural networks [15]	Neural network method	forward = LSTM(128); backward = LSTM (128); learning_rate = 0.0001; rho = 0.9; optimizer = "rmsprop"

Note that we did not extensively search for best parameters but manually found near optimal ones for L1 models. Exhaustive grid search is infeasible for such a large dataset because it is extremely time consuming.

Second Level Activity Recognition. In second level activity recognition, we adopt the bagging technique in machine learning. Specifically, we randomly chose 5 subsets of predictions from the first level and applied the master algorithm to train the second level (L2) models. Three algorithms including XGB, ETC, and ANN were used in the second phase. The final prediction was the weighted average of all L2 models. The details of these models will be presented in the next sections. The difference between our bagging approach and the traditional model is that we used different algorithms for bagging, while the traditional model applies the same algorithm for all subsets of the training data.

5 Performance Evaluation

We performed stratified 10-fold cross validation for performance evaluation. There are 17,354 features in total, 16,124 training and 16,600 testing instances. In this section, we compare the predictive power of each model based on Brier score in both first and second level models. Additionally, we study and discuss the importance of each feature.

5.1 Location Prediction Model

Figure 4a shows the performance of location models on the feature set A. We tried different algorithms including XGB, ETC, RFC, LoR, KNN, ANN, and SVM with other feature sets for location prediction. Additionally, we also applied stacking to improve the performance of the location models. We found that even if we were able to improve the performance of location models, there was not much gain in the activity recognition models. The experimental results show that the ensemble algorithms XGB, ETC, and RFC are the best in terms of Brier, accuracy, log loss, and F1 scores where XGB is the best performer with an F1 score of 0.9250; and ETC and RFC are the first and second runner up with F1 scores of 0.9208 and 0.9201, respectively. For the experiments in the next section, we chose the ETC model with feature set A for location prediction because its predictions not only make more contribution to HAR but are also fast for training.

5.2 First Level Activity Recognition Model

Figure 3a shows the mean of 10-fold cross validation Brier scores of the first level models for all feature sets where each cell represents the Brier score of an algorithm (column) on a feature set (row). Clearly, XGBoost (XGB) outperforms all other algorithms. Especially, it performs the best and the second

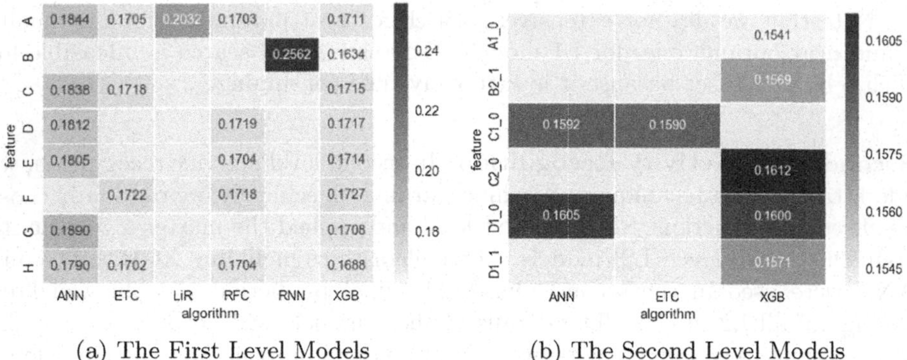

(a) The First Level Models (b) The Second Level Models

Fig. 3. Cross validation Brier score

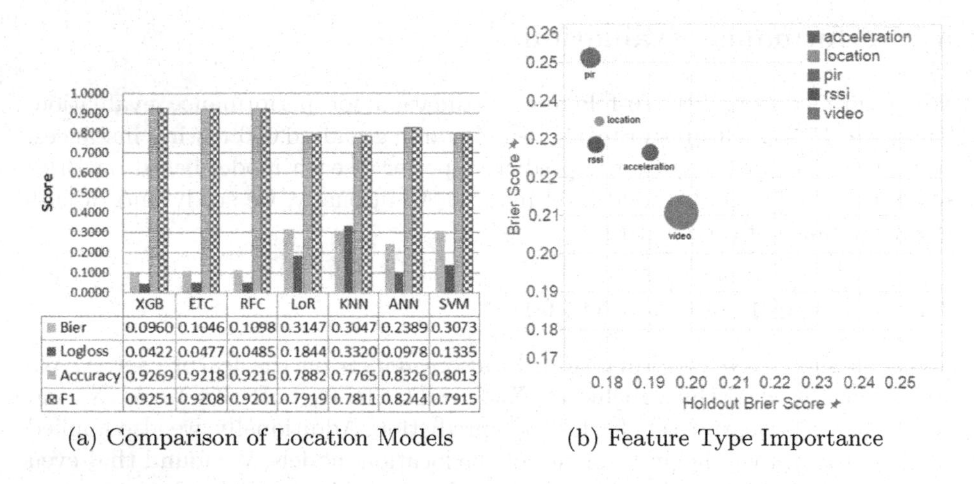

(a) Comparison of Location Models (b) Feature Type Importance

Fig. 4. Location model performance and feature type importance

best on feature sets B and H with Brier score of 0.1634 and 0.1688, respectively. The runner up is Extra Trees (ETC) with a Brier score of 0.1702. Similarly, Random Forest (RFC) has nearly the same result as ETC. We also carried out the experiments with neural networks. In this task, we found that Multi-Layer Perceptrons (MLP/ANN) perform worse than ensemble models. We also tried Recurrent Neural Network (RNN) to capture the historical activities but it did not perform better than the baseline KNN.

5.3 Second Level Activity Recognition Model

Figure 3b shows the mean of 10-fold cross validation Brier score of L2 models. In this phase, we focus mainly on three algorithms: XGB, ANN, and ETC. The experimental results show that XGB outperforms the other two algorithms. The best Brier score obtained is 0.1541 on feature set A1_0 including all L1 predictions. Compared to those of L1 models, the best L2 model works better than the L1 models with a margin of 0.0093 in terms of the Brier score. We also randomly sampled L1 predictions to obtain another 5 feature sets and then trained L2 models. Our winning submission is a linear combination of all L2 model predictions that have the testing Brier score of 0.1346. This means that our solution can make 9 out of 10 correct predictions compared to human-labeled descriptions. Given the complexity of our model, one may express concern about the modeling complexity. Depending on the requirements on accuracy and running time, it is possible to create a trade-off between complexity and running time.

5.4 Feature Importance Study

To verify the importance of each data type, we studied the performance of each type of feature including acceleration, RSSI, PIR, and location as shown in Fig. 4b. We carried out 10-fold cross validation by selecting only one type of feature, *e.g.*, video, and excluding the rest. The performance results were plotted against the number of features where the size of the bubbles is proportional to the number of features. Obviously, video data is the most useful for activity recognition. Using solely video features, we could achieve a Brier score of 0.2108 which is the best compared to other individual types of data. However, if we did not use video data and combined all the other four, the Brier score would be 0.1975. This means that

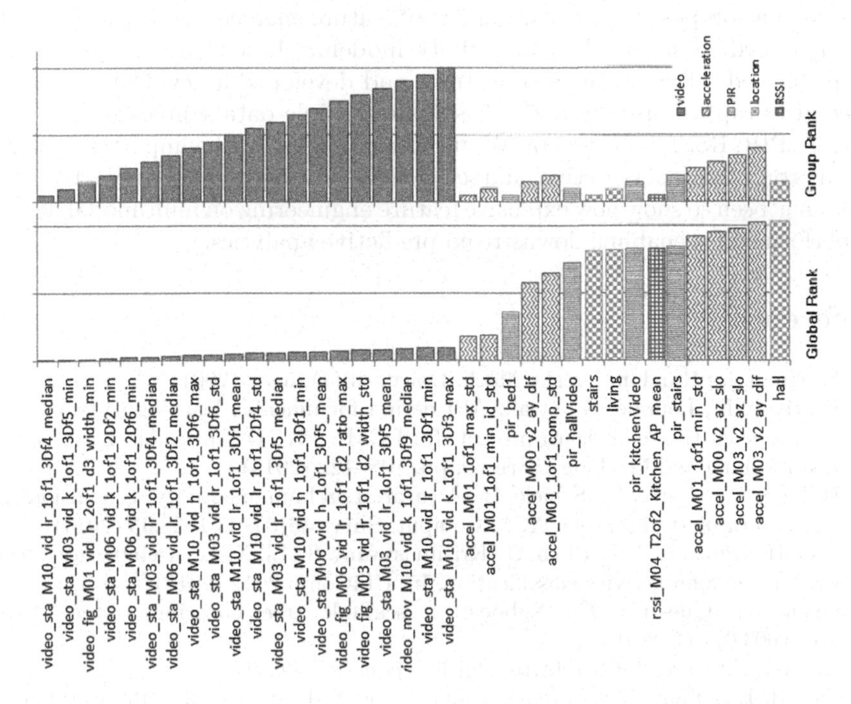

Fig. 5. Top 35 features (best view in color) (Color figure online)

video data alone would work worse than the combination of other data. Moreover, regarding the efficiency, the location feature set is the best performer. With only 9 features, it works much better than PIR data and is slightly worse than RSSI and acceleration data.

Top Features. Besides feature group/subset importance, we also investigated the role of individual features. Due to space limitations, we only list the most important ones in this section. Figure 5 shows the top-35 features with global and group ranks where camera/video predictors are dominant in the list with 19 features in the top-20. The feature naming convention is as follows: data source + sta/fig (if any) + preprocessing (if any) + attribute operator/feature name. For example, the best feature is calculated from video_lr (video data from living room) based on the preprocessed set $M10$ and attribute (z coordinate for the bottom right back corner of the 3D bounding box) using the 'median' operator. The rest of the features can be interpreted similarly.

6 Conclusion

In this paper, we presented our location-aware framework for human activity recognition which is one of the winning solution of a data science challenge organized by DrivenData in conjunction with the European Conference on Machine Learning and Principles and Practice of Knowledge Discovery in Databases conference. The proposed approach consists of feature engineering, feature selection, location prediction, and human activity modeling based on multimodal data. We generated a large number of features and developed a new feature selection method to capture user activities based on multiple data sources such as acceleration, PIR, RSSI, and camera. We further investigated the importance of these features on various perspectives and selected the top features. The objective of this paper has been to show how extensive feature engineering on multimodal data can be performed for enabling downstream predictive analytics.

References

1. Breiman, L.: Random forests. Mach. Learn. **45**(1), 5–32 (2001)
2. Buitinck, L., Louppe, G., et al.: API design for machine learning software: experiences from the scikit-learn project. In: ECML PKDD Workshop: Languages for Data Mining and Machine Learning, pp. 108–122 (2013)
3. Bulling, A., Blanke, U., Schiele, B.: A tutorial on human activity recognition using body-worn inertial sensors. ACM Comput. Surv. **46**(3), 33:1–33:33 (2014)
4. Cao, H., Nguyen, M.N., Phua, C., Krishnaswamy, S., Li, X.-L.: An integrated framework for human activity classification. In: UbiComp 2012 (2012)
5. Chen, T., Guestrin, C.: Xgboost: a scalable tree boosting system. CoRR, abs/1603.02754 (2016)
6. Chollet, F.: Keras (2015). https://github.com/fchollet/keras
7. Fan, R.-E., Chang, K.-W., Hsieh, C.-J., Wang, X.-R., Lin, C.-J.: Liblinear: a library for large linear classification. J. Mach. Learn. Res. **9**, 1871–1874 (2008)

8. Jiang, W., Yin, Z.: Human activity recognition using wearable sensors by deep convolutional neural networks. In: MM 2015 (2015)
9. Lafferty, J.D., McCallum, A., Pereira, F.C.N.: Conditional random fields: probabilistic models for segmenting and labeling sequence data. In: ICML 2001, pp. 282–289 (2001)
10. Liu, G., Nguyen, T.T., Zhao, G., Zha, W., Yang, J., Cao, J., Wu, M., Zhao, P., Chen, W.: Repeat buyer prediction for e-commerce. In: KDD 2016 (2016)
11. Lu, C., Fu, L.: Robust location-aware activity recognition using wireless sensor network in an attentive home. IEEE Trans. Autom. Sci. Eng. **6**(4), 598–609 (2009)
12. Nguyen, T.T., Chang, K., Hui, S.C.: Two-view online learning. In: Tan, P.-N., Chawla, S., Ho, C.K., Bailey, J. (eds.) PAKDD 2012. LNCS, vol. 7301, pp. 74–85. Springer, Heidelberg (2012). doi:10.1007/978-3-642-30217-6_7
13. Plötz, T., Hammerla, N.Y., Olivier, P.: Feature learning for activity recognition in ubiquitous computing. In: IJCAI 2011 (2011)
14. Rabiner, L.R.: Readings in speech recognition. In: A Tutorial on Hidden Markov Models and Selected Applications in Speech Recognition, pp. 267–296. Morgan Kaufmann Publishers Inc., San Francisco (1990)
15. Schuster, M., Paliwal, K.: Bidirectional recurrent neural networks. Trans. Sig. Proc. **45**(11), 2673–2681 (1997)
16. Twomey, N., Diethe, T., Kull, M., Song, H., Camplani, M., Hannuna, S., Fafoutis, X., Zhu, N., Woznowski, P., Flach, P., Craddock, I.: The SPHERE challenge: activity recognition with multimodal sensor data. arXiv preprint arXiv:1603.00797 (2016)
17. Yang, J., Nguyen, M.N., San, P.P., Li, X., Krishnaswamy, S.: Deep convolutional neural networks on multichannel time series for human activity recognition. In: IJCAI 2015 (2015)
18. Zhang, M., Sawchuk, A.A.: A feature selection-based framework for human activity recognition using wearable multimodal sensors. In: BodyNets 2011 (2011)

Demos

SWYSWYK: A New Sharing Paradigm for the Personal Cloud

Paul Tran-Van[1,2,3(✉)], Nicolas Anciaux[1,2], and Philippe Pucheral[1,2]

[1] Inria Saclay-Île-de-France, 1 rue d'Estienne d'Orves, 91120 Palaiseau, France
{paul.tran-van,nicolas.anciaux,philippe.pucheral}@inria.fr
[2] DAVID Lab, University of Versailles, 45 av. Etats-Unis, 78035 Versailles, France
[3] Cozy Cloud, 158 rue de Verdun, 92800 Puteaux, France

Abstract. Pushed by recent legislation and smart disclosure initiatives, the Personal Cloud emerges and holds the promise of giving the control back to the individual on her data. However, this shift leaves the privacy and security issues in user's hands, a role that few people can properly endorse. This demonstration illustrates a new sharing paradigm, called SWYSWYK (*Share What You See with Who You Know*), dedicated to the Personal Cloud context. It allows each user to physically visualize the net effects of sharing rules and automatically provides tangible guarantees about the enforcement of the defined sharing policies. The usage and internals of SWYSWYK are demonstrated on a running prototype combining a commercial Personal Cloud platform, Cozy, and a secure hardware reference monitor, PlugDB.

Keywords: Personal cloud · Privacy-by-design · Access control · Data security

1 Introduction

The ever increasing centralization of personal data on servers exacerbates the risk of privacy leakage due to piracy and opaque business practices. Today, a rebalancing of personal data management is occurring worldwide thanks to legislation evolution [1] and smart disclosure initiatives (e.g., blue and green buttons in the US, MesInfos in France). This enables individuals to get their personal data back from companies or administrations and organize it in a Personal Information Management System (PIMS) [2] and share it with applications and users under their control.

But empowering citizens to leverage their personal data leaves the privacy and security issues in user's hands, a paradox if we consider the weaknesses of individuals' defenses in terms of computer security and ability to administer sharing policies. Existing sharing models [3] are geared towards central authorities and their secure enforcement requires a deep expertise, out of reach of individuals. Conversely, decentralized tools (e.g., Web of Trust models or FOAF dissemination rules [4–6]) put on individuals the burden of defining manually each basic sharing rule and leave them on their own to manage complex cryptographic protection against piracy [7]. This often

G. Cong et al. (Eds.): ADMA 2017, LNAI 10604, pp. 839–845, 2017.
https://doi.org/10.1007/978-3-319-69179-4_59

leads to consider data sharing as an intractable burden, letting desperate owners either define far too permissive policies [8] or delegate the administration of their PIMS to centralized service providers. The circle would come back around, with service providers now in possession of the complete individual's digital history.

This demonstration proposes an answer to solve this issue. It capitalizes upon a new paradigm called SWYSWYK (*Share What You See with Who You Know*) helping the PIMS owner to visually check and sanitize the net effect of a sharing policy over her data [9]. A reference architecture providing tangible guarantees about the enforcement of SWYSWYK policies has been discussed in [10]. We demonstrate how the SWYSWYK paradigm can be put in practice, by combining an open-source PIMS platform, Cozy[1], with a reference monitor embedded in secure hardware, PlugDB[2].

2 SWYSWYK Baseline

SWYSWYK is not yet another access control model. Rather, the access control policy is defined by the PIMS platform. It simply does the assumption that the sharing granularity is the document and that every shareable document is made viewable by the PIMS owner. We do not accept a smaller granularity as it could make the visualization difficult. Every user (called subject hereafter) the owner wants to interact with is also assumed to correspond to a PIMS viewable document (e.g., a contact record). The third and last assumption is that the access control policy is materialized by a set of Access Control List (ACL, or permissions) of the form <*s, d, a*>, where *s* and *d* respectively refer to a subject and a document stored in the PIMS, and *a* is an action granted to *s* on *d*.

The PIMS owner has the ability to check these ACLs and freely filter out those which presumably hurt her privacy thanks to administration tools detailed next. This principle gives substance to the Share What You See with Who You Know (SWYSWYK) principle. This is in frontal opposition with approaches where sharing policies are defined by a set of potentially complex rules, evaluated on the fly by an opaque reference monitor. The logic of a SWYSWYK reference monitor can be trivially understood by anyone: operation *a* on *d* is granted to *s* iff $(s, d, a) \in ACL$.

The tricky point of the SWYSWYK paradigm lies in the detection and validation of suspicious ACLs. Indeed, permissions are created through a genuine access control model, provided by the PIMS, on which no security assumption can be made.

The global ACL validation process works as follows. First, the genuine sharing policy is translated into a materialized set of candidate ACL named ACL^*. Second, suspicious ACLs are detected and put in quarantine, in a set named $ACL^?$, waiting for the decision of the PIMS owner. Non suspicious ACLs are directly integrated in the set ACL^+, the unique set to be considered by the reference monitor to grant or deny accesses to documents. Third, the PIMS owner sanitizes the set of suspicious ACLs on a case-by-case basis. She visualizes the net effect of suspicious ACLs in $ACL^?$ and decides to store them in ACL^+ if she considers them innocuous or in ACL^- otherwise.

[1] https://cozy.io/en/.

[2] https://project.inria.fr/plugdb/.

We propose two mechanisms to automatically detect suspicious ACLs and feed $ACL^?$ from the content of ACL^*. The first mechanism is based on an *Advisor* process identifying elements of ACL^* which are contradictory to past decisions. This mechanism is based on the assumption that owners exhibit a rather stable data disclosure behavior over time [11]. The second mechanism uses *watchdog triggers* highlighting ACLs concerning sensitive documents (e.g., "which new subjects have access to my medical records?"), sensitive subjects (e.g., "which new documents can be seen by my manager?") or sensitive associations (e.g., "which new authorizations my colleagues have on my family photos?"). This mechanism is further detailed in [10].

3 SWYSWYK Architecture

The objective of this architecture is to protect the owner's data by construction against any form of confidentiality attacks. Presented in Fig. 1, it distinguishes three main parts with different assumptions in terms of trustworthiness: (i) an *untrusted environment (UE)* on which no security assumption is made for the code nor for the data, (ii) an *isolated environment (IE)* on which general purpose code can be run with the guarantee that it cannot leak any information but with no guarantee about the soundness and honesty of its output (i.e., code can be corrupted) and (iii) a *Secure Execution Environment (SEE)* which runs only certified core programs and protects data and code against snooping and tampering. In this demonstration, the *UE* is represented by a personal computer, with a Cozy instance running on it, using an Internet connection. Cozy is a representative open-source PIMS suite, gathering personal data from multiple sources. The *IE* is a Raspberry Pi 3 without any network connection. Finally, the *SEE* is played by PlugDB, a secure and open hardware/software platform developed at Inria. It combines a smartcard to store cryptographic secrets, a microcontroller (MCU) running a relational database engine [12] and a microSD flash card storing the database with crypto-protection against snooping and tampering. It communicates with both the *UE* (WiFi IEEE 802.11n) and the *IE* (High Speed USB 2.0).

PIMS Data System. In Cozy, one can install web app created by any developer or third-party on which none security assumption can be made. It is then part of the untrusted environment *UE*. All documents of the PIMS need then be stored encrypted in this area to protect them against confidentiality attacks.

Reference Monitor. The reference monitor executes the *Allowed* function which grants or denies access. It must be part of the secure core of the architecture and embedded into the *SEE* to guarantee that it cannot be bypassed, observed nor corrupted by any external application. It acts as an incorruptible doorkeeper.

Administration Console. The administration console is used to help the PIMS owner to perform the ACL validation task. This console runs the *watchdog triggers* over ACL^* and puts suspicious ACLs in quarantine in $ACL^?$. The administration console must be trusted, but cannot be entirely executed inside the *SEE*. Indeed, it involves interactions with the owner through a GUI and requires displaying the content of

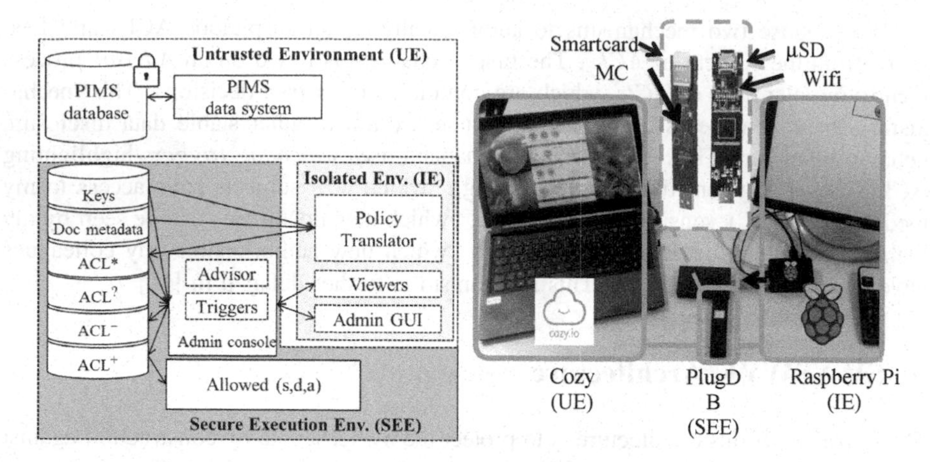

Fig. 1. Demonstration platform.

documents and subjects. Thus, the Administration GUI must be isolated in the *IE* to prevent any information leakage.

Internal Data Structures. The ACL^*, $ACL^?$, ACL^+ and ACL^- sets, the document metadata and the encryption keys must all be stored inside *SEE* for obvious security reasons, but also for performances issues, as storing them in the *UE* would incur prohibitive decryption and integrity costs. Each ACL set is stored as a bipartite graph to avoid any combinatorial explosion from large sharing rules. This allows the access control to remains *consistent* by construction (the decision is unique), *complete* (the decision always exists) and can be evaluated in *logarithmic time*.

4 Demonstration Scenario

The first part of the demonstration (see Fig. 2, steps 1–4) shows the utility of SWYSWYK in terms of privacy protection[3]. We use a personal cloud populated by Cozy applications with a set of predefined documents and sharing rules, to which the attendees can connect as Alice (the owner). A remote personal cloud instance, identified as Bob (a subject), is also pre-installed. The attendees first browse Alice's Cozy, and see contact files with pictures representing subjects (among which Bob and Boss, the manager of Alice) and a set of general purpose pictures (among which photos of Alice's 'swollen belly' to be shown to her doctors). The privacy expectations of Alice are that (i) her medical pictures are not shared with anybody and (ii) only innocuous documents are shared with her manager.

The attendees use the 'Files' application on Alice's Cozy and create a new sharing rule through the interface. They are then invited to go in the Administration GUI, to look at the existing sharing rules, represented as logic-based predicates on documents'

[3] A video of the demonstration is available at : http://wanda.inria.fr/CIKM/cikm.ogg.

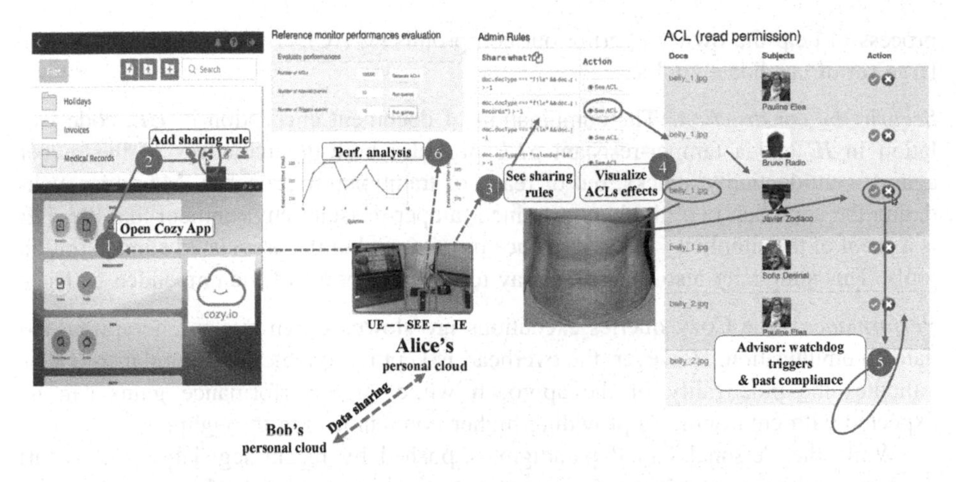

Fig. 2. Demonstration scenario and GUI.

metadata. Unsurprisingly, this task requires a deep expertise, out of reach of the regular user as the number of rules increases. Alternatively, the GUI shows the corresponding set of visualizable ACLs, where attendees can discover that Bob has a read access to compromising pictures of Alice-confirmed when connecting to Bob's personal cloud. However, the size of the ACL set proscribes any exhaustive 'manual' check. The attendees then activate the *Advisor* module to identify suspicious ACLs. They also create (or choose predefined) *watchdog triggers* to automatically detect appearance of sensitive objects (e.g., medical pictures) or subjects (e.g., Boss) in the produced ACLs. As a result, the attendees detect further ACLs hurting Alice's privacy, which can be rejected with direct effect on Bob's Cozy.

The second part of the demonstration (Fig. 2, steps 1–4 and step 5) focuses on the security properties and shows what is happening 'under the hood' at rule creation and execution time. The attendees play the attacker role and add a malicious rule hurting Alice privacy. The GUI shows what is running in the three environments, where and when data is decrypted, keys are stored and access decisions are taken.

The third part of the demonstration (Fig. 2, step 6) focuses on performance, scalability and compliance with constrained secure execution environments like PlugDB. We use an ACL generator, producing large sets of ACLs combining existing subjects and objects. The performances of the reference monitor are plotted along with detailed statistics about execution times, cryptographic impact and I/O costs.

5 Conclusion

This demonstration illustrates the three following properties attached to the SWYSWYK paradigm.

Usability. The focus of the demonstration is on validating and sanitizing the resulting set of ACLs. It highlights the effectiveness of *watchdog triggers* and the *Advisor* process to help the owner filtering out compromising ACLs, even when applied to a large set of candidate ACLs.

Security by construction. The combination of document encryption in *UE*, code isolation in *IE* and a tamper-resistant *SEE* provides built-in guarantees to the owner against confidentiality attacks, out of reach of traditional approaches. Moreover, validating the approach in a highly constrained tamper-resistant environment like PlugDB is a proof of the simplicity of the reference monitor and of the associated administration tools. This simplicity also opens the way to a formal proof of the embedded code.

Performance. The Cozy queries executions are slowed down due to encryption and data communication. However, the overhead is kept reasonable for a regular use. This validates the practicality of the approach while large performance gains can be expected with environments providing higher communication throughput.

While the Personal Cloud paradigm is pushed by recent legislation and smart disclosure initiatives, finding new ways to intuitively and securely share personal data is paramount. We hope that this work actively contributes to this challenge.

References

1. Regulation (EU) 2016/679 of the European Parliament and of the Council of 27 April 2016 on the protection of natural persons with regard to the processing of personal data and on the free movement of such data
2. Abiteboul, S., André, B., Kaplan, D.: Managing your digital life. Commun. ACM (CACM) **58**(5), 32–35 (2015)
3. Bertino, E., Ghinita, G., Kamra, A.: Access control for databases: concepts and systems. Found. Trends Databases **3**(1–2), 1–148 (2011)
4. Bellavista, P., Giannelli, C., et al.: Peer-to-peer content sharing based on social identities and relationships. IEEE Internet Comput. **18**(3), 55–63 (2013)
5. Carminati, B., Ferrari, E., Perego, A.: Rule-based access control for social networks. In: Meersman, R., Tari, Z., Herrero, P. (eds.) OTM 2006. LNCS, vol. 4278, pp. 1734–1744. Springer, Heidelberg (2006). doi:10.1007/11915072_80
6. Van Kleek, M., Smith, D.A., Shadbolt, N., et al.: A decentralized architecture for consolidating personal information ecosystems: The WebBox. In: PIM (2012)
7. Wang, F., Mickens, J., Zeldovich, N., Vaikuntanathan, V.: Sieve: cryptographically enforced access control for user data in untrusted clouds. In: USENIX Symposium on Networked System Design and Implementation (2016)
8. Liu, Y., Gummadi, K.P., Krishnamurthy, B., Mislove, A.: Analyzing facebook privacy settings: user expectations vs. reality. In: Proceedings of ACM SIGCOMM Conference on Internet Measurement Conference, pp. 61–70 (2011)
9. Tran-Van, P., Anciaux, N., Pucheral, P.: A new sharing paradigm for the personal cloud. In: Lopez, J., Fischer-Hübner, S., Lambrinoudakis, C. (eds.) TrustBus 2017. LNCS, vol. 10442, pp. 180–196. Springer, Cham (2017). doi:10.1007/978-3-319-64483-7_12
10. Tran-Van, P., Anciaux, N., Pucheral, P.: SWYSWYK: a privacy-by-design paradigm for personal information management systems. In: To Appear at the 26th International Conference on Information Systems Development (2017)

11. Roth, M., Ben-David, A., Deutscher, D., Flysher, G., Horn, I., et al.: Suggesting friends using the implicit social graph. In: Proceedings of the 16th ACM SIGKDD International Conference on Knowledge Discovery and Data Mining, pp. 233–242 (2010)
12. Anciaux, N., Bouganim, L., Pucheral, P., Guo, Y., Le Folgoc, L., Yin, S.: MILo-DB: a personal, secure and portable database machine. Distrib. Parallel Databases **32**(1), 37–63 (2014)

Tools and Infrastructure for Supporting Enterprise Knowledge Graphs

Sumit Bhatia[1](✉), Nidhi Rajshree[2], Anshu Jain[2], and Nitish Aggarwal[2]

[1] IBM Research, New Delhi, India
sumitbhatia@in.ibm.com
[2] IBM Research, San Jose, USA
{nidhi.rajshree,anshu.n.jain}@us.ibm.com, nitish.aggarwal@ibm.com

Abstract. We demonstrate EKG, a collection of tools and back-end infrastructure for creating custom, domain specific knowledge graphs. The toolkit is geared toward enterprises and government organizations where domain specific knowledge graphs are often not available. During the demo, audience members will be able to ingest their own documents and instantiate their own knowledge graphs and update them in real time. We will also present a demo app built using the toolkit consisting of more than 30 million entities and 192 million edges in order to demonstrate the kind of applications that could be built using the proposed toolkit. The app can be used to answer questions like *who are the relevant persons named Steve in context of apple computers?*, or *who are the most important persons related to Barack Obama in context of healthcare reforms act?* The functionalities of the toolkit are also exposed through REST APIs making it easier for developers to use the capabilities in their own applications.

1 Introduction

Semantic Knowledge Bases such as Knowledge Graphs play a crucial role in modern day data and knowledge management applications by offering a consolidated, concise view of the knowledge present in diverse, and often unstructured data sources. While publicly available Knowledge bases such as DBPedia [1], Freebase [4], Yago [7], etc. have been used for various applications, they represent a generic view of the World and are not suitable for developing solutions to problems often encountered by enterprises and government organizations. For example, a pharmaceutical company may require a Knowledge Base representing interactions between gene, proteins, and drugs for accelerating drug development [6]. Development of such domain-specific enterprise knowledge graphs is expensive, time consuming and requires significant human efforts and domain expertise on part of developers. Further, enterprises often have to deal with a continuous incoming stream of new data and it is crucial that the underlying knowledge graphs are constantly updated to reflect this changing knowledge. In this demonstration, we demonstrate **EKG** – a suite of tools and back-end infrastructure to assist in development of such **E**nterprise **K**nowledge **G**raphs.

G. Cong et al. (Eds.): ADMA 2017, LNAI 10604, pp. 846–852, 2017.
https://doi.org/10.1007/978-3-319-69179-4_60

The proposed set of tools offers organizations *(i)* tools to extract entities and relationships of interest from unstructured documents using machine learning and rule based extractors; *(ii)* back-end infrastructure to store the extracted knowledge graph and associated metadata; *(iii)* mechanism to incrementally add to and update the graph as new documents become available; and *(iv)* API based access to a collection of analytic methods to query and retrieve the knowledge graph.

2 System Architecture

The major components of the proposed system are illustrated in Fig. 1 and are described in more detail in the following subsections.

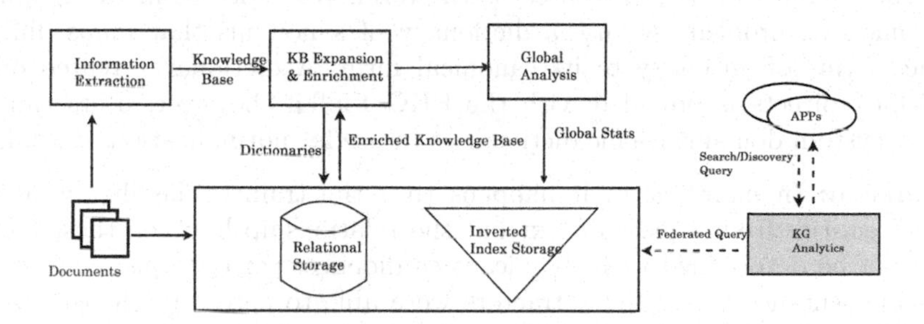

Fig. 1. System architecture

2.1 Information Extraction Module

The input to to the system is a collection of unstructured text documents that are processed via an information extraction pipeline that extracts entities and relationships between the entities. For this extraction, the system uses SIRE (**S**tatistical **I**nformation and **R**elation **E**xtraction) toolkit [5] that deploys a Maximum Entropy classifier using lexical, syntactic, and semantic features to extract entities and relationships from text. SIRE has been successfully used for information extraction in multiple domains such as news domain, healthcare, etc. Further, we also use SystemT[1], a declarative rules based information extraction system where the end-users can specify custom information extraction rules suitable for their domain of interest by using SystemT's Annotation Query Language (AQL).

2.2 Knowledge Expansion and Enrichment Pipeline

The baseline knowledge graph output by the information extraction pipeline is then passed through the following post-processing operations in the expansion and enrichment pipeline.

[1] https://en.wikipedia.org/wiki/IBM_SystemT.

Noise Removal: Since the entities and relationships are extracted automatically using trained classifiers and rules specified by SystemT, often there is some noise in the output such as entity names containing punctuation marks or other special characters due to errors in extraction (*Barack Obama, Steve Jobs,* etc.) Such errors are corrected using a set of replacement filters that use regular expressions to find and replace such errors. The system provides a set of about 800 filters for this task and users can either chose from them or specify custom regular expressions to suite their task.

Entity Normalization: It may happen that the same entity is mentioned by different synonymous surface forms in different documents that causes the same entity to be represented as different entities corresponding to different surface forms in the graph. For example, *Barack Obama*, *Barack H. Obama*, and *Barack Hussain Obama* can be represented as three different entities in the graph. To overcome this problem, we use a dictionary of synonyms that maps different surface forms of an entity to its canonical form. A dictionary created out of dbPedia redirects is provided with the EKG toolkit, however, users can also specify custom domain specific dictionaries to use for normalization, if available.

Expansion: In many cases, it happens that the trained classifier is able to extract entities from a piece of text but the relationship between these entities could not be determined with significant confidence. For example, consider the following sentence where the extractors were able to correctly identify *Obama* and *Hillary Clinton* as two entities, but failed to identify the relationship between them.

... In 2008, Obama was nominated for president, a year after his campaign began, and after a close primary campaign against Hillary Clinton ...

In such cases, the system creates a *colocation* relationship between the two identified entities and adds it to the graph. This expansion step is turned on by default to minimize the loss of useful information, however, users can turn this feature off if so desired.

2.3 Global Analysis

The enriched and expanded graph is then analyzed and several frequently required important statistics such as edge counts (number of times a relationship was observed), number of documents in which an entity or relationship was observed, etc. are computed. Further, we also compute a context model for each node (entity) in the graph. The context for an entity e consists of a language model approximated by all the terms surrounding the mentions of e in the text as well as a term vector consisting of all entity names connected with e in the graph. This context model provides an approximate representation of the *context* in which the entity e appears in the corpus. This context model is used by the analytics engine as described in Sect. 2.5.

2.4 Storage Back-End

The enriched and expanded graph along with pre-computed statistics and context models is then stored in a federated backend consisting of a *(i)* relational database to store the entity relationship tuples, optional domain-specific dictionaries provided by the user, and the global statistics as described above; and *(ii)* a SOLR[2] store to store the input text corpus and the context models for entities.

2.5 Analytics Engine

In addition to offering tools and infrastructure for creating and storing knowledge graphs, the EKG suite also offers a collection of methods for querying the graph for exploring entities and their relationships. Following are the major query APIs offered by the EKG toolkit.

Context Sensitive Entity Search: Given a query string and a few context terms, the API returns a ranked list of entities relevant in the given context. Due to the space constraints, we refer the reader to our previous work [3] where the probabilistic model for ranking entities in a given context has been described in detail. Further, the screenshots in Fig. 2 illustrate the different results produced with changing context for the same input token *larry*.

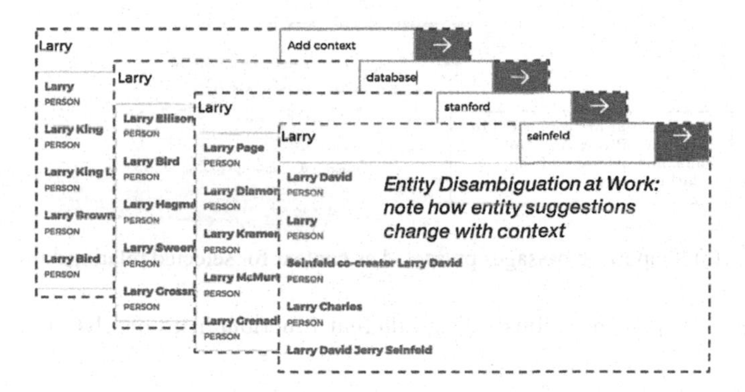

Fig. 2. Ranked list of relevant entities shown to the user under different contexts for the input token *larry*.

Relationship Search and Ranking: This API can be used to search for relationship information about one or more entities and to explore connections between different entities. The API offers different relationship search and ranking strategies to enable more fine-tuned entity exploration. For example, users can search for relationships of *Osama Bin laden* ranked by popularity, or they

[2] http://lucene.apache.org/solr/.

can perform a context sensitive relationship search for *Osama Bin laden* in context of *geronimo.* Figure 3 illustrate these examples. As can be noted in Fig. 3c, the users can also query and retrieve the supporting evidence for selected relationships. For details of the relationship search algorithms, we direct the reader to our previous work [2].

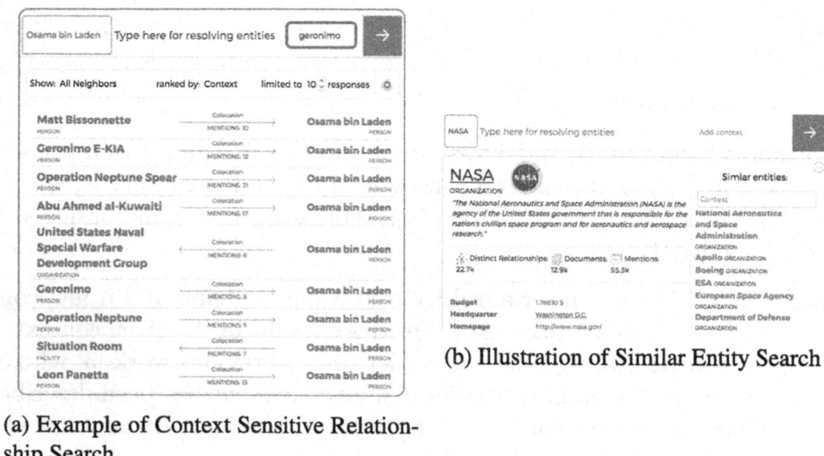

(a) Example of Context Sensitive Relationship Search

(b) Illustration of Similar Entity Search

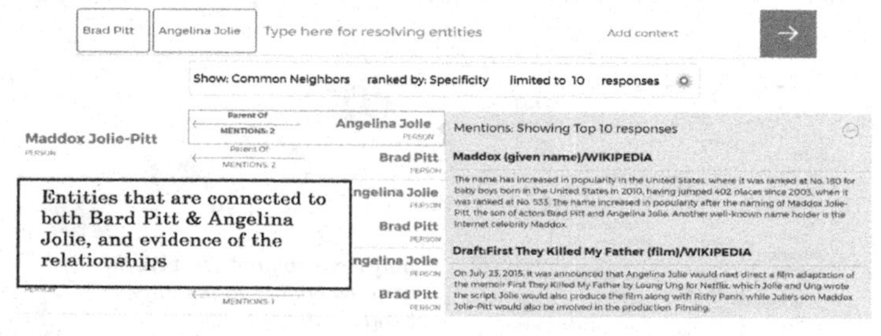

(c) Supporting passages presented as context for selected relationships

Fig. 3. Screenshots illustrating different functionalities of EKG toolkit.

Similar Entity Search: This API allows users to search for entities similar to a given entity and thus enables them to further their exploration. We use the context models for entities as described above to find entities that are observed in similar contexts in the input text corpus to determine similarity between two entities. Figure 3b illustrates the working of similar entity search with *NASA* as the input entity.

2.6 EKG REST APIs

All the operations that have been described above are exposed to the end-user through RESTful web service enabling end-users to ingest their own documents on demand, extract entities and relationships, create and update the knowledge graph, and query the graph using the analytics APIs. The organizations can thus set up their own custom knowledge graphs and incorporate this domain specific knowledge in multiple data and knowledge management applications, thereby reducing cost and complexity of enterprise knowledge management.

3 Demonstration Set Up and Requirements

We will demonstrate the capabilities of the EKG toolkit by means of a web service running on our organization's servers. We will only require a working internet connection to connect to our organization's VPN network to access the web service. Our demonstration will consist of two parts. In the first part, members of the audience will be able to ingest their own documents (text from a web page, or a passage typed by them) and create their own instances of knowledge graph representing knowledge extracted from their documents. We will show how the system is able to handle this on demand ingestion of documents and how the statistics and state of the graph is updated in real time, a crucial requirement for various organizations. Further, users will be able to play with all the functionalities like adding custom filters (Sect. 2.2) for data cleaning, and query APIs to see how to query the graph. For the second part, we will present a demo app using a knowledge graph constructed from text of all articles in Wikipedia. This graph contains more than 30 millions entities and 192 million distinct relationships in comparison to 4.5 million entities and 70 million relationships in DBpedia. Using this app, users will be able to query the graph and search for entities, relationships, and play with different search and ranking strategies as described in Sect. 2.5. The purpose of this app is to convey the capability of the proposed system to scale to graphs with tens of millions of nodes and edges, and thus, its suitability for organizations working with large amounts of data. Further, while the REST APIs are more geared towards app developers, a demo app also offers audience a visual means to explore and experiment with different functionalities offered by the proposed system.

4 Conclusion

We proposed to demonstrate the EKG toolkit that enables end-users to ingest their data, extract entities and relationships, and create knowledge graphs that could then be used in multiple knowledge management applications. Users can create custom annotators and can specify rules for information extraction using AQL and can also specify different post-processing rules for improving the quality of information extraction output. The proposed architecture is also optimized to handle incremental ingestion of data and offers a suite of query APIs that different apps can use to retrieve relevant information from the graph.

References

1. Auer, S., Bizer, C., Kobilarov, G., Lehmann, J., Cyganiak, R., Ives, Z.: DBpedia: a nucleus for a web of open data. In: Aberer, K., et al. (eds.) ASWC/ISWC 2007. LNCS, vol. 4825, pp. 722–735. Springer, Heidelberg (2007). doi:10.1007/978-3-540-76298-0_52
2. Bhatia, S., Goel, A., Bowen, E., Jain, A.: Separating wheat from the chaff – a relationship ranking algorithm. In: Sack, H., Rizzo, G., Steinmetz, N., Mladenić, D., Auer, S., Lange, C. (eds.) ESWC 2016. LNCS, vol. 9989, pp. 79–83. Springer, Cham (2016). doi:10.1007/978-3-319-47602-5_17
3. Bhatia, S., Jain, A.: Context sensitive entity linking of search queries in enterprise knowledge graphs. In: Sack, H., Rizzo, G., Steinmetz, N., Mladenić, D., Auer, S., Lange, C. (eds.) ESWC 2016. LNCS, vol. 9989, pp. 50–54. Springer, Cham (2016). doi:10.1007/978-3-319-47602-5_11
4. Bollacker, K., Evans, C., Paritosh, P., Sturge, T., Taylor, J.: Freebase: a collaboratively created graph database for structuring human knowledge. In: SIGMOD, pp. 1247–1250 (2008)
5. Castelli, V., Raghavan, H., Florian, R., Han, D.J., Luo, X., Roukos, S.: Distilling and exploring nuggets from a corpus. In: SIGIR, p. 1006 (2012)
6. Nagarajan, M., et al.: Predicting future scientific discoveries based on a networked analysis of the past literature. In: KDD 2015, pp. 2019–2028 (2015)
7. Suchanek, F.M., Kasneci, G., Weikum, G.: YAGO: a core of semantic knowledge. In: Proceedings of the 16th International Conference on World Wide Web, pp. 697–706. ACM (2007)

An Interactive Web-Based Toolset for Knowledge Discovery from Short Text Log Data

Michael Stewart[1(✉)], Wei Liu[1(✉)], Rachell Cardell-Oliver[1], and Mark Griffin[2]

[1] School of Computer Science and Software Engineering, The University of Western Australia, Perth, Australia
michael.stewart@research.uwa.edu.au, {wei.liu,rachel.cardell-oliver}@uwa.edu.au
[2] School of Management and Organisations, The University of Western Australia, Perth, Australia
mark.griffin@uwa.edu.au

Abstract. Many companies maintain human-written logs to capture data on events such as workplace incidents and equipment failures. However, the sheer volume and unstructured nature of this data prevent it from being utilised for knowledge acquisition. Our web-based prototype software system provides a cohesive computational methodology for analysing and visualising log data that requires minimal human involvement. It features an interface to support customisable, modularised log data processing and knowledge discovery. This enables owners of event-based datasets containing short textual descriptions, such as occupational health & safety officers and machine operators, to identify latent knowledge not previously acquirable without significant time and effort. The software system comprises five distinct stages, corresponding to standard data mining milestones: exploratory analysis, data warehousing, association rule mining, entity clustering, and predictive analysis. To the best of our knowledge, it is the first dedicated system to computationally analyse short text log data and provides a powerful interface that visualises the analytical results and supports human interaction.

Keywords: Knowledge discovery · Visualisation · Unstructured data mining

1 Introduction

Unstructured text is often included alongside structured data within company databases. In the mining industry, for example, written descriptions of accidents may be included alongside structured fields that hold information relating to the context of an accident. Examples of such a description are as follows:

`Upon exiting ute, IP tripped over wire and sprained left ankle.`
`Operator was traveling down the decline, travelled over a corragation and jared his back.`

G. Cong et al. (Eds.): ADMA 2017, LNAI 10604, pp. 853–858, 2017.
https://doi.org/10.1007/978-3-319-69179-4_61

Traditional data mining techniques often only focus on utilising numerical, ordinal and nominal data, i.e. structured fields such as dates, locations and age groups. Unstructured textual descriptions are often ignored. However, these textual descriptions contain a vast amount of invaluable information. By analysing these descriptions it may be possible to determine, for example, that loose wire on the ground is a common cause of sprained ankles. Employing data analysts to analyse log descriptions is an expensive undertaking that requires an immense amount of time, especially with large datasets.

Despite the urgent need for a system capable of analysing domain specific textual descriptions alongside the structured data, no such system exists to the best of our knowledge. Many general purpose text processing toolkits are available including programmable interfaces such as NLTK[1], Apache UIMA[2], and GATE[3]. However, these toolkits are not directly usable by domain experts. Moreover, to achieve better performance on short text, new algorithms need to be developed based on these APIs. Recently, many researchers have targeted the analysis of social media data [1], but log data has gone largely unnoticed even though it presents similar technical challenges.

In light of this, we present a web-based prototype that:

- Effectively processes log data to provide useful results that may be acted upon in the real world.
- Visualises the results as intuitively as possible so that they may be utilised by domain experts.

With a comprehensive interface the system is capable of customisable, modularised log data processing and knowledge discovery. New workflows can be built by turning on and off certain processing modules. Five primary tasks of data mining, namely exploratory analysis, data warehousing, association rule mining, entity clustering and predictive analysis are supported in the current prototype.

2 System Overview

Our system incorporates a number of data mining techniques in order to analyse and visualise log data. As shown in Fig. 1, upon receiving a new dataset, the system cleans the data and places it into a database. In addition, a knowledge base constructed by domain experts provides the concept hierarchies present within the data (such as entity categories).

The architecture of the system enables five key data mining techniques [2] to be performed. *Exploratory analysis* involves visualising the data so that domain experts may investigate the landscape of the data and gain insights prior to delving into more complex processing. *Data warehousing* consolidates further analysis by maintaining a concept hierarchy of the entities contained within

[1] NLTK. http://www.nltk.org/.
[2] Apache UIMA Project. https://uima.apache.org/.
[3] GATE. https://gate.ac.uk/.

the data. This stage determines which categories each of the entities within the data belong to. *Association rule mining* finds significant relationships between the categories within the data warehouse [3]. *Entity clustering* aims to cluster similar entities together, enabling the categorisation of new entities. Finally, *Predictive analysis* combines all of these techniques in order to make predictions about new data based on historical data. Examples of each analytical stage are described with further details and screenshots in Sect. 3.2.

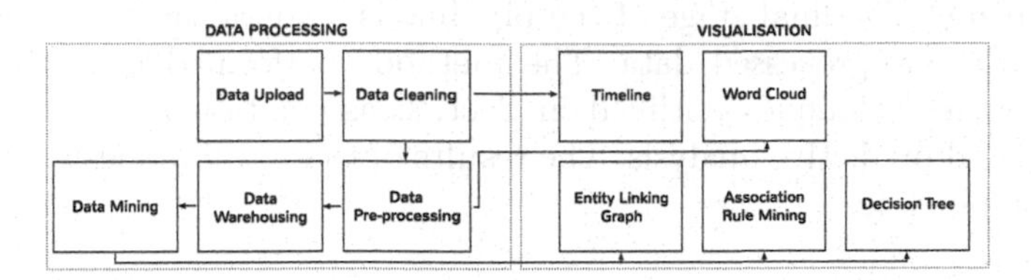

Fig. 1. The system architecture of our prototype implementation.

3 Prototype Description

The dataset used in our prototype tracks workplace accidents in the mining industry by storing textual descriptions alongside structured fields. The system is currently hosted on Nectar[4], a cloud-based hosting platform.

3.1 Data Processing

The data processing functionality is written in Python 2.7. All natural-language based tasks such as tokenisation, POS-tagging and noun-phrase chunking are performed using NLTK[5].

Data Upload. The first stage in the pipeline is an interface for uploading data. Data owners may use this web-based interface to submit their dataset to the server, which sends the dataset through the pipeline.

Data Cleaning. The next step is to clean the uploaded data so that the effectiveness of downstream analysis is maximised. The system performs lexical normalisation, which aims to correct every non-standard word in a dataset to its canonical form [4].

Data Pre-processing. This component transforms the data into an appropriate representation for the data warehousing system. This involves using several natural language processing techniques, including tokenisation, POS tagging, noun-phrase chunking and entity recognition. The output of this component is suitable for analysis/visualisation by several of the later pipeline components.

[4] Nectar. https://nectar.org.au/research-cloud/.
[5] NLTK. http://www.nltk.org/.

Data Warehousing. The data warehousing component utilises the user-specified, domain-dependent concept hierarchy to classify entities into different categories. The concept hierarchy enables categories to act as subclasses of other categories, such as `leg` being a subclass of `body_part`. The entity recognition performed within this stage forms the basis for the data mining techniques present in subsequent stage of the pipeline.

Data Mining. The final stage of the pipeline is to perform data mining techniques on the pre-processed data. The methods performed here directly correspond to the techniques outlined in Sect. 2: association rule mining, entity clustering, and predictive analysis. The results of these techniques are visualised later in the pipeline.

3.2 Visualisation

Our system is visualised through an interactive web-based application. It is written in Node.js. The majority of the visualisations were implemented in D3.js[6]. Several visualisations utilised jsTree[7]. The Word Cloud visualisation made use of d3-cloud[8], and the Decision Tree visualisation was created using treant.js[9].

Timeline for Exploratory Data Analysis. The first visualisation generated by the system after receiving a new dataset is an expandable and collapsible Timeline, shown in Fig. 2a. This component creates a histogram-like chart which plots the number of events per day against the days of the year.

Each dot represents a data record. The details of the record are available when the mouse is hovering over a dot. The colour of the dot in our example represents the severity of injury. Users may aggregate the data based on weeks, months, or years, simulating drill-down/roll-up operations native to online analytical processing (OLAP) systems.

The main purpose of this visualisation is to facilitate exploratory analysis by allowing users to quickly view the data in a temporal format.

Word Cloud. The Word Cloud enables users to quickly view the noun phrases and relation phrases within their dataset. Phrases that are more common than others appear larger in the visualisation. In order to display the phrases in the word cloud, the dataset is first processed using natural language processing techniques including tokenisation and noun and relation phrase chunking.

Like the timeline, this visualisation also facilitates exploratory analysis. From the word cloud, domain experts can easily see that the main focus of these logs is on `Injured Person`. `Operator`, `worker`, `employee` and `pain` are also important terms in our dataset.

---

[6] D3.js. https://d3js.org/.
[7] jsTree. https://www.jstree.com/.
[8] D3 Cloud. https://github.com/jasondavies/d3-cloud.
[9] Treant-js. https://github.com/fperucic/treant-js.

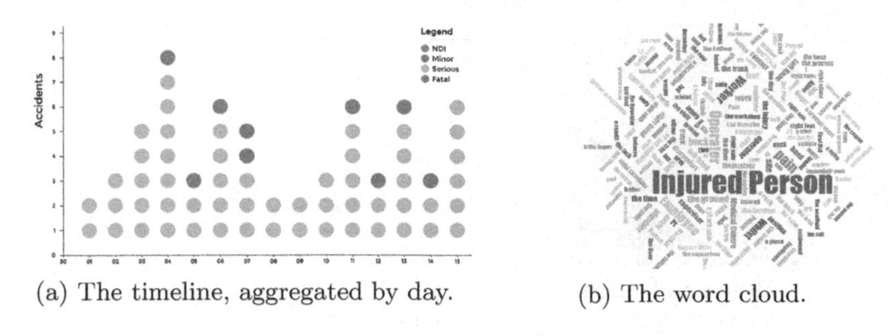

(a) The timeline, aggregated by day. (b) The word cloud.

Fig. 2. The exploratory analysis visualisations.

Association Rule Mining. The association rule mining visualisation simply visualises the results obtained by the respective technique. These results may be filtered so that only rules pertaining to a particular entity appear. This enables users to focus on uncovering information relating to a particular entity.

The colours of each entity in the visualisation represent the base entity classes in the data, as specified by domain experts. Every member of a concept tree (such as `back`, `neck` and `arm`) appear with the same colour in the visualisation. At this stage the entities are determined using a dictionary-based method, which tags entities directly matching any category in the concept hierarchy. In the future we aim to use entity recognition in order to provide better results.

As an example, the highest-ranked rule in our dataset states that whenever the entities `operator`, `serious` and `haul_truck` appear in the same record, there is a 62.5% chance that the record will also contain the entities `neck` and `back`. In other words, operators of haul trucks involved in serious injuries are likely to injure their neck and/or back.

Entity Linking Graph. The entity linking graph, as shown in Fig. 3, displays the links between entities in the data. Every entity in the concept hierarchy is represented by a node, and entities within the same concept tree are clustered together. Entities that are considered by the system to be "linked" (i.e. the entities that co-occur in the same record) are connected by an edge. The weight of each edge is the number of times two distinct entities are connected.

Domain experts are able to conduct more detailed analysis by clicking on an entity node and holding down the mouse button. This hides any nodes not linked to the selected entity, as shown in Fig. 3b. The user may, for example, select the `Haul_truck` entity and can easily view the entities related to it.

The strength of this visualisation lies in its ability to facilitate knowledge discovery by domain experts. By interacting with the visualisation it is possible to quickly discover links between entities that were previously obscured by the sheer volume of text in the original dataset.

Decision Tree. The final visualisation is the decision tree. The goal of this component is to provide a means for users to conduct predictive analysis.

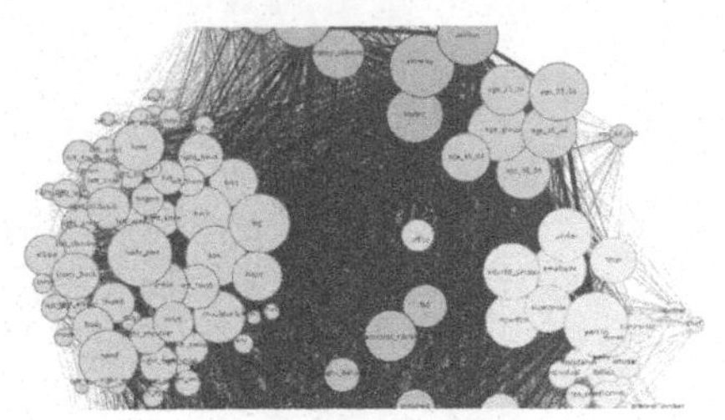

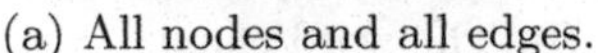

(a) All nodes and all edges.

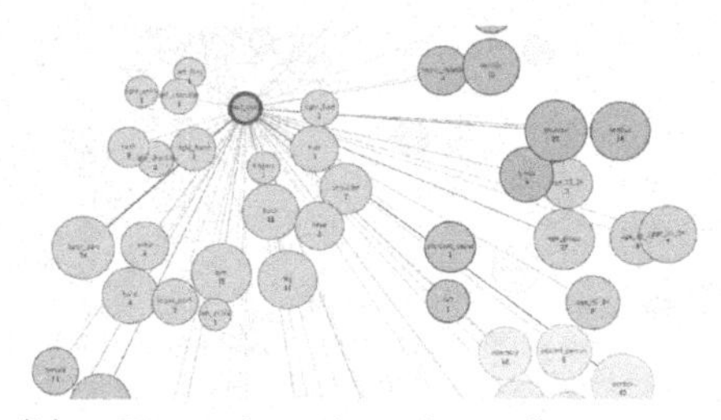

(b) User-selected node and its associates.

Fig. 3. The entity linking graph visualisation.

In the future, this component will allow users to upload new data to see how it is classified by the tree. For example, a user may upload a potential accident description to see how likely it is to result in a serious injury.

4 Conclusion

In this paper we present a prototype system that effectively processes log data and visualises the results as clearly as possible. We have introduced a web-based toolset for knowledge discovery from log data. Our system processes data using a number of data mining techniques, and features an interactive user interface that allows domain experts to easily analyse their data. This system enables owners of log data, such as occupational health & safety officers and machine operators, to quickly identify latent knowledge in their data that was not previously acquirable.

Acknowledgements. This research was funded by an Australian Postgraduate Award Scholarship and a UWA Safety Net Top-up Scholarship.

References

1. Baldwin, T., Kim, Y.B., de Marneffe, M.C., Ritter, A., Han, B., Xu, W.: Shared tasks of the 2015 workshop on noisy user-generated text: twitter lexical normalization and named entity recognition. In: ACL-IJCNLP 2015, vol. 126 (2015)
2. Han, J., Pei, J., Kamber, M.: Data Mining: Concepts and Techniques. Elsevier, New York (2011)
3. Agrawal, R., Imieliński, T., Swami, A.: Mining association rules between sets of items in large databases. ACM Sigmod Rec. **22**, 207–216 (1993). ACM
4. Sproat, R., Black, A.W., Chen, S., Kumar, S., Ostendorf, M., Richards, C.: Normalization of non-standard words. Comput. Speech Lang. **15**(3), 287–333 (2001)

Carbon: Forecasting Civil Unrest Events by Monitoring News and Social Media

Wei Kang[1(✉)], Jie Chen[1], Jiuyong Li[1], Jixue Liu[1], Lin Liu[1], Grant Osborne[2], Nick Lothian[2], Brenton Cooper[2], Terry Moschou[2], and Grant Neale[2]

[1] University of South Australia, Mawson Lakes, SA 5095, Australia
{wei.kang,jie.chen,jiuyong.li,jixue.liu,lin.liu}@unisa.edu.au

[2] Data to Decisions CRC, Kent Town, SA 5067, Australia
{grant.osborne,nick.lothian,brenton.cooper,terry.moschou, grant.neale}@d2dcrc.com.au

Abstract. Societal security has been receiving unprecedented attention over the past decade because of the ubiquity of online public data sources. Much research effort has been taken to detect relevant societal issues. However, forecasting them is more challenging but greatly beneficial to the entire society. In this paper, we present a forecasting system named Carbon to predict civil unrest events, e.g., protests and strikes. Two predictive models are implemented and scheduled to make predictions periodically. One model forecasts through the analysis of historical civil unrest events reported by news portals, while the other functions by detecting and integrating early clues from social media contents. With our web UI and visualisation, users can easily explore the predicted events and their spatiotemporal distribution. The demonstration will exemplify that Carbon can greatly benefit the society such that the general public can be alerted in advance to avoid potential dangers and that the authorities can take proactive actions to alleviate tensions and reduce possible damage to the society.

Keywords: Civil unrest · Predictive models · Open source data

1 Introduction

Societal security has great impact on daily lives of the public and the stability of a society. Great attention has been paid to security incidents thanks to instant news reports and the widespread use of social media. Nowadays, people can read "hot-off-the-press" emergency reports instantly via online news portals, while social media users can even smell the emergence of incidents earlier before their occurrences. Much effort has been invested in detecting events or generating summaries from social media data [4–6,8]. Compared with detecting, however, forecasting them could be much more desirable, as it allows the public to be alerted prior to dangers and enables the authorities to take proactive actions to alleviate tensions and minimise disruption. Some researchers tried to make forecasts with public data to predict crowd behavior [3]. Researchers from Virginia

G. Cong et al. (Eds.): ADMA 2017, LNAI 10604, pp. 859–865, 2017.
https://doi.org/10.1007/978-3-319-69179-4_62

Tech has built EMBERS to forecast civil unrest events such as protests in 10 Latin American countries [1,7]. As an intelligence project supported by IARPA[1], other than the published papers, however, plenty of details of EMBERS are still unclear and kept confidential, and the system is not accessible by external users. Besides, it focuses on forecasting only for Latin American countries.

In this paper, we have built a system named Carbon to forecast civil unrest events for Australia and some other Asia-Pacific countries by monitoring and analysing news and social media. To process millions of civil unrest related documents each day, Carbon has been built on Apache Spark[2] to provide real-time and scalable data processing, analysing and event forecasting. Note that civil unrest forecasting is more challenging for Asia-Pacific countries, esp. Australia, where such events are often less frequent and on smaller scales. To tackle the challenges, we propose a novel and effective time-series model and improve the planed protest model in EMBERS for fine-grained predictions.

Carbon ingests open source data, mainly news articles and Twitter/Facebook streams, to capture precursory clues for civil unrest events. Our news analysts search through popular news portals every day and take down reported civil unrest events as Gold Standard Records (GSRs), which are then used as the ground truth to build and evaluate our models. Each GSR represents a reported event, e.g., a protest, with attributes such as the event date, reported date, location, predefined event type (e.g., political or economic issues), predefined population group (e.g., education, labor) and description. We also purchase Twitter data from GNIP[3] continuously to avoid the Twitter API rate limits and to collect as much civil unrest related data as possible to enhance the predictiveness of our system. Carbon is currently aimed at Australia and nearby countries. However, with our generic system design and solutions, it can be easily extended to other regions.

To predict civil unrest events, we propose a GSR based model which utilises underlying patterns of historical GSRs, and another model which leverages civil unrest indicators extracted from social media streams. These models are designed to work complementarily. That is, the GSR based model makes use of evolutionary features of different types of historical events, and the other model analyses social media precursory clues. We notice that, although some events can be predicted by both models, most of them are captured by one model only, indicating that the two models can complement each other to provide a greater coverage.

Since predictions are made to forecast future events, the evaluation of the predictions cannot be conducted until GSRs are collected for the corresponding predicted time period. A background job is scheduled weekly in Carbon to evaluate the precision and recall of those predictions. A prediction is considered correct only if all its attributes (mainly the date or time range, location, event type and population group) match the corresponding attributes of some GSR within the examined time period. In addition, we compute a lead time for

[1] https://www.iarpa.gov/.
[2] http://spark.apache.org/.
[3] https://gnip.com/.

each true prediction, i.e., how many days in advance the prediction is produced before the corresponding event is reported on news portals. The quantitative experimental results are summarised in Table 1.

The targeted audience includes both the public and authorities, who will have a deeper understanding of the importance of a civil unrest forecasting system to the maintenance of the security and stability of a society. We will demonstrate how to explore the predictions through a web UI with three views, i.e., the Predictions List showing recent predictions with details such as model name, generation/predicted event date, location, probability, supporting evidence, etc., and the Predictions Map and Timeline which visualise the geographical and temporal distribution of the predictions respectively.

Our major contributions include: (1) we have built a system which forecasts rather than detects civil unrest events for countries where civil unrest events are less frequent; (2) we have introduced two predictive models which make use of different types of knowledge (i.e., evolutionary trends and social media precursory clues of civil unrest events respectively) and work complementarily; (3) the predictions are of great value for the benefit of both the general public and the authorities.

2 System Architecture

As is shown in Fig. 1, the architecture of Carbon consists of three major components – the data storage, the data processing and modelling, and the Carbon UI. The data processing and modelling component in the middle is the core of Carbon. Spark jobs are scheduled and submitted periodically to perform day-to-day operations, such as continual ingestion of open source data, data enrichment and feature extraction (including the inference of Twitter/Facebook users' locations based on their profiles and check-ins, the conversion of a relative day, e.g., next Monday, to an absolute date, etc.), inverted index building and so on.

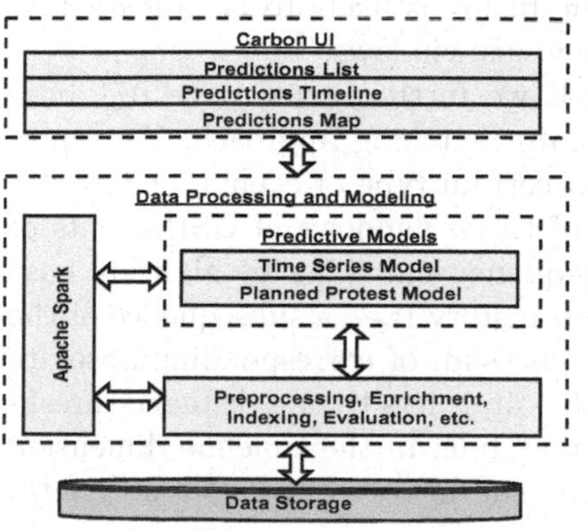

Fig. 1. Architecture of Carbon

Table 1. Experimental results

Model	Precision	Recall	Lead time
Time-series or TS (0/1)	0.42	0.27	5
TS (approx.)	0.42	0.55	5
TS (1 month)	0.8	0.52	5
PPM	0.38	0.94	9

The predictive models which are designed to work complementarily are submitted to run at regular intervals by a scheduler. The output predictions are stored in the database and presented in the web UI, and will be scheduled later for evaluation when GSRs are gleaned for the predicted time period.

3 Predictive Models

3.1 Time-Series Model

The time-series model predicts the future by leveraging both historical evolutionary patterns and recent trends of events. It first sorts the GSR events ranging from t_{start} to t_{end} in chronological order, and divides them into equally sized (e.g., one week long) windows $w_1, w_2, ..., w_n$ such that each window contains events falling in the corresponding time range. With the n windows, our aim is to predict whether certain events will happen in window w_{n+1} by exploring historical events based on a group of base patterns. A base pattern is produced by examining GSR events in a few, say 3, recent windows to capture the latest trends of a certain type of events. For instance, if a series of protests was about immigration officers calling for higher salary and it happened in windows w_{n-2} and w_n but not w_{n-1}, we can derive a time-series base pattern $(1, 0, 1)$, where 1 indicates the occurrence of a protest in corresponding windows and 0 otherwise, to capture recent trend of this type of protests. To make predictions, we need to generate all possible base patterns in recent windows. Once having the base patterns ready, we then scan GSR events window by window to figure out the number of occurrences of the same patterns in history. For each base pattern *bp*, we obtain the numbers of cases that the same type of events happened or did not happen respectively in the subsequent window when there are consecutive windows matching *bp* in history, and then estimate the probability of the corresponding event to happen in window w_{n+1}. We have adopted the idea of higher order Markov chains in this model, meaning the prediction of w_{n+1} depends on multiple precedent windows $w_n, w_{n-1}, ...$ instead of only the most recent window w_n because the occurrence of an event in the future is likely to be triggered by similar events that happened in multiple previous windows.

To enhance the sensitivity of the model, we further extend the 0/1 base pattern matching approach to an approximate matching approach. We represent a base pattern using the frequency of a certain type of events, $(1, 0, 4)$ for instance, to match against the frequencies of the n windows of GSR events of the same type. We support approximate frequency matching by allowing base pattern $(1, 0, 4)$ to be matched with some sub-history (i.e., a subsequence of the GSR history), say $(..., 2, 0, 5, ...)$, as long as the sum of corresponding absolute frequency differences, i.e., $|2-1| + |0-0| + |5-4|$, is less than a distance threshold. Besides, we also support approximate matching in the timeline dimension by allowing $(1, 0, 4)$ to be matched with some sub-history of a different length, say $(..., 2, 0, 0, 5, ...)$. A combined difference is computed and compared with the threshold to take into account the differences in both the frequency and timeline dimensions, which provides a fine-grained comparison between a base pattern and sub-histories by matching their signal strengths and durations with certain tolerance.

As shown in Table 1, the experimental study has verified that the approximate matching approach can significantly improve the average recall. As a trade-off, if we gradually expand the prediction time window from one week to one month, the average precision will continuously increase to 0.8 while the average recall slightly drops to 0.52.

3.2 Two-Phase Planed Protest Model

Although most types of events occur from time to time, there are still certain types which never appeared before or cannot be modelled by the GSR based model. As such, we have also introduced a *two-phase* planned protest model (PPM) which clusters social media textual data to generate predictions with strong evidence. Our PPM is an extension of the planned protest model in [7] to overcome the difficulty in distinguishing different predictions generated for the same location and event date.

PPM applies two clustering phases over the indicators, which are the enriched data containing the original contents (e.g., Tweets) and inferred phrase lists. A list often contains seed keywords and related lemmas (e.g., "good" is the lemma of "better"), inferred future dates and locations. The indicators are filtered to English only, and binned into date and location groups. In the first phase, we extract cleaned (i.e., with unicode symbols, RT blocks, quotes, etc. removed) textual Tweet features first and maintain them using a token/count vectoriser. Next, we estimate an epsilon density measure using a nearest neighbour max absolute distance and apply it in DBSCAN [2] to cluster Tweet based indicators whose textual contents are similar. In the second phase, we add new data sources (e.g., Facebook URLs) to existing Tweet clusters based on the URLs contained in the Tweets, and merge related Tweet clusters together if they all reference the same URL (e.g., a news article). In the end, these clustered indicators are output as predictions if they cross over a configurable threshold. The performance of PPM can be found in the last row of Table 1.

4 Demonstration

In the demonstration, we will exhibit Carbon, our civil unrest forecasting system, which has been producing predictions since June 2016. We will elaborate the system design, predictive models and predictions, such that users can obtain an in-depth understanding of how the system effectively generates predictions and why the predictions it produces can greatly benefit the society.

We will also introduce the system interface, where we provide user admin functions to grant proper privileges to a new user. Users can log in to see the main interface (cf. external snapshots[4]), where on the left panel users can click

[4] https://www.dropbox.com/s/7pwjnj97r46abmo/carbonUI.pdf?dl=0.

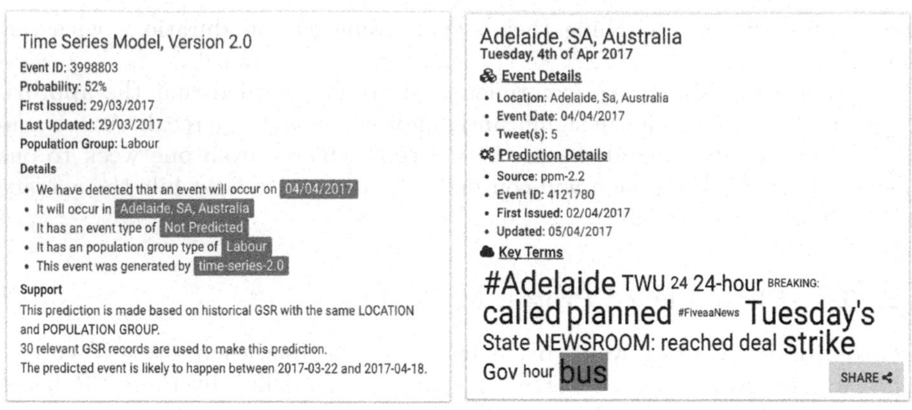
Time Series Model, Version 2.0
Event ID: 3998803
Probability: 52%
First Issued: 29/03/2017
Last Updated: 29/03/2017
Population Group: Labour
Details
We have detected that an event will occur on 04/04/2017
It will occur in Adelaide, SA, Australia
It has an event type of Not Predicted
It has an population group type of Labour
This event was generated by time-series-2.0
Support
This prediction is made based on historical GSR with the same LOCATION and POPULATION GROUP.
30 relevant GSR records are used to make this prediction.
The predicted event is likely to happen between 2017-03-22 and 2017-04-18.
Adelaide, SA, Australia
Tuesday, 4th of Apr 2017
Event Details
Location: Adelaide, Sa, Australia
Event Date: 04/04/2017
Tweet(s): 5
Prediction Details
Source: ppm-2.2
Event ID: 4121780
First Issued: 02/04/2017
Updated: 05/04/2017
Key Terms
#Adelaide TWU 24 24-hour BREAKING:
called planned #FiveaaNews Tuesday's
State NEWSROOM: reached deal strike
Gov hour bus
SHARE

(a) Prediction issued by Time-series Model (b) Prediction issued by PPM

Fig. 2. Example predictions

on one of the three views, i.e., the Predictions List, Map and Timeline, while on the right details of the selected view will be presented. At the top of each view is a section where users can specify a time range and choose one or both of the models to explore the predicted events.

The Predictions List displays the detailed predictions which are likely to happen in the coming few weeks in chronological order. As an example, Fig. 2 shows two predictions, issued by the time-series and PPM models respectively, regarding the same bus drivers strike planned for 4 April 2017 in Adelaide. It was reported on 1 April that up to 50,000 commuters would face great chaos after bus drivers voted for a 24-hour strike, which could halt a third of Adelaide Metro bus services[5]. The time-series model issued the prediction on 29 March, 6 days before the planned strike, based on 30 historical GSRs, and predicted "labour" as its population group which referred to the bus drivers. Meanwhile, the PPM model also predicted the same event on 2 April based on 5 Tweets, from which keywords were extracted and visualised in word cloud. Although the strike was called off owing to an in-principle agreement between the bus service operator and the workers union right before it was about to take place, similar events are not always avoidable. Had the strike happened, great chaos could hit the city, let alone the possibility that it might have triggered conflicts and other violent events. Therefore, forecasting strikes and other civil unrest events can be vital and greatly beneficial to the public and authorities for them to take proactive actions to avoid possible loss and disruption.

Different from the List view, the Predictions Map and Timeline views integrate multiple predictions and visualise their spatiotemporal distributions over a map and a histogram timeline. By hovering the mouse over a circle on the map or a bar in the timeline, users will see integrated information about a

[5] http://www.adelaidenow.com.au/news/south-australia/09a3a63b361a785fabc949828148025e.

location/date, including the number of predictions, their corresponding models and probabilities. Users can gain insight into safety condition of different places by observing the distribution of reported and predicted civil unrest events. The observations could serve as guidance for travel planning.

References

1. Doyle, A., Katz, G., Summers, K., Ackermann, C., Zavorin, I., Lim, Z., Muthiah, S., Zhao, L., Lu, C.T., Butler, P., et al.: The EMBERS architecture for streaming predictive analytics. In: IEEE BigData, pp. 11–13 (2014)
2. Ester, M., Kriegel, H., Sander, J., Xu, X.: A density-based algorithm for discovering clusters in large spatial databases with noise. In: SIGKDD, pp. 226–231 (1996)
3. Kallus, N.: Predicting crowd behavior with big public data. In: WWW, pp. 625–630 (2014)
4. Kang, W., Tung, A.K., Chen, W., Li, X., Song, Q., Zhang, C., Zhao, F., Zhou, X.: Trendspedia: an internet observatory for analyzing and visualizing the evolving web. In: ICDE, pp. 1206–1209 (2014)
5. Kang, W., Tung, A.K., Zhao, F., Li, X.: Interactive hierarchical tag clouds for summarizing spatiotemporal social contents. In: ICDE, pp. 868–879 (2014)
6. Nguyen, D.T., Jung, J.J.: Real-time event detection on social data stream. Mob. Netw. Appl. **20**(4), 475–486 (2015)
7. Ramakrishnan, N., Butler, P., Muthiah, S., Self, N., Khandpur, R., Saraf, P., Wang, W., Cadena, J., Vullikanti, A., Korkmaz, G., et al.: 'Beating the news' with EMBERS: forecasting civil unrest using open source indicators. In: SIGKDD, pp. 1799–1808 (2014)
8. Zhou, X., Chen, L.: Event detection over twitter social media streams. VLDB J. **23**(3), 381–400 (2014)

A System for Querying and Analyzing Urban Regions

Wee Boon Koh(✉) and Xiaolei Li(✉)

School of Computer Science and Engineering, Nanyang Technological University, Singapore, Singapore
wkoh014@e.ntu.edu.sg, lixl@ntu.edu.sg

Abstract. We develop a new interactive visualization system to support the visualization of different aspects of a region as well as querying and analyzing similar land uses. The main contributions of this work include an urban region query framework and an analysis of using the social media and traditional census data to identify similar areas. Two example potential applications of our system are given as follows: (1) Our system can be employed by city planners to analyze and observe identical land uses, assisting them in making development objectives; (2) Our system can also be used by business owners to observe similar urban regions for potential areas of expansion.

Keywords: Urban analytics · Smart city · Urban systems · Similarity measures

1 Introduction

Effective land use planning is essential for countries where land is scarce. In most of such countries, residential zones are composed of high-rise buildings with a mixture of different functional facilities and spaces. Budget is another important consideration for land use planning. Intuitively, a multi-storey building costs much more than a single floor house due to the materials and time required to construct. Given the budget limitation, it is unfeasible to put all the development efforts into a single neighbourhood. On the other hand, an evenly distributed development effort may have a negative impact on the neighbourhoods that require more attention. A more appropriate solution is to analyze all neighbourhoods and focus the development efforts on areas that are less matured and have room for expansion. One traditional way of analyzing these neighbourhoods include observing the population census in each area. However, the information provided by existing systems on the market is often limited and they usually only provide basic reporting purposes. In the era of the big data, it is desirable to be able to analyze these neighbourhoods using a combination of data related to these areas. For example, a city planner might want to know whether there are sufficient health care facilities in a neighbourhood where most residents are elderly. In such cases, a ratio of elderly and health care facilities in a neighbourhood can be used as an indication.

G. Cong et al. (Eds.): ADMA 2017, LNAI 10604, pp. 866–871, 2017.
https://doi.org/10.1007/978-3-319-69179-4_63

From a commercial perspective, it is also essential for business owners to understand the demographics of a neighbourhood. For example, a restaurant owner might want to open a shop in a neighbourhood with demographics that best fit his target market. Similarly, a business owner might want to open additional shops in similar neighbourhoods. An urban region query system can allow these business owners to analyze and query for these demographics and use it as an indicator for the potential areas to open new shops.

Objectives. We expect that our urban region query system can be used for different purposes. Therefore, instead of adopting a rigid way of measuring the similarity of urban regions, we propose a flexible way of computing the similarity. Many factors may affect the results that are perceived as relevant by a user. For example, two regions may be similar in terms of the population demographics but dissimilar in terms of the facilities. It is essential for the urban region query system to be able to customize the aspects of an urban region for similarity computation when identifying similar regions.

The objective of this work is to come up with an urban region query system that is able to find similar areas and provide analysis on the result. In particular, the first objective is to address how to query similar urban land regions. The second objective is to analyze the different aspects of urban land regions that make them similar to one another.

Contributions. The first contribution of this work is the query framework to identify similar urban regions. In this work, we consider several aspects of an urban region for measuring the similarity of two regions and we use a weight-based approach to measure similarity. This is the first work that considers the different aspects and measures the similarity of regions from the urban region search perspective. The intuition for doing so is that individual users have different views on whether two urban regions are similar, which is often based on the single or multiple aspects of that area. In this work, the main technical challenge is to find the appropriate data points in one group to compare with another. For example, we use topic models to mine topics for each region, where each generated topic is represented by a distribution over words. However, the topics generated for different distributions are likely to be different. For any two regions, we use the most similar topic terms in each topic found in each region to compare two topics of two regions.

The second contribution is the analysis of the suitability of urban and social media data for region similarity. In this work, we propose that geospatial social media data, such as geotagged tweets, can be used to identify similar urban land regions.

2 Related Work

There are many forms of urban data. One such example is the census. However, there has been an increasing number of studies that circle around the use of urban and geospatial social media data in recent years, such as the taxi trips data [5], Sina Weibo data [1], Foursquare data [4] and tweets [6]. There also exist studies [2,3] that focus on data collection from a controlled environment and may not necessarily be sufficient to justify their analysis in urban settings. Another observation made from these studies is the possibility of including social media data in city planning and policy making. However, analysis of a single urban data like taxi trips would be limited. A more desirable approach will be to combine multiple data sources for analysis.

There also exist work on searching a region based on user queries, such as the work [7]. Our problem is different in that we aim to search similar regions for a given region.

3 System Design

We collected four types of data for this work. The first dataset consists of the 2,938 region boundaries from city planners in Singapore. The second set of data consists of 5,040,007 tweets gathered between 24th June 2014 and 21st September 2015 in Singapore. The third set of data contains 15,864 points of interests (POI) in Singapore. The last set of data consists of the population census by age and gender for each of the region planned by the city planners.

A region is similar to another in many different ways. Moreover, the similarity level is perceived differently by individuals. Therefore, this work proposes a weight-based query framework as illustrated in Fig. 1.

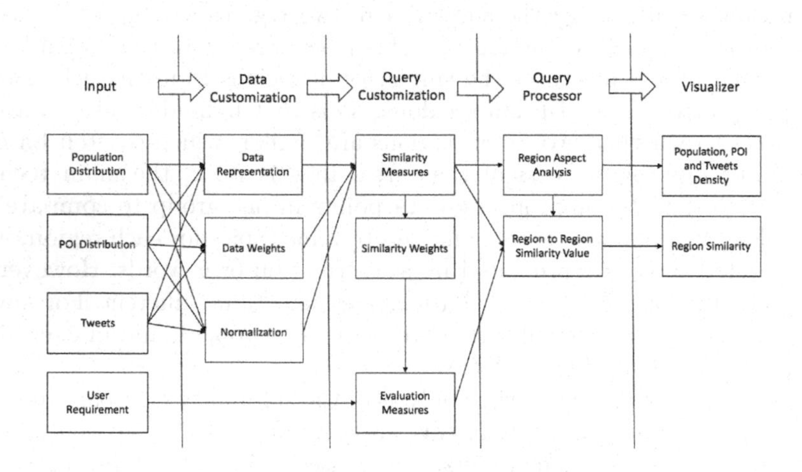

Fig. 1. Proposed query framework

The proposed framework places emphasis on the flexibility of allowing users to customize their queries. We assume that users of our system have sufficient knowledge on the different similarity measures and their limitations. With that knowledge, it is possible for users to assign weights to different aspects of measuring region similarity such that the similarity function fits their requirement.

In the query framework, users can assign weights to different aspects of a region. The idea behind is that a user may want to place emphasis on certain aspect during a query. In this work, we consider three aspects of a region, namely, tweets, POI and the population. The weight-based similarity measure formula, for considering two aspects of a region, is shown in Eq. 1. If there are more than two aspects, the user will be required to set additional weights $w_1, w_2, \ldots, w_k$ where k is the number of aspects and $\sum_{i=1}^{k} w_i = 1$.

$$Sim(a_i, a_j) = w_1(Sim1(a_{i_1}, a_{j_1})) + (1 - w_1)(Sim2(a_{i_2}, a_{j_2})) \tag{1}$$

- w_1 is a user-defined parameter for the first similarity measure
- A is the collection of all the regions, $a_i, a_j \in$ A
- a_{i_1} and a_{j_1} are 1st aspect of the region i and j
- a_{i_2} and a_{j_2} are 2nd aspect of the region i and j
- Sim1 refers to the first similarity measure
- Sim2 refers to the second similarity measure

To evaluate the effectiveness of the query, users are asked to annotate the relevancy of the results generated by the system. This is achieved by asking users to give a score between 0 to 5, where 0 is not relevant and 5 for most relevant, for each aspect for each result returned by the system. This list is stored and used to evaluate similar future queries from the same user. The two evaluation measures used in this work are nDCG and precision. Two observations were made from our experiments. Firstly, combining topic aspects of tweets with the POI or the population aspect will give higher precision and nDCG values than if only either was considered. Secondly, the average precision and nDCG values are the highest when considering all three aspects.

The system integrates multiple commonly used commercial platforms and libraries. This is to widen the number of potential user groups. The developed system demonstrates the use of R scripts in the proposed query framework with a scalable non-SQL JSON-based database, MongoDB. In addition, the system

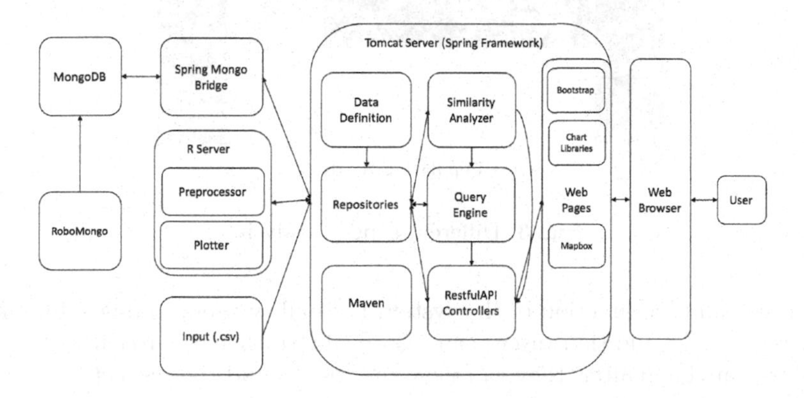

Fig. 2. System architecture

uses Maven and Spring framework for quick deployment and development. The web interface is developed using the Bootstrap responsive framework to allow users to use the system on devices of varying screen sizes. For visualization, the system uses the Chart.js library for interactive charts. Lastly, MapBox and Leaflet libraries are used for plotting updated urban maps. The architecture of the system is shown in Fig. 2.

4 System Functions

The first core function of the system is the analysis of different aspects of an urban region. For example, suppose geotagged tweets are used as an indicator for similar urban regions. In this case, it may be desirable to display the terms and topic distributions in that region. On the population census perspective, especially for the aging population, it may be essential for city planners to know the ratio of health care facilities to the number of elderly in the region. For growing population, the ratio of educational facilities to the number of schooling teens should also be considered. Figure 3 shows the screen shots of the system showing the analysis for three different aspects of an urban region.

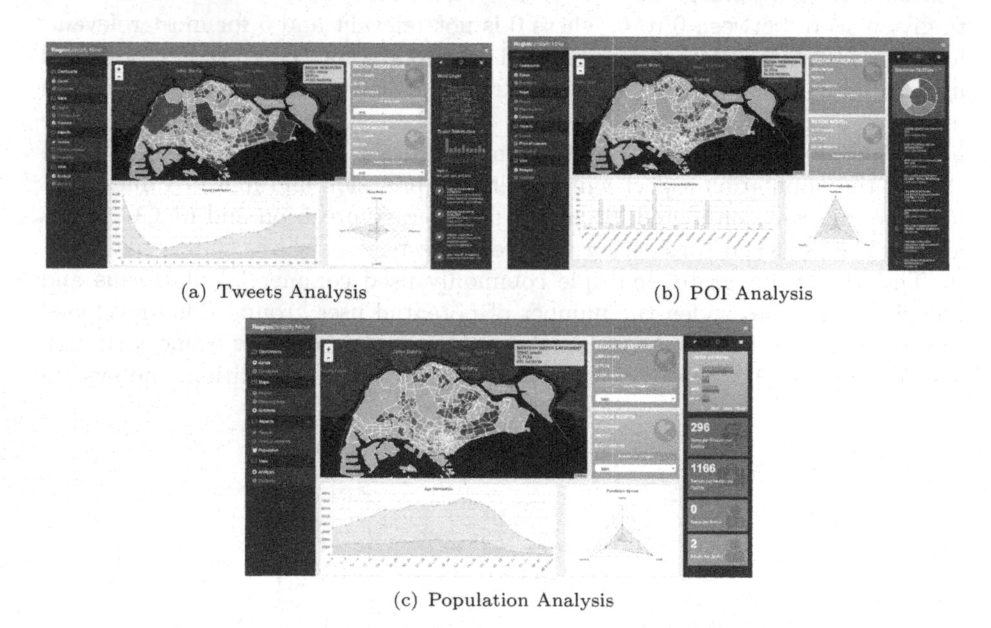

(a) Tweets Analysis

(b) POI Analysis

(c) Population Analysis

Fig. 3. Different aspect analysis

The second core function of the system is to allow users to query for similar urban regions. In addition, users can also evaluate their approach in this part of the system. Thereafter, they can view the results and the respective precision and nDCG values. Figure 4 shows the screen shots of the system for the region query analysis.

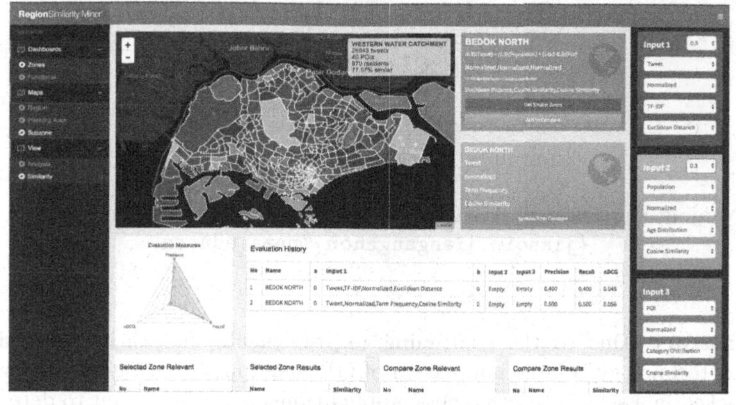

(a) Region Query Analysis

(b) Query Results

Fig. 4. Similar region query

References

1. Jendryke, M., Balz, T., McClure, S.C., Liao, M.S.: Putting people in the picture: combining big location-based social media data and remote sensing imagery for enhanced contextual urban information in Shanghai. Comput. Environ. Urban Syst. **62**, 99–112 (2017)
2. Yoshimura, Y., Krebs, A., Ratti, C.: Noninvasive bluetooth monitoring of visitors' length of stay at the Louvre. IEEE Pervasive Comput. **16**, 26–34 (2017)
3. Kontokosta, C.E., Johnson, N.: Urban phenology: toward a real-time census of the city using Wi-Fi data. Comput. Environ. Urban Syst. **64**, 114–153 (2017)
4. Agryzkov, T., Mart, P., Tortosa, L., Vincent, J.F.: Measuring urban activities using foursquare data and network analysis: a case study of Murcia (Spain). Int. J. Geogr. Inf. Sci. **31**, 100–121 (2017)
5. Shin, D.: Urban sensing by crowdsourcing: analysing urban trip behaviour in Zurich. Int. J. Urban Reg. Res. **40**, 1044–1060 (2016)
6. Anantharam, P., Barnaghi, P., Thirunarayan, K., Sheth, A.: Extracting city traffic events from social streams. ACM Trans. Intell. Syst. Technol. **6**, 43:1–43:27 (2015)
7. Feng, K., Cong, G., Bhowmick, S.S., Peng, W., Miao, C.: Towards best region search for data exploration. In: Proceedings of 2016 International Conference on Management Data (SIGMOD), pp. 1055–1070 (2016)

Detect Tracking Behavior Among Trajectory Data

Jianqiu Xu(✉) and Jiangang Zhou

Nanjing University of Aeronautics and Astronautics, Nanjing, China
{jianqiu,jiangangzhou}@nuaa.edu.cn

Abstract. Due to the continuing improvements in location acquisition technology, a large population of GPS-equipped moving objects are tracked in a server. In emergency applications, users may want to detect whether a target is tracked by another object. We formulate the tracking behavior by continuous distance queries in trajectory databases. Index structures are developed to improve the query performance. Using real trajectories, we demonstrate answering continuous distance queries in a database system and animating moving objects fulfilling the distance condition in the user interface. The result benefits mining the interesting behavior among trajectory data and answering distance join queries.

1 Introduction

The rise of GPS-equipped mobile devices has led to the emergence of big trajectory data. A large amount of historical trajectory data has become available for emerging applications such as traffic monitor and location-based services. Real time tracking has been studied to efficiently track an object's trajectory in real-time [12]. However, so far little attention has been paid to detect the tracking behavior over historical movement. That is, given a query trajectory o_q and a distance threshold d, we aim to find whether there is any object keeping some distance to o_q at each time point of o_q. We formulate the problem by continuous distance queries over trajectory data in which users define a threshold to return objects within a distance (e.g., 500 m) to the query.

Consider an example in Fig. 1. There are five trajectories $\{o_1, o_2, o_3, o_4, o_5\}$ and the task is to find whether o_3 is tracked by another object during $[t_1, t_2]$. Suppose that a short distance d is defined, e.g., 500 m. In the example, we will find o_4 following o_3. Other objects are within the distance to o_3 but only for a short time period. This will not be treated as tracking behavior. To find the *tracker*, we need to compute the time-dependent distance between trajectories and determine whether the period fulfilling the distance condition contains each time point of the query trajectory. This is not a simple task because the precise distance needs to be determined. One may think of using the continuous nearest neighbor query to find the tracking behavior, but such a query will return objects with small distances at each piece of time. We need to figure out the precise distance and find whether there are objects that always keep a certain distance to the target rather than only at a short period.

G. Cong et al. (Eds.): ADMA 2017, LNAI 10604, pp. 872–878, 2017.
https://doi.org/10.1007/978-3-319-69179-4_64

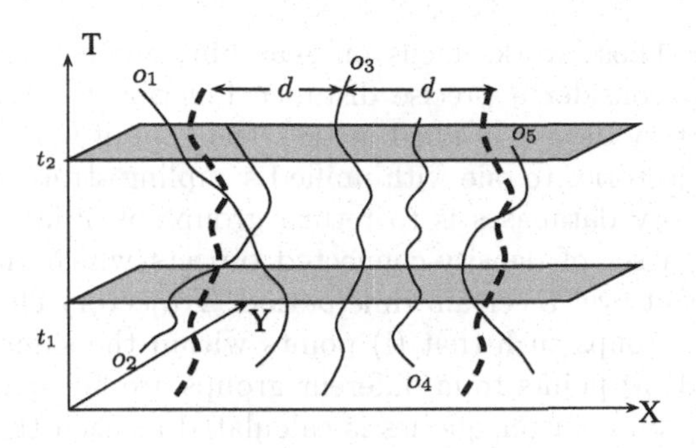

Fig. 1. Detect tracking behavior

In the literature, a lot of effort has gone to process k nearest neighbor queries in which a distance function is defined to return k objects with the smallest distance to the target. Due to diverse spatial environments, e.g., free space [8], road network [13] and obstacle space [5], different distance functions are used. The distance is a static value if a time point is considered and becomes a time-dependent function if the continuous query over a time period is considered. The latter is non-trivial because the distance varies over time such that returned objects change at certain points. In some special applications, the tracking behavior is helpful to find interesting objects that cannot be discovered by nearest neighbor queries. For example, to look for the tracker or travelers with common routes, we would like to search the object that always keeps a certain distance to the target rather than the nearest object at certain time points. On one hand, the nearest object to the target may change at some points or places. On the other hand, the nearest object is usually not the tracker because of being easily exposed.

In the demo, we detect the tracking behavior by using continuous distance queries. To be general, the query is of three forms in terms of distance parameters. We are able to search objects within or out of a certain distance to the target. To efficiently answer the query, several trajectory indexes are provided in the system such as 3D R-tree and TB-tree. We propose a novel index structure that combines the grid index and R-tree. Given a query trajectory, one quickly calculates the cells within the query distance. During the R-tree traversal, we make use of the index structure to prune the space that cannot contribute to the result. Real datasets are used in the demonstration scenario for continuous distance queries and distance join queries.

The rest of the paper is organized as follows. We review the related work in Sect. 2, formulate the problem and introduce the solution in Sect. 3, demonstrate continuous distance queries in Sect. 4, followed by conclusions in Sect. 5.

2 Related Work

In the literature, tremendous efforts have been made on querying trajectories including nearest neighbors [6,8], similarity search [4,17] and pattern discovery [10,14]. Those works focus on searching some targets *close* to the query, but do not consider a precise distance function to evaluate the query. *Calibrating* trajectory data is studied in [17], the goal of which is to transform heterogeneous trajectories to one with unified sampling strategies. Discoverying convoys in trajectory databases is to return groups of objects such that each group consists of a set of density-connected objects which should satisfy the distance requirement over a certain time period. Trajectory clustering [9,11,15] also aims to form groups such that (i) points within the same group are close to each other, and (ii) points from different groups are far apart. However, the distance in convoy and cluster queries is calculated at each time point but not a time-dependent function as we use for processing continuous queries. In addition, discovery of convoys and clusters in trajectory database shows the behavior for a group of objects. In contrast, we aim to find whether a target is tracked by another object, which is an *individual* behavior.

The *closest-point-of-approach join* is studied in [2,18], the task of which is to return all object pairs. Each pair of trajectories has the distance less than a threshold at some point in time. This is not a continuous query and cannot be used to detect the tracking behavior. Two objects close to each other at some point in time do not mean that one is tracked by another. Probably this is treated as *passby* or *overtaken.* We generalize the distance query by considering a time interval such that the distance between two trajectories is less than a certain value at each time point during the query.

3 The Framework

3.1 Problem Definition

Let the database $\mathcal{O}$ be a set of trajectories, each of which consists of a sequence of temporal units. Each unit represents the movement over a time interval by recording start and end locations. Locations between them are estimated by interpolation. Given two trajectories $o_1, o_2 \in \mathcal{O}$, we let $dist(o_1, o_2, t)$ return the distance between o_1 and o_2 at time point t.

Definition 1 *(Tracking behavior). Let $T(o)(o \in \mathcal{O})$ return the time period of a trajectory. Given a query trajectory $o_q \in \mathcal{O}$ and a distance d, we define o_q's tracker by*

$$Tracker(o_q) \in \mathcal{O} : \forall t \in T(o_q), dist(o_q, Tracker(o_q), t) < d$$

We generalize the query by defining a distance range, i.e., $d = [d_1, d_2]$. If $d_1 = 0$ and $d_2 > 0$, this is used to find the tracking behavior. If $0 < d_1 < d_2$, we can return objects between d_1 and d_2 to the target which may also be trackers. If $d_1 > 0$ and $d_2 = \infty$, objects that are further than a certain distance to the target are found and can be used to exclude suspicious objects.

3.2 The Solution

An outline of the solution is provided in Fig. 2. To efficiently find trajectories within a certain distance to the target, an index structure is essentially needed. We have implemented well established trajectory indexes including TB-tree [16], 3D R-tree and Grid index [3]. We perform a traversal on the indexes to retrieve trajectories that approximately belong to the result and then do the exact distance computation. The distance function over a time period is represented by a parabola function. We will receive pieces of distance functions and split trajectories at certain points to restrict the movement fulling the query condition. The method is able to find the tracking behavior but can be further optimized.

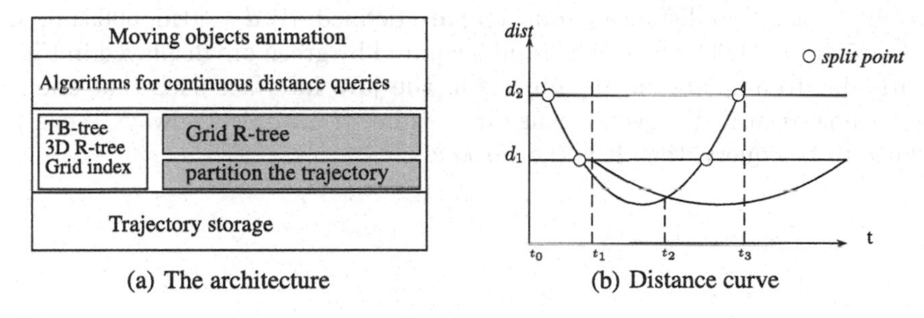

Fig. 2. An overview

To enhance the performance, we propose an index structure that combines the grid index and R-tree, as shown in Fig. 3. The 2D space is partitioned into a set of equal-size cells and trajectories are decomposed according to cells. That is, each trajectory is split into pieces and each piece is limited to a cell. We sort trajectory pieces by cell id, time and the spatial box. Each leaf R-tree node only contains trajectories from the same cell. The query procedure will make use of the cells to prune the search space. We first determine the cells in which the query trajectory is located. Since cells have the same size, we can quickly calculate *target* cells which are within the specified distance to the query trajectory. *Target* cells will be used to

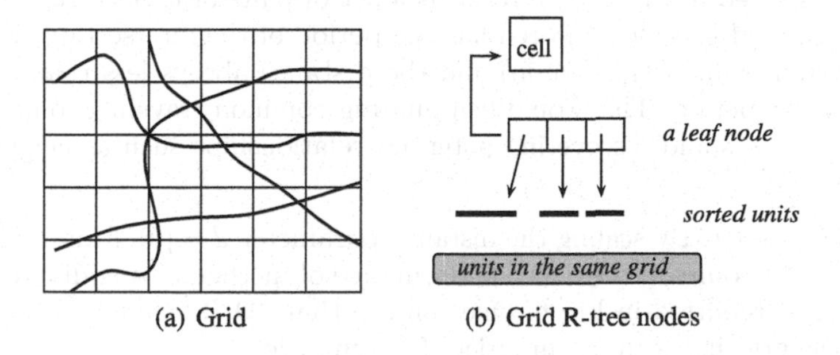

Fig. 3. Grid R-tree

prune R-tree nodes that do not cover *target* cells because only trajectories located in *target* cells will contribute to the result.

4 Demonstration

The implementation is developed in an extensible database system SECONDO [7] and program in C/C++. We use real datasets from a data company DataTang [1] including 1,675,667 GPS records of Beijing taxis. There are 22,269 trajectories in total.

In the demonstration, we randomly select a trajectory from the dataset and search trajectories keeping the specified distance to the query during its whole life time. Two distance parameters are defined: (i) $d = [0\,\text{m}, 5000\,\text{m}]$; and (ii) $d = [5000\,\text{m}, 20000\,\text{m}]$ and the results colored by green are displayed in Fig. 4. We are able to animate moving objects in the java interface such that one can observe how returned objects change over time. If an object always keeps the distance to the query, then it is the *tracker*.

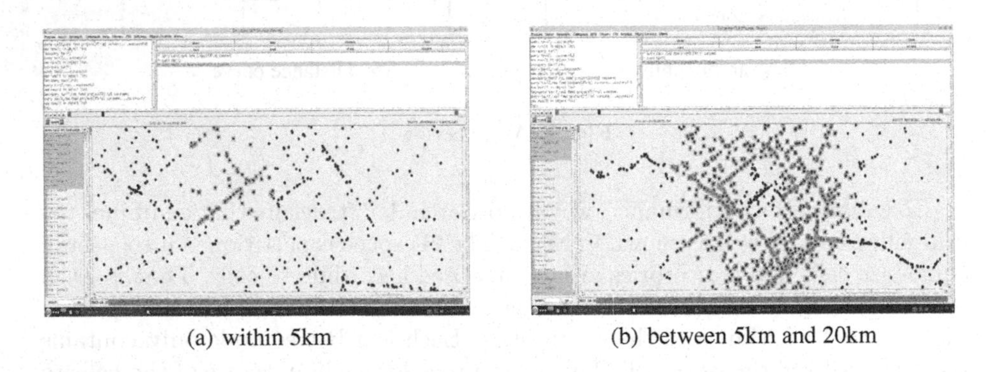

(a) within 5km (b) between 5km and 20km

Fig. 4. Continuous distance queries (Color figure online)

Distance join queries. We also demonstrate distance join queries over trajectories, as illustrated in Fig. 5. The result is a set of pairs of trajectories such that each pair colored by green and red has the period of the intersection time more than a certain value (e.g., 15 min) and the distance always less than a threshold during the period. This would help finding common traveling routes among different travelers and discovering potential relationships such as neighbor and colleague.

Index performance. By scaling the distance parameter $d = \{[0,\, 5\,\text{km}],\, [0,\, 10\,\text{km}],\, [0,\, 20\,\text{km}]\}$, we compare the query performance of methods using different index structures, as reported in Fig. 6. One can see that 3D R-tree and TB-tree outperform the grid index up to an order of magnitude.

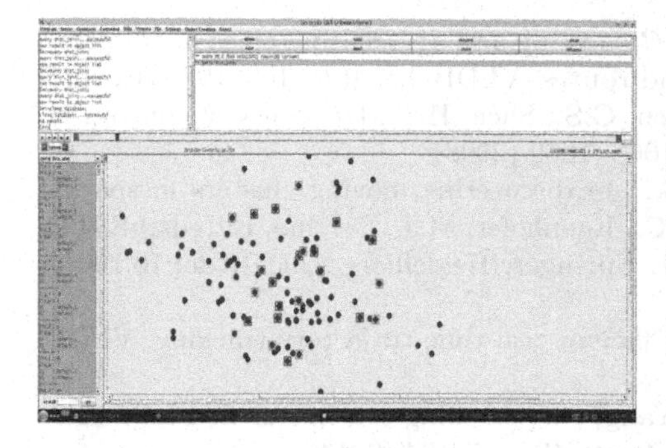

Fig. 5. Distance join queries (Color figure online)

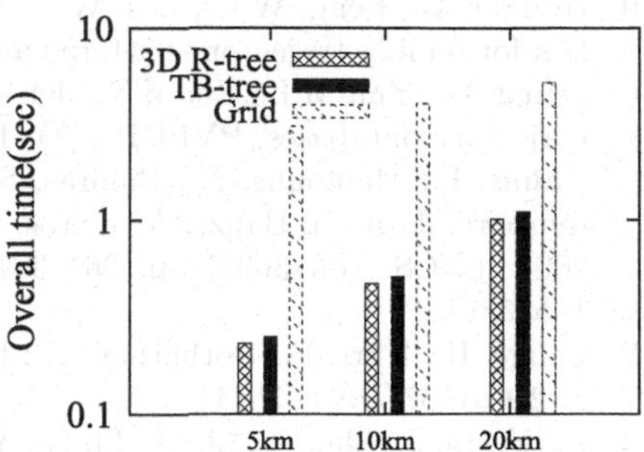

Fig. 6. Performance comparison

5 Conclusions

We study detecting the tracking behavior over trajectory data and formulate the problem by continuous distance queries. The framework of processing the queries is introduced including partitioning the data, building index structures, developing query algorithms and animating moving objects in the user interface. We demonstrate answering continuous distance and distance join queries in a prototype database system.

The future work is to evaluate the system performance by using big trajectory data and flexibly visualize a large number of trajectories in the user interface.

Acknowledgment. This work is supported by NSFC under grant numbers 61300052 and the Fundamental Research Funds for the Central Universities NO. NZ2013306.

References

1. http://factory.datatang.com/en/ (2006)
2. Arumugam, S., Jermaine, C.: Closest-point-of-approach join for moving object histories. In: ICDE, p. 86 (2006)
3. Chakka, V.P., Everspaugh, A., Patel, J.M.: Indexing large trajectory data sets with SETI. In: CIDR (2003)
4. Chen, L., Özsu, M.T., Oria, V.: Robust and fast similarity search for moving object trajectories. In: SIGMOD, pp. 491–502 (2005)
5. Gao, Y., Zheng, B.: Continuous obstructed nearest neighbor queries in spatial databases. In: ACM SIGMOD, pp. 577–590 (2009)
6. Gao, Y., Zheng, B., Chen, G., Li, Q.: Algorithms for constrained k-nearest neighbor queries over moving object trajectories. GeoInformatica **14**(2), 241–276 (2010)
7. Güting, R.H., Behr, T., Düntgen, C.: SECONDO: a platform for moving objects database research and for publishing and integrating research implementations. IEEE Data Eng. Bull. **33**(2), 56–63 (2010)
8. Güting, R.H., Behr, T., Xu, J.: Efficient k-nearest neighbor search on moving object trajectories. VLDB J. **19**(5), 687–714 (2010)

9. Hung, C.C., Peng, W.C., Lee, W.C.: Clustering and aggregating clues of trajectories for mining trajectory patterns and routes. VLDB J. **24**(2), 169–192 (2015)
10. Jeung, H., Yiu, M.L., Zhou, X., Jensen, C.S., Shen, H.T.: Discovery of convoys in trajectory databases. PVLDB **1**(1), 1068–1080 (2008)
11. Kalnis, P., Mamoulis, N., Bakiras, S.: On discovering moving clusters in spatio-temporal data. In: Bauzer Medeiros, C., Egenhofer, M.J., Bertino, E. (eds.) SSTD 2005. LNCS, vol. 3633, pp. 364–381. Springer, Heidelberg (2005). doi:10.1007/11535331_21
12. Lange, R., Dürr, F., Rothermel, K.: Efficient real-time trajectory tracking. VLDB J. **20**(5), 671–694 (2011)
13. Li, Y., Li, J., Shu, L., Li, Q., Li, G., Yang, F.: Searching continuous nearest neighbors in road networks on the air. Inf. Syst. **42**, 177–194 (2014)
14. Li, Z., Ding, B., Han, J., Kays, R.: Swarm: mining relaxed temporal moving object clusters. PVLDB **3**(1), 723–734 (2010)
15. Pelekis, N., Tampakis, P., Vodas, M., Panagiotakis, C., Theodoridis, Y.: In-DBMS sampling-based sub-trajectory clustering. In: EDBT 2017, pp. 632–643 (2017)
16. Pfoser, D., Jensen, C.S.: Novel approaches in query processing for moving object trajectories. In: VLDB, pp. 395–406 (2000)
17. Su, H., Zheng, K., Wang, H., Huang, J., Zhou, X.: Calibrating trajectory data for similarity-based analysis. In: SIGMOD, pp. 833–844 (2013)
18. Zhou, P., Zhang, D., Salzberg, B., Cooperman, G., Kollios, G.: Close pair queries in moving object databases. In: ACM-GIS, pp. 2–11 (2005)

Author Index

Printed in the United States
By Bookmasters